Water-Soluble Vitamins

D0477898

Vitamin C (mg)	Thiamin (mg)	Riboflavin (mg)	Niacin (mg NE)[f]	Vitamin B$_6$ (mg)	Folate (µg)	Vitamin B$_{12}$ (µg)	Calcium (mg)	Phosphorus (mg)	[Mag]nesium (mg)	Iron (mg)	Zinc (mg)	Iodine (µg)	[Sele]nium (µg)
30	0.3	0.4	5	0.3	25	0.3	400	300	40	6	5	40	10
35	0.4	0.5	6	0.6	35	0.5	600	500	60	10	5	50	15
40	0.7	0.8	9	1.0	50	0.7	800	800	80	10	10	70	20
45	0.9	1.1	12	1.1	75	1.0	800	800	120	10	10	90	20
45	1.0	1.2	13	1.4	100	1.4	800	800	170	10	10	120	30
50	1.3	1.5	17	1.7	150	2.0	1200	1200	270	12	15	150	40
60	1.5	1.8	20	2.0	200	2.0	1200	1200	400	12	15	150	50
60	1.5	1.7	19	2.0	200	2.0	1200	1200	350	10	15	150	70
60	1.5	1.7	19	2.0	200	2.0	800	800	350	10	15	150	70
60	1.2	1.4	15	2.0	200	2.0	800	800	350	10	15	150	70
50	1.1	1.3	15	1.4	150	2.0	1200	1200	280	15	12	150	45
60	1.1	1.3	15	1.5	180	2.0	1200	1200	300	15	12	150	50
60	1.1	1.3	15	1.6	180	2.0	1200	1200	280	15	12	150	55
60	1.1	1.3	15	1.6	180	2.0	800	800	280	15	12	150	55
60	1.0	1.2	13	1.6	180	2.0	800	800	280	10	12	150	55
70	1.5	1.6	17	2.2	400	2.2	1200	1200	320	30	15	175	65
95	1.6	1.8	20	2.1	280	2.6	1200	1200	355	15	19	200	75
90	1.6	1.7	20	2.1	260	2.6	1200	1200	340	15	16	200	75

Estimated Safe and Adequate Daily Dietary Intakes of Selected Vitamins and Minerals[a]

Vitamins

Category	Age (years)	Biotin (µg)	Pantothenic Acid (mg)
Infants	0-0.5	10	2
	0.5-1	15	3
Children and	1-3	20	3
adolescents	4-6	25	3-1
	7-10	30	4-5
	11+	30-100	4-7
Adults		30-100	4-7

Trace Elements[b]

Category	Age (years)	Copper (mg)	Manganese (mg)	Fluoride (mg)	Chromium (µg)	Molybdenum (µg)
Infants	0-0.5	0.4-0.6	0.3-0.6	0.1-0.5	10-40	15-30
	0.5-1	0.6-0.7	0.6-1.0	0.2-1.0	20-60	20-40
Children and	1-3	0.7-1.0	1.0-1.5	0.5-1.5	20-80	25-50
adolescents	4-6	1.0-1.5	1.5-2.0	1.0-2.5	30-120	30-75
	7-10	1.0-2.0	2.0-3.0	1.5-2.5	50-200	50-150
	11+	1.5-2.5	2.0-5.0	1.5-2.5	50-200	75-250
Adults		1.5-3.0	2.0-5.0	1.5-4.0	50-200	75-250

[a]Because there is less information on which to base allowances, these figures are not given in the main table of RDA and are provided here in the form of ranges of recommended intakes.
[b]Since the toxic levels for many trace elements may be only several times usual intakes, the upper levels for the trace elements given in this table should not be habitually exceeded.

FOUNDATIONS AND CLINICAL APPLICATIONS OF

NUTRITION

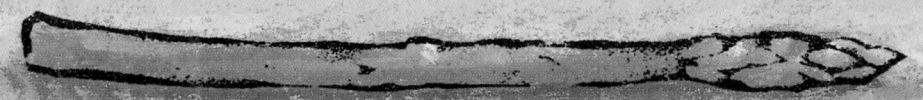

A Nursing Approach

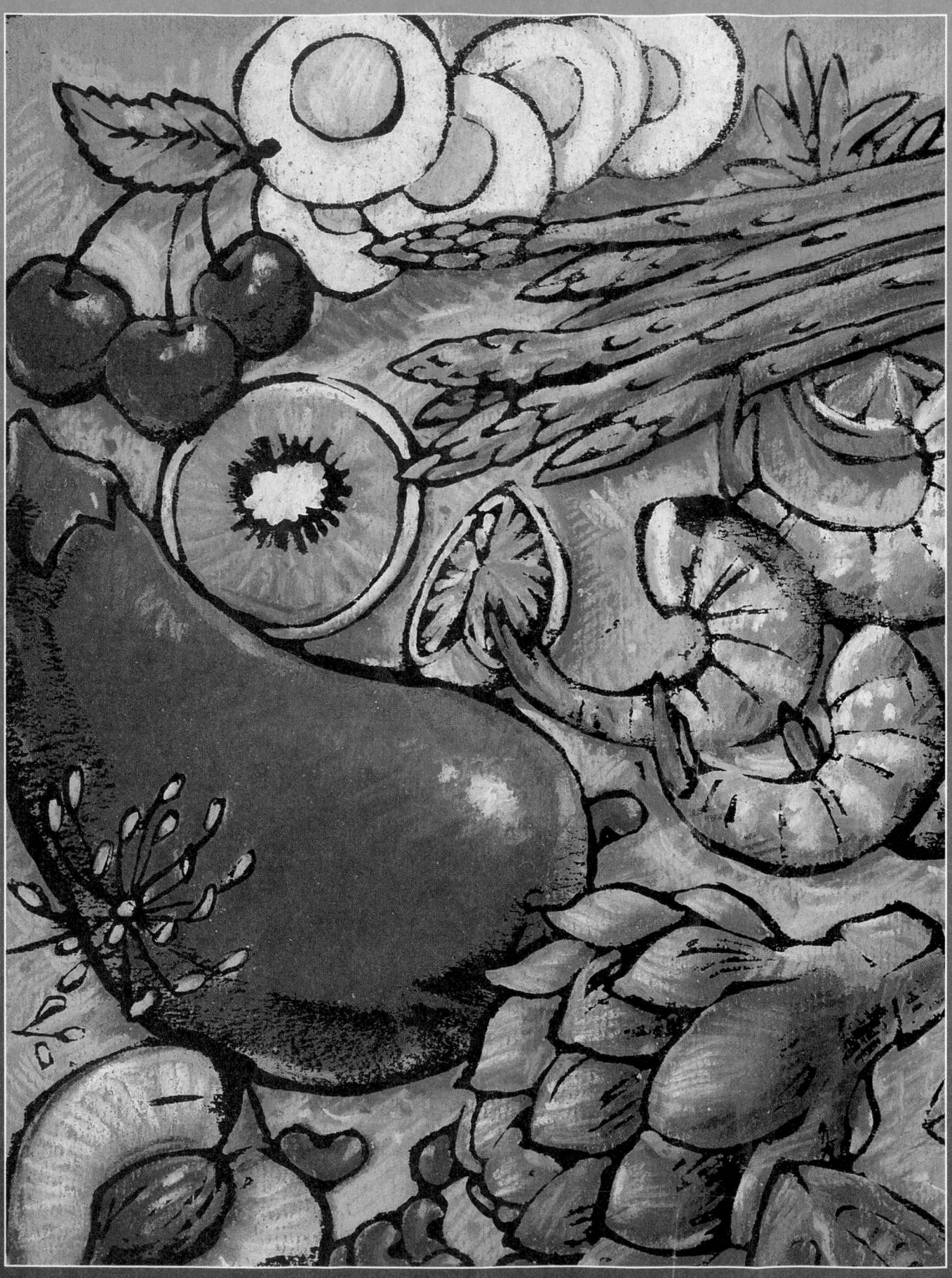

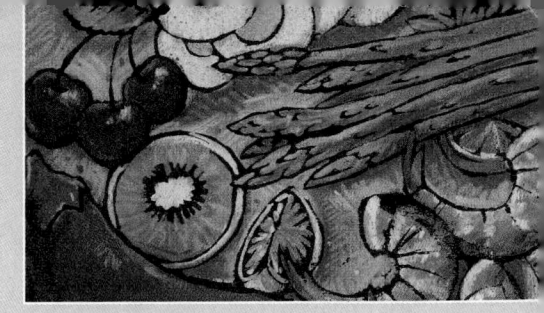

FOUNDATIONS AND CLINICAL APPLICATIONS OF
NUTRITION

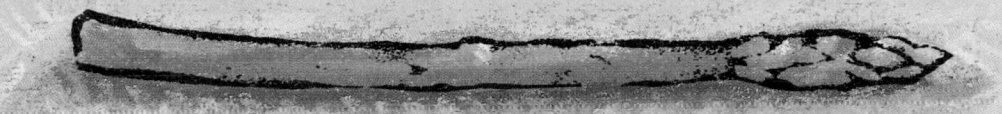

A Nursing Approach

MICHELE GRODNER, EdD, CHES
Associate Professor and Nutrition Coordinator
Department of Community Health
William Paterson College
Wayne, New Jersey

SARA LONG ANDERSON, PhD, RD
Assistant Professor and Director, Didactic Program in Dietetics,
Department of Animal Science, Food, and Nutrition
Southern Illinois University at Carbondale
Carbondale, Illinois

SANDRA DeYOUNG, PhD, RN
Professor and Chairperson
Department of Nursing
William Paterson College
Wayne, New Jersey

with 181 *illustrations*

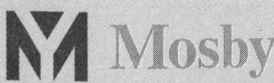 Mosby

St. Louis Baltimore Boston Carlsbad Chicago Naples New York Philadelphia Portland
London Madrid Mexico City Singapore Sydney Tokyo Toronto Wiesbaden

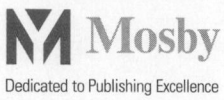

Mosby

Dedicated to Publishing Excellence

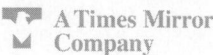

A Times Mirror
Company

Publisher: James M. Smith
Senior Acquisitions Editor: Vicki Malinee
Managing Editor: Janet Russell Livingston
Developmental Editor: Terry Eynon
Project Manager: Carol Sullivan Weis
Production Editor: Karen Rehwinkel
Designer: Sheilah Barrett
Manufacturing Supervisor: David Graybill
Cover and Part Opener Illustrations: Viv Eisner Hess

Printed in the United States of America

Composition by TSI Graphics.
Printing/Binding by Von Hoffmann Press, Inc.

Mosby-Year Book, Inc.
11830 Westline Industrial Drive
St. Louis, MO 63146

International Standard Book Number 0-8151-4041-X

95 96 97 98 99 / 9 8 7 6 5 4 3 2 1

CONTRIBUTORS

Elaine Asp, PhD
Associate Professor,
Department of Food Science and Nutrition,
University of Minnesota, St. Paul, Minnesota
Section on Consumer Food Decision Making in Chapter 2, Personal and Community Nutrition

Sharron Dalton, PhD, RD
Associate Professor,
Department of Nutrition and Food Studies,
New York University, New York, New York
Chapter 5, Fats

Marian L. Stone Neuhouser, BS, RD
Interdisciplinary Program in Nutritional Sciences,
University of Washington, Seattle, Washington
Chapter 11, Life Span Health Promotion: Pregnancy, Lactation, and Infancy

Ellen Parham, PhD, RD
Professor,
Department of Human and Family Resources,
Northern Illinois University, DeKalb, Illinois
Chapter 10, Management of Body Fat Levels

Jaime Ruud, MS, RD
Sports Nutrition Consultant,
International Center for Sports Nutrition, Lincoln, Nebraska
Chapter 9, Energy Supply and Fitness

Bonnie Worthington-Roberts, PhD
Professor,
Interdisciplinary Program in Nutritional Sciences,
University of Washington, Seattle, Washington
Chapter 11, Life Span Health Promotion: Pregnancy, Lactation, and Infancy

To the courageous souls who attempt to cross boundaries to collaborate for the health of us all.

Michele Grodner

To everyone who believes in me.

Sara Long Anderson

To my parents: examples of integrity, hard work, persistence, and love.

Sandra DeYoung

PREFACE

The basis of effective preventive, acute, and rehabilitative health care is collaboration. As we recognize how the physical and psychological dimensions of health are interconnected, we realize that all health professionals need an interdisciplinary understanding of the health needs of both individuals and communities. This interconnection challenges the nursing profession to prepare professionals who are competent and comfortable in clinical institutional settings that serve individuals and their families, as well as in community settings where the focus is on the health status of groups. The nutrition and dietetics profession is challenged to provide other health professionals with an understanding of nutrition that will allow them to support the strategies of successful nutrition intervention.

Foundations and Clinical Applications of Nutrition: A Nursing Approach meets these challenges by bridging the worlds of nursing and nutrition. With a solid background in basic nutrition, nurses will understand the dietary modifications that are designed to maintain and restore health. Consequently, this nutrition text considers wellness from the personal and professional perspective of nurses. Each topic in nutrition is discussed both as it relates to the nurse's individual, personal knowledge and to the professional knowledge nurses need to serve patients and clients in various institutional and community settings. (Reflecting an emphasis on wellness, individuals being cared for by health professionals for health maintenance are referred to as clients. Those who are ill or recuperating from illness are referred to as patients.)

Health care professionals also need to be concerned with their own dietary patterns. Nursing practice demands stamina and well-being. Recognizing the personal nutrition needs of nurses, this book provides a basis of optimum nutrition strategies that can be applied to our lifestyles and those of our families. Client education is a fundamental responsibility of nursing. We can be role models for the positive effects of enhanced nutritional lifestyles as we teach our clients about nutritional wellness.

Nurses interact daily with patients around the issues of food and nutrition. As managed health care and home health services increase nationwide, the role of nurses expands. To highlight the role of nutrition intervention as corollary treatment for clinically diagnosed disorders, the term *medical nutrition therapy* replaces the term *diet therapy*. Nutrition is increasingly recognized as an integral component of health maintenance and rehabilitation. Thus the influence of nurses in the larger community expands, and the importance of reinforcement of nutrition intervention by nurses is highlighted. Medical nutrition therapy provides control while patients are in the hospital setting, but patients need a personal foundation of information to use when they leave the hospital. The overall goal of patient care is to empower patients to take responsibility for their own nutrition status. Patient education provides the lifestyle strategies that enable individuals to develop their own healthful dietary patterns.

AUDIENCE

This book is designed primarily for a nursing audience studying nutrition and medical nutrition therapy. Secondary audiences are health education and health science students. The book is also an ideal reference for nurses, nurse practitioners, and other health care professionals in all manners of health care settings.

Although the book is designed for a one-semester course, it can be adapted for a basic nutrition course, using Part One, Wellness, Nutrition, and the Nursing Role; Part Two, Nutrients, Food, and Health; and Part Three, Health Promotion Through Nutrition and Nursing Practice. Part Four, Overview of Diet Therapy, can then be used as a future reference for medical nutrition therapy.

APPROACH

Most nutrition and diet therapy texts attempt to reach several groups, such as nutrition and dietetics majors and nursing students. In contrast, nursing students are the only target audience of this text. This narrowed focus allows us to emphasize the skills applicable to nursing practice. Information needed by dietetics majors but not by nurses is omitted. We recognize that nurses do not prescribe or develop "diets" for patients. Instead, skills essential for nursing professionals if they are to implement and educate patients and clients about prescribed dietary patterns are emphasized.

FEATURES

Integrated nursing content. Every aspect of nutrition is tied to the nursing experience within a framework of providing holistic patient care to achieve wellness. Carefully constructed boxes on The Nursing Role demonstrate the continual application of the nursing process to each content area. Skill-building is maximized through Teaching Tools and other pedagogical strategies.

Most current dietary recommendations. The latest guidelines and their rationales are included, offering students tools with which to interpret ever-changing information, as well as the competence to make well-informed personal and professional decisions. Updated Food Exchange Lists (1995) and the Renal Diet from the American Dietetic Association and the American Diabetes Association appear in Appendixes B and K.

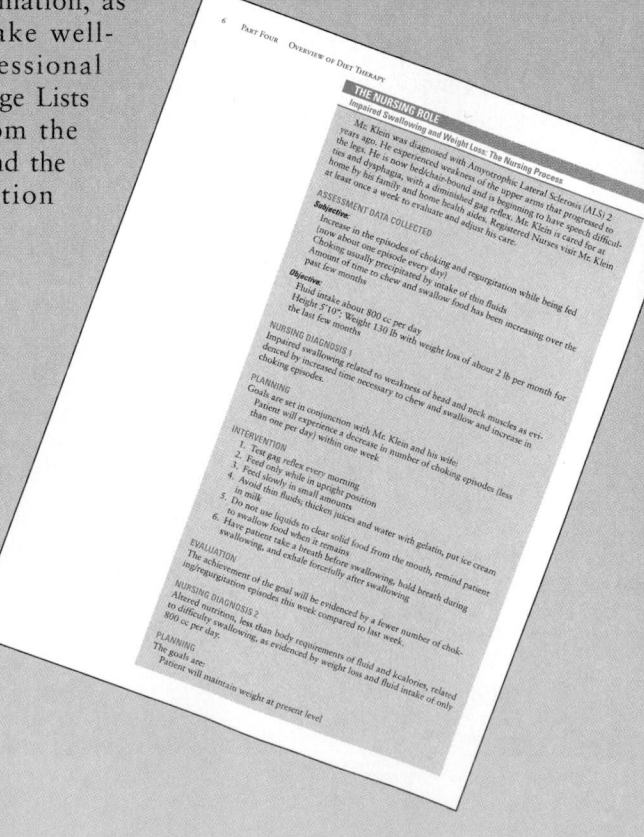

Lifespan approach. Vital information on age-related variations gives students the background knowledge needed to modify assessments when caring for individuals in varying age groups. Lifespan content is indicated with this special icon 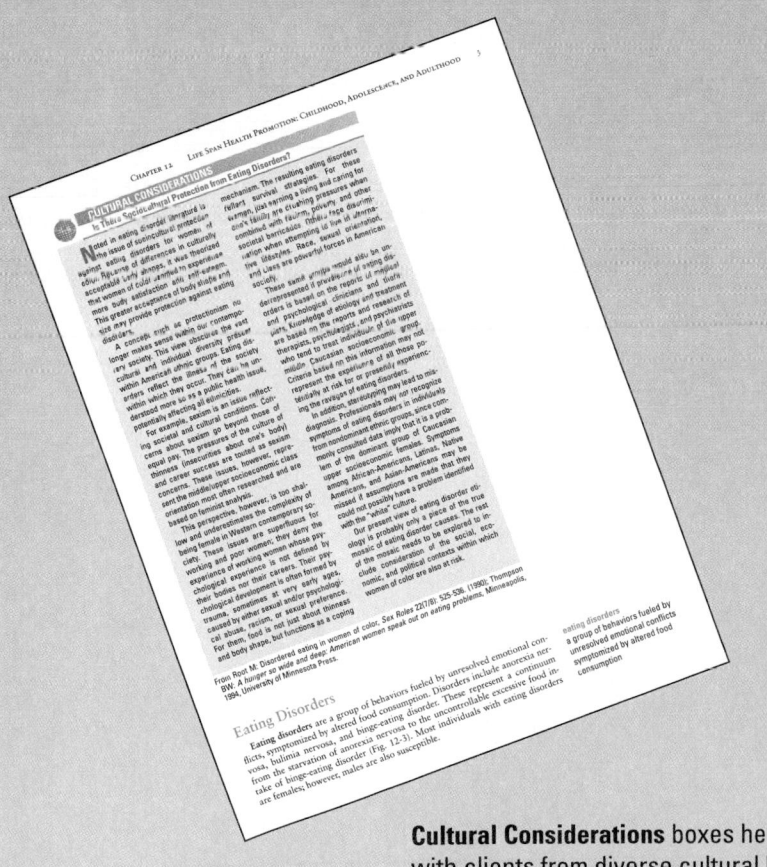 throughout the text.

Cultural awareness. Cultural Considerations boxes highlight multicultural issues to help students approach, interview, and assess patients from diverse cultural backgrounds. Appendix M presents cultural dietary patterns of different ethnic groups, allowing nurses to focus on the specific populations with whom they work.

Innovative approach to weight. The chapter on Management of Body Fat Levels emphasizes total fitness and wellness rather than body weight, equipping nurses to educate and care for persons of all sizes.

Conversational writing style. Nutrition is an engaging topic. The writing style of this book reflects the authors' philosophy that serious topics can be presented in a clear, conversational style that can make the study of nutrition enjoyable as well as rewarding.

Current food labeling requirements. Practical information on reading and understanding food labels provides applications to promote wellness.

Incorporation of Healthy People 2000. Healthy People 2000 nutrition priorities, introduced in Chapter 1 and discussed when relevant, integrate personal nutrition goals with national objectives for communities. This framework clarifies how the nutritional status of our communities reflects individual nutritional health.

Cultural Considerations boxes help students work with clients from diverse cultural backgrounds.

PEDAGOGY

Supportive learning aids appear in every chapter. Margin definitions of key terms, Wellness and Nutrition charts, chapter summaries, and current references all enhance students' efforts to study more effectively. A comprehensive glossary supports the marginal definitions. Additionally, the following pedagogical features support the text's holistic, interdisciplinary approach to nutrition in nursing settings and present related information in interesting and thought-provoking ways:

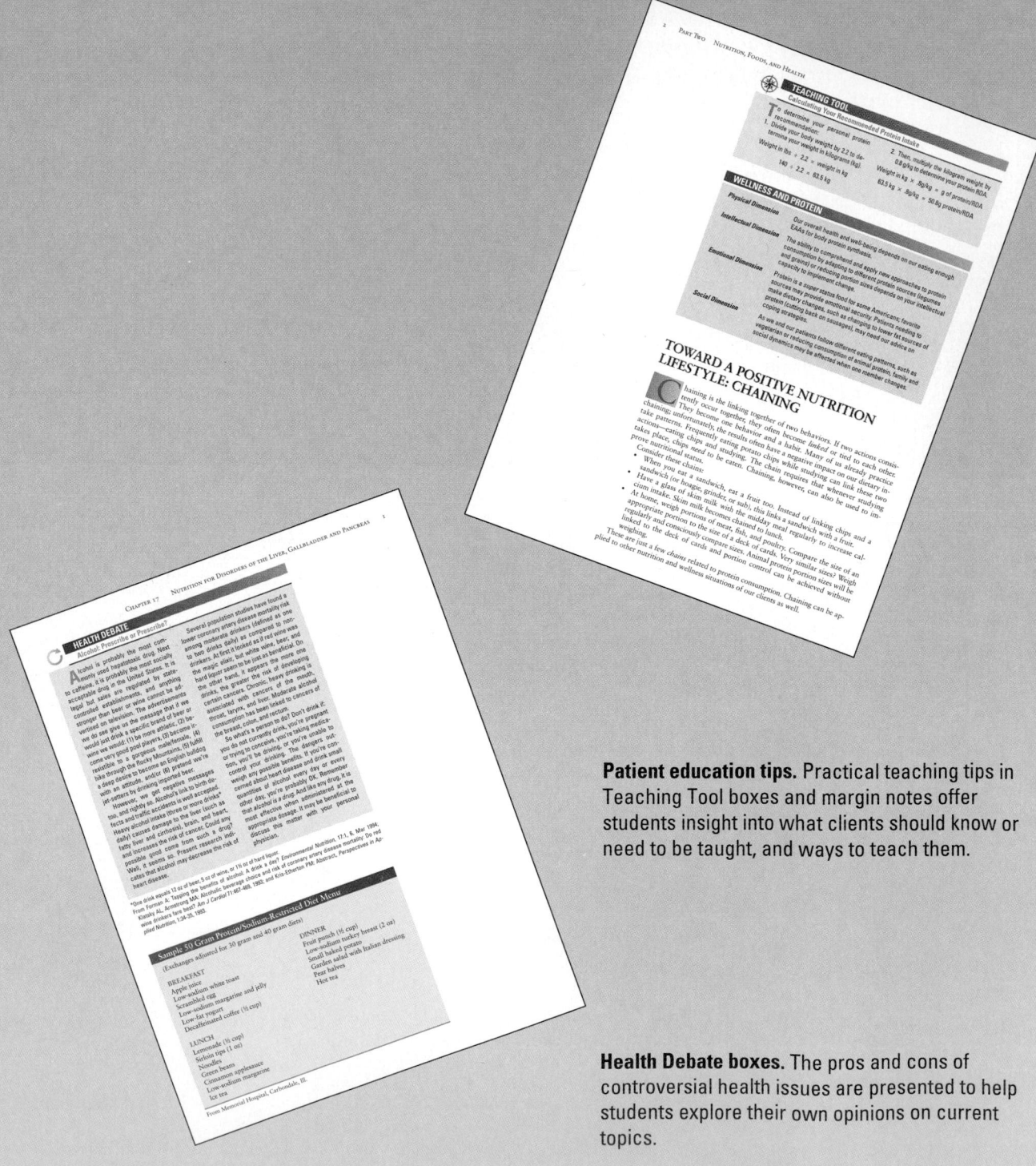

Patient education tips. Practical teaching tips in Teaching Tool boxes and margin notes offer students insight into what clients should know or need to be taught, and ways to teach them.

Health Debate boxes. The pros and cons of controversial health issues are presented to help students explore their own opinions on current topics.

Social Issue boxes. Highlighting aspects of health and nutrition of national and international communities provides important social and global perspectives.

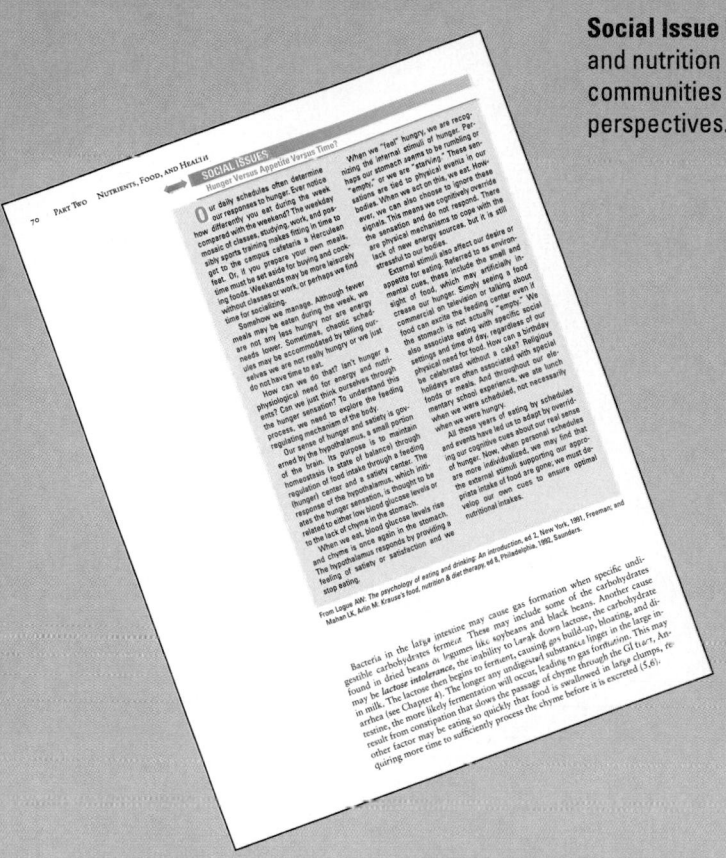

Myth boxes. Common fallacies, accompanied by the facts, help readers overcome their own as well as patients' misconceptions about nutrition.

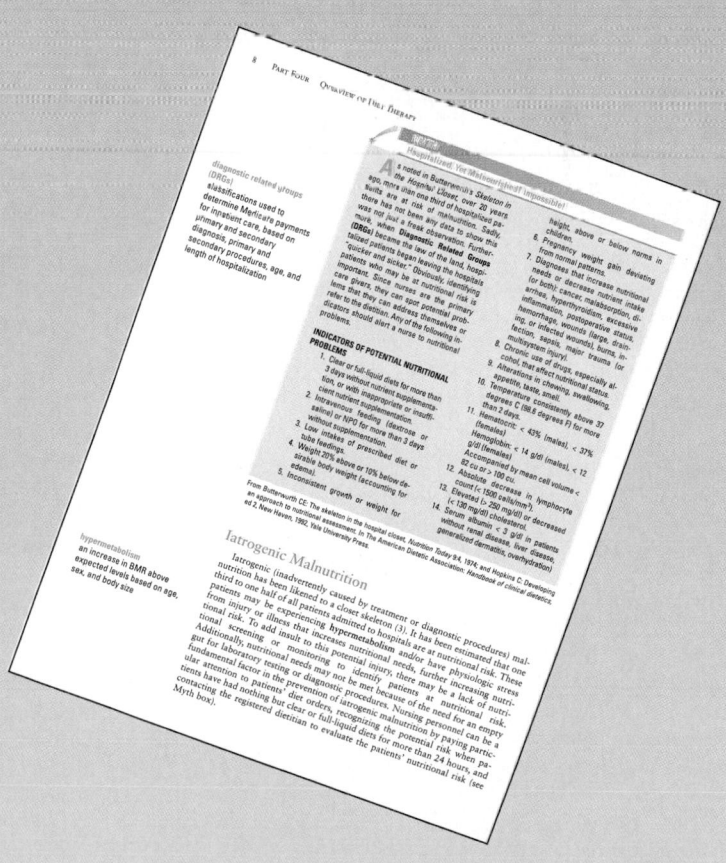

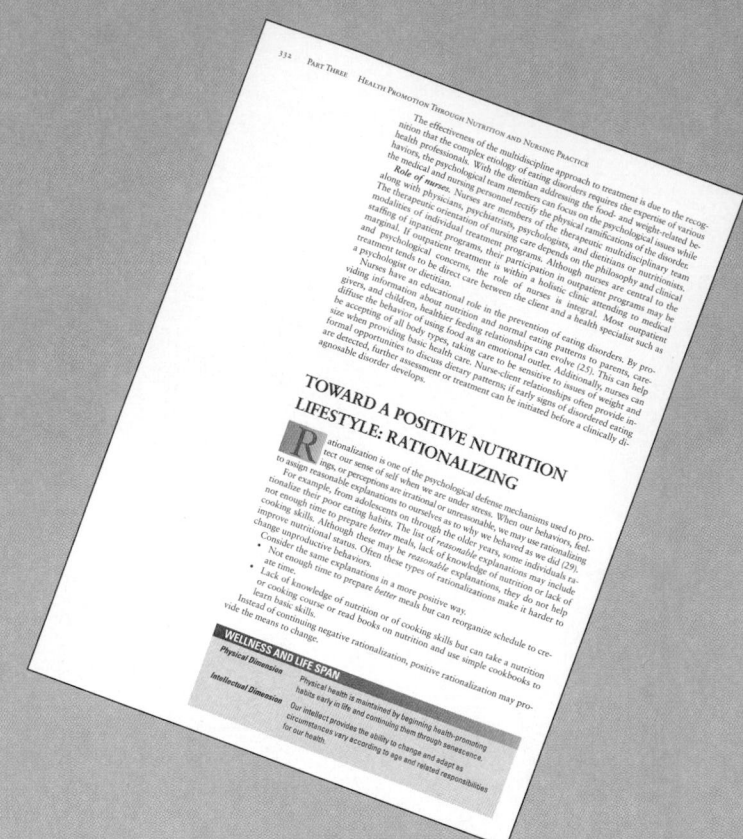

Toward a Positive Nutrition Lifestyle section. The psychosocial strategies presented in this section (appearing in Parts I, II, and III), promote self-efficacy in students and their patients.

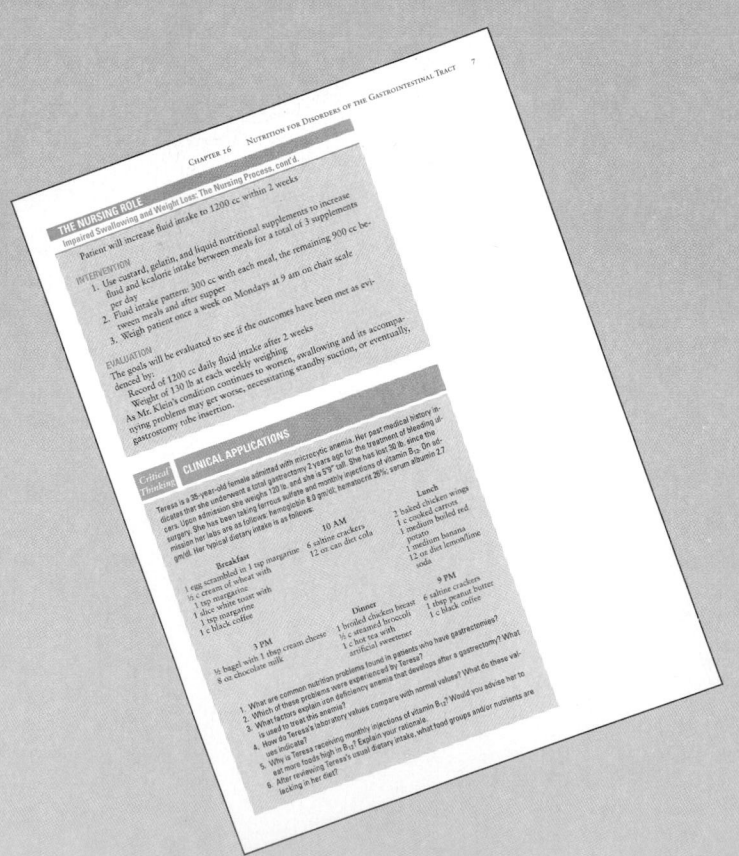

Clinical Applications. Critical thinking skills are enhanced by Clinical Application boxes in all chapters of Part IV, Overview of Diet Therapy. Responding to case study scenarios allows students to synthesize what they've learned by applying their knowledge to actual clinical situations. In addition, certain Nursing Role boxes and Health Debate boxes exercise critical thinking skills. (Answers to the critical thinking questions, including answers for all Clinical Application boxes, appear in the back of the text.)

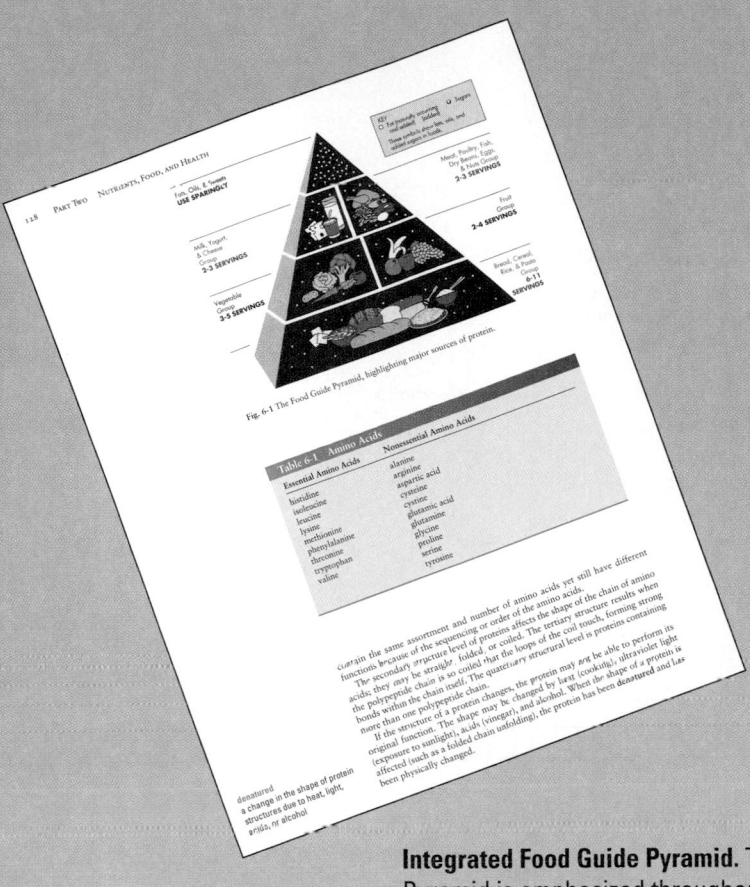

Integrated Food Guide Pyramid. The Food Guide Pyramid is emphasized throughout the text as a guide for self-education and as a tool for teaching patients about balanced diets.

SUPPLEMENTARY MATERIALS

A complete ancillary package accompanies this text, including an instructor's manual and test bank, a computerized test bank,* and a student study guide, including NCLEX-RN-style questions. Transparency acetates,* as well as a series of videotapes* and videodiscs,* support the text visually. Nutri-Trac diet analysis software allows students to input food intake and physical activities, promoting active learning.

*Available to qualified adopters.

ACKNOWLEDGMENTS

Our appreciation to the contributing authors who offered their unique perspectives on their areas of nutritional expertise: Elaine Asp, PhD; Sharron Dalton, PhD, RD; Marian L. Stone Neuhouser, BS, RD; Ellen Parham, PhD, RD; Jaime Ruud, MS, RD; and Bonnie Worthington-Roberts, PhD.

Our gratitude to the reviewers who considered every nutrition detail and concept from the beginning of Chapter 1 to the last words of Chapter 21. Many of the revisions that strengthen this text reflect reviewers' suggestions.

REVIEWERS

Janet Azar, RN, MNEd
Tidewater Community College
Portsmouth, Virginia

Merilyn Hunter, MS
Garland County Community College
Hot Springs, Arkansas

Janet Keen, RN, MS, CEN, CCRN
Gordon College
Barnsville, Georgia

Linda L. Lilley, RN, MS
Old Dominion University School of Nursing
Norfolk, Virginia

Joan Magee, MS
Henry Ford Community College
Dearborn, Michigan

Bruce Rengers, PhD, RD
University of Northern Colorado
Greeley, Colorado

Nancy Scott
Wenatchee Valley Community College
Wenatchee, Washington

Mary Jane Ward, RN, PhD, FAAN
University of Oklahoma Health Sciences Center
Oklahoma City, Oklahoma

SPECIAL ACKNOWLEDGMENTS

This book has had a long and winding road from conception to realization. Initial thanks to Chris Rodgers, now with Times Mirror, who was sure that there was a text inside of MG before a word was ever written. Our appreciation to the supportive staff at Mosby. Thanks to Jim Smith, Publisher, for overseeing the transition and evolution of this project and to Vicki Malinee, Senior Acquisition Editor, who quickly sensed what was different about the book. Special appreciation to Janet Livingston, our final Managing Editor, who easily took over supervision of this book during its final stages. We are most indebted to Terry Eynon, who switched from our Managing Editor to our Developmental Editor. Her ability to devote her full attention to this text accounts for its smoothness of format and consistency of style. Our joy of sharing life experiences during the development of this book will probably be a one-of-a-kind experience.

Thanks also to Sheilah Barrett, for a beautiful design that enhances the learning experience, and to Carol Sullivan Weis, Project Manager, and Karen Rehwinkel, Production Editor, who guided us quickly and expertly through a complex production process but never lost sight of the importance of details.

Finally, thanks to our friends and especially our families, who endured our late hours, lonely meals, and delayed celebrations. Now no one will need to ask, "Have you finished THAT book yet?"

As authors of this text, we represent a collaboration of expertise in nutrition, education, dietetics, and nursing. As we formulated and implemented this book, we continually asked ourselves: "What do nurses need to know about nutrition? How would they apply this knowledge to their patients and clients?" We hope we have succeeded in answering these questions.

Michele Grodner
Sara Long Anderson
Sandra DeYoung

CONTENTS IN BRIEF

CONTENTS

FOUNDATIONS AND CLINICAL APPLICATIONS OF

NUTRITION

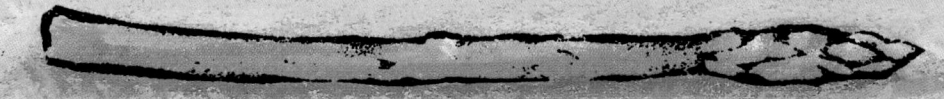

A Nursing Approach

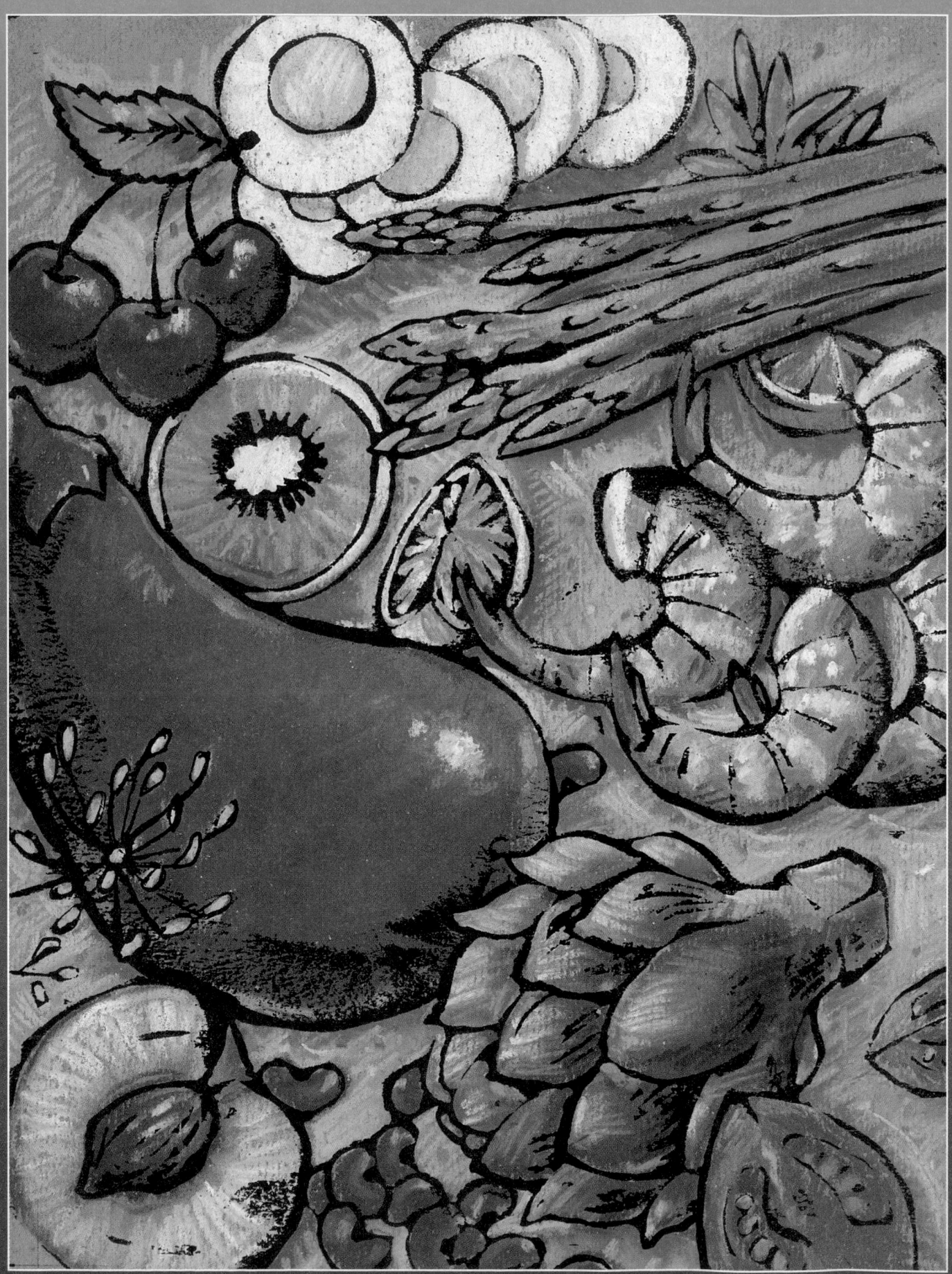

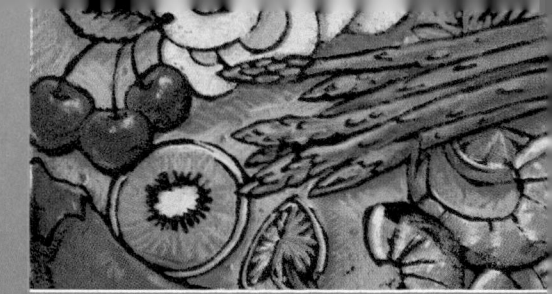

PART ONE

Wellness, Nutrition, and the Nursing Role

Chapter 1

WELLNESS NUTRITION

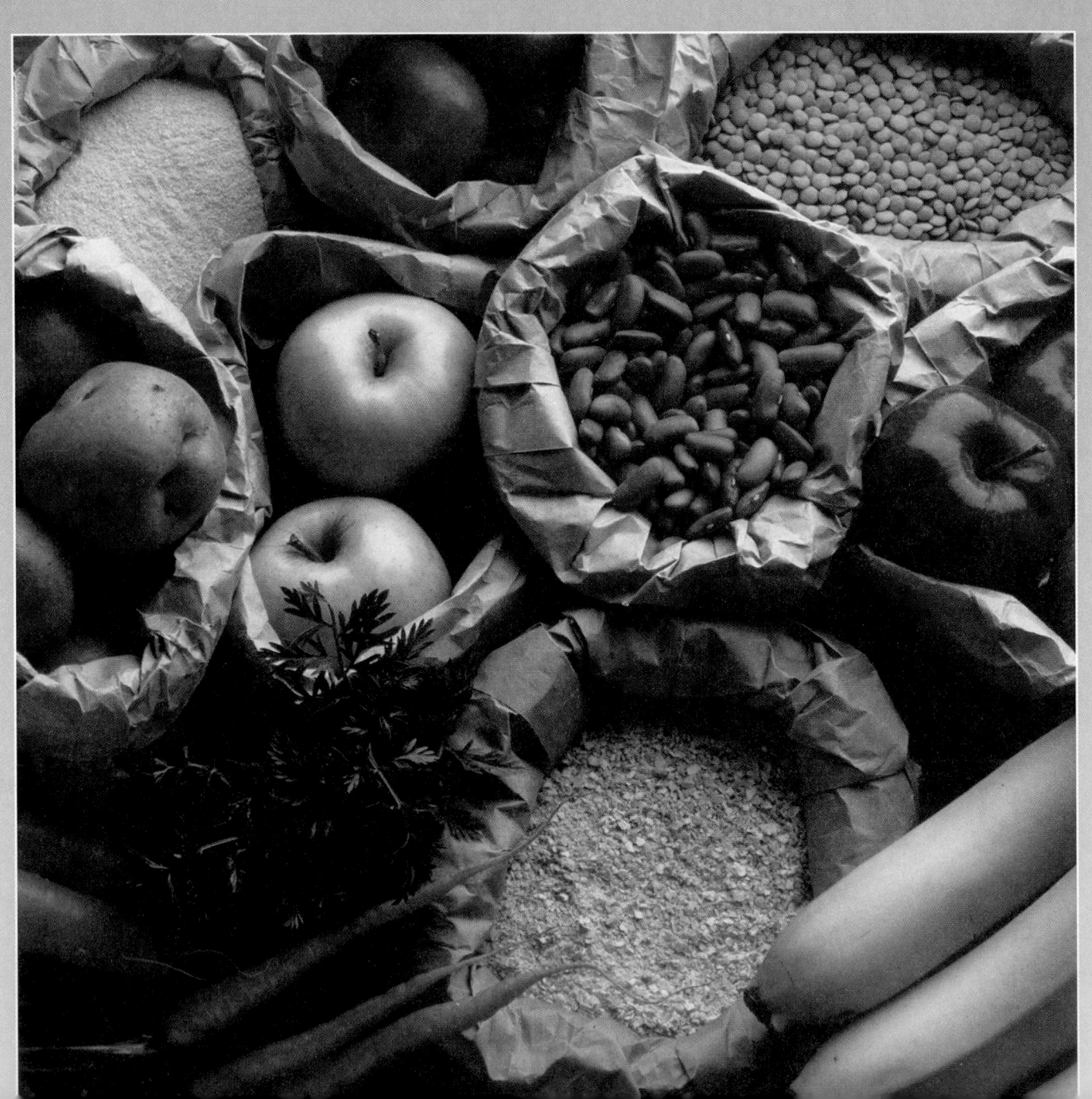

Wellness is a lifestyle in which we strive to enhance our level of health. Achieving wellness is a continuous, never-ending journey. This text provides knowledge, strategies, and techniques about food, nutrition, and health. These tools allow us and our clients to achieve wellness through personal nutrition lifestyles.

Nutrition is a "hot topic" that generates interest easily; everyone seems to have an opinion about what to eat and concerns about their own eating styles. The public is flooded with knowledge and techniques related to health promotion through nutrition. This education of the public occurs in three different forms: formal, nonformal, and informal. *Formal* education is purposefully planned for implementation in a school setting. *Nonformal* education takes place through organized teaching and learning events in such places as hospitals, community centers, and clinics. *Informal* education encompasses a variety of educational experiences that occur through daily activities. These experiences may include watching television, reading newspapers and magazines, and conversing with other people (1).

The most effective education, however, results in behavior change. Nurses, through formal, nonformal, and informal educational interactions, can introduce knowledge and strategies for personal lifestyle choices that consider the social context of the patients' lives (2). Formal education may be conducted by school nurses teaching health courses; topics can be approached through the health issues of the ethnic and cultural groups of the school population. Nonformal education occurs when associations such as the American Heart Association and hospital wellness programs teach courses on risk-reducing lifestyle changes; these courses are usually open to the community-at-large. Informal education takes place when a nurse chats with a patient and her family, explaining the purpose of the dietary modifications recommended for the patient's particular disorder.

Never before have we had so much information about the effects of our personal behavior patterns on our level of health. Changing (or maintaining) our patterns of behaviors and therefore our lifestyles is the key to achieving wellness. Many social, community, and occupational forces affect our ability to change. Strategies and techniques ease our ability to modify our personal behaviors.

Modifying behaviors means changing lifestyles. Since this text is about food and nutrition, patterns of behaviors affecting the foods we choose to eat constitute our nutrition lifestyles. Our nutrition lifestyles won't all be the same. Some of us are caught in extremely hectic work/college/sports schedules; we're lucky to find time to eat at all. Others find that our original families are still the center of our eating patterns; our families, however, may not have adopted recent recommendations to decrease the risks of diet-related diseases. Many of us are part of new social settings on campus and need to deal with the artificial schedules and menus of school cafeterias. What we do have in common is the ability to improve our nutrition lifestyles.

As health care professionals, we need to be concerned with our own nutritional patterns, as well as those of our clients. To reflect a health promotion perspective, individuals being cared for by health professionals to maintain health are referred to as "clients." Those who are ill or recuperating from illness are called "patients."

Enhancing personal health provides the stamina and well-being to fulfill the rigorous demands of nursing practice. A fundamental responsibility of nursing is client education. As we teach our clients about nutritional wellness, we also function as role models for the positive effects of enhanced nutritional lifestyles.

DEFINITION OF HEALTH

In the past, health was often defined as the absence of disease or illness. Since then, modern medicine has conquered a number of life-threatening diseases such as smallpox and polio. Public health measures of pasteurization and sanitation have reduced the risk of foodborne and environmental hazards. As concern over the physical status of the human body has lessened, we've been able to consider other aspects of the qualities of health.

Health is now understood to be a complex concept best represented by five physical and psychological dimensions (3). The five dimensions include the following:

Physical health: the efficiency of the body to function appropriately, to maintain immunity to disease, and to meet daily energy requirements.

Intellectual health: the use of intellectual abilities to learn and to adapt to changes in one's environment.

Emotional health: the capacity to easily express or suppress emotions appropriately.

Social health: the ability to interact with people in an acceptable manner and to sustain relationships with family members, friends, and colleagues.

Spiritual health: the cultural beliefs that give purpose to human existence. This belief may be found through faith in the teachings of organized religions, in an understanding of nature or science, or in an acceptance of the humanistic view of life.

Health is the merging and balance of the five dimensions. This holistic view incorporates many aspects of human existence. Using this definition of health allows for more individualized assessment of health status. As we evaluate our health and the health of our clients in relation to each dimension, some dimensions will be stronger than others.

Role of Nutrition

Nutrition is the study of nutrients and the processes by which they are used by the body. **Nutrients** are chemicals in foods that are required by the body for energy, growth, maintenance, and repair. Some nutrients are *essential*; they cannot be made by the human body and must be provided by foods.

Since the primary role of nutrients is to provide the building blocks for the efficient functioning and maintenance of the body, nutrition may appear to belong only within the physical health dimension. But the effects of nutrients and their sources on the other health dimensions are far-reaching. Nutrition is the cornerstone of each health dimension.

Physical health is extremely dependent on the quantity of nutrients available to the body. The human body, from skeletal bones to minute amounts of hormones, is composed of nutrients in various combinations.

health
the merging and balance of five physical and psychological dimensions of health: physical, mental, emotional, social, and spiritual

nutrition
the study of essential nutrients and the processes by which nutrients are used by the body

nutrients
chemicals in foods that are required by the body for energy, growth, maintenance, or repair

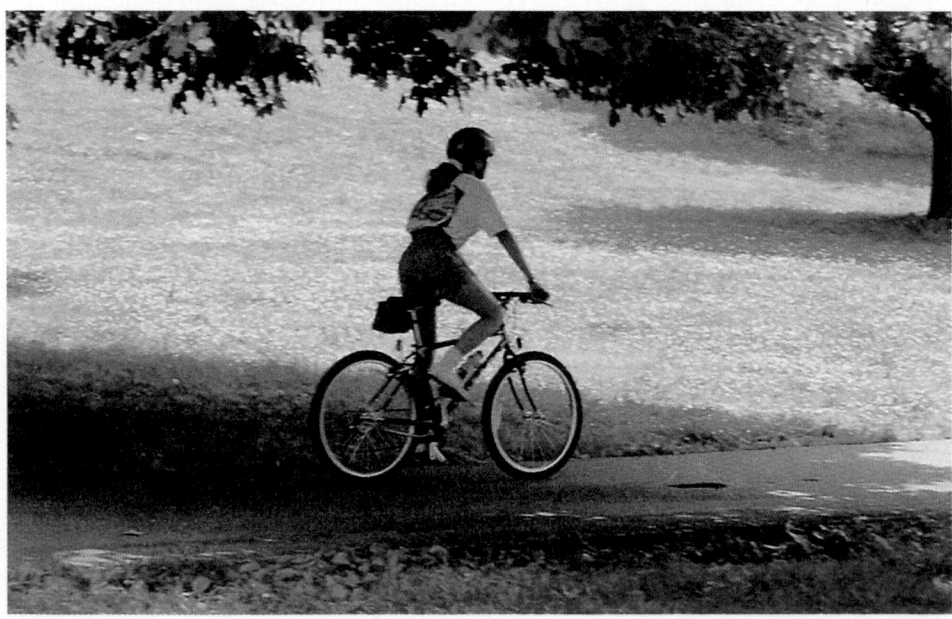

Physical health benefits from a good diet.

Intellectual health relies on a well-functioning brain and central nervous system. Nutritional imbalances can affect intellectual health, for example, as in iron deficiency anemia. Although milk is an excellent source of protein, calcium, and phosphorus, it is a negligible source of iron. Some young children drink so much milk that it affects their appetite for other foods such as meats, chicken, legumes, and leafy green vegetables, which are good sources of iron. Iron-deficiency may result. The cognitive abilities of children who are iron-deficient may be affected, possibly leading to learning problems in the classroom.

Emotional health may be affected by poor eating habits that result in hypoglycemia or low blood glucose levels. Low blood glucose occurs normally in anyone who is physically hungry. When the body's need for food is ignored (when we miss meals because of poor planning or are too busy to eat), feelings of anxiety and confusion and trembling may be experienced. Emotions may be harder to control when we feel this way. Although blood glucose levels may affect our emotions, there are, of course, other factors influencing emotional health.

Social health situations often center around food-related occasions, ranging from holiday feasts to everyday meals. Nutritional status is sometimes affected by the quality of our relationships with family and friends. Are family meals an enjoyable experience or a tense ordeal? How might this affect a person's dietary intake?

Spiritual health often has ties to foods. Several religions prohibit the consumption of specific foods. Many followers of Islam and Judaism adhere to the dietary laws of their religions. Both forbid consumption of pork-related products. Seventh Day Adventists follow an ovo-lacto vegetarian dietary pattern, consuming only plant foods plus dairy products and so do not consume meat, fish, or poultry. In India, cows are viewed as sacred animals that are not eaten but revered as a source of sustenance (milk), fuel (burning of feces), power (as a work animal) and fertilizer (manure).

HEALTH PROMOTION

The goal of **health promotion** is to increase the level of health of individuals, families, groups, and communities. In community and occupational health settings, health promotion strategies implemented by nurses often focus on lifestyle changes that will lead to new positive health behaviors. Development of these behaviors may depend on knowledge, techniques, and community supports.

Knowledge: Learning new information about the benefits or risks of health-related behaviors.

Techniques: Applying new knowledge to everyday activities; developing ways to modify present lifestyles.

Community supports: Availability of environmental or regulatory measures to support new health promoting behaviors within a social context.

health promotion
strategies to increase the level of health of individuals, families, and communities

Role of Nutrition

Healthy People 2000, a document prepared by the US Public Health Service of the Department of Health and Human Services outlines national health promotion and disease prevention objectives for Americans. These health objectives are to be achieved by the year 2000. One of the three broad goals is to "increase the span of healthy life for Americans" (4). Nutrition is a priority area for achieving this goal, as evidenced by the inclusion of 21 nutrition-related objectives (Table 1-1).

One nutrition objective is that individuals reduce their intake of dietary fat to an average of 30% or less of total caloric intake (4). To achieve this through health promotion strategies, health professionals need *knowledge* of the relationship

Table 1-1   Healthy People 2000: Nutrition Objectives

Category	Objectives
Health status	1. Reduce heart disease deaths to no more than 100 per 100,000 people. 2. Reverse the rise in cancer deaths to achieve a rate of no more than 130 per 100,000 people. 3. Reduce overweight to a prevalence of no more than 20% among people ages 20 years and older and no more than 15% among adolescents ages 12 through 19 years. 4. Reduce growth retardation among low-income children ages 5 years and younger to less than 10%.
Risk reduction	5. Reduce dietary fat intake to an average of 30% of calories or less and average saturated fat intake to less than 10% of calories among people ages 2 years and older. 6. Increase complex carbohydrate- and fiber-containing foods in the diets of adults to five or more daily servings for vegetables (including legumes) and fruits and to six or more daily servings for grain products. 7. Increase the proportion of overweight people ages 12 years and older who have adopted sound dietary practices combined with regular physical activity to attain an appropriate body weight to at least 50%. 8. Increase calcium intake, so at least 50% of youth ages 12 through 24 and 50% of pregnant and lactating women consume three or more servings daily of foods rich in calcium and at least 50% of people ages 25 years and older consume two or more servings daily. 9. Decrease salt and sodium intake, so at least 65% of home meal preparers prepare foods without adding salt, at least 80% of people avoid using salt at the table, and at least 40% of adults regularly purchase foods modified or lower in sodium. 10. Reduce iron deficiency to less than 3% among children ages 1 through 4 years and among women of childbearing age. 11. Increase to at least 75% the proportion of mothers who breastfeed their babies in the early postpartum period and to at least 50% the proportion who continue breastfeeding until their babies are 5 to 6 months old. 12. Increase to at least 75% the proportion of parents and caregivers who use feeding practices that prevent baby bottle tooth decay. 13. Increase to at least 85% the proportion of people ages 18 years and older who use food labels to make nutritious food selections.
Services and protection	14. Achieve useful and informative nutrition labeling for virtually all processed foods and for at least 40% of fresh meats, poultry, fish, fruits, vegetables, baked goods, and ready-to-eat carry-away foods. 15. Increase the availability of processed food products that are reduced in fat and saturated fat to at least 5000 brand items. 16. Increase to at least 90% the proportion of restaurants and institutional food service operations that offer identifiable low-fat, low-calorie food choices, consistent with the Dietary Guidelines for Americans. 17. Increase to at least 90% the proportion of school lunch and breakfast services and child care food services with menus that are consistent with the nutrition principles in the Dietary Guidelines for Americans. 18. Increase to at least 90% the proportion of school lunch and breakfast services by people ages 65 years and older who have difficulty in preparing their own meals or are otherwise in need of home-delivered meals. 19. Increase to at least 75% the proportion of the nation's schools that provide nutrition education from preschool through twelfth grade, preferably as part of quality school health education. 20. Increase to at least 50% the proportion of worksites with 50 or more employees that offer nutrition education and/or weight management programs for employees. 21. Increase to at least 75% the proportion of primary care providers who provide nutrition assessment and counseling and/or referral to a qualified nutritionist or dietitian.

From US Department of Health and Human Services: *Healthy people 2000: National health promotion and disease prevention objectives,* US Public Health Service Pub No 91-50212, Washington, DC, 1990, US Government Printing Office.

between the fat consumption and the risk of developing coronary artery disease, certain cancers, and obesity; which foods are high in fat; and effective ways to translate technical information to the public. *Techniques* include teaching clients the skills of how to shop for and cook foods that contain lower levels of fat. *Community supports* involve recognition of supermarkets stocking low-fat food alternatives, restaurants offering low-fat entrees, friends and family providing social support, and the media publicizing the relationship between coronary artery disease, cancer, and dietary fat intake.

DEFINITION OF WELLNESS

 ellness is a **lifestyle** (pattern of behavior) that enhances each of the five dimensions of health. Individuals engaged in wellness lifestyles feel a sense of competency and achievement in their ability to modify their behaviors to increase or maintain positive levels of health.

Hectic contemporary schedules may seem to interfere with efforts to achieve wellness. The aim is to strive for wellness even if the path may seem more like a roller coaster than a smooth uphill climb (Fig. 1-1). At times, clients may falter in their efforts, but the key is to renew positive behaviors as soon as possible.

wellness
a lifestyle that enhances our level of health

lifestyle
a pattern of behaviors

◄► SOCIAL ISSUE
Healthy People 2000

The purpose of *Healthy People 2000* is to create a blueprint for American health professionals to follow. This blueprint provides agreed upon health goals for many segments of our population. For example, a community health nurse specializing in adolescent and young adult health does not need to spend time and resources to determine appropriate objectives. The objectives are already stated in *Healthy People 2000*.

How will this affect your health as a student? Health and nutrition education programs on your campus may already focus on these objectives. Some of the objectives affecting college students of all ages are to reduce sedentary lifestyles, increase cal-

cium intake, reduce total dietary fat intake, decrease levels of alcohol consumption, and assure availability of nutrition assessment and counseling. Primary health providers of the college health center may address objectives of adequate immunizations, clinical services for HIV and other sexually transmitted diseases, and access to primary medical services. Counselors and psychologists of the mental health or counseling centers address the objectives to reduce the incidence of suicide and eating disorders.

So although you may not have read the original document of *Healthy People 2000*, campus health professionals are attempting to improve your health and well-being.

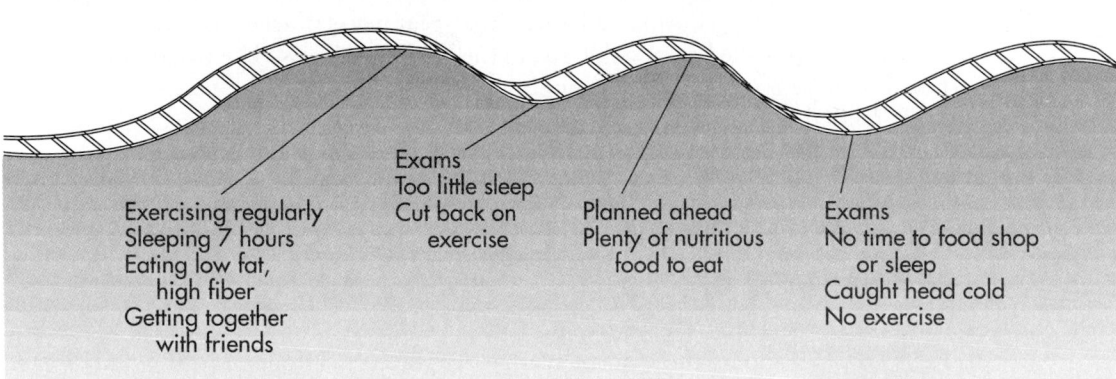

Fig. 1-1 Wellness effort roller coaster.

Role of Nutrition

"Wellness nutrition" approaches food consumption as a positive way to nourish the body. This approach focuses on ways to organize our lives so that we can more easily follow an eating pattern designed to enhance health status. Consuming a diet based on lower fat/higher fiber and moderate caloric consumption is then not a chore, but an affirmation of our competency to care for ourselves. Conveying this approach to our patients is a nursing challenge.

DISEASE PREVENTION THROUGH NUTRITION

disease prevention
the recognition of a danger to health that could be reduced or alleviated through specific actions or changes in lifestyles behaviors

Disease prevention is the recognition of a danger to health that could be reduced or alleviated through specific actions or changes in lifestyle behaviors. The hazard may be due to disease, lifestyle or genetic factors, or an environmental threat. The three classifications of disease prevention are primary, secondary, and tertiary (5). Disease prevention has strong ties to nutrition.

Primary prevention consists of activities to avert the initial development of a disease or poor health. A primary disease prevention approach is to eat a variety of foods to avert nutrient deficiencies. Adopting a low-fat, high-fiber eating style before diet-related health problems develop is another form of primary prevention.

Secondary prevention involves early detection to halt or reduce the effects of a disease or illness. Some diseases cannot be prevented, but early detection can minimize negative health effects. Secondary prevention strategies are useful in reducing the effects of chronic diet-related diseases. Controlling the intake of certain nutrients can decrease the severity of some disorders. Some individuals with high blood pressure or hypertension are sodium-sensitive, and simply reducing the amount of sodium consumed can decrease blood pressure levels and bring the disorder under control. Since hypertension is a risk factor for coronary artery disease, strokes, and renal disease, reduction of blood pressure through decreased sodium consumption is a secondary prevention strategy.

Tertiary prevention occurs after a disorder develops. The purpose is to minimize further complications or to assist in the restoration of health. These efforts may involve continued medical care. Often, learning more about the disorder is helpful for patients and their families. Tertiary prevention frequently involves diet therapy. Direct treatments of many disorders have a dietary component. Some of these disorders include ulcers, diverticulitis, and coronary artery disease; they often occur during the middle and older years of adulthood. Other disorders may affect food intake and the ability of the body to absorb nutrients. For example, chemotherapy for cancer sometimes has side effects of nausea and loss of appetite. Nutrition counseling during and after these treatments is necessary so that patients are as well-nourished as possible to aid the healing process. The five dimensions of health can be an excellent teaching tool in promoting health and preventing diseases related to nutrition (see box).

OVERVIEW OF NUTRIENTS WITHIN THE BODY

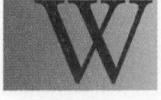**W**hat are these nutrients that are the cornerstone of health and disease prevention? What do they do to make them so important? Why can't we just take a nutrient pill?

TEACHING TOOL
Dimensions of Health

To broaden a patient's understanding of health, use the five dimensions of health. Describe the dimensions and then discuss with the patient each that pertains to his nutrition and health situation. By exploring other aspects of health, besides physical health, a person can then use all of his resources to restore his overall level of well-being.

Wellness Through the Five Dimensions of Health

Physical health: efficient body functioning
Intellectual health: use of intellectual abilities
Emotional health: ability to control emotions
Social health: interactions and relationships with others
Spiritual health: cultural beliefs about the purpose of life

Table 1-2   Known Essential Nutrients

Nutrient	Source
Carbohydrates	Glucose
Lipids (fats)	Linoleic acid
	Linolenic acid
Protein	Amino acids
	Histidine, Isoleucine, Leucine, Lysine, Methionine, Phenylalanine, Threonine, Tryptophan, Valine
Vitamins	Fat-soluble vitamins
	A (retinol), D (cholecalciferol), E (tocopherol), K
	Water-soluble vitamins
	Thiamin, Riboflavin, Niacin, Pantothenic acid, Biotin, B-6 (pyridoxine), B-12 (cobalamin), Folate, C (ascorbic acid)
Minerals	Major minerals
	Calcium, Phosphorus, Sodium, Potassium, Sulfur, Chlorine, Magnesium
	Trace minerals
	Chromium, Cobalt, Copper, Fluorine, Iodine, Iron, Manganese, Selenium, Zinc
Water	

Nutrient Categories

Nutrients can be divided into the following six categories:

carbohydrates	vitamins	lipids (fats)
minerals	protein	water

Nutrients may be either essential or nonessential, depending on whether the body can manufacture them. When the body requires a nutrient for growth or maintenance but lacks the ability to manufacture amounts sufficient to meet the body's needs, the nutrient is **essential** and must be supplied by the foods in our diet. Table 1-2 lists the essential nutrients needed in our diet. Other nutrients that the body can make on its own are called **nonessential**.

The functions of essential nutrients in the body include aiding growth and repair of body tissues, regulating body processes, and providing energy. Some nutrients are diverse in their impact, while others have very specific functions.

Only carbohydrates, proteins, and lipids are nutrients that provide energy. Whereas carbohydrates primarily contribute only energy, proteins and lipids are also essential for the growth and repair of body tissues and are required for regulating body processes. Although vitamins and minerals cannot provide energy, they do have indirect roles as catalysts for the body's use of nutrients for energy. Each vitamin serves a different specific function related to regulation of body processes. Minerals and water also regulate body processes and are required for growth and maintenance of tissues.

FOOD, ENERGY, AND NUTRIENTS

While the discussion so far focuses on nutrients, we must remember that nutrients are found in foods. Since foods usually contain a mixture of nutrients, we often categorize a food based on the most predominate nutrient found in the food. A bagel is a carbohydrate food and contains mostly complex carbohydrates, although it also contains protein, water, small amounts of vitamins and minerals, and an even smaller amount of lipids or fat (6) (Fig. 1-2).

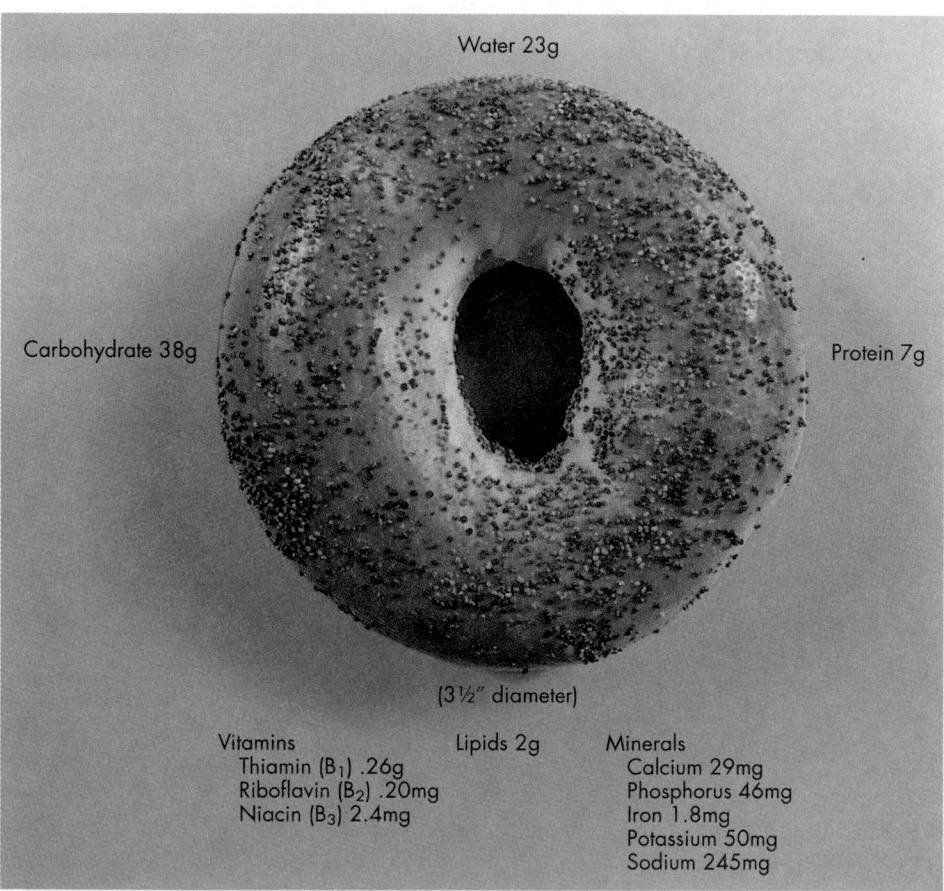

Fig. 1-2 Most foods contain a mixture of nutrients. (Data from USDA: Nutritive value of foods, *Home and Garden Bulletin* 72, 1991.)

The gold mine of nutrients found in foods is why taking a nutrient-specific pill will not provide for all the necessities of the human body.

Energy

Let's consider the energy-containing nutrients of carbohydrates, protein, and lipids. These contain energy because they are organic. Being organic means that they are composed of a structure consisting of hydrogen, oxygen, and carbon. Organic compounds are produced by living or once-living things, including plants and animals. The carbon-containing structure identifies these nutrients as being organic. When these nutrients are oxidized (burned in the body), energy is released and available for use by the cells. Although vitamins are also organic, the human body cannot use energy from them. Only carbohydrates, proteins, and lipids are energy-yielding nutrients.

The energy released from food is measured in kilocalories (thousands of calories) or calories. Technically a calorie is the amount of heat necessary to raise the temperature of a gram of water 1-degree Celsius. When someone asks how much energy is in an 8-ounce glass of skim milk, the correct response is 90,000 calories or 90 kilocalories. For numerical simplicity, we commonly refer to the calories in a food rather than use the correct term of kilocalories. To assure accuracy, the term *kilocalories* will be used throughout this text, abbreviated as "kcalories" or "kcal."

Energy-yielding nutrients provide different amounts of energy (Table 1-3). Carbohydrates and protein each provide 4 kcalories per gram. Lipids contain more than twice as much energy and provide 9 kcalories per gram. The kcalorie content of a specific food, for example, a bagel, is based on the amount of carbohydrate, lipid, and protein energy contained in the food (Fig 1-3). When we consume energy-yielding foods, we are usually ingesting other nutrients as well, including vitamins, minerals, and water.

Another energy-yielding substance is alcohol. Alcohol provides 7 kcalories per gram. But alcohol is not considered a nutrient because although it does provide

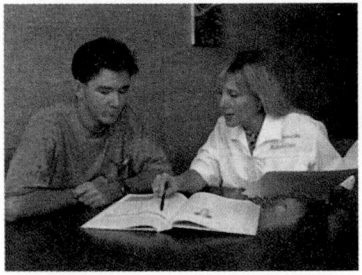

Nutrition is an integral part of health care education.

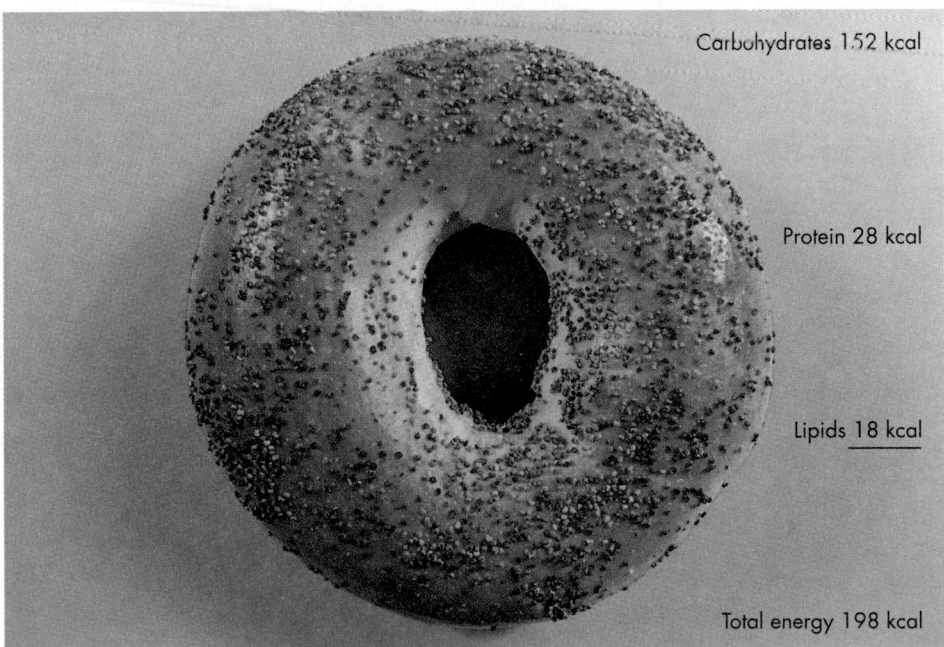

Carbohydrates 152 kcal

Protein 28 kcal

Lipids 18 kcal

Total energy 198 kcal

Fig. 1-3 A food's kcalorie content is based on the energy-yielding nutrients it contains. (Data from USDA: Nutritive value of foods, *Home and Garden Bulletin* 72, 1991.)

Table 1-3 Kcaloric values	
Nutrient	Kcal value/gram
Carbohydrates	4
Protein	4
Lipids (fats)	9
Alcohol	7

energy, the body treats it as a toxin. Breaking down or metabolizing alcohol is not only stressful to the body but also uses essential nutrients that could be better used to nourish the body.

Although protein, lipids, and carbohydrates do provide energy, they and the other three nutrient categories of vitamins, minerals, and water also have other important functions. A brief introduction to each nutrient category follows.

CARBOHYDRATES

simple: sugar.

Carbohydrates are a major source of fuel. They consist of simple carbohydrates, often called sugars, and complex carbohydrates that include starch and fiber. Simple carbohydrates are found in foods such as white sugar, fruits, and milk. Complex carbohydrates are found in cereals, grains, pastas, fruits, and vegetables. All, except fiber, are broken down to units of glucose, which is one of the simple carbohydrates. Glucose provides the most efficient form of energy for the body, particularly for muscles and the brain.

Fiber cannot be broken down by the human digestive system, therefore it doesn't provide energy. Instead, fiber just passes through the body. Although fiber is not an essential nutrient, consuming fiber is necessary for good health. Dietary fiber provides several beneficial effects on the digestive and absorptive systems of the body. These effects range from preventing constipation to reducing the incidence of colon cancer.

PROTEINS

Proteins, in addition to providing energy, perform an extensive range of functions in the body. Some of these functions include roles in the structure of bones, muscles, enzymes, hormones, blood, the immune system, and cell membranes. Proteins are formed by the linking of amino acids in various combinations. Twenty amino acids are required to create all the necessary proteins to maintain life. Some are formed by the body, others are called essential amino acids and must be consumed in foods. The nine essential amino acids are found in animal and plant sources. Animal sources include meat, fish, poultry, and some dairy products such as milk and cheeses. Plant sources include grains, legumes (peas and beans that contain protein), seeds, nuts, and small amounts in many vegetables.

Even though protein is important nutritionally, eating too much protein can be a problem. Eating substantially more than the recommended amounts of protein does not produce superhumans. Instead, our physical systems can become overworked. Excess protein is broken down to amino acids. The amino acids are then used for energy or broken down further and excreted through the kidneys in urine.

FATS

Fats are the most dense form of energy available in foods and as stored energy in our bodies. But fats, or lipids, serve other purposes, such as functioning as a component of all cell structures, having a role in the production of hormones, and providing padding to protect body organs. Essential fatty acids and the fat-soluble vitamins A, D, E, and K are found in food lipids. And it's the fats in foods that make certain foods taste so appealing!

Lipids are divided into three categories: triglycerides, phospholipids, and sterols. Triglycerides are called saturated, monosaturated, or polyunsaturated fats based on the types of fatty acids they contain. Fatty acids are carbon chains of varying lengths and degree of hydrogen saturation. The most common phospholipid is lecithin; among sterols we hear most about cholesterol. Although we consume lecithin and cholesterol in our foods, our bodies manufacture them as well.

Fats and cholesterol are often in the news. Saturated fats or triglycerides found in some fat-containing foods and dietary cholesterol are associated with increased blood lipid levels. Elevated blood lipid levels, whether formed by our bodies or consumed in dietary sources, are a risk factor for the development of coronary artery disease. Saturated fats and to a certain extent polyunsaturated fats have also been associated with increased risk for certain cancers. Coronary artery disease and cancer are serious public health diseases affecting millions of North Americans. Consequently, medical and health professionals emphasize the need to reduce our intake of foods containing fats and cholesterol.

VITAMINS

Vitamins are compounds that indirectly assist other nutrients through the complete processes of digestion, absorption, metabolism, and excretion. Thirteen vitamins are needed by our bodies and each has a specific function. As noted earlier, vitamins provide no energy but assist in the release of energy from carbohydrates, lipids, and proteins.

Vitamins are divided into two classes based on their solubility (ability to dissolve) in water. The water-soluble vitamins are the B vitamins (thiamin, niacin, riboflavin, folate, cobalamin [B_{12}], pyridoxine [B_6], pantothenic acid, biotin) and vitamin C. The fat-soluble vitamins are vitamins A, D, E, and K.

Vitamins are found in many foods; fruits and vegetables are particularly good sources. Since some foods are better sources of specific vitamins, eating a variety of foods is the best way to consume sufficient amounts.

MINERALS

In our bodies, minerals serve structural purposes such as in bones and teeth, and they are found in body fluids. Minerals in body fluids affect the nature of the fluids, which in turn influence the functioning of muscles and the central nervous system. Sixteen essential minerals are divided into two categories of major minerals and trace minerals. Although this distinction is based on the quantity required by the body, all are equally important.

Minerals are plentiful in fruits, vegetables, dairy products, meats, and legumes. Although minerals are indestructible, some may be lost through food processing. For example, when whole wheat flour is processed or refined to white flour, minerals such as phosphorus and potassium are lost and are not replaced.

WATER

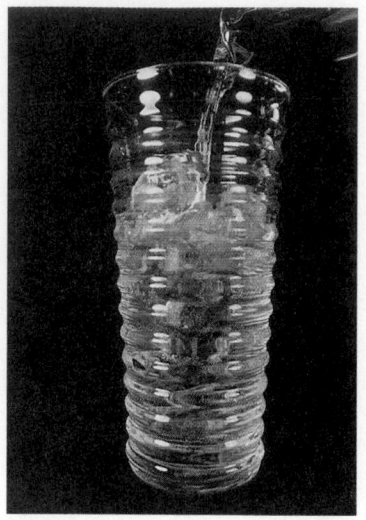

The need for water is more urgent than the need for any other nutrient.

dietary standards
a guide to adequate nutrient intake levels against which to compare the nutrient values of foods consumed

Recommended Dietary Allowances (RDAs)
average daily intake levels of essential nutrients that meet the nutritional needs of almost all healthy individuals

Water is a major part of every tissue of our bodies. We can live only a few days without water. Water functions as a fluid in which substances can be broken down and reformed for use by our bodies. As a constituent of blood, water also provides a means of transportation for nutrients to and from cells.

Many of us probably do not drink enough water or liquids to best meet the needs of our bodies. We should consume the equivalent of about eight to ten cups a day from foods and beverages (7). Awareness of the value of water consumption is growing as bottled water companies heavily advertise their products to the public. Although public water supplies are safe, bottled waters have become a fashionable alternative to other beverages. These products seem to offer convenience and status against which tap water can't compete. Although more money may be spent on bottled water than is necessary, the health benefits are still achieved.

DIETARY STANDARDS

Simply knowing which nutrients are essential to life is not sufficient. We need to know how much of each nutrient to consume to be assured of basic good health. Similarly, eating foods without awareness of their nutrient value does not assure an adequate intake of nutrients. **Dietary standards** provide a bridge between knowledge of essential nutrients and food consumption. Dietary standards provide a guide of adequate nutrient intake levels against which to compare the nutrient values of foods consumed.

Requirement Versus Allowance

A *requirement* is the amount of a nutrient that must be consumed to prevent deficiency symptoms. It is the minimum level needed to provide for basic physiological functioning of our bodies. An *allowance* is the amount of a nutrient that must be consumed to maintain good health. An allowance "allows" for variation in individual needs and supplies enough of a nutrient to provide for possible nutrient storage in our bodies. Since dietary standards aim to provide nutrient guidelines for health, rather than just the absence of deficiency symptoms, allowances are used to create dietary standards for the levels of nutrient intake.

Recommended Dietary Allowances

The **Recommended Dietary Allowances** (RDAs) are average daily intake levels of essentials nutrients that meet the nutritional needs of almost all healthy individuals (7). These standards are set by the members of the Food and Nutrition Board of the National Academy of Sciences-National Research Council. To incorporate the most recent scientific knowledge, the Board revises the RDAs every 5 to 10 years. The current RDA table can be found inside the front cover of this book.

The RDAs recommend allowances for 19 nutrients. Seventeen different levels are set for each nutrient based on age, gender, and physiological needs of growth or pregnancy. When deciding the RDA level for each nutrient, members of the Food and Nutrition Board consider the average person's requirement for the nutrient and the amount of variability of the level among the population. For example, the requirement for vitamin C is 10 mg. This level prevents the symptoms of scurvy, a disorder that results from vitamin-C deficiency. However, some individuals may be protected at levels of 5 mg while others may require 15 mg. This variability is considered when setting the allowance for vitamin C at 60 mg.

Another factor taken into account is the efficiency with which the body uses the nutrient. How absorbable is the nutrient? How well can our bodies use it? For example, we cannot efficiently absorb the iron in foods. The human body absorbs only about 10% of the iron we eat, regardless of the amount we consume. With that fact in mind, the RDA for iron is set at a level 10 times what we need to account for its absorption rate. Once absorbed, the iron is efficiently used and even recycled within the body to be used again.

An additional concern is the existence of **precursors**, which are substances that the human body can convert to a nutrient. One of these substances is beta carotene. Beta carotene is responsible for the deep orange and yellow colors in many fruits and vegetables. It can be transformed by our bodies into vitamin A and is an important source of the nutrient. The RDA for vitamin A takes this alternative source of the vitamin into account.

precursor
a substance that the human body can convert to a nutrient

Margin of safety

Since the RDAs are allowances rather than minimum requirements, a reasonable amount is added when setting each recommended level. This amount provides an additional safety factor referred to as "the margin of safety," which means that the RDAs are about 30% higher than most individuals need.

RDAs are intended to be general guidelines rather than specific requirements.

The RDAs are designed to meet the needs of most healthy individuals. Those with special nutritional needs, such as those suffering from disease, injury, or other medical conditions, may have nutrient needs that are higher than the RDAs. In addition, the RDAs are not set to reflect potential disease prevention or pharmacological roles of essential nutrients (see box).

Use of the RDAs

The RDAs are used widely throughout the US food systems. Uses include the following:

- Planning meals for large groups such as the military.
- Creating dietary standards for governmental food assistance programs such as the Women, Infants and Children (WIC) and Food Stamp programs.

HEALTH DEBATE
Politics of Recommended Dietary Allowances

Nutrient deficiencies were a health issue when the RDAs were created. The problem of deficiencies, however, has decreased. Now more concern exists about the relationship between our dietary intake and the development of chronic diseases such as cancer and heart disease.

When the 1985 RDA committee met, the members recommended revisions reflecting new data on vitamin requirements. According to these data, the RDA levels of vitamins A and C could be reduced and still safely assure basic health needs. At the same time, new data were presented to the health care community showing that people who eat more foods containing vitamins A and C are less likely to develop cancer.

When the 1985 RDA committee recommendations (including lower RDA for vitamins A and C) were first proposed, they were not accepted by the National Research Council. Some members were concerned that lowering the vitamin A and C levels would be detrimental to the health of the nation. The National Research Council viewed the RDA goal of basic good health to also include primary prevention against disease, not just against deficiencies.

The concerns of both groups were not resolved until 1989 when the tenth edition of the RDAs was released. Although other recommendations of the 1985 committee were adopted, the levels of vitamins A and C basically stayed the same (higher than necessary to safely assure basic health needs).

What do you think? Should the RDAs only reflect nutrient levels to prevent deficiencies or also provide for preventive health needs?

- Interpreting food consumption information on individuals and populations. Although originally intended only for analysis of the diets of large groups of people, they can be used for individuals if compared with an average intake over a period of time. The intake of a single day does not have to meet the recommended levels. A comparison with the RDA does not determine nutritional status but is only one of several measurements used to assess nutritional status.
- Meeting national nutrition goals such as those listed in *Healthy People 2000*.
- Developing new food products such as imitation products that duplicate the nutrient values of the original.
- Providing guidelines for nutrition labeling of foods. The 1968 RDAs are used to create the labeling standard called the Daily Reference Values. These values were formerly the US Recommended Dietary Allowances and are based on the highest RDAs of any category except for pregnancy and lactation.

Additional Standards

For some essential nutrients, no RDA has been established. Either the exact required levels for these nutrients are not known or consuming enough of the nutrient is not a problem. For some other essential nutrients, the Food and Nutrition Board develops two additional standards: (1) Estimated Safe and Adequate Daily Dietary Intakes (ESADDI) of Selected Vitamins and Minerals and (2) Median Heights and Weights and Recommended Energy Intake (7).

While the RDAs are listed as specific quantities, the ESADDIs of selected vitamins and minerals give ranges of intake. A range is suggested because sufficient information exists to estimate the range of the requirement but not enough is known to set a specific RDA. This approach recognizes the importance of the nutrients but reflects our limited knowledge.

The Median Heights and Weights and Recommended Energy Intake standard presents average heights and weights of Americans. The energy intake recommendations are an average of the need for each category. A margin of safety is not added to avoid recommending potentially excessive intakes of energy; consuming too much energy may be a primary cause of obesity.

In contrast to these standards, minimum requirements for electrolytes are presented separately in the Estimated Sodium, Chloride, and Potassium Minimum Requirements of Healthy Persons (7). This standard addresses the recognized need for these nutrients but reflects that our knowledge is insufficient to recommend even ranges of intake. Only the minimum amounts required by our bodies to maintain health are listed.

Standards Around the World

Other countries have developed dietary standards based on energy needs, food supply, or environmental factors affecting their populations. In addition, the Food and Agriculture Organization of the United Nations with the World Health Organization has developed a dietary standard that would meet the practical needs of healthy adults worldwide (8).

Why aren't nutrient recommendations the same for every country or population? After all, the needs of the human body must be the same around the world. The difference lies in the definitions and purposes of nutrient recommendations.

Standards may be designed to provide the basic amount of a nutrient to prevent deficiency symptoms or to supply sufficient amounts for basic good health. These amounts may differ substantially based on the nature of the nutrient such as whether it is stored in the body. In addition, health professionals of a nation or organization may interpret the same scientific data differently, arriving at various recommended amounts.

Whether a standard is set to provide for just basic nutrient needs may depend on the availability of food. In the United States, where access to food is easy and the supply plentiful, the setting of nutrient recommendations higher than minimum levels is reasonable; most citizens have access to foods to meet those levels. In parts of the world where the food supply is more limited, the immediate goal would be for as many individuals as possible to be supplied with basic needs to prevent deficiencies.

Some values differ from the US standards based on the most common sources of nutrients worldwide. For example, most of the world relies heavily on plant protein sources, while North Americans use mainly animal sources. Recommended protein levels reflect this difference.

Ultimately, all standards are simply guidelines. Even when set at a specific amount, standards represent a range of the requirement of the nutrient. Individual needs may vary, so consuming enough food to meet the basic amounts should be each person's nutritional goal.

ADEQUATE EATING PATTERNS

Knowing the RDAs makes nutrition seem simple. Just eat enough of the RDA nutrients and good health seems assured. However, we don't eat nutrients, we eat foods. For an eating pattern to be considered adequate, the foods we eat must provide all the essential nutrients plus fiber and energy. An adequate eating pattern takes into account assortment, balance, and nutrient density (Figs. 1-4 to 1-6).

No single food contains all the nutrients essential for optimum health. An adequate eating pattern incorporates an assortment of foods.

NUTRITIONAL ASSESSMENT

Nutritional assessment is the process of determining nutritional status and nutrient deficiencies. A deficiency severe enough to cause overt changes in the body may be either a primary nutrient deficiency due to an inadequate intake of a nutrient or a secondary nutrient deficiency caused by the body's inefficient use of the nutrient once it is absorbed.

There are two levels of nutritional assessment. One level evaluates dietary intake or the foods we eat to determine the quantities of nutrients consumed as compared to the RDA standard. The other level evaluates dietary intake but also considers how the body uses the nutrients for growth and maintenance of health. Several methods of evaluation may be used. A brief introduction to nutritional assessment follows. Chapter 15 contains a detailed nursing orientation for comprehensive nutritional assessment to be used as a basis for medical nutritional therapy.

Assessment of Dietary Intake

The RDAs offer guidelines for safe and appropriate levels of nutrients to be consumed by individuals or provided in the food supply. If a person's intake does not meet RDA levels, however, his diet is not necessarily deficient because the RDAs do not reflect the use of nutrients by individual bodies. Nor do they take into account overconsumption of specific nutrients, health problems, or environmental influences. So when evaluating nutritional status, a healthcare worker may note whether a patient's dietary intake meets the RDA standard but should not base the evaluation solely on a comparison with the RDAs. A complete nutritional assessment is necessary to evaluate a person's nutritional status.

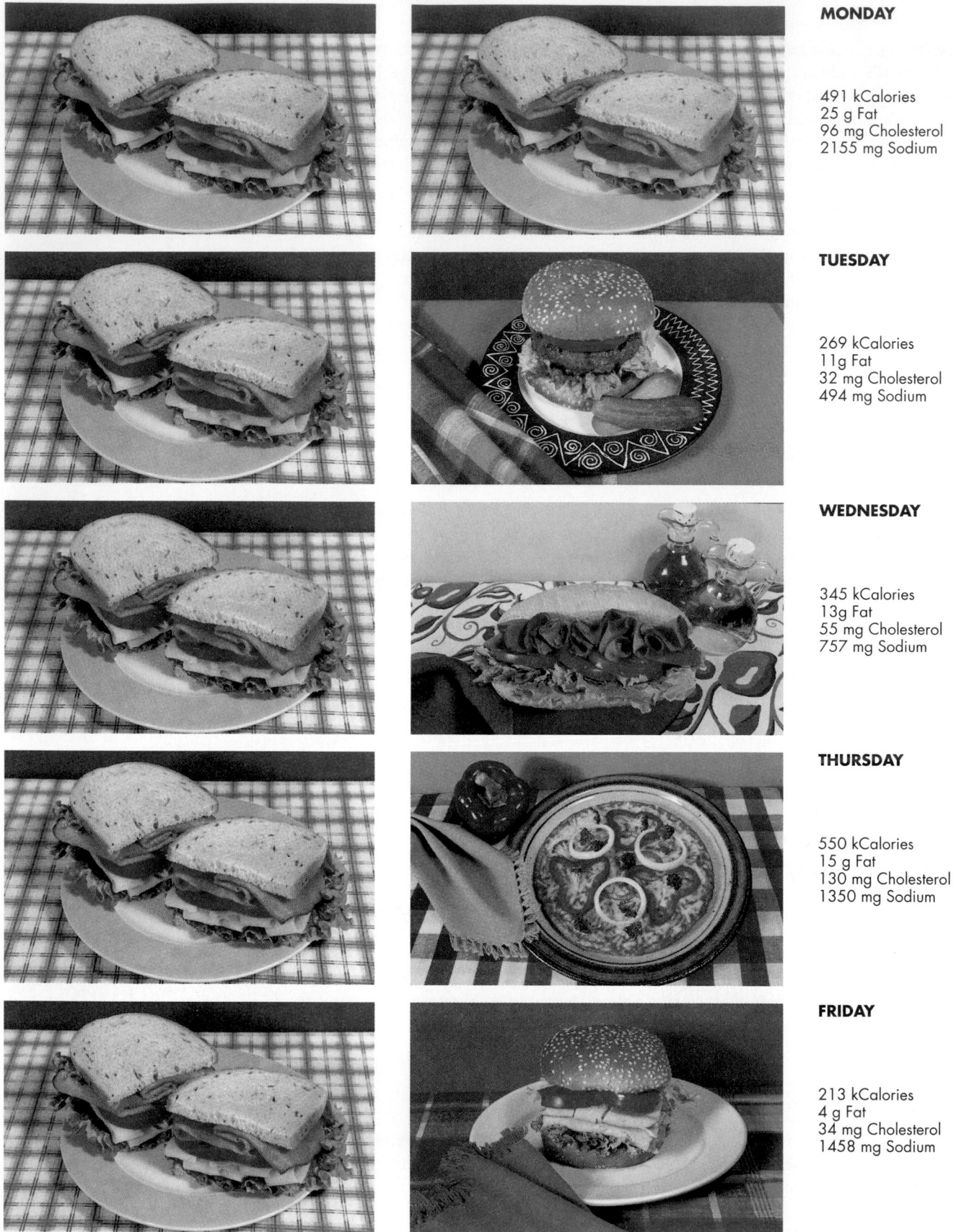

MONDAY

491 kCalories
25 g Fat
96 mg Cholesterol
2155 mg Sodium

TUESDAY

269 kCalories
11g Fat
32 mg Cholesterol
494 mg Sodium

WEDNESDAY

345 kCalories
13g Fat
55 mg Cholesterol
757 mg Sodium

THURSDAY

550 kCalories
15 g Fat
130 mg Cholesterol
1350 mg Sodium

FRIDAY

213 kCalories
4 g Fat
34 mg Cholesterol
1458 mg Sodium

Fig. 1-4 An adequate eating pattern incorporates an assortment of foods. Eating a ham and cheese sandwich (HCS) every day may seem like a quick lunchtime solution, but an assortment of selections (AS) over a 5-day period provides a daily average of fewer calories (491 kcal HCS vs. 354 kcal AS), less fat (25 g HCS vs. 14 g AS), less cholesterol (96 mg HCS vs. 70 mg AS), and less sodium (2155 mg HCS vs. 1243 mg AS). (Data from USDA: Nutritive value of foods, *Home and Garden Bulletin 72*, 1991.)

Estimates of food consumption are often used to determine the nutritional status of individuals and populations. Sometimes if the dietary intake is not sufficient, undernutrition, overnutrition, or malnutrition may be diagnosed.

Undernutrition is the underconsumption of energy or nutrients based on RDA values. This means either not eating enough food to take in all the essential nutrients or eating enough food for energy but choosing foods that are lacking certain nutrients. In the United States, some women do not consume enough of the vitamin folate, even though the rest of their nutrient intake is adequate.

Overnutrition is consuming too many nutrients and too much energy compared to RDA levels. More nutrients and energy are eaten than the body needs to function well. North Americans generally overconsume saturated fats, which is a risk factor for the development of heart disease.

undernutrition
the underconsumption of energy or nutrients based on RDA values

overnutrition
consumption of too many nutrients and too much energy compared with RDA levels

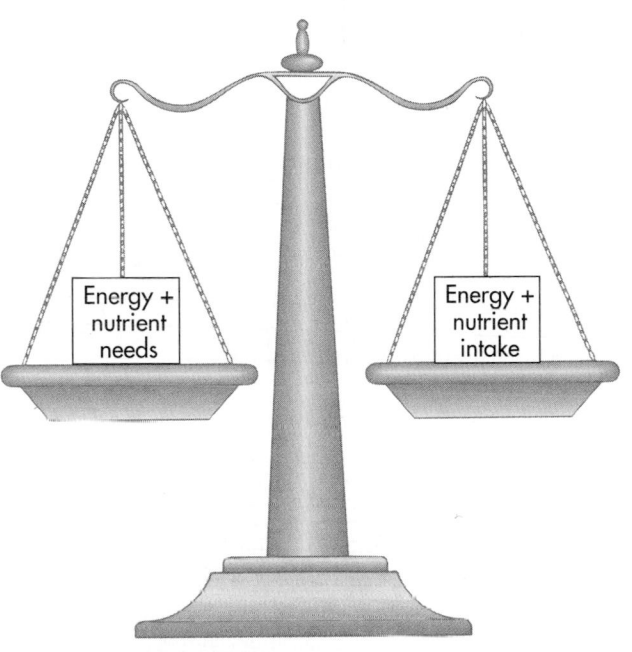

Fig. 1-5 A balance of nutrients in the diet helps to ensure adequacy.

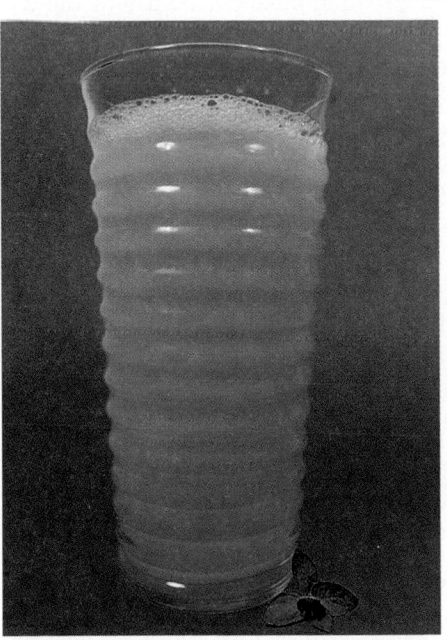

Orange juice: 12 oz, 120 kcal
Nutrients:

Phosphorus	63 mg
Potassium	744 mg
Iron	.75 mg
Sodium	3 mg
Calcium	40 mg
Vitamin A	75 re
Thiamin (B$_1$)	.33 mg
Riboflavin (B$_2$)	.15 mg
Niacin	1.5 mg
Vitamin C	186 mg

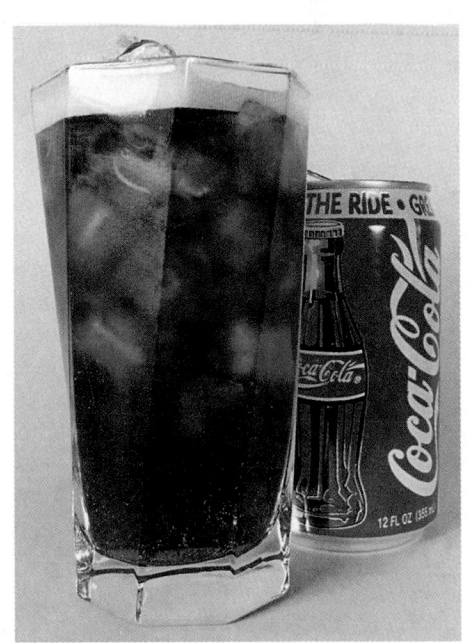

Soda: 12 oz, 160 kcal
Nutrients:

Phosphorus	52 mg
Potassium	7 mg
Iron	.2 mg
Sodium	18 mg

Fig. 1-6 The more nutrients and the fewer kcalories a food provides, the higher its nutrient density. (Data from USDA: Nutritive value of foods, *Home and Garden Bulletin* 72, 1991.)

malnutrition
an imbalanced nutrient and
energy intake

Malnutrition is an imbalanced nutrient and energy intake. It is an umbrella term that includes the undernutrition of too few nutrients or energy nutrient intake and overnutrition of excess consumption. An obese man who consumes an excessive amount of kcalories is malnourished because his intake is off balance. His intake does not equal his energy output. In contrast, a college student who is constantly dieting for slimness or sports, consuming below the RDA for nutrients and energy, is also malnourished.

Portraits of malnutrition

Not all those who are malnourished resemble famine victims. The effects of long-term famines represent extreme forms of malnutrition (see Chapter 6). Lesser degrees of malnutrition are all around us. Consider the nutritional status of hospital patients, the elderly, and chronic alcohol users.

For hospital patients, the nature of an illness combined with medications may affect appetite and the absorption of nutrients. The effects of malnutrition may be thought due to the illness rather than improper nutrient intake. Clinical nurses are trained to detect hospital malnutrition in acute care settings.

The elderly may be at risk for malnutrition. They may not be able to afford fresh fruits and vegetables or may be unable to get to the supermarket regularly because of transportation difficulties. Dental and other health problems may make chewing or digesting foods difficult. Social factors may affect appetite as well. Cooking for one and eating alone are not very appealing and may affect food intake. Home health nurses must be alert to the social and economic factors that may be contributing to malnutrition in the elderly.

Individuals who excessively consume alcohol and who may still be functional and working or attending college are often malnourished because alcohol replaces nutrient-dense foods; alcohol affects the gastrointestinal tract and so impairs absorption of nutrients. The health needs of chronic alcohol abusers may be noticed by nurses in community and occupational health centers.

It is hard to imagine malnutrition happening close to home, especially when we shop in supermarkets overflowing with food products. Although hidden malnutrition among these groups is not as severe, it does affect their health and productivity.

Diet evaluation

Ways to gather data on the food a person eats may include the use of the 24-hour recall, a food record, and a diet history (9). The 24-hour recall is a report on what an individual ate during the previous 24-hour period. The information is usually gathered in a personal interview or by telephone. A food record is created by the individual measuring and recording the amount and kind of food and drink consumed during a certain time period. It is somewhat time consuming because the individual needs to be willing to keep careful notes on intake and to use measuring utensils to provide accuracy. A diet history is an approximate representation of a person's eating habits over a long period of time. The data are gathered through interviews or questionnaires. None of these methods is totally accurate. They depend on good memories and recording skills and accurate measurements. But at present, they are the most convenient ways to collect data on dietary intake.

Once the data are collected, they can be analyzed through a number of available computer dietary analysis programs and compared with the RDA for that individual. When this analysis is performed on a group of individuals who are representative of the larger population, we can then estimate the nutritional status of a population based on the dietary intake analysis.

Assessment of Nutritional Status

Assessing nutritional status uses several methods of evaluation. Each method provides different data by which to assess nutritional status. Specific instructions for implementing these methods are in Chapter 15.

Since the methods for assessing nutritional status involve dietary, clinical, and biochemical analyses, collaboration by a multidisciplined health team is usually required. In addition to dietary evaluations conducted by dietitians, methods may include the following:

- A clinical examination performed by a primary health provider, nurse, or dietitian to note outward signs of nutritional health.

This includes physical examination through observations of the eyes, mucous membranes, skin, hair, mouth, teeth, and tongue. Clinical observations are limited in value because overt symptoms of nutrient deficiencies would not become apparent until late stages of deficiencies. In addition, some of the symptoms observed could be due to other conditions besides dietary deficiencies. Therefore a client's medical history from medical records or through direct interview and a social history are also important data to consider.

- Biochemical analysis of samples of body tissues, such as blood and/or urine tests, to assess how the body is using nutrients.

If the blood level of a nutrient is low, it could mean either that the dietary intake was low, the nutrient was consumed but was poorly absorbed, or the individual has a higher than average requirement for the nutrient. Iron is a nutrient that can be assessed through blood levels. Urine analysis can reveal the efficiency with which our bodies use glucose and protein and excrete other nutrients. Although the actual tissue samples would be drawn by a primary health provider, nurse, or technician, a dietitian would complete the nutritional analysis and interpretation of the results.

- Anthropometric measurements, such as measuring the height, weight, and limb circumference of an individual and comparing those dimensions with national standards, to determine healthy growth patterns.

Body composition may also be used to determine percentages of lean body mass and body fat levels. In addition to height, weight, and limb circumference, skinfold measurements are often used to assess body fat composition. Skill gained through careful practice is necessary to minimize the margin of error in taking body measurements. Before an assessment of this kind of data is completed, a family history should be conducted. Heredity, of course, plays a role in the growth patterns and final height and weights we achieve.

Through consideration of data from clinical, biochemical, and anthropometric measurements, the nutritional status of individuals can be determined. As with dietary assessment, if these analyses are performed on enough individuals who are representative of the total population, the nutritional status of nations can be estimated.

Nurses who are providing maintenance health care to nonhospitalized clients may implement a limited form of dietary evaluation as a screening procedure. For example, community and home health nurses who may not have access to computer analysis when conferring with clients can compare the results of the 24-hour recall or food record to the recommended servings of the Food Guide Pyramid (see Fig. 2-2) or, if the client is receiving medical nutritional therapy, to a prescribed diet. Clients can then use this form of quick assessment to periodically check the status of their intake. This quick assessment does not, however, provide the same in-depth analysis as the comprehensive nutritional assessment performed by a dietitian working with a multidisciplinary health team.

What's in a Name?

Who is the nutrition specialist—the dietitian or the nutritionist? They both are; the difference is in the type of training and credentialing completed after majoring in foods and nutrition on the college or university level.

A **registered dietitian (RD)** is a professional trained in foods and the management of diets (dietetics) who is credentialed by the Commission on Dietetic Registration of the American Dietetic Association. Credentialing is based on completion

registered dietitian (RD)
a professional trained in foods and the management of diets (dietetics) who is credentialed by the Commission on Dietetic Registration of the American Dietetic Association; credentialing is based on completion of a BS degree from an approved program, clinical and administrative training, and passing a registration examination

of a BS degree from an approved program, clinical and administrative training, and passing a registration examination. Continuing education is mandatory for continued registration. Registered dietitians may also have advanced training in specialized areas of medical nutritional therapy.

A **nutritionist** is a professional who has completed academic degrees of BS, MS, EdD, or PhD in foods and nutrition. In some states, nutritionist is a legally defined and licensed title; a nutritionist may also be an RD.

Similar to nurses, dietitians and nutritionists practice in a variety of health care settings. Clinical dietitians and nutritionists focus on the therapeutic needs of individuals and their families in institutional settings such as hospitals, long-term care facilities, and rehabilitation centers. Others work in community-based practice settings as community nutritionists, dietitians and educators; they may concentrate on health promotion and disease prevention in addition to therapeutic issues. Public health nutritionists attend to diet-related health issues of the larger community to include state, national, and international nutrition concerns.

nutritionist

a professional who has completed academic degrees of BS, MS, EdD, or PhD in foods and nutrition

TOWARD A POSITIVE NUTRITION LIFESTYLE: SELF-EFFICACY

Achieving wellness is an ongoing process. We all experience times when meeting our personal dietary goals is easy, and other times when it seems as if we will never regain a sense of control over our nutritional lifestyles. These "ups and downs" are all part of the process of achieving wellness.

To support our pathway toward achieving wellness, this section in each chapter will feature psychosocial strategies to enhance positive self-efficacy. Self-efficacy is our perception of our ability to have power over our lives and behaviors. Positive self-efficacy means believing that personal behaviors can be changed and one has control over one's life. Negative self-efficacy refers to feeling as if one is powerless with little control over circumstances. A sense of positive self-efficacy is essential for attaining and then maintaining nutritional lifestyles for optimum health. These strategies may be applicable in our own life situations or may be useful for our clients as they, too, strive for enhanced self-efficacy.

SUMMARY

Health is the merging and balance of physical, intellectual, emotional, social, and spiritual dimensions. Nutrition, the study of essential nutrients and the ways they are used by the body, is a cornerstone of each health dimension. To improve health and nutrition, health promotion strategies can be implemented. These strategies often rely on knowledge, techniques, and community supports to initiate and maintain lifestyle behaviors to enhance health. Wellness is a lifestyle through which the five dimensions of health are further enhanced. "Wellness nutrition" approaches food consumption as a positive way to nourish the body.

The essential nutrients that must be obtained from foods are divided into six categories: carbohydrates, proteins, fat, vitamins, minerals, and water. These nutrients aid growth and repair of body tissues, regulate body processes, and provide energy. Some nutrients are diverse in their impact, whereas others have very specific functions. This chapter explores how the recommended daily levels of essential nutrients are determined. To prevent nutrient deficiencies, dietary standards have been developed to provide guidelines about sufficient nutrient intakes. The Recommended Dietary Allowances (RDAs) are the US standard.

Nutritional assessment determines nutritional status and nutrient deficiency in individuals. The techniques include two levels of assessment: evaluation of the quality of nutrients consumed and the body's use of nutrients for growth and maintenance of health.

THE NURSING ROLE
Holistic Assessment and Nutrition: The Nursing Process

The Nursing Process can be applied to patients' nutritional needs as it can be to all human needs. This section in most chapters includes assessment, planning, intervention, and evaluation of some aspect of nutritional or diet therapy needs. Nursing diagnoses, when given, are usually based on the North American Nursing Diagnosis Association (NANDA) diagnoses such as "Nutrition, altered: less than body requirements" or "Knowledge deficit" or "Fluid volume deficit." The Nursing Process box in some chapters addresses only portions of the process, such as critical thinking, assessment, or diagnosis.

The nurse, whether hospital staff nurse, home health nurse, occupational health nurse, or nurse practitioner, is in a unique position regarding patients' nutritional needs. Although the nurse may not be as expert as the dietitian, it is the nurse who does a holistic assessment of each patient and who diagnoses strengths and weaknesses in nutrition lifestyle. Intervention may follow in the form of reinforcement, teaching, consultation with the primary health provider, or referral to a dietitian.

The nurse who has a thorough knowledge of basic nutrition will never underestimate the importance of diet in maintaining health and in recovery from disease or injury.

REFERENCES

1. Thomas PR, ed: *Improving America's diet and health: From recommendations to action*, Washington, DC, 1991, National Academy Press.
2. Burns CM: Toward healthy people 2000: The role of the nurse practitioner and health promotion, *J Am Acad Nurse Pract* 6(1): 29-35, 1994.
3. Payne WA, Hahn DB: *Understanding your health*, ed 4, St. Louis, 1995, Mosby.
4. US Department of Health and Human Services, Public Health Service: *Healthy people 2000: National health promotion and disease prevention objectives*, Washington, DC, 1990, US Government Printing Office.
5. Greene W, Simon-Mark B: *Introduction to health education*, Prospect Heights, Ill, 1990, Waveland Press.
6. Pennington J: *Bowes & Church's food values of portions commonly used*, ed 15, Philadelphia, 1989, Lippincott.
7. Food and Nutrition Board, National Research Council: *Recommended dietary allowances*, ed 10, Washington, DC, 1989, National Academy Press.
8. Food and Agricultural Organization/World Health Organization/UN University: *Energy and protein requirements*, Rome, 1985, Food and Agricultural Organization.
9. National Research Council: *Diet and health: Implications for reducing chronic disease risk*, Washington, DC, 1989, National Academy Press.

Chapter 2

PERSONAL AND COMMUNITY NUTRITION

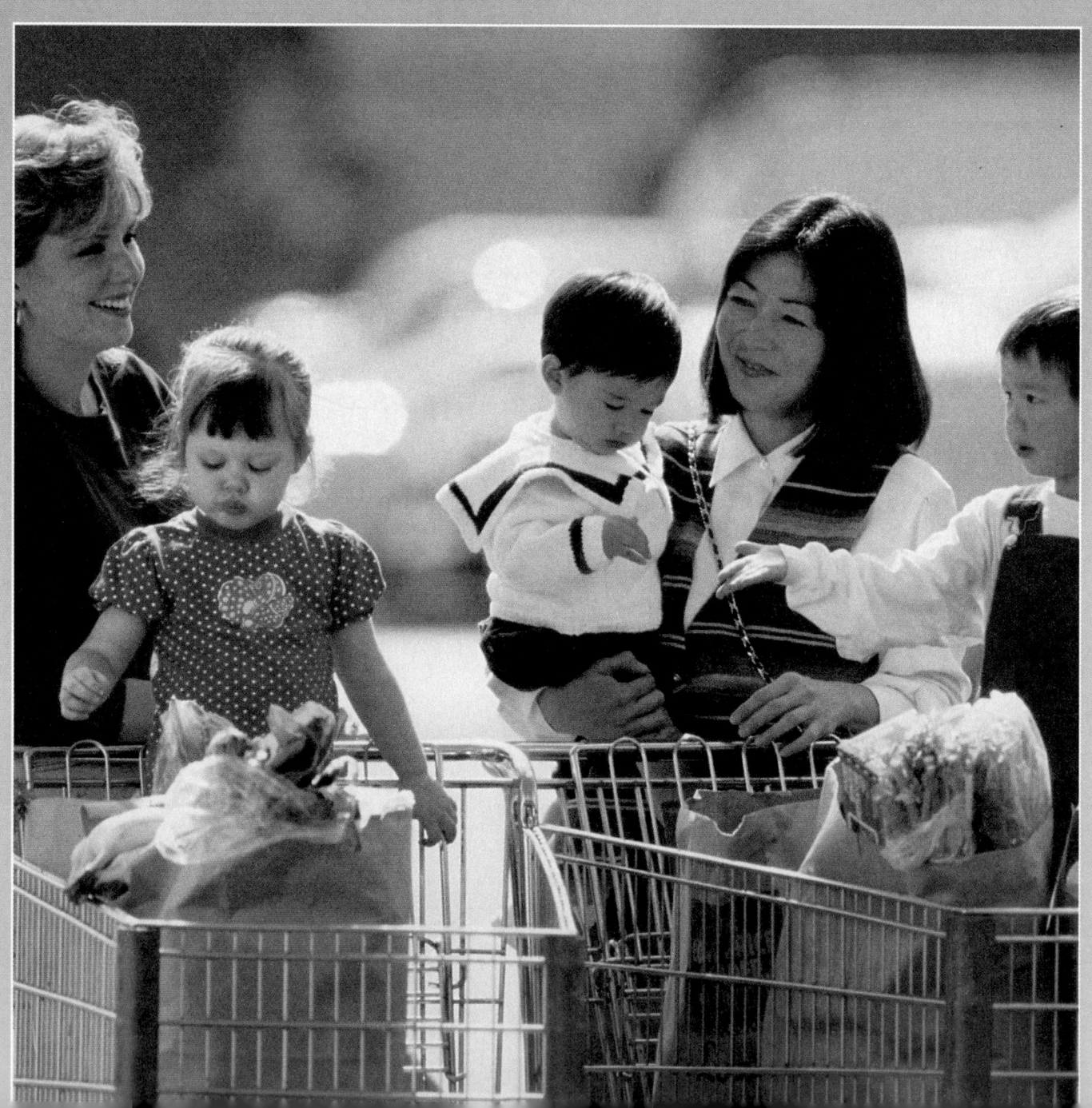

Have you ever thought about who is responsible for your health? Perhaps you thought of your parents, spouse, or significant other. Or possibly you have always taken your health for granted, not as something to actively work toward improving or maintaining. What of the health of the community in which you live or work? Have you ever considered the health status of the residents of your town or college community?

In the foreword to *Healthy People 2000*, the US Secretary of Health and Human Services urges us as a nation to develop "a culture of character" through which we take responsibility for our personal health and the health of our communities-at-large (1). This chapter considers strategies for improving our health by taking charge of our personal nutrition and becoming aware of nutrition issues of our communities."

ROLE IN WELLNESS

The decisions individuals make about the food they eat determine their health and wellness. Health professionals frequently give advice about appropriate foods for clients to consume. Therefore it is important for nurses in institutional and community settings to understand how a person's food behavior is influenced by personal factors and community issues affecting food availability, consumption and expenditure trends, consumer information, and food safety. Effects of these personal and community factors on consumers' food decisions are some of the major topics of this chapter.

PERSONAL NUTRITION

Ultimately, as adults, we each are responsible for the quality of our dietary intake. Although external forces may affect our everyday food choices, we can decide to have the internal self-awareness to consciously modify those forces. To be accountable for our nutritional status and health may require adjusting some personal goals to allow time to work on achieving a wellness lifestyle.

Food Selection

The foods we select to eat are affected by our food preferences, food choice, and food liking. While these terms reflect similar food-related behaviors, they are quite different (2).

Food preferences are those foods we choose to eat when all foods are available at the same time and in the same quantity. Factors affecting preferences include genetic determinants and environmental effects. Genetic factors include inborn desires for sweet and salty tasting flavors. One recent study of taste receptors noted that, to some people, vegetables like broccoli and brussels sprouts taste bitter and so are avoided, whereas other people find their flavors enjoyable (3). Consumption of cruciferous vegetables, such as broccoli and brussels sprouts, is associated with a decreased risk of developing certain cancers (4). If some people avoid them because of perceived bitter taste, will they be more at risk for cancers?

Environmental effects are learned preferences that are the result of cultural and socioeconomic influences. We often adjust our choices to those we are around. An indirect influence is the media, particularly television. Television advertising is a potent force influencing the foods we prefer and buy. Programs also spread messages as to food and lifestyle preferences of different socioeconomic groups. A television show about a working class family presents images of food intake associated with a lower socioeconomic status—dinner might be franks and beans. In another show an upper socioeconomic family might sit down to a meal of baked salmon and salad. Each unintentionally sends messages about appropriate food intake for individuals belonging to each group.

food preferences
the foods we choose to eat when all foods are available at the same time and in the same quantity

Health promotion issues are tied to **food preferences.** If recommendations call for changes in foods rooted in genetic determinants, the motivation for change needs to be different than if the food preference is environmentally learned. New preferences can be learned; genetic preferences are more difficult to change.

Food choice concerns the specific foods convenient to choose when we are actually ready to eat; rarely are all our preferred foods available at the same time to satisfy our preferences. Food choices are restricted by convenience. With hectic lifestyles, we tend to avoid foods that take long to prepare. Instead, we often repeatedly choose foods that are easy to prepare and eat, regardless of their nutritional value. Cost is also a factor. We sometimes weigh cost benefits against time benefits. If a food costs more but saves us time, we may choose it. Or we may decide that a food item, even if nutrient dense, costs too much money for the benefits received. Again, nutritional value may not be a prime concern affecting food choice.

food choice
the specific foods that are convenient to choose when we are actually ready to eat

food liking
foods we really like to eat

Food liking considers which foods we really like to eat. We may prefer to eat foods that enhance our health, but we like to eat chocolate layer cake. We are constantly weighing all the factors of preference, choice, and liking when we select the foods we eat. Ultimately, these three types of food behaviors greatly affect individual nutritional status (2).

It is the small steps we take that eventually lead to cumulative change. As we study different aspects of food and nutrition, we will present suggestions that will move us and our clients towards significant change. These suggestions will lead to the formation of new personal food habits.

COMMUNITY NUTRITION

The nutritional status of our communities is a reflection of our individual nutritional health. Perhaps the most significant factor affecting nutritional status of communities is economic (see box). Having sufficient funds to purchase adequate food supplies is a necessity. Public health nutrition efforts to prevent nutrient deficiencies include the US government's food stamp program. This program provides individuals and families below certain income levels with coupons to use to purchase nutritious foods. Another is the Special Supplemental Food Program For Women Infants and Children (WIC). The WIC program provides medical care, nutrition counseling, and supplemental foods to women who are pregnant or breastfeeding and infants and children up to the age of 5 who are at nutritional risk. Both programs have a significant impact on improving the nutritional status of those who participate. Additional government programs are discussed in Chapter 12.

Another level of public health nutrition is aimed at the nutrient excesses of our dietary intake. In the late 1970s, a new era in nutrition recommendations began in the United States. Rather than focusing on nutrient deficiencies as a cause of poor health, health professionals began to notice that the cause of an increasing amount of chronic illness was possibly tied to an excessive intake of certain nutrients such as saturated fats, cholesterol, sodium, and sugars. As knowledge of diet-related diseases of heart disease, hypertension, cancer, diabetes, osteoporosis, and obesity increases, several sets of dietary recommendations from different government agencies and voluntary health and scientific associations have been released to address this issue. Each has served a different purpose, but all have led to consensus in recommendations for maintaining general good health (4-7). Recommendations

SOCIAL ISSUE
Implementing Dietary Guidelines: Easier Said Than Done

As most of us become familiar with the Dietary Guideline recommendations and the Food Pyramid, we probably reflect on the different food choices available to us and what changes we could most easily implement. But many low-income and unemployed individuals and families don't have the luxury of deciding among a variety of available foods. Instead, their problem is one of food security.

Food security is the difficulty of obtaining enough food. The available financial resources of these households may not be able to stretch far enough to provide sufficient quantities of high-quality foods. A recurring strain for these families is to provide enough food for their children and themselves; sometimes they may all experience hunger.

In this context, the definition of hunger is not just the physiological need for food. Instead, a social definition of hunger is being unable to have access to enough food to feel nourished and satisfied.

Although government programs like Food Stamps and WIC and private non-profit food banks do fill hunger gaps, they are not often sufficient to provide enough food for all of those in need. When clients are struggling to adopt new dietary guidelines, keep in mind the range of food choices easily available.

From Senauer B, Asp E, Kinsey J: *Food trends and the changing consumer*, St. Paul, Minn, 1991, Eagan Press.

from these studies have been issued as national goals. All point to reduced intake of saturated fat, total fat, cholesterol, sodium, and excessive kcalories and an increased intake of fiber, complex carbohydrates, fruits, and vegetables. These goals form the basis of health promotion efforts to implement primary, secondary, and tertiary prevention strategies. Education at the community level to reach as many individuals and families as possible has been a challenge for health professionals.

Dietary Guidelines for Americans

In response to the dietary recommendations, the US Department of Agriculture (USDA) and Department of Health and Human Services (USDHHS) in 1977 developed *Dietary Guidelines for Americans*. These guidelines, revised in 1985 and in 1990, contain general suggestions regarding food selection for healthy Americans over age 2 (Fig. 2-1) (8).

Lifestyle applications

Certainly, your clients would like to follow the Dietary Guidelines, but how? Their busy schedules barely allow time for any food at all? Have them consider the following suggestions:

- In the morning, choose dry cereals and bread products (such as English muffins) that contain whole grains and alternate or mix with less-fiber favorites. If no time can be found for breakfast, stock up on juice packs to drink and portable fruit such as apples or bananas to eat on the way to class or work. Throw some into backpacks or briefcases for a quick snack.
- Be creative with vending machine selections. Choose lower-fat and lower-sugar selections: raisins, bagel chips, pretzels (rub off excess salt), popcorn, and even some plain cookies or crackers. Some vending machines stock small cans of tuna fish, yogurts, and fruits. Contact the staff responsible for filling the vending machines to request healthier selections.
- If lunch and dinner are on the run and fast food drive-throughs are the only option, select lower-fat items such as grilled chicken sandwiches or plain hamburgers. Don't have French fries or milkshakes (unless low-fat) every time but alternate with salads and low-fat milk or juice.
- Perhaps lunch and dinner are in a college or employee cafeteria. Try to select turkey, chicken (without skin), fish, and lean beef dishes. Include bread, a grain (rice or pasta), several vegetables, and salad. Try fruit for dessert; it's good with some frozen low-fat yogurt, if available.

Leading causes of death in the United States
1. Heart disease*
2. Cancers*
3. Stroke*
4. Accidents*
5. Lung diseases
6. Pneumonia and influenza
7. Diabetes
8. Suicide†
9. Homicide
10. Chronic liver disease†

From National Center for Health Statistics: Annual summary, 39(13), 1990.

*Causes in which diet played a part.

†Causes in which alcohol plays a part.

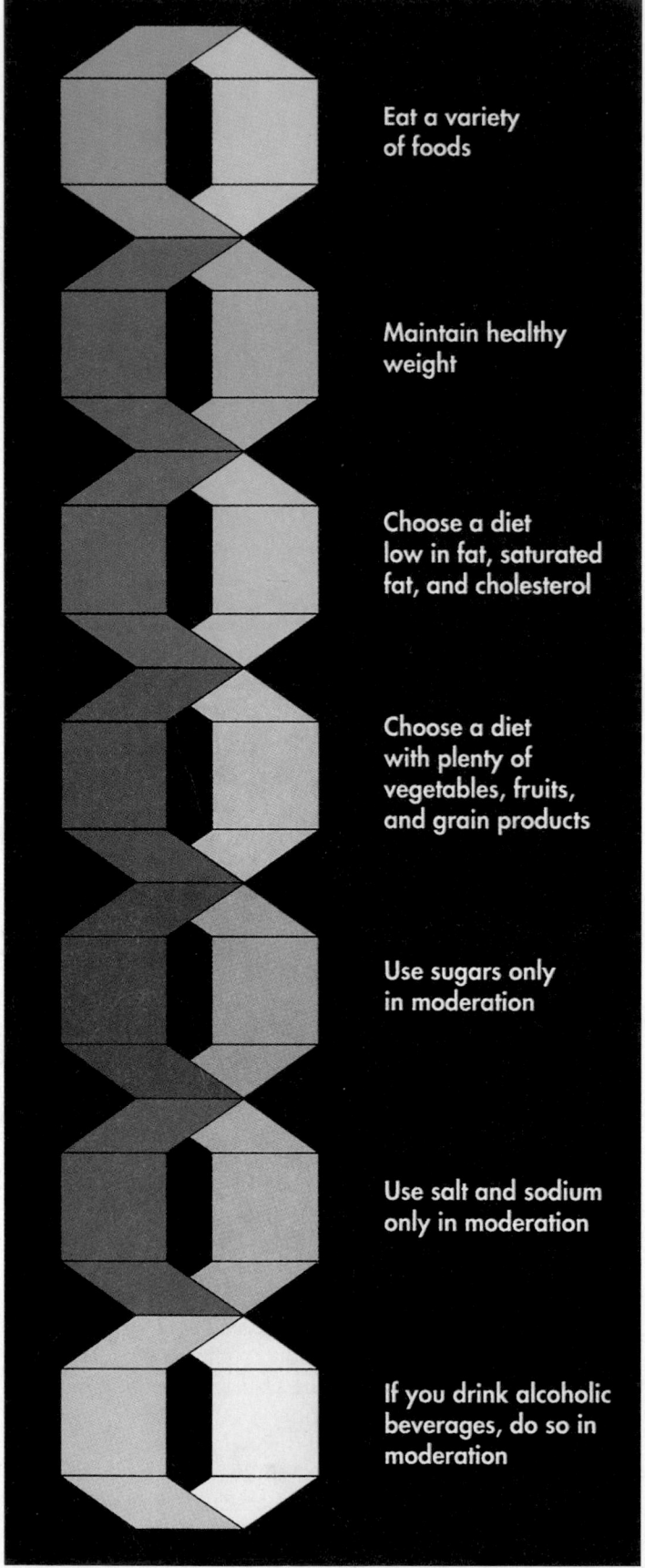

Fig. 2-1 The recommendations made by the current version of Dietary Guidelines for Americans.

- Maybe you don't really eat "meals," but eat snacks throughout the day. This is called "grazing." It is possible to graze and follow the *Dietary Guidelines* by choosing wholesome foods, instead of candy bars and soda. Bagels (with just a little cream cheese), yogurt, fruits, yogurt shakes, pretzels, pizza (but not every day because of high-fat cheese), and dry cereals with milk are high-quality grazing foods that are often available.

So next time your clients are food shopping or grabbing a snack or meal, have them stop a moment and consider the best choices possible!

Food Guides

Now that we are armed with the latest nutrient recommendations, we can apply this knowledge to the way we eat every day. Since we think about what food to eat, rather than which nutrients, these nutrient recommendations are most useful when translated to real food. To help us do this, food guides have been developed.

The food guide pyramid

The Food Guide Pyramid (Fig. 2-2) is designed to help us follow most of the *Dietary Guidelines for Americans* (9). Developed by the USDA and released in 1992, it is a guide to the amounts and kinds of foods that we should eat daily to maintain health and to reduce our risks of developing diet-related diseases.

As an outline of what to eat, the Food Guide Pyramid presents five major food groups: bread, cereal, rice, and pasta group (6 to 11 servings); vegetable group (3 to 5 servings); fruit group (2-4 servings); milk, yogurt, and cheese group (2-3 servings); and meat, poultry, fish, dry beans, eggs, and nuts group (2-3 servings). The small tip of the Pyramid is for fats, oils, and sweets. There is no serving number suggested for these; we are advised to consume these in small quantities.

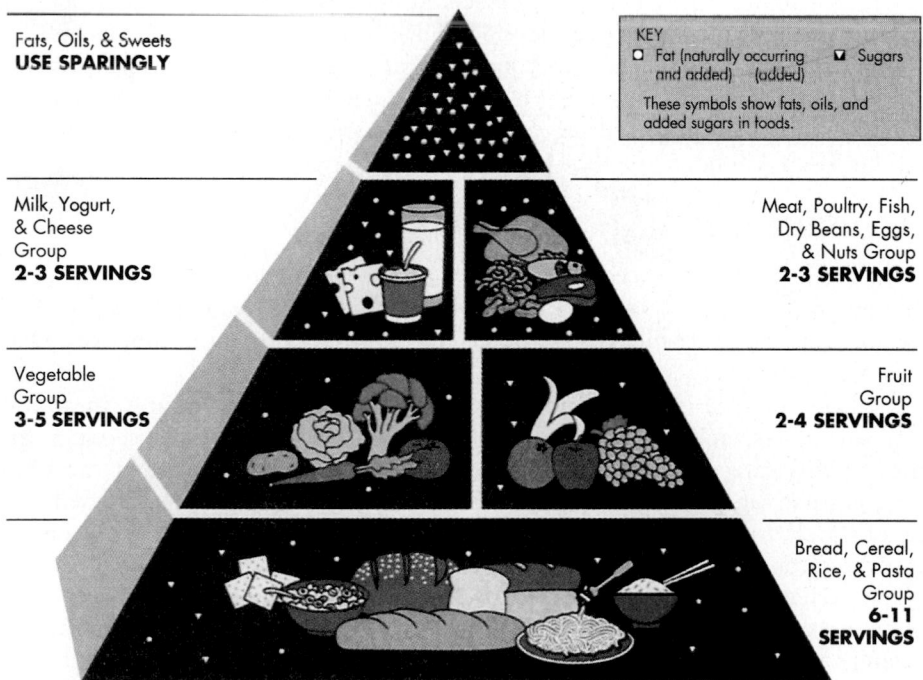

Fig. 2-2 The Food Guide Pyramid: A guide to daily food choices.

Each food group is visually displayed to represent the number of servings we should eat daily; the number is a range of servings. This range takes into account our different energy needs and our personal food preferences. Everyone should eat at least the lowest number of servings for each group. By doing so, we consume an adequate quantity of essential nutrients.

The Pyramid allows us to choose between foods containing different levels of fats or lipids, fiber, and sodium. To use the Pyramid as a guide for choosing a low-fat, high-fiber meal pattern, we also need to understand the effect of food preparation on the fat and fiber content of meals. By arming ourselves with more information about the foods we choose and how we prepare them, we can develop an optimum meal pattern. This textbook provides this information in the chapters discussing fats, carbohydrates, and sodium (a mineral). The Food Guide Pyramid is used as a Teaching Tool in Chapter 4.

5 a day program

Perhaps you've noticed banners and brochures in your local supermarket proclaiming "5 a Day—for Better Health" and other posters advising increased consumption of fruits and vegetables. The banners are part of the National 5 a Day for Better Health program. This program is the first government and private industry partnership to improve our health and is a collaborative effort of the National Cancer Institute/National Institutes of Health and the Produce for Better Health Foundation, a nonprofit consumer education foundation funded by the fruit and vegetable industry (10).

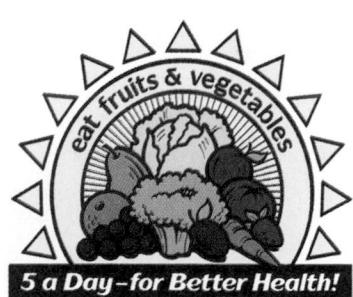

The purpose of the program is to increase our consumption of fruits and vegetables to at least five servings a day. By doing so, goals of the *Dietary Guidelines for Americans, Healthy People 2000,* and other dietary recommendations may be achieved.

Research shows that only 9% of Americans consume the recommended five servings a day (10), although this amount is the minimum number recommended in the Food Guide Pyramid. By focusing on only fruits and vegetables, this guide becomes an easy way to decrease intake of fats since fruits and vegetables are naturally low in fat. With five servings of fruits and vegetables each day, increased consumption of fiber, vitamin C, and beta-carotene will also occur. These nutrients, in addition to their functions as essential nutrients, are recognized as having the potential to reduce the risk of developing heart disease and certain cancers.

Although it may be difficult for you and your clients to determine the percentage of daily dietary fat consumed, it is easy to count the number of servings of fruits and vegetables. If more fruits and vegetables are eaten everyday, appetites for high-fat foods will be smaller (see Sample Menu).

Sample day of how to do 5 a Day
Breakfast: orange juice (1), oatmeal, toast, coffee with milk
Snack: orange or apple (2)
Lunch: turkey hero sandwich with lettuce and tomato (3), skim milk
Snack: popcorn and ice tea
Dinner: lemon pepper catfish, baked potato (4), broccoli (5), tossed green salad (6), French bread with butter or margarine, skim milk

Exchange Lists

The food guides refer to eating a number of servings of specific foods daily, but what is a serving size? A resource for serving sizes is the *Exchange Lists for Meal Planning,* published by the American Dietetic Association and the American Diabetes Association (11) (see Appendix B).

Foods are divided into three different groups or lists: carbohydrates, meat and meat substitutes, and fats. Each list or exchange contains sizes of servings for foods of that category; each serving size provides a similar amount of carbohydrate, protein, fat, and kcalories (kcal). The carbohydrate group is subdivided into lists of starch, fruit, milk, other carbohydrates, and vegetables. The meat and meat substitute group is sorted by fat content (see box).

The exchange lists were first developed for use by persons with diabetes. A dietitian can create an appropriate dietary program prescribing the number of kcalories and units of each exchange category to be consumed daily, as well as a plan for when they should be eaten. By using the exchange lists, an individual is able to choose favorite foods from each list while controlling the amount and kind of carbohydrates consumed throughout the day.

Exchange List		
Group	Fat	kCalories
CARBOHYDRATE		
Starch	1 or less	80
Fruit	—	60
Milk		
skim to whole	0-8	90-150
Other	varies	varies
Vegetables	—	25
MEAT/MEAT SUBSTITUTE		
Very lean	0-1	35
Lean	3	55
Medium	5	75
High fat	8	100
FAT	5	45

New guidelines for individuals with diabetes, published by the American Dietetic Association, de-emphasize prescribed calculated kcaloric diets using only the exchange lists (12). The focus is now on adapting dietary intake to meet individual metabolic nutrition and lifestyle requirements (see Chapter 19).

Since the exchange lists encourage variety while helping to control kcalories and grams of carbohydrates, protein, and fats, these lists have been adapted to meet the needs of weight reduction programs and medical nutrition therapy planning. The Food Pyramid also utilizes the concept of units of servings by recommending a range of servings for each food category. A difference is that the Food Pyramid categorizes by food groups such as dairy foods and grains and cereals foods, rather than by nutrients.

Criteria for Future Recommendations

Although we expect the present recommendations to provide sound advice for quite a while, other organizations may issue their own guidelines in the future. Which guidelines should we follow? Should we change our eating habits and revise client dietary recommendations for each new study? Or since it all gets so confusing, should new recommendations just be ignored?

Criteria for evaluating future dietary guidelines and recommendations follow:

1. *Consider the source of the nutrition advice.* Are the recommendations from a federal government agency? If so, the work of these agencies is usually reviewed by health and nutrition professionals before release to the public. If the advice is from a private nonprofit group, is the group nationally recognized? A number of well-respected organizations are devoted to prevention and treatment of specific diseases, such as the American Heart Association, American Cancer Society, and American Diabetes Association. In addition, there are professional associations including the Society For Nutrition Education and the American Dietetic Association that specialize in the relationship of nutrition and health. (See Appendix C for a complete listing of organizations.)

2. *Assess the comprehensiveness of the recommendations.* Do the recommendations address only one health problem? If so, is that a health problem that affects your clients? Would following these recommendations have any negative effects? Would a category of nutrients be underconsumed? Recommendations that address several health issues are usually more complete and provide an increased level of prevention.

3. *Evaluate the basis of the recommendations.* How were the recommendations determined? The present recommendations are based on many research studies on the relationships between diet and diseases. If new recommendations are issued, are they based on the results of new studies? If so, how many and what kinds of studies? Collecting this type of information means more than just listening to a 2-minute radio announcement or a 5-minute television report. Some newspapers contain in-depth evaluations of research; others just skim the surface. It may be necessary to read the original study in the library or to discuss the recommendations.

4. *Estimate the ease of application.* Can the recommendations be easily adopted? Are they presented in terms of foods (easier to apply) or nutrients (harder to apply)? Is a degree in nutrition needed to understand the recommendations?

CONSUMER FOOD DECISION MAKING

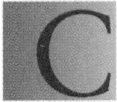ommunity supports can have an impact on the quality of personal nutrition. Primary are the consumer decisions made daily when buying food to be prepared in the home or when eating out.

Food Selection Patterns

The reasons people choose the foods they do are tracked by the Food Marketing Institute, an international organization of food retailers and wholesalers, in annual surveys of US food shoppers (13). Since 1988, survey responses show that taste is the factor consistently considered "very important" to the most (approximately 90%) shoppers when they select food. Next, nutrition, price, and product safety are rated as "very important" factors by approximately 75% of shoppers. Other factors thought "very important" by less than 50% of the shoppers surveyed are storability, recyclable product packaging, ease of preparation, and food-preparation time.

Awareness of the rationale for food purchasing decisions and knowledge of the changing patterns of food consumption are useful for nurses as we assist patients to modify their individual dietary patterns.

Food Consumption Trends

Food consumption trends reflect the food decisions Americans have made in the past. Tracking these trends since 1909 has been the responsibility of the USDA. Following the trends for specific foods as they fluctuate yearly also reveals information about food substitutions. These substitutions may include variations in the processing of a product. New technologies may result in new types of food products that affect overall consumption patterns for food categories. A prime example is the change from fresh to frozen concentrated juices due to new processing technologies (14).

Fruits and vegetables

Overall, total fruit (fresh and processed) and vegetable consumption is increasing (14). Trends since 1909 show that both total fruit consumption and fresh fruit consumption peaked in the 1940s, decreased to a low in the early 1960s, and have been gradually increasing since then. Vegetable consumption, except potatoes, shows a steady increase since 1909. Potato consumption decreased overall since 1909, although increases occurred since the 1960s because new processing technologies produced a variety of convenient processed potato products for consumers. Among these products are the baked potatoes and French fries that are popular in fast food outlets and other eating places.

As a result of this greater demand for fruits and vegetables, food stores increased their availability by adding a large number of new products to their produce departments. Increased imports make it possible to market a greater variety of fresh fruits and vegetables throughout the year. Processed fruit consumption also increased because of technological improvements in processing such as freezing fruit juice. Frozen fruit consumption shows moderate increases since the late 1940s when the processing technologies to make these products became available. Canned juice consumption also increased in the 1980s, with an accompanying decrease in consumption of chilled juice because aseptic packaging technology makes it possible to market convenient single-serving juice boxes that do not need refrigeration. Changes in the form in which fruits and vegetables are sold have increased their availability, convenience, and potential for consumption; examples include prepared items in the produce section of supermarkets and salad bars in both restaurants and food stores.

Dietary guidelines and health recommendations have been encouraging everyone to eat more fruits and vegetables to reduce the risk of diet-related disorders (4). As discussed previously, the "5 a Day" program targets this issue by recommending five servings of fruits and vegetables daily to help prevent cancer and other chronic diseases (10). Consumers appear to be hearing this message. Heightened consumer awareness of these health issues has contributed to the recent trend in increased fruit and vegetable consumption.

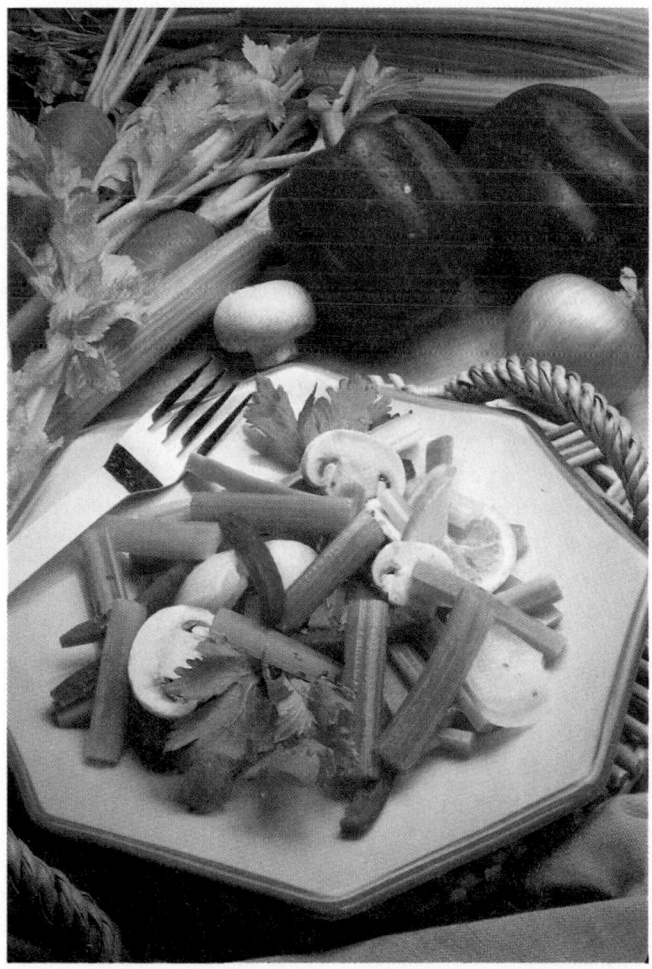

Choose fruits and vegetables each day to reduce the risk of diet-related diseases.

Cereals and grains

Flour and cereal product consumption decreased since 1909, but that trend shows a reversal since the mid-1980s (14). Increases in breakfast cereal consumption in recent years contributes to this rise. These products have qualities in demand by today's consumers; they are convenient, may contain fiber, are good sources of nutrients, and are low in calories. The placement of cereal products at the base of the Food Guide Pyramid with substantial serving increases recommended (6 to 11 servings) makes it likely that the consumption of cereals and cereal-based foods will continue to increase (15).

Meat, poultry, and fish

Meat, poultry, and fish consumption increased since 1909, while egg and dairy product consumption decreased (14). When meat, poultry, and fish are considered individually, the data show that beef consumption has decreased since the mid-1970s, pork remains at a constant level, poultry shows a dramatic increase, and fish has increased slightly. The substitution of poultry for beef and decreases of egg and dairy product consumption reflect not only changes in prices but also changes in consumer preferences, demographics, and health concerns. Changes in fish consumption show how technology affects the availability of forms of a food. Fresh and frozen fish consumption increased with the development of refrigerated and frozen storage, while consumption of cured fish decreased, especially between 1909 and the 1930s.

Dairy products

Although dairy product consumption decreased overall since 1909, a reversal of that trend started in the early 1980s. Increased consumption of frozen dairy products, cheese, and lowfat milk is noted, while consumption of whole milk decreased. Another example of technological effects on product availability is the change in frozen dairy product consumption. Improved freezing and frozen storage technologies and new ingredients for frozen dairy products such as fat replacers, sugar substitutes, and stabilizers greatly expand choices. Differences in the type of milk consumed are attributed to concern about fat in the diet and a population with a decreasing percentage of children.

Sweeteners

Overall, sweetener consumption has been increasing since 1909, but the types of sweeteners are changing (14). Consumption of cane and beet sugars decreased, while corn and noncaloric sweetener consumption increased. These changes occurred because technologies associated with the production of corn sweeteners from corn starch and the manufacturing of noncaloric sweeteners reduced their costs so they can compete economically with sugars and corn sweeteners. Other issues of sweeteners are discussed in Chapter 4.

Beverages

Beverage consumption trends show increases in soft drinks and juices (14). Alcoholic beverage consumption increased at about the same rate as soft drinks until the 1980s when it stabilized and began to decrease. Decreases have occurred in milk and coffee consumption. Tea consumption has remained stable through the years.

Implications of food consumption trends

Food consumption trends have an impact on the nutritional status of the US population. Increased consumption of fruits and vegetables is ideal for reducing risk factors associated with diet-related chronic diseases. Generally, however, many of us need to learn how to cook the wider variety of vegetables now available in the

CULTURAL CONSIDERATIONS
Salsa Surpasses Ketchup!

Whether slathered over French fries, poured on hamburgers, or dabbed over eggs, ketchup has been a part of American cuisine as long as records have been kept! Ketchup sales, however, have been recently surpassed by Mexican-style salsa. As a food product category, salsas include taco, picante, enchilada, and other chili-style sauces. Salsas, especially the tomato relish, seem to have a wider range of uses than traditional ketchup. Besides use as dips with chips and vegetables, salsas serve as sauces on foods, as marinade bases, as toppings on salads and cooked potatoes, and other inventive purposes.

How and why did this happen? It may be due to a rise in the health consciousness of Americans. As we strive to reduce our intake of fat and sodium, turning from fat-laden meats and highly processed foods to poultry, fish, and vegetarian dishes, we still want intense flavors to spark our taste buds. Salsas, while providing that spark, also add novelty to foods with little or no fat content, which is welcomed by food manufacturers, as well as consumers.

In addition to Mexican cuisine, Italian and Asian cuisines continue to be popular ethnic foods of Americans. These foods tend to be healthier than traditional American foods because they usually dilute or extend the meat, poultry, or fish protein sources with a cereal food—spaghetti, rice, or corn— to which vegetables and flavorful sauces are added. Trends indicate that Thai, Indian, Caribbean, Greek, Japanese, and Eastern European foods also are in demand in the United States.

Other Latino (besides Mexican), Asian, and Indian seasonings are showing up in all kinds of fresh, frozen, and packaged products in supermarkets and on restaurant menus. The dishes created are not necessarily authentic, but are adaptations for Americans that reflect "ethnic flavor profiles." These modifications of authentic ethnic foods and the combination of foods from different ethnic cuisines in the same meal are also becoming trends in the food service industry. Indian foods provide vegetarian dishes for those who demand flavorful, low-fat alternatives. One supplier of Thai foods has combined ethnic foods by marketing Thai tortilla chips and Thai salsas in peanut, ginger, cilantro, and mango flavors.

Travel and media make our world smaller and our foods more universal!

From O'Neill M: New mainstream: Hot dogs, apple pie and salsa, *New York Times* March 11, 1992; Sloan AE: The explosion of multicultural cuisine, *Food Technology* 48(3):74-76, 1994; Fusaro D: Changing demographics serve up new ethnic foods, *Prepared Foods* 163(5):22-28, 1994.

---

supermarkets so they taste and look good. Similarly, since consumption of cereals and grains is beginning to rise, we need suggestions about new ways to prepare different kinds and forms of grains to meet the dietary recommendations of six to eleven servings a day.

Overall, animal sources of protein appear to be decreasing. Within the meat, poultry, and fish category, beef consumption decreased while poultry and fish consumption increased in recent years. The message to reduce dietary fat intake is affecting meat consumption. But how poultry and fish are prepared is also important. The cooking method determines the final dietary fat content. Health benefits are greatest when we choose low-fat cooking methods. Some popular ethnic cuisines also extend meat, poultry, or fish by combining these protein sources with cereals, grains, vegetables, and sauces (see box).

Dairy product trends reflect dietary recommendations for lower fat products. The consumption of whole milk, the fluid milk highest in fat content, is decreasing, and at the same time the consumption of low-fat and nonfat products is increasing with the wide array of new products in the marketplace. Consumption of frozen dairy products remained quite stable in recent years. Sweetener and beverage consumption trends affect the nutritional status depending on whether the type of sweetener or beverage chosen lowers intake of more nutrient-dense foods and drinks.

Although these trends reflect per capita consumption patterns based on the total population, it is our individual food choices that have the greatest influence on our personal level of wellness.

Effective Food Buying Styles

This chapter is full of information about consumer decisions, but how to apply it? How do you and your clients become better shoppers? The first step is to tailor a shopping style to one's particular situation. Consider the following questions to formulate the most effective approach to food shopping (16):

1. *What is your food budget?* A food budget should take into account funds needed to keep a moderate amount of food in the house as well as money spent on meals away from home.
2. *For whom do you buy food?* Buying food for a single young adult is very different than for a family. Lifestyles of household members affect the number and types of meals served.
3. *Are there special dietary needs to be considered?* We all have food preferences based on ethnicity, habits, chronic illness, or ethical views such as vegetarianism. Each affects food buying selections.
4. *How often do you shop? Do you have a shopping schedule?* Each household works best with a shopping plan—perhaps weekly, every 2 weeks, or simply when needed on the way home from school or work.
5. *Where can you shop?* Different types of stores provide a range of services and products. Limited assortment warehouse stores are good for bulk supplies; conventional supermarkets, superstores, and super warehouse stores are valuable for fresh produce, perishables, and basic grocery items; specialty stores offer the unique; and convenience stores save the day!

CONSUMER INFORMATION AND WELLNESS

The more information consumers have about the food we eat the better we can choose foods that will contribute to our wellness. Unfortunately, as consumers, we need to use a food product before we can decide whether we like it. Economists call this type of product an "experience good" (14). But foods are also "credence goods" in that we cannot evaluate their impact on our health until some time after they have been eaten. Therefore it is hard for consumers to evaluate attributes of foods before we buy and use them.

Food Labeling

Food labels are the best way for us as consumers to see how individual foods fit our nutritional needs. Their purpose is to "help consumers choose more healthful diets, and to offer an incentive to food companies to improve the nutritional qualities of their products"(16).

Food labeling for processed foods in the United States is based on standards established under authority of the 1990 Nutrition Labeling and Education Act. Although nutrition labeling is mandatory for most processed products, it is voluntary for fresh meat, poultry, fish, milk, eggs, and produce. An example of the label for processed foods is shown in Fig. 2-3.

The "Nutrition Facts" panel must list the quantities of energy (kcalories), fat, and specific other nutrients in a serving:

- Total food energy
- Food energy from fat

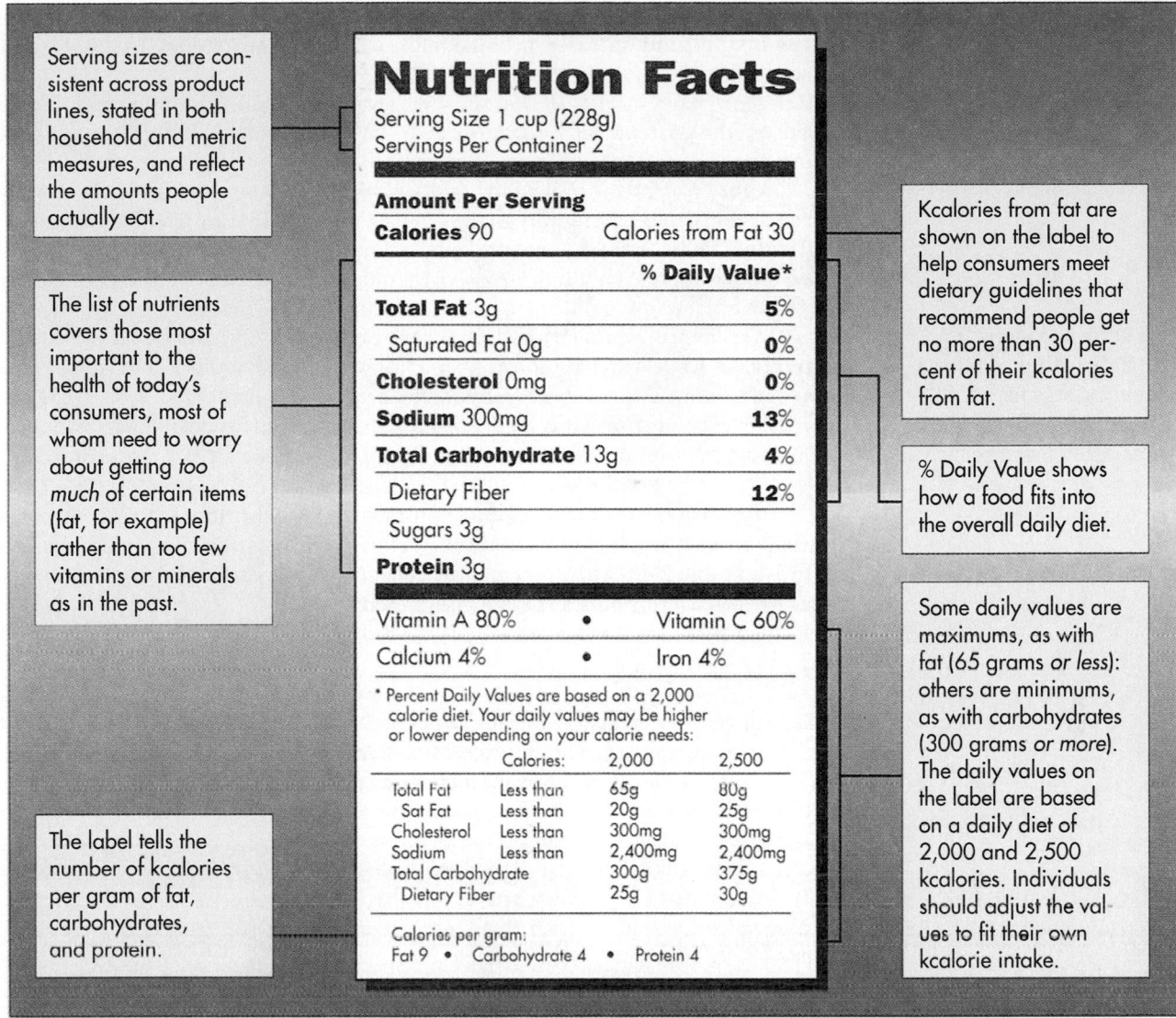

Fig. 2-3 An example of the food label format that currently is mandatory in the United States.

- Total fat
- Saturated fat
- Cholesterol
- Sodium
- Total carbohydrates
- Dietary fiber
- Sugars
- Protein
- Vitamin C
- Calcium
- Iron

The "% Daily Values" information, based on a 2000 kcalorie diet, is intended to show consumers how much of a day's ideal intake of a particular nutrient they are eating. Daily values for selected nutrients and food components are also given at the bottom of the label for a 2500 calorie diet. **Daily values** are based on either of two sets of reference values: Reference Daily Intakes or Daily Reference Values,

Daily Values

a system for food labeling composed of two sets of reference values: Reference Daily Intakes and Daily Intake Values

Reference Daily Intakes
a set of daily nutrient values for protein, vitamins, and minerals based on allowances of the 1968 RDAs

Daily Reference Values
a set of daily nutrient and food constituent values for which there are no RDAs, including fat, fiber, cholesterol, and sodium

depending on the nutrient or food component. The reference values are used primarily by food and nutrition professionals, while the daily values are used by consumers.

Reference daily intakes (RDIs) set standards for protein, vitamins, and minerals based on the current US Recommended Daily Allowances (US RDAs). The US RDAs were created for nutrition labeling and are set on the highest 1968 RDAs of any category except for pregnancy and lactation. RDIs are the basis for the standards of the federal programs that provide nutritional support. The five sets of RDI values categorized by age and physiological state are adults and children 4 years old and older; children 1 to 4 years old; infants 1 year old or younger; and pregnant or lactating women.

Daily reference values (DRVs) are for nutrients and food constituents for which there are no RDAs, including fat, fiber, cholesterol, and sodium. DRVs have been developed because these food components are important to health, as recognized by current recommendations for minimum or maximum intakes. Fiber recommendations are minimum values and cholesterol recommendations are a maximum value.

Uniform definitions for food descriptors such as light, low-fat, and others for nutrient content claims are now clearly defined and must be consistently used for all foods (Table 2-1). This information helps consumers trying to control their intakes of specific nutrients and food components.

To help clients evaluate food labels, use the Teaching Tool on p. 41.

Health claims

Health claims that relate a nutrient or food to risk of a disease or health-related condition now appear on food labels. Only health claims approved by the FDA may be used. So far, those allowed include a relationship between (17): a diet with

Table 2-1   Food Descriptors

Free
Contains only a tiny or insignificant amount of fat, cholesterol, sodium, sugar, and/or calories. For example, a "fat-free" product will contain less than 0.5 grams of fat per serving.

Low
"Low" in fat, saturated fat, cholesterol, sodium, and/or calories; can be eaten fairly often without exceeding dietary guidelines. So "low in fat" means no more than 3 grams of fat per serving.

Lean
Contains less than 10 grams of fat, 4 grams of saturated fat, and 95 mg of cholesterol per serving. "Lean" is not as lean as "Low." "Lean" and "Extra Lean" are USDA terms for use on meat and poultry products.

Extra Lean
Contains less than 5 grams of fat, 2 grams of saturated fat, and 95 mg of cholesterol per serving. Leaner than "Lean," "Extra lean" is still not as lean as "Low."

Reduced, Less, Fewer
Contains 25% less of a nutrient or calories. For example, hotdogs might be labeled "25% less fat than our regular hot dogs."

Light/Lite
Contains one third fewer calories or one half the fat of the original. "Light in Sodium" means a product with one half the usual sodium.

More
Contains at least 10% more of the Daily Value of a vitamin, mineral, or fiber than usual single serving.

Good Source of
Contains 10% to 19% of the Daily Value for a particular vitamin, mineral, and fiber in a single serving.

TEACHING TOOL

Just the Facts — Using Labels to Teach Nutrition

Present clients with three boxes of cereal or Nutrition Facts labels from three cereal products. Choose products that are diverse. For example, include a heavily presweetened cereal, a lightly sweetened cereal, and one with no added sweeteners. Ask the following questions:

Which has the most kcalories per serving? This may be affected by weight, volume of the cereal (popped with air) and the density of added ingredients like raisins.

Which has the largest serving size? Servings sizes are the same by weight for all products in a food category.

Which contains the most dietary fat? Fat is not an issue with cereals, except for granola.

Which contains the most sodium? Some cereals contain about 300 mg, which is high for sodium-sensitive clients.

Which contains the most added sugars? Added sugars can range from none to 13 grams per serving.

How many calories come from sugars? Multiply the number of grams of sugars by 4 kcalories. By dividing this number into the total serving, you can determine the percentage of sugar content.

Which contains the most fiber? Fiber content can range from none to about 5 grams per serving.

As your study of nutrition continues, you may add other questions and be able to relate client responses to preventive heath issues of diet-related diseases or to address specific dietary needs of a patient's medical nutrition therapy.

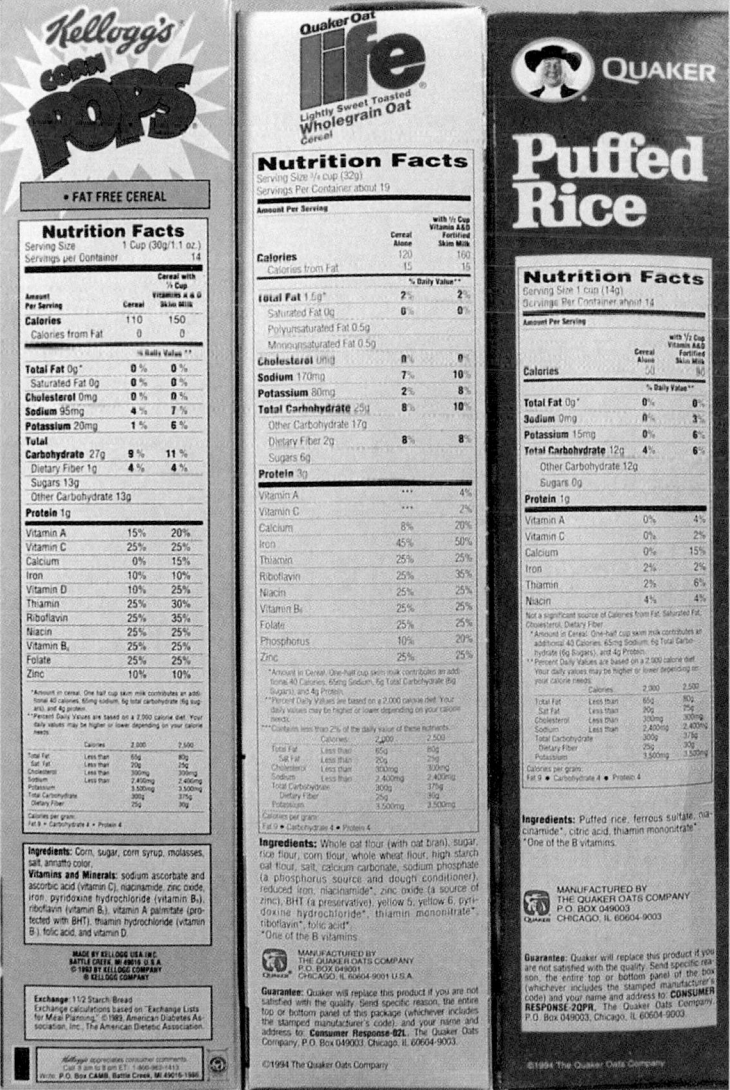

sufficient calcium and lower risk of osteoporosis; a diet low in total fat and decreased risk of some cancers; a diet low in saturated fat and cholesterol and reduced risk of coronary heart disease; a diet high in fiber-containing fruits, vegetables, and grain products and decreased risk of some cancers; a diet high in fruits, vegetables and grain products containing fiber and decreased risk of coronary heart disease; a diet low in sodium and reduced risk of hypertension; a diet high in fruits and vegetables and decreased risk of some cancers; and sufficient intake of folic acid and reduced risk of neural tube defects. This information helps consumers select those foods that can keep them healthy and well.

Food Safety Decisions

Food safety is influenced by community decisions and personal behaviors. We expect the larger community such as government agencies to supervise the production and preparation of food products to assure the safety of the foods we purchase. But once we, as consumers, purchase food products, we then take the responsibility for properly handling foods to prevent foodborne illness.

These concerns apply equally in the nursing setting. Our clients are also consumers. Our recommendations regarding nutritional intake are "translated" by our clients when they become consumers. As we advise about nutrition concerns, public and personal food safety is also an issue.

The knowledge, attitudes, perceptions, and concerns consumers have about food safety affect the food decisions they make. There is enormous concern by consumers and the food industry that the US food supply be safe. To have a safe food supply, it is essential that each sector of the food chain (producers, manufacturers, wholesalers, food stores, food service outlets, and consumers) follow correct food handling procedures.

Recent data show that consumers have confidence in the safety of the food supply and in their ability to select safe food products. Some 73% of food shoppers are completely or mostly confident that the food available in supermarkets is safe. In terms of taking responsibility for the safety of the food they buy, nearly twice as many shoppers (38%) take this responsibility individually compared to the 21% who rely on food manufacturers and the 20% who rely on the government to make sure foods are safe (13).

Communication about food safety between consumers and food safety professionals is difficult, however, because their food safety concerns differ (14). One concern of food shoppers in recent years is the perception that "residues such as pesticides and herbicides" are serious health hazards. Seventy-nine percent of food shoppers who rated their concerns regarding health hazards in the food supply for a Food Marketing Institute survey consider these residues a serious health hazard. However, when these shoppers were asked in the survey what they perceive as threats to food safety, only 13% listed pesticides/residues/insecticides/herbicides. In explaining this finding, the Food Marketing Institute states: "An item considered to be a serious hazard in and of itself, for example, might be seen as little or no threat because it is perceived to occur rarely or at very low levels in the actual food supply." Other items considered a serious health hazard by food shoppers are "antibiotics and hormones in poultry and livestock" by 55%; "nitrites in foods" and "irradiated foods" by 35%; "additives and preservatives" by 23%, and "artificial coloring" by 19% (13).

Food safety professionals on the FDA staff, however, rank "microbiological contaminants" highest as a health hazard (14). Other health hazards that concern food professionals are "malnutrition, diet, and disease," "environmental contaminants," "naturally occurring toxins in foods," and "food additives" in that order. Although they use different terms to describe the problem, food shoppers also are concerned about microbiological contaminants (13). Nearly half (46%) of food shoppers list food spoilage as a food safety threat. Shoppers' concerns about spoilage include "freshness/long shelf life/expiration dates" by 20%; "spoilage/germs" by 18%; "quality control/improper shipping, handling, etc." by 9%; and "bacteria/contamination" by 8%. It is not yet clear how consumers ultimately will respond to genetically modified foods or what kind of labeling may be required on such products (see box).

Risk analysis and food safety

Setting risk standards is difficult because it requires evaluation of trade-offs and "placing a value on reduced pain and suffering and the saving of human lives" (14). Approaches being used to set risk standards for food safety are primarily based on keeping substances out of the food supply (14, 18). These include the "zero risk" standard of the Delaney Clause for food additives, the "de minimus" standard covering substances with a low level of risk, the "no significant risk" standard of California's Proposition 65 (Safe Drinking Water and Toxic Enforcement Act), and the "risk-benefit" standard of the Federal Insecticide, Fungicide, and Rodenticide Act (FIFRA) (14).

The "zero risk" standard of the **Delaney Clause** applies specifically to food additives and dates back to the 1958 Food Additives Amendment to the Federal Food, Drug and Cosmetic Act of 1938, the major law regulating food safety (14, 18). This clause states "no additive shall be deemed to be safe if it is found to induce cancer when ingested by man or animal, or if it is found, after tests which are appropriate for the evaluation of the safety of food additives, to induce cancer in man or animal" (14). This amendment also shifts the responsibility for proving the

Delaney Clause
the 1958 Food Additives Amendment to the federal Food, Drug and Cosmetic Act of 1938 that bans any intentional food additive found to induce cancer in man or animal

HEALTH DEBATE
Biotechnology: Consumer Risk or Benefit?

No, biotechnology does not mean that the androids are coming! Instead, the most recent form of food biotechnology is controlled modification of the genetic structure of foods at the molecular level to improve nutrient content, increase crop or animal yield, inhibit spoilage, and otherwise enhance desirable characteristics of food products.

Traditional biotechnological efforts resulted in random mutations from crossbreeding of plants or animals. These changes seem to have shown little risk to consumers or the environment. But the new molecular biotechnology raises concerns by some consumers and scientists even though risks are decreased compared to traditional biotechnology.

Presently, one gene of the thousands found in tomatoes has been altered by molecular biotechnology in the new Flavr Savr tomato approved for marketing by the FDA. This alteration allows the tomato to ripen on the vine for best flavor by inactivating the enzyme that causes a tomato to soften during ripening. Therefore shelf life of the tomatoes is extended both in the retail store and at home. Because of this added value, these tomatoes are expected to sell at a higher price than regular tomatoes. Data show that Flavr Savr tomatoes are safe, based on field, safety, and nutritional tests. What if other tomato genes are manipulated? When is a tomato no longer a tomato?

Additional questions need to be considered as other food products are genetically modified. Will such changes increase the supply and availability thereby lowering the price of nutritious foods? An example is the increased milk yield from cows treated with bovine somatotropin (BST). Another is the use in cheesemaking of pure chymosin enzyme from molecular biotechnology rather than the more expensive rennet from calves' stomachs. The FDA has approved both of these products of biotechnology.

How would lower prices affect the farmers who grow the crops or whose cows produce the milk? If these genetic manipulations keep prices high by producing "status" perfect quality products such as the Flavr Savr tomato, who gains? Or are these scientific developments simply a continuation of the food biotechnology timeline started when milk was first pasteurized to destroy bacteria? What's your opinion?

From Hardy RWF: Biotechnology and food, *Contemporary Nutrition* 19(2):1994.

safety of food additives from the government to the food manufacturer wishing to use the additive(s).

Additives considered safe and used when the Amendment went into effect are on a Generally Recognized As Safe (GRAS) list; new additives are added as their safety is established. However, because of questions regarding the safety of additives on the original GRAS list when methods of analysis became more sensitive and could detect lower and lower levels of these substances, a comprehensive review of the list and all chemicals added to food was recently completed by the Federation of American Societies for Experimental Biology (FASEB).

Additives used for their functional properties in foods during processing, that is, to improve food quality in some way, are called **intentional** or **direct food additives** and those that inadvertently become a part of a food at some time as it passes through the food system are called **indirect** or **unintentional food additives** (18). Direct additives are used to improve, maintain, and stabilize food quality; to increase availability across the country and lengthen storage time; to increase convenience; to decrease waste; and to stabilize or increase nutrient content (18). Table 2-2 lists selected intentional GRAS food additives. Indirect additives include pesticide and herbicide residues, animal drugs, processing aids, and packaging constituents that migrate from the package into the food. Regardless of their source, indirect additives seem to be of greatest concern to consumers (14,18).

The "de minimus" risk standard essentially proposes ignoring very small risks and suggests that a "hazard should not cause more than one additional death per one million people over their lifetimes" (14). The "no significant risk" of California's Proposition 65 established a standard that no more than one additional death per one hundred thousand people over their lifetimes should be caused by a hazard. These standards are difficult to establish because they depend on extrapolating data from animal tests and applying them to humans, and also are influenced by the susceptibility of humans and the extent of their exposure to a substance.

The "risk-benefit" approach of the FIFRA involves "balancing the risks and benefits to society from an activity or use of a substance" (14). In this case, risks to human health and to the environment are balanced against the economic benefits sustained by the use of insecticides, fungicides, and rodenticides. However, like the other approaches being used to set risk standards, risk-benefit estimates for foods are limited by the unavailability of reliable quantitative data to use in the analysis.

Foodborne Illness

From the practical standpoint of keeping people well, the importance of microbiological contaminants must be acknowledged by consumers and professionals; both groups need to work together to help prevent foodborne illness. In addition to the discomfort, these illnesses cause greater economic costs in terms of lost time at work and productivity than most people can imagine. Unfortunately, the incidence of foodborne illness in the United States is increasing, according to the federal Centers for Disease Control and Prevention, which keeps statistical data on these illnesses (18). Since many cases of foodborne illness are not reported, federal agencies must rely on estimates to define the size of the problem. The FDA estimates an annual incidence of from 25 to 81 million cases of foodborne illness. And foodborne illness is estimated to cost up to $8.4 billion annually (18).

Food can become contaminated with bacteria, molds, parasites, and viruses during production, processing, transporting, storage, and retailing and in the home (14,18). Although the entire food distribution system may contribute to foodborne illness, improper handling of food in the home is a commonly overlooked source of contamination and growth of microorganisms causing illness. The severity of foodborne illness varies with the microorganism, the susceptibility of the person, and the amount of bacteria or enterotoxin ingested. Information about sources, symptoms, and special control recommendations for common bacterial infections and intoxications are outlined in Table 2-3.

intentional food additives
substances purposely added during manufacturing to food products

incidental additives
substances that inadvertently contaminate processed foods

Table 2-2   Intentional Food Additives

Nutrients
  Fat replacers
  Iodide in some salt
  Sugar replacers
  Vitamins A and D
Processing Aids
  Anticaking agents
  Conditioners
  Dough strengtheners
  Drying agents
  Emulsifiers
  Enzymes
  Firming agents
  Flour treatments
  Formulation aids
  Leavening agents
  Lubricants
  Propellants
  Solvents
  Stabilizers
  Surface agents
  Surface finishing
  Synergists
  Texturizers
  Thickening agents
Preservatives
  Antimicrobials
  Antioxidants
  Curing and pickling agents
  Fumigants
  Humectants
  Oxidizing and reducing agents
  Sequesterants
Appearance and Flavor Enhancers
  Clarifying agents
  Color
  Flavor enhancers
  Flavoring agents
  Foam inhibitors
  Foaming agents
  Nonnutritive sweeteners
  Nutritive sweeteners

As the palates of Americans become used to exotic sensations, the Japanese meal of sushi, raw fish with vinegared rice, is ordered more often in the growing number of Japanese restaurants. Unless the fish is served fresh and free of parasites, though, Anisakid nematode parasites can be a problem when eating raw fish. Sushi is not a dish to prepare at home. It has been thought to be safest when prepared by experienced Japanese chefs. Licensing of sushi chefs, however, is not mandatory in the United States; therefore they are not required to meet the strict standards of licensed chefs. Recent research has shown the prevalence of parasites in sushi in the Seattle area, thus confirming that experienced sushi chefs do not discard infected fish (19). As a precaution, patients with reduced immune system disorders and other at-risk clients should consider avoiding raw fish and animal foods such as sushi and shashimi (raw fish only). Regardless, these foods should not be an everyday treat, but can be safely enjoyed in moderation.

Table 2-3 Foodborne Illnesses

Illness	Organism	Foods	Symptoms	Precautions
Botulism	*Clostridium botulinum*	Underprocessed low-acid canned food (pH > 4) such as vegetables, meat, poultry, fish; particularly home-canned food; cured and smoked fish in air-tight packages	Occur 12-36 hrs after eating food containing the toxin; dizziness, weakness, double vision, hoarseness, thirst; death occurs from paralysis of the diaphragm	Toxin unstable to heat; boil home-canned, low-acid foods 10 minutes before even tasting; be aware that canned tuna, mushrooms, and soups eaten cold have caused botulism when not heated before use; when canning vegetables, meat, poultry and fish at home, be sure to follow USDA directions for canning in a pressure canner; if botulism illness is suspected, seek medical help and anti-toxin immediately
Campylobac-teriosis	*Campylobacter jejuni*	Drinking water, raw and undercooked poultry, raw milk, raw hamburger, raw clams	Occur 2-5 days after eating contaminated food; diarrhea that may be bloody, abdominal pain, fever, vomiting; may cause meningitis, urinary infections; infants and males under 45 yrs vulnerable	Sanitary food handling practices; adequate cooking and preservation methods that use heat, dehydration, salt, acid; avoid anaerobic (no oxygen) and partially anaerobic conditions (very little oxygen) in packaging and storage
Listeriosis	*Listeria monocytogenes*	Milk, cheese, ice cream, sausage, leafy vegetables from fields fertilized with contaminated manure, raw meat and poultry, water	Occur 1-12 days after eating contaminated food; illness similar to flu with nausea, fever, headache; may develop into meningitis or infection similar to mono-nucleosis; most serious for infants, pregnant women, persons with immune problems	Sanitary food handling practices; be careful not to cross-contaminate raw foods or cooked foods with raw foods; use pasteurized milk and make sure foods from animal sources are adequately cooked; difficult to control growth once contaminated because organism is not well controlled by refrigeration or preservation methods commonly used
Pathogenic *Escherichia coli* food-borne illness	*Escherichia coli*	Raw ground beef, possibly chicken, and imported soft cheeses from unsanitary handling of food and unsanitary processing equipment	Different with each strain of organism; some cause infection, some produce toxins that cause illness along with infection; can be fatal; *Escherichia coli* 0157:H7 recently implicated in illness and death; most frequent symptoms include bloody diarrhea, cramps, fever, chills, dehydration, kidney problems	Sanitary food handling during processing and in the home; cook ground beef to well-done stage; do not eat undercooked meat or poultry with any red or pink color; avoid cross-contamination between meat and other foods via cutting boards, counter surfaces, preparation equipment, or knives

Table 2-3   Foodborne Illnesses, cont'd.

Illness	Organism	Foods	Symptoms	Precautions
Perfringens foodborne illness	*Clostridium perfringens*	Meat, gravies, casseroles, mostly from food service items held warm for a long time	Occur 8-24 hrs after eating the contaminated food; illness lasts about a day; toxin released by the organism growing in intestine causes cramps, diarrhea	Refrigeration immediately after cooking; avoid foods held for long periods in steam tables and cold or reheated meat that has previously been cooked; spores are heat resistant and may not be destroyed by cooking
Salmonellosis	*Salmonella*	Eggs, poultry, raw milk, meats, other foods from cross-contamination	Occur 12-24 hrs after eating contaminated food; nausea and vomiting, cramps, diarrhea, chills, fever; most serious for infants, elderly, persons with chronic diseases	Sanitary
Staphylococcal foodborne illness	*Staphylococcus aureaus*	Found on skin and transmitted to foods requiring handling in preparation such as salads, cream filling in baked products and pies, milk contaminated after pasteurization, poultry, ham, salad-based sandwich fillings	Occur 2-3 hours after eating the food containing the toxin; nausea, vomiting, diarrhea, cramps, fever, chills; sensitivity of individuals varies	Avoid contaminating the food; refrigerate food to decrease possibility of microorganism growth and toxin formation; toxin is not destroyed by heat, so cooking or boiling the contaminated food does not make the food safe to eat
Vibriosis	*Vibrio parahaemolyticus*	Raw seafood and fish	Occur 2-48 hrs after eating the contaminated food; flu-like symptoms—nausea, vomiting, diarrhea, fever, chills, cramping	Adequate cooking or drying of seafood and fish; low temperatures of refrigeration and freezing retard growth but may not destroy the microorganisms

From Jones JM: *Food safety,* St. Paul, Minn, 1992, Eagan Press; and American Home Economics Association: *Handbook of food preparation,* ed 9, Dubuque, Iowa, 1993, Kendall/Hunt.

What could be more wholesome and healthful than fresh cider straight from the cider mill? Well, a number of folks who sipped cider at an apple farm in Massachusetts learned otherwise when they fell victim to a pathogenic type of *Escherichia coli (E. coli)* bacteria and experienced gastrointestinal distress. It seems that apples used for cider are often those that have fallen to the ground and have blemishes. The problem is that those apples may come in contact with animal feces and manure fertilizer; unless the apples are washed well or the cider is pasteurized or preserved with sodium benzoate, this contamination can lead to illness (21).

Some types of *E. coli* are normally found in the human intestinal system; they are responsible for producing vitamins B_{12} and K if needed and for limiting the growth of other undesirable bacteria. But we have few defenses against the pathogenic *E. coli* 0157:H7, which was found in a batch of meat distributed to a number of restaurants in the Northwest United States in 1993. When cooks at a fast food restaurant chain undercooked hamburgers containing this *E. coli* organism, 4 children died and about 500 people became ill. The bacteria attacked the intestinal walls, allowing the effects to then spread to other parts of the body, particularly the kidneys. Cooking the meat to a "well-done" stage with no trace of redness would have destroyed the *E. coli* bacteria (21). As a result of this outbreak, the USDA has recently revised the internal temperature to which meat should be cooked in restaurants and in the home.

Personal food safety

Although government inspection programs should guard against these episodes, as an aspect of personal responsibility for our nutrition, we must adhere to safe food handling procedures in the home and follow food safety guidelines when we eat away from home. Here are some recommendations (18):

- Sanitary food handling in the home means clean hands for the food preparer, clean equipment, and clean surroundings, including cutting boards and countertops.
- Wash hands with soap and hot water before preparing and cooking foods.
- Wash cutting boards, utensils, and/or countertops that come in contact with uncooked meats, poultry, or fish with hot soapy water with a disinfectant in it.
- Do not place cooked foods on unwashed surfaces where uncooked foods have been prepared because they will become contaminated with the microorganisms on these surfaces.
- Bacteria are destroyed by cooking, but bacteria from uncooked foods on unwashed surfaces can reinfect any cooked food placed on them.
- Keep foods either colder than 40° F or hotter than 140° F. The "danger zone" for rapid growth of microorganisms is within this temperature range. Foods can easily fall into this zone at a picnic or a pot-luck meal.
- Refrigerate cooked foods immediately after meals or after they are cooked. DO NOT cool to room temperature and then refrigerate.
- Boil all home-canned vegetables, meats, poultry and fish for 10 minutes before even tasting.
- Marinades used with uncooked meats, poultry, and fish should be discarded or boiled after marination is completed; bacteria is not destroyed until heated.
- Cook all meat, poultry, shellfish, and fish to the well-done stage.
- Do not eat or taste any uncooked foods containing raw eggs, including cookie and cake batters. They could contain *Salmonella*.
- NEVER use a recipe that calls for raw eggs and is not cooked or baked after addition of the eggs. And when making homemade ice cream, be sure to cook the eggs by making a soft custard; do not use raw eggs in the mixture to be frozen.
- Microwave cooking can be tricky—and dangerous. NEVER store defrosted and/or partially cooked meats and poultry. Cook them completely to the well-done stage first, and then eat or refrigerate.
- When food shopping, choose perishable foods (those from the refrigerator or freezer cases) last and get them home as soon as possible. Don't leave them sitting in the car while doing other errands.
- Never buy or use foods in a bulging can, cracked jar, or bulging lid. Damage to containers may have allowed botulism to develop. Don't taste to determine if spoiled; this toxin is extremely dangerous!

We tend to be casual about food preparation. After all, we eat all the time! However, sometimes being too relaxed allows for these bacterial and viral contaminations to occur. In our homes, we must implement basic food safety procedures when preparing and storing foods; in food retail markets and food service facilities, we count on the expertise and supervision of public health officers to enforce regulations providing for safe food availability.

Nurses need to recognize our role in providing safe foods to patients. When handling foods for patients, care needs to be taken to prevent contamination by using the tactics of food handlers such as hand washing before serving or assisting patients with their meals.

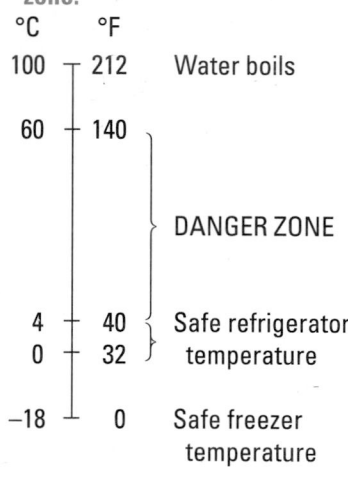

Keep food out of the danger zone:

°C	°F	
100	212	Water boils
60	140	
		DANGER ZONE
4	40	Safe refrigerator
0	32	temperature
−18	0	Safe freezer temperature

Food preservation to control foodborne illness

Through the years, many methods have been developed and used to preserve food for future use by controlling decomposition and microbial growth that could lead to foodborne illness. Besides drying and dehydration, which limit moisture in the food, methods developed include canning, refrigeration and freezing, pasteurization, curing and smoking, modified atmosphere packaging, aseptic packaging, and irradiation. In canning, heat is used to destroy microorganisms; in pickling, salt, acid (vinegar), and usually heat control microbial growth; and in jellies and jams, sugar is the preservative. Refrigeration and freezing limit the growth of microorganisms by the use of cold temperatures. Pasteurization employs heat to destroy pathogenic organisms in milk and other undesirable ones in other foods. The use of various salts and smoke cure and preserve meat, poultry, and fish. Modified atmosphere packaging provides an atmosphere of various gases within the package that helps control microbial growth to preserve the food. Aseptic packaging preserves food and prevents contamination by placing food products that are sterilized separately from the packaging into sterilized containers, which are immediately sealed.

Irradiation is a food preservation technology that is beginning to be used not only to control the microorganisms that cause foodborne illness but also to increase international and domestic food trade. By decreasing economic losses caused by food spoilage, insects, sprouting, and changes associated with ripening, irradiated products can travel further (18,22). Irradiation involves exposure of food to gamma irradiation using cobalt-60 or cesium-137 or to an electron beam from electron accelerators (17,21). The machine sources may be the least controversial of the sources of radiation because they are independent of nuclear energy, and so there is no radioactive waste. Extensive testing has shown that irradiated foods are wholesome, do not become radioactive, and provide consumers with a reduced risk of foods contaminated with microorganisms that cause foodborne illness (18,23,24).

Food is now irradiated in 37 countries, with 26 of these using irradiation for foods and ingredients used commercially (22). The foods most often irradiated are spices and dried vegetable seasonings. With banning or potential banning of fumigants now used for these foods, as well as for fresh fruits and vegetables, dried fruits, tree nuts, and cocoa beans, it is anticipated that irradiation will increase. The use of irradiation for poultry products is a specific example of efforts to control salmonellosis and campylobacteriosis (22).

In the United States, irradiation was approved early in the 1960s to control sprouting in white potatoes and insects in wheat and wheat flour; early in the

irradiation
a procedure by which food is exposed to radiation that destroys micro-organisms, insect growth, and parasites that could spoil food or cause illness

Fig. 2-4 The "radura" symbol must be carried by all foods that have been treated with radiation, although it need not be carried by processed foods that include irradiated ingredients.

1980s for spices and dried vegetable seasonings; in 1986 to destroy *Trichinella spiralis* parasites in pork, control insects in foods, and delay ripening and sprouting of fresh fruit and vegetables; and in 1992 for poultry pathogens (23).

Irradiated whole foods (as opposed to foods containing irradiated ingredients) in the United States must be labeled as "Treated with Radiation" or "Treated by Irradiation" and display the international symbol for irradiated foods (Fig. 2-4) (18,23,24).

TOWARD A POSITIVE NUTRITION LIFESTYLE: LOCUS OF CONTROL

D o things just happen to you? Does it seem as if school, family, or society affects what you do without your input? Or do you feel that you have control over what takes place? Do you have a life plan (or weekly plan) that you follow?

locus of control
the perception of one's ability to control life events and experiences

Locus of control is the perception of one's ability to control life events and experiences. Having an internal locus of control means feeling as if you can influence the forces with which you come in contact. You have an inner sense of your ability to guide life events. An external locus of control is defined as the perception of not being able to control what happens to you and that outside forces have power over what you experience.

Let's apply these concepts to your style of making food choices when shopping. In particular, consider the nutritional implications of locus of control. If you have an internal locus of control, you may develop a basic plan of the types of nutritious foods to be purchased during a shopping trip. You may make a few unplanned purchases, but they would be limited in number. You feel in control of your choices. Having an external locus of control means that you might start out with a shopping list, but you are probably easily swayed by in-store promotions, coupons, and even colorful packaging to select products not on your list. You often buy more than needed because so much "looked good."

Awareness of our type of locus of control allows us to develop strategies to improve our food decisions. Individuals with an internal locus of control tend to develop their own approaches for changing food-related behaviors; those with an external locus of control may need a structured program or group support to provide guidance to modify their food behaviors.

WELLNESS AND PERSONAL/COMMUNITY NUTRITION

Physical Dimension	Following the Food Guide Pyramid and 5 a Day may reduce risk of diet-related diseases. Implementing food safety strategies decreases foodborne illness.
Intellectual Dimension	Consumer decisions about food purchases and application of food safety recommendations depend on reasoning abilities.
Emotional Dimension	Our emotions may affect our ability to be flexible when adopting suggested guideline changes. If we (or our clients) have problems, will we view ourselves as "failures"?
Social Dimension	Social skills will be tested as we (and our clients) interact with family and friends while attempting to follow the guidelines. Can we be role models for others without being perceived as threatening?

SUMMARY

This chapter considers factors of personal and community nutrition. Food preferences, food choices, and food liking greatly influence the foods we choose and so affect our overall nutritional status. As knowledge of the relationship between diet and disease increases, public health approaches to diet-related disease prevention have been formulated to encourage us to select foods, not just for their nutrient and energy content but with primary disease prevention value as well. Food guides have been created to implement the dietary recommendations on a daily basis. These guides address the concerns of nutrient adequacy and primary disease prevention. The Food Guide Pyramid and 5 a Day program are easy to follow to improve our nutritional intake.

Food consumption trends in the United States are an indication of changes in the American diet. Consumption trends for most foods can be followed from 1909. These trends for fruits and vegetables; cereals and grains; meat, poultry and fish; dairy products; sweeteners; and beverages reflect the availability and food choices of per capita consumption. This information helps us to translate nutrients into food categories and to attend to consumer needs and issues when advising clients or patients.

Providing consumers and health professionals with more information about foods through food labels increases the probability that decisions made and advice given about which foods to eat will be based on nutrition as well as on taste, and thus will contribute to health and wellness. Food safety is of concern because of its potential to eliminate, or at least substantially decrease foodborne illness as more is learned about the various causes of this illness. Knowledge of how bacteria, molds, parasites, and viruses can be problems in the food supply helps us to understand how to control these problems in order to stay well.

THE NURSING ROLE

Dietary Teaching: The Nursing Process

Most nurses are concerned with nutrition at the individual and family levels. Some, however, especially public health nurses, may also become involved in community nutrition. Whether we are working with individuals or groups, the nurse's role is heavily weighted toward dietary teaching. To determine learning needs, the nursing process is applied to individual or group nutritional patterns as follows.

ASSESSMENT FACTORS

Objective

Knowledge of:
   RDA
   Height/weight/energy intake recommendations
   Protein/fat/carbohydrate ratios
   Food Guide Pyramid
   Dietary contributions to preventing chronic diseases
Ability to pay for food
Access to government food programs

Subjective

Food preferences, choices, and likings
Interest in changing dietary patterns
Motivation to persevere with needed changes

Continued.

THE NURSING ROLE, cont'd.
Dietary Teaching: The Nursing Process

NURSING DIAGNOSIS

The data may reveal that nutritional status is adequate. Although the North American Nursing Diagnosis Association (NANDA) has not yet approved such a diagnosis, it could be stated as "Satisfactory nutrition lifestyle related to adequate knowledge and availability of appropriate foods as evidenced by positive health status" or the approved diagnosis, "Effective individual management of therapeutic regimen related to adequate knowledge of diet as evidenced by compliance with prescribed therapeutic diet." If a nutritional problem becomes evident, the nurse must determine the exact nature of it. For example, "Altered nutrition, less than body requirements, related to lack of knowledge about Food Guide Pyramid principles as evidenced by insufficient vegetable and fruit intake."

PLANNING

Goals may be set for individuals or groups. A measurable goal that might be appropriate for an individual with the diagnosis above is, "Mr. Green will increase daily intake of fruits and vegetables to 5 servings." A goal for a group of clients in a senior citizens center might be, "The group will demonstrate understanding of Food Guide Pyramid principles."

INTERVENTION

Interventions should be aimed at reinforcing positive behaviors or altering the causes of problems. In the case of Mr. Green, actions might include the following:
1. Show and explain the Food Guide Pyramid.
2. Describe health risks of inadequate fruit and vegetable intake.
3. Help client select appropriate foods from a list of choices.

EVALUATION

Each goal should be evaluated for how well the desired outcomes were met. Evaluation approaches that can be used for dietary teaching include the following:
Short verbal quizzes
Having the learner select appropriate food choices
Evaluating a follow-up food record for a week's intake

REFERENCES

1. US Department of Health and Human Services, Public Health Service: *Healthy people 2000: National health promotion and disease prevention objectives*, Washington, DC, 1990, US Government Printing Office.
2. Logue AW: *The psychology of eating and drinking: An introduction*, ed 2, New York, 1991, Freeman.
3. Drewrowski A: Genetics of task and smell. In Simpoulos AP, Child B, eds: *Genetic variation and nutrition: World review of nutrition and diet*, Basel, 1990, Karger.
4. Food and Nutrition Board, National Research Council: *Diet and health: Implications for reducing chronic disease risk*, Washington, DC, 1989, National Academy Press.
5. Senate Select Committee on Nutrition and Human Needs: *Dietary goals for the United States*, ed 2, Washington, DC, 1977, US Government Printing Office.
6. American Heart Association: *Dietary guidelines for healthy American adults: A statement for physicians and health professionals*, Dallas, 1991, The Association.

7. Nixon DW: *Nutrition and cancer: American Cancer Society guidelines, programs and initiatives,* Atlanta, 1990, American Cancer Society.

8. US Department of Agriculture and US Department of Health, Education and Welfare: *Nutrition and your health: Dietary guidelines for Americans,* ed 3, Home and Garden Bulletin 232, Washington, DC, 1990, USDA.

9. USDA Human Nutrition Information Service: *The food pyramid,* Home and Garden Bulletin 249, Washington, DC, 1992, US Government Printing Office.

10. National Cancer Institute/National Institutes of Health: *5 a day for better health: A baseline study of Americans' fruit and vegetable consumption,* Rockville, Md, 1992, The Institute.

11. American Diabetes Association and American Dietetic Association: *Exchange lists for meal planning,* rev, Alexandria, Va, 1995, American Dietetic Association.

12. Nutrition recommendations and principles for people with diabetes mellitus, *J Am Diet Assoc* 94:504-506, 1994.

13. Food Marketing Institute: *Trends '93: Consumer attitudes & the supermarket 1993,* Washington, DC, 1993, The Institute.

14. Senauer B, Asp E, Kinsey J: *Food trends and the changing consumer,* St. Paul, Minn, 1991, Eagan Press.

15. Salsbury B: *Cut your grocery bills in half! Supermarket survival,* Washington, DC, 1983, Acropolis.

16. Food and Drug Administration: *FDA backgrounder: The new food label,* Washington, DC, 1992, US Government Printing Office.

17. Kurtzweill P: Food label close-up, *FDA Consumer* 28(3):15-20, 1994.

18. Jones JM: *Food safety,* St. Paul, Minn, 1992, Eagan Press.

19. *Food Chem News,* May 9, 1994.

20. Besser RE et al: An outbreak of diarrhea and hemolytic uremic syndrome from *Escerichia coli* 0157:H7 in fresh-pressed apple cider, *JAMA* May 5, 1993.

21. Foulke JE: How to outsmart dangerous *E. coli* strain, *FDA Consumer* 28(1):7-11, 1994.

22. Loaharanu P: Cost/benefit aspects of food irradiation, *Food Technology* 48(1):1, 4-108, 1994.

23. Morrison RM: Food irradiation still faces hurdles, *Food Review* 15(3):11-15, 1994.

24. Mason J: Food irradiation: Let's move ahead, *Am Fam Phys* 47:1064, 1993.

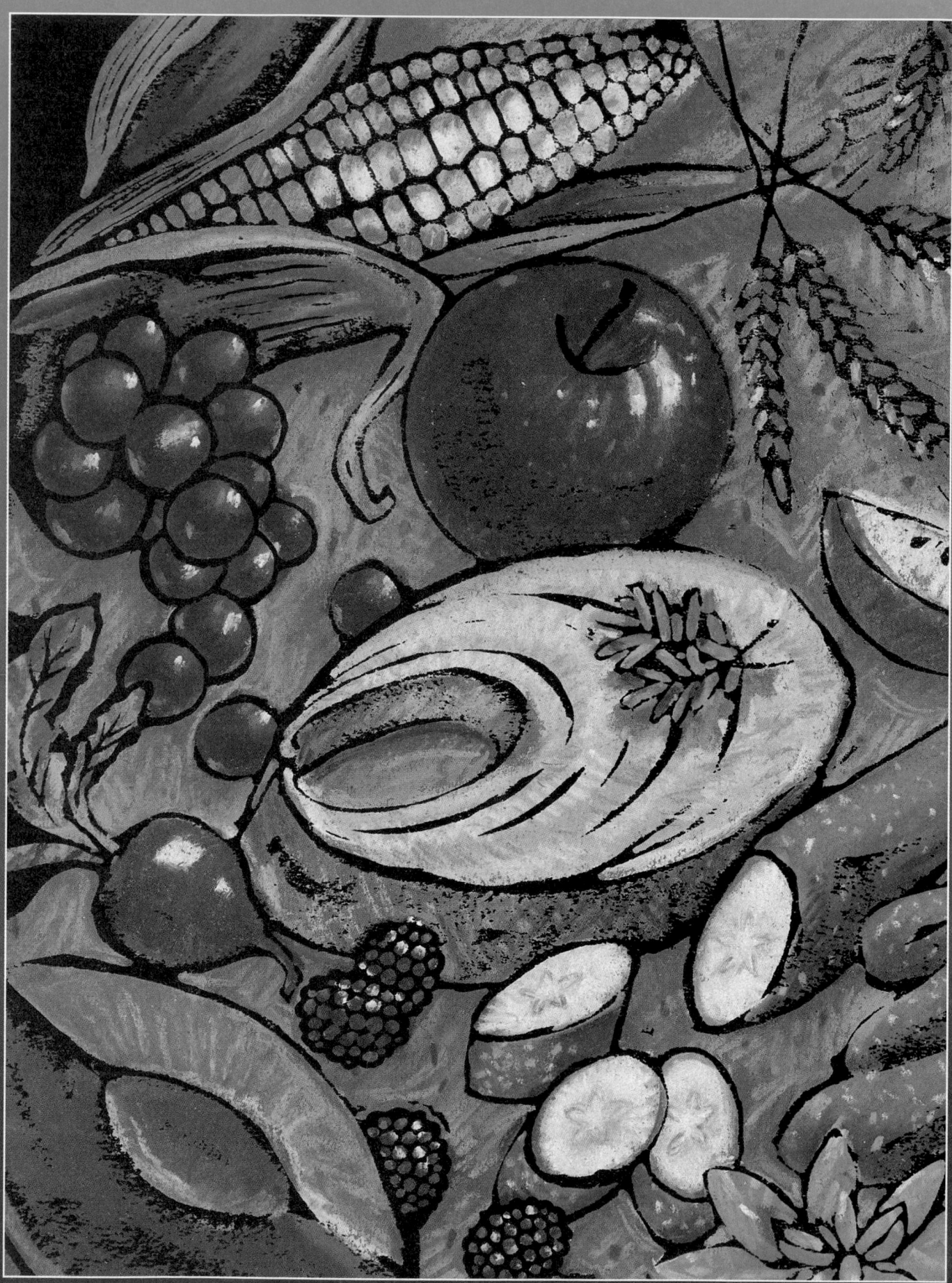

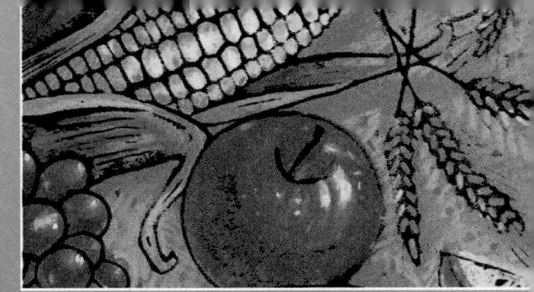

PART TWO

Nutrients, Food, and Health

Chapter 3

DIGESTION, ABSORPTION, AND METABOLISM

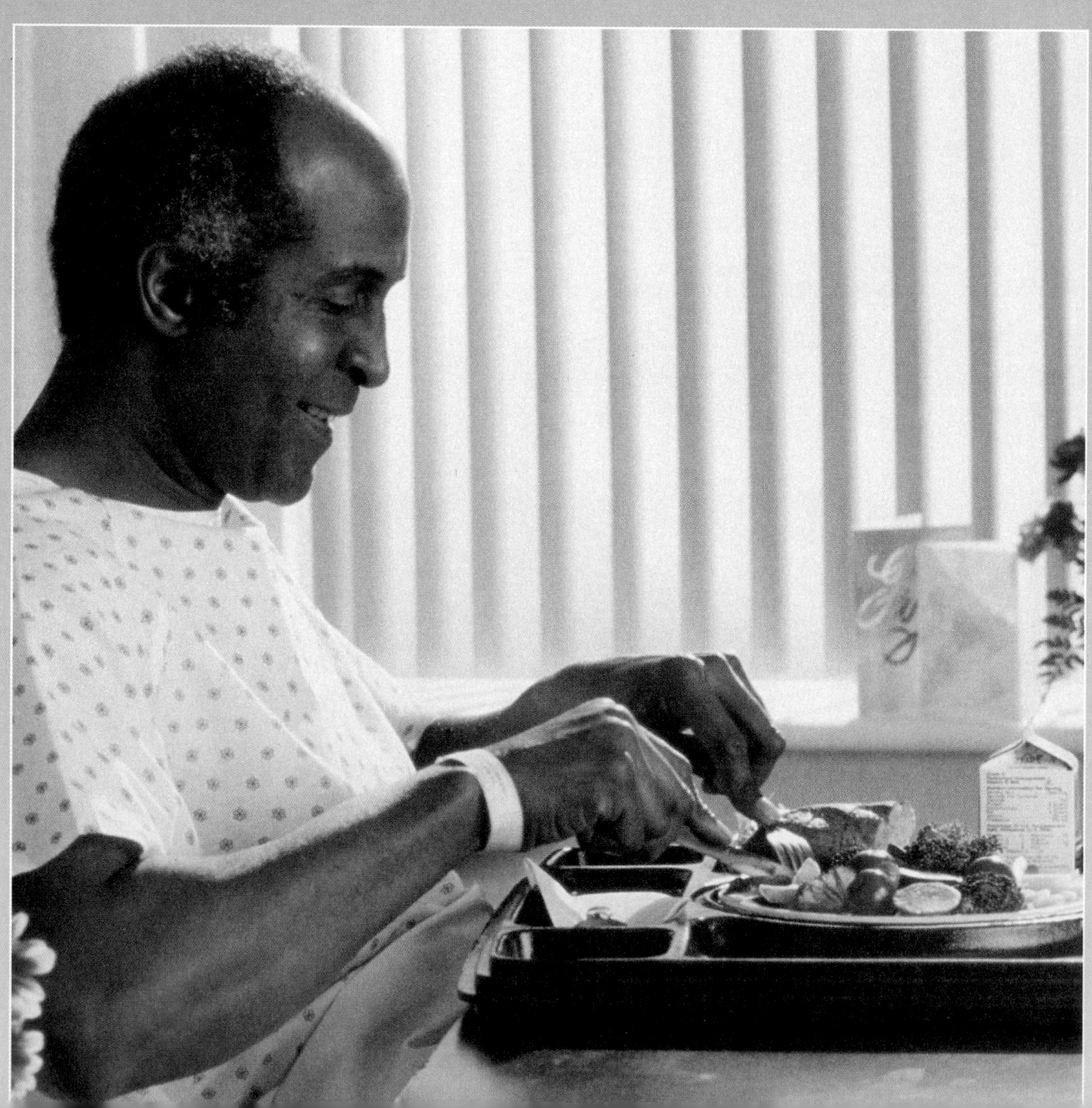

ROLE IN WELLNESS

Gulping down breakfast on the way to class or work, skipping lunch, and then eating dinner late may not seem to affect the health status of adults. However, if this kind of eating pattern becomes routine, not only does it begin to affect health status, it also characterizes an individual's lifestyle.

The health of the body is based on the nutrients available to support growth, maintenance, and energy needs. Inadequate nutritional intake can affect our body's ability to use the foods we consume. The digestive system, responsible for processing foods, depends on our nutrient intake for its maintenance. Although the body is quite resilient, we stress our physical limits when we adopt habits that do not support optimal health. A primary way to decrease our risk of future disease and achieve wellness is to use our lifestyle choices to support positive health behaviors.

This chapter presents a brief orientation to the processes of digestion, absorption, and metabolism. These processes work together to provide all body cells with energy and nutrients.

DIGESTION

The main organs of the digestion system (Fig. 3-1 and Table 3-1) form the **gastrointestinal (GI) tract** or alimentary canal, creating an open tube that runs from the mouth to the anus. Everything we eat is processed through the GI tract. The **digestive system** prepares ingested nutrients for digestion and absorption and protects against consumed microorganisms and toxic substances (1). To achieve these functions a series of processes occur. These processes of ingestion, digestion, absorption, and elimination depend on the motility or movement of the GI wall and the secretions of digestive juices and enzymes (2).

The movement of the food mass through the GI tract is controlled to enhance digestion and absorption. During passage through the GI tract, more than 95% of carbohydrate, fat, and protein ingested is absorbed. Some minerals, vitamins, and trace elements may be less absorbed (1).

Digestion occurs due to combined muscular and chemical actions. Two kinds of digestion, mechanical and chemical, take place as food substances move through the GI tract. **Mechanical digestion** is the crushing and twisting effect of teeth and muscles that divides and mixes foods with digestive juices in the GI lumen (open space of the tube) and exposes intestinal mucosa to enhance absorption of nutrients. This digestion includes the muscular actions of peristalsis and segmentation that propel the food mass through the digestive system. **Peristalsis** is the rhythmic contractions of muscles causing wavelike motions moving food down the tract. **Segmentation** is the forward and backward muscular action that assists in controlling the movement of the food mass.

Muscular actions depend on the four layers of tissues that form the tube of the GI tract (Fig. 3-2). The **mucosa** layer is composed of mucous membrane and forms the inside layer. Under the mucosa is the **submucosa,** which is a layer of connective tissue. Digestion depends on the blood vessels and nerves of the submucosa to regulate digestion. Surrounding the submucosa is a thick layer of muscle tissue called the **muscularis.** The outermost layer of the GI wall is made of serous membrane called **serosa,** which is actually the visceral layer of the peritoneum lining the abdominal pelvic cavity and covering organs (2).

The coordination of these muscle layers provides the varied movements required for digestion. Essentially, muscular action controls the movement of the food mass through the GI tract. Churning action within a segment of the GI tract

gastrointestinal (GI) tract
the main organs of the digestive system that form a tube that runs from the mouth to the anus

digestive system
a series of organs that function to prepare ingested nutrients for digestion and absorption

digestion
the process through which foods are broken down into smaller and smaller units to prepare nutrients for absorption

mechanical digestion
the crushing and twisting effects of teeth and peristalsis that divide foods into smaller pieces

peristalsis
the rhythmic contractions of muscles causing wavelike motions moving food down the GI tract

segmentation
the forward and backward muscular action that assists in controlling food mass movement through the GI tract

mucosa
the inside GI muscle tissue layer composed of mucous membrane

submucosa
a layer of connective muscle tissue under the mucosa

muscularis
a thick layer of muscle tissue surrounding the submucosa

serosa
the outermost layer of the GI wall, made of serous membrane

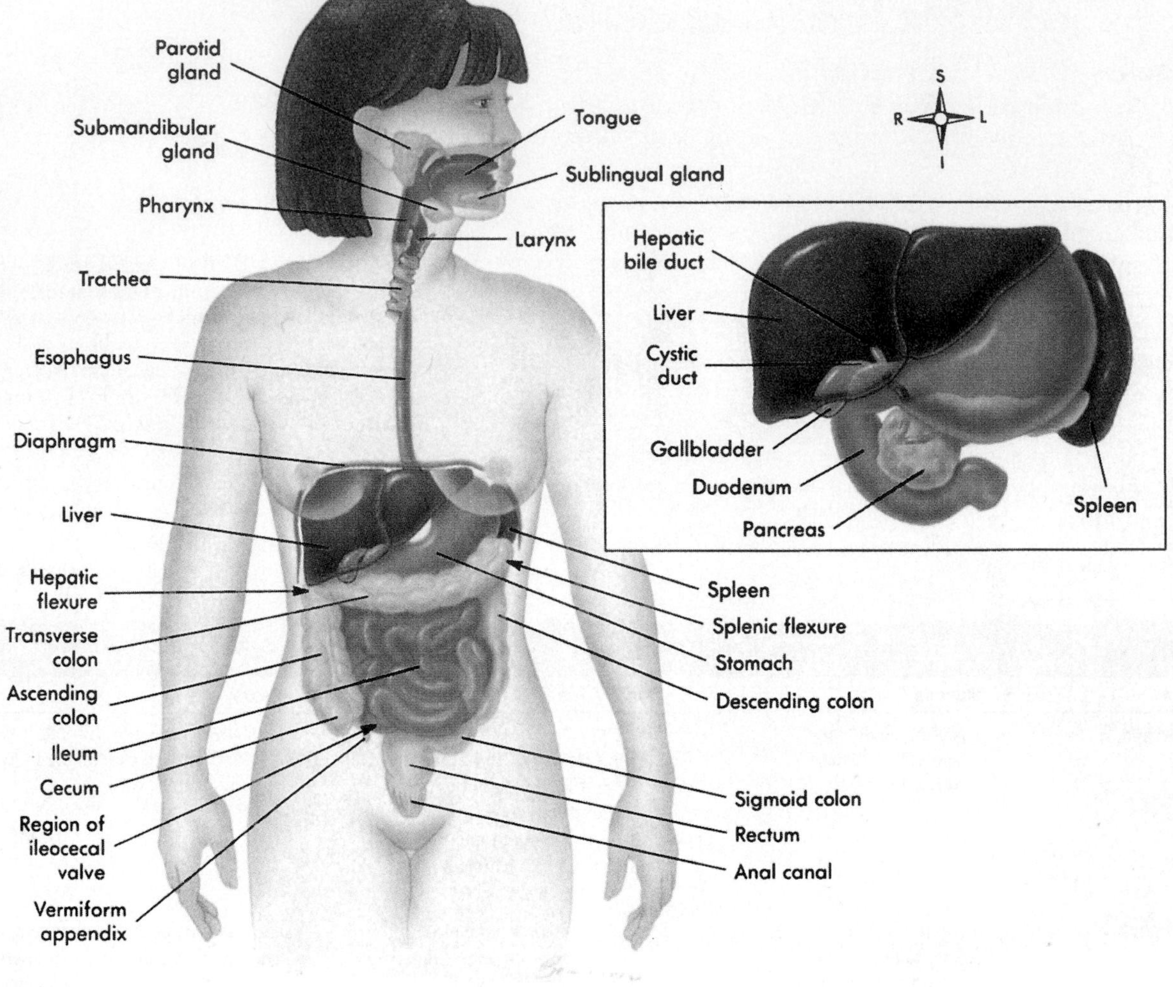

Parotid gland

Submandibular gland

Pharynx

Trachea

Esophagus

Diaphragm

Liver

Hepatic flexure

Transverse colon

Ascending colon

Ileum

Cecum

Region of ileocecal valve

Vermiform appendix

Tongue

Sublingual gland

Larynx

Spleen

Splenic flexure

Stomach

Descending colon

Sigmoid colon

Rectum

Anal canal

S
R ◆ L
I

Hepatic bile duct

Liver

Cystic duct

Gallbladder

Duodenum

Pancreas

Spleen

Fig. 3-1 Digestive system.

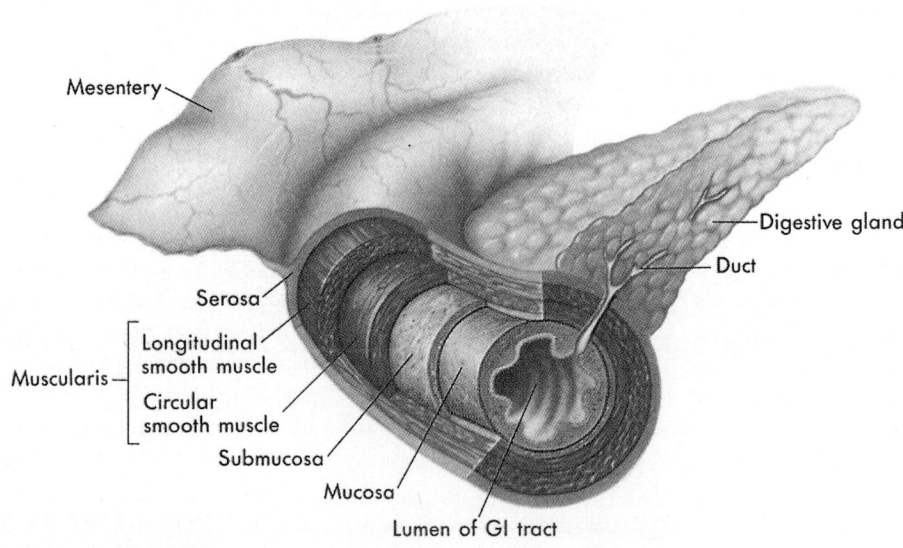

Mesentery

Serosa

Muscularis

Longitudinal smooth muscle

Circular smooth muscle

Submucosa

Mucosa

Lumen of GI tract

Digestive gland

Duct

Fig. 3-2 Muscle layers of the GI tract.

Table 3-1   Digestive System Organs

SEGMENTS OF THE DIGESTIVE TRACT

Mouth
Oropharynx
Esophagus
Stomach
Small intestine
 Duodenum
 Jejunum
 Ileum
Large intestine
 Cecum
 Colon
  Ascending colon
  Transverse colon
  Descending colon
  Sigmoid colon
Rectum
Anal canal

ACCESSORY ORGANS

Salivary glands
 Parotid
 Submandibular
 Sublingual
Tongue
Teeth
Liver
Gallbladder
Pancreas
Vermiform appendix

allows secretions to mix with food mass. Circular muscles surround the GI tube. Rhythmic contractions of these muscles cause wavelike motions of peristalsis, moving food downward. Longitudinal muscles run parallel along the GI tube. The combined effect of the circular and longitudinal muscles causes segmentation as a forward and backward movement. Sphincter muscles are stronger circular muscles that act as valves to control the movement of the food mass in a forward direction. In effect, sphincter muscles prevent reflux by forming an opening when relaxed and closing completely when contracted. The cardiac sphincter is between the esophagus and stomach; the pyloric sphincter is between the stomach and small intestine; the ileocecal sphincter is between the small intestine and large intestine; and the anal sphincter controls the release of feces.

Digestive secretions, gastric juices, and enzymes perform **chemical digestion** by altering chemical composition of food as it moves through the digestive tract. This process breaks food substances into smaller particles to expose nutrients for absorption. Some gastric juices provide the acidity of the stomach to assist certain enzymes to function effectively. As agents of chemical digestion, enzymes are specific in action, working only on individual classes of nutrients and changing substances from one form to a simpler form. Enzymes are "organic catalysts" formed from protein structures; they function at specific pHs and are continually created and destroyed. Specific enzymes are required for energy release and digestion and to add or remove carbon dioxide.

Regulating the release of gastric juices and enzymes, **hormones** act as messengers between organs to cause the release of needed secretions; in digestion, hormones affect the secretions from the stomach, intestines, and gallbladder. These secretions

chemical digestion
the chemical altering effects of digestive secretions, gastric juices, and enzymes on food substance composition

hormones
substances that act as messengers between organs to cause the release of needed secretions

Table 3-2	Digestive Processes
Mechanism	**Description**
Ingestion	Process of taking food into the mouth, starting it on its journey through the digestive tract
Digestion	A group of processes that break complex nutrients into simpler ones, thus facilitating their absorption; *mechanical digestion* physically breaks large chunks into small bits; *chemical digestion* breaks molecules apart
Motility	Movement by the muscular components of the digestive tube, including processes of mechanical digestion; examples include *peristalsis* and *segmentation*
Secretion	Release of digestive juices (containing enzymes, acids, bases, mucus, bile, or other products that facilitate digestion); some digestive organs also secrete endocrine hormones that regulate digestion or metabolism of nutrients
Absorption	Movement of digested nutrients through the GI mucosa and into the internal environment
Elimination	Excretion of the residues of the digestive process (feces) from the rectum, through the anus; defecation

From Thibodeau GA, Patton KT: *Anatomy and physiology*, ed 2, St. Louis, 1993, Mosby.

may slow or speed digestion, as well as affect the pH levels of gastric juice. Overall, the mechanical and chemical actions work together to complete the process of digestion. Table 3-2 summarizes the primary mechanisms of the digestive system. Details of carbohydrate, protein, and lipid digestion follow in specific chapters.

The Mouth

Are you hungry? Thinking about your favorite food? Is your mouth watering? Our mouths really do "water" when we think about or begin to eat foods. Only it is not actually water we sense, but a thin mucus-like fluid, saliva.

saliva
the secretions of the salivary glands of the mouth

Saliva is the term for the secretions of the salivary glands of the mouth. There are three salivary glands and each produces a different type of secretion. The parotid glands create watery saliva that supplies enzymes; the submandibular glands produce mucus and enzyme components; and the sublingual glands, the smallest, create a mucous type of saliva. A reflex mechanism controls these secretions. Food in the mouth stimulates chemical and mechanical digestion. Saliva not only moistens the foods we are chewing but also contains amylase, an enzyme that begins the process of breaking down starches.

Another digestive process occurring in the mouth depends on teeth. Teeth rhythmically tear and pulverize food. The enamel covering teeth is the hardest substance in the body and so protects teeth from the harsh effects of chewing. The tongue assists by guiding food into chewing positions and then leads the pulverized food into the esophagus. Another function of the tongue is that it contains taste buds. Over 2000 taste buds are responsible for our sensations of sweet, bitter, sour, and salty when tasting foods.

As toddlers, we have the highest number of taste buds and a higher degree of taste sensitivity, so bland foods are more appealing. The number of taste buds declines as we grow older, explaining why the elderly have diminished taste sensitivity. Elderly clients may need to be encouraged to avoid using too much salt, particularly if they have hypertension or cardiac disorders (2).

Combined with our taste bud sensations is our sense of smell. The two combined actually account for the perception (and enjoyment) of the flavors of different kinds of foods. Our positive or negative response to specific foods affects our food choices (3).

bolus
a masticated lump or ball of food ready to be swallowed

Portions of the pulverized or masticated food get formed into the shape of a ball called a **bolus**. Our tongues effortlessly form the bolus, which is swallowed and then passes by the epiglottis and into the esophagus within about 5 to 7 seconds. The epiglottis is a flap of tissue that closes over the trachea to prevent the bolus from entering the lungs.

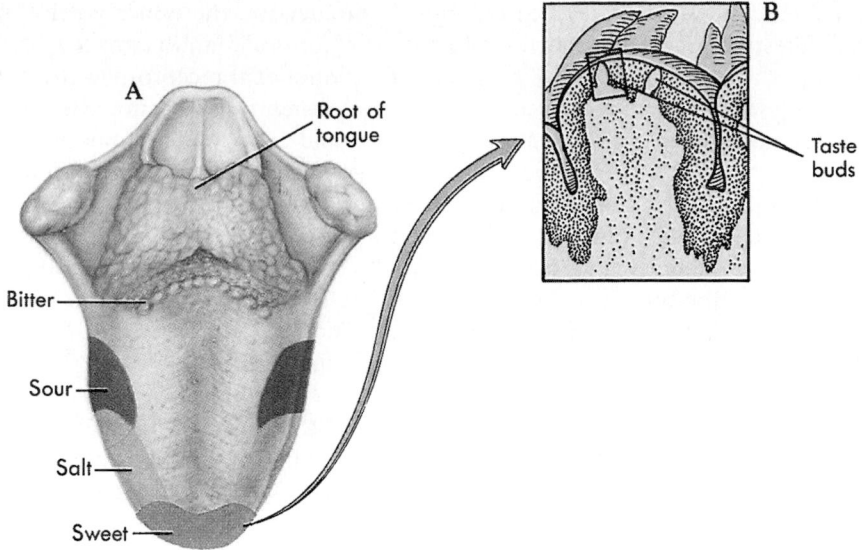

Fig. 3-3 **A,** Areas of sensations of sweet, bitter, sour, and salty. **B,** A detailed site of a taste bud.

The Esophagus

The esophagus is a muscular tube through which the bolus travels from the mouth to the stomach. The process begins at the top of the esophagus as peristalsis, the involuntary movements of circular and longitudinal muscles, begins and draws the bolus further into the GI tract. This mechanical action further breaks down the size of foodstuff and increases exposure to digestive secretions. At the bottom of the esophagus, the cardiac sphincter controls the movement of the bolus from the esophagus into the stomach. It also prevents the acidic contents of the stomach from moving upward back through the esophagus.

The Stomach

The bolus enters the fundus, the upper portion of the stomach that connects with the esophagus. The other divisions of the stomach include the body, or center portion, and the pylorus, the lower portion. The stomach wall contains gastric mucosa containing gastric pits. At the base of the pits are the gastric glands whose chief cells create gastric juice, a mucous fluid containing digestive enzymes, and parietal cells that secrete stomach acid, called hydrochloric acid.

Gastric secretions occur in three phases: cephalic, gastric, and intestinal (2). The cephalic phase is referred to as the "psychic phase," since mental factors can stimulate **gastrin,** a hormone. In the gastric phase, gastrin increases the release of gastric juices when the stomach is distended by food. The third phase is the intestinal phase in which the gastric secretions change as chyme passes through to the duodenum. Gastric secretions are inhibited by exocrine and nervous reflexes of gastric inhibitory peptides, secretin, and cholescystokinin-pancreozymin (CCK), a hormone secreted by intestinal mucosa.

Gastric motility or movement of food mass through the stomach requires 2 to 6 hours. The churning and mixing of the food mass with gastric juices creates a semiliquid mixture called **chyme.** When chyme enters the pylorus section of the stomach, it causes distention and the release of the hormone gastrin. Gastrin sends a message that hydrochloric acid is needed to continue the breakdown of chyme. As hydrochloric acid is released from the stomach lining, thick mucus is also secreted to protect the stomach walls from the harsh hydrochloric acid.

From the plate to the cell: food transit times

Chewing and swallowing	Depends on texture and quantity
Esophagus	5-7 seconds
Stomach	2-6 hours
Small intestine	About 5 hours
Large intestine	9-16 hours
TOTAL	16-27 hours ingestion to elimination

gastrin
a hormone that increases the release of gastric juices; secreted by stomach mucosa

chyme
a semiliquid mixture of food mass

Every 20 seconds, chyme is released into the duodenum, the upper portion of the small intestine; this action is controlled by the hormonal and nervous system mechanism of enterogastric reflex. This consists of duodenal receptors in the mucosa that are sensitive to the presence of acid and distention. The impulses over sensory and motor fiber in the vagus nerve cause a reflex restriction of gastric peristalsis. The gastric inhibitory peptide released in response to fats in the duodenum decreases peristalsis of stomach muscles and slows chyme passage.

The combined action of mechanical digestion (the strong muscular movements of peristalsis) and chemical digestion (the effects of the gastric juices) works to prepare nutrients for the process. Chyme is kept in the stomach by the actions of the pyloric sphincter, which slowly releases it into the duodenum.

Functions of the stomach include holding food for partial digestion; producing gastric juice; providing muscular action, which, combined with gastric juice, mixes and tears food into smaller pieces; secreting the intrinsic factor for vitamin B_{12} absorption; releasing gastrin; and by the acidity of its secretions assisting in destruction of pathogenic bacteria that may have inadvertently been consumed (2).

The Small Intestine

The chyme entering the duodenum soon moves through to the jejunum and ileum of the small intestine. Intestinal motility, due to peristalsis and segmentation, takes about 5 hours for chyme to pass through the small intestine. Segmentation in the duodenum and upper jejunum mixes chyme with digestive juices from the pancreas, liver, and intestinal mucosa. Peristalsis is controlled by intrinsic stretch reflexes and initiated by CCK, the hormone secreted by intestinal mucosa.

In the small intestine, the nutrients in chyme are completely prepared for absorption. The small intestine is the major organ of digestion; the final stages of digestion occur in the small intestine. Since it is also the site of almost all of the absorption of nutrients, the intestinal lining must be able to accommodate the actions of both digestion and absorption. The intestinal walls are covered with a thin layer of mucus to protect them from digestive juices. But the walls are also adapted to enhance the absorption process. Fingerlike projections, **villi,** greatly increase the mucosal layer available for absorption of nutrients (Fig. 3-4). On the villi are hairlike projections called *microvilli.* These also enhance absorption by their structure and movements.

As chyme enters the small intestine, hormones begin sending messages that regulate the release of digestive juices to continue the process of digesting chyme. Some hormones are provided by the small intestine; several are released by other organs into the small intestine. These secretions include enzymes from the small intestines, bile produced in the liver, and digestive juices from the pancreas.

One of the first hormones released by the small intestine is **secretin.** This hormone causes the pancreas to send bicarbonate to the small intestine to reduce the acidic content of the chyme. As the acidic level decreases, other pancreatic juices enter and begin their work. Another hormone secreted by the small intestine is **cholecystokinin-pancreozymin (CCK);** it functions to initiate pancreatic exocrine secretions, act against gastrin by inhibiting gastric HCl secretion, and activate the gallbladder to contract, causing bile to be released into duodenum.

Bile, secreted by the liver and stored in the gallbladder, is released to emulsify fats, aiding in the digestion of lipids. The liver is always secreting bile. CCK and secretin spur the gallbladder to release bile for digestion of fats. In addition, the small intestine produces enzymes to assist in the digestive process. Although much of the chyme is absorbed, the rest, usually consisting of fiber, minerals, and water, passes through the next sphincter, the ileocecal valve, into the large intestine (ascending colon).

villi
fingerlike projections on the walls of the small intestine

secretin
a hormone secreted by the small intestine that causes the pancreas to release bicarbonate to the small intestine

cholecystokinin-pancreozymin (CCK)
a hormone that initiates pancreatic exocrine secretions, acts against gastrin, and activates the gallbladder to release bile; secreted by the small intestine

bile
a substance that emulsifies fats to aid the digestion of lipids; produced by the liver and stored in the gallbladder

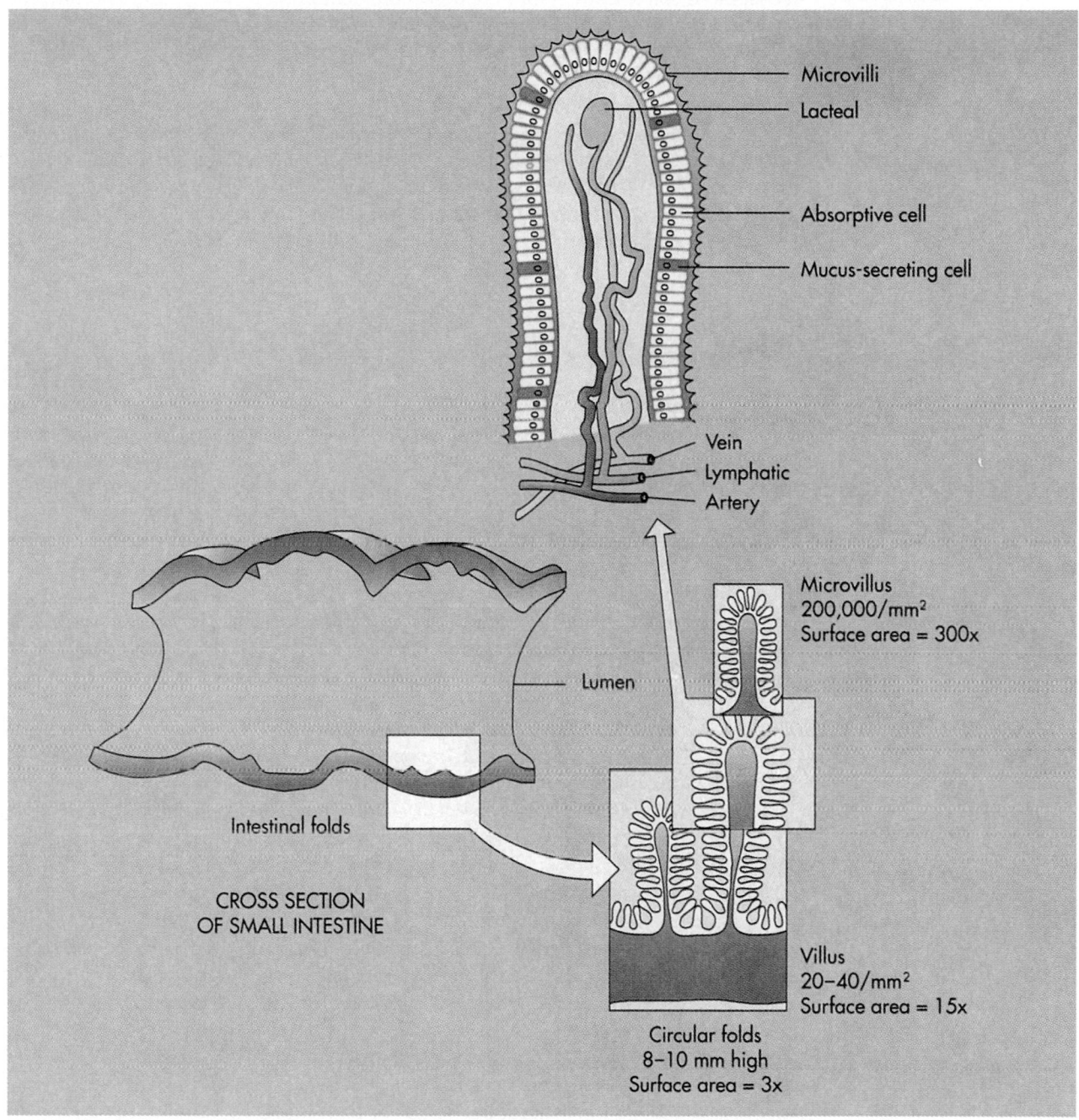

Fig. 3-4 Structure of the intestinal wall. The circular folds, villi, and microvilli multiply the surface area and enhance absorption.

The Large Intestine

The large intestine consists of the cecum, colon, and rectum. The cecum is a blind pocket, so the mass bypasses it entering the ascending colon, leading into the transverse colon that runs across the abdomen over the small intestine to the descending colon. The descending colon extends down the left of the abdomen into the sigmoid colon leading into the descending colon on to the rectum and into the anal canal; finally, any remaining mass passes out through the anus. The journey through the large intestine takes about 9 to 16 hours.

In the large intestine or colon, final absorption of any available nutrients, usually water and some minerals, occurs. Bacteria residing in the large intestine produce several vitamins, which are then absorbed. Water is withdrawn from the fibrous mass, forming solidified feces. Mucous glands in the intestinal wall create a mucus that lubricates and covers feces as it forms. Again, peristalsis continues to move substances through the GI tract, resulting in the excretion of feces from the colon through the anus, the last sphincter muscle of the GI tract.

ABSORPTION

absorption

the process by which substances pass through the intestinal mucosa into the blood or lymph

Even though the food mass has possibly spent several hours in the tube of the GI tract, it is not yet actually inside the body until its nutrient components are absorbed. **Absorption** is the process by which substances pass through the intestinal mucosa into the blood or lymph. Transport processes provide the means for nutrients to actually pass through the wall of the small intestine. These include passive diffusion and osmosis, facilitated diffusion, energy-dependent active transport, and engulfing pinocytosis (Fig. 3-5).

Passive diffusion and osmosis occur when pressure is equal on both sides of the intestinal wall, allowing molecules to travel through capillaries. Facilitated diffusion takes place when, despite positive pressure flow, molecules may be unable to pass through membrane pores unless aided. Specific integral membrane protein supports the movement by bringing the larger nutrient molecules through the capillary membrane. Energy-dependent active transport happens when fluid pressures work against the passage of nutrients. As an active process, energy is required. This energy is supplied by the cell and a "pumping" mechanism, which are assisted by a special membrane protein carrier. Engulfing pinocytosis takes place when a substance, either fluid or nutrient, contacts the villi membrane, which then surrounds the substance creating a vacuole encompassing the substance. Passing through the cell cytoplasm, it is then released into the circulatory system (4).

The amounts of vitamins and minerals absorbed depend on our body's storage levels and immediate need for these nutrients. Nutrients such as fats, carbohydrates, and protein are easily absorbed regardless of the level of need. The structure of the small intestine, the site of almost all nutrient absorption, allows for efficient absorption to occur. The microvilli are extremely sensitive to the exact nutrient needs of our bodies. Their wavelike motions, caused by peristalsis, result in the most exposure of the nutrient-laden chyme to the absorbing cells. This exposure allows needed nutrients to leave the GI tract and pass through the microvilli cells. At this point, the nutrients are truly "inside" our bodies.

Various factors may affect absorption of nutrients. Combinations of naturally occurring substances such as fiber or binders may move nutrients through the GI tract too quickly for optimum absorption to occur. Individual nutrient absorption and other issues of bioavailability are addressed in other chapters. The relationship between food and drug absorption is also an important issue of medical treatment. Ingesting medications with food may decrease the absorption rate of the medica-

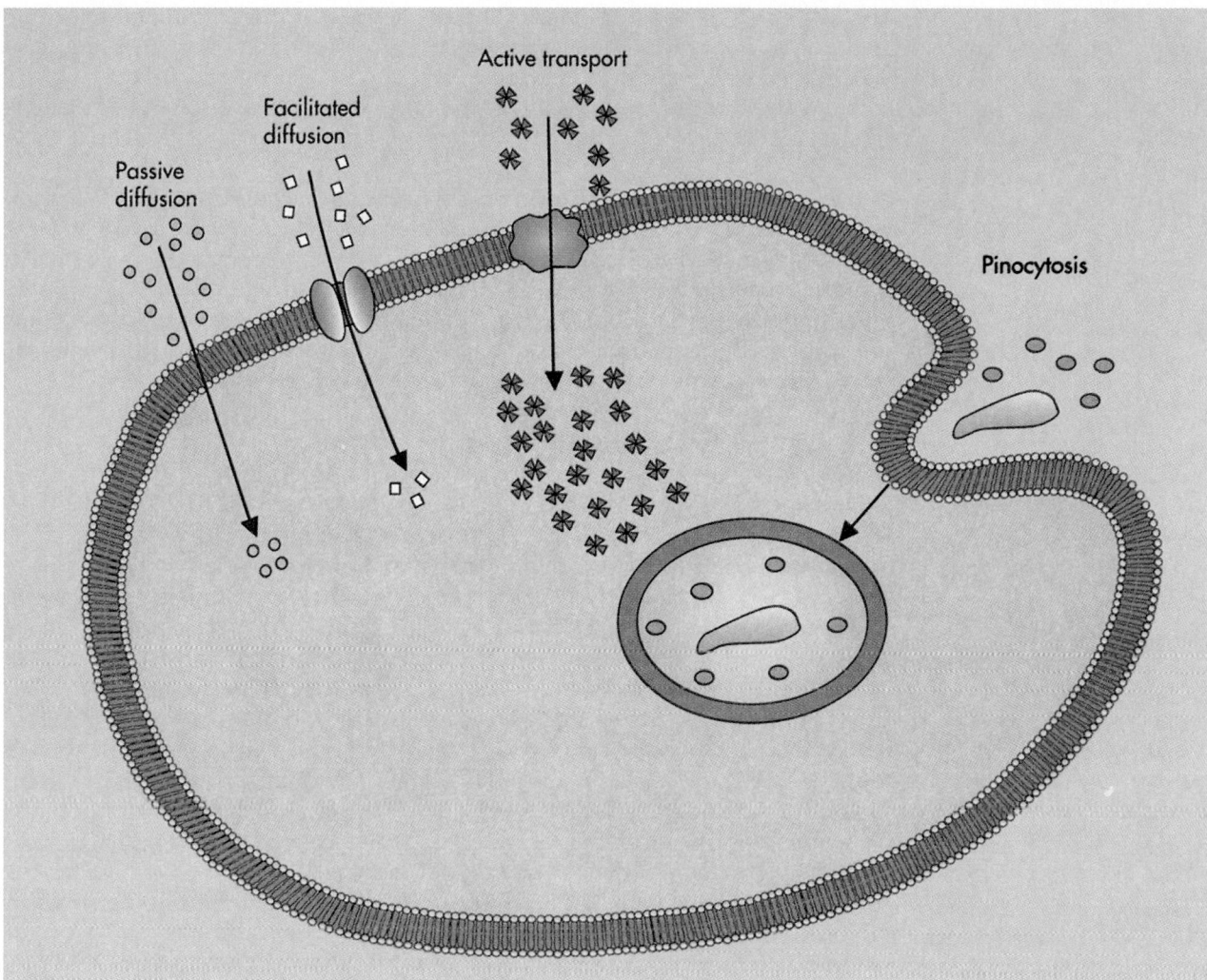

Fig. 3-5 Methods of absorption. *Passive diffusion*, the movement of molecules from a region of high concentration to low concentration; *facilitated diffusion*, the movement of molecules by a carrier protein across the cell membrane from a region of high to low concentration; *active transport*, the movement of molecules and ions by means of a carrier protein against fluid pressures that require the expenditure of cellular energy; *pinocytosis*, the engulfment of molecules by the cellular membrane folding inward and pinching off to form an intracellular vesicle.

tion and may also interfere with the absorption of other nutrients contained in the food consumed. This issue is explored in depth in Chapter 14.

Once "inside" our bodies, the nutrients enter the circulatory systems of the bloodstream or lymphatic system. The general circulatory or blood system receives absorbed protein, carbohydrates, and most vitamins and minerals and transports these nutrients throughout the body. The lymphatic system, a secondary circulatory system, receives lipids and fat-soluble vitamins. The nutrients travelling in the lymphatic system are deposited into the bloodstream near the heart. All nutrients then circulate throughout the body in the blood, providing for the nutrient requirements of cells.

Soon after entering the bloodstream, nutrients pass by the liver. This allows the liver to have "first choice" of the available nutrients. The liver is a powerhouse organ that provides a wide variety of services and substances; thus its nutrient needs are a priority. From there, the bloodstream's journey of nutrients continues to the heart to also give it a prime nutrient selection. The journey then continues through the circulatory system to all cells. Some nutrients end up in nutrient storage sites of the body. These sites include the bones, liver, and kidney. Other nutrients, if not discarded or used by cells, are filtered out of the blood by the kidneys to be reabsorbed or excreted in urine.

Elimination

The expulsion of feces or body waste products is called defecation. When the rectum is distended due to waste accumulation, the reflex to defecate occurs. The residue may include substances unable to be digested by human enzymes such as cellulose and other dietary fibers and connective tissue from meat collagen. Undigested fats may combine with dietary minerals such as calcium and magnesium and form residue. Additional residue may include water, bacteria, pigments, and mucus. Fig. 3-6 summarizes the functions of the digestive system.

Digestive Process Across the Lifespan

Over the course of the lifespan, the main and accessory organs of digestion develop and change. The immature GI tract, particularly the intestinal mucosa of young infants, may allow intact proteins to be absorbed without complete digestion occurring. This incomplete digestion may result in an allergic response by the immune system and is part of the reason for delaying the introduction of solid foods such as cereals until the GI tract has matured sufficiently. Another age-related condition is lactose intolerance in which the body ceases to produce lactase, the enzyme that breaks down the milk carbohydrate of lactose. For some people, this occurs once the primary growth need for nutrients contained in milk is met. For others, this may not occur until adulthood or not at all. Conditions of the middle years include gallbladder disease and peptic ulcers (sores that may occur on the epithelial surfaces of the stomach or small intestine). Older years may be marked by problems of constipation and diverticulosis, which may be related to decreased peristalsis combined with decreased physical activity and worsened by chronic low dietary fiber consumption (2).

METABOLISM

metabolism

a set of processes through which absorbed nutrients are used by the body for energy and to form and maintain body structures and functions

I t is hard to imagine that a lunch of tuna on rye bread will actually end up being part of the cells of the body. Fortunately, the human body is able to transform the nutrients of the sandwich into substances usable by cells. **Metabolism** is a set of processes through which absorbed nutrients are used by the body for energy and to form and maintain body structures and functions. The two main processes of metabolism involve catabolism and anabolism. Catabolism is the breakdown of food components into smaller molecular particles, causing the release of energy as heat and chemical energy (2). Anabolism is the process of synthesis from which substances are formed, such as new bone or muscle tissue. Both processes happen within cells at the same time.

When nutrients finally reach individual cells, they may be chemically changed through anabolism to help form new cell structures or to create new substances such as hormones and enzymes. Some vitamins and minerals assist in the use of other nutrients within the cell. They act as catalysts or coenzymes to initiate and support the transformation and use of carbohydrates, proteins, and lipids. Other nutrients may be used as energy to continue life-supporting processes. These processes include the energy needed to support DNA reproduction and create proteins and other molecules, nerve impulses, and muscle contractions. Some energy is stored in a ready-to-use state. Specific metabolic functions of individual nutrients are discussed in later chapters.

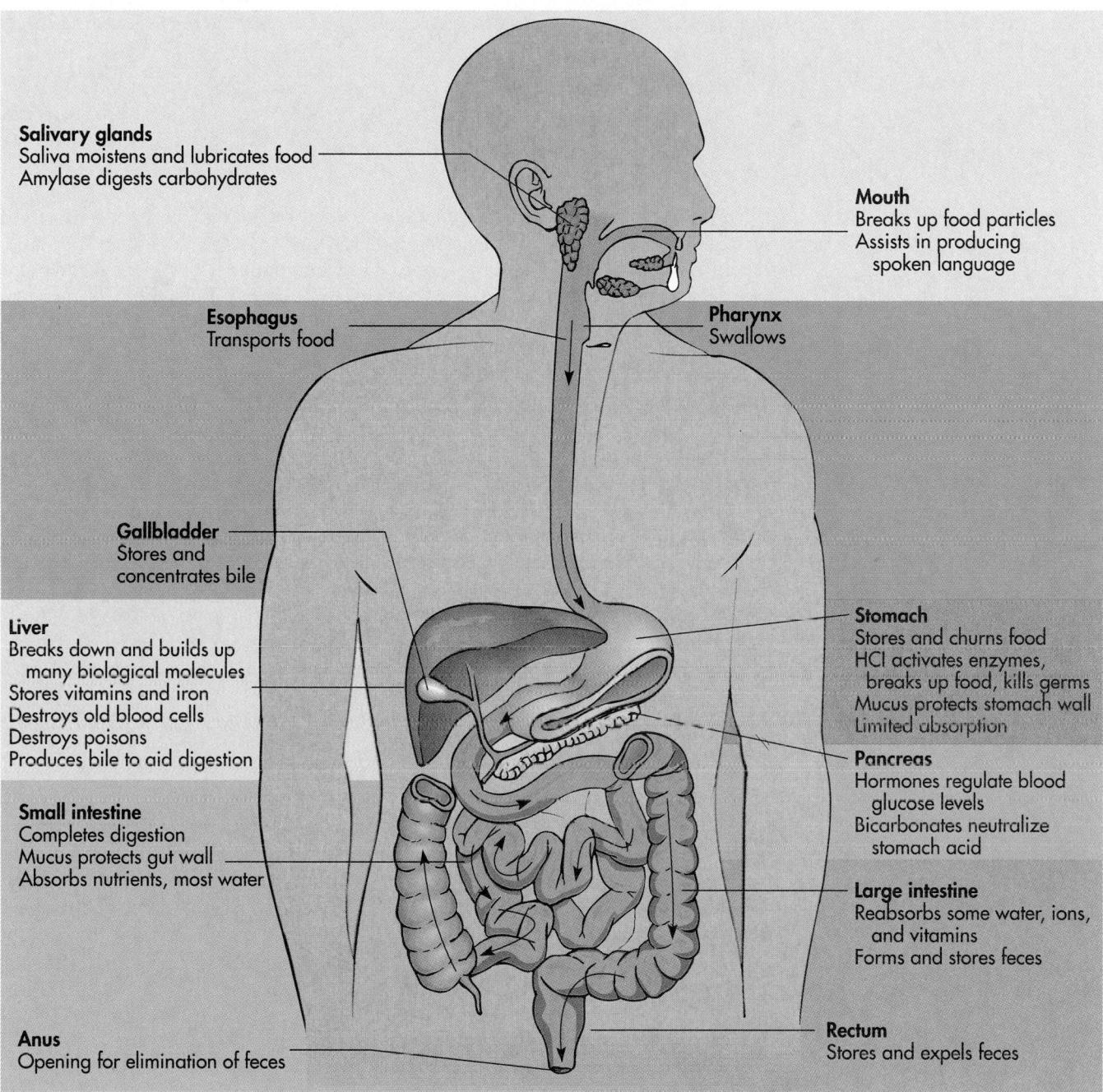

Salivary glands
Saliva moistens and lubricates food
Amylase digests carbohydrates

Mouth
Breaks up food particles
Assists in producing
    spoken language

Esophagus
Transports food

Pharynx
Swallows

Gallbladder
Stores and
concentrates bile

Stomach
Stores and churns food
HCl activates enzymes,
    breaks up food, kills germs
Mucus protects stomach wall
Limited absorption

Liver
Breaks down and builds up
    many biological molecules
Stores vitamins and iron
Destroys old blood cells
Destroys poisons
Produces bile to aid digestion

Pancreas
Hormones regulate blood
    glucose levels
Bicarbonates neutralize
    stomach acid

Small intestine
Completes digestion
Mucus protects gut wall
Absorbs nutrients, most water

Large intestine
Reabsorbs some water, ions,
    and vitamins
Forms and stores feces

Anus
Opening for elimination of feces

Rectum
Stores and expels feces

Fig. 3-6 Summary of digestive organ functions.

Waste products from metabolism are discarded by the cells and wind up circulating in the blood. They are then excreted through the lungs, the kidneys, or large intestine. The lungs release excess water and carbon dioxide. The kidneys filter and excrete metabolic waste and excess vitamins and minerals but reabsorb nutrients that the body needs to retain. Waste products may also be discarded through the large intestine in feces.

Fortunately, we do not have to consciously control these processes. Our responsibility is to provide an adequate selection of nutrients through the foods we choose to eat and to eat those foods in a way that enhances the functioning of the GI tract.

Metabolism Across the Lifespan

Metabolic changes are most noticed later in life as the amount of food energy required decreases in relation to lowered metabolic rates. Nutrient needs, however, remain constant. Our challenge as we (and our clients) enter the middle years and beyond is to meet nutrient needs while maintaining or reducing our kcaloric needs to equal actual metabolic use. Recognition of this change can forestall the unexpected weight gain that appears to accompany aging in the United States.

OVERCOMING BARRIERS

Some of our lifestyle behaviors affect the functioning and health of our GI tracts and so influence our nutritional status. Some common GI tract health problems are due to the everyday decisions we make but which we can change. Prevention suggestions and treatment strategies for some common GI tract health problems follow.

Heartburn

heartburn
a burning sensation felt in the esophagus caused by stomach reflux

Heartburn, fortunately, has nothing to do with the health of our hearts. Instead, it is a burning sensation felt in the esophagus when food, which has already been passed to the stomach, refluxes or passes back up through the cardiac sphincter into the esophagus. The esophagus is not lined with mucus as is the stomach, so the acidic mixture of food burns the walls of the esophagus and it hurts!

Prevention and treatment strategies aim at reducing the amount of pressure in the stomach so that the cardiac sphincter is not opened by excess pressure from stomach contents. A primary approach is not to overeat so that the stomach can easily accommodate its contents. Other strategies include avoiding the following (5,6):

- Constipation: straining to defecate affects the contents of the stomach by creating additional pressure.
- Lying down shortly after eating: resting or sleeping with a full stomach may push contents against the cardiac sphincter. Wait several hours after a meal before lying flat or keep head and shoulders elevated when reclining.
- High-fat meals: slow emptying of the stomach from eating high-fat food increases the chance of reflux.
- Tight clothing: wearing restrictive clothing around the waist and midriff affects the functioning of the stomach and may increase stomach pressure.
- "Eating on the run": eating meals while under stress or trying to do other activities at the same time may cause food not to be chewed enough. Big clumps of foods in the stomach force the stomach muscles to react strongly, which may cause reflux (see box).
- Certain foods and drinks: consuming either chocolate, alcohol, peppermints, spearmints, liqueurs, or possibly caffeine, tomatoes, and citrus fruits and juices.
- Some medications: taking certain medications regularly may initiate heartburn. If experiencing heartburn often and taking birth control pills, antihistamines, tranquilizers (such as Valium), or any drug regularly, check with the primary care provider. Heartburn could be caused by these medications.

If these strategies are not helping and heartburn is common, consult a primary care provider.

Cool heartburn heat by avoiding
alcohol
caffeine
chocolate
citrus fruit
citrus juice
high-fat food
liquor
peppermint
spearmint
tomato

Vomiting

Although vomiting is not usually related to lifestyle behaviors, it is a common digestive disorder worthy of review. **Vomiting** is reverse peristalsis. Instead of food moving down the GI tract, the peristalsis muscles move the contents of the stomach back through the esophagus and forcefully out the mouth. It is an involuntary muscular action that we cannot easily control. Often it is painful; the contents of the stomach already consist of a mixture of food and acidic gastric juices that burns the unprotected esophagus.

Vomiting is a way of the body protecting itself. Perhaps an intruding virus or toxin has entered the GI tract; vomiting removes the offending substance. Mixed messages regarding the body's sense of equilibrium during air or sea travel can result in motion sickness, of which vomiting may be a symptom.

Dehydration is a concern when vomiting is continuous. Vomiting causes a loss of fluid and electrolytes such as magnesium, potassium, and sodium, which stresses the functioning of the body. Infants are at particular risk for dehydration since more of their bodies consist of fluids (5). A primary care provider should be consulted to determine the cause of vomiting and to recommend treatment.

Also at medical risk are individuals who use vomiting as a way to control their weight and are suffering from eating disorders such as anorexia nervosa and bulimia. Repetitive self-induced vomiting can injure the esophagus and wear away the enamel of teeth (7). Anyone practicing this kind of self-destructive behavior should consult a primary care provider or mental health professional as soon as possible (see Chapter 13).

vomiting
reverse peristalsis

Intestinal Gas

Annoying, embarrassing, and offensive are all terms that come to mind when intestinal gas or **flatus** is the subject. Actually, everyone's body produces and releases gas from the lower intestinal tract. Most gas leaves the GI tract without our awareness because it is odorless. Sometimes if the gas passes through too quickly, it is quite noticeable!

flatus
intestinal gas

SOCIAL ISSUES
Hunger Versus Appetite Versus Time?

Our daily schedules often determine our responses to hunger. Ever notice how differently you eat during the week compared with the weekend? The weekday mosaic of classes, studying, work, and possibly sports training makes fitting in time to get to the campus cafeteria a Herculean feat. Or, if you prepare your own meals, time must be set aside for buying and cooking foods. Weekends may be more leisurely without classes or work, or perhaps we find time for socializing.

Somehow we manage. Although fewer meals may be eaten during the week, we are not any less hungry nor are energy needs lower. Sometimes, chaotic schedules may be accommodated by telling ourselves we are not really hungry or we just do not have time to eat.

How can we do that? Isn't hunger a physiological need for energy and nutrients? Can we just think ourselves through the hunger sensation? To understand this process, we need to explore the feeding regulating mechanism of the body.

Our sense of hunger and satiety is governed by the hypothalamus, a small portion of the brain. Its purpose is to maintain homeostasis (a state of balance) through regulation of food intake through a feeding (hunger) center and a satiety center. The response of the hypothalamus, which initiates the hunger sensation, is thought to be related to either low blood glucose levels or to the lack of chyme in the stomach.

When we eat, blood glucose levels rise and chyme is once again in the stomach. The hypothalamus responds by providing a feeling of satiety or satisfaction and we stop eating.

When we "feel" hungry, we are recognizing the internal stimuli of hunger. Perhaps our stomach seems to be rumbling or "empty," or we are "starving." These sensations are tied to physical events in our bodies. When we act on this, we eat. However, we can also choose to ignore these signals. This means we cognitively override the sensation and do not respond. There are physical mechanisms to cope with the lack of new energy sources, but it is still stressful to our bodies.

External stimuli also affect our desire or appetite for eating. Referred to as environmental cues, these include the smell and sight of food, which may artificially increase our hunger. Simply seeing a food commercial on television or talking about food can excite the feeding center even if the stomach is not actually "empty." We also associate eating with specific social settings and time of day, regardless of our physical need for food. How can a birthday be celebrated without a cake? Religious holidays are often associated with special foods or meals. And throughout our elementary school experience, we ate lunch when we were scheduled, not necessarily when we were hungry.

All those years of eating by schedules and events have led us to adapt by overriding our cognitive cues about our real sense of hunger. Now, when personal schedules are more individualized, we may find that the external stimuli supporting our appropriate intake of food are gone; we must develop our own cues to ensure optimal nutritional intakes.

From Logue AW: *The psychology of eating and drinking: An introduction,* ed 2, New York, 1991, Freeman; and Mahan LK, Arlin M: *Krause's food, nutrition & diet therapy,* ed 8, Philadelphia, 1992, Saunders.

Bacteria in the large intestine may cause gas formation when specific undigestible carbohydrates ferment. These may include some of the carbohydrates found in dried beans or legumes like soybeans and black beans. Another cause may be *lactose intolerance,* the inability to break down lactose, the carbohydrate in milk. The lactose then begins to ferment, causing gas build-up, bloating, and diarrhea (see Chapter 4). The longer any undigested substances linger in the large intestine, the more likely fermentation will occur, leading to gas formation. This may result from constipation that slows the passage of chyme through the GI tract. Another factor may be eating so quickly that food is swallowed in large clumps, requiring more time to sufficiently process the chyme before it is excreted (5,6).

Generally, however, we can probably decrease intestinal gas through some simple changes of food-related behaviors. Here are some suggestions:

- If making dietary changes to increase fiber intake, gradually add more fibrous foods like dried beans to allow your system to adjust.
- Notice the effects of drinking milk. If a problem occurs, consider eating other milk-related products such as yogurt, cheese, or lactose-reduced milk.
- Increase fluid intake and consume sufficient amounts of fiber to prevent constipation.
- Take the time to consider which foods may be problematic. Each person's cause of flatulence may be different.
- Finally, eat slower and chew foods more thoroughly.

Constipation

There is no clear definition of constipation. It is usually considered as difficulty and discomfort associated with defecation. Individuals may interpret these terms differently and may vary in their natural urge to defecate. Not everyone needs to pass a bowel movement daily. Normal functioning ranges from once a day to every 3 days. Generally, **constipation** is recognized as straining to pass hard, dry stools (5,6,8).

The causes of constipation are usually related to lifestyle behaviors that can easily be changed. The following strategies address these behaviors:

- Choose foods that are high in fiber, particularly insoluble fiber like wheat bran. Whole grain breads, fruits, and vegetables are important foods to consume. Fiber provides bulk that softens the stool and makes elimination easier.
- Listen to body signals and follow a schedule that allows time for a bowel movement to occur. Ignoring the natural urge to defecate causes feces to remain in the colon longer. This allows more water to be withdrawn, resulting in harder, drier feces.
- Exercise regularly. Lack of exercise can lead to a loss of tone to the muscles of the lower GI tract.
- Drink enough liquids. Fluid intake should be approximately 8 to 10 cups a day. Most of us need to consciously remember to drink water or other liquids to fulfill this need.
- Relax. Stress tightens muscles throughout the body and may inhibit proper bowel functioning.
- Consume regular meals. The body works best with an intake of nutrients and fiber throughout the day.

Constipation caused by lifestyle behaviors should respond to these strategies. If using these strategies does not relieve constipation, consult a primary care provider to rule out more serious disorders (see box).

Diarrhea

Diarrhea is the passing of loose, watery bowel movements. The contents of the GI tract move through too quickly to allow water to be absorbed in the large intestine. Diarrhea may be caused by bacterial or viral infections (stomach virus or intestinal flu), lactose intolerance, spoiled foods, or even stress (2,5). An occasional bout is not a problem. But if diarrhea continues, too much fluid and electrolytes may be lost and dehydration is possible. Efforts should be made to drink enough fluids to replace those lost. This is particularly a concern for infants and the elderly who are most at risk for dehydration; their fluid levels are delicately maintained. Infants cannot easily communicate their thirst, and a greater proportion of their bodies consist of fluid; the excessive loss of fluid has serious consequences of electrolyte imbalance and distorted ability to maintain body temperature and

constipation
straining to pass hard, dry stools; slow movement of feces through colon

diarrhea
frequent passing of loose, watery bowel movements

HEALTH DEBATE
Laxative Use: By Prescription Only?

Laxatives are classified as over-the-counter (OTC) drugs, which means they can be purchased without a prescription. This allows individuals the opportunity for self-care for minor health discomforts. Some OTC drugs, when misused, allow individuals to often inappropriately self-medicate. Laxatives are among those drugs that are often misused.

Laxatives stimulate the colon by increasing peristalsis or causing water to be pulled into the colon to increase the bulk of feces. Those that increase peristalsis are stimulant cathartics (Ex-Lax and Correctal) that act by irritating intestinal mucosa. Laxatives that increase the bulk of feces are referred to as bulk-forming (Naturacil and Metamucil); the water that is absorbed by the high-fiber laxative increases and softens feces, which facilitates elimination. Both actions replicate what fibrous foods and sufficient fluids do. Although the action of laxatives seems harmless, the long-term effects are not. The following four issues must be considered regarding use of laxatives:

1. Using laxatives regularly to relieve constipation prevents underlying health problems from being diagnosed. Serious health disorders such as blockages from tumors or colon cancer might be masked by misuse of laxatives.

2. Laxative use can become a habit. The muscles of the lower GI tract become addicted to the effect of laxatives. Eventually after weeks and months of laxative use, the muscles are unable to respond on their own. They depend on stimulation from laxatives to initiate bowel movements.

3. Unfortunately, laxatives are too easily abused. Use of laxatives is not a weight-loss technique. Some individuals who are obsessed with their body weight have misconceptions about laxatives. They believe that by taking laxatives after eating, the food just eaten will leave the body without being absorbed and so will not cause weight gain. This is not the case. Most of the caloric value of food is still absorbed, but what is lost are vitamins and minerals, particularly calcium. These nutrients need to be in the digestive system longer to be absorbed. Often, laxative abuse is a symptom of anorexia nervosa or bulimia. The abuse may consist of taking laxatives several times during a day. The physical effects of the laxative drugs may cause additional health problems. Addiction to laxatives requires medical assistance as soon as possible.

4. Most cases of constipation can be resolved by lifestyle changes as suggested in this chapter. By relying on a drug to alleviate a health problem, we are not taking responsibility for maintaining our own health.

Primary care providers may recommend the use of laxatives to relieve constipation that results from drug interactions, therapeutic dietary restrictions, or specific medical conditions. Most use of laxatives, however, is self-prescribed.

If laxatives are often misused, should they be available as an OTC drug or only by prescription? What do you think?

From Mahan LK, Arlin, M: *Krause's food, nutrition & diet therapy*, ed 8, Philadelphia, 1992, Saunders; and Payne WA, Hahn DB: *Understanding your health*, ed 4, St. Louis, 1995, Mosby.

functions. Among the elderly, the ability to detect thirst may be diminished; disorientation, sometimes assigned to senility, may actually be a sign of dehydration that if not diagnosed may further deteriorate health. Since it is a symptom of illness, diarrhea that lasts more than 2 days should be discussed with a primary care provider to uncover the actual cause.

TOWARD A POSITIVE NUTRITION LIFESTYLE: CONTRACTING

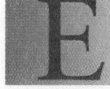

Ever make a bet? Contracting is similar to making a bet with a friend, only the object of the bet is a health behavior! A contract is a specific agreement with yourself, or between you and a friend, spouse, or other relative.

The agreement represents your willingness to attempt to change a health-related behavior. The advantage to contracting is that the goal or behavior change is clearly defined and observable. You also decide on a specific period of time within which to achieve the goal. And as with a bet, you determine a reward or penalty for not completing the contract. By practicing a new health-related behavior for a specific period of time, the expectation is that the change will be permanent.

A contract with yourself might be to drink eight glasses of water a day for a week to relieve constipation. The change to increase fluid intake is a behavior you can directly control and observe. Although the aim is to alleviate constipation, that may not be a behavior you can consciously change, although risk factors can be reduced. At the end of the week, your reward could be to see a movie with a friend, whereas the penalty might be to clean out your messy bedroom closet. (Yes, contracts with oneself are much easier to break!)

Perhaps you have noticed that you regularly work through lunch and eat at your desk. The result is that heartburn has become a regular discomfort, and a discussion of remedies is often the topic of work breaks. A coworker complains that she seems unable to break her habit of buying a high-calorie Danish pastry with her coffee each morning. You could contract with her that for the next 2 weeks you will eat lunch away from your desk, either in the employee cafeteria or at a local restaurant. She contracts with you that she will buy fruit instead of a Danish pastry for her morning snack. If you both complete the contracts, a reward could be to lunch together at a special restaurant. If only one person completes a contract, the penalty could be for the "loser" to pack a brown bag lunch for a week for the "winner."

Contracting is applicable to many aspects of contemporary lifestyles and is limited only by our imagination.

WELLNESS AND BODY FUNCTIONS

Physical Dimension	The GI tract is the first stop to maintain body functioning; unless nutrients in foods are digested and absorbed, life cannot continue!
Intellectual Dimension	The decision and follow through to change lifestyle behaviors to positively improve health in relation to digestive disorders is an aspect of intellectual health.
Emotional Dimension	Several disorders of the GI tract are tied to our emotional state and the ability to handle stress; constipation, diarrhea, and heartburn may be due to emotional health effects of lifestyle behaviors.
Social Dimension	Reducing the causes of intestinal gas guards against socially embarrassing moments. Again, our food choices and styles of eating may affect the level of flatus experienced. Negativity associated with body smells is defined by society and so affects our social dimension of health.

SUMMARY

The processes of digestion, absorption, and metabolism work together to provide all body cells with energy and nutrients. Within the digestive system, all foods are digested. The organs forming the gastrointestinal (GI) tract include the mouth, esophagus, stomach, small intestine, and large intestine or colon. Peristalsis, segmentation, and the action of sphincter muscles regulate the movement of foodstuff through one organ to the next. Other structures support the digestive system including the teeth, tongue, salivary glands, liver, gallbladder, and pancreas. They assist with mechanical digestion (chewing) and chemical digestion (producing or storing secretions).

The main site of nutrient absorption is the small intestine. Once absorbed, nutrients are truly "inside" the body. Nutrients then enter the circulatory system of the bloodstream or lymphatic system and become available to all cells. When the nutrients reach the cells, they may be metabolized. The metabolic changes allow the nutrients to fulfill many cell functions.

Some common GI tract health problems are due to lifestyle behaviors that can be changed. Prevention suggestions and treatment strategies for heartburn, intestinal gas, and constipation consider the effect of lifestyle behaviors. Although vomiting and diarrhea are not usually related to lifestyle, each has an impact on the functioning of the GI tract.

THE NURSING ROLE
Using Your Skills in Informal Situations

As a student nurse and ultimately a licensed nurse, you may often be approached by patients and their families, by neighbors, friends, and your own family for advice on common health problems. As your nursing judgment grows, you will gain confidence in distinguishing situations where general health advice can be given from situations that require referral to another health care professional.

The GI health problems discussed in this chapter are the kinds of problems about which people feel comfortable seeking the advice of a nurse. For example, someone may ask which OTC remedy you recommend for heartburn. Although you may suggest one or two products, this is a good opportunity for you also to engage in some health teaching about the prevention of heartburn and to use your assessment skills to determine if this "heartburn" could be a sign of cardiac disease.

It's amazing how, even in a social situation, people you don't know very well confide very personal information just because you are a nurse. A good example of this is the problem of constipation. Some people will describe the details of their malady, as well as a long history of their home remedies. You might wish you didn't know such intimate information about people you contact only socially. However, in some situations you can give very brief but helpful information about dietary solutions to the problem or make arrangements to talk to the person in more detail at a more suitable time.

It doesn't always take a lot of time to give valuable advice about health and wellness, and it can make a big difference in the life of the questioner.

REFERENCES

1. Greene HL, Moran JR: The gastrointestinal tract: Regulator of nutrient absorption. In Shils ME, Olson JA, Shike M, eds: *Modern nutrition in health and disease,* ed 8, Philadelphia, 1994, Lea & Febiger.
2. Thibodeau GA, Patton KT: *Anatomy & physiology,* ed 2, St. Louis, 1993, Mosby.
3. Logue AW: *The psychology of eating and drinking: An introduction,* ed 2, New York, 1991, Freeman.
4. Williams SR: *Essentials of nutrition and diet therapy,* ed 6, St. Louis, 1994, Mosby.
5. Mahan LK, Arlin M: *Krause's food, nutrition & diet therapy,* ed 8, Philadelphia, 1992, Saunders.
6. University of California, Berkeley: *The wellness encylopedia,* Boston, 1991, Houghton Mifflin.
7. Mitchell JE: Bulimia: Medical and physiological aspects. In Brownell KD, Foreyt JP, eds: *Handbook of eating disorders,* New York, 1989, Basic Books.
8. Food and Nutrition Board, National Research Council: *Diet and health: Implications for reducing chronic disease risk,* Washington, DC, 1989, National Academy Press.

Chapter 4

CARBOHYDRATES

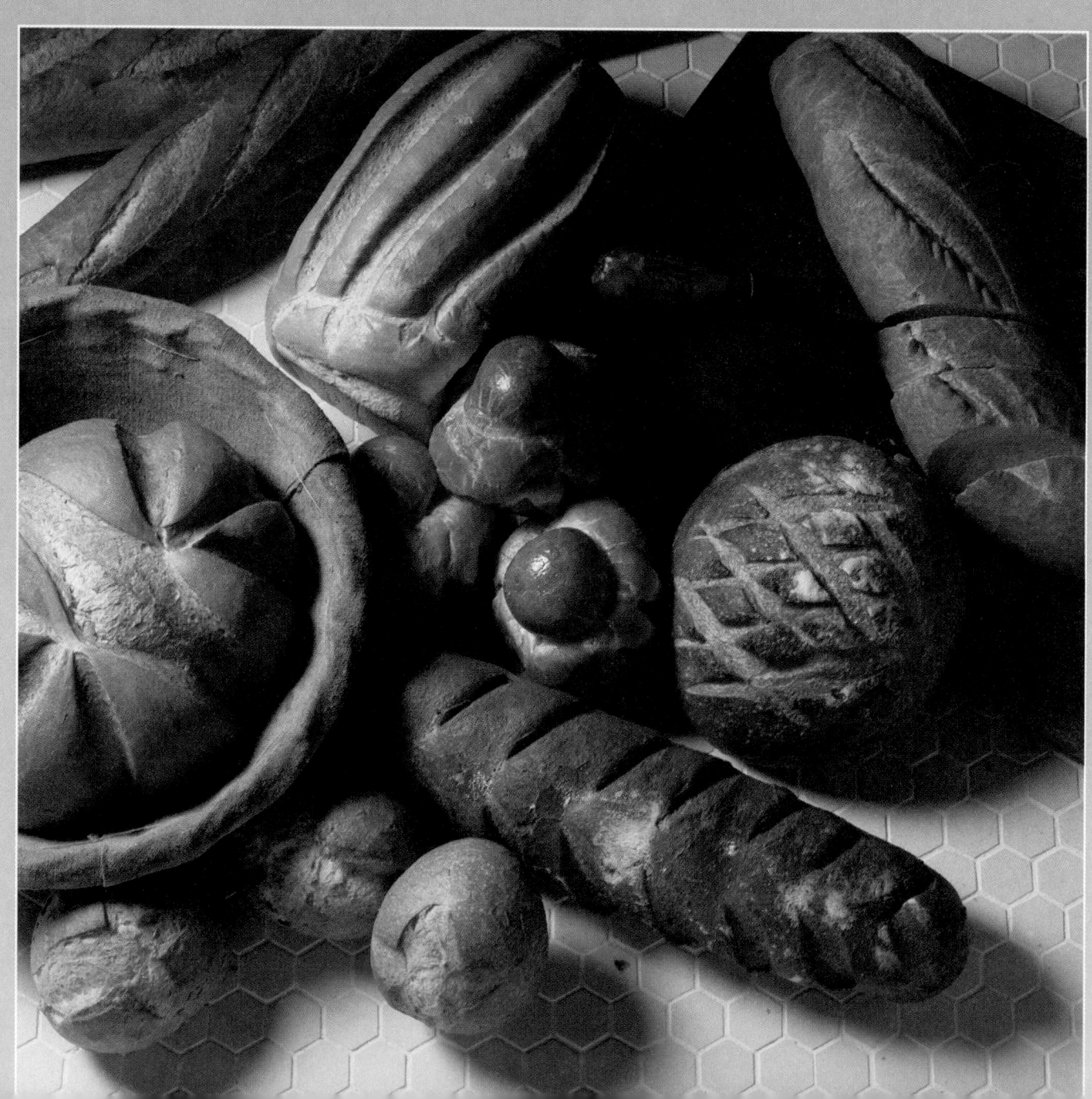

ROLE IN WELLNESS

Nature has provided us with an excellent source of energy—carbohydrates. Found primarily in plants, carbohydrates are a convenient and economical source of calories for people throughout the world. Carbohydrates include simple carbohydrates such as glucose and sucrose and the complex carbohydrates of starch and dietary fiber. Each serves a distinct role in nourishing our bodies.

In addition to being a source of energy, some carbohydrates are also sweetening agents. When carbohydrate sweeteners are found naturally in foods such as in fruits, they are also accompanied by essential nutrients. The sweetness makes eating nutrient-dense foods even more enjoyable. Some carbohydrates also supply dietary fiber. Although dietary fiber is not a required nutrient, it is important for good health.

The energy value of carbohydrates was discovered in 1844 (1). The recognition that increasing our consumption of carbohydrates provides preventive health benefits is more recent. Increased levels of complex carbohydrates appear to reduce risk factors of chronic diet-related disorders such as heart disease, diabetes, and some cancers (2). *Diet and Health* recommends that we consume at least 55% of our total kcaloric intake (about 300 to 375 grams a day) as primarily complex carbohydrates (2). *Healthy People 2000* concurs as follows:

> Increase complex carbohydrate and fiber-containing foods in the diets of adults to 5 or more daily servings for vegetables (including legumes) and fruits, and to 6 or more daily servings for grain products.

This advice is reflected in the Food Guide Pyramid. The five to six servings of fruits and vegetables and six to eleven servings of bread, cereal, rice, and pasta provide adequate amounts of complex carbohydrates (Fig. 4-1).

FOOD SOURCES

The carbohydrates we consume are primarily from plant sources. As plants grow, they capture energy from the sun and chemically store it as carbohydrates. This process, photosynthesis, depends on water from the earth, carbon dioxide from the atmosphere, and chlorophyll in the plant leaves to create carbohydrates.

All **carbohydrates** are organic compounds composed of carbon, hydrogen, and oxygen in the form of simple carbohydrates or sugars. When linked together, these simple sugars form three sizes of carbohydrates: monosaccharides, disaccharides, and polysaccharides (Fig. 4-2).

carbohydrates
organic compounds composed of carbon, hydrogen, and oxygen

Monosaccharides are composed of a single carbohydrate unit. Glucose, fructose, and galactose are monosaccharides.

Disaccharides consist of two single carbohydrates bound together. Sucrose, maltose, and lactose are disaccharides.

Polysaccharides consist of many units of monosaccharides joined together. Starch and fiber are food sources of polysaccharides, whereas glycogen is a storage form in the liver and muscle.

The three sizes of carbohydrates are divided into two classifications: *simple carbohydrates* (monosaccharides and disaccharides) and *complex carbohydrates* (polysaccharides) (Table 4-1). Both are valuable sources of carbohydrate energy. There are differences, however, between the health value of simple and complex carbohydrates found in the foods we consume. Although simple carbohydrates primarily provide energy in the form of glucose, fructose, and galactose, complex carbohydrates may also provide fiber in addition to glucose.

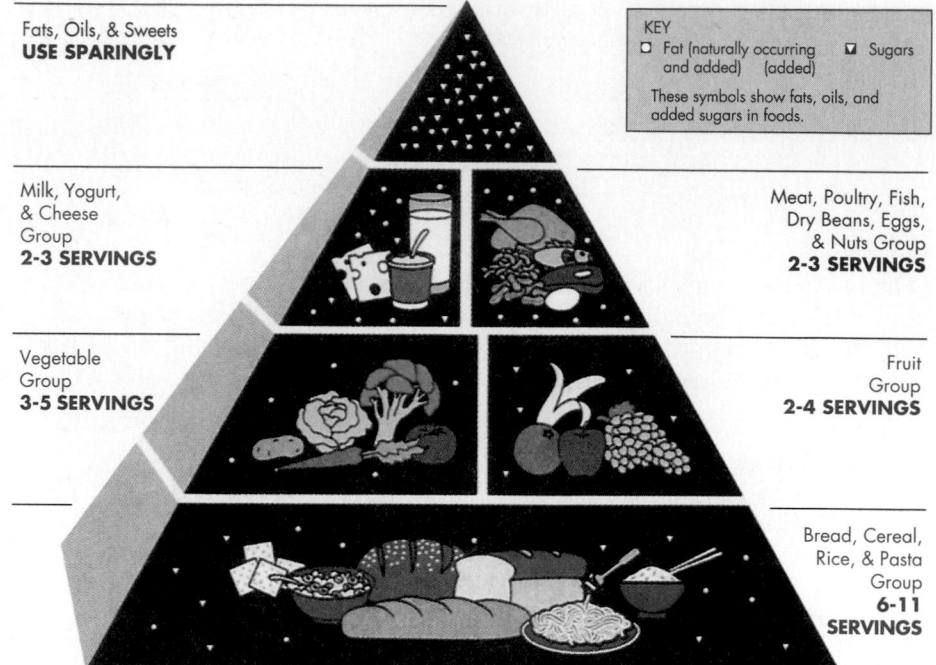

Fig. 4-1 The Food Guide Pyramid, highlighting sources of complex carbohydrates.

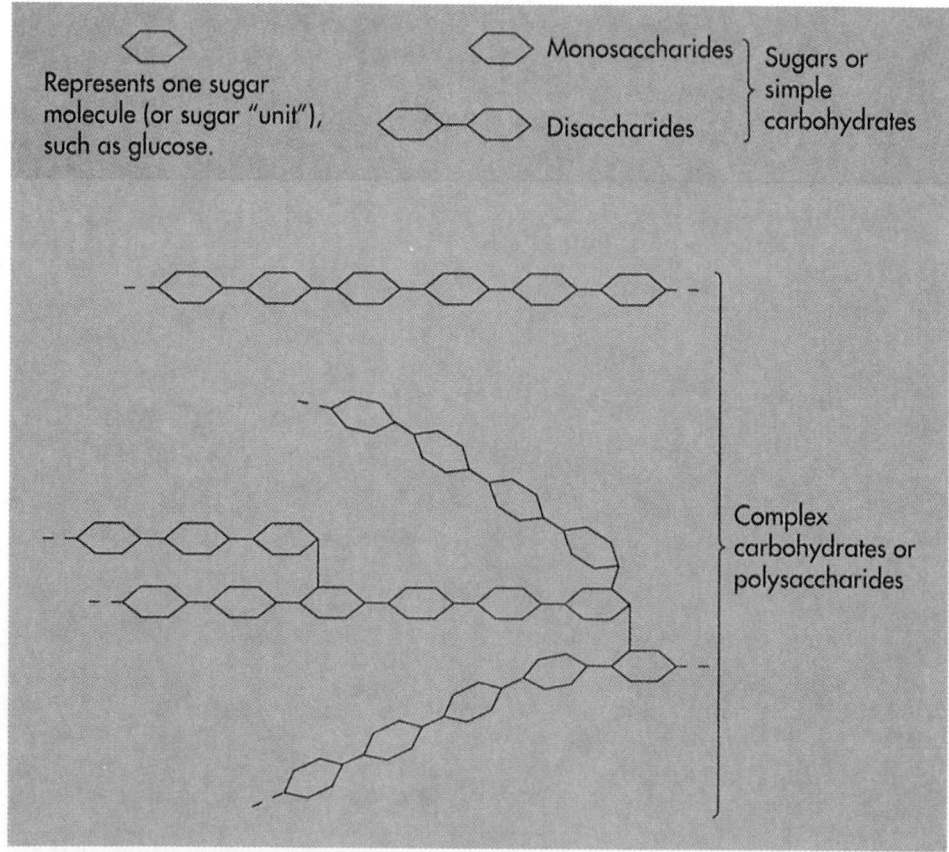

Fig 4-2 Structure of monosaccharides, disaccharides, and polysaccharides.

Table 4-1 Dietary Carbohydrates		
Carbohydrate Type	Common Names	Naturally Occurring Food Sources
SIMPLE		
Monosaccharides		
Glucose	Blood sugar	Fruits, sweeteners
Fructose	Fruit sugar	Fruits, honey, syrups, vegetables
Galactose	—	Part of lactose, found in milk
Disaccharides		
Sucrose (glucose + fructose)	Table sugar	Sugar cane, sugar beets, fruits, vegetables
Lactose (glucose + galactose)	Milk sugar	Milk and milk products
Maltose (glucose + glucose)	Malt sugar	Germinating grains
COMPLEX		
Polysaccharides		
Starches (strings of glucose)	Complex carbohydrates	Grains, legumes, potatoes
Fiber (strings of monosaccharides, usually glucose)	Roughage	Legumes, whole grains, fruits, vegetables

SIMPLE CARBOHYDRATES

Monosaccharides

Glucose, often called blood sugar, is the form of carbohydrate most easily used by our bodies. It is the **simple carbohydrate** that circulates in our blood and is the main source of energy for our central nervous systems and brains. Glucose is rapidly absorbed into the bloodstream from the intestine, but needs insulin to be taken into the cells where energy is released.

Fructose is the sweetest of the sugars. Although fruits and honey contain a mixture of sugars, including sucrose, fructose provides the characteristic taste of fruits and honey. After absorption from the small intestine, fructose circulates in the bloodstream. When it passes through to the liver, liver cells rearrange fructose into glucose.

Galactose is rarely found in nature by itself but is part of the disaccharide lactose, the sugar found in milk. Absorbed like fructose, galactose is converted to glucose by the liver.

simple carbohydrates
monosaccharides and disaccharides

Disaccharides

Sucrose is formed from the pairing of units of glucose and fructose. We know it as table sugar. Sugar cane and sugar beets are two sources. Since it contains fructose, sucrose is quite sweet. It is found naturally in fruits. Sucrose has a special place in our history of food consumption and is further explored as a special disaccharide.

Maltose is created when two units of glucose are linked. It is available when cereal grains are about to germinate and the plant starch is broken down into maltose. The vast majority of maltose in human nutrition is created from the breakdown of starch in the small intestine. Maltose is of particular value in the production of beer and other malt beverages. When maltose ferments, alcohol is formed.

Lactose is composed of glucose and galactose. It is sometimes called milk sugar because it is the primary carbohydrate in milk.

monosaccharides
a sugar composed of a single carbohydrate unit; glucose, fructose, and galactose are monosaccharides

Sugar—a Special Disaccharide

The term *sugar* is a word with many meanings. Sugar may refer to the simple carbohydrates (**monosaccharides** and **disaccharides**). Sucrose, the disaccharide

disaccharides
a sugar formed by two single carbohydrate units bound together; sucrose, maltose, and galactose are disaccharides

Table 4-2   The Sweetness of Sugars and Sugar Substitutes

Sweetener	Relative Sweetness* (Sucrose = 1.0)	Sources
SUGARS		
Lactose	0.2	Dairy products
Glucose	0.7	Corn syrup
Sucrose	1.0	Table sugar, most sweets
Invert sugar†	1.3	Some candies, honey
Fructose	1.2-1.8	Fruit, honey, some soft drinks
SUGAR ALCOHOLS		
Sorbitol	0.6	Dietetic candies, sugarless gum
Mannitol	0.7	Dietetic candies
Xylitol	0.9	Sugarless gum
ALTERNATIVE SWEETENERS		
Aspartame	180-200	Diet soft drinks, diet fruit drinks, sugarless gum, powdered diet sweetener, pudding, gelatin, yogurt
Acesulfame K	200	Sugarless gum, diet drink mixes, powdered diet sweetener, puddings, gelatin, yogurt
Saccharin (sodium salt)	300-700	Diet soft drinks

Modified from American Dietetic Association, 1993.
*On a per gram basis.
†Sucrose broken down into glucose and fructose.

naturally found in many fruits, is also called sugar. White table sugar refers to sucrose extracted from sugar cane and sugar beets. Or sugar may be an umbrella term covering numerous kcaloric sweetening agents used in our food production system, although US commercial law defines sugar as sucrose. There is a distinction between how the term "sugar" is used on a label versus its use by a biologist, chemist, or nutritionist. Often, blood glucose levels are referred to as blood sugar levels. It's important that we, as health professionals, be aware that our clinical use of the term may confuse clients.

Concerns about sugar center around three issues: sources in the food supply, consumption levels, and health effects.

Sources

Sugar in our food supply may include the following kcaloric sweeteners: refined white sugar, brown sugar, dextrose, fructose, high fructose corn syrup, honey, maple syrup, and molasses (Table 4-2). All forms of sugar are chemically similar; each provides kcalories and most do not contain any other nutrients. Blackstrap molasses does contain iron, but other more nutrient dense sources of iron are easily available. Honey, which seems less processed than other sweeteners, provides only a trace of minerals and therefore is as nonnutritious as any other sweetener.

Consumption levels

Our national intake of refined white sugar has declined, while consumption of high fructose corn syrup (HFCS) has greatly increased. In the 1970s, a process was perfected through which HFCS, a very sweet-tasting syrup, can be made from corn syrup. HFCS is less expensive to produce than refined sugar and is sweeter as well. Used extensively in food manufacturing, it has replaced refined white sugar in many products such as in soft drinks. (3)

Health effects

The health concerns regarding sugar consumption include nutrient displacement, dental caries, and related issues of obesity, diabetes, and hyperactivity.

Does it matter to our bodies what the source is of the sweet taste? It depends. A major health concern is nutrient displacement. Displacement happens when whole foods, which are minimally processed, are not eaten and are replaced by foods containing added sugars. If we are eating candy and soda instead of a sandwich and juice for lunch, we are losing a number of important nutrients (Fig. 4-3).

Foods and drinks with added sugars often contain empty kcalories that provide few nutrients. Since all forms of sugar are chemically similar, the sucrose in fruits is actually the same as the sucrose in a creme-filled doughnut. The difference, however, is that naturally occurring vitamins, minerals, and fiber available in the fruit are not available in the doughnut. The doughnut's empty kcalories can replace kcalories from other foods that might contain a natural sweetener and also provide vitamins, minerals, protein, complex carbohydrates, and fiber. Consumption of excessively sugared food does not support wellness goals since it probably replaces other more nutrient-dense foods.

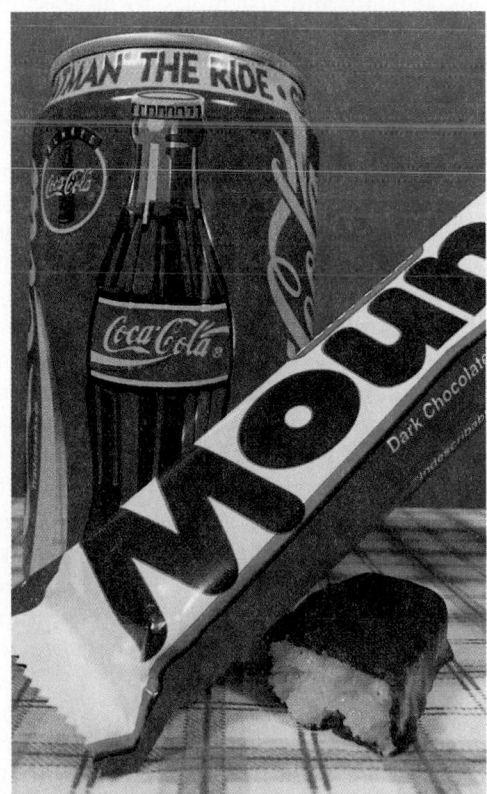
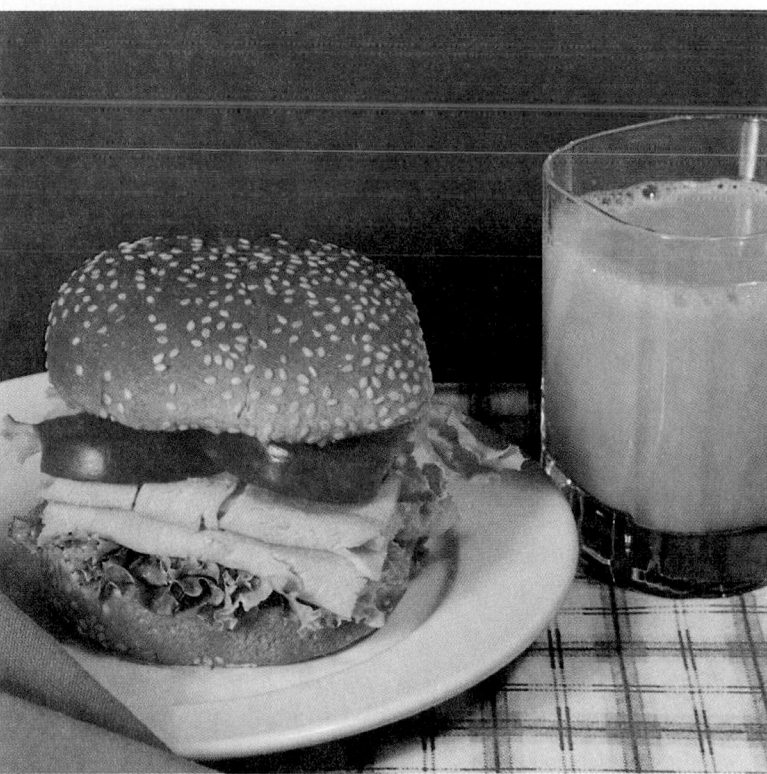

Fig. 4-3 Consuming products with added sugars (**A**) can displace more nutrient-dense foods (**B**).

Dental caries are related to eating concentrated sweets and sticky carbohydrates. Sugar supports the growth of bacteria that promote the formation of plaque. Plaque leads to tooth decay. Ways to decrease this risk are to eat sweets at the end of meals rather than between meals and to monitor the quantity and frequency of sugar intake. Optimal dental hygiene reduces plaque formation and promotes dental health.

High sugar intakes are sometimes thought to be the cause of obesity, but this is not usually true. Obesity may be due to an excess intake of kcalories stored as body fat; however, the source of kcalories does not make a difference. Often, sugared foods are also high in fat. Since fat is the most energy dense nutrient, fat intake may be more of a risk factor than sugar intake.

Similarly, there is no relationship between the level of sugar intake and increased risk of developing non–insulin-dependent diabetes mellitus (NIDDM) (2). Persons with diabetes are counseled to restrict their intake of concentrated sweets to assist the regulation of insulin needs once the disorder is confirmed. However, consumption of sweets does not cause the disorder. These issues become complicated because obesity is a risk factor for NIDDM. Health concerns related to obesity and NIDDM are explored in Chapters 10 and 18.

A myth that sugar consumption by children produces hyperactivity and/or disorders such as attention-deficient disorders (ADD) continues to be perpetuated. Controlled research studies have consistently failed to support this assertion. More than likely, excessively active behavior is related to the occasions at which sugared foods such as cake and candy are ingested (4). If children regularly consume excessive amounts of refined sugar, their overall dietary intake may be nutritionally deficient, possibly resulting in altered behaviors.

So how much sugar is okay? Moderate amounts are acceptable when our diets are low in fat and high in fiber. The *Dietary Guidelines for Americans* suggests consuming sugars in moderation (See Chapter 2). *Diet and Health* recommendations do not directly address consumption of simple sugars. By following the recommendations to increase consumption of fruits and vegetables to at least five servings a day and complex carbohydrates to six servings a day, however, we can reduce our intake of simple sugars.

Other Sweeteners

sugar alcohols
nutritive sweeteners related to carbohydrates that provide 4 kcalories per gram; include sorbitol, mannitol, and xylitol

alternative sweeteners
nonnutritive sweeteners (or artificial sweeteners) synthetically produced to be sweet-tasting but provide no nutrients and few if any kcalories; include aspartame, saccharin, and acesulfame K

Other available sweeteners are sugar alcohols and alternative sweeteners. **Sugar alcohols** are nutritive sweeteners because they provide 4 kcalories per gram. They occur naturally in fruits and include sorbitol, mannitol, and xylitol. **Alternative sweeteners** are nonnutritive substances produced to be sweet-tasting that provide no nutrients and few if any kcalories. Aspartame and saccharin are commonly used alternative sweeteners.

Sugar alcohols have several advantages. They are less cariogenic than sucrose. In contrast to carbohydrate sugars, sugar alcohols do not encourage the growth of bacteria in the mouth that leads to tooth decay. Although chemically related to carbohydrates, sugar alcohols are absorbed more slowly than carbohydrates. The longer absorption time leads to a slower rise in blood glucose levels. Persons with diabetes may be able to consume moderate amounts of these sweeteners and still control their blood glucose levels. The gastrointestinal (GI) tract, however, needs more time to convert the sugar alcohols to glucose compared with other simple sugars. If large quantities of sugar alcohols are consumed, they may begin to ferment in the intestinal tract and cause diarrhea (5).

Alternative sweeteners, also referred to as artificial sweeteners, are manufactured to be sweetening agents in food products. Their function is to replace naturally sweet kcaloric substances such as sugar, honey, and other sucrose-containing substances. Alternative sweeteners most commonly used in the United States are aspartame, saccharin, and acesulfame potassium (K) (5).

Aspartame is formed by the bonding of the amino acids phenylalanine and aspartic acid. When consumed, aspartame is digested and absorbed as two separate amino acids (6). Although aspartame contains the same kcalories as sucrose, much less aspartame is needed to get the same sweet taste because it is 180 to 200 times sweeter than sucrose. This provides so few kcalories that aspartame can be considered a non-kcaloric sweetener (7). Used in a wide variety of products such as soft drinks, cereals, chewing gum, frozen snacks, and puddings, aspartame is consumed throughout the world.

A number of studies have shown aspartame to be safe, yet about 500 individuals reported side effects thought attributable to aspartame consumption. The Centers for Disease Prevention and Control investigated these concerns and concluded that the relationship between the symptoms and aspartame consumption was not strong enough nor clear enough to warrant aspartame restriction (8,9).

However, individuals with the disorder **phenylketonuria (PKU)** should not consume aspartame; their bodies cannot break down excess phenylalanine and its buildup causes medical problems. All products containing aspartame have a warning label to alert individuals with PKU. This warning should apply to pregnant women as well. Since the fetus would be exposed to excess phenylalanine before the presence of PKU could be determined, the safest approach is to restrict consumption of aspartame during pregnancy.

The general adult population is advised to keep daily aspartame consumption for a 132 lb person at or below 50 milligrams per kilogram body weight (the equivalent of 83 packets of Equal, an aspartame product) or 14 12-oz cans of aspartame-sweetened soda (5). Aspartame, when added to products, is most often listed by its original brand name of Nutrasweet.

Saccharin has had a stormy history since it was accidentally discovered more than 100 years ago (10). The storm began when some animal studies indicated an association between excessive saccharin consumption and the development of bladder cancer (10). In 1977 the Food and Drug Administration (FDA) proposed a ban of saccharin. Many Americans were upset that the only available non-kcaloric sweetener was to be banned. The public outcry was so great that Congress, in an unusual move, created a moratorium to prevent the ban from occurring. In addition, Congress passed legislation requiring all products containing saccharin to clearly state a warning that the consumption of saccharin may be hazardous to health.

The danger from saccharin is probably minimal. The risk of bladder cancer does not appear to apply to humans since no noticeable increase of bladder cancer has occurred. It is expected that the moratorium will continue, and saccharin will remain available for consumption.

Compared with other alternative sweeteners, saccharin has a bitter aftertaste. To mask this, it is often used in combination with other alternative sweeteners. Saccharin is still valuable because it is extremely sweet—300 to 700 times as sweet as sucrose (10).

Acesulfame K, marketed by the trade name Sunette, The Sweet One, received FDA approval in 1988. Synthetically produced, it tastes 200 times sweeter than sucrose, but is not digestable by the human body and therefore provides no kcalories. Although acesulfame K has approval to be used in a variety of products from chewing gums to nondairy creamers, so far its use has been limited. One advantage of this product over aspartame is that it can be used for baking. Heat does not affect its sweetening ability, whereas heat destroys the sweet taste of aspartame (11). Persons who must severely limit potassium intake because of medical nutritional therapy for renal disorders should consult a registered dietitian about acceptable levels of acesulfame K.

Other artificial sweeteners are awaiting FDA approval. Altimore and sucralose are in the process of safety evaluations (12). Others are waiting for reapproval. Cyclamate, a sweetener used in Canada, appeared in the United States for only a

aspartame
a nonnutritive sweetener formed by bonding the amino acids of phenylalanine and aspartic acid

phenylketonuria (PKU)
a genetic disorder in which the body cannot break down excess phenylalanine

saccharin
a nonnutritive sweetener

acesulfame K
a nonnutritive sweetener

20-year period until it was banned in 1970 (13). At that time the FDA determined that cyclamate consumption caused bladder cancer in animals. Although reevaluation of the data revealed that the risk to humans is minimal, the ban is still in effect; however, it is being appealed (5).

Sweet Decisions

Should you consume foods with *real* sugar or *artificial* sugar? Which is better? Which is worse? There are no clear answers, but here is a way to decide. A concept used with food safety issues is a benefits/risks analysis. Does the benefit of consuming a substance outweigh the risk? This analysis can be applied to the decision of whether to consume artificial sweeteners.

Benefits of consuming artificial sweeteners include experiencing a sweet taste with lower kcalories and less cariogenic effect than sucrose. Many people believe these sweeteners are an important part of their weight reduction effort. For most, however, the *saved* kcalories are often replaced by consuming other kcaloric foods (14). In other words, individuals who successfully lose weight and maintain that weight loss do not depend on artificial sweeteners. Instead, changes in exercise and food selection behaviors are the basis of the weight change.

Risks associated with use of artificial sweeteners involve safety concerns. This is a difficult issue to sort out. Since sucrose in the form of white table sugar has been used for thousands of years, we essentially have a large scale study of its safety for humans. In contrast, artificial sweeteners have existed only for a century or less. Since they are not naturally formed in plants or animals, safety must be determined through research studies.

The research process is difficult. Rather than using humans as test subjects, researchers use animals. The test animals are given extremely large doses of the artificial sweeteners and are followed by researchers for several generations of their species. If the physiology of the animals is affected, particularly in regard to cancerous tumors, the substance may be regarded as too dangerous for consumption by humans. The difficulty is that the extremely large doses given to the animals are not replicating the amounts that would be typically consumed by humans. Questions raised include is the substance causing the tumor or is the excessive quantity interfering with normal cell function? Also, how many animals need to be affected for a substance to be considered dangerous and in what animal generation of the experiment? Who is funding the studies? If the company manufacturing the substance is paying, will that affect the interpretation of the results? These are difficult questions with which health scientists and FDA officials grapple.

The FDA is also charged with implementing the Delaney Clause. This law states that if a substance is shown to cause cancer at any level of intake, the substance must be banned from the American food supply. This was the situation when saccharin was to be banned. This is an area, however, in which we can make a personal decision whether to consume products containing artificial sweeteners. Based on our analysis of the benefits and risks, we can decide if our wellness goals are better met by consuming a moderate amount of sucrose or a reasonable intake of artificially sweetened products.

polysaccharide
a carbohydrate consisting of many units of monosaccharides joined together; starch and fiber are food sources and glycogen is a storage form in the liver and muscles

complex carbohydrates
polysaccharide of starch and fiber

COMPLEX CARBOHYDRATES: POLYSACCHARIDES

P olysaccharides are many units of monosaccharides held together by different kinds of chemical bonds. These types of bonds affect the ability of the body to digest **polysaccharides** and therefore account for the classification of polysaccharides as **complex carbohydrates**.

Starch

All starchy foods are plant foods. Starch is the storage form of plant carbohydrate. The strings of glucose that form starch are broken down by the digestive tract to provide glucose. Food sources of starch include grains, legumes, and some vegetables and fruits. Grains are the best source of starch. Grains provide more carbohydrates than any other food category (2). Grains are consumed in many forms and include wheat, oats, barley, rice, corn, and rye. The overall health value of processed grain products differs based on their sugar, fat, and fiber content.

Breads, bagels, breakfast cereals, pasta, pancakes, grits, oatmeal, and other cooked cereals provide high quality complex carbohydrates. These grain products may also contain fiber if made with whole grains. Depending on the spreads and toppings served, they may also be low in fat. Main dish items such as pizza, rice casseroles, and pasta mixtures create another category of complex carbohydrate foods. Other foods such as crackers, cakes, pies, cookies, and pastries also provide carbohydrates but often contain considerable amounts of added sugar and fats; they should be eaten in moderation.

Legumes or beans are another significant source of complex carbohydrates. They are low in fat and are also an excellent source of fiber, iron, and protein. Available dried, canned, or frozen, beans can be easily incorporated into commonly eaten foods.

Multicultural influences have expanded our exposure to inexpensive and versatile legumes. Mexican foods feature kidney beans as an ingredient of tacos and

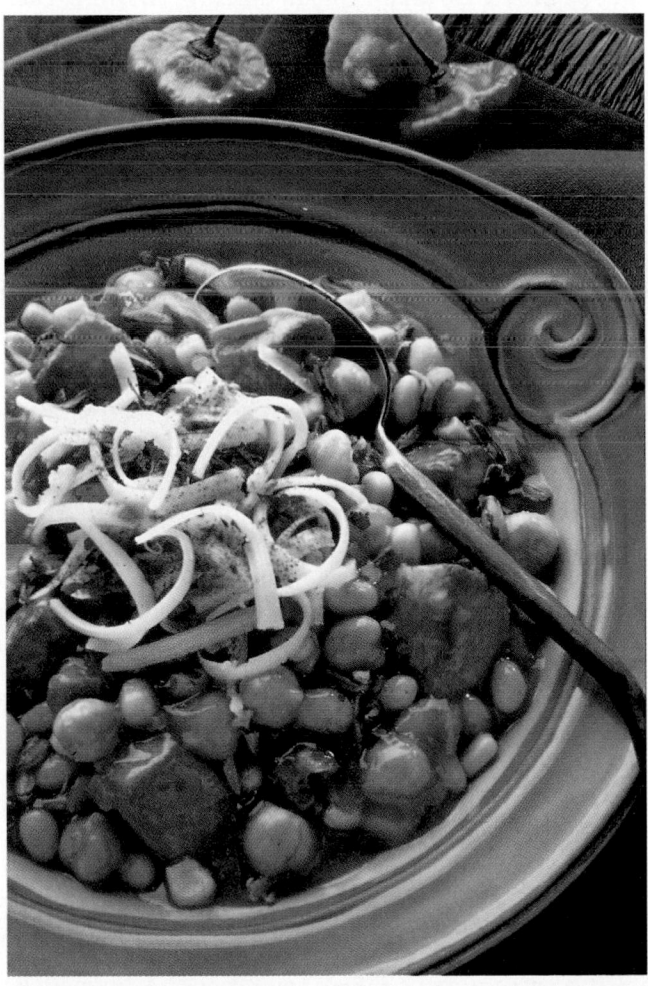

Ethnic cuisines can provide a source of complex carbohydrates and variety in our diets.

chili. Puerto Rican and Caribbean meals highlight rice and beans in savory sauces. Hearty Italian style soups often depend on white and kidney beans combined with pasta. An African influence is reflected in dishes combining black-eyed peas with meats or green vegetables. Hummus, a chick pea paste dip of Middle Eastern heritage, is often served at parties with pita bread or vegetables.

Among vegetable sources of starch, potatoes lead the way. We consume potatoes in so many ways that we sometimes forget their humble "roots." As a root vegetable, the potato is a powerhouse of complex carbohydrates, fiber, vitamins, and even some protein. Unfortunately, some of the ways we prepare potatoes undo their positive health benefits. Most potatoes are processed into products loaded with fat and sodium. Nutritionally, potato chips have little in common with baked potatoes. The best health value is to eat potatoes in the least processed form. Instead of French fries, choose a baked potato or prepare mashed potatoes with skim milk and a small amount of margarine.

Other starchy root vegetables include parsnips, sweet potatoes, and yams. Sweet potatoes and yams provide the same nutrients as white potatoes plus significant amounts of beta carotene. Carrots and some varieties of squash such as acorn and butternut also provide starch and beta carotene. Beta carotene, a substance the body can convert into vitamin A, may have a protective effect against some forms of cancer (2).

Fiber

Fiber, like starch, also consists of strings of simple sugars. Unlike starch, however, fiber cannot be broken down by human digestive enzymes. **Dietary fiber** consists of substances in plant foods that, for the most part, cannot be digested by humans. We do not produce digestive juices strong enough to break down the bonds holding the simple carbohydrates of most plant fibers, so fiber "passes through" our bodies without providing kcalories or nutrients. Its texture provides bulk that thickens chyme and eases the work of the gastrointestinal (GI) muscles that regulate movement of the food mass.

Although human digestive juices cannot digest fiber, microflora that normally reside in the colon utilize fiber as a medium for microbial fermentation, resulting in the synthesis of vitamins and the formation of short chain fatty acids (SCFA). Several vitamins, including vitamin K, biotin, B_{12}, folate, and thiamin, are synthesized by the bacteria that reside in the colon. Only vitamin K and biotin can be absorbed in sufficient amounts from the colon to be significant; the other vitamins are absorbed from the small intestine so that the synthesized vitamins are not bioavailable (15). The SCFA that are produced can be absorbed and used for energy by the mucosa of the colon, thereby maintaining the health of the colon epithelial cells (15). Fecal matter bulk is also increased by the effects of SCFA.

Dietary fiber actually refers to several kinds of carbohydrate substances from different plant sources; all serve similar functions in the human body. Dietary fibers are divided into two categories based on their solubility in fluids. **Soluble dietary fibers,** which dissolve in fluids, include pectin, mucilage, guar gum, and other related gums. Soluble fiber thickens substances. Insoluble dietary fibers do not dissolve in fluids and therefore provide structure and protection for plants. Some **insoluble dietary fibers** are cellulose and hemicellulose. Lignin, considered a dietary fiber, is composed of chains of alcohol rather than carbohydrate.

Foods are sometimes classified based on the predominate type of fiber they contain. Oatmeal is a very good source of soluble fiber because oat bran, part of the whole oatmeal grain, is particularly high in soluble fiber. But the whole grain is a good source of insoluble fiber as well. Although Table 4-3 specifically lists foods containing soluble and insoluble dietary fiber, many fiber-rich foods contain some of each kind of fiber. For example, an apple is a source of the soluble dietary fiber pectin, which is part of the inside "stuff" of the apple. An apple is also a source of

dietary fiber
polysaccharides in plant foods that cannot be digested by humans

soluble dietary fibers
dietary fibers that dissolve in fluids

insoluble dietary fibers
dietary fibers that do not dissolve in fluids

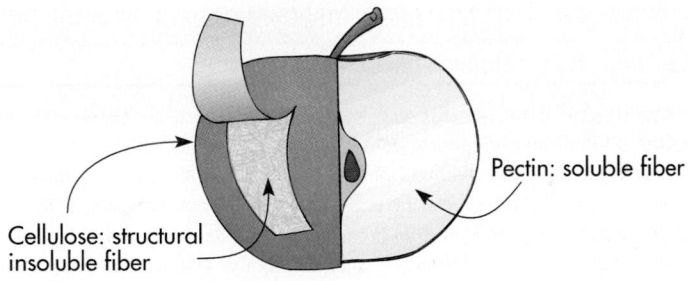

Cellulose: structural
insoluble fiber

Pectin: soluble fiber

Fig. 4-4 In an apple, insoluble fiber (cellulose) inside and in the skin provides structure, and
soluble fiber (pectin) inside adds substance.

Table 4-3 Fibers and Food Sources	
Fibers	**Food**
INSOLUBLE	
Cellulose	Whole grains, brown rice, buckwheat groats,
Hemicellulose	whole wheat flour, whole wheat pasta, oatmeal, unrefined
Lignin	cereals, vegetables, wheat bran, seeds, popcorn, nuts,
	peanut butter, leafy green vegetables such as broccoli
SOLUBLE	
Pectin	Kidney beans, split peas, lentils, chick peas (garbanzo
Mucilage	beans), navy beans, soybeans, apples, pears, bananas,
Guar and other gums	grapes, citrus fruits (oranges and grapefruits), oat bran,
	oatmeal, barley, corn, carrots, white potatoes

cellulose, an insoluble dietary fiber that forms the structure of the apple and gives it its characteristic shape (Fig. 4-4). Popcorn is another source of insoluble dietary fiber that has been with us for a long time (see box).

Health effects

All the health benefits of fiber improve the physical functioning of the human body. The benefits are not directly nutritional but allow the body to function at a more efficient level. Each of the disorders listed below may develop due to genetic predisposition, environmental factors, and/or lifestyle behaviors. However, a low consumption of dietary fiber seems to increase the risk of developing these disorders. Since eating sufficient fiber appears to be a preventive factor, we consider the benefits of fiber on primary disease prevention.

Primary prevention aims to avert the initial development of a disorder or health problem. The risk of developing obesity, constipation, hemorrhoids, diverticular disease, and colon cancer may be decreased by regularly consuming sufficient amounts of fiber.

Obesity. Eating high fiber foods seems to make weight control easier. The volume of fibrous foods makes us feel fuller, so less food is consumed. Often, fibrous foods replace those that are higher in fat and kcalories. Regularly eating foods high in fiber and low in fat may reduce or prevent obesity.

Constipation. Fiber, particularly insoluble fiber such as wheat bran and whole grains, prevents the dry, hard stools of constipation (see Chapter 3). A sufficient fiber intake assures larger, softer stools that are easier to eliminate. Less straining during elimination also reduces the risk of developing hemorrhoids (enlarged veins in the anus) and diverticular disease.

CULTURAL CONSIDERATIONS
The "Pop" Heard Through the Centuries

Next time you're at the movies digging into a giant tub of popcorn, appreciate one of the tastier contributions of Native Americans to our food supply. Five thousand years ago, popping corn was first created over an open fire. The delectable popcorn added variety to ways to prepare corn, a mainstay of the Native American diet. Gifts of popcorn necklaces were made by the Indians of the Caribbean in the 1500s and the Aztecs used popcorn in religious ceremonies. And what would Thanksgiving have been without some popped corn—compliments of the Wampanoag tribe.

Today, special varieties of corn have been developed for their "popping" characteristics. When heated, water in the corn kernel creates steam. This steam, unable to escape through the heavy skin of the kernel, causes an explosion that exposes the white starchy center. Fortunately, the skin remains attached to the starch, which makes popcorn an excellent source of dietary fiber.

Although all popcorn provides dietary fiber, some of the ways it is prepared negate this health benefit. Popcorn laden with butter and covered with salt is not a healthful snack. Nor is a batch popped with the aid of oil, even if vegetable oil is used. Microwaveable packets of popcorn are equally deceiving since they contain oil and other additives. We also may easily be mislead into eating more than we should, since each bag contains four servings that most of us devour singlehandedly.

Instead, return to the native style—fresh air-popped corn. Air popping appliances and microwave containers eliminate the need for oil. Better toppings include sodium-reduced salt, garlic powder, or Cajun spices. While devouring your wholesome snack, remember to acknowledge the inventiveness of Native Americans.

From Elkort M: *The secret life of food,* Los Angeles, 1991, Jeremy P. Tarcher.

Diverticular disease. Diverticular disease is a disorder primarily afflicting people in their 50s and 60s. Some 30% to 40% of Americans over the age of 50 are estimated to have the disorder (2). It begins, however, earlier in life because of a consistently low intake of dietary fiber.

Diverticular disease affects the large intestine. Pockets (diverticula) develop on the outside walls of the intestine, as shown in Fig. 4-5. Low-fiber diets may create increased internal pressure from segmentation muscles attempting to move the food mass since the bulk of fiber is not available. This pressure may then weaken intestinal muscles. Weakened muscles are more at risk for the formation of diverticula. If feces gets caught in the pockets, bacteria may develop and cause serious and painful inflammation (diverticulitis). Medical treatment and nutritional therapy are necessary and are discussed in Chapter 19.

Colon cancer. Eating enough dietary fiber may also reduce the risk of developing colon cancer. Two risk factors related to fiber intake are a high dietary fat intake and exposure to carcinogenic substances in the GI tract (16).

The higher our fat intake, the more at risk we are for colon cancer. By eating more fiber, we tend to eat less fat. Fiber foods tend to replace foods that are high in fat. Since foods containing fiber are bulkier, they seem to fill the stomach quicker, providing satiety sooner and with less kcalories than foods containing fat.

Consumption of sufficient fiber speeds the movement of substances through the GI tract, reducing exposure of the colon to potential carcinogens (2,16). In particular, the longer feces sit in the large intestine or colon the greater the chance for carcinogenic substances to form and affect the colon. The larger bulk of feces formed by fiber intake also acts to dilute the substances, further reducing risk.

Ongoing laboratory research has led to speculation that the SCFA (also referred to as volatile fatty acids) produced by the fermentation of fiber in the colon may have a role in protecting colon cells from cancer and may inhibit cholesterol synthesis. These roles, although still being explored, may reveal further physiological benefits of dietary fiber.[15]

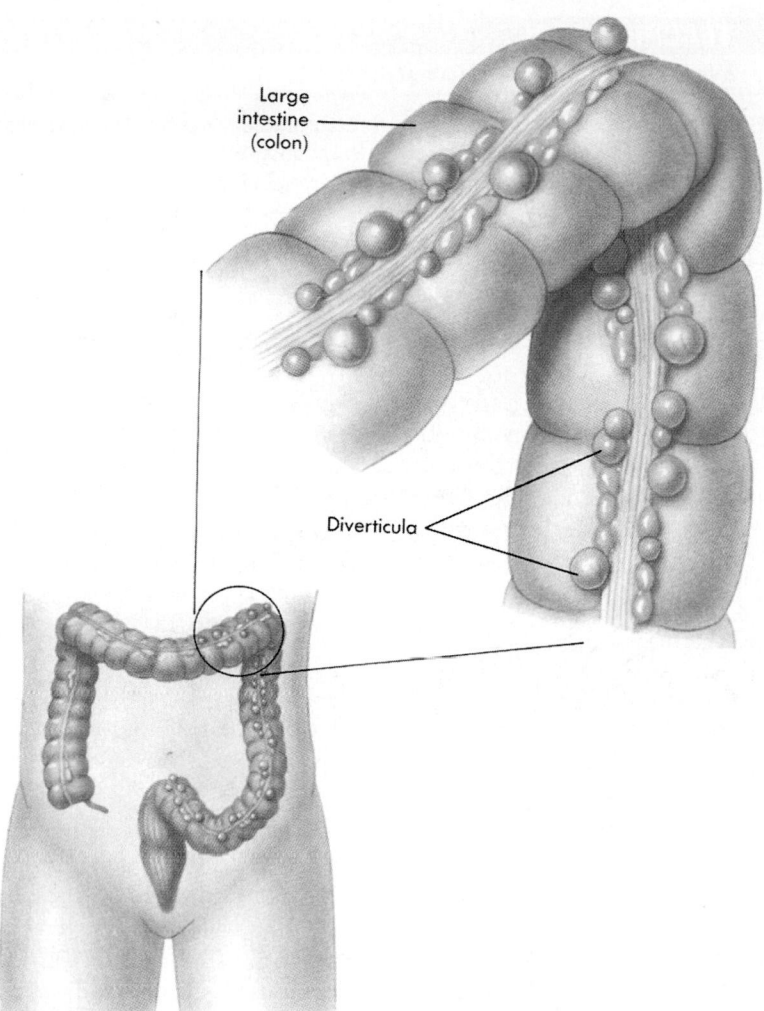

Fig. 4-5 Diverticulosis in the colon. A low-fiber diet increases the risk for this disorder.

Heart disease. Two heart disease risk factors are high blood cholesterol and increased lipid levels. (See Chapter 5 for recommended levels.) Increasing dietary fiber consumption can lower blood cholesterol and lipid levels two ways. One is for fiber foods to replace higher fat foods, particularly those containing dietary cholesterol and saturated fats. In the second, soluble fiber such as pectin (citrus fruits and apples), guar gum (legumes), and oat gum (oat bran) binds lipids and cholesterol as they move through the intestinal tract (17,18). Since fiber is not digested, neither are the bound lipids and cholesterol, and less cholesterol and lipids are available to the bloodstream.

Diabetes control. Dietary fiber intake may help persons with diabetes to stabilize blood glucose levels. Diabetes mellitus affects the body's ability to regulate blood glucose levels. When fiber is consumed, particularly soluble fiber, glucose may be absorbed more slowly. The slower absorption rate of glucose may keep blood glucose within acceptable levels (19).

Consuming increased amounts of dietary fiber may seem to decrease the risk for developing certain diseases; however, reduced risk may not be due to the increased dietary fiber but to other dietary changes. By eating more foods containing fiber, we may reduce our intake of high-fat foods. It may be the lower fat intake that reduces the risk not the higher dietary fiber intake.

TEACHING TOOL
What's Your Fiber Score Today?

Although the foods below are particularly good sources of dietary fiber, many other foods — all fruits and vegetables — contain smaller amounts that add up by the day's end. Does your typical intake meet the recommended levels of 20 to 35 grams per day?

About 2 g/serving	About 3 g/serving	About 4 g or more/serving
apricot	apple with skin	baked beans
banana	corn	bran cereals
blueberries	orange	kidney beans
broccoli	pear	lentils
cantaloupe	peas	navy beans
carrot	potato with skin	whole wheat spaghetti
cauliflower	raisins	
grapefruit	shredded wheat cereal	
oatmeal	strawberries	
peach		
pineapple		
rye crisp		
whole wheat bread		
whole wheat cereals		

From Lanza E, Butrum R: A critical review of food fiber analysis and data, *J Am Diet Assoc* 86(6):732-739, 1986.

When the recommended increase of dietary fiber intake is fulfilled by fiber-containing foods, there tend to be few health risks. Problems may develop when fiber supplements or other forms of processed or purified fiber, such as oat or wheat bran, are consumed in large quantities. When used as a supplement, excessive quantities of purified fiber can overwhelm the GI tract and lead to blockages in the small intestine and colon (20). This is a serious medical condition that fortunately is a rare occurrence.

Bioavailability of minerals may be lowered by the presence of fiber-containing foods. Some fibers and/or substances in whole grains such as phytates and oxalates may bind minerals, making them unable to be absorbed. However, higher fiber dietary patterns tend to also be higher in mineral content, therefore absorption of minerals remains adequate (20).

As fiber passes through the GI tract it provides a number of health promoting services that are still being discovered. Some foods that contain fiber also contain an assortment of essential nutrients. That is why it's best to get our fiber from real foods rather than from supplements.

Since some benefits do vary between soluble and insoluble fiber, should daily intakes of each kind of fiber be calculated? Not at all. Increase total dietary fiber to recommended levels slowly by gradually substituting whole grain foods, fresh fruits, and vegetables for some lower fiber foods (see box). This allows the body to adjust to the additional fiber, reducing the possible formation of intestinal gas.

Food sources and issues

Although the functions of fiber are important for optimum health, there is not an RDA for dietary fiber. Since fiber is not absorbed, it does not serve a nutrient function in the body and so does not meet the definition of an RDA nutrient.

An optimal recommended intake of dietary fiber is 20 to 35 grams per day (19). Most Americans consume much lower levels of fiber; we often average only 12 grams of fiber per day (21). This is due to several factors. Many Americans do not consume enough fruits and vegetables on a daily basis. Somehow, high protein and fat dietary intakes have pushed fruits and vegetables out of our meal patterns. Possibly the most significant factor is that most Americans regularly eat foods made with refined grains from which dietary fiber has been removed.

Unrefined Versus Refined Grains

Unrefined grains are prepared for consumption containing their original components. These grains are really seeds or kernels that include all the nutrients necessary to support plant growth and are segmented inside the kernel to be used when needed. **Whole grain products** refer to food items made using all the edible portions of kernels.

In contrast, **refined grains** have been taken apart. Only portions of the edible kernel are included in refined grain products. Although both unrefined and refined grain products are good sources of complex carbohydrates, other nutritional qualities of the whole grain are lost when grains are refined. Grains most often refined are wheat, rice, oats, corn, and rye.

To better understand how the nutrients are lost, consider the wheat kernel shown in Fig. 4-6. The kernel consists of three nutrient-containing components. The outer layer, bran, is an excellent source of cellulose dietary fiber and also contains magnesium, riboflavin, niacin, thiamin, vitamin B_6, and some protein.

The germ found in the base of the kernel contains a wealth of nutrients to support the sprouting of the plant. Some of these include thiamin, riboflavin, vitamin B_6, vitamin E, zinc, protein, and wheat oil (polyunsaturated vegetable oil).

The endosperm, the largest component of the kernel, contains starch, the prime energy source for the sprouting plant. It also contains protein and riboflavin, but much smaller amounts of niacin, thiamin, and B_6.

When flour is refined, the bran and germ are removed; the bran affects the physical lightness of the flour and the oil in the germ may spoil, reducing the shelf life of the flour. Only the starchy endosperm is used to mill refined flour. Since flour is the mainstay of grain products, the loss of nutrients to the population is significant. In the 1940s it was determined that deficiencies of thiamin, riboflavin, niacin, and iron occurred because of the refining process. To counteract this loss those four nutrients were added back to flour. Now, flour with these specific nutrient additives is referred to as enriched flour. **Enrichment** is the replacement of nutrients to their original levels that were lost during processing. Athough the four lost nutrients are replaced, other vitamins, minerals, and fiber originally in whole wheat

unrefined grains
grains prepared for consumption containing all edible portions of kernals

whole grain products
food items made using unrefined grains

refined grains
grains that contain only some of the edible kernal

enrichment
returning nutrients that were lost because of processing to their original levels

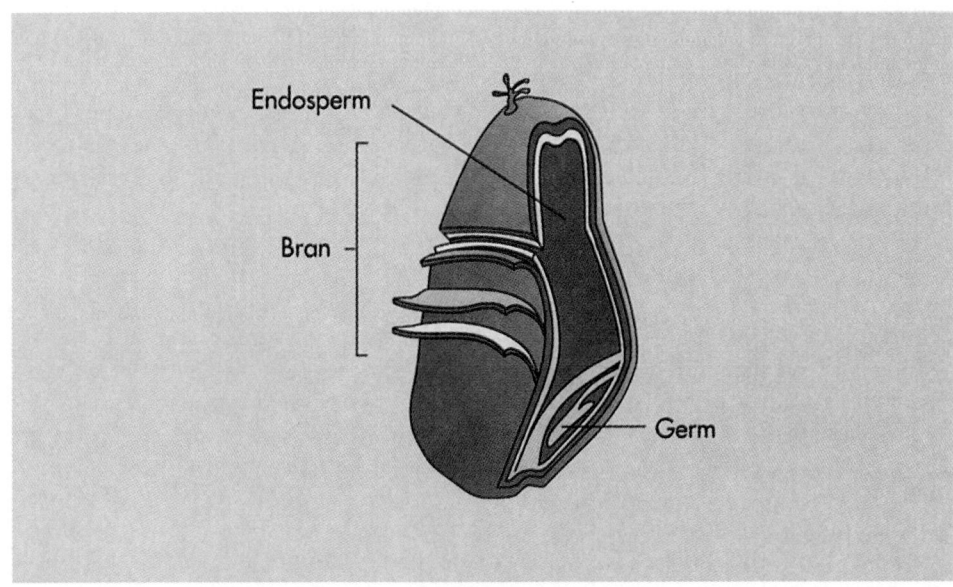

Fig. 4-6 Inside a wheat kernel.

HEALTH DEBATE

If Dietary Fiber is so Important, Should Grain Products be Allowed to be Refined?

This chapter highlights the health benefits of eating the recommended levels of fiber. Also emphasized are nutrition losses that occur when fruits, vegetables, and grains are processed or refined. The process of refining can lead to the extensive loss of fiber and various nutrients. Although some nutrients are replaced, some such as dietary fiber are not.

If health benefits of dietary fiber and nutrients are so valuable, should there be government regulations to restrict or prohibit the removal of valuable nutrients and dietary fiber? Several of the diseases associated with low fiber intake are chronic diseases. Treating these long-term diseases places a burden on the entire American health care system. Is it fair for all of us to bear the financial burden of those not consuming the most healthful form of foods available? Should there be a law against the processing of whole grains? Should white flour production be restricted?

Or is the availability of white (or wheat) and whole wheat products sufficient? Is it our "freedom of choice" to be able to select among different food products even though some are more beneficial to health than others?

What do you think?

are not. Zinc, magnesium, vitamin E, and dietary fiber are not returned to the refined white flour. Consequently, any product made with enriched white flour is still nutritionally inferior to whole wheat flour (see box).

The preference for refined complex carbohydrates may be changing. The health benefits of dietary fiber have been so newsworthy and the focus of such intensive advertising that consumer perception of fiber has evolved from a negative selling point to a positive one (22). Twenty years ago, if products claimed to be high in fiber or made from whole grains, sales would decline. Today, high-fiber food items are among the better sellers in categories such as cereals and breads (22).

CARBOHYDRATE AS A NUTRIENT WITHIN THE BODY

Function

Carbohydrates provide energy, fiber, and naturally occurring sweeteners (sucrose and fructose). The roles of fiber and carbohydrate sweeteners have already been explored in this chapter. Since energy is the only real *nutrient* function of carbohydrates, further consideration of this role is necessary.

Carbohydrates supply energy in the most efficient form for use by our bodies. If enough carbohydrate is provided to meet the energy needs of the body, protein can be spared or saved to use for specific protein functions. This service of carbohydrates is referred to as the protein-sparing effect of carbohydrates.

When adequate amounts of carbohydrates are available, both carbohydrates and small amounts of fats are used for energy. When there are not enough carbohydrates available, fat is metabolized, resulting in the formation of ketones, intermediate products of fat metabolism. Low levels of ketones can easily be disposed of by the body without distress. If carbohydrate levels continue to be insufficient to meet energy demands, increased levels of ketones overwhelm the physiological system and ketoacidosis develops; ketoacidosis affects the pH balance of the body, which can be lethal if uncontrolled. Although lipids and proteins can, if necessary, provide energy for most bodily needs, the brain and nerve tissues function best on glucose from carbohydrates.

Digestion and Absorption

Our food sources of carbohydrates tend to be disaccharides (sugars) and polysaccharides (starches). The gastrointestinal (GI) tract has the role of digesting carbohydrates into monosaccharides to be easily absorbed.

The digestive process begins in the mouth. Mechanical digestion breaks food into smaller pieces and mixes the carbohydrate-containing food with saliva containing amylase, called ptyalin. This begins the hydrolysis of starch into simpler carbohydrate intermediary forms of dextrin and maltose. In the small intestine, intestinal enzymes and specific pancreatic amylase work on starch intermediary products to continue the breakdown to monosaccharides. Enzymes specific for disaccharides (lactase for lactose, sucrase for sucrose, maltase for maltose) are secreted by the small intestine's brush border cells, which then hydrolyze disaccharides into monosaccharides. Generally following an active absorption process (one that requires energy input), these monosaccharides are taken up by absorptive cells in the small intestine. Once glucose, fructose, and galactose enter the villi, they are transported via the portal blood circulatory system to the liver. The liver removes fructose and galactose, converting them to glucose. This glucose may be used immediately for energy or for glycogen formation, a storage form of carbohydrate, that provides an always ready source of energy. Fig. 4-7 summarizes carbohydrate digestion.

Glycogen: Storing Carbohydrates

Glycogen is carbohydrate energy stored in the liver and in muscles. The amount held in the muscles of an adult is 150 grams (600 kcalories); 90 grams (360 kcalories) is stored in the liver. Retrieved as needed for energy, glycogen is quickly broken down by enzymes to produce a surge of energy. The process of converting glucose to glycogen is **glycogenesis**.

Glycogen levels can be significantly increased through physical training and dietary manipulations (see Chapter 9). It is still considered a relatively limited source of energy compared to the amounts of energy stored in body fat (23).

glycogen
carbohydrate energy stored in the liver and in muscles

glycogenesis
the process converting glucose to glycogen

Metabolism

A primary aspect of carbohydrate metabolism is the maintenance of blood glucose homeostasis at a level between 70 to 120 mg/dL. Sources of blood glucose, the most common sugar circulating in the blood, may be from carbohydrate as well as from noncarbohydrate sources. Dietary starches and simple carbohydrates provide blood glucose after digestion and absorption; glycogen stored in the liver and muscle tissue is converted back to glucose in a process called **glycogenolysis**. Intermediate carbohydrate metabolites are also a source of blood glucose. The metabolites include lactic acid and pyruvic acid, which occur when muscle glycogen is used for energy.

Noncarbohydrates can also provide blood glucose. **Gluconeogenesis** is the process of producing glucose from fat and protein. It is not as efficient as using carbohydrate directly for glucose. As fat is metabolized into fatty acids and glycerol (discussed in Chapter 5), the smaller glycerol portion can be converted by the liver into glycogen, which is then available for glucose needs through glycogenolysis. Protein may also be a source of glucose and is composed of numerous combinations of amino acids. Some of these are glucogenic amino acids; if not used for protein structures, they can be metabolized to form glucose.

glycogenolysis
the process converting glycogen back to glucose

gluconeogenesis
the process producing glucose from fat and protein

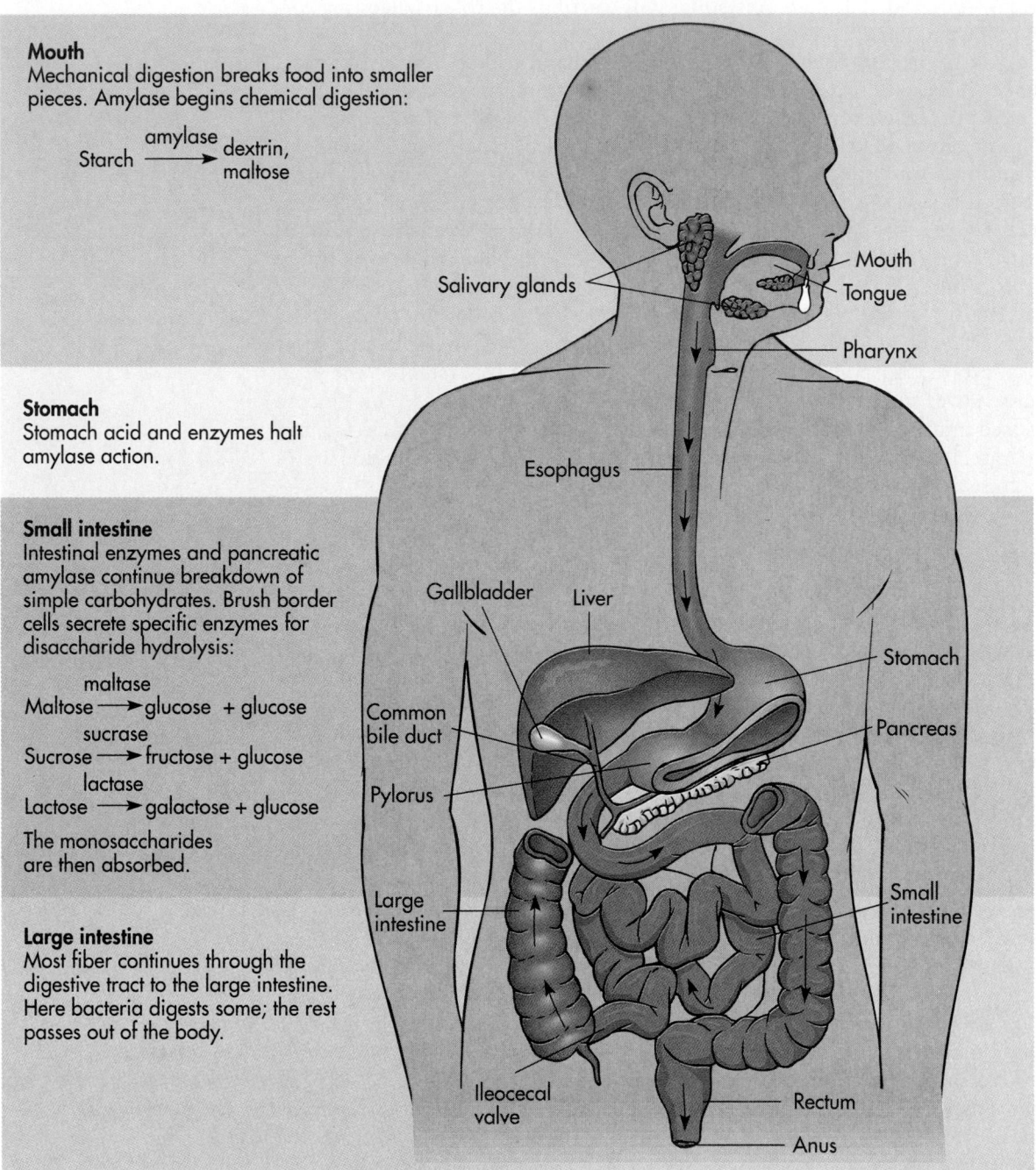

Mouth
Mechanical digestion breaks food into smaller pieces. Amylase begins chemical digestion:

$$Starch \xrightarrow{amylase} dextrin, maltose$$

Stomach
Stomach acid and enzymes halt amylase action.

Small intestine
Intestinal enzymes and pancreatic amylase continue breakdown of simple carbohydrates. Brush border cells secrete specific enzymes for disaccharide hydrolysis:

$$Maltose \xrightarrow{maltase} glucose + glucose$$
$$Sucrose \xrightarrow{sucrase} fructose + glucose$$
$$Lactose \xrightarrow{lactase} galactose + glucose$$

The monosaccharides are then absorbed.

Large intestine
Most fiber continues through the digestive tract to the large intestine. Here bacteria digests some; the rest passes out of the body.

Salivary glands
Mouth
Tongue
Pharynx
Esophagus
Gallbladder
Liver
Stomach
Common bile duct
Pancreas
Pylorus
Large intestine
Small intestine
Ileocecal valve
Rectum
Anus

Fig. 4-7 Summary of carbohydrate digestion and absorption.

CULTURAL CONSIDERATIONS
The Missing Enzyme

A number of adults throughout the world are unable to easily digest the lactose found in milk. This condition, *lactose intolerance*, occurs when the body does not produce enough lactase, a digestive enzyme that breaks lactose into glucose and galactose. When the lactose sits in the large intestine, bacteria begin to ferment the undigested lactose, causing diarrhea, bloating, and increased gas formation.

Lactase deficiency may be due to a primary or secondary cause. Primary lactose intolerance is caused by a genetic factor that limits the ability to produce lactase. Although small amounts of lactose can often be tolerated, the level of lactase produced cannot be enhanced. The condition is common among Asians (Asian-Americans), Africans (African-Americans), Hispanics (Hispanic-Americans), Latinos, and Native

Americans. Most likely, being able to tolerate quantities of lactose as an adult is abnormal, whereas lactase deficiency is normal.

One explanation for lactose intolerance is that the ability to digest milk is an age-related ability. Consider that the milk of mammals, including humans, was intended for the young to consume during periods of major growth with the ability to do so diminishing as the biological need is lessened as maturity is reached.

Sometimes secondary lactose intolerance occurs when a chronic gastrointestinal illness affects the intestinal tract, reducing the amount of lactase produced (See Chapter 19). Even a bout of an intestinal virus or flu can cause temporary lactose intolerance. Most of these individuals recover and are again able to digest lactose.

From Erikson RS: Disaccharidase insufficiency and other disorders of carbohydrate digestion. In Gitnick G, ed: *Principles and practice of gastroenterology and hepatology,* New York, 1988, Elsevier; Ketchmer N: The significance of lactose intolerance. In Paige SM and Bayless TM, ed: *Lactose digestion: Clinical and nutritional implications,* Baltimore, 1982, The Johns Hopkins University Press; and Scrimshaw NS and Murray EB: Lactose intolerance and milk consumption, *Am J Clin Nutr,* 1988; 48(suppl):1083-1159.

Blood glucose is a source of energy to all cells. Glucose may be used immediately as energy or converted to glycogen or fat; both conversions provide energy for the future. Although glycogen can be converted back to glucose, the conversion of glucose to fat is irreversible. Glucose cannot be formed again, but is stored as fat and if needed, metabolized later as fat, even though its original source was carbohydrate.

Glucose is essential for brain function and cell formation, particularly during pregnancy and growth. Since the body can form glucose through gluconeogenesis from protein and fat, glucose technically is not an essential nutrient. Gluconeogenesis can provide some, but not enough glucose to meet essential needs if dietary carbohydrate is insufficient. To compensate, as discussed previously, ketone bodies can be used for energy. **Ketone bodies** are created when fatty acids are broken down for energy without the availability of carbohydrates. This process of fat metabolism is incomplete. If carbohydrate continues to be insufficient, a buildup of ketones results, causing ketosis to occur.

Blood glucose regulation

Metabolism of glucose and regulation of blood glucose levels are controlled by a sophisticated hormonal system. **Insulin,** a hormone produced by the beta cells of the islets of Langerhans, functions to lower blood glucose levels. It does so by enhancing the conversion of excess glucose to glycogen through glycogenesis or to store as fat in adipose tissue through the functions of lipoprotein. Insulin also eases the absorption of glucose into the cells so use as energy is increased.

As insulin functions to lower blood glucose levels, other hormones raise glucose levels. Two hormones with this function, **glucagon** and **somatostatin,** are produced by the pancreas. Glucagon stimulates conversion of liver glycogen to glucose,

ketone bodies
a breakdown product of fatty acid catabolism

insulin
a hormone produced by the pancreas that regulates blood glucose levels

glucagon
a pancreatic hormone that releases glycogen from the liver

somatostatin
a hormone produced by the pancreas and hypothalamus that inhibits insulin and glucagon

TEACHING TOOL
Lacking Lactose? No Problem!

Lactose intolerance is not an illness and should not undermine a person's sense of wellness. To assure adequate consumption by clients (without the use of supplements) of nutrients usually consumed in lactose-containing dairy products (especially calcium, riboflavin, and vitamin D), consider suggesting the following to clients:

- Experiment with different portion sizes of lactose-containing foods to determine individual levels of tolerance; small amounts up to ½ cup consumed throughout the day can often be tolerated.
- Use over-the-counter lactase-enzyme tablets when consuming dairy products (presently available as Lactaid, Lactrase, DairyEase, and others).
- Purchase lactose-reduced dairy products such as fluid milk, ice cream, and soft cheeses.
- Consume foods high in nutrients found in lactose-containing foods; high calcium foods include broccoli, eggs, kale, spinach, tofu, shrimp, canned salmon, and sardines with bones.
- Consume hard cheeses (in moderate amounts because of fat content) that contain lower lactose levels such as Swiss, cheddar, Muenster, Parmesan, Monterey, and provolone.
- Avoid softer cheeses (or experiment to learn level of tolerance) including ricotta, cottage cheese, mozzarella, neufchatel, and cream cheese (see Appendix D for lactose content of foods).
- Test tolerance of different brands of yogurt; lactose levels may vary according to processing variations. Generally, lactase bacteria in yogurt culture hydrolyses some of the lactose.
- Consider supplementation if these dietary modifications are not achieved; consult with a nutritionist for an appropriate supplement.

From Nelson JK et al: *Mayo Clinic diet manual*, ed 7, St. Louis, 1994, Mosby.

assisting the regulation of glucose levels during the night; somatostatin, secreted from the hypothalamus and pancreas, inhibits the functions of insulin and glucagon. Several adrenal gland hormones also have a role in raising blood glucose levels. *Epinephrine* enhances the fast conversion of liver glycogen to glucose. *Steroid hormones* function against insulin and promote glucose formation from protein. Produced by the pituitary gland, *growth hormone* and *adrenocorticotropic hormone (ACTH)* function as insulin inhibitors. The thyroid hormone *thyroxine* affects blood glucose levels by enhancing intestinal absorption of glucose and releasing epinephrine.[24]

OVERCOMING BARRIERS

As we eat throughout the day, our bodies respond to the available glucose and easily adjust to provide glucose during the hours between food intake. For some of us, however, these regulating mechanisms malfunction. When this happens, the effect of food consumption on blood glucose levels needs to be considered to avoid sudden rises and falls in blood glucose levels. The two conditions most related to carbohydrate metabolism are hypoglycemia and diabetes mellitus. These conditions are introduced here; nutritional therapy for diabetes mellitus is detailed in Chapter 19.

Hypoglycemia

Hypoglycemia, or low blood glucose level, is a symptom of an underlying disorder; it is not a disease. We may all experience hypoglycemia when we haven't eaten for a few hours and are beginning to feel hungry. If we don't eat, our bodies switch to an alternative source of energy. This causes the release of epinephrine and glucagon, which act to make the liver glycogen available for energy. For some individuals, the transition to this energy source or the experience of hypoglycemia may be uncomfortable, causing rapid heartbeat, sweating, weakness, anxiety, and hunger.

If these symptoms occur regularly, even when an individual is eating well, a primary health care provider should be consulted. The underlying cause of hypoglycemia needs to be determined. Some health problems for which hypoglycemia may be a symptom are over-production of insulin by the pancreas, which excessively lowers blood glucose levels, and intestinal malabsorption of glucose or insufficient glucose storage (glycogen) in the liver. Other disorders may have symptoms similar to hypoglycemia. A tumor on the adrenal gland may cause excessive amounts of epinephrine to be released or a circulatory problem may affect blood flow to the brain, thus causing the confusion, headaches, and other symptoms often associated with hypoglycemia.

Symptoms similar to chronic hypoglycemia may also occur when patterns of food intake are erratic or when we simply don't eat enough. True hypoglycemia is rare (25). If hypoglycemia is suspected, dietary intake patterns are analyzed. Is the day full of concentrated sweets and sodas? This would cause an excessive release of insulin that could then lead to a low blood glucose response. That is not true hypoglycemia. Instead a mix of carbohydrate and protein foods should be eaten throughout the day and hypoglycemic symptoms will probably decrease. However, if the best efforts at diet control do not eliminate hypoglycemic episodes, medical advice should be sought.

hypoglycemia
blood glucose levels that are below normal values

Diabetes Mellitus

Whereas hypoglycemia involves low blood sugar, diabetes is concerned with very high blood glucose levels or **hyperglycemia. Diabetes mellitus** is a disorder of carbohydrate metabolism characterized by hyperglycemia caused by insulin that is either ineffective or deficient. The impact of diabetes is that the energy supply of glucose keeps circulating in the bloodstream; it is not available in sufficient quantities to support the energy needs of the cells.

There are several types of diabetes:

Insulin-dependent diabetes mellitus

In **insulin-dependent diabetes mellitus (IDDM),** the pancreas produces no insulin at all. Insulin must be provided through daily insulin injections to control blood glucose levels. IDDM tends to occur early in life, caused by viral or autoimmune destruction of the area of the pancreas responsible for insulin production; genetic factors may also be associated with IDDM. This disorder is not risk related. We cannot prevent nor develop IDDM by our dietary intake or lifestyle behaviors. When the disorder occurs, lifelong treatment depends on dietary intake that balances food intake with insulin injection and on lifestyle behaviors to reduce the complications of IDDM. Individuals with IDDM are more at risk for heart disease and kidney disorders.

Non–insulin-dependent diabetes mellitus

In **non–insulin-dependent diabetes mellitus (NIDDM),** the pancreas produces some insulin, but it is ineffective and unable to meet the needs of the body. Risk is related to genetic, environmental, and lifestyle factors. The risk of developing

hyperglycemia
elevated blood glucose levels (> 120 mg/dl)

diabetes mellitus
a disorder of carbohydrate metabolism characterized by hyperglycemia caused by insulin that is either defective or deficient

insulin-dependent diabetes mellitus (IDDM)
a form of diabetes mellitus in which the pancreas produces no insulin at all

non–insulin-dependent diabetes mellitus (NIDDM)
a form of diabetes mellitus in which the pancreas produces some insulin that is defective and unable to serve the complete needs of the body

NIDDM increases with family history, age, weight, and caloric intake. NIDDM is associated with advancing age, being overweight, and consuming excess kcalories. If family members have NIDDM, adopting preventative lifestyle behaviors as young adults can reduce the risk of developing this disorder later in life. Preventive lifestyle behaviors include exercising regularly and eating a moderately kcaloric, high-fiber, low-fat diet to avoid weight gain as we grow older. Both of these behaviors also work to treat NIDDM as well.

Gestational diabetes mellitus

gestetional diabetes mellitus (GDM)
a form of diabetes occurring most commonly after the 20th week of gestation

Gestational diabetes mellitus (GDM) may occur during pregnancy when blood glucose levels remain abnormally high. This form of diabetes may affect the health and development of the fetus as well as the health of the mother (26). Although it seems as if the pregnancy triggers the diabetic response in some women, studies show that some women who develop gestational diabetes tend to develop NIDDM later in life. Many exhibit several of the risks factors of NIDDM before pregnancy and so are predisposed to develop diabetes. (27). To limit the negative impacts of GDM, which if not controlled may lead to pregnancy-induced hypertension, premature birth, large fetus size, and other birth complications, routine screening for diabetes is part of quality prenatal care (28).

Dietary modifications are an important part of controlling diabetes. This is accomplished through individually developed dietary prescriptions based on metabolic nutrition and lifestyle requirements. Basic changes include reduced intake of simple sugars such as white table sugar and syrups. These are replaced by more complex carbohydrates and a balanced intake of nutrients, particularly carbohydrates, throughout the day. To make implementation easier, Registered Dietitians use the Exchange List to assist clients with diabetes with meal planning. The Exchange List (see Appendix B) was first developed for diabetic meal planning, but has become a basic tool for almost all food guides and dietary recommendations (29).

TOWARD A POSITIVE NUTRITION LIFESTYLE: TAILORING

Consider what a tailor does. A tailor takes a bolt of cloth and by cutting, shaping, and sewing fits a garment to the exact measurements of a person. Tailoring as a behavior change technique takes a health recommendation and by "cutting," "shaping," and "sewing" fits the recommendation to the limitations or requirements of our lifestyles.

Strong recommendations to increase our fiber intake are made in this chapter. Ideally, fiber intake should be 25 to 35 grams a day. The most efficient means of intake would be to replace all refined grain products with whole grain products. But is that possible considering contemporary lifestyles? Often we are not able to control available food choices and so we have difficulty changing our behavior to implement this type of recommendation. By tailoring the recommendation or goal to our individual lifestyles, we can succeed. Here's some tailoring in practice.

- Overwhelmed by the thought of eating only whole grain foods? Decide to eat more whole grain products for breakfast and dinner eaten at home, when control is easier.
- No time to cook vegetables? Prepare or order salads and keep fresh fruits of any kind handy.
- When possible, choose fiber-rich foods for lunch; but be realistic since foods available at the cafeteria or coffee shop are limited.
- Family holiday dinner, special event, or vacation? Enjoy what's served. Then resume a regular fiber-rich dietary pattern when back to work or school.

While the goal is to increase fiber intake, the objective is to *fit* positive dietary choices and habits to the shape of our nutrition lifestyles.

WELLNESS AND BODY FUNCTIONS

Physical Dimension	Depends on our ability to provide our bodies with enough carbohydrate kcalories for energy and complex carbohydrates and fiber consumption for optimum body functioning.
Intellectual Dimension	Issues related to the role of carbohydrates often are in the headlines. Our ability to process research findings and decide the level of impact on our foods choices reflects our level of intellectual or reasoning health.
Emotional Dimension	For some of us, emotional health may depend on being able to distinguish hypoglycemic symptoms. If we are aware of our personal response to normal hypoglycemia, can we then distinguish *real* emotional issues from those caused by hypoglycemia?
Social Dimension	Social groups can support change or make them even harder to achieve. Will you or your client feel comfortable pulling out a snack of a banana (good fiber source) while chocolate bars are being unwrapped?

SUMMARY

Carbohydrates are composed of carbon, hydrogen, and oxygen. There are three sizes of carbohydrates: monosaccharides (glucose, fructose, and galactose), disaccharides (sucrose, maltose, and lactose), and polysaccarides (starch and dietary fiber). These three sizes are divided into the two categories of simple carbohydrates (monosaccharides and disaccharides) and complex carbohydrates (polysaccharides).

Primarily found in plant foods, carbohydrates are an abundant food source of energy and dietary fiber. Glucose is the carbohydrate form through which energy circulates in the bloodstream. Blood glucose levels are naturally regulated through hormonal systems that aim to keep the body in balance. Hypoglycemia and diabetes mellitus may occur when these systems cannot regulate glucose within normal levels. In contrast to glucose, dietary fiber does not provide energy. Although dietary fiber is a carbohydrate, it is not digestible by humans. The health benefits of consuming sufficient quantities of dietary fiber, however, are significant.

The best food energy sources of carbohydrates are grains, legumes, and starchy root vegetables. Dietary fiber is available in many foods such as fruits, vegetables, and whole grain products. Dietary fiber and other nutrients are often lost when foods, particularly grains, are processed.

The most recent dietary guidelines recommend the increased consumption of complex carbohydrates. The Food Pyramid suggests 6 to 11 servings of grains and 5 to 9 servings of fruits and vegetables. The intent is to reduce our fat intake by increasing intake of starch and dietary fiber. By following these guidelines, our risk of developing diet-related diseases will be decreased.

THE NURSING ROLE
Fiber Case Study: The Nursing Process

Alice is a 15-year-old who visits a nurse practitioner's (NP) office for a physical examination before joining the high school soccer team. In collecting the health history, the NP finds that Alice usually has a bowel movement every 3 days. Although Alice doesn't complain of constipation, the NP is concerned that these data may be indicative of a pattern leading to constipation. Further data are needed and are collected quickly by means of interviewing Alice.

ASSESSMENT DATA COLLECTED
Subjective
Small, hard stool
No difficulty defecating
Fiber intake minimal; prefers white bread and low fiber cereals and vegetables
Fluid intake of 6 to 7 glasses per day

NURSING DIAGNOSIS
Altered health maintenance, related to lack of knowledge, as evidenced by inadequate fiber intake.

PLANNING
The NP sets this goal with Alice:
Increase fiber-rich foods by 3 servings per day

INTERVENTION
1. Explain the importance of fiber
2. Give a handout on types and sources of fiber
3. Explore food likes and preferences to determine high fiber foods acceptable to Alice
4. Encourage Alice to add 1 serving per day every 2 weeks until 3 servings per day have been added to daily intake

EVALUATION
Call Alice in 2 months to see if the goal of an increase in fiber intake has been met as evidenced by intake of 3 servings of fiber rich food per day.

REFERENCES

1. Dolan JP, Adams-Smith WN: *Health and society: A documentary history of medicine,* New York, 1978, The Seabury Press.
2. Food and Nutrition Board, National Research Council: *Diet and health: Implications for reducing chronic disease risk,* Washington, DC, 1989, National Academy Press.
3. Glinsmann WH, Irausqoin H, Park YK: Evaluation of health aspects of sugars contained in carbohydrate sweeteners: Report of Sugars Task Force, 1986, *J Nutr* 116:S1-S216, 1986.
4. Guthrie HA, Picciano MF: *Human nutrition,* St. Louis, 1995, Mosby.
5. American Dietetic Association: Appropriate use of nutritive and non-nutritive sweeteners: Technical support paper, *J Am Diet Assoc* 87(12):1690-1693, 1987.
6. Steglink LD: Aspartame: Review of the safety issues, *Food Technology,* 41:119-122, July 1987.

7. Holmer B, Kedo A, Shazer WR: FDA approves four new aspartame uses, *Food Technology* 41:41-44, July 1987.

8. Tollefson L, Barnard R: An analysis of FDA passive surveillance reports of seizures associated with consumption of aspartame, *J Am Diet Assoc* 92(5):598-601, 1992.

9. Centers for Disease Control: Evaluation of consumer complaints related to aspartame use, *MMWR* 33(43):605, 1985.

10. Bakal A: Saccharin functionality and safety, *Food Technology* 41:117-118, Jan 1987.

11. US Food and Drug Administration: New sweetener approved, *FDA Consumer* 22:4, 1988.

12. Jacobson MF, Lefferts LY, Garland AW: *Safe food: Eating wisely in a risky world,* Los Angeles, 1991, Living Planet Press.

13. Miller WT: The legacy of cyclamate, *Food Technology* 41:116, Jan 1987.

14. Chen LA, Parham ES: College students' use of high-intensity sweeteners is not consistently associated with sugar consumption, *J Am Diet Assoc* 91(6):686-691, 1991.

15. Goldin BR, Lichetenstein AH, Gorbach SL: Nutritional and metabolic roles of intestinal flora. In Shils ME, Olson JA, Shike M, eds: *Modern nutrition in health and disease,* ed 8, Philadelphia, 1994, Lea & Febiger.

16. Reddy B et al: Effect of dietary fiber on colonic bacterial ezymes and bile acids in relation to colon cancer, *Gastroenterology* 102(5): 1475-82, 1992.

17. Kashtan H et al: Wheat-bran and oat-bran supplements' effects on blood lipids and lipoproteins, *Am J Clin Nutr* 55(5):976-80, 1992.

18. Whyte JL, McArthur R, Topping D, Nestel P: Oat bran lowers plasma cholesterol level in mildly hypercholesterolemic men, *J Am Diet Assoc* 92(4):446-9, 1992.

19. American Dietetic Association: Position of the American Dietetic Association: Health implications of dietary fiber/technical support paper, *J Am Diet Assoc* 88(2):216-220, 1988.

20. Schneeman BO, Tietyen J: Dietary fiber. In Shils ME, Olson JA, Shike M, eds: *Modern nutrition in health and disease,* ed 8, Philadelphia, 1994, Lea & Febiger.

21. Lanza E et al: Dietary fiber intake in the US population, *Am J Clin Nutr* 46:790-797, 1987.

22. Senauer B, Asp E, Kinsey J: *Food trends and the changing consumer,* St Paul, Minn, 1991, Eagan Press.

23. MacDonald I: Carbohydrates. In Shils ME, Olson JA, Shike M, ed: *Modern nutrition in health and disease,* ed 8, Philadelphia, 1994, Lea & Febiger.

24. Williams SR: *Essentials of nutrition and diet therapy,* ed 8, St. Louis, 1994, Mosby.

25. Parlady J et al: Blood glucose measurements during symptomatic episodes in patients with suspected postprandial hypoglycemia, *N Engl J Med* 321:1421-1425, 1989.

26. Gabbe SF: Gestational diabetes mellitus, *N Engl J Med* 315:1025-1026, Oct 1986.

27. Wyngaarden JB: Gestational diabetes may be unrelated to pregnancy, *JAMA* 250:3406, Dec 1988.

28. Association of Family Physicians: Screening recommendations for gestational diabetes mellitus, *Am Fam Phys* 45:352, Jan 1992.

29. American Diabetes Association and American Dietetic Association: *Exchange lists for meal planning,* Alexandria, Va, 1995, American Dietetic Association.

Chapter 5

FATS

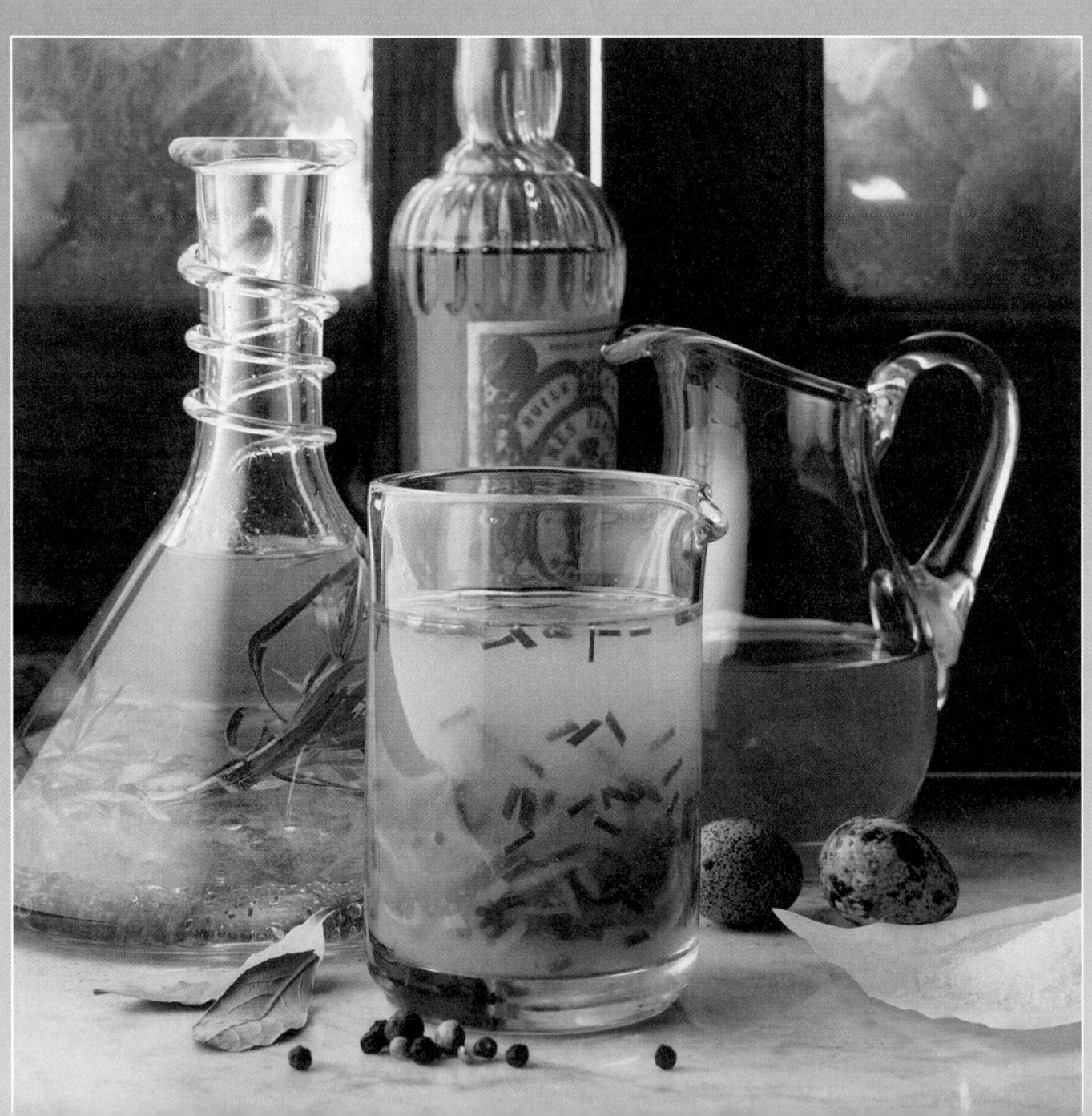

ROLE IN WELLNESS

Some people fear fat. We may have friends who have so called *fat attacks*. These attacks are reported to be both a craving for tasty, fatty foods and worrying about the way fat appears on the body. Fat is not always an enemy. Fat is valuable and necessary to health. It is important to learn about fat in food, what the fat we eat does in our bodies, and how it can be both helpful and harmful to our health.

Fats actually refer to the chemical group of lipids. Lipids are divided into three classifications: fats or triglycerides and the fat-related substances of phospholipids and sterols. About 95% of the lipids in foods and in our bodies is in the form of fat as *triglycerides*, the largest class of lipids that may be in the form of fats (somewhat solid) or oils (liquid). The other two lipid classifications are the fat-related substances of *phospholipids* and *sterols*. Lecithin is the best known phospholipid; cholesterol is the best known sterol. All are organic, composed of carbon, hydrogen, and oxygen, and cannot dissolve in water.

FUNCTIONS

The functions of lipids divide into two categories; some functions are through characteristics of lipids in foods and others are related to the physical health of our bodies.

Food Functions

Source of energy

Fat is the most dense form of stored energy in both food and in our bodies. This means that gram for gram food fat, in the form of triglycerides, can produce over twice the energy in kcalories as carbohydrate or protein. For example, a gram of nearly pure fat such as butter provides over twice the kcalories as a gram of nearly pure carbohydrate such as sugar or a gram of nearly pure protein such as dried, lean fish.

An important point to be aware of from this example is that these three foods are comparable by weight because they are described as *nearly pure*. The weight of food is generally not a good guide to the amount of carbohydrate, protein, fat, or kcalories in a food. There are two reasons for this: (1) the water content of foods varies and results in a significant difference in the weight of individual foods, and (2) most foods are a mixture of water and the three energy nutrients—carbohydrate, protein, and fat—with their varying kcalorie density.

Palatability

Fat makes food smell and taste good. Deep fat fried potatoes outrank all other vegetable choices among North Americans. Bread with butter (or margarine), salad with dressing, desserts with cream: fat makes these foods taste pleasant for many people. For patients who are anorectic because of illness, strategically adding small amounts of fats to meals may increase their nutrient intake.

Satiety

Fat helps prevent hunger between meals. Because it is kcalorically dense, fat slows down digestion and makes us feel full and satisfied; we call this *satiety*.

Food processing

Certain qualities of lipids, aside from nutritional purposes, make them a valuable resource for the processing of foods. The use of processed fats helps keep the

emulsifier
a substance that works by being soluble in water and fat at the same time

essential fatty acids
polyunsaturated fatty acids that cannot be made in the body and must be consumed in the diet

fat in food products from turning rancid. Lecithin, a phospholipid, has an extensive role as an **emulsifier**. These functions, which will be described in more detail, also increase our overall intake of lipids.

Nutrient source

Some fats contain or transport the fat-soluble nutrients of vitamins A, D, E, and K and the **essential fatty acids (EFAs)**, linoleic and linolenic fatty acids.

These essential fatty acids, components of fat triglycerides, are necessary materials for making compounds such as prostaglandins that regulate many body functions including blood pressure, blood clotting through platelet aggregation, gastric acid secretions, and muscle secretions. The overall strength of cell membranes depends on EFAs. Overt deficiency symptoms of EFAs include skin lesions and scaliness (eczema) due to increased permeability leading to membrane breakdown throughout the body (Fig. 5-1). Inflammation of epithelial tissue and increased susceptibility to infections throughout the body are also possible.

Since the minimum amount of EFA required is contained in only about 2 teaspoons of polyunsaturated vegetable oil, deficiencies of EFAs were thought to be rare. However, deficiencies have been noted in elderly patients with peripheral vascular disease (a potential complication of diabetes mellitus), in patients with fat malabsorption, and/or in patients receiving treatment for protein malnutrition with diets low in fat and high in protein. Individuals recovering from serious accidents and burns are also at risk (1). It is possible that individuals striving to achieve extremely low dietary fat intake could develop EFA deficiencies.

Physiological Functions

Stored energy

Body fat cells contain *nearly pure* fat also in the form of triglycerides. This means a pound of adipose tissue, the storage depot of body fat, could produce about 3500 kcalories as energy. Because glucose stored in our bodies as glycogen is stored with water, carbohydrate is a more clumsy form of stored energy than body fat. **Adipose tissue** provides important fuel during illness or times of food restriction and is a major energy source for muscle work. When female adipose tissue or body fat levels decreases below 20%, reproductive capabilities may be compromised.

adipose tissue
stored form of fat (mainly triglycerides) in the body

Organ protection

Stored fat safely cushions and protects body organs during bumpy activities such as impact aerobics or riding a toboggan.

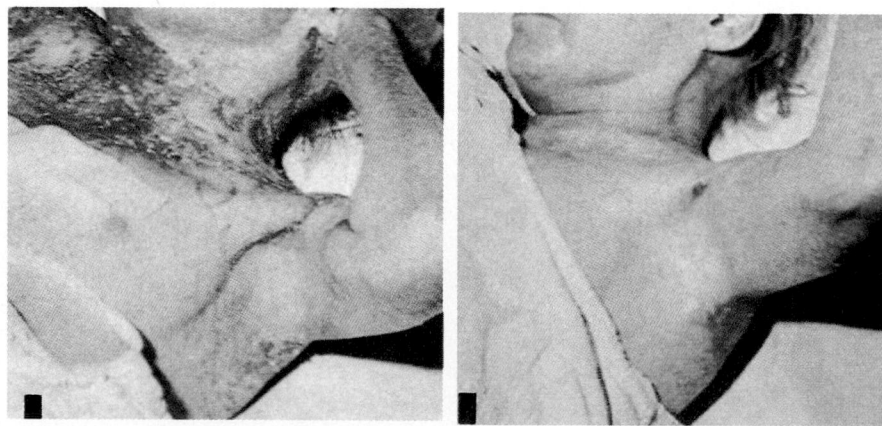

Fig. 5-1 A, Essential fatty acid deficiency. Patients receiving fat-free parenteral nutrition have developed biochemical abnormalities and skin lesions as shown here. **B,** Resolution in same patient after 2 weeks of treatment.

Temperature regulator

The fat layer just under our skin serves as insulation to regulate body temperature.

Transmission of nerve impulses

Fat layers around nerve fibers allow for transmission of nerve impulses.

Functions of Phospholipids and Sterols

So far, we have discussed the major roles of triglycerides. Phospholipids are important as part of erythrocyte plasma membrane and body cell membrane structure and serve as emulsifiers, keeping fats dispersed in body fluids.

Lecithins are the main phospholipids. Lecithin is a constituent of lipoproteins, which are carriers or transporters of lipids, including fats and cholesterol in the body. This characteristic has earned lecithin a reputation for carrying fat and cholesterol away from plaque deposits in the arteries. Although lecithin does play a role in transporting fat and cholesterol, supplementary lecithin from sources outside of the body does not help make the body's transportation system more efficient. Instead, dietary lecithin is simply digested and used by the body as any other lipid.

Sterols as a lipid group are critical components of complex regulatory compounds in our bodies and provide basic material to make bile, vitamin D, sex hormones, and cells in brain and nerve tissue. Cholesterol in particular is a vital part of all cell membranes and nerve tissues and serves as a building block for hormones. When exposed to ultraviolet light, a cholesterol substance in our skin can be converted to vitamin D by the kidneys and liver. The liver synthesizes cholesterol to make bile, the emulsifying substance necessary to absorb dietary lipids.

STRUCTURE AND SOURCES OF LIPIDS

Fats: Saturated and Unsaturated

Triglycerides are compounds consisting of three fatty acids and one glycerol molecule (Fig. 5-2). The glycerol portion is derived from carbohydrate, but it is a very small part compared with the fatty acids that may be alike or different from each other. Fatty acids can be made of long or short chains of carbon atoms. Each carbon atom has four bonding sites or imaginary arms where it can attach to other atoms. To form a carbon chain, one site on each side of the carbon bonds to a neighboring carbon, as if one arm on each side were outstretched to form a chain. Because these atoms have four arms, the two extra arms each attach to a hydrogen atom, which makes the chain saturated with hydrogen.

If a hydrogen atom is removed from two neighbor carbons, freeing the extra arm on each, the carbons are bonded to each other at two sites. The two arms on the same side both clasp the two arms of the neighboring carbon, forming a double bond. We call this an unsaturated carbon chain because there is a possibility that hydrogen could come along and saturate the chain by breaking one set of clasped arms and attaching to them. In foods, this is sometimes done artificially through the process of **hydrogenation,** which forces hydrogen atoms to break a double bond and attach to the carbons, creating a saturated fat. Hydrogenation is discussed in the section on processed fats.

All natural fats are mixtures of different types of fatty acids. Most plant oils contain some saturated fatty acids, and animal fats contain amounts of polyunsaturated fats (Fig. 5-3). The predominate type of fat in a food determines its category.

Saturated fatty acids have single bonded carbon chains that are fully saturated because hydrogen atoms are attached to all available bonding sites. Palmitic acid (16 carbons atoms) (Fig. 5-4, *A*), a saturated fatty acid, is contained in meats,

triglycerides
the largest class of lipids found in food and body fat; composed of three fatty acids and one glycerol molecule

hydrogenation
breaking a double bond on a fatty acid carbon chain and saturating it with hydrogen

saturated fatty acid
a fatty acid with carbon chains completely saturated or filled with hydrogen

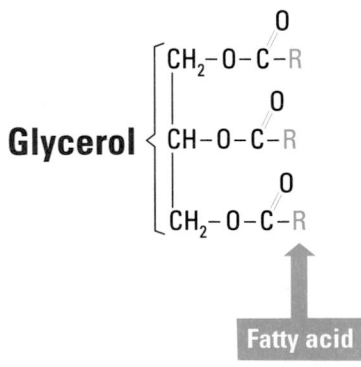

Fig. 5-2 Structure of triglyceride.

Dietary fat	Cholesterol (mg/tbsp)	Breakdown of fatty acid content (normalized to 100%)			
Canola oil	0	6%	22%	10%	62%
Safflower oil	0	10%	77%	Trace-	13%
Sunflower oil	0	11%	69%		20%
Corn oil	0	13%	61%	1%-	25%
Olive oil	0	14%	8%	-1%	77%
Soybean oil	0	15%	54%	7%	24%
Margarine	0	17%	32%	-2%	49%
Peanut oil	0	18%	33%		49%
Vegetable shortening	0	28%	26%	-2%	44%
Palm oil	0	49%		9%	37%
Palm kernel oil	0	81%		2%-	11%
Coconut oil	0	87%		2%-	6%
Lard	12	41%	11%	-1%	47%
Beef fat	14	52%	3%-	-1%	44%
Butter fat	33	66%	2%-	-2%	30%

Polyunsaturated fat

☐ Saturated fat   ☐ Linoleic acid   ☐ Monounsaturated fat

☐ Alpha-linolenic acid

Fig. 5-3 Comparison of dietary fats in terms of cholesterol, saturated fat, and the most common unsaturated fats.

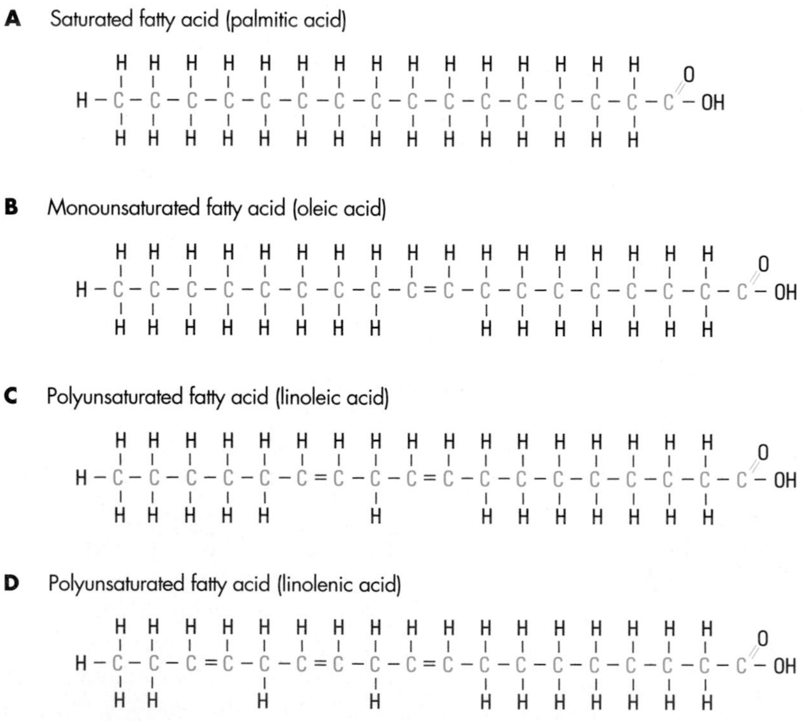

A   Saturated fatty acid (palmitic acid)

B   Monounsaturated fatty acid (oleic acid)

C   Polyunsaturated fatty acid (linoleic acid)

D   Polyunsaturated fatty acid (linolenic acid)

Fig. 5-4 Examples of fatty acids found in foods.

butterfat, shortening, and vegetable oils. Other saturated fatty acids include stearic (18 carbon atoms), myristic (14 carbon atoms), and lauric (12 carbon atoms) (2). Additional food sources of saturated fatty acids are primarily animal including beef, poultry, pork, lamb, luncheon meats, egg yolks, and dairy products (milk, butter, and cheeses); the only plant sources are palm and coconut oils (often called tropical oils) and cocoa butter.

Unsaturated fatty acids have one or more unsaturated double bonds along the carbon chain. If a carbon chain has only one unsaturated double bond, it is a **monounsaturated fatty acid**. Oleic acid (Fig. 5-4, *B*) is the main monounsaturated fatty acid in foods. Dietary sources include olive oil, peanuts (peanut butter and peanut oil), and canola oil.

If a carbon chain has two or more unsaturated double bonds, it is a **polyunsaturated fatty acid (PUFA)**. Food sources include vegetable oils (corn, safflower, wheat germ, canola, sesame, and sunflower), fish, and margarine.

PUFAs are categorized by the location of the unsaturation in the molecular structure of the fatty acid. Two categories of polyunsaturated fatty acids, omega-6 and omega-3, contain two fatty acids, (linolenic and linoleic) that our bodies cannot manufacture; these acids are essential fatty acids and must be provided by dietary intake. The characteristic that distinguishes them from other PUFAs is the position of the final double bond in relation to the end of the carbon chain. The final double bond is at the sixth carbon from the omega end of the chain in **linoleic acid** (Fig. 5-4, *C*), the main member of the omega-6 family. The first double bond is at the third carbon atom from the omega end in **linolenic acid** (Fig. 5-4, *D*), the main member of the omega-3 family.

Americans consume an abundance of linoleic acid because we eat large amounts of vegetable oils such as margarine, salad dressing, and in prepared foods. Another source of linoleic acid may be animal foods; for example, although poultry fat is predominately saturated, it also contains some PUFA, including linoleic acid.

On the other hand, linolenic acid is associated with fish consumption because that is how it was first recognized as important in health. A low death rate from heart disease among the native people of Greenland and Alaska, in spite of a very high-fat diet, was traced to the oils in deep-water fish, the staple in their diet (3). One of the main omega-3 fatty acids in fish is **eicosapentaenoic acid (EPA)**, which is derived from linolenic acid. Fish are more efficient in this conversion of fatty acids than humans. Omega-3 fatty acids appear to lower the risk of heart disease by reducing the blood clotting process; clots can cause blockages in the arteries if plaques exist. Although consuming extra omega-3 fatty acids is likely to have little effect on blood cholesterol levels, it may reduce the risk of clots that may cause a myocardial infarction (heart attack).

Certain fish provide more omega-3 fatty acids than others. Good sources include tuna, salmon, bluefish, halibut, sardines, and lake trout. Table 5-1 lists additional sources. Eating fish twice a week or using canola oil, another source of linolenic acid, should provide an adequate balance between sources of omega-6 and omega-3 fatty acids, although the best balance is still unknown.

Eskimos consume 4 to 5 grams of EPA daily (3), about the amount in 1½ to 3 lbs of certain deep water fish. Because it is unlikely that most Americans will consume this quantity of fish, fish oil supplements of these fatty acids are manufactured. However, questions about proper dosages, safety, and side effects have not been resolved yet. For now, the best approach is to increase consumption of foods containing these potentially important fatty acids.

Phospholipids

Phospholipids are similar to triglycerides except they have only two fatty acids; the third spot contains a phosphate group. Phospholipids, found in every cell, are manufactured by the body, so they are not essential nutrients. Lecithin, the main

monounsaturated fatty acid
a fatty acid containing a carbon chain with one double bond

polyunsaturated fatty acid (PUFA)
a fatty acid containing one or more double bonds on the carbon chain

linoleic acid
an essential polyunsaturated fatty acid with the first double bond located at the sixth carbon atom from the omega end

linolenic acid
an essential polyunsaturated fatty acid with the first double bond located at the third carbon atom from the omega end

eicosapentaenoic acid (EPA)
the main omega-3 fatty acid in fish

phospholipids
lipid compounds that form part of cell walls and act as a fat emulsifier

Food	Total Lipid as Omega-3 (%)	
OILS		GRAMS/OZ*
Menhaden	23	6.9
Salmon	22	6.6
Cod liver	20	6.0
Canola	10	3.0
Soybean	7	2.1
Butterfat	2	0.6
Corn	1	0.3
FISH		GRAMS/4 OZ
Cod	42	0.3
Shrimp	38	0.5
Tuna	30	2.3
Pink salmon	29	1.0
King crab	20	0.6
Mackerel	17	1.8-2.6
Herring	6	1.0-2.0

Table 5-1   Food Sources of Omega-3 Fatty Acids

*1 oz = 2 tablespoons; 1 oz provides 246 kcal.

phospholipid, contains two fatty acids, with the third spot filled by a molecule of choline plus phosphorus. In the body, lecithin's function as an emulsifier is to work by being soluble in water and fat at the same time.

Lecithin from soybeans is used in food processing to perform an emulsification role. In egg yolks, lecithin is the versatile ingredient in mayonnaise that prevents separation of vinegar and oil. Lecithin is also used in manufacturing chocolates to keep the cocoa butter and other ingredients combined, and in cakes and other bakery products to maintain freshness.

Sterols

sterols
fat-like class of lipids that serve vital functions in the body

Sterol structures, including cholesterol, are carbon rings intermeshed with side chains of carbon, hydrogen, and oxygen, which makes them more complex than triglycerides. Like phospholipids, sterols are synthesized by the body and are not essential nutrients. For example, if dietary cholesterol is not consumed, the liver will produce the amount required for body functions.

Generally, dietary cholesterol accounts for about 25% of the cholesterol in the body. The rest, which is made in the liver, seems to be produced in relation to how much is needed. Food sources of cholesterol are only animal and include beef, pork, chicken, bacon, luncheon meats, eggs, and dairy products (milk, butter, and cheeses); plant foods do not contain cholesterol.

FAT INTAKE AND ISSUES

Awareness of the fat content of foods is steadily growing. Whether we are consuming a sophisticated gourmet feast or chowing down hot dogs and hamburgers at a summer barbecue, the fat levels of our meals may be of interest. Concerns about fat in our diets center around health issues of excessive intake of energy, excessive fat intake that replaces other nutrients, and the relationship between dietary fat intake and the development of chronic diet-related diseases. Some lipids consumed in foods are essential to our bodies to achieve wellness.

Fat content of foods

High-fat foods are always high-calorie foods. This is because fats are the most concentrated source of food energy, supplying nine calories per gram; carbohydrates and proteins supply four calories per gram. Since most foods contain a mixture of nutrients, we can identify the fat content of food by the number of fat grams in a serving or the percent of Daily Value of recommended fat intake in a serving. Nutritional labels on packaged food contain this information.

The *Diet and Health* dietary guidelines advise that we eat 30% or less of our kcaloric intake from fats with 10% or less of kcalories from saturated fats (4). Based on the Daily Values, total fat intake for an average daily kcaloric intake ranging from 2000 to 2500 kcalories should range from 80 to 65 grams or less (720 to 585 kcalories or less), and saturated fat should be 25 to 20 grams or less (225 to 180 kcalories or less). More health benefits may accrue at fat intake levels of 20% to 25%, but the *Diet and Health* guidelines take a moderate approach to fat reduction. The individual foods we eat daily may have a higher or lower fat content, but overall we should average 25% to 30% of kcaloric fat intake from all the foods we eat each day (see box).

How do we measure the fat in foods without labels such as fresh foods, home-cooked recipes, and restaurant items? One way is to classify foods into groups according to fat content. The Food Guide Pyramid illustrates the density of fat in different food groups by the concentration of symbols for fat in each section (Fig. 5-5). There are few fat symbols in the bottom sections for bread and cereal, fruits, and vegetables, and many more in the three top sections for dairy foods; meat, fish, and nuts; and added fats. Of course there are some exceptions to these guidelines. Half an avocado contains 15 grams of fat and 150 calories, about 90% fat. Six medium shrimp contain 2 grams of fat and 150 calories, less than 2% fat. Grams of fat in examples from different food groups are listed in the margin.

Detecting dietary fat

Some fats are visible; others invisible. Visible fat is fairly easy to find and control; just cut off the white fat on the outside of a steak and measure the butter or sour cream on the baked potato. Invisible fat is harder to measure. Fat in milk, cheese, and yogurt is nearly impossible to see, but many people learn to taste the difference between whole and low-fat dairy products. In addition, dairy foods are all labeled so fat content is known. Some foods give other clues that they contain fat. Press a napkin on a slice of pizza, a Danish pastry, or an egg roll. Look for oil around the edge of stir-fried Chinese food.

Examples of fat in food servings

Butter/Margarine	1 Tbs	11 g
Salad dressing	1 Tbs	7 g
Mayonnaise	1 Tbs	11 g
Cream cheese	1 Tbs	10 g
Carrots	½ cup	trace
Broccoli	½ cup	trace
Potato, baked	1	trace
French fries	10	8 g
Apple	1	trace
Orange	1	trace
Banana	1	trace
Fruit juice	1 cup	trace
Rice or Pasta	½ cup	trace
Bagel	1	trace
Muffin	1 medium	6 g
Danish pastry	1 medium	13 g
Skim milk	1 cup	trace
Low-fat milk	1 cup	5 g
Whole milk	1 cup	8 g
American cheese	2 oz	18 g
Cheddar cheese	1½ oz	14 g
Frozen yogurt	½ cup	2 g
Ice milk	⅓ cup	3 g
Ice cream	⅓ cup	7 g
Lean beef	3 oz	6 g
Poultry	3 oz	6 g
Fish	3 oz	6 g
Ground beef	3 oz	16 g
Bologna (2 slices)	1 oz	16 g
Egg	1	5 g
Nuts (⅓ cup)	1 oz	22 g

TEACHING TOOL
Calculating Your Daily Fat Intake

Here's how to calculate your daily grams of fat:

1. Use the Recommended Energy Intake chart in Chapter 9 to determine your appropriate energy needs for the day. Multiply that number of kcalories by 0.25 for 25% fat or .30 for 30% fat intake.

2. Divide that number by 9, since each gram of fat has 9 kcalories. For example, if you consume 1800 kcal. a day and want to get 25% of those kcal. from fat: 0.25 × 1800 = 450. Then divide 450 by 9 to get 50 grams of fat. Energy needs for the day _____ kcal. × .30 = _____ kcal. fat intake/day. _____ kcal. fat intake/day ÷ 9 kcal. = _____ grams of fat/day.

3. Next, check food labels and/or use Food Composition Tables (Appendix A) for the grams of fat per food serving. You then can compare the sum of the fat grams consumed with the recommended levels for your particular energy needs.

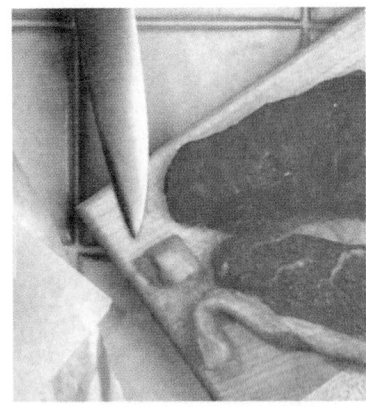

Trim meat before cooking to reduce your fat intake.

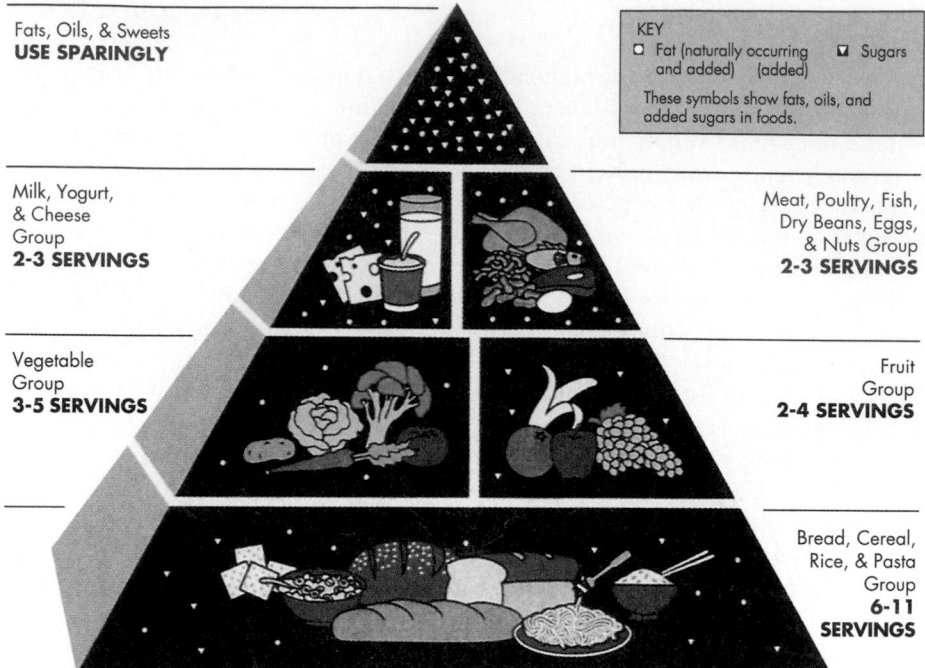

Fig. 5-5 The Food Guide Pyramid, highlighting major sources of fat. Note that the fat symbol also appears in the Vegetable and Bread, Cereal, Rice, and Pasta Groups; be alert to fat hiding in individual items in these food groups. For example, an avocado contains about 40 grams of fat.

Be aware of general characteristics that signal the level of fat in foods. Some cooking methods, such as deep frying, add fat. The way you usually eat a prepared food may also increase fat intake, such as spreading butter or oil on bread rather than just dipping it in soup. Whether eating in or dining out, the amount of food you regularly select from high-fat animal sources such as meat and cheese compared with the amount of food you consume from low-fat grains, vegetables, and fruit affects total dietary fat consumption levels.

An objective of *Healthy People 2000* is for 90% of restaurants and institutional food service operations to "offer identifiable low-fat, low-calorie food choices, consistent with the *Dietary Guidelines.*" Encourage clients to identify healthy menu choices when eating away from home.

The cuisines of China and Italy are based on rice, pasta, and bread. When prepared with small amounts of fat and eaten with little fatty meat and plenty of vegetables, these cultural food patterns are excellent examples of healthful diets. Yet, when Chinese and Italian foods are prepared to please the American palate, large amounts of fat are used in cooking or added in ingredients such as cheese (see box).

Compare the percentage of fat in U.S. and Chinese diets (Fig. 5-6). Note that the incidence of heart disease and overweight is higher among Americans than among people who live in China and in the Mediterranean countries (5,6).

Fast, but High-Fat Foods

Contemporary lifestyles sometimes leave little room for meal planning and preparation. Often we may find ourselves heading for the nearest fast-food restaurant or

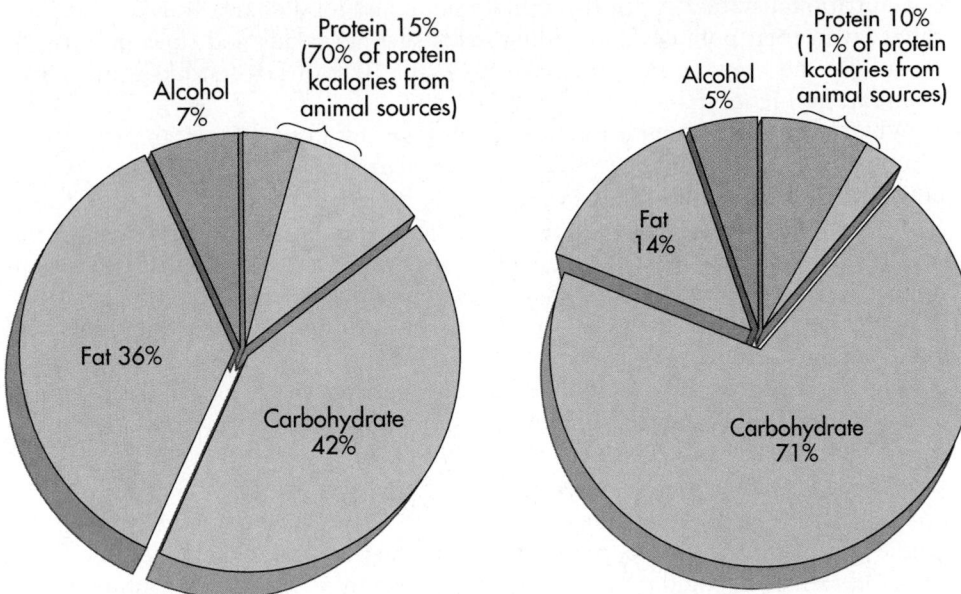

Fig. 5-6 The higher fat and lower carbohydrate intakes by Americans versus those of the Chinese may account for differences in heart disease and prevalence of overweight within these populations. (Data from the China-Cornell-Oxford Project on Nutrition, Health, and Environment, Cornell University.)

CULTURAL CONSIDERATIONS
Choosing Lower Fat Ethnic Dishes

Perhaps you've grown up eating rice and beans, homemade lasagna, or Chinese take-out. Regardless of who prepares the food, Americans are consuming more international foods than ever before. We have a smorgasbord of ethnic foods from which to choose. Chinese, Indian, Mexican, and Greek dishes have become commonplace.

We may assume, however, that since these foods are different and exotic, they are healthier for us. After all, aren't hamburgers and hot dogs, all-American favorites, the worst offenders for our health? Although we won't let them off the fat hook, some ethnic delights aren't much better.

The Chinese foods eaten in America would be considered far too rich (and high in fat) by the Chinese; they are reserved for banquets and even then eaten in moderation. To enhance the healthfulness of prepared Chinese foods, avoid fried dishes, especially egg rolls, and make rice the centerpiece of your meal. Top the rice with moderate portions of entrees of chicken or seafood mixed with vegetables.

Italian dishes of pasta and gravy (tomato sauce) are healthful but begin to be problematic when teamed with sausage, meatballs, fried breaded meats, and layers of cheeses, or if tomato sauce is replaced by a cream Alfredo sauce. Each adds substantial amounts of saturated fats. Be aware of portion sizes and focus on large portions of pasta served with smaller servings of the high-fat foods.

Mexican and Latino foods are sometimes made with lard, a heavily saturated animal fat, and with fatty portions of pork. These negatives, however, are somewhat offset by the generous (and delicious) use of beans, rice, and soft tortillas made from corn or wheat. When possible, avoid or reduce the use of lard; vegetable oils are a good substitute. Generally the less fat used, the healthier the entree. For example, a taco made with a soft tortilla contains less fat than one made with a hard tortilla which has been fried. And be sure to pile on lots of lettuce, tomatoes and salsa!

Become familar with the exotic tastes of international cuisines. By doing so, you'll be able to assist clients in understanding the fat content of their ethnic favorites. Just remember that the palatability of fat is a worldwide phenomenon, so choose wisely.

snack bar as we dash off to school or work. What impact do these meals have on our nutritional status? A positive trend among fast-food chains is using less saturated fat in fried potatoes and adding items such as salads and skim milk to the menu. On the negative side, between 40% and 50% of fast-food kcalories come from fat, far higher than the recommended 30%.

When we study the major food contributors of fat in the American diet, the list is topped by hamburgers, cheeseburgers, meat loaf, and hot dogs. Whole milk beverages including shakes are next, followed by doughnuts, cookies, and cake. Cheese and salad dressings provide about equal amounts, followed by fried potatoes (7). It is no surprise that the majority of fat in the American diet happens to appear in menu favorites served in fast-food restaurants. It also turns out that the majority of fat in these foods happens to be saturated, with hamburgers and cheeseburgers leading the pack.

One may wonder why some foods that are fast to fix such as apples, oranges, and bananas are not considered fast foods, nor are they sold in fast-food restaurants. The answer probably has to do with the fact that fat lends a seductive flavor to fast-food favorites.

How can you lower fat intake? First, start early to include children and the whole family in food buying, preparation, and the practice of having low-fat foods on hand. Lots of people prefer fast food because they don't have fresh or partly prepared foods ready to cook. Teaching children at an early age to learn cooking skills from simple recipes, videos, and with friends has been shown to establish low-fat food preferences early. Studies show that people are more likely to adopt low-fat diets if eating partners or families do the same (8).

Second, most major secondary and tertiary health care settings have an active dietitic department, often geared to pediatrics and family practice. Programs offered may include healthy cooking classes for children and/or their parents, or nutrition and wellness classes. Providing lists of such programs is a valuable resource for clients.

Third, never say never. It is okay to include some high-fat foods in food plans because they taste good. If a mixture of low- and high-fat foods is eaten, preferences for both are developed; this automatically controls overdoing the fatty foods. The Teaching Tool is packed with other strategies for fast but low-fat eating patterns.

Preserving Fats in Foods

Processed fats and oils: hydrogenated and emulsified

A problem with unsaturated fats in foods is that oxygen attacks the unsaturated double bonds (oxidation), causing damage that makes them rancid; rancid fats have an odor, bad flavor, and may cause illness. One way to reduce vulnerability to oxidation is to artificially saturate the fatty acids by adding hydrogen at the double bonds. This process of hydrogenation makes the fat solid and more stable. When vegetable oil, which is polyunsaturated, is completely hydrogenated, it becomes a white, waxy or plastic-like substance called vegetable shortening. Since it is saturated with hydrogens, the body processes it as if it were a saturated fat. The ingredient list on a product label can truthfully note that the product contains only vegetable oil, but the Nutrition Facts box lists the amount of saturated fat the product contains, regardless of its source.

Often, food manufacturers only partially hydrogenate fats. Then the process turns oil into margarine or other usable forms. Depending on the amount of hydrogenation, some margarines are more spreadable than others. This means that tub margarine, compared with the stick variety, usually has more liquid unsaturated oil mixed in with the partially hydrogenated fat. Partially hydrogenated fats are used in a wide variety of food products.

TEACHING TOOL
But Fast Fatty Foods are so Convenient . . .

Our advice to clients needs to be realistic—that means accepting that most people occasionally eat at fast-food restaurants. Rather than attempting to dissuade them, give clients these tools for making lower-fat selections.

Advice about reducing fat intake sounds good when we have the time to prepare wholesome meals. If you are one of the harried millions rushing between school, work, and extracurricular activities, cooking advice sounds like a foreign language. Here are reality-based fast-food restaurant strategies for reducing fat intake while eating quickly.

• Avoid deep-fried fish and chicken sandwiches. Although fish and chicken are lower in fat and cholesterol than beef, when they are breaded and fried more fat is soaked up than in a hamburger. Choose grilled chicken sandwiches and, if possible, remove the high-fat sauces.

• Always order a side salad and/or top sandwiches with lettuce and tomato.

• Try the junior size of the specialty sandwiches. Particularly for lunch, we don't need to eat half our daily intake of calories in one meal.

• Order quarter-pound hamburgers plain, without cheese or bacon. Enough fat calories will be saved to occasionally order fries—a small portion, of course!

• Order a plain baked potato as a side dish. Top with a small amount of butter or just eat it plain with a bit of salt and pepper.

• Salad bars can be deceiving. Fat lurks in salad dressing, mayonnaise-based cole slaw, and potato and macaroni salads. Go heavy on the lettuce, carrots and other sliced vegetables, beans, and fruits. Put salad dressing in a small pile. Dip your fork into the dressing, then into the salad. This gives you the same taste, but less fat.

Eat quickly, but smartly.

Sometimes the solution to one problem causes another problem. Although it stabilizes fat, hydrogenation sometimes changes the structure of fatty acids, from *cis* fatty acids to *trans* fatty acids. Most fatty acids in natural foods are in the *cis* form, but margarine and vegetable shortening contain high concentrations of *trans* fatty acids. Controversy over the impact of *trans* fatty acids in relation to cancer vulnerability and elevated blood cholesterol levels, has confused the public.

Before completely deciding that butter is better, consider that even though tub margarines are fairly high in *trans* fatty acids, they usually have less than many commercially made foods such as French fries, potato chips, and bakery products made from partially hydrogenated vegetable oils. On the other hand, of the 37% of kcalories consumed as fat by Americans, only 3% to 4% of total kcalories come from *trans* fatty acids. This may not be of any practical importance.

Meanwhile, until conclusive recommendations are developed by major government agencies and health organizations, we should continue to consume *trans* fatty acids without health concerns and continue moderating our overall fat intake. Guidelines currently suggest that a priority is to reduce overall food fat to 30% of total kcalories; less fat means less *trans* fatty acids as well. This means eating less margarine, French fries, potato chips, cakes, and cookies, as well as fatty meat and ice cream.

cis fatty acids
cis indicates the configuration of the double bond in a natural oil

trans fatty acids
fatty acids with unusual double-bond structures caused by hydrogenated unsaturated oils

Antioxidants

Another way to preserve polyunsaturated fats without hydrogenation is through the use of antioxidant additives. These substances block oxidation, or the breakdown of double bonds by oxygen. Food manufacturers can use either natural or synthetic forms of antioxidants. Natural sources include vitamin E (tocopherol) and vitamin C (ascorbic acid). Their use not only helps to preserve foods but also adds essential vitamins. Synthetic forms consist of the food additives of butylated hydroxyanisole (BHA) and butylated hydroxytoluene (BHT). These forms are used in packaging as well, which also helps to prevent the oxidation of the foods.

Food Cholesterol Versus Blood Cholesterol

Cholesterol is a waxy substance found in all tissues in humans and other animals. Thus all foods from animal sources such as meat, eggs, fish, poultry, and dairy products contain cholesterol. The highest sources of cholesterol are egg yolks and organ meats (liver and kidney). No plant-derived food contains cholesterol; not even avocado, which is very high in fat. People often misunderstand this because they confuse food (dietary) cholesterol with blood cholesterol.

A high level of cholesterol in the blood is a risk factor for coronary artery disease. In order to understand blood cholesterol levels, the role of lipoproteins, specialized transporting compounds, needs clarification. Lipoproteins are compounds that contain a mix of lipids, including triglycerides, fatty acids, phospholipids, cholesterol, and small amounts of other steroids and fat-soluble vitamins, that are covered with a protein outer layer. The outer layer of protein allows the compound to move through a watery substance like blood. Lipoproteins, along with apoproteins, transport fats in the circulatory system (9).

The amount of fat and protein determines the density or weight of the lipoprotein. The more fat and lipid substances, the lower the density (or lighter) the compound. Four forms of these compounds are most important for understanding the route of cholesterol in the body; they are chylomicrons, very low-density lipoproteins, low-density lipoproteins, and high-density lipoproteins.

Chylomicrons transport absorbed fats from the intestinal wall to the liver cells. Fats are then used for synthesis of lipoproteins. **Very low-density lipoproteins (VLDLs)** leave the liver cells full of fats and lipid components to transfer newly made (endogenous) triglycerides to the cells. **Low-density lipoproteins (LDLs)** form from VLDLs as density is reduced as fats and lipids are released on their journey through the body. LDLs carry cholesterol throughout the body to tissue cells for various functions. In contrast to the delivery functions of the first three lipoproteins, **high-density lipoproteins (HDLs)** are formed within cells to remove cholesterol from the cell, bringing it to the liver for disposal.

A total blood cholesterol reading reflects the level of cholesterol contained in LDL and HDL. To get a clearer assessment of cholesterol activity in the body, the individual levels of LDL and HDL are valuable. The risk of coronary artery disease associated with blood cholesterol levels is presented in Table 19-1. LDL levels reflect the amount of cholesterol being brought to cells that has the potential to be dropped off along the way to clog vessels and arteries, contributing to plaque formation while HDL is removing cholesterol from the circulatory system. Removal of cholesterol is a positive action reducing risk.

Health guidelines generally recommend a dietary cholesterol intake of 300 mg or less per day. Table 5-2 lists the cholesterol content of selected foods. However, the major culprit that raises blood cholesterol is not dietary *food cholesterol,* but too much *food fat* (dietary triglycerides), particularly saturated fats; food cholesterol alone makes a minor difference for most people (10). Too much food cholesterol becomes a problem when it is eaten in conjunction with very high-fat diets (11). Sometimes, this extra cholesterol may be dropped off, staying in the vessels and arteries. This extra cholesterol becomes a problem when the diet is high in fat, particularly saturated fat; it is a factor involved in **plaque** buildup, called **atherosclerosis** or coronary artery disease (Fig. 5-7).

One reason for the confusion is the way food is cooked and eaten. Eggs, for example, are high in cholesterol and are often cooked and served with high-fat bacon or sausage. The combined meal of eggs and bacon then gets a bad reputation for raising blood cholesterol. The fact is that the large amount of fat in bacon and sausage is more likely to raise blood cholesterol than the food cholesterol in eggs. Shrimp are high in cholesterol, but low in fat. That is, low in fat if the shrimp are steamed or broiled, not encased in a deep-fat fried coating. Of course, moderation is recommended when eating eggs or shrimp.

very low-density lipoproteins (VLDLs)
lipoproteins made of the largest proportions of cholesterol that carry fats and cholesterol to body cells

low-density lipoproteins (LDLs)
lipoproteins made of large proportions of cholesterol that carry fats and cholesterol to body cells

high-density lipoproteins (HDLs)
lipoproteins made of large proportions of proteins that carry fats and cholesterol from body cells to the liver

plaque
deposits of fatty substances, including cholesterol, that attach to arterial walls

atherosclerosis
accumulation of plaques that result in blockage in the arteries

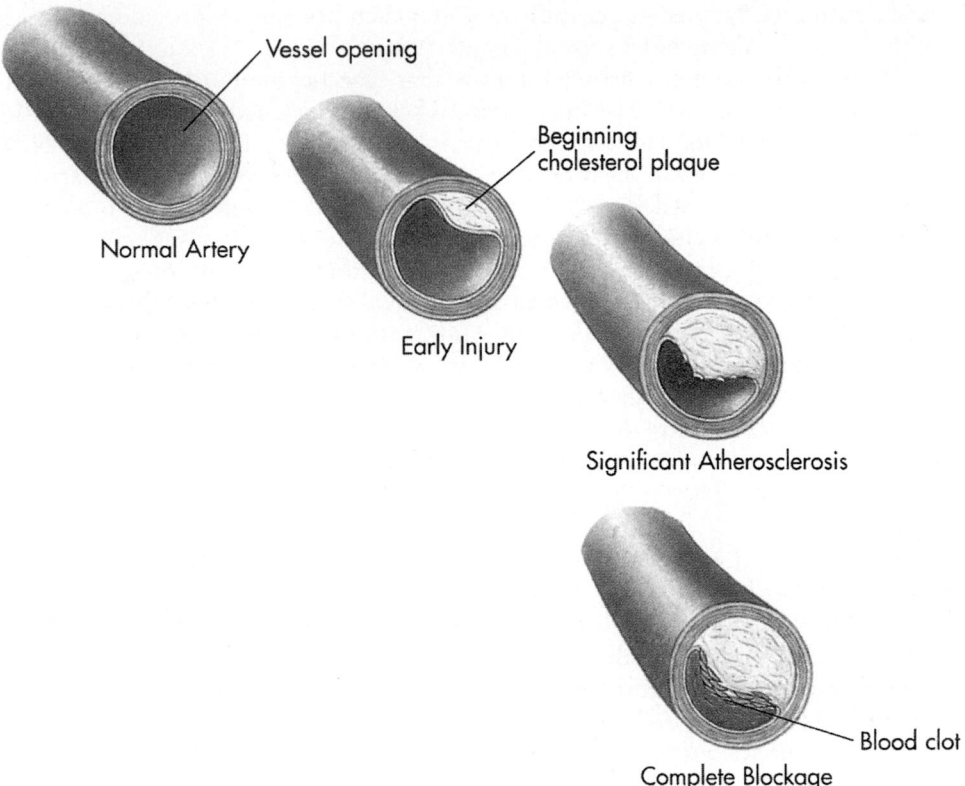

Fig. 5-7 Development of atherosclerosis.

Table 5-2 Cholesterol Content of Selected Foods*		
Food	Amount	Cholesterol (mg)
Milk, nonfat/skim	1 cup	4
Mayonnaise	1 Tbsp	8
Cottage cheese, lowfat/2%	1/2 cup	10
Milk, lowfat/2%	1 cup	18
Cream cheese	1 oz	28
Hot dog[†]	1	29
Ice cream, 10% fat	1/2 cup	30
Cheddar cheese	1 oz	30
Butter	1 Tbsp	31
Milk, whole	1 cup	33
Clams, fish fillets, oysters	3 oz	50-60
Beef,[†] pork[†], poultry	3 oz	70-85
Shrimp	3 oz	166
Egg yolk[†]	1	213
Beef liver	3 oz	410

*In ascending order.
[†]Leading contributors of cholesterol to US diet.

Another source of confusion is that cooking oils made from corn, safflower, and soybeans are often labeled as cholesterol free. Of course they are cholesterol free; only foods from animals contain cholesterol. Yet vegetable oils are virtually 100% food fat, and large amounts of dietary fat can also raise blood cholesterol.

In addition to the amount of fat, another characteristic of food fat that causes it to affect blood cholesterol differently is whether the fat is saturated or unsaturated. That is, whether the fat is mostly made of saturated or unsaturated fatty

We usually classify beef and chocolate as cholesterol-raising foods. Stearic acid is a major long chain saturated fatty acid in beef fat and cocoa butter (the fat that gives chocolate its appealing *mouth feel*). Stearic acid does not seem to raise blood cholesterol levels by itself (13), but because of other fatty acids in the beef and chocolate that do raise blood cholesterol, the entire food is assigned to the cholesterol raising category. Although growers are trying to manipulate animal feed, we can do little to alter the mixture of fatty acids in beef fat. However, we might seek chocolate products that are not made with added saturated fatty acids such as butter fat, coconut, and hydrogenated fats.

acids. Saturated fatty acids generally raise blood cholesterol by providing the liver with the best *building blocks* for making cholesterol.

A rule of thumb many people follow is that blood cholesterol is raised by eating solid saturated fats, lowered by unsaturated liquid fats, and not affected by monounsaturated fats. However, this rule is oversimplified for two reasons. First, food fats are a mixture of the three types. Second, although saturated fatty acids as a group raise cholesterol, some individual ones do not. Therefore even though we classify food fats as cholesterol raising (butter), cholesterol lowering (corn oil), or neutral (olive oil), these guidelines are based on the proportion of specific fatty acids in each food and how much each individual fatty acid affects blood cholesterol. The accompanying box clears up some confusion over the finer points of fat.

Researchers have studied individual fatty acids as well as combinations regarding their effects on blood cholesterol (12). We discuss these effects in the section on Fats as a Nutrient Within the Body.

Synthetic Fats and Fat Replacers

Many people dream about eating brownies and ice cream, magically stripped of fat, but still richly satisfying in taste and texture. Although surveys show that sugar substitutes have not reduced the amount of sugar we consume, optimists hope fat substitutes will reduce fat in our diets. Scientists are working to develop reduced-fat or fat-free substances that replace fat yet retain the taste and *mouth-feel* of fat in foods (14).

Fat replacers, as they are called, generally are classified two ways: already existing in nature or synthesized in the laboratory. The naturally occurring ones do not change chemically and thus require less rigorous testing before the Food and Drug Administration (FDA) allows them to be used in foods. One type is produced by heating and then blending protein from milk and/or eggs in a process called microparticulation. Simplesse is an example. Food applications include ice cream, frozen yogurt, and salad dressings, but not baked or deep-fried foods.

Carrageenan, a carbohydrate extracted from seaweed, has been used for centuries to thicken foods. Added to lean ground beef, carrageenan yields moist, juicy cooked meat with the texture of higher-fat beef. Similar gum-like products from

---

MYTH

No-Cholesterol Potato Chips Must Mean Fat Free!

Have you ever noticed how some food packages proclaim that the contents are cholesterol free? Often, this give us the impression that the products are reformulated to be healthier than their old version. We might then be tempted to buy the products. But are they really cholesterol free?

Many of us still associate dietary cholesterol with being our only lipid concern in foods. Fats tend to have a greater impact on health than dietary cholesterol. To be a savvy consumer, read ingredient labels and be aware of some finer points of *fat* education.

• Hydrogenated vegetable oils—corn, soybean, and cottonseed—are cholesterol-forming saturated fats often used to prepare potato and corn chips.

• Tropical oils of palm, palm kernel, and coconut are the only naturally saturated fat

plant source. Found in many food products, they should be consumed only occasionally. (Popcorn popped in tropical oils recently came under fire; many movie theater chains now offer air-popped popcorn in addition to traditionally prepared popcorn.)

• Margarines are cholesterol-free if made from vegetable oils, but still contain the same number of calories as butter; both are about 100% lipid. Margarines, however, contain unsaturated fatty acids. Note that the level of hydrogenation used to form the margarine affects the amount of saturated fatty acids contained. Use label information to select the least saturated product.

Advise clients to check the labels of foods regularly eaten; a cholesterol-free product might not be as healthy as it seems.

oats, corn, and potatoes are under development and would provide lower kcalorie fat-like properties in food.

Fat replacers made in the laboratory and not digested in the human body are being extensively tested. Olestra, a combination of sucrose and fatty acids, resembles standard fats and oils in many ways, including the ability to withstand frying and baking at high temperatures. The characteristics of Olestra are very attractive to manufacturers and consumers. These characteristics include the sensory properties of taste and texture, the no calorie value because of the body's inability to digest it, and the reduced absorption of fat and cholesterol from the intestine. The FDA has not yet approved Olestra for human consumption.

As the story of fat replacers continues to unfold we need to study their effect on people's food choices. Will we be mislead into thinking that low or no-fat foods automatically are low kcalorie? Many fat-reduced foods will increase the amounts of other ingredients, such as carbohydrates, and not result in low kcalorie items. Will use of reduced-fat, nonessential foods result in eating less balanced diets? And do we really know the long-term effects of eating fat replacers?

One of the objectives of *Healthy People* 2000 addresses the development of lower-fat food products:

> Increase to at least 5000 brand items the availability of processed food products that are reduced in fat and saturated fat (15).

Although replacers may play an important role in meeting this objective, the most prudent and health-promoting approach is for products to be reformulated or initially developed without the use of fat replacers so that products contain lower fat ingredients but still taste good. Research studies suggest that eating a low-fat diet can lead to a decrease in the preference for fat (16). Is it possible that fat replacers could undermine this healthful change? Nutritionists and scientists undoubtedly will continue to seek answers in order to make our fat-free brownie and ice cream dreams come true.

FATS AS A NUTRIENT WITHIN THE BODY

Digestion

Mouth

The mouth's only digestive process is mechanical, as teeth masticate fatty foods.

Stomach

Mechanical digestion continues through the strong actions of peristalsis. Fat-splitting enzymes (lingual lipase and gastric lipase) hydrolyze fatty acids from triglycerides.

Small intestine

Fats entering the duodenum initiate the release of cholecystokinin (CCK) hormone from the duodenum walls. CCK, as described in Chapter 3, then sparks the gallbladder to release bile into the small intestine. The bile emulsifies fats to facilitate digestion. Mechanical digestion through muscular action allows for increased exposure of the fat globules and pancreatic lipase. This enzyme is the primary digestive enzyme breaking triglycerides into fatty acids, monoglycerides, and glycerol molecules. Note that fats may not be completely broken down. Some may also pass through without being digested or absorbed (17). Fig. 5-8 summarizes digestion of triglycerides.

Triglycerides are composed of long chains of fatty acids; to aid fat digestion in those patients with malabsorption, synthetically manufactured medium chain triglycerides (MCT) may be incorporated into a patient's dietary intake. MCT may not completely replace dietary fats since they do not contain EFAs.

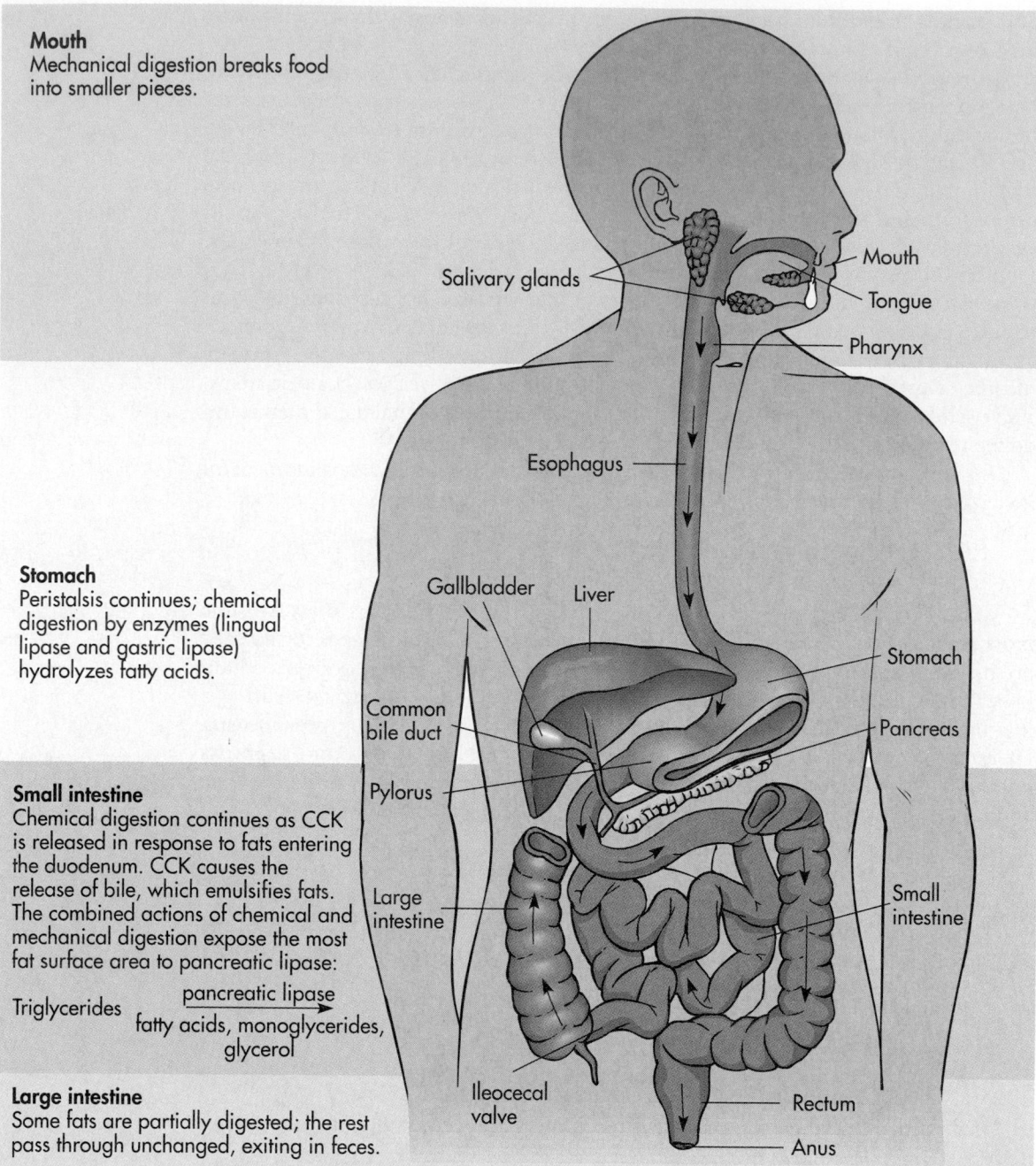

Mouth
Mechanical digestion breaks food into smaller pieces.

Stomach
Peristalsis continues; chemical digestion by enzymes (lingual lipase and gastric lipase) hydrolyzes fatty acids.

Small intestine
Chemical digestion continues as CCK is released in response to fats entering the duodenum. CCK causes the release of bile, which emulsifies fats. The combined actions of chemical and mechanical digestion expose the most fat surface area to pancreatic lipase:

Triglycerides $\xrightarrow{\text{pancreatic lipase}}$ fatty acids, monoglycerides, glycerol

Large intestine
Some fats are partially digested; the rest pass through unchanged, exiting in feces.

Salivary glands — Mouth
Tongue
Pharynx
Esophagus
Gallbladder   Liver
Stomach
Common bile duct
Pancreas
Pylorus
Large intestine
Small intestine
Ileocecal valve
Rectum
Anus

Fig. 5-8 Summary of fat digestion and absorption.

Absorption

Fatty acids, monoglycerides, and cholesterol are assisted by bile salts to move from the lumen to the villi for absorption. *Micelles,* created by bile salts encircling lipids, aid diffusion through the membrane wall. When through the membrane wall, fatty acids and glycerol combine back into triglycerides. These triglycerides are incorporated into **chylomicrons,** containing fats and cholesterol coated with protein, to allow travel through the lymph system to the blood circulatory system toward the hepatic portal system and the liver. Some glycerol and any short- and medium-chain fatty acids are absorbed directly into the blood capillaries leading to the portal vein and liver.

chylomicrons
the first lipoproteins formed after absorption of lipids from food

In the blood, the triglycerides in the chylomicrons are broken down into fatty acids and glycerol with assistance from an enzyme called lipoprotein lipase. Most of the fatty acids released by the breakdown of chylomicrons are taken up by muscle cells, adipose cells, and other cells in the vicinity (18). Cells can use the absorbed fatty acids immediately as fuel, or they can reform them into triglycerides to be stored as reserve energy supplies.

Metabolism

Lipid metabolism consists of several processes. Catabolism (breakdown) of lipids for energy involves the hydrolysis of triglycerides into two-carbon units that become part of **acetyl coenzyme A (acetyl CoA)**. The acetyl CoA then enters the series of reactions known as the **TCA cycle**, eventually leading to the oxidation of the carbon and hydrogen atoms derived from fatty acids (or carbohydrates or amino acids) to carbon dioxide and water with the release of energy as adenosine triphosphate (ATP) (19).

If fat catabolizes very quickly because of a lack of carbohydrate for energy, the liver cells form intermediate products called ketone bodies. These ketone bodies accumulate in the blood, causing a condition called **ketosis.**

Anabolism (synthesis) of lipids, or **lipogenesis,** results in the formation of triglycerides, phospholipids, cholesterol, and prostaglandins for use throughout the body. Triglycerides and phosphates form from fatty acids and glycerol or from excess glucose or amino acids; extra carbon, hydrogen, and oxygen from any source can be converted to and stored as triglycerides in adipose tissues, so we can gain fat from foods other than fat (17).

Lipid metabolism is regulated mainly by insulin, growth hormone, **adrenocorticotropic hormone (ACTH)**, and **glucocorticoids** (17).

OVERCOMING BARRIERS

Health concerns about our dietary fat intake fall into several categories: energy intake, reduced intake of other nutrients because of dietary fat consumption, and the relationship between dietary fat intake and diet-related diseases.

Energy Intake

Foods that contain significant amounts of dietary fat will naturally provide more kcalories than other lower-fat foods. Although high-fat treats are fine occasionally, indulging too often or not even realizing which foods are fat-laden, can result in consumption of too many kcalories. These kcalories may end up stored as body fat in adipose tissues.

Fat is even more efficient at being stored than is carbohydrate or protein, which means that we may gain more body fat eating fat kcalories than eating the same number of carbohydrate kcalories (20). The evidence for this comes from studying people who eat low-fat, but high-kcalorie diets as discussed earlier. A likely explanation for this is that the energy cost to convert dietary fat to body fat requires only 3% of the calories consumed; carbohydrate requires 23% of the energy consumed to be converted to body fat. For many individuals struggling with moderate or even excessive weight, awareness of their dietary fat intake sources can make a difference. By gradually reducing fat intake, energy intake lessens and weight maintenance becomes easier to achieve.

acetyl coenzyme A
important intermediate byproduct in metabolism formed from the breakdown of glucose, fatty acids, and certain amino acids

TCA cycle
cellular reactions that liberate energy from fragments of carbohydrates, fats, and protein; also known as the tricarboxylic acid cycle or Krebs cycle

ketosis
a condition in which the absence of plasma glucose results in partial oxidation of fatty acids

lipogenesis
anabolism (synthesis) of lipids

adrenocorticotropic hormone (ACTH)
an adrenal cortex hormone that stimulates secretion of more hormones

glucocorticoid
an adrenal cortex hormone that affects food metabolism

Extreme Dietary Fat Restrictions

Dietary intake of fat can also get too low. Although general population recommendations are for fat consumption to be 30% or less of our kcalorie intake, Dr. Dean Ornish developed a regimen to reverse coronary artery disease that is based on a dietary fat intake of 10% or less of kcaloric intake. An intake this low, based on a primarily vegetarian dietary pattern, may be difficult for most Americans to maintain; adequate intake of EFAs must also be provided. Most Americans who are at risk for coronary artery disease would most likely achieve beneficial results at 20% dietary fat kcaloric intake.

Our health warnings about fat intake can also be taken too seriously and interpreted too intensely, creating health hazards through the life span. Infants and young children depend on dietary fats and cholesterol for the formation of brain and nerve tissue. Cases of failure to thrive have been reported when parents restricted the intake of dietary fats by their infants (21). Dietary fats should not be restricted for children under 2 years of age. After that, a prudent diet with recommended levels of fats can be followed. Persons afflicted with the eating disorder of anorexia nervosa envision their bodies as being fat and, even though they are emaciated, often focus on their dietary fat consumption. They may reduce dietary fat intake to dangerously low levels through the erroneous belief that fat consumption at any kcaloric level would make them fat. Among the elderly, fear of dietary fat and cholesterol may cause malnutrition. Some have become so focused on the potential negative effects of cholesterol on the health of their hearts that their food intake is overly restrictive of all nutrients. Although our dietary fat and cholesterol intake impacts the course of coronary artery disease, it is most potent during the early and middle years of adulthood, rather than in the later years of life.

Reduced Intake of Other Nutrients

Even if dietary fat consumption does not result in weight gain, foods high in fat tend not to contain much dietary fiber and may be low in other nutrients. Not consuming enough dietary fiber, as noted in Chapter 4, is a risk factor for several chronic conditions. The seductive nature of foods containing fats may lead us to crave these foods and neglect others. The best guarantee toward achieving the goal of nutritional wellness is to consume a balanced intake of nutrients, based on recommended guidelines, through consumption of at least five to seven servings of naturally low-fat fruits and vegetables per day.

Dietary Fat Intake and Diet-related Diseases

Too much fat in the American diet is directly related to several chronic diseases such as coronary artery disease and certain types of cancer. High-fat diets are indirectly related to NIDDM and hypertension. Health guidelines to prevent and treat these diseases call for less dietary fat than average Americans eat. *Diet and Health* daily recommendations are to eat a total fat intake of 30% or less of kcalories, saturated fatty acid less than 10% of kcalories, and less than 300 mg cholesterol. U.S. surveys indicate we actually eat daily 37% of kcalories as total fat, 14% as saturated fat, and about 370 mg of cholesterol (2). Consider how this affects our risk for these diet-related diseases.

Coronary artery disease

The relationship between coronary artery disease and dietary fat intake, particularly of saturated fats, seems strong. Based on the effects of saturated fat and cholesterol intake on blood cholesterol levels, a high-fat diet is a risk factor for the development of coronary artery disease.

Compared with recommended guidelines (see Table 19-1), over 50% of Americans have high or borderline high blood cholesterol levels. An elevated blood cholesterol count is considered a signal for risk of coronary artery disease and a potential heart attack, especially when the ratio of LDL to HDL is high. We also have good evidence that eating lots of saturated fat is related to high blood cholesterol and, conversely, eating mostly monounsaturated fats is related to low blood cholesterol and low rate of heart disease deaths (22). Yet, what exactly is the connection between saturated fat and heart disease?

The suggested steps in the theory linking saturated fat to heart disease go like this. First, large amounts of saturated fat produce more LDL to circulate in the blood. Second, the cholesterol carried in the LDL is more likely to be attacked by oxygen, which in turn attracts big scavenger cells called **macrophages.** Third, the macrophages consume the oxidized material that accumulates in a modified form, called foam cells. Fourth, the foam cells cluster under the lining of the artery wall forming bulges that cause fatty streaks, which is the first event in plaque formation. Finally, the foam cells produce chemicals that further damage and cause changes that produce artery clogging plaque. Saturated fat started the whole thing off by requiring too many LDL *buses* to carry it around. To reduce the amount of LDL, we should eat less saturated fat. If we eat more saturated fat than we need, the gradual buildup of plaque as atherosclerosis is likely to follow. Also, some people seem to be more disposed than others to this series of events leading to atherosclerosis.

macrophages
cells that are able to surround, engulf, and digest micro-organisms and cellular debris; big scavenger cells

Geneticists have claimed discovery of a gene they say could account for the characteristics of what is called an *atherogenic profile,* which describes an estimated 30% of the U.S. population. These characteristics include upper-body obesity, low concentration of HDL, and a preponderance of LDL fatty compounds in the blood (23). This finding suggests that some people may indeed be predisposed to atherosclerosis and heart disease.

Since we cannot control our heredity, the main goal for all, regardless of genes, is prevention to lower the risk factors for atherosclerosis and heart disease that are under our control. High blood cholesterol, especially LDL cholesterol, is one risk factor that can be affected by diet, mainly by reducing total fat intake and particularly saturated fatty acids. Blood cholesterol level is just one of several risk factors. Other widely known risk factors are cigarette smoking, sedentary lifestyle, stress, overweight, alcohol consumption, and hypertension. Experts stress the importance of reducing each risk factor to prevent or reduce the symptoms of heart disease.

Cancer

An association may also exist between high dietary fat consumption and increased risk for a variety of cancers including colon and prostate cancer. It may be that diets high in fat and low in fruits and vegetables limit the body's ability to prevent cancer cell formation. Is fat a cancer promoter? Or do substances in fruits and vegetables such as antioxidants protect cells from cancerous mutations?

In spite of evidence from both Japan and China that low-fat diets appear to be related to a low incidence of breast cancer, a large and well-designed study of 89,000 American women found no evidence that a diet low in fat or high in fiber protects against breast cancer (24). Research will continue to seek answers to the potential link between dietary fat intake and breast cancer.

NIDDM and hypertension

NIDDM and hypertension are indirectly related to dietary fat intake. Both of these disorders may stress the circulatory system; a high dietary fat intake may further limit the functioning of the circulatory system through the potential development of atherosclerosis. Also, these disorders are managed better when weight moderation is achieved; dietary fat reduction may enhance this process.

Medical nutritional therapy for these disorders is detailed in Chapters 19, 20, and 22.

TOWARD A POSITIVE NUTRITION LIFESTYLE: GRADUAL REDUCTION

It's the subject of television situation comedies. One member of the family becomes a health food fanatic, serving blades of grass, sprouts, and weird mixtures of soybeans, nuts and who knows what. And what is the immediate response of the sitcom family? Disgust and rebellion, of course.

As we make recommendations to our clients to reduce their fat intake (and perhaps for ourselves and our families, too), consider that often the most effective way to achieve permanent change is through gradual reduction. That's the mistake made by the TV character, too many changes too quickly.

An action plan for gradual reduction of dietary fat intake could include the following:

1. For one week, record all food and beverages consumed.
2. Based on reading this chapter, assess which foods are likely to be high fat. Particularly note if one high-fat food item, such as whole milk, is consumed often or if a certain meal or snack regularly includes fatty foods. Perhaps scrambled eggs and bacon are eaten almost every morning for breakfast, and an afternoon coffee break always includes either a sweet Danish pastry or a huge, buttery muffin.
3. The next week choose one item and either reduce consumption or replace it with a lower-fat substitute. Instead of whole milk, use 2% or 1% fat milk, or replace the coffee break treat with an English muffin with a bit of butter or margarine and jelly.
4. The following week, select another food item or meal and make a simple substitution.

This process can continue with small changes—gradual reductions—resulting in major reductions in dietary fat intake.

WELLNESS AND FATS

Physical Dimension	Consuming dietary fats is necessary for essential fatty acids, for energy, and for fat-soluble vitamins. Excessive intake may increase risk of obesity and diet-related diseases.
Intellectual Dimension	As research continues on the role of dietary fats in health and disease, intellectual skills are necessary to assess the type of dietary fat modification most appropriate for our personal and client health needs.
Emotional Dimension	How we emotionally approach nutritional lifestyle change for ourselves and our clients to decrease fat intake, possibly restricting consumption of favorite foods, affects success. Can these emotions be expressed or are changes simply disregarded because they make us feel uncomfortable?
Social Dimension	Are relationships of family and friends based on sharing high-fat meals? Can you or your clients refuse to take part without jeopardizing relationships or making others feel defensive? Can food preparation suggestions to lower fat content be made without seeming overly critical?

SUMMARY

L ipids include fats and fat-related substances that are divided into three classifications. About 95% of the lipids in foods and in our bodies is in the form of fat as triglycerides, the largest class of lipids. The other two lipid classifications are the fat-related substances of phospholipids and sterols. Lecithin is the best known phospholipid; cholesterol is the best known sterol. All are organic, composed of carbon, hydrogen, and oxygen, and cannot dissolve in water.

Functions of lipids fall into two categories: food value and physiological purposes in the body. Food value functions include that fat is the most dense form of stored energy in both food and in our bodies. Foods containing fat smell and taste good and provide satiety. Fat-soluble nutrients—vitamins A, D, E, K, and linoleic and linolenic fatty acids, the essential fatty acids—are available through foods. Physiological functions include that stored fat provides a backup energy supply, cushions body organs, and serves to regulate body temperature.

Phospholipids are part of body cell membrane structure and serve as emulsifiers. Cholesterol, a sterol, has a role in the formation of bile, vitamin D, sex hormones, and cells in brain and nerve tissue.

Triglycerides are compounds made of three fatty acids and one glycerol molecule. The fatty acids may be saturated, monounsaturated, or polyunsaturated depending on their number of double bonds. Phospholipids are similar to triglycerides except they have only two fatty acids; the third spot contains a phosphate group. Sterol structures, including cholesterol, are carbon rings intermeshed with side chains of carbon, hydrogen, and oxygen. All three types of lipids can be manufactured in our bodies. The only exceptions are two fatty acids, linolenic and linoleic fatty acids, found in triglycerides; these cannot be formed by the body and are essential nutrients.

Digestion of lipids occurs mainly in the small intestine; absorption depends on the transportation of lipids through the lymph and blood circulatory systems. Lipids travel through the body in lipoprotein packages containing triglycerides, protein, phospholipids, and cholesterol, but differ according to the proportions or ratio of these ingredients. Low density lipoproteins (LDLs) and high density lipoproteins (HDLs) are found in the blood. Containing cholesterol, their levels may serve as medical markers of one of the risks of coronary artery disease.

Health concerns about our dietary fat intake fall into several categories including appropriate energy intake, reduced intake of other nutrients because of excessive dietary fat consumption, and the relationship between dietary fat intake and diet-related diseases.

THE NURSING ROLE
Critical Thinking and the Nursing Process

To arrive at thorough and accurate assessments, nursing diagnoses, and goals, you must apply critical thinking skills. That means you must analyze information, evaluate your assumptions, identify patients' misconceptions, and use logical thought processes to determine cause and effect relationships.

Bring your critical thinking skills to bear on the following situations and questions and, if necessary, go back into the chapter to find clues to the answers.

1. A patient tells you she has lowered fat intake in her diet by switching from beef to chicken. What else would you have to ask this patient before accepting her conclusion that she has lowered fat intake?

Continued.

THE NURSING ROLE, cont'd.
Critical Thinking and the Nursing Process

2. A friend complains that although he eats *a lot*, he is always *starving* between meals. What might account for that?

3. A man who has heart disease tells you that he has *clogged arteries* in his heart. He says if he can reduce his cholesterol intake he knows he can get the problem under control. Is he correct? Why or why not?

4. What would happen to a child who ingested well below the recommended daily amount of fat?

5. A teenager thinks that just drinking skim milk instead of whole milk is adequate fat control for her age. Is this a true assumption?

6. Is it possible to eat fats that contain only high-density lipoproteins?

7. Is reducing sugar and carbohydrates in your diet the most efficient way to reduce calories?

8. The wife of a patient with diabetes tells you that she has adhered to cooking a low-fat diet for her husband by trimming external fat from meat and serving skim milk. What other assessments would you have to make to decide if her husband's fat intake is appropriate?

REFERENCES

1. Linsheer WG, Vergroesen AJ: Lipids. In Shils ME, Olson JA, Shike M, eds: *Modern nutrition in health and disease,* ed 8, Philadelphia, 1994, Lea & Febiger.

2. Woteki CE, Thomas PR, eds: *Eat for life,* Washington, DC, 1992, National Academy of Sciences.

3. Harris WS: Fish oils and plasma lipid and lipoprotein metabolism in humans: A critical review, *J Lipid Res* 30:785-807, 1989.

4. Food and Nutrition Board, National Research Council: *Diet and health: Implications for reducing chronic disease risk,* Washington, DC, 1989, National Academy Press.

5. Junshi C et al: *Diet, lifestyle, and mortality in China,* Oxford, United Kingdom, 1990, Oxford University Press.

6. Varela G, Moreiras O: Mediterranean diet, *Cardiovascular Risk Factors* 1:313-321, 1991.

7. Block G et al: Nutrient sources in the American diet: Quantitative data from the NHANES II survey, *Am J Epidemiol* 122:27-40, 1985.

8. Shattuck AL, White E, Kristal AR: How women's adopted low-fat diets affect their husbands, *Am J Public Health* 82:1244-1250, 1992.

9. Williams SR: *Essentials of nutrition and diet therapy,* ed 6, St. Louis, 1994, Mosby.

10. Hegsted DM, Ausman LM, Johnson JA: Dietary fat and serum lipids: An evaluation of the experimental data, *Am J Clin Nutr* 57:875-883, 1993.

11. Grundy SM, Denke MA: Dietary influences on serum lipids and lipoproteins, *Lipid Res* 31:1149-1172, 1990.

12. Menskink RP, Katan KB: Effect of dietary fatty acids on serum lipids and lipoproteins: A meta-analysis of 27 trials, *Arterioscler Thromb Vasc Biol* 12:911-916, 1992.

13. Menskink RP: Effects of the individual saturated fatty acids on serum lipids and lipoprotein concentration, *Am J Clin Nutr* 57(suppl):711S-715S, 1993.

14. Position of the American Dietetic Association: Fat replacements, *J Am Diet Assoc* 91:1285-1288, 1991.

15. US Department Health and Human Services, Public Health Service: *Healthy people 2000: National health promotion and disease prevention objectives,* Washington, DC, 1990, US Government Printing Office.

16. Rolls BJ, Shide DJ: The influence of dietary fat on food intake and body weight, *Nutr Rev* 50:283-290, 1992.

17. Thibodeau GA, Patton KT: *Anatomy & physiology,* ed 2, St. Louis, 1993, Mosby.

18. Murray RK et al: *Harper's biochemistry,* ed 22, Norwalk, Conn, 1993, Appleton & Lange.
19. Guthrie HA, Picciano MF: *Human nutrition,* St. Louis, 1995, Mosby.
20. Bennet C: Short-term effects of dietary fat ingestion on energy expenditure and nutrient balance, *Am J Clin Nutr* 55:1071-1077, 1992.
21. Pugliese MT et al: Parental health beliefs as a cause of failure to thrive, *Pediatrics* 80(2):175-181 Aug 87.
22. National Institutes of Health: *NIH consensus statement: Triglyceride, high density lipoprotein and coronary heart disease,* Washington, DC, 1992.
23. Nishina PM et al: Linkage of atherogenic lipoprotein phenotype to the low density lipoprotein receptor locus on the short arum of chromosome 19, *Proceedings of the National Academy of Sciences, USA* 89:708-712,1992.
24. Willet WC et al: Dietary fat and fiber in relation to risk of breast cancer, JAMA 268:2037-2044, 1992.

Chapter 6

PROTEIN

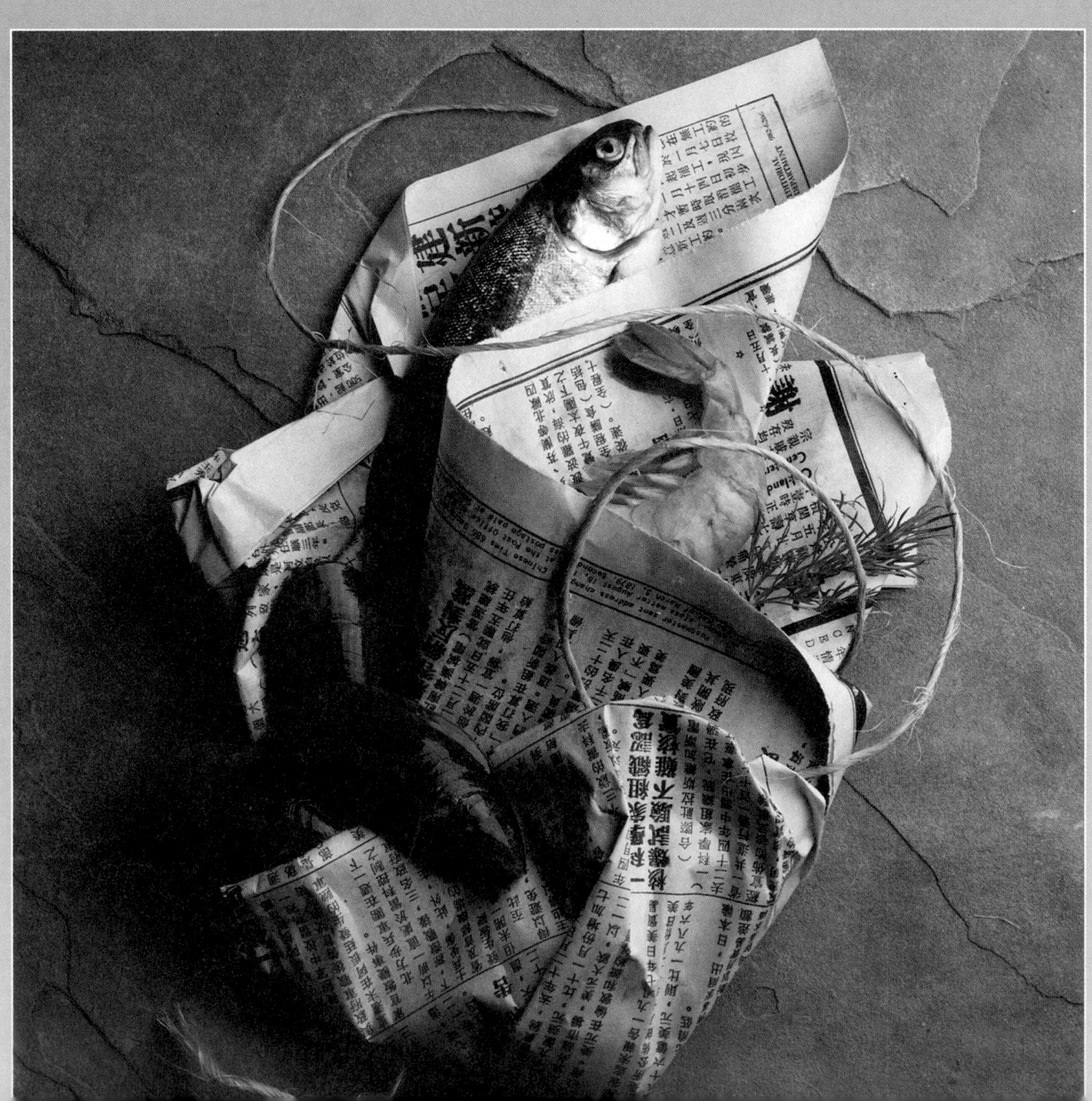

ROLE IN WELLNESS

"A chicken in every pot!" was the campaign motto used by Republican candidates during the 1928 elections. At that time, being able to afford animal protein on a daily basis was the mark of a high standard of living and an assurance of good health. Today the motto might be "rice and beans for us all!" We now know that there are many sources of protein available in our food supply. Some offer advantages over others by being lower in fat and higher in other nutrients such as complex carbohydrates and fiber.

Protein in food is our only source of amino acids, which are absolutely necessary to make the thousands of proteins that form every aspect of the human body. No wonder protein, which is plentiful in our food supply, has gained the status of a *super* nutrient for Americans. We expect that the more protein we eat, the stronger our immune system will be, the less we will weigh, and the more muscles we will develop.

Although proteins formed by our bodies do have a role in those functions, the amounts we consume are often greater than we need. Awareness of protein sources and portion sizes is important as we work toward achieving health promotion goals to decrease our risk of diet-related diseases (Fig. 6-1).

STRUCTURE OF PROTEIN

Proteins are formed by the linking of many smaller molecules of amino acids. **Amino acids,** like glucose, are organic compounds made of carbon, hydrogen, and oxygen. However, amino acids also contain nitrogen, which clearly distinguishes protein from other nutrients.

There are 20 amino acids from which all proteins are made that are required by both plants and animals. The human body is able to manufacture some of the amino acids for its own protein-building function, but nine amino acids cannot be made by the cells of the body. Therefore these **essential amino acids** must be eaten in food, digested, absorbed, and then brought to cells by circulating blood. The other 11 are **nonessential amino acids (NEAA)** (Table 6-1). They can be created by the liver as long as structural components, including nitrogen, from other amino acids are available to use for NEAA formation.

Each cell constructs or synthesizes the proteins it needs. In order to build proteins, the cell must have access to all 20 amino acids. This available supply of amino acids is in the metabolic amino acid pool. The **amino acid pool** is a warehouse that is constantly resupplied with essential (from dietary intake) and nonessential (synthesized in the liver) amino acids. It allows the cell to build proteins easily.

Protein Composition

The functions of proteins are closely related to their structures. The complex composition of proteins is best understood through four structural levels: primary, secondary, tertiary, and quaternary (1) (Fig. 6-2).

The primary structure of protein composition is determined by the number, assortment, and sequence of amino acids in polypeptide chains. Amino acids are linked together by peptide bonds to form a practically unlimited number of proteins. The peptide bond occurs at the point at which the carboxyl group of one amino acid is bound to the amino group of another amino acid. The 20 amino acids form chains that may contain any combination or assortment of amino acids. This allows for thousands of different proteins to be formed. Two proteins may

---

proteins
organic compounds formed from chains of amino acids

amino acids
organic compounds containing carbon, hydrogen, oxygen, and nitrogen

essential amino acids
amino acids that cannot be manufactured by the human body

nonessential amino acids (NEAA)
amino acids manufactured by the human body

amino acid pool
the assortment of amino acids available to cells

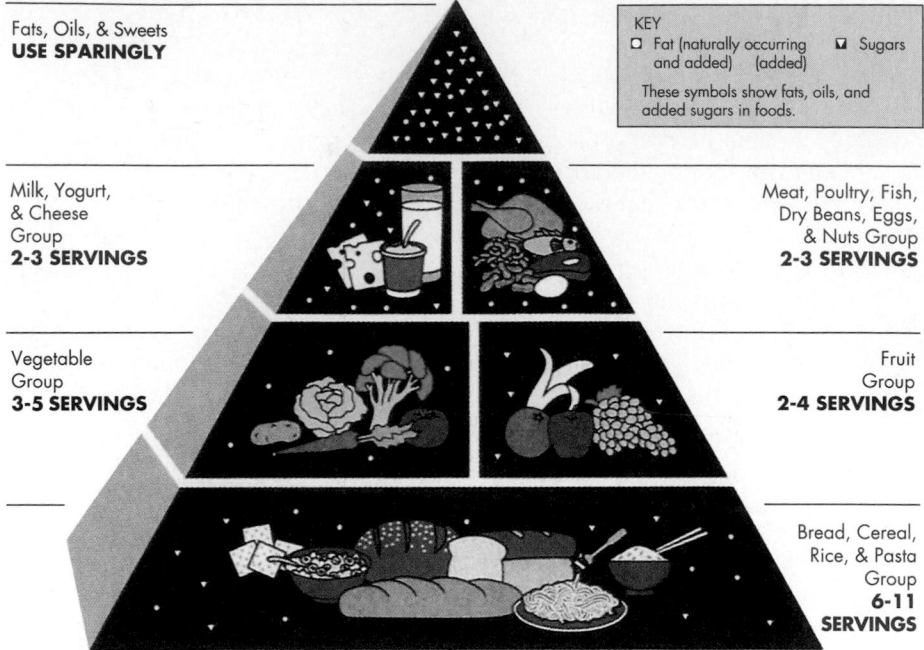

Fig. 6-1 The Food Guide Pyramid, highlighting major sources of protein.

Table 6-1 Amino Acids	
Essential Amino Acids	**Nonessential Amino Acids**
histidine	alanine
isoleucine	arginine
leucine	aspartic acid
lysine	cysteine
methionine	cystine
phenylalanine	glutamic acid
threonine	glutamine
tryptophan	glycine
valine	proline
	serine
	tyrosine

contain the same assortment and number of amino acids yet still have different functions because of the sequencing or order of the amino acids.

The secondary structure level of proteins affects the shape of the chain of amino acids; they may be straight, folded, or coiled. The tertiary structure results when the polypeptide chain is so coiled that the loops of the coil touch, forming strong bonds within the chain itself. The quaternary structural level is proteins containing more than one polypeptide chain.

If the structure of a protein changes, the protein may not be able to perform its original function. The shape may be changed by heat (cooking), ultraviolet light (exposure to sunlight), acids (vinegar), and alcohol. When the shape of a protein is affected (such as a folded chain unfolding), the protein has been **denatured** and has been physically changed.

denatured

a change in the shape of protein structures due to heat, light, acids, or alcohol

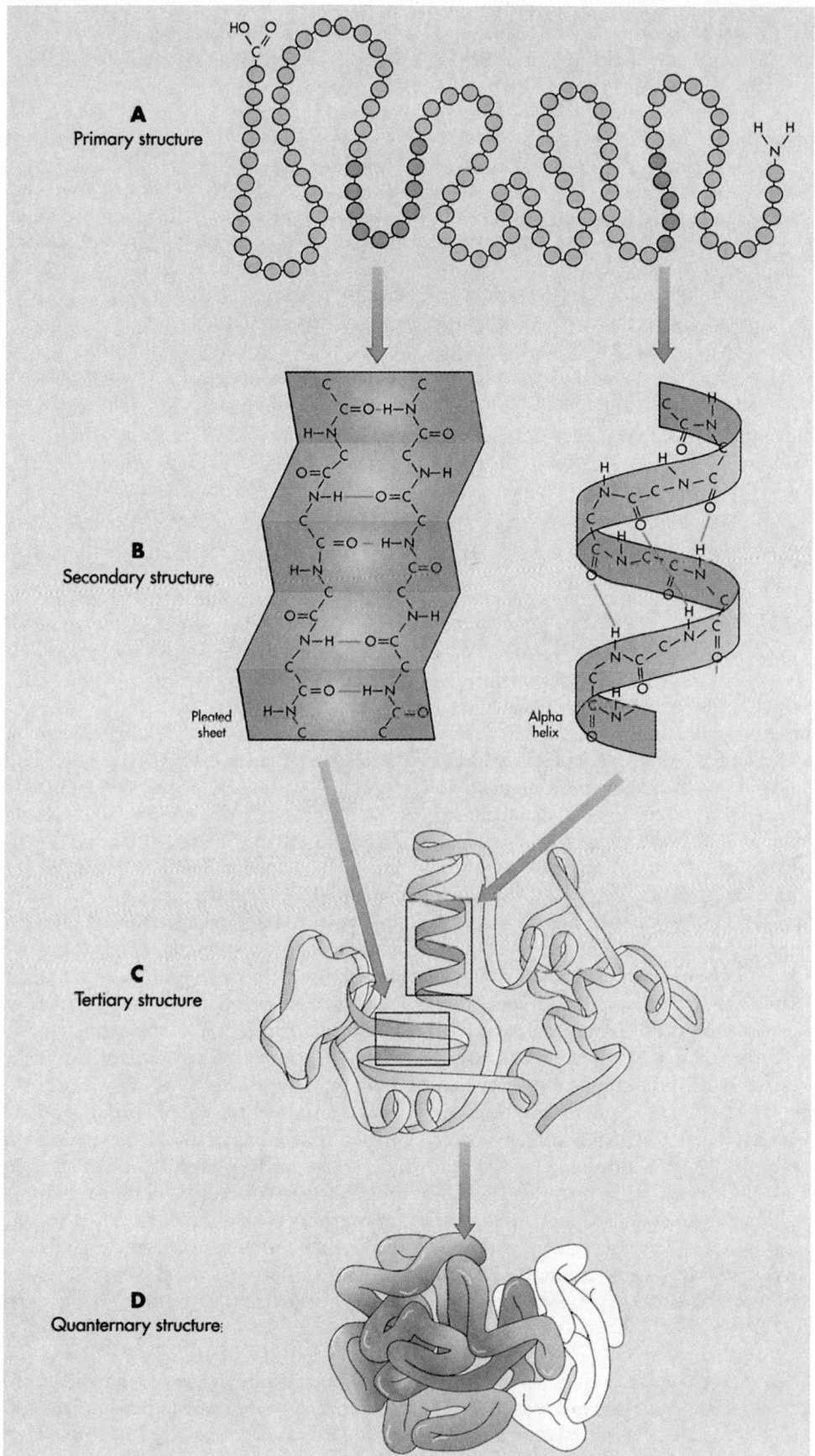

Fig. 6-2 Structural levels of protein. **A,** Primary structure: determined by number, kind, and sequence of amino acids in the chain; **B,** Secondary structure: hydrogen bonds stabilize folds of helical spirals; **C,** Tertiary structure: globular shape maintained by strong intramolecular bonding and by stabilizing hydrogen bonds; **D,** Quaternary structure: results from bonding between more than one polypeptide unit.

An example of denaturing a food protein is the change that occurs when the white of an uncooked egg (a clear liquid) is beaten. The clear liquid turns white, foamy, and stiff. The protein in the egg has been denatured; however, it is still a valuable source of amino acids. The amino acids are not affected, only the shape of the chain has been changed.

Inside the body, denaturing of proteins is controlled by mechanisms that keep the internal body environment from getting too basic or too acidic. Either extreme can lead to the denaturation of vital proteins within the body. Body temperature also affects the protein structure of the body. High fevers can become lethal as protein structures within the body become denatured. When body proteins are denatured, they cannot perform their original functions.

Although uncontrolled denaturation can be dangerous, it is helpful for digestion. Denaturing changes the three-dimensional structure of a protein, providing more surface area on which digestive juices act to release the amino acids of the food proteins.

FUNCTIONS

roteins created in our bodies perform numerous functions, including the following:

- Growth and maintenance
- Creation of communicators and catalysts
- Immune system response
- Fluid regulation
- Acid-base balance
- Transportation

Growth and Maintenance

Each body cell contains proteins. All growth depends on a sufficient supply of amino acids. The amino acids are needed to make the proteins required to support muscle, tissue, and bone formation.

Maintaining our bodies also requires a constant supply of amino acids. There is a continual turnover of body cells, which are composed of protein. The cells break down and must immediately be replaced. Each replacement cell requires the formation of additional protein.

Also needed for growth and maintenance is the protein collagen, found throughout the body. Collagen forms connective tissues such as ligaments and tendons and acts as a glue to keep the walls of the arteries intact. In addition, collagen has a role in bone and tooth formation. First, collagen forms a framework structure that is then filled with minerals such as calcium and phosphorus. Synthesis of scar tissue also depends on collagen. Other structures such as hair, nails, and skin are composed of similar protein substances.

Creation of Communicators and Catalysts

Many vital substances produced by our bodies are formed of protein. Some hormones are proteins. Hormones act as communicators to alert different parts of the body of changes or to regulate functions of organs. Insulin, a hormone that directs cells to take in glucose, is a protein. Enzymes are also proteins. When necessary, enzymes are catalysts that trigger chemical reactions or biological changes to occur within the body. Each enzyme has a specific target; consequently, numerous enzymes continually are being formed.

Blood clotting depends on protein substances as well. Twelve factors must be in place for blood to clot when injury has occurred; several of the factors, such as fibrogen, are composed of protein.

Immune System Response

The defense system of our bodies depends on proteins produced in response to foreign virus and bacteria that invade our bodies. The proteins, or antibodies, are specific to each intruder. If sufficient levels of amino acids are not available to form these antibodies, we may have difficulties maintaining our health. Our overall immunological response, our resistance to disease, depends on proteins formed within our bodies.

Fluid Regulation

Water is balanced among three compartments in the body: intravascular (within veins and arteries), intracellular (inside cells), and interstitial (between cells). Proteins and minerals attract water, creating osmotic pressure. As proteins circulate through our bodies, they maintain body fluid balance by keeping water appropriately divided among the three compartments.

Acid-Base Balance

Some reactions occurring within the body lead to the release of acidic substances; others cause basic matter to enter the fluids of the body. Because the chemical structure of amino acids combines an acid (the carboxyl group [COOH]) and base (amine), an amino acid can function either as an acid or base depending on the pH of the medium it is in. This means that proteins can buffer the effects of fluids to maintain a safe acidic level in body fluids. The ability of protein to regulate the balance between the acidic and base characteristics of fluids is called the *buffering effect* of protein. This function is crucial to protect all proteins in the body. If fluids become either too acidic or too basic, the shape of proteins is altered or denatured. Denatured proteins are not able to perform their usual functions.

Consider that many of the constituents of blood are protein based. If their functions are affected, the result can be lethal. Instead, proteins maintain a delicate pH level to assure the proper functioning of all body systems.

Transportation

Proteins are able to transport nutrients and other vital substances throughout our bodies. For individual cells, proteins act as *pumps,* assisting the movement of nutrients in and out of cells. Nutrients, including lipids, minerals, and vitamins, are carried by proteins such as lipoproteins in blood, which allows the nutrients to be available to all parts of the body. Hemoglobin, a special carrier composed of protein, transports oxygen in blood. Oxygen is stored in our muscles in another protein carrier, myoglobin. These protein barriers, hemoglobin and myoglobin, are essential for a well-functioning body.

FOOD SOURCES

Quality of Protein Foods

The proteins in foods are categorized by the essential amino acids they contain. **Complete protein** contains all nine essential amino acids in quantities that best

complete proteins
proteins containing all nine essential amino acids

Table 6-2	Sources of Complete and Incomplete Proteins
Foods Containing Complete Proteins	Foods Containing Incomplete Proteins
fish	cereals
shellfish	ready-to-eat
chicken	oatmeal
turkey	wheatena
duck*	grains
beef*	wheat
lamb*	rice
pork*	corn
eggs*	oats/oatmeal
soybeans (tofu)	barley
cheese	spaghetti/pasta
hard cheeses*	bagels
cheddar	bread
Muenster	legumes
Swiss cheese	black-eyed peas
soft cheeses	lentils
cottage cheese†	beans
ricotta†	peanuts/peanut butter
milk†	chick peas
ice milk/reduced fat ice cream	split peas
yogurt†	broccoli
frozen yogurt	potatoes
	green peas
	leafy green vegetables

*Possible high-fat source of protein.
†Protein in skim, 2%, and whole milk products.

support growth and maintenance of our bodies. Animal-related foods, including meat, poultry, fish, eggs, and most dairy products contain complete protein. Soybeans are the only plant source that provide all nine essential amino acids. Foods that contribute the best balance of essential amino acids and the best assortment of nonessential amino acids for protein synthesis are **high quality protein** foods. The two highest quality protein foods are eggs and human milk. The egg is of high quality since it contains all the necessary nutrients to support life. Human breast milk is the perfect food; its nutrient profile is ideal for human growth.

Incomplete protein lacks one or more of the nine essential amino acids. These proteins will not provide a sufficient supply of amino acids and will not support life (Table 6-2). Many plant foods contain considerable amounts of incomplete proteins. Some of the better sources are grains and legumes.

The essential amino acids that incomplete proteins lack are referred to as **limiting amino acids.** The limiting amino acid reduces the value of the protein contained in the food. Unless the limiting amino acid is consumed in other foods, the amino acid pools inside the cells would be missing some of the essential amino acids. Protein production within the cell would be affected, and fewer proteins could be formed. Consequently, limiting amino acids reduces the number of proteins that can be made by our bodies. Generally, we consume a sufficient mix of complete and incomplete proteins, so this is not a health problem. Only those who adopt a dietary pattern restricting certain types of protein foods are at risk for an imbalanced intake.

high quality protein
a food containing the best balance and assortment of essential and nonessential amino acids for protein synthesis

incomplete proteins
proteins lacking one or more of the essential amino acids

limiting amino acid
the essential amino acid or amino acids that incomplete proteins lack

Table 6-3   Food Combinations That Provide Complete Proteins

Grains + Legumes = Complete Protein	Grains or Legumes + Animal Protein (small amount) = Complete Protein
Examples	**Examples**
peanut butter sandwich	chili with beans and cornbread
tacos with refried beans	ready-to-eat cereal with skim milk
rice and beans	cheese sandwich
split pea soup with croutons	pasta with cheese
falafel (chick-pea balls) on pita bread	rice pudding
lentil soup with rye bread	French toast
baked beans with bread	pancakes (made with milk and/or eggs)
	tuna casserole

Complementary Proteins

By eating different kinds of plant foods throughout the day, the total protein intake will equal that of complete proteins found in animal-related products. The advantages to complementing proteins are that plant foods cost less and tend to contain less fat; consuming less dietary fat is a prevention strategy for several chronic diet-related diseases.

A balance of amino acids is required throughout the day for protein synthesis. A sufficient assortment of essential amino acids is provided without planning if both animal and plant protein foods are eaten. If animal foods are not eaten, more care is required to assure that limiting amino acids are consumed. Combinations of plant foods that provide all the essential amino acids are grains (such as wheat or rice) with legumes (such as kidney beans or chick peas), and grains or legumes with small amounts of animal protein from dairy, meat, poultry, or fish (Table 6-3).

Measures of Food Protein Quality

Many foods contain protein, however, the value of specific foods as protein sources varies. Perhaps the protein contained is incomplete or is difficult to digest (bound tightly to fiber). If food proteins are not digested, the amino acids can't be absorbed to nourish our bodies.

Several methods are used to analyze the quality of proteins in food, including biological value and protein efficiency ratio. **Biological value** measures how much nitrogen from a protein food is retained by the body after digestion, absorption, and excretion. This measurement of nitrogen balance reveals how available the protein of that food is to the human body. An egg has the highest reference protein score of 100; all of the egg protein can be used. It has become a standard against which all other food proteins are judged. Fish has a score of 75 to 90, and corn, which contains protein but also has lower amino acid ratios, has a score of 40 (2).

The other method for assessing protein quality is **protein efficiency ratio (PER)**. Using this method, rats are fed a set amount of protein and then, based on weight gain, the physiological value of the food protein consumed is determined (2). The FDA uses this process to determine protein levels listed on food labels.

$$PER = \frac{\text{Weight gain}}{\text{Protein intake}}$$

biological value
a method to determine the quality of food protein by measuring the amount of nitrogen kept in the body after digestion and absorption

protein efficiency ratio (PER)
a method to determine the quality of food protein by comparing weight gain to protein intake

Protein RDA

The RDA for protein provides for sufficient intake of the essential amino acids and enough total protein to provide the amino groups needed to build new NEAAs. Other factors that affect the RDA for protein are age, gender, physiological state, and sources of protein (3).

TEACHING TOOL
Calculating Your Recommended Protein Intake

To determine your personal protein recommendation:

1. Divide your body weight by 2.2 to determine your weight in kilograms (kg).

Weight in lbs ÷ 2.2 = weight in kg

140 ÷ 2.2 = 63.5 kg

2. Then, multiply the kilogram weight by 0.8 g/kg to determine your protein RDA.

Weight in kg × .8g/kg = g of protein/RDA

63.5 kg × .8g/kg = 50.8g protein/RDA

HEALTH DEBATE
Amino Acid Supplements

Bodybuilders focus on muscles, muscles, muscles! Unfortunately, many believe that since muscles are composed of protein, excessive amounts of protein must be eaten. However, just eating protein does not build muscles. Working a muscle develops and strengthens it when adequate protein is present in the diet.

There is also a mistaken belief that certain nonessential amino acids, such as arginine and ornithine, should be taken as supplements. The perception is that they have special abilities to enhance muscle development. However, studies show that amino acids taken as supplements are ineffective for increasing lean body mass.

When ingested, these supplements are treated as any other protein source of amino acids. Too much of any one may prevent absorption of another required amino acid since they compete for the same absorption sites. Consuming too much of any one could result in a deficiency of another.

Once a supplement is absorbed, the liver views any protein supplement as a source of amino acids. The supplemental amino acids will not necessarily be directed to muscle development. They may just be converted to other nonessential amino acids. Or, if too much protein or too few kcalories are consumed, amino acids will be used for energy immediately or stored as body fat.

Some bodybuilders also illegally use drugs to pump up muscles. These drugs, such as anabolic steroids, produce dangerous emotional and physical side effects. Amino acid supplements that are perceived to build muscles, even though ineffective, are less dangerous than steroids. Should this misperception continue to be fostered as a safer option? Should bodybuilders use drugs at all? What do you think?

From Christensen HN: Amino acid nutrition: A two-step absorptive process, *Nutr Rev* 51(4):95-100, 1993; and Williams M: Ergogenic and ergolytic substances, *Medicine & Science in Sports & Exercise* 24(9Xsupplement):S344-348, 1992.

Age affects protein requirements because when growth occurs, such as during childhood, a greater percentage of dietary intake of protein is needed compared with adulthood. Growth results in additional muscle and tissues, all of which require the amino acids contained in dietary protein. Theoretically, the elderly may require lower levels of protein since muscle mass is reduced as we age; protein utilization may also be affected by variables of decreased physical activity, illness, and chronic use of medications. However, few studies exist to confirm a lower requirement, so the protein RDA for adults age 50 and over is the same as for younger adults (3). Gender differences also affect protein needs. Males tend to have more lean body mass or muscle than females. Lean body mass requires more protein for maintenance.

Certain physiological states require different amounts of nutrients, for example pregnancy and lactation. Pregnant women should consume additional protein to meet the needs of the growing fetus as well as those of their own bodies. RDA recommendations for protein are 20% higher (from 50 grams to 60 grams) for pregnant women. **Lactation,** the production of breast milk, also requires consumption of additional protein. Breast milk contains high quality protein that is formed from

lactation
the production of breast milk

amino acids provided by the woman. The protein RDA for lactation is even higher than during pregnancy (from 50 grams to 65 grams). Special circumstances of serious physical illness, wound healing, fevers (increased metabolic rate), or unusual stress may also increase protein needs.

The type of food sources also affects the amount of protein needed. In the United States, most of the protein eaten is complete protein from animal sources. These sources are considered when the RDA for protein is set. Other countries rely on more plant sources of incomplete proteins, so worldwide recommendations, such as those of the World Health Organization, differ from the US guidelines.

The RDA for protein is 0.8 g/kg (or 2.2 lb). For an *average* adult male, the RDA is 58 to 63 grams; for an *average* adult female, the RDA is 46 to 50 grams (see the RDA Table inside the front cover). Recent research suggests that recommended levels for athletes are 1.0 to 1.5g/kg body weight. Since most Americans eat more protein than recommended, even athletes tend to easily meet protein recommendations (4). Determine your recommended protein intake using the formula in the box on p. 134.

VEGETARIANISM

Vegetarian dietary patterns have long been a part of human history. Instead of animal protein sources, vegetarian dietary patterns focus on plant proteins to provide essential amino acids. The **vegan dietary pattern** consists of plant foods including grains, legumes, fruits, vegetables, seeds, and nuts; no animal-related products are eaten. The **lacto-vegetarian dietary pattern** includes all the foods of the vegan plus dairy products such as milk, cheese, yogurt, and butter. The **ovo-lacto vegetarian dietary pattern** incorporates eggs into the lacto-vegetarian assortment of foods.

Why Vegetarianism?

Vegetarian dietary patterns may be followed to achieve health, spiritual, economic and/or environmental benefits. The health benefits are similar to those of a low-fat, high-fiber diet and consist of reduced risk of coronary artery disease, non–insulin-dependent diabetes, gastrointestinal disorders, and certain cancers (5).

Since animal foods are our primary source of saturated fat and only source of cholesterol, plant-based vegetarian dietary patterns tend to be lower in total fat and cholesterol. This reduced intake, combined with the high fiber content of plant foods, often results in lower blood cholesterol levels. In addition, the body weight of individuals following vegetarian dietary patterns is generally lower. This also reduces the risk of developing hypertension and diabetes.

The spiritual rationale for some individuals who are vegetarians is based on the belief in nonharming. Several religions, including Hinduism and Seventh-Day Adventists, see the consumption of animal flesh as being unhealthy or polluting the body. Other vegetarians do not follow a formal religion, but believe strongly in the protection of animal rights and are opposed to the slaughter of animals for human consumption.

The economic approach addresses the belief that animal-related products cost more than plant protein foods, not only financially but in terms of costs to our natural environment as well. Livestock and other domesticated animals are inefficient producers of protein. Although protein foods from cattle and chicken are of high quality, many pounds of grains are used by these animals to produce one pound of edible food. Some people maintain that by eating from lower on the food chain—eating more plant foods—there will be less waste and limited environmental impact on our natural resources.

vegan dietary pattern
a food plan consisting of only plant foods

lacto-vegetarian dietary pattern
a food plan consisting of only plant foods plus dairy products

ovo-lacto vegetarian dietary pattern
a food plan consisting of only plant foods plus dairy products and eggs

Vegetarian Drawbacks

The vegetarian dietary pattern has several drawbacks. The most critical affects vegans. The vegan dietary pattern can provide all the essential nutrients except vitamin D and B_{12}.

Most dietary vitamin D is consumed through milk fortified with the vitamin. Since vegans do not consume any dairy products, this source of vitamin D is diminished. However, vitamin D is available through synthesis during exposure of the skin to direct sunlight. This source was thought to be adequate for adults and children, but recent reports reveal that rickets, the vitamin D deficiency disorder, has been diagnosed among some infants and young children of vegetarian African-American Muslims (6). The children were well-fed, but dietary sources of vitamin D were negligible. Even maternal breast milk may be low in vitamin D if not consumed in dietary form. It is possible that the combination of dressing young children in heavy clothing (restricting exposure of the skin to the sun) and darker skin pigmentation (which also reduces vitamin D synthesis) places some children at risk for vitamin D deficiency.

Sources of vitamin B_{12} are all animal-related. By excluding animal-related foods, including milk, sources of B_{12} are simply not available. Symptoms of vitamin B_{12} deficiency take years to appear and may cause permanent damage to the central nervous system. Vegans should take B_{12} supplements to insure adequate intake.

Other nutrients for which vegans could be deficient are iron and zinc, minerals usually consumed in meat, fish, and poultry. Calcium levels may also be low if dairy products are excluded; few plants are good sources of calcium. These nutrients are available in a well-planned vegan diet of whole foods. But if the vegan dietary pattern is poorly implemented and depends on refined and processed foods, nutrients may be lacking.

Another drawback pertains to the dimension of social health. Social health is the ability to interact with people in an acceptable manner and to sustain relationships with family members, friends, and colleagues. Those following a vegetarian dietary pattern often find themselves rationalizing their behaviors to others. It can sometimes be tricky to do so without alienating others—especially while they are in the midst of a steak dinner. Perhaps the simplest approach is to emphasize the health benefits gained by adopting a vegetarian dietary pattern.

To ensure that a vegetarian dietary pattern is healthful necessitates learning about protein complementing and new ways of preparing meatless dishes. Simply replacing meat with lots of cheese won't result in any health benefits. In fact, the fat content of a cheese dish is probably higher than a lean meat dish. The most helpful approach is to read vegetarian cookbooks that not only provide recipes, but often include vegetarian nutrition information as well.

Vegetarianism for the 90s

Other terms have evolved to describe semi-vegetarian dietary patterns. In addition to the nonanimal flesh foods consumed by ovo-lacto vegetarians, pesco-vegetarians consume small amounts of fish. Eating limited quantities of chicken is a pollo-vegetarian dietary pattern. These titles do not reflect the original ideals of vegetarianism. They are representative of new dietary patterns evolving in response to health issues of the 1990s.

These health issues center around the risk of developing one or more of the chronic diet-related diseases: coronary artery disease, cancer, non–insulin-dependent diabetes, and hypertension. Risk is reduced as dietary fat intake is lowered. A major source of fat in our diets is our consumption of animal protein foods. Reducing levels of this category of dietary fat lowers risk for chronic diet-related diseases. By doing so, the health promotion goals of *Healthy People 2000* and the *Diet and Health* recommendations are being achieved.

DIETARY PATTERNS OF PROTEIN

S o what should we eat for protein? No longer do we need to be confined to a meat and potatoes mentality when it comes to protein. The healthiest approach is to eat mixed sources of protein—animal and plant sources. The mix provides an excellent assortment of essential amino acids plus sufficient *building block* materials for constructing nonessential amino acids. By eating fewer animal protein foods, dietary fat intake is reduced. By eating more plant protein foods, more dietary fiber is taken in.

Restructuring the Dinner Plate

If asked to plan a *balanced* meal, what would the plate look like? Perhaps animal protein (meat, fish, or poultry), vegetables (broccoli and a salad), and a grain (bread). But how much room on the plate would each portion take up?

Before reading this chapter, the plate would most likely look like that in Fig. 6-3. Notice how meat is the centerpiece taking up the most space on the plate. Is this large portion of chicken necessary? Not at all.

A 6-oz serving of chicken provides about 53 grams of protein. Add to that amount the protein in the bread (3g), potato (4g), broccoli (2g), salad (1g), and skim milk (8g), and the total protein intake from one meal alone is 71 grams. Since we eat protein throughout the day, no one meal needs to provide all our protein. Instead, the balance of the meal needs to be restructured. Since each component of the meal contains protein, whether from animal or plant sources, portion quantities can shift and still provide plenty of protein. An adequate serving of protein is about the size of a deck of cards or the size of your palm. Notice in Fig. 6-4 how the chicken, reduced to 3 oz, is no longer the focus of the plate. Each item occupies a more equal space on the plate. The protein total is still high at 48 grams.

By spreading protein intake throughout the food groups, the objectives of the Food Guide Pyramid are being met. The first plate (Fig. 6-3) provides: 1 serving of grains, 2 servings from the vegetable group, 0 servings of fruit, 1 serving of dairy, and 2 servings from the meat/beans/eggs group. The second plate (Fig. 6-4)

Use the concept of the deck of cards and the restructured meal to visually display to clients appropriate animal-protein portion sizes.

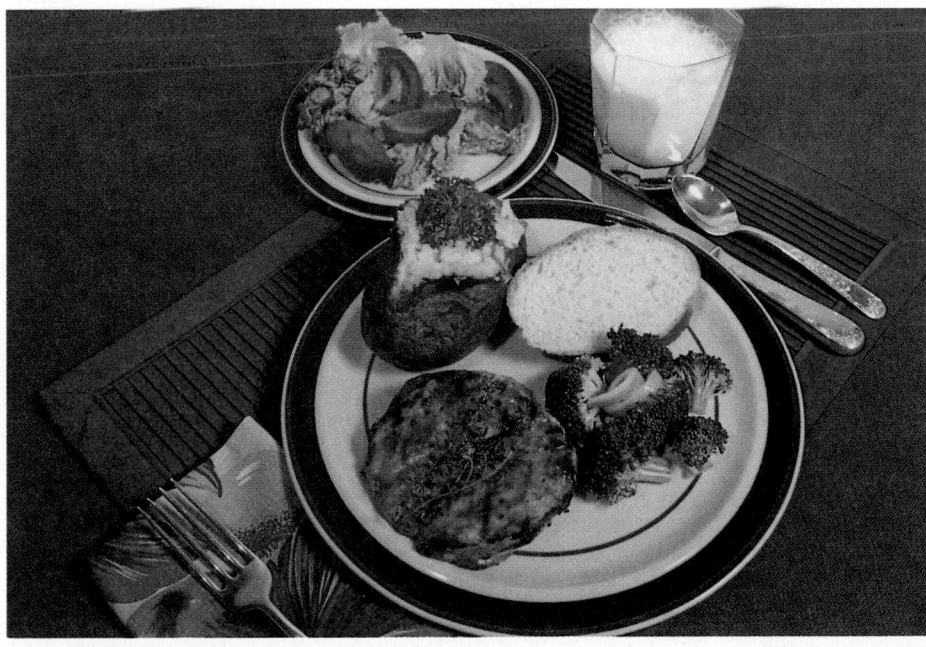

Fig. 6-3 A balanced meal?

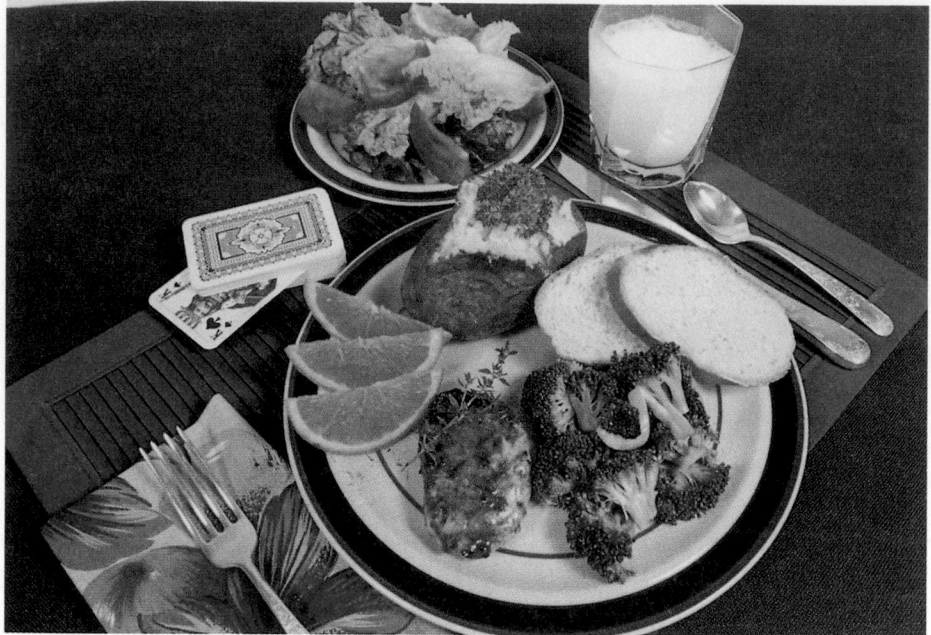

Fig. 6-4 A restructured meal.

provides: 2 servings of grains, 4 servings of vegetables, 1 serving of fruit, 1 serving of dairy, and 1 serving of protein. The new plate provides more complex carbohydrates from grains, fruits, and vegetables while still providing sufficient amounts of protein.

PROTEIN AS A NUTRIENT WITHIN THE BODY

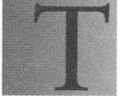he proteins we consume in foods are not the same proteins used by our bodies. Actually, the only nutrient role protein in foods serves is to provide amino acids, the building blocks of all proteins.

Digestion and Absorption

proteases
protein enzymes

Due to the complex structure of proteins, a number of protein enzymes or **proteases** produced by the stomach and pancreas are required to hydrolyze proteins into smaller and smaller peptides until individual amino acids are ready for absorption (Fig. 6-5).

Mouth

Only mechanical digestion of protein occurs in the mouth. Mastication breaks protein-containing food into smaller pieces that mix with saliva passing through to the stomach.

pepsinogen
the inactive form of pepsin

Stomach

Pepsinogen, an inactive form of the gastric protease **pepsin,** is secreted by the stomach mucosa. Pepsin becomes activated when it mixes with hydrochloric acid, also produced by stomach secretions. It then begins the process of protein hydrol-

pepsin
the gastric protease

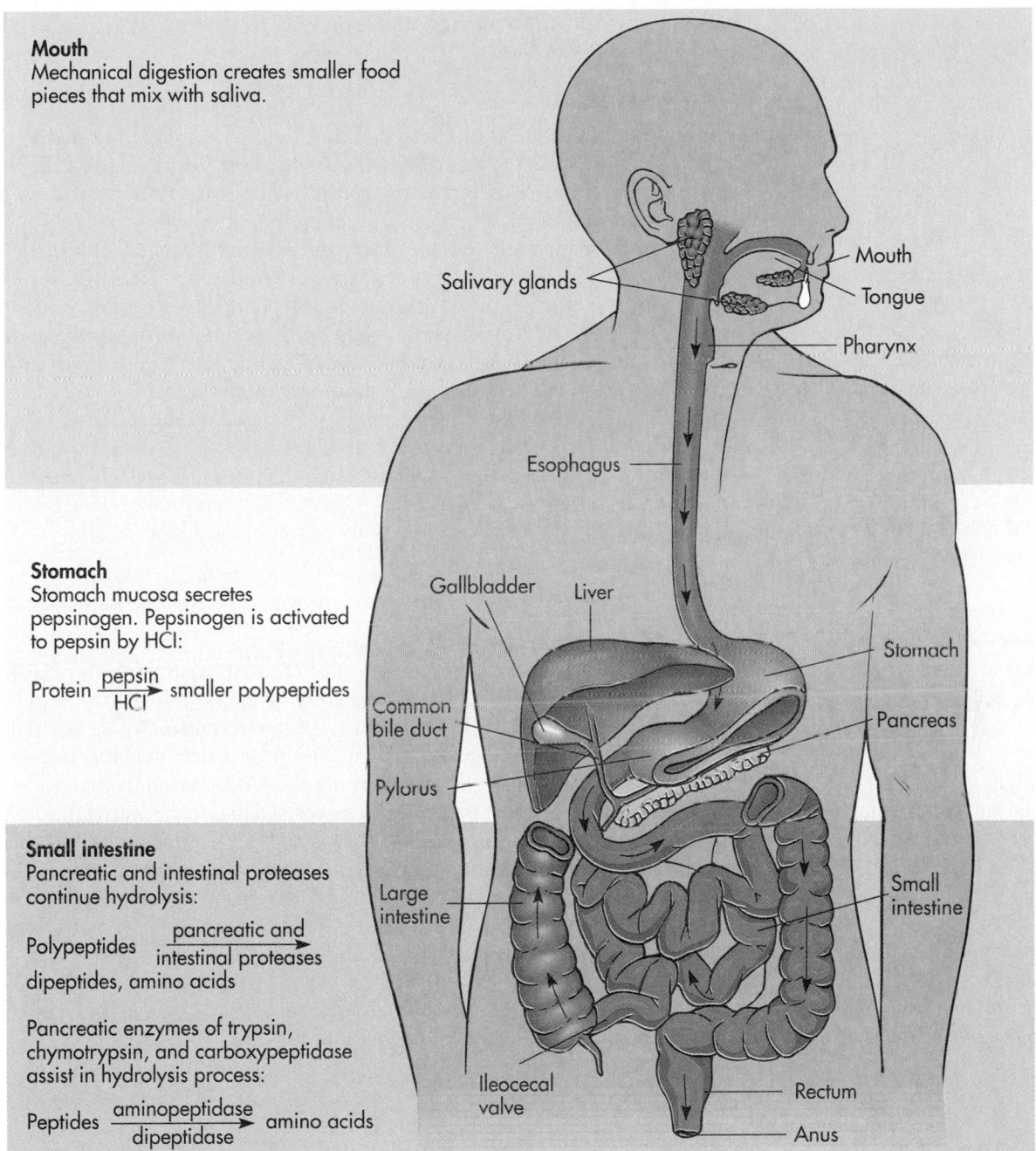

Mouth
Mechanical digestion creates smaller food pieces that mix with saliva.

Stomach
Stomach mucosa secretes pepsinogen. Pepsinogen is activated to pepsin by HCl:

Protein $\xrightarrow[\text{HCl}]{\text{pepsin}}$ smaller polypeptides

Small intestine
Pancreatic and intestinal proteases continue hydrolysis:

Polypeptides $\xrightarrow[\text{intestinal proteases}]{\text{pancreatic and}}$ dipeptides, amino acids

Pancreatic enzymes of trypsin, chymotrypsin, and carboxypeptidase assist in hydrolysis process:

Peptides $\xrightarrow[\text{dipeptidase}]{\text{aminopeptidase}}$ amino acids

Salivary glands, Mouth, Tongue, Pharynx, Esophagus, Gallbladder, Liver, Stomach, Common bile duct, Pancreas, Pylorus, Large intestine, Small intestine, Ileocecal valve, Rectum, Anus

Fig. 6-5 Summary of protein digestion and absorption.

ysis by uncoiling the protein chains and breaking the bonds linking the amino acids of the protein peptide bonds. The result is smaller-sized polypeptides, rather than single amino acids or dipeptides, because of the limited time pepsin has to *work over* the large polypeptides. The polypeptides pass through to the small intestine for further hydrolysis.

Renin, an important gastric protease, is only produced during infancy and childhood. It functions with calcium to thicken or coagulate the milk protein casein; this slows the movement of milk nutrients from the stomach, allowing additional digestion time (7).

Small intestine

In the small intestine, pancreatic and intestinal proteases continue the hydrolysis of polypeptides. As these smaller peptides touch the brush cells of the intestinal walls, peptidases are released, which complete the hydrolyses of protein into absorbable units of individual amino acids and dipeptides.

The primary pancreatic enzyme is **trypsin.** It is first secreted as *trypsinogen,* an inactive form. The intestinal hormone *enterokinase* activates trypsinogen into trypsin, which continues the hydrolysis of polypeptides. Two other pancreatic enzymes assist in the hydrolysis process; **chymotrypsin** hydrolyzes polypeptides into dipeptides, and **carboxypeptidase** breaks polypeptides and dipeptides into amino acids. Two intestinal peptidases are **aminopeptidase,** which releases free amino acids from the amino end of short chain peptides, and **dipeptidase,** which completes the hydrolysis of proteins to amino acids.

Absorption of amino acids occurs through the intestinal walls by means of competitive active transport that requires vitamin B_6 (pyridoxine) as a carrier. Since amino acids are water soluble, they easily pass into the bloodstream.

Metabolism

To understand the importance of protein metabolism in the growth and maintenance of the body, consider that most protein functions are a result of protein *anabolism* (synthesis) in cells. Hormones have a major role in the regulation of protein metabolism. Anabolism is enhanced by the effect of growth hormone (from the pituitary gland) and the male hormone testosterone. Hormones affecting the *catabolism* (break down) of proteins are the glucocorticoids that are enhanced by ACTH; both of these hormones are secreted from the adrenal cortex. This process releases proteins in the cells to break down to amino acids and then travel in the bloodstream, contributing to an available pool of amino acids (Fig. 6-6).

The liver cells begin the process of catabolism through deamination. **Deamination** results in an amino acid (NH_2) group breaking off from an amino acid molecule, resulting in one molecule each of ammonia (NH_3) and a keto acid. Liver cells convert most of the ammonia to **urea,** which is later excreted in urine. The keto acid may enter the TCA cycle to be used for energy or, through gluconeogenesis and lipogenesis, be converted to glucose and fat (1).

Nitrogen Balance

Nitrogen-balance studies are used to determine the protein requirements of the body throughout the life cycle and to assign value to protein quality of foods determining biological value (2). Since nitrogen (**N**) is a primary component of protein, the body's use of protein can be determined by comparing the amount of nitrogen entering the body in food protein with the nitrogen lost from the body in feces and urine.

N lost or excreted from the body may be endogenous **N** (from catabolism of body protein), metabolic **N** (from intestinal cells), or exogenous **N** (from dietary proteins). **N** in feces may be metabolic and exogenous, (from cells and dietary

---

trypsin
the primary pancreatic protease

chymotrypsin
a pancreatic protease that hydrolyzes polypeptides into dipeptides

carboxypeptidase
a pancreatic protease that hydrolyzes polypeptides and dipeptides into amino acids

aminopeptidase
an intestinal peptidase that releases free amino acids from the amino end of short chain peptides

dipeptidase
an intestinal peptidase that completes the hydrolysis of proteins to amino acids

deamination
a process through which an amino acid group breaks off from an amino acid molecule resulting in molecules of ammonia and keto acid

urea
product of ammonia conversion produced during deamination

nitrogen-balance studies
measurement of the amount of **N** entering the body compared to the amount excreted

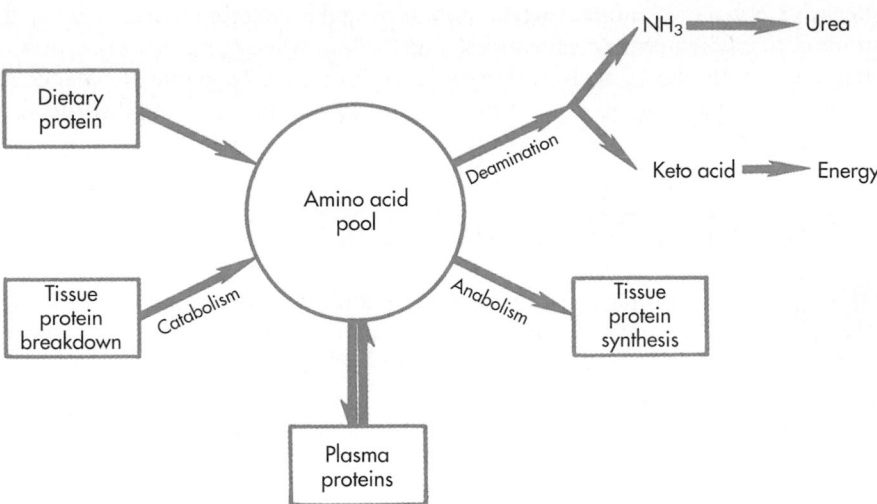

Fig. 6-6 The body's equilibrium depends on a balance between the rates of protein breakdown (catabolism) and protein synthesis (anabolism).

Genetic Disorders

A genetic disorder with a protein link is *phenylketonuria* (**PKU**). This disorder is characterized by the inability to use or break down excess phenylalanine, an essential amino acid. The excess phenylalanine circulating inside the body can cause various health problems. Individuals with this disorder follow a limited protein diet to control the intake of phenylalanine.

Another genetic protein disorder is *sickle cell disease*, which affects the shape of red blood cells. Because of abnormalities of the hemoglobin molecule, the red blood cell is curved or *sickled* rather than round. The sickled shape can cause these blood cells to clog small blood vessels. This can be painful, may cause damage to internal organs such as the kidneys and heart, and may lead to frequent infections throughout the body. Early screening can prevent secondary infections with long-term penicillin treatment (9).

Having the sickle cell disease trait is not the same as having the disease itself. Both parents have to have the trait for a child to be at risk. Even then, there is only a one-in-four chance of developing the disorder. Sickle cell disease may occur in any ethnic group, but is more common among Africans and African-Americans; some states screen all infants to determine susceptibility.

proteins) and in urine from endogenous and exogenous (from catabolism of body proteins and dietary proteins) (8).

An individual is in **N** equilibrium or zero **N** balance if the amount of nitrogen consumed in foods equals the amount excreted. This occurs in normal, healthy adults when nitrogen in food protein (input) to the body equals the nitrogen leaving the body (output). Since adults are no longer growing, the nitrogen entering the body is not needed to build new tissue but simply to maintain the body.

Positive **N** balance occurs when more nitrogen is retained in the body than excreted. The nitrogen is used to form new cells for growth or healing. This occurs in children who are growing and in pregnant women who require additional nitrogen (and protein) for the growth of the fetus. Individuals recovering from illness or injury may be in positive **N** balance as the body heals.

Negative **N** balance happens when more nitrogen is excreted from the body than is retained from dietary protein sources. This occurs when there is a breakdown of proteins within the body, such as in muscles and organs. Negative **N** balance may be due to aging, physical illness, extreme stress, starvation, or eating disorders.

OVERCOMING BARRIERS

Malnutrition, caused by an inadequate intake of energy and/or protein, is discussed in depth in this chapter. Since the functions of protein are so wide-ranging, malnutrition—whether due to an inadequate intake of energy or of protein—affects many vital body functions that depend on an adequate supply of protein.

Malnutrition

malnutrition
an imbalanced nutrient and/or energy intake

Malnutrition, the imbalance of nutrient intake, encompasses a range of conditions from over-consumption of nutrients to extreme under-consumption. This discussion concerns the conditions related to under-consumption of nutrients. Under-consumption can result in nutrient deficiencies that range from marginal to severe starvation. Marginal deficiencies occur when lower than recommended levels of nutrients are regularly consumed. Although obvious signs of specific nutrient deficiencies may not be visible, the level of wellness and ability to function at an optimum level are compromised. As the other nutrient categories of vitamins and minerals are studied, specific symptoms of deficiencies will be explored.

Starvation has become a catch-all term. Although we may say "we're starving" when we've missed a meal, our *starvation* in no way compares with the meaning of the term to those who truly do not have access to sufficient quantities of high-quality food. The technical term for starvation is **protein energy malnutrition (PEM)**. PEM is an umbrella term for malnutrition caused by the lack of protein, energy, or both.

protein energy malnutrition (PEM)

malnutrition caused by the lack of protein, energy, or both

PEM affects populations around the world. Almost 150 million children under 5 years old are affected by PEM (10). In young children, PEM can cause permanent disabilities because most brain growth occurs during the early years of life. Extreme PEM results in the conditions of marasmus and kwashiorkor (Fig. 6-7).

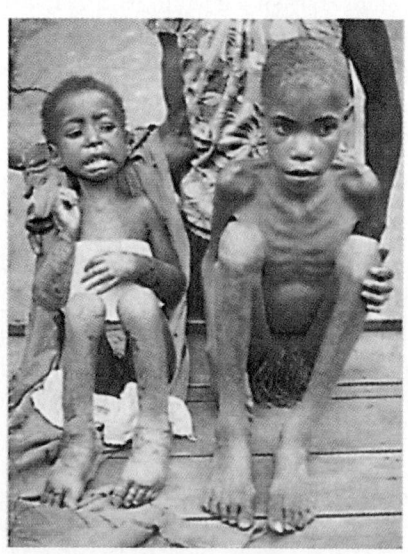

Fig. 6-7 Children suffering from kwashiokor (*left*) and marasmus (*right*) as a result of inadequate energy intake.

These disorders can be fatal because of decreased resistance to infections; the body, lacking protein, is unable to create sufficient quantities of antibodies to support the immune system.

Marasmus is malnutrition caused by a lack of sufficient energy (kcalorie) intake. An individual with marasmus is extremely thin; skin seems to hang on the skeletal bones. Fat stores that normally fill out the skin have been used for energy to maintain minimum body functioning. In addition, muscle mass is also reduced, having been used for energy as well with nutrients not available to rebuild it. If the condition continues, damage may occur to major organs such as the heart, lungs, and kidneys. Marasmic children will not grow. If the condition occurs between 6 and 18 months of age, the time during which the most brain development occurs, permanent brain damage may result.

In contrast to marasmus, the symptoms of kwashiorkor give the appearance of more than sufficient fat stores in the stomach and face. **Kwashiorkor** is malnutrition caused by a lack of protein while consuming adequate energy. The swollen belly and full cheeks of kwashiorkor are due to edema (water retention). Edema occurs because protein levels in the body are so low that protein is not available to maintain adequate water balance in the cells and fluid accumulates unevenly. When adequate nutrition is provided, the fluid is no longer retained. Instead of a full belly and round cheeks, the loss of fat stores becomes apparent and the skin hangs loosely, similar to marasmus. An individual with kwashiorkor is apathetic and experiences muscle weakness and poor growth.

Without sufficient protein, lipids produced by the liver are unable to leave the liver and accumulate there. The liver becomes fatty and unable to function well. Even hair quality is affected, since protein is the main constituent of hair. Curly hair becomes straight, hair falls out easily, and the pigmentation changes.

The definition of kwashiorkor is evolving. Kwashiorkor was identified as a disorder that develops when very young children are switched from breast milk to solid foods. Although they are consuming enough calories, it seems as if their protein intake is too low for the needs of their growing bodies (11). Based on these observations, kwashiorkor is defined as malnutrition caused by protein deficiency while consuming adequate energy.

This definition, however, does not explain why other children and adults develop marasmus instead of kwashiorkor. As researchers continue to study the disorder, they have noticed that the symptoms of kwashiorkor are similar to those of aflatoxin poisoning. Aflatoxin is a mold that develops when grains are stored under poor conditions of heat and humidity. Eating grains affected by aflatoxin can affect liver function, even leading to liver cancer (12).

The liver produces nonessential amino acids, without which protein synthesis throughout the body is limited. If liver function is reduced, as with aflatoxin poisoning, then the production of protein-related structures and substances is decreased. Compared with healthier children and adults, it appears that when malnourished children consume aflatoxin-tainted grains, their weakened bodies are not able to fight off the effects of aflatoxin to their livers. It is possible that these complications lead to the development of kwashiorkor (12).

Malnutrition factors

Malnutrition is often caused by a number of factors affecting food availability. Although poverty tends to be a dominant influence, other forces also affect the development of malnutrition. These include biological, social, economic, and environmental factors (Table 6-4).

Biological factors affect the ability of the body to use nutrients. Economic effects encompass the ability to purchase food, but also consider the structure of a country's economy and access to employment. Environmental factors directly affect the availability of food as related to crop production and food safety. Lack of education, social isolation, and the rippling effects of underemployment seem to be

marasmus
malnutrition caused by a lack of energy (kcalorie) intake

kwashiorkor
malnutrition caused by a lack of protein while consuming adequate energy

Table 6-4   Malnutrition Factors

BIOLOGICAL FACTORS
- Maternal malnutrition before or during pregnancy and/or lactation
- Infections that may affect nutrient absorption
- Chronic diarrhea as both a cause and effect of malnutrition
- Toxins such as aflatoxin
- Lack of food, particularly protein

SOCIAL FACTORS
- Ignorance of nutrient needs of children, resulting in inappropriate weaning foods
- Child abuse and neglect
- Eating disorders, particularly anorexia nervosa
- Drug abuse affecting the ability to care for oneself appropriately
- Social isolation of the elderly, leading to an inability to purchase and prepare adequate quantities of food
- Alcoholism (kcalories from alcohol replace consumption of nutrient-dense foods)
- Wars/civil strife disrupting normal social and food production systems

ECONOMIC FACTORS
- Poverty and socioeconomic status
- Unemployment
- Under-education
- Political strife affecting distribution of wealth and land ownership

ENVIRONMENTAL FACTORS
- Polluted water, reducing food production and directly impacting the health of populations
- Famine caused by droughts and/or crop failures
- Improper farming techniques

malnutrition factors throughout the world, regardless of the overall wealth of nations. Health and economic support systems provided throughout the life cycle may prevent the development of factors affecting food availability.

Groups at risk in North America

Most people in North America are well-nourished, although growing numbers of homeless individuals living in shelters or other temporary sites are at risk for varying levels of malnutrition (13). Without access to cooking facilities nor the funds to purchase adequate quantities of foods, these individuals are at nutritional risk (14). In response to this crisis, food pantries and soup kitchens have been established by nonprofit and charitable groups to distribute food and meals. Also at risk are the working poor, whose incomes barely cover basic expenses of housing, utilities, and health care and leave little for food purchases (15).

 Another group at risk is the elderly. Although their nutritional concerns will be covered in depth in Chapter 12, consider that the physical and financial limitations of the elderly may reduce their ability to purchase and prepare wholesome meals. When these issues are also compounded by social isolation, the situation of the elderly becomes serious.

Hospital patients and those with chronic illnesses such as AIDS and cancer are also at risk for PEM, even while under medical care. This is called *hospital malnutrition*. This condition may be due to not consuming enough food, side effects from the illness, and/or medications that reduce the body's ability to absorb nutrients. Weight loss may be attributed to the illness rather than to lack of nutrients. The patient seems *sicker*, but is actually malnourished and not absorbing the nutrients needed to heal and recover.

Primary care providers, nurses, and dietitians all play a collaborative role in preventing, identifying, and treating hospital malnutrition. Astute nursing assessment may uncover early signs of malnutrition or factors predisposing a patient to

"Finish all that food on your plate. Children in India are starving." Parents used to tell their children this quite often. And countless numbers of children tried to figure out how their finishing their vegetables would help to feed children in a far-away land. Of course, parents wanted their children not to waste food and to appreciate their good fortune. However, many children probably believed that by finishing their food they were somehow helping those hungry children.

With today's technology we can have no illusions about the plight of others. We get complete, immediate reports of devastation caused by wars and famines. Reports of hunger among the homeless and the elderly are televised. If only finishing the food on our plates would help.

So what can we do? Here are some ideas.

AS INDIVIDUALS
- Be well informed. Learn about hunger in your backyard. All communities have those who are in need.
- Volunteer to help in a local soup kitchen.
- Create a food drive at holidays; donate foods to a food bank.
- Let local politicians know of your concerns; give a voice to the voiceless.

CAMPUS ORGANIZATIONS (POLITICAL, SOCIAL AND RELIGIOUS)
- Include a service component to the group's mission.
- Support World Food Day sponsored by the United Nations and other organizations.
- Ask local anti-hunger agency representatives to speak to campus groups.
- Incorporate volunteer time as part of an initiation process or as a commitment of all members.

From Contra Costa County Hunger Task Force: *Hunger in the midst of affluence,* Pleasant Hill, Calif, 1993, Contra Costa County Health Service Department.

it. Dietitians work not only with individual patients, but also with the health care industry to develop new products and technologies designed to either prevent or reduce the incidents of PEM among hospital patients (16). The box above gives ideas on how to help reduce malnutrition at the community level.

Chronic hunger

Although famines and wars affect the nutritional status of people throughout the world, the population of North America has not experienced this extreme of deprivation. Instead, **chronic hunger,** defined as a continual experience of undernutrition (not enough food to eat), has become the norm for a subset of our population. This subset is growing as the economies of North America tighten, causing government food and welfare programs to be unable to provide an appropriate safety net to prevent and alleviate chronic hunger (14). Instead, more individuals and families are faced with a consistent lack of opportunities to improve their standard of living and most importantly their health.

chronic hunger
a continual experience of undernutrition

TOWARD A POSITIVE NUTRITION LIFESTYLE: CHAINING

Chaining is the linking together of two behaviors. If two actions consistently occur together, they often become *linked* or tied to each other. They become one behavior and a habit. Many of us already practice chaining; unfortunately, the results often have a negative impact on our dietary intake patterns. Frequently eating potato chips while studying can link these two actions—eating chips and studying. The chain requires that whenever studying takes place, chips *need* to be eaten. Chaining, however, can also be used to improve nutritional status.

Consider these chains:

- When you eat a sandwich, eat a fruit too. Instead of linking chips and a sandwich (or hoagie, grinder, or sub), this links a sandwich with a fruit.
- Have a glass of skim milk with the midday meal regularly to increase calcium intake. Skim milk becomes chained to lunch.
- At home, weigh portions of meat, fish, and poultry. Compare the size of an appropriate portion to the size of a deck of cards. Very similar sizes? Weigh regularly and consciously compare sizes. Animal protein portion sizes will be linked to the deck of cards and portion control can be achieved without weighing.

These are just a few *chains* related to protein consumption. Chaining can be applied to other nutrition and wellness situations of our clients as well.

WELLNESS AND LIPIDS

Physical Dimension	Our overall health and well-being depends on our eating enough EAAs for body protein synthesis.
Intellectual Dimension	The ability to comprehend and apply new approaches to protein consumption by adapting to different protein sources (legumes and grains) to reducing portion sizes depends on your intellectual capacity to implement change.
Emotional Dimension	Protein is a *super* status food for some Americans; favorite sources may provide emotional security. Patients needing to make dietary changes, such as changing to lower fat sources of protein (cutting back on sausages), may need our advice on coping strategies.
Social Dimension	As we and our patients follow different eating patterns, such as vegetarian or reducing consumption of animal protein, family and social dynamics may be affected when one member changes.

SUMMARY

Proteins consist of chains of amino acids. Amino acids are organic compounds made of carbon, hydrogen, oxygen, and nitrogen. There are 20 amino acids from which all proteins are made. The body can manufacture some, but not all of the amino acids. Essential amino acids cannot be made by the body; these nine amino acids are needed from food. The other 11 nonessential amino acids can be created by the liver. All are available to the cells through the amino acid pool to allow proteins to be synthesized.

The proteins in foods are categorized by the essential amino acids they contain. Complete proteins contain all nine essential amino acids, while incomplete proteins lack one or more of the essential amino acids.

The proteins in foods are not the same as those used by our bodies. During digestion, food protein is broken down to amino acids. Once absorbed, the amino acids circulate in the blood to build new proteins. The new proteins are used to perform numerous functions, including growth and maintenance, creation of essential substances, immune system response, fluid regulation, acid-base balance, and transportation of nutrients and other substances in the body. Malnutrition resulting in PEM, marasmus, and kwashiorkor is a world-wide concern.

THE NURSING ROLE

Protein Case Study: The Nursing Process

Roy is a 69-year-old homeless man who comes to a walk-in clinic with leg ulcers that he says he has had for several months and that continue to increase in diameter. He is obviously poorly nourished. He says he eats what he can find on the street and sometimes goes to the city food center for the homeless for a hot meal. The nurse cleans Roy's leg ulcers, and the physician orders laboratory tests that rule out diabetes but include some other abnormal results.

ASSESSMENT DATA COLLECTED

Subjective

Minimal intake of meat, eggs, or complete protein foods
Lack of appetite
Fatigue

Objective

Height 6'2"
Weight 140 lb
Muscle atrophy in extremities bilaterally
Decreased muscle strength
Poor skin turgor
Hair dull and thin
Slight ankle edema bilaterally
Hepatomegaly
Leg ulcer healing delayed
Laboratory results:
    Total serum protein 5.4 (norm 6.6-7.9 Gm/dl)
    Serum albumin 3.1 (norm 3.3-4.5 Gm/dl)
    Serum transferrin 200 (norm 220-400 ug/dl)

NURSING DIAGNOSIS

Altered nutrition, less than body requirements of protein, related to lack of money and food availability as evidenced by delayed healing of leg ulcers and underweight status.

PLANNING

Specific realistic goals and outcomes for Roy include:
    Roy will express understanding of the importance of protein and the variety of food sources of protein
    Healing of leg ulcers within 3 months
    Weight gain of 5 lb in 3 months

INTERVENTION

1. Teach Roy about protein and dietary sources of protein.
2. Supply Roy with cans of high protein supplements at each clinic visit.
3. Apply wet-to-dry dressings and antibiotic ointment to leg ulcers during clinic visits twice a week.
4. Encourage Roy to move into the local shelter for the homeless at least until leg ulcers heal.

Continued.

THE NURSING ROLE, cont'd.
Protein Case Study: The Nursing Process

5. Encourage Roy to eat at least one meal per day in the shelter or city food center.
6. Contact the city shelter to secure a place for Roy and give them dates of clinic visits.

EVALUATION

Each goal should be evaluated to see if the outcome has been fully or partially met as evidenced by:

After four clinic visits, client describing high protein food sources he has eaten each day

Decrease in diameter of leg ulcers in one month and healing in 3 months

Weight gain of at least 5 lb in 3 months

REFERENCES

1. Thibodeau GA, Patton KT: *Anatomy & physiology*, ed 2, St. Louis, 1993, Mosby.
2. Crim MC, Munro HN: Proteins and amino acids. In Shils ME, Olson, JA, Shike M, eds: *Modern nutrition in health and disease*, ed 8, Philadelphia, 1994, Lea & Febiger.

3. Food and Nutrition Board/National Research Council: *Recommended dietary allowances,* ed 10, Washington, DC, 1989, National Academy Press.

4. Ruud J: *Protein,* Lincoln, Neb, 1990, International Center For Sports Nutrition and the US Olympic Committee.

5. American Dietetic Association: Position of the American Dietetic Association: Vegetarian diets, *J Am Diet Assoc* 93(11):1317-1319, 1993.

6. Tortorella K: Rickets, a relic shows up again, *New York Times* sec 13:1, March 12, 1995.

7. Williams SR: *Essentials of nutrition and diet therapy*, ed 6, St. Louis, 1994, Mosby.

8. Whitney EN et al: *Understanding normal and clinical nutrition*, ed 4, St Paul, Minn, 1995, West.

9. Agency for Health Care Policy and Research: *Sickle cell disease guidelines,* Silver Spring, Md, 1993, US Public Health Service.

10. Udani PM: Protein energy malnutrition (PEM), brain and various facets of child development, *Indian J Pediatr* 59:165-186, March-April 1992.

11. Solomons NW, Molina S, Bluw J: Weanling diarrhea: A case report, *Nutr Rev* 48(5):212-215, 1990.

12. Ramjee G et al: Aflatoxins and kwashiokor in Durban, SA, *Annual Trop Paedai* 12(3):241-7, 1992.

13. Wolgamuth JC et al: Wasting malnutrition and inadequate nutrient intakes identified in a multiethnic homeless population, *J Am Diet Assoc* 92(7):834-842, 1992.

14. Lenhart NM, Raad MH: Demographic profile and nutrient intake assessment of individuals using emergency food programs, *J Am Diet Assoc* 89(9):1288-1292, 1989.

15. Nestle M, Guttmacher S: Hunger in the US, *J Nutr Ed* 24: 18S-21S, January/February Supp 1992.

16. Coats KG et al: Hospital-associated malnutrition: A reevaluation 12 years later, *J Am Diet Assoc* 93(1):27-33, 1993.

Chapter 7

VITAMINS

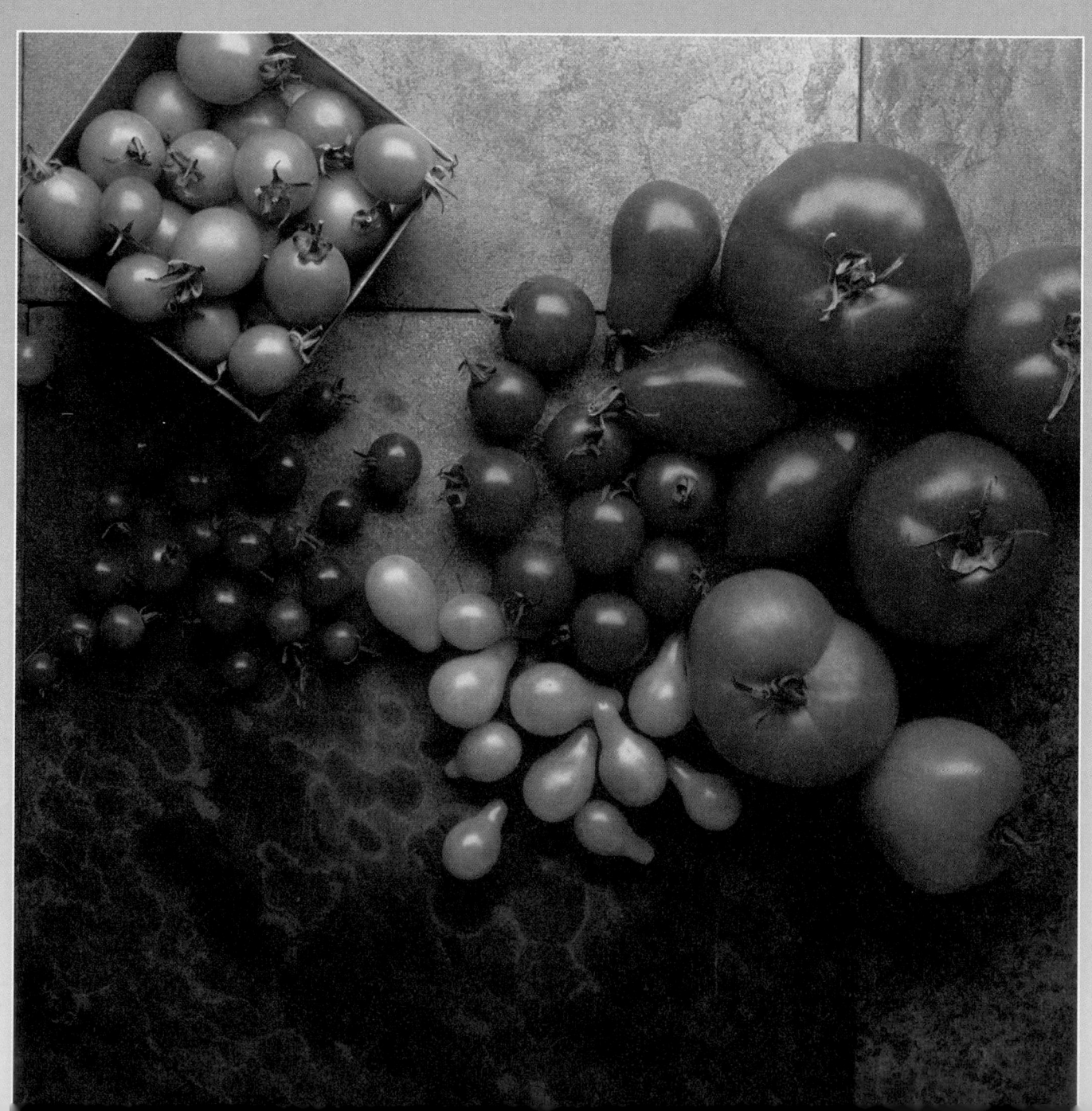

ROLE IN WELLNESS

Vitamins seem to have a magical aura. Take enough and you'll have more energy and be healthier, smarter, and even better looking. If only it were so easy. Although vitamins are essential for life, they are only one of many factors required for wellness.

Knowledge of the existence of vitamins is recent; the discovery of vitamins slowly evolved, beginning in the early part of this century. The focus of research was to discover the amounts of vitamins needed to prevent deficiency symptoms and diseases that undermined the health and well-being of populations throughout the world. The American Recommended Dietary Allowance (RDA) guide for vitamins reflects the requirements necessary to prevent deficiencies as well as toxicity from overdoses.

The scientific view of vitamins, however, is in flux. Additional effects of vitamin use are surfacing as more is learned about the functions of vitamins as antioxidants and hormone-like substances. Some vitamins and related substances such as carotenoids may reduce the risk of developing certain chronic diseases. Clearly defined answers are not yet available; however, information is emerging that points to relationships between foods high in vitamins and a lower incidence of disease.

Vitamins are organic molecules that are required in very small amounts. They usually are not synthesized by our bodies, and thus are essential nutrients that must be provided through dietary intake. Each vitamin performs a specific metabolic function.

As vitamins are discussed, note that some are referred to by specific names or by letters and numbers. Each vitamin has a history that affects how we refer to it today. In 1929 vitamin K was discovered by Henrik Dam in Copenhagen, Denmark. It was the only substance able to halt a hemorrhagic disease in which blood does not coagulate. Dam named the vitamin *K* for the Danish word *koagulation*. In another case, several B vitamins were isolated into the same test tube labeled B, and we now have vitamins numbered B_1, B_2, and B_3. In the 1970s the science community decreed that all vitamins should be called by their formal biochemical titles. The public and many health professionals still refer to the simpler letter and number names for vitamins. Both the formal and informal names are used in this chapter.

Vitamin RDAs are stated for each vitamin in this chapter. Because there are 17 different RDAs based on age, gender, and physiological need, only the RDAs for male and female young adults, ages 19 to 24, are included for each vitamin unless special circumstances surrounding the need for a vitamin warrant discussion of other age or physiological RDAs. The RDA Table is located inside the front cover of this book; the Canadian Recommended Nutrient Intake (RNI) Table is in Appendix F.

A primary deficiency of a vitamin occurs when the vitamin is not consumed in sufficient amounts to meet physiological needs. A secondary deficiency develops when absorption is impaired or excess excretion occurs, limiting bioavailability. Most deficiencies are detected through clinical and biochemical assessment; specific diagnostic and laboratory procedures are beyond the scope of this text and are available elsewhere (1).

Although vitamin deficiencies are no longer common among Americans, subgroups are at risk. Because of their increased needs, pregnant women are often at risk for marginal deficiencies of essential vitamins. The elderly may also be at risk because of decreased absorptive ability and limited economic and physical resources for food availability. Poverty is an overwhelming factor affecting the nutritional status of children as well as adults. Chronic alcohol and drug abuse not only alters psychological and mental capacities, but limits the body's ability to absorb and use essential vitamins. People dealing with long-term chronic disorders that

vitamin

essential organic molecules needed in very small amounts for cellular metabolism affect the total body response, such as AIDS or liver or kidney disorders, also have special vitamin concerns.

Toxicities of vitamins rarely occur naturally from food consumption. Instead, inappropriate use of supplements may be toxic to our bodies. Vitamins have been studied for their physiological effect or basic need for health maintenance. The recommended levels reflect this knowledge. Use of vitamin supplements at megadose levels is equivalent to a pharmacological effect, with potential drug-like physical responses. A megadose is 10 times the RDA for a specific nutrient. Vitamins have not been studied to determine function and safety at these levels. Extensive use without guidance can be problematic.

VITAMIN CATEGORIES

Vitamins are divided into two categories based on their solubility in solutions. Water-soluble vitamins dissolve or disperse in water; they are vitamin C and the B complex vitamins (thiamin, riboflavin, niacin, folate, pyridoxine, vitamin B_{12}, biotin, and pantothenic acid). Fat-soluble vitamins dissolve in fatty tissues or substances; they are vitamins A, D, E, and K.

Solubility characteristics affect how vitamins are absorbed and transported in the body. Water-soluble vitamins are easily absorbed in the small intestine, then pass into the bloodstream for circulation throughout the body. Fat-soluble vitamins follow the more complicated route of other fat-containing substances; bile is

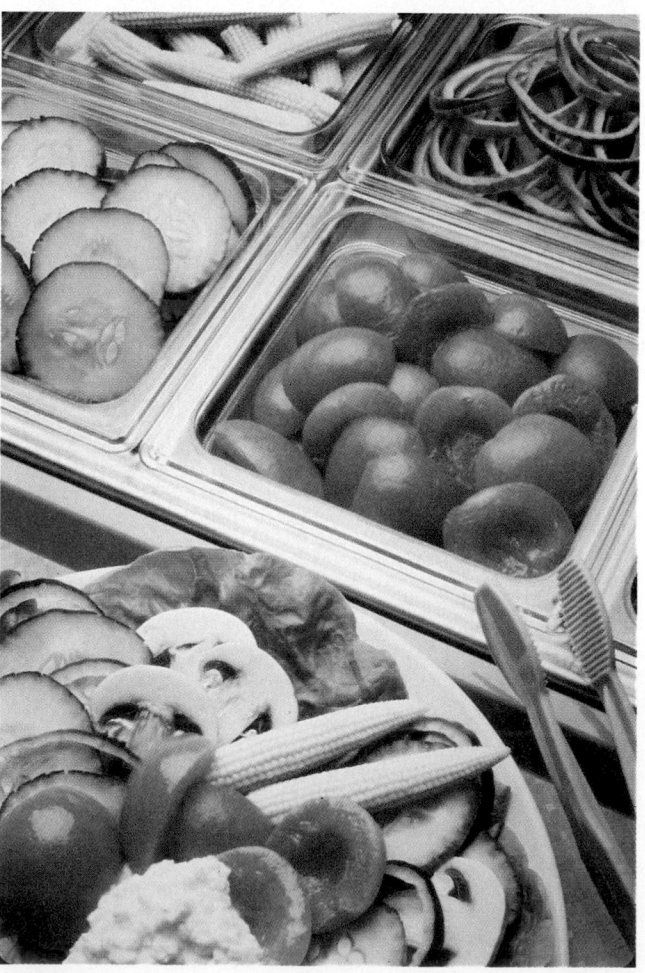

Although vitamins are in almost all foods, fruits and vegetables are especially rich sources.

required for absorption from the small intestine. Fat malabsorption problems may also lead to potential deficiencies of fat-soluble vitamins.

The water solubility of the B vitamins and vitamin C allows for minimal storage of any excess vitamin consumed; tissues may be saturated with these vitamins, but they usually are not stored. Deficiencies can develop quickly, within weeks. We need to consume these vitamins on a daily basis. Excesses are generally not toxic and are simply excreted in urine. However, damage may result if vitamin levels are chronically high due to supplementation.

If we consume more than the daily requirement of a fat-soluble vitamin, our bodies store the excess rather than excreting it. The RDAs for fat-soluble vitamins account for this storage capacity. Although storage is expected in organs such as the liver and spleen, other fatty tissues in the body can also retain excessive amounts of fat-soluble vitamins. Overloading the storage capabilities can be toxic and produce illness; toxicity rarely comes from excessive dietary intake but from improper use of vitamin supplements.

FOOD SOURCES

Vitamins are in almost all foods, yet no one food group is a good source of all vitamins. Fresh fruits and vegetables are particularly rich sources. Others include legumes, whole grains, and animal foods of meat, fish, poultry, eggs, and dairy products. Even the almost pure fats of vegetable oils and butter provide vitamins E and A, respectively. Although this does not mean we should consume these products for the vitamin content, it does mean that we have a wide range of foods to choose from for our vitamin nutrition.

It is always best to consume vitamins from foods sources. Although synthetic forms of vitamins will perform vitamin functions, there may be other factors in foods that also provide benefits. For instance, broccoli and other cruciferous vegetables have recently been found to contain a wide variety of chemicals including sulforaphane, a **phytochemical.** Sulforaphane appears to block the growth of tumors in animals (2).

phytochemicals
nonnutritive substances in plant-based foods that appear to have disease-fighting properties

WATER-SOLUBLE VITAMINS

Thiamin (B1)

For centuries, a mysterious disease afflicted people throughout Asia of all ages and status. The disease so wasted muscles that sufferers trying to stand would cry out, "beri beri," meaning "I can't! I can't!" in Thai. This phrase, **beriberi,** became the name of a serious disease resulting from thiamin deficiency. In the 1890s it was discovered that beriberi resulted from consumption of hulled (white) rice, and that unhulled (brown) rice prevented or cured this disease. Later, researchers found that thiamin in the hulls of whole grains prevents or cures beriberi.

beriberi
a severe chronic deficiency of thiamin characterized by muscle weakness and pain, anorexia, mental disorientation, and tachycardia

Function

The main function of thiamin is to serve as a **coenzyme** in energy metabolism; it also has a role in nerve functioning related to muscle actions.

coenzyme
a substance that activates an enzyme

Recommended intake and sources

The RDA recommends that men and women consume 1.5 mg and 1.1 mg per day, respectively. The amount of thiamin required increases as the metabolic rate rises. Those engaged in rigorous physical activity burn more energy, so they require more thiamin.

Lean pork, whole or enriched grains and flours, legumes, seeds, and nuts are good sources of thiamin. As a water-soluble vitamin, some thiamin can be lost in food processing or when foods are cooked at home (3). Thiamin may be leached into cooking fluid or destroyed by heat. Generally, however, most of us consume sufficient amounts of thiamin.

Deficiency

Thiamin deficiency alters the nervous, muscular, gastrointestinal, and cardiovascular systems (3). A severe, chronic deficiency results in beriberi characterized by **ataxia** (muscle weakness and loss of coordination), pain, anorexia, mental disorientation, and **tachycardia** (rapid beating of the heart) (Fig. 7-1). **Wet beriberi** manifests with edema, affecting cardiac function by weakening the heart muscle and vascular system. **Dry beriberi** affects the nervous system, producing paralysis and extreme muscle wasting. Marginal deficiencies may occur, producing psychological disturbances, recurrent headaches, extreme tiredness, and irritability (3).

Beriberi still occurs in areas of the world such as Asia, where the staple food is a highly polished rice that is low in thiamin. The practice of repeatly washing the milled rice results in further loss of thiamin. Very high intakes of raw fish can also produce beriberi. Raw fish naturally contains an enzyme, thiaminase, that destroys thiamin. This does not affect those of us who occasionally enjoy sushi or sashimi, Japanese specialities of raw fish.

In the United States, enrichment of refined flour has virtually eliminated thiamin deficiency. However, persons who are chronic alcohol users may develop thiamin deficiency due to decreased food intake and reduced intestinal absorption coupled

ataxia
muscle weakness and loss of coordination

tachycardia
rapid beating of the heart

wet beriberi
thiamin deficiency with edema affecting cardiac function by weakening of heart muscle and vascular system

dry beriberi
thiamin deficiency affecting the nervous system producing paralysis and extreme muscle wasting

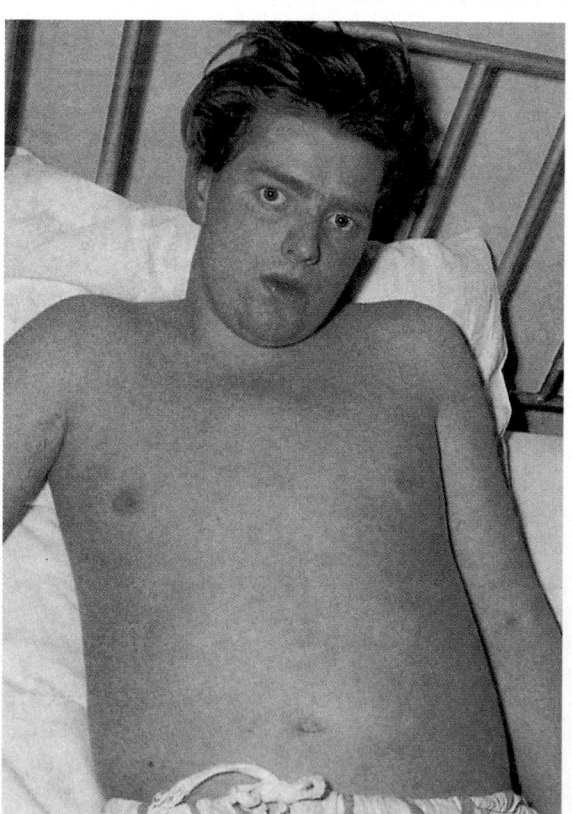

Fig. 7-1 Wet beriberi. This patient with chronic alcoholism has edema up to his chest.

CULTURAL CONSIDERATIONS
Cuban Crisis

In the spring of 1993 a harsh economy and natural disasters played havoc with Cuba's food supply. The breakup of the Soviet Union dissipated a valuable trade network for Cuba. This, combined with the devastating effects of a tropical storm, severely limited the variety of foods available. The consequence? A disease resulting in vision loss and numbness caused by nerve damage spread primarily among men. The *New York Times* headlines were startling, "Twenty-six thousand Cubans partly blinded."

There is speculation that the epidemic was caused by nutritional deficiencies of thiamin and/or folate. These deficits were exacerbated by consumption of home-brewed rum. The rum required thiamin to detoxify the alcohol, further decreasing the available thiamin for body functions. Folate levels declined as supplies of folate-containing foods diminished. Increased reliance on naturally available foods such as cassava root, and the popularity of cigarettes among 95% of Cuban men further affected folate availability. Both are high in cyanide, which uses up folate stores in the body. The epidemic was brought under control as the Cuban government distributed vitamin supplements to provide the missing nutrients.

From Altman LK: 26,000 Cubans partly blinded; cause is unclear, *New York Times* May 21, 1993:A7, and Community Nutrition Institute: Epidemic, *Nutrition Week Newspaper* 22:8 June 11,1993.

with an additional need for thiamin by the liver to detoxify alcohol (see box). A severe deficiency may cause a cerebral form of beriberi, called **Wernicke-Korsakoff syndrome.** It is the most common disorder of the central nervous system because of the effects of alcohol on nutritional status (4). The loss of memory, extreme mental confusion, and ataxia exhibited by persons with chronic excessive alcohol ingestion may be due to the effects of this thiamin deficiency syndrome. Clinically, care must be taken when a malnourished person is given parenteral fluids containing glucose. Parenteral fluids should contain a mix of B vitamins; otherwise the marginal thiamin levels of nutritionally depleted individuals, combined with a sudden increase of glucose to the brain, can initiate Wernicke-Korsakoff syndrome, regardless of the level of alcohol intake.

Others at risk for thiamin deficiency include renal patients undergoing dialysis, patients receiving parenteral nutrition, and individuals with a genetic disorder affecting thiamin use (3).

Wernicke-Korsakoff syndrome cerebral form of beriberi affecting the central nervous system

Toxicity

Excess thiamin is excreted in urine. Although thiamin is nontoxic, there is no rationale for supplementation in healthy people. In acute care settings, supplemental thiamin and other B vitamins may be recommended for individuals with chronic excessive alcohol consumption. Advice generally is to take a daily multivitamin containing B vitamins.

Riboflavin (B₂)

Do you ever wonder why milk is sold in opaque cardboard containers? These containers protect riboflavin from exposure to light. Riboflavin is sensitive to ultraviolet rays in sunlight and artificial light; much of the riboflavin is destroyed if milk, an excellent source of riboflavin, is sold in clear glass or plastic receptacles. Why risk loss of a valuable vitamin?

Function

Like thiamin, riboflavin's main function is as a coenzyme in the release of energy from nutrients in every cell of the body.

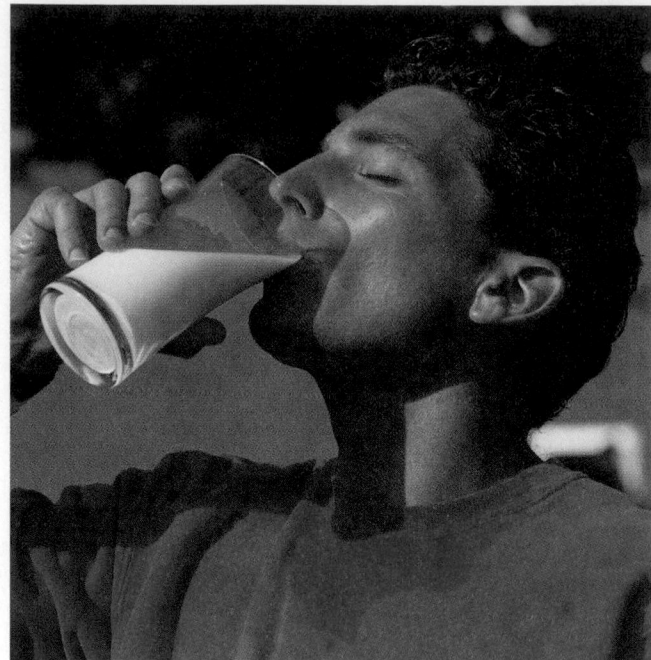

Milk is the major source of riboflavin in the United States.

Recommended intake and sources

The RDA for riboflavin is 1.7 mg for men and 1.3 mg for women. The body's need is related to total calorie intake, energy needs, body size, metabolic rate, and growth rate. Conditions requiring increased protein also require increased riboflavin, such as during wound healing or the growth periods of childhood, pregnancy, and lactation.

Riboflavin is found in both plant and animal foods, but in the United States milk is a major source, with small amounts coming from other foods such as enriched grain. Good plant sources are broccoli, asparagus, dark leafy greens, whole grains, and enriched breads and cereals. Rich sources of animal origin include dairy products, meats, fish, poultry, and eggs.

As mentioned, riboflavin is sensitive to light and irradiation. It can also be lost in cooking water, but is heat stable.

Deficiency

Ariboflavinosis is the name given to a group of symptoms associated with riboflavin deficiency. The lips become swollen; cracks develop in the corners of the mouth (**cheilosis**). The tongue becomes swollen and purplish-red (**glossitis**). Seborrheic dermatitis, a skin condition characterized by greasy scales, may occur in the regions of the ears, nose, and mouth. Riboflavin deficiency may also affect the availability and use of pyridoxine and niacin.

Nutritional deficiencies tend to be multiple rather than single, and it is difficult to separate symptoms. For example, esophageal cancer is associated with deficiencies of riboflavin and zinc, particularly in Africa, Iran, and China (5).

Toxicity

Toxicity to riboflavin has not been reported (6). Absorption of riboflavin tends to be limited under normal circumstances; excessive absorption is extremely unlikely (7).

ariboflavinosis
a group of symptoms associated with riboflavin deficiency

cheilosis
inflammation of the mucous membrane of the mouth and lips (angular stomatitis) caused by riboflavin and other B vitamin deficiencies

glossitis
inflammation of the tongue

Niacin (B₃)

Niacin occurs naturally in two forms, nicotinic acid and niacinamide. It's hard to imagine, but before niacin was identified people who were actually suffering from niacin deficiency were so psychologically disoriented that they were sent to mental institutions for treatment. Niacin deficiency can bring on a psychosis that dissipates once sufficient quantities are consumed.

Function

Niacin is involved as a cofactor with many enzymes, especially those involved in energy metabolism; it is critical for glycolysis and the TCA cycle.

Recommended intake and sources

Niacin is available in foods as the active vitamin or as its precursor, the amino acid tryptophan. That is, tryptophan can be converted to niacin and some niacin can be provided this way. Diets adequate in protein are adequate in niacin.

Niacin requirements are measured in niacin equivalents (NE), reflecting the body's ability to convert tryptophan to niacin. Sixty milligrams of tryptophan are needed to form 1 mg of niacin, both of which equal 1 mg NE. The RDA recommends that men and women consume 19 mg NE and 15 mg NE per day, respectively.

Protein-containing foods are good sources of both niacin and tryptophan. Meats, poultry, fish, legumes, enriched cereals, milk, and even coffee and tea are sources of niacin (8).

Deficiency

Pellagra, the niacin deficiency disorder, is characterized by the 3 Ds: (8)

1. Diarrhea: Damage to the gastrointestinal tract affects digestion, absorption, and excretion of food, leading to glossitis, vomiting, and diarrhea.
2. Dermatitis: A symmetrical scaly rash occurs only on skin exposed to the sun (Fig. 7-2).
3. Dementia: As the central nervous system becomes affected in severe deficiencies, confusion, anxiety, insomnia, and paranoia develop.

pellagra
the deficiency disorder of niacin characterized by diarrhea, dermatitis, and dementia

Early in this century, pellagra was common in the southern United States among the poor who subsisted on corn-based diets. The niacin in corn is in a bound form that is unavailable for absorption, and many persons subsisting on low incomes had such a limited intake of protein food that neither tryptophan nor preformed niacin was available. Since the discovery of the cause of pellagra, flours have been enriched with niacin and the incidence of pellagra has decreased dramatically. In the United States, pellagra may still occur among persons with chronic excessive alcohol ingestion, although in Africa and Asia pellagra occurs among the general population.

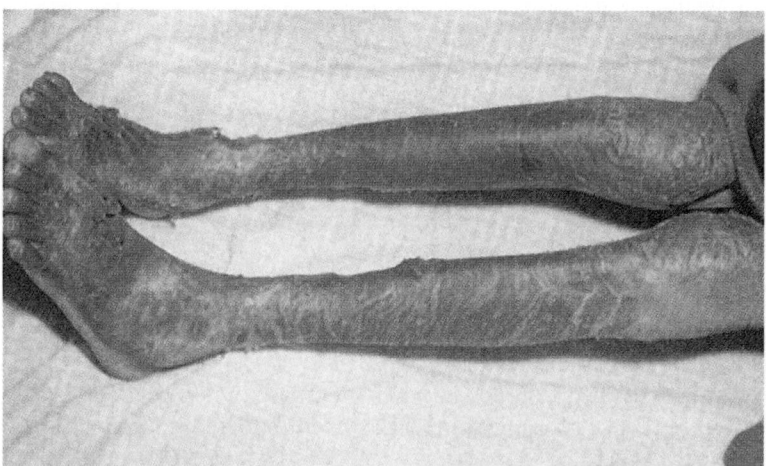

Fig. 7-2 Dermatitis in a patient suffering from pellagra.

Toxicity

When consumed in megadoses, preformed niacin and nicotinic acid (but not niacinamide) vasodilate the vascular system, producing a flushing effect throughout the body. A pharmacological dose is 3 to 9 grams of niacin, compared with the RDA of 19 mg NE. Niacin has been used therapeutically because megadoses may lower total cholesterol and LDL and increase HDL (5). These therapeutic doses, however, must be medically administered to guard against liver damage and related gout and arthritic reactions.

Pyridoxine (B$_6$)

Vitamin B$_6$ and *pyridoxine* are generic terms representing a group of related chemicals. The three main members are pyridoxine, pyridoxal, and pyridoxamine. All three forms can be converted to the coenzyme pyridoxal phosphate (PLP) for use in the body.

Function

In the form of PLP, the major function of vitamin B$_6$ is as a coenzyme in the metabolism of amino acids and proteins. These reactions are involved in the formation of neurotransmitters and are essential for proper functioning of the nervous system. PLP is essential for hemoglobin synthesis. It is required for the conversion of tryptophan to niacin. It also serves as a coenzyme for fatty acid and carbohydrate metabolism.

Recommended intake and sources

The RDA for vitamin B$_6$ is 2.0 mg for men and 1.6 mg for women. These amounts are based on protein intake.

This vitamin is widespread in foods. Particularly good sources include whole grains and cereals, legumes, and chicken, fish, pork, and eggs.

Deficiency

A deficiency of vitamin B$_6$ rarely occurs alone, but accompanies low intakes of other B vitamins as well. Symptoms include dermatitis, altered nerve function, weakness, poor growth, convulsions, and microcytic anemia (small red blood cells deficient in hemoglobin).

Of the numerous drugs that affect the bioavailability and metabolism of vitamin B$_6$, oral contraceptive agents (OCAs) may be among the most widely used. Women taking OCAs containing estrogen may have an increased B$_6$ need. Additionally, OCAs taken before conception may result in low B$_6$ plasma concentration in the mother during pregnancy and lactation; low maternal body stores can cause a vitamin B$_6$ deficiency in the newborn (9).

Prolonged use of such drugs as isoniazid (for tuberculosis), penicillamine (for lead poisoning, cystinuria, Wilson's disease, sclerosis, and rheumatoid arthritis), cycloserine (for tuberculosis), and hydralazine (for hypertension) may require vitamin B$_6$ supplements to reduce neurological side effects and prevent deficiency during treatment (10).

Toxicity

Vitamin B$_6$ has sometimes been prescribed to relieve the symptoms associated with PMS (premenstrual syndrome); there is not adequate data, however, to support this treatment. Although doses of 10 mg, an amount often prescribed, are most likely not harmful even considering the RDA of 1.8 mg, long-term supplementation in megadose gram quantities has been reported to cause ataxia and sensory neuropathy.

Folate

Folate, like other B vitamins, actually consists of several similar compounds. One of these compounds was originally extracted from spinach and was given the name *folic acid,* from the Latin word *folium* or leaf. Folic acid was discovered in 1945 during the search for the nutritional factor responsible for control of pernicious anemia. We now know that vitamin B_{12}, rather than folic acid, is the nutrient that cures **pernicious anemia.** Folic acid and its related compounds, however, play a role in other essential biological processes. The terms *folate, folic acid, folacin,* and *pteroylglutamic acid* (PGA) are often used interchangeably.

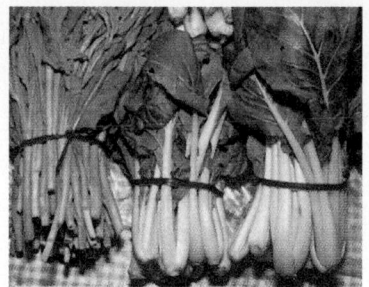

Leafy green vegetables are rich in folate.

Function

Folate acts as a coenzyme in reactions involving the transfer of one-carbon units during metabolism. As such, it is required for the synthesis of amino acids, which are the building blocks of protein, and for the synthesis of DNA and RNA. Blood health also depends on folate to form the heme portion of hemoglobin. For the active form of folate to be maintained for use in the body, vitamin B_{12} must be available.

Attention recently focused on the role of folate in the proper formation of fetal neural tubes (11). Neural tube birth defects affect brain and spinal cord development, resulting in the disorders of spina bifida and anencephaly. **Spina bifida** is a congenital defect of the spinal column causing the spinal cord to be unprotected. This results in a range of disabilities including paralysis and incontinence. With **anencephaly,** a congenital defect in which the brain does not develop, death occurs shortly after birth. Although these disorders result from a combination of genetics and environment, adequate folate levels during the first month after conception appear to greatly reduce these serious birth defects. Unfortunately, women of childbearing age are sometimes marginally deficient in folate. They may not know they are pregnant during the first few crucial months during which neural tubes of the fetus form.

spina bifida
a congenital defect of the spinal column causing the spinal cord to be unprotected, resulting in a range of disabilities including paralysis and incontinence

anencephaly
a congenital defect in which the brain does not develop; death occurs shortly after birth

Recommended intake and sources

The RDA reflects that some folate is stored in the liver, but generally daily supplies are needed. Physiological state greatly affects folate need. Although the RDA for males is 200 mcg and is 180 mcg for females, recommended levels jump to 400 mcg during pregnancy because of an increased blood supply, and 280 mcg for lactation needs.

In 1992 the US Public Health Service recommended that women of childbearing age increase their folate intake to 400 mcg. The increased levels could be provided by natural sources, fortified foods, or supplements (11) (Table 7-1). In October 1993 the FDA proposed folate fortification of all bread and grain products (12). This proposal is under consideration, although concerns exist as to the efficacy of

Table 7-1　Food Sources of Folate	
Food	**Micrograms** **(per 100 g of food—3.5 oz)**
Dark-green leafy vegetables	120–160
Other vegetables	40–100
Fruits (particularly citrus)	50–100
Beans (legumes)	50–300
Whole grains	60–120
Breakfast cereals	100 or 400

From Williams RD: FDA proposes folic acid fortification, *FDA Consumer* May 1994.

fortifying bread products for this target group of women and to potential hazards of toxicities for the general population.

Folate is widely available in foods, particularly in leafy green vegetables, legumes, ready-to-eat cereals, and some fruits and juices. Folate is affected by heat, oxidation, and ultraviolet light; processing and cooking of fresh foods reduce the amount of folate available. Folate is found in many foods containing ascorbic acid (vitamin C), such as oranges and orange juice. Ascorbic acid protects folate from oxidation. Diets deficient in one are often deficient in the other (11).

Deficiency

Cells whose normal activities require rapid cell growth and division are particularly sensitive to folate deficiency. Examples include red blood cells and the cells lining the gastrointestinal tract. Folate deficiency results in megaloblastic anemia. This is a form of anemia characterized by large red blood cells that cannot carry oxygen properly. Other deficiency symptoms include glossitis, diarrhea, irritability, absentmindedness, depression, and anxiety (11,13).

Eating one fresh fruit or one fresh vegetable per day provides enough folate to prevent deficiency in the average adult.

Deficiency may result from any condition that requires cell division to speed up, including infection, cancer, burns, blood loss, gastrointestinal damage, and pregnancy. Presently about one third of pregnant women worldwide are affected by folate deficiency (13). Other groups at risk include those with a limited intake and variety of food, including elderly people with low incomes and persons with chronic excessive alcohol ingestion. Alcoholic cirrhosis often results in both liver damage, which interferes with storage and metabolism of folate, and excessive losses of the vitamin in feces and urine (14).

Numerous medications may affect folate absorption or be antagonistic to folate. These drugs include anticonvulsants, oral contraceptives, aspirin, cancer chemotherapy agents, sulfasalazine, nonsteroidal antiinflammatory medications, and antacids. Long-term use of any medication may affect the body's use of nutrients; folate is one that is particularly vulnerable.

Before folate supplementation, the absence of vitamin B_{12} deficiency must be established. Therapy with folate in the presence of vitamin B_{12} deficiency will favorably improve blood profiles, decreasing megaloblastic anemia, while damage to the central nervous system from lack of B_{12} continues.

Toxicity

Excess folate intake is not recommended or warranted. There is a lack of data available to assess the effects of fortification or widespread supplementation. Megadoses may mask the presence of pernicious anemia, discussed under Cobalamin.

Cobalamin (B_{12})

Cobalamin and *vitamin B_{12}* are used as generic terms to refer to a group of cobalt-containing compounds. The common pharmaceutical name, used widely in supplements, is *cyanocobalamin*.

Function

Two cobalamins function as vitamin B_{12} coenzymes in humans. The B vitamin folate depends on vitamin B_{12} for its transport and storage. The metabolism of fatty acids and amino acids also requires vitamin B_{12}.

Recommended intake and sources

intrinsic factor
a substance produced by stomach mucosa that is required for vitamin B_{12} absorption

Absorption of vitamin B_{12} relies on an intrinsic factor. The **intrinsic factor** is produced by stomach mucosa. Both vitamin B_{12} and the intrinsic factor must be present for absorption. Recommended levels take into account that some vitamin B_{12} is stored in the liver. The RDA for young adults is 2.0 mcg daily.

Foods of animal origin are the only reliable sources of vitamin B_{12}; meat, fish, poultry, eggs, and dairy products are all good sources. One glass of skim milk provides .93 mcg of vitamin B_{12}. The vitamin has been reported to be found in legumes (nodules on roots) because of bacteria formation in soil, but they are not a reliable source. Vegans must supplement their intake with vitamin B_{12} supplements or use fortified products.

Deficiency

Deficiencies of B_{12} are usually secondary deficiencies. **Pernicious anemia** (from B_{12} deficiency) or megaloblastic anemia (from related folate dysfunction) occurs. Additional neurological effects develop because of damage to the spinal cord as myelin synthesis affects brain, optic, and peripheral nerves (13).

Elderly persons are more at risk for deficiency because of a naturally occurring reduction in production of the intrinsic factor by the stomach mucosa; most older persons, however, remain within normal range. For those who do become deficient, injections to bypass intestinal absorption are warranted. Noted particularly among this population are neuropsychiatric symptoms including delusions and hallucinations without anemia (15). These symptoms can be misdiagnosed as senility or other illnesses.

As discussed in relation to folate supplementation, folate levels may disguise a B_{12} deficiency. Blood hematologic damage is masked by folate, but neurological damage continues (13).

Toxicity

Toxicity to vitamin B_{12} has not been noted, but there are no benefits to large doses unless deficiency exists.

Biotin

Biotin, a member of the B vitamin complex, is needed in tiny amounts by humans.

Function

Biotin assists in the transfer of carbon dioxide from one compound to another, playing an important role in carbohydrate, fat, and protein metabolism.

Recommended intake and sources

Biotin is synthesized in the lower GI tract by bacterial microorganisms. However, the amount produced and its bioavailability are unknown. Although biotin is produced in the body, it is still an essential nutrient. (The human body does not produce biotin, but bacteria hosted in the gut do.) It must also be consumed in foods.

No RDAs have been established for biotin. The estimated safe and adequate daily dietary intake (ESADDI) is 30 to 100 mcg.

Biotin is widespread in foods. The richest sources are liver, kidney, peanut butter, egg yolks, and yeast.

Deficiency

Naturally occurring biotin deficiency in people eating a typical North American diet is unknown. Experimentally, symptoms of biotin deficiency include a scaly red skin rash, hair loss, loss of appetite, depression, and glossitis (16).

Biotin deficiency has been produced by consumption of large amounts of avidin, a protein in raw egg whites that binds biotin. You would need to consume many raw egg whites for this to occur; *Salmonella* poisoning would probably strike first. Avidin is denatured by heat, so cooked egg whites pose no problem to biotin status.

Antibiotics are known to reduce the number of biotin-producing bacteria. Also, clients receiving long-term intravenous feeding are prone to biotin deficiency, so their feeding mixtures should contain biotin.

pernicious anemia
inadequate red blood cell formation caused by a lack of intrinsic factor in the stomach with which to absorb vitamin B_{12}

Toxicity

There is no known toxicity.

Pantothenic Acid

Pantothenic acid gets its name from its presence in all living things (from the Greek *pantothen* meaning *from all sides*).

Function

The principal active form of pantothenic acid is a part of coenzyme A (CoA for short). Therefore it is required for the metabolism of carbohydrates, fats, and protein.

Recommended intake and sources

There are no RDAs for pantothenic acid. Instead an ESADDI of 4 to 7 mg has been established.

Pantothenic acid is widespread in foods and easily consumed in whole grain cereals, legumes, meat, fish, and poultry.

Deficiency

Deficiencies do not naturally occur in humans.

Toxicity

Doses of up to 10 grams daily have been administered with no ill effects. Researchers have reported that daily doses of 10 to 20 grams may produce diarrhea or water retention.

Vitamin C

Vitamin C is almost a household word. It's hard to believe that it was isolated as a nutrient only around 1930. The discovery of vitamin C is associated with the search for the cause of **scurvy,** a potentially fatal disease that weakens and causes inflammation of the body's connective tissues. As early as the eighteenth century, it was known that eating certain foods, particularly citrus fruits, could control scurvy, but the actual substance responsible for *gluing* the cells together was not determined until Albert Szent-Gyorgy and Glen King isolated it in 1928 and 1930, respectively (17). One of the two active forms of vitamin C is ascorbic acid, meaning *without scurvy*.

Function

Vitamin C functions as an antioxidant and as a coenzyme. It can perform different functions in various situations. Collagen formation for bone matrix, teeth, cartilage, and connective tissue depends upon ascorbic acid. Vitamin C provides the cement that holds structures together. Wound healing, which necessitates the formation of new tissue, also requires vitamin C.

As an antioxidant, vitamin C protects folate, vitamin E, and polyunsaturated substances from destruction by oxygen as they move throughout the body. An **antioxidant** is a compound that guards others from damaging oxidation by being oxidized itself. Vitamins C and E also work together as antioxidants to destroy substances released as cells age, are oxidized, and/or become damaged. Their work may prevent free radical damage to vascular walls, thereby limiting the development of atherosclerotic plaques.

Among its other functions, vitamin C enhances the absorption of nonheme iron, found in plant foods. Thyroid and adrenal hormone synthesis requires vitamin C. Several conversion processes depend on vitamin C; these include tryptophan to serotonin, cholesterol to bile, and folate to its active form.

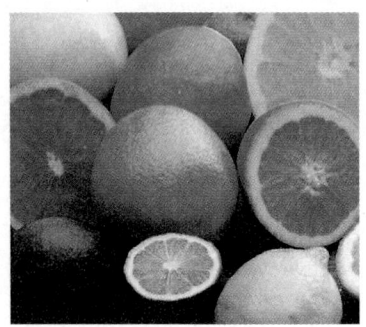

Although citrus fruits are well known for being rich in vitamin C, vegetables such as green peppers, cauliflower, and broccoli are also nutrient-dense sources.

scurvy
extreme vitamin C deficiency disorder characterized by inflammation of connective tissues, gingivitis, muscle degeneration, bruising, and hemorrhaging as the vascular system weakens

antioxidant
a compound that guards other compounds from damaging oxidation

Vitamin C may have a role in reducing the risk of cancer development. Epidemiologic studies have uncovered an association between levels of dietary intake of vitamin C and incidence of cancer in the stomach, esophagus, and colon (5). Since these studies are of dietary intakes of populations, it is not yet known whether the effects are due to vitamin C or to other, as yet unidentified components of foods containing vitamin C.

Recommended intake and sources

The RDA for vitamin C has varied from 45 mg to 60 mg for adults. Presently the RDA is 60 mg. Recommendations world-wide vary; the minimum requirement to prevent symptoms of scurvy is 10 mg. The amount recommended daily to provide enough circulating vitamin C for tissue saturation for good health is open to interpretation.

As more is learned about vitamin C functions, recommendations customized to specific disease and lifestyle behaviors will be determined. For example, cigarette smokers have lower circulating levels of vitamin C compared to nonsmokers, regardless of their dietary intake of vitamin C. The metabolic use of vitamin C by smokers is twice that of nonsmokers. Recognizing this deficit, smokers are advised to increase their vitamin C intake from the 60 mg RDA to 100 mg daily (6).

> Recommend that clients who smoke consume 100 mg rather than 60 mg of vitamin C daily.

Fruits and vegetables provide 95% of the vitamin C we consume. Many foods are excellent sources; some of them include citrus fruits, red and green peppers, strawberries, tomatoes, potatoes, broccoli, and other green leafy vegetables. Servings sizes to meet the RDA are listed in Table 7-2.

Some foods and drinks are fortified with vitamin C. Ready-to-eat cereals have added vitamin C (about 25% of the daily values) and other vitamins not naturally found in grains. Additional vitamin C, often 100% of the daily values, is added to the small amounts naturally found in apple and grape juice.

Vitamin C is destroyed by air, light, and heat. Fruit juices should be stored in an airtight container that holds only the amount that can be consumed in a short time. The vitamin C content of cooked foods can be maximized by cooking in the minimal amount of water or, even better, by microwaving (see box).

Deficiency

Although vitamin C deficiency is rare in Western developed countries, it may still occur among persons who are chronic alcohol and drug users, whose dietary intakes are extremely poor. Elderly persons may have marginal intake because of difficulty in obtaining and preparing fresh foods. These at-risk groups may experience other vitamin and mineral deficiencies as well.

Scurvy represents the extreme result of vitamin C deficiency. The symptoms are tied to the functions of vitamin C in the body. As the glue-like substance of

Table 7-2 RDA Serving Sizes of Vitamin C (RDA = 60 mg)		
Food	**Serving**	**Vitamin C**
Broccoli	½ cup	58 mg
Brussel sprouts	½ cup	48 mg
Cantaloupe	1 cup	68 mg
Grapefruit	½ fruit	47 mg
Kiwifruit	1 piece	75 mg
Orange	1 piece	80 mg
Orange juice	¾ cup	93 mg
Peppers, green or red	½ cup	64 mg
Strawberries	¾ cup	64 mg

Data from Pennington JAT: *Bowes & Church's food values of portions commonly used,* ed 16, Philadelphia, 1994, Lippincott.

TEACHING TOOL
Vegetable Victories

We may focus on teaching clients what vitamins do in their bodies, but this education is pointless unless they relate the information to the foods they actually eat. Some of our clients, who may be willing to experiment with preparing foods (particularly vegetables) in a more nutrient-retaining manner, may be at a loss as to how to proceed. We cannot assume that everyone has grown up naturally knowing how to steam broccoli.

Clients need assistance in achieving vegetable victories. What is a vegetable victory? It's when individuals figure out how they most enjoy eating a particular vegetable and learn how to cook it so it still retains the most nutrients possible. With vegetables, most of those nutrients are vitamins, mainly water-soluble vitamins. Since water-soluble vitamins are in the liq-

uid parts of vegetables, if vegetables are cooked or boiled (please don't) the vitamins are either leached into the cooking water or may even be destroyed by the heat. What to do? Below are some preparation pointers.

Nutritional value is reduced by air, heat, water and light. To prevent loss from air exposure, use plastic containers to store vegetables, and cook with lids. To limit vitamin forfeiture from water-related preparation, cook vegetables with as little water as possible, or use vegetable cooking water in soups or sauces. To reduce destruction from light, keep vegetables in dark places; most should be stored in the refrigerator. To reduce heat damage to vitamins, keep vegetables cool and cook only until they are crisp by microwaving, stir-frying, or lightly steaming.

From Clark N: *The New York City Marathon cookbook,* Nashville, Tenn, 1994, Rutledge Hill Press.

---

collagen is not replaced, tissues throughout the body degenerate. Gingivitis causes gums to bleed, and teeth come loose; joints and limbs ache from muscle degeneration and lack of new connective tissue formation; bruising and hemorrhages occur as the vascular system weakens, and plaques form as a result of the vascular damage. Death ultimately occurs as functioning of all body systems disintegrates.

Marginal deficiency symptoms may manifest as gingivitis, poor wound healing, inadequate tooth and bone growth or maintenance, and increased risk of infection as the integrity of tissues throughout the body becomes compromised.

Toxicity

The bulk of evidence does not support the theory that vitamin C reduces the incidence of the common cold. Taking supplemental vitamin C, however, can decrease the duration and reduce the severity of the symptoms (18).

Toxicity from foods high in vitamin C does not occur even if we consume cups of fresh strawberries washed down with a quart of orange juice. Chronic supplement intakes of megadoses from 1 gm to 15 gm may result in cramps, diarrhea, nausea, kidney stone formation, and gout. The effects of anticlotting medication may also be affected (5).

Taking supplements of vitamin C seems so benign, but the body adapts to protect itself from harm. If continually inundated with excessive vitamin C, the body develops a mechanism that destroys much of the extra vitamin C circulating in the body. A rebound effect may occur if, after taking megadoses for several months or more, an individual abruptly stops supplementation and consumes a quantity closer to the RDA. The protective mechanism of the body is still in gear and continues to destroy vitamin C. An individual may develop symptoms of scurvy even though the RDA amount is being consumed. A newborn exposed to vitamin C megadoses in utero may experience this rebound effect. Although the rebound effect may not occur in every case, withdrawal from vitamin C megadoses should be gradual, over a period of 2 to 4 weeks.

Table 7-3 provides a quick reference to water soluble vitamins.

Table 7-3   Water-Soluble Vitamins

Vitamin	Function	Clinical Issues (Deficiency/Toxicity)	Requirements	Food Sources
Thiamin (B$_1$)	Coenzyme energy metabolism; muscle nerve action	Deficiency: beriberi (ataxia, disorientation, tachycardia); marginal (headaches, tiredness); wet beriberi (edema); dry beriberi (nervous system): Wernicke-Korsakoff syndrome (alcoholism)	Men: 1.5 mg Women: 1.1 mg	Lean pork, whole or enriched grains and flours, legumes, seeds, and nuts
Riboflavin (B$_2$)	Coenzyme energy metabolism	Deficiency: ariboflavinosis with cheilosis, glossitis, seborrheic dermatitis	Men: 1.7 mg Women: 1.3 mg	Milk/dairy products; meat, fish, poultry, and eggs; dark leafy greens (broccoli); whole and enriched breads and cereals
Niacin (B$_3$) (nicotinic acid and niacinamide) precursor: tryptophan	Cofactor to enzymes involved in energy metabolism; glycolysis and TCA cycle	Deficiency: pellegra Toxicity: vasodilation, liver damage, gout, and arthritic reactions	Men: 19 mg NE Women: 15 mg NE	Meats, poultry, and fish; legumes; whole and enriched cereals; milk
Pyridoxine (B$_6$)	Forms coenzyme pyridoxal phosphate (PLP) for energy metabolism; CNS; hemoglobin synthesis	Deficiency: dermatitis, altered nerve function, weakness; anemia; OCAs decrease B$_6$ levels Toxicity: ataxia, sensory neuropathy	Men: 2.0 mg Women: 1.6 mg	Whole grains/cereals, legumes, poultry, fish, pork, eggs
Folate (folic acid, folacin, PGA)	Coenzyme metabolism (synthesis of amino acid, heme, DNA, RNA); fetal neural tube formation	Deficiency: megaloblastic anemia, many drugs affect folate use Toxicity: megadoses may mask pernicious anemia	Men: 200 mcg Women: 180 mcg Pregnancy: 400 mcg Lactation: 280 mcg	Widely available leafy green vegetables, legumes, ascorbic acid-containing foods
Cobalamin (B$_{12}$)	Transport/storage of folate; metabolism of fatty acids/amino acids	Deficiency: pernicious anemia, CNS damage	Adults: 2.0 mcg	Animal sources
Biotin	Metabolism of carbohydrate, fat, and protein	Deficiency: produced by avidin and long-term antibiotics	Adults: 30 to 100 mcg ESADDI	Liver, kidney, peanut butter, egg yolks, intestinal synthesis
Pantothenic acid	Part of Coenzyme A	Deficiency: not possible	Adults: 4-7 mg ESADDI	Widespread in foods
Vitamin C	Antioxidant, coenzyme, collagen formation, wound healing, iron absorption, hormone synthesis	Deficiency: scurvy Toxicity: cramps, nausea, kidney stone formation, gout, (1 to 15 g), rebound scurvy	Adults: 60 mg	Fruits/vegetables (citrus fruits, tomatoes, peppers, strawberries, broccoli)

ESADDI, Estimated Safe and Adequate Daily Dietary Intake.

FAT-SOLUBLE VITAMINS

Vitamin A

Each year about 250,000 children enter a world of permanent darkness (5). The cause? Extreme vitamin A deficiency so damages corneas that blindness occurs. This could be prevented by just a few cents worth of vitamin A per year, but in areas of the world where food is scarce there is little money for preventive health measures.

Function

Vitamin A is a group of compounds that function to maintain skin and mucous membranes throughout the body. Specific activities that depend on vitamin A are vision, bone growth, functioning of the immune system, and normal reproduction. Our eyes depend on visual purple, technically called rhodopsin, to be able to adjust to light variations. Rhodopsin is formed from retinal, a vitamin A substance, and opsin, a protein. Without enough vitamin A, rhodopsin cannot be formed and the retina cannot easily respond to light changes; **night blindness** develops (Fig. 7-3). Bone growth involves a process of remodeling that reshapes as well as enlarges the skeleton. Reshaping requires vitamin A to *undo* existing bone. Vitamin A maintains integrity of epithelial tissues throughout the body, providing protection against infections and assuring optimum function. Hormone-like effects of vitamin A appear to be tied to cell synthesis for reproductive purposes.

Recommended intake and sources

Vitamin A is measured as retinol equivalents (RE). The RDA, based on providing optimum storage of vitamin A in the liver, is 1000 RE for men and 800 RE for women. RE incorporates both the preformed, active forms of vitamin A called retinoids (found in animal foods) and the precursor forms of vitamin A called carotenoids (found in plant foods). The carotenoid beta carotene is the primary source of vitamin A from plant foods.

Since vitamin A (a fat-soluble vitamin) is stored in the body, daily doses are not necessary but are desirable. Deficiency of other nutrients affects the absorption and use of vitamin A (19). Nutrients are interdependent, and imbalances of specific nutrients affect the functioning of others.

Natural preformed vitamin A is found only in the fat of animal-related foods; these include whole milk, butter, liver, egg yolks, and fatty fish. Carotenoids are found in deep green, yellow, and orange fruits and vegetables. The best sources include broccoli, cantaloupe, sweet potatoes, carrots, tomatoes, and spinach (Table 7-4). High consumption of carotenoids recently has been associated with decreased risk of certain cancers and other chronic diseases (see box).

When fats are removed from animal-related foods, preformed vitamin A is also lost. To maintain traditional sources of the vitamin, lowfat, skim, and nonfat milks are fortified with vitamin A. Other products that are fortified include margarine (which often replaces butter, a natural source of vitamin A), and ready-to-eat cereal, a staple food product that is commonly fortified with a number of nutrients.

Deficiency

Vitamin A deficiency is either primary, caused by lack of dietary intake, or secondary, the result of chronic fat malabsorption. As liver storage becomes depleted, symptoms develop. The effects are closely tied to vitamin A functions. Ocularly, **xerophthalmia** incorporates a range of symptoms manifested by night blindness progressing to a hard, dry cornea (keratinization) or **keratomalacia,** resulting in complete blindness. The degeneration of the epithelial tissues protecting the eye itself leads to the effects of xerophthalmia. Compromised epithelial tissues also result in respiratory infections, diarrhea, and other gastrointestinal disturbances. Overall, the immune system is endangered; for children especially, a minor illness

nightblindness
the inability of the eyes to readjust vision from bright to dim light caused by vitamin A deficiency

xerophthalmia
a condition caused by vitamin A deficiency ranging from night blindness to keratomalacia; may result in complete blindness

keratomalacia
a condition caused by vitamin A deficiency in which the cornea becomes dry and thickens from the formation of hard protein tissue

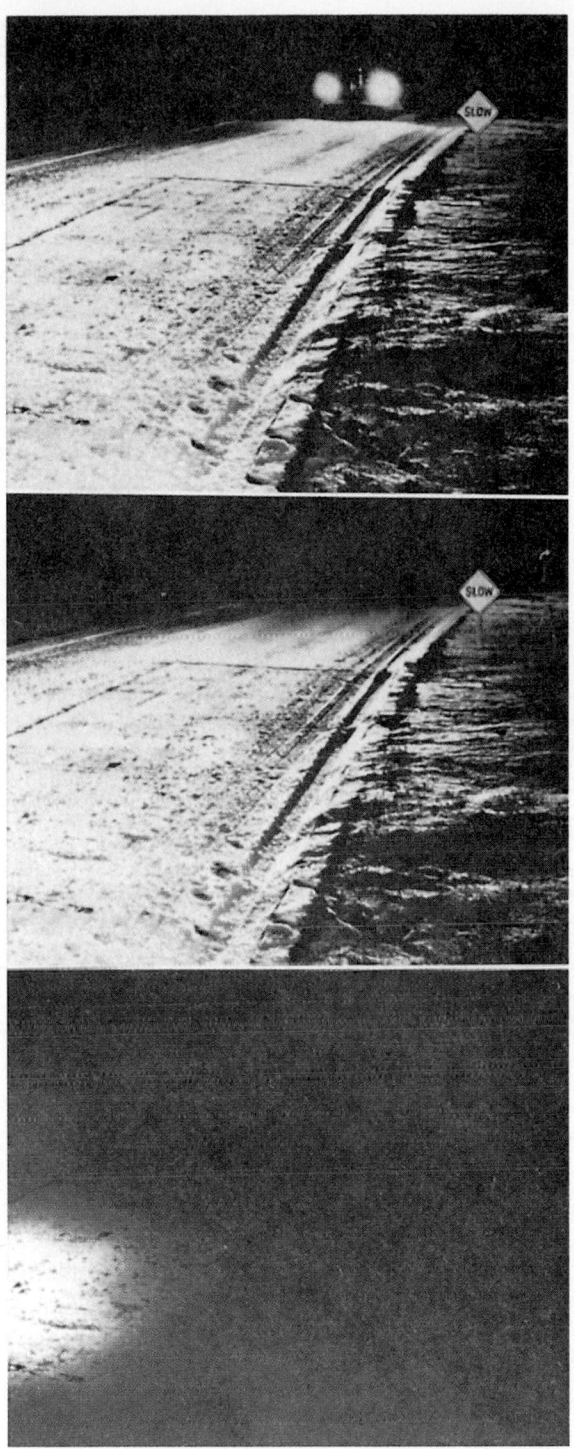

Fig. 7-3 Night blindness. These photographs simulate the eyes' slow response to a flash of light at night.

or a bout of measles may be deadly. Growth is inhibited because of lack of vitamin A-dependent proteins for bone growth.

In the United States, individuals experiencing chronic fat malabsorption would be at risk for vitamin A deficiency as well as deficiencies of other fat-soluble vitamins. These nutrients would be incorporated into their overall medical nutrition therapy plans. Although marginal vitamin A deficiency is possible, overt deficiencies are rare. Deficiency is a health threat in parts of the world where food availability is limited.

HEALTH DEBATE

Antioxidants: A Medical Wonder?

Beta-carotene, a precursor for vitamin A, functions as an antioxidant in the body. Antioxidants appear to protect the maturing body from the effects of free radicals on cell structure; this protection may reduce the risk of developing cancer and heart disease.

Free radicals include oxidizing agents such as singlet oxygen. Oxygen is usually found as molecular oxygen (O_2), which is stable. However, it can occur as a single oxygen atom and is quite unstable, ready to hook up with other substances. Any substance *hooked up* with the singlet oxygen is destroyed. Free radicals are formed as part of metabolic processes in cells or from the effects of environmental pollutants on the body. Pollutants may include exposure to smoke, ozone, car exhaust, cigarette smoke, and sunlight.

Antioxidant nutrients, which also include vitamin C and vitamin E, can be thought of as cellular lifeguards. Like any lifesaver,

antioxidants can be viewed as protecting membranes and other cell components, including DNA. This protection may prevent damage by the free radicals. Instead of the cellular components being oxidized by free radicals, the antioxidant is oxidized.

The controversy over antioxidants is whether we can consume sufficient amounts through our dietary intake of foods, particularly from fruits and vegetables. Medical experts disagree as to whether supplementation with antioxidants should be recommended. Those in favor of supplementation maintain that the amount of antioxidants needed for disease prevention is more than Americans could reasonably consume from foods. Those opposed believe supplementation is premature and has associated risks such as iron overload from large doses of vitamin C. More research is needed before general recommendations to the public are advocated. Table 7-5 lists sources of the major antioxidants.

From Mermel VL et al: Antioxidants: The basics, *Nutri News* Spring 1994.

Table 7-4	Vitamin A/Beta-Carotene Sources*	
Food	**Serving**	**Vitamin A/Beta-Carotene**
Apricots	3 medium	277 RE
Butternut squash	½ cup cooked	714 RE
Carrots	1 whole	2025 RE
	½ cup cooked	1915 RE
Cantaloupe	1 cup	516 RE
Liver (beef)	3½ oz	10,000 RE
Spinach	½ cup cooked	737 RE
Sweet potato	1 whole baked	2488 RE
Red pepper	1 whole	422 RE

Data from Pennington JAT: *Bowes & Church's food values of portions commonly used*, ed 16, 1994, Lippincott.
*RDA = 1000 RE for men; 800 RE for women.

Vitamin A supplements taken internally will not cure or improve acne and are toxic in excess.

The acne medications Accutane and Retinaid are nonnutritive sources of vitamin A that cause birth defects when used by pregnant women. Advise women who take either of these drugs to use a highly reliable birth control method.

Toxicity

Hypervitaminosis A occurs only from preformed vitamin A from either an acute or chronic intake of supplements. Most food sources of preformed A do not contain high enough levels to ever result in toxicity. The only exception noted is polar bear liver. Explorers who feasted on polar bear liver developed hypervitaminosis A; in fact, the way we learned about the toxic effects of vitamin A was through their misfortune (5). Apparently, the livers of hibernating animals store an extraordinary quantity of vitamin A to provide sufficient amounts for a long winter without nourishment. When humans consume the preformed vitamin A of these livers, the quantity is toxic.

Toxicity does not occur from the carotenoid precursor in foods. If carotenoids are consumed in excess, either from foods or supplements, the skin takes on an orange hue, which dissipates when carotenoid consumption is reduced.

Table 7-5   Antioxidants

Antioxidant	Antioxidant Functions	Major Food Sources	Adult RDA	Daily Recommended Supplementation
Beta-carotene (pre Vitamin A)	May decrease risk of some cancers and CAD	Sweet potatoes, winter squash, carrots, red bell peppers, dark green vegetables, apricots, mangos, canteloupe	No RDA (1 sweet potato = 15 mg, 1 carrot = 10 mg)	6-15 mg, nontoxic, higher doses may give skin a harmless orange cast
Vitamin C	May decrease risk of risk of certain cancers and CAD	Kiwi, citrus fruits, berries, cantaloupe, honeydew, bell peppers, tomatoes, cabbage family vegetables	60 mg (1 kiwi = 150 mg 1 cup broccoli = 115 mg, 1 orange = 70 mg)	250-500 mg, more may cause diarrhea
Vitamin E	May decrease risk of cancer and CAD; may also prevent or delay cataracts	Vegetable oil, nuts, seeds, margarine, wheat germ, olives, leafy greens, avocado, asparagus	12 IU for women; 15 IU for men (1 tbsp oil = 12 IU, 1 tbsp margarine or 1 oz nuts = 3 IU)	200-400 IU daily for all adults, higher doses may cause headaches and diarrhea

Modified from University of California at Berkeley Wellness Letter, Jan 1994. In *Nutri-News* Spring 1994:6.

Immediate symptoms of vitamin A toxicity include blistered skin, weakness, anorexia, vomiting, headache, joint pain, irritability, and enlargment of the spleen and liver; long-term effects include bone abnormalities and liver damage (20).

Vitamin D

With sufficient exposure to ultraviolet light or sunshine, the body can manufacture its own supply of vitamin D by converting a form of cholesterol in the skin. Because vitamin D can be produced by the body, it is technically a hormone. However, when vitamin D is supplied by the diet, it is technically a vitamin. Regardless of how it is classified, vitamin D is a substance that is necessary for a variety of the body's regulating processes as well as normal development of bones and teeth.

Function

Intestinal absorption of calcium and phosphorus depends on the action of vitamin D. This vitamin also affects bone mineralization and mineral homeostasis by helping to regulate blood calcium levels.

Recommended intake and sources

The RDA for vitamin D is 10 mcg.

Vitamin D is available through body synthesis or from dietary sources. Cholecalciferol, the active form of vitamin D, can be synthesized; ultraviolet irradiation from sunlight affects the vitamin D precursor, 7-dehydrocholesterol, in our skin, and this cholesterol derivative is transformed by the liver and kidneys into cholecalciferol. The amount of vitamin D produced depends on length of exposure to ultraviolet irradiation, atmospheric conditions, and skin pigmentation. Geographical regions and seasons that are particularly cloudy and rainy diminish the quantity of vitamin D synthesized. Darker skin pigmentation also reduces the effect of radiation on the skin, as does sun screen and concealing clothing. Aging may lessen the amount of vitamin D to be formed from sunlight exposure (5).

The few sources of natural preformed vitamin D are the fat of the animal-related foods of butter, egg yolks, fatty fish, and liver. Milk, although containing fat, is not a good source; it is, however, a good vehicle for vitamin D fortification because it contains calcium and phosphorus, which need vitamin D for absorption. Since vegans consume no animal foods, they may require supplements or regular sunlight exposure to assure formation of cholecalciferol. Appropriate guidance should be sought from a physician or dietitian.

Deficiency

A deficiency of vitamin D can lead to the disorders of **rickets** (Fig. 7-4) and **osteo-malacia.** Because of insufficient mineralization of bone and tooth matrix, rickets in children leads to malformed skeletons characterized by bowed legs unable to bear body weight, oddly angled rib bones and chests, and abnormal tooth formation. In adults, osteomalacia or *bad bones* is characterized by soft bones that are at risk for fractures.

Rickets has been thought to rarely occur among well-nourished populations, but recent reports reveal that among well-fed African-American children of families following the dietary and dress customs of the Muslim faith, the risk of rickets has increased (21). The increased risk is due to several factors including darker pigmentation, having children wear heavier clothing that limits exposure of the skin to vitamin D synthesis, and limited consumption of dietary sources of fortified vitamin D dairy products by children or women who are breastfeeding infants. Health care providers initially misdiagnosed cases of rickets among these children, since the disease is more common in instances of famine, neglect, malabsorption, or restricted dietary intakes (21).

Among older adults who may also have a diminished ability to produce vitamin D, osteomalacia may develop when marginal intakes of vitamin D and/or calcium exist for a number of years; the first outward symptom may unfortunately be a fractured hip.

The use of sedatives and tranquilizers as well as anticonvulsant therapy in persons with epilepsy also has been associated with increases in the incidence of rickets and osteomalacia (14).

Another disorder of the skeleton is **osteoporosis.** As with osteomalacia, osteoporosis is a condition in which bone density is reduced and the remaining

rickets
a childhood disorder caused by vitamin D or calcium deficiency leading to insufficient mineralization of bone and tooth matrix

osteomalacia
an adult disorder caused by vitamin D or calcium deficiency characterized by soft, demineralized bones

osteoporosis
a multifactorial disorder in which bone density is reduced and remaining bone is brittle, breaking easily

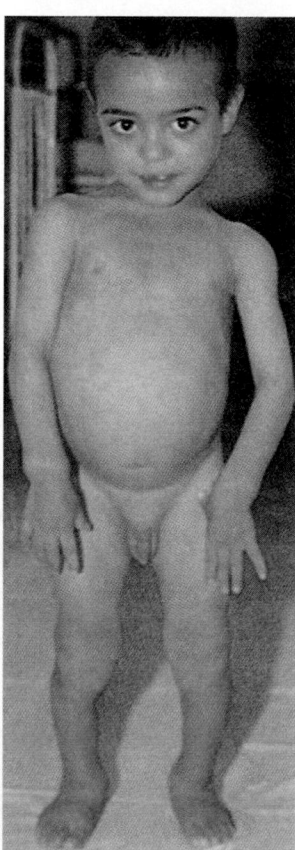

Fig. 7-4 Rickets. This child has characteristic bowed legs.

bone is brittle and breaks easily. Since vitamin D is crucial for absorption of calcium and the mineralization of bone, chronic vitamin D deficiency may be one of the risk factors of this disorder. Osteoporosis is discussed in detail in Chapter 8.

Outright deficiency of vitamin D is rare in the United States, since milk and related food products are fortified. Deficiency is a concern when a lack of exposure to sunlight occurs, either because of environmental limitations or cultural clothing customs that conceal the body, or in the elderly or persons with disabilities who may be unable to get outdoors and/or be malnourished. These conditions may require vigilance in the consumption of fortified dietary sources, or supplements may be appropriate (5).

Toxicity

High intakes of vitamin D can result in *hypercalcemia* (high blood levels of calcium) and *hypercalciuria* (high calcium level in urine), which affect kidneys and may cause cardiovascular damage. Toxicity symptoms occur in people whose diet contains as little as five times the RDA, making vitamin D the most toxic of vitamins.

Vitamin E

During the 1970s vitamin E supplements were a popular aphrodisiac. Male virility, in particular, was thought to be enhanced by taking extra vitamin E. There was only one problem. Vitamin E increased the libido of male rats, not of humans. Research conducted on rats about the effects of vitamin E noted that male rats were able to reproduce better with additional intake of vitamin E. Although research conducted on rats is often applicable to humans, in this instance the results could not be generalized to humans. However, vitamin E is an essential nutrient performing vital functions; we are still learning more about its role in relation to disease prevention.

Function

Vitamin E acts as an antioxidant, protecting polyunsaturated fatty acids and vitamin A in cell membranes from oxidative damage by being oxidized itself. This function is particularly important in protecting the integrity of lung and red blood cell membranes, which are exposed to large amounts of oxygen. Other antioxidative functions of vitamin E are performed as part of a system in conjunction with selenium and ascorbic acid (vitamin C).

Recommended intake and sources

Vitamin E is the name given to a family of compounds called tocopherols, which are found in plants. Alpha-tocopherol is the most widely occurring form of tocopherol and is also the most active for vitamin E. Vitamin E is measured in terms of alpha-tocopherol equivalents (α-TE). The RDA for vitamin E is 10 mg α-TE for men and 8 mg α-TE for women. A positive relationship exists between dietary intake of polyunsaturated fats and vitamin E requirements; as our dietary intake of polyunsaturated fats increases, we need more vitamin E to protect the integrity of the polyunsaturated fats from oxidation as they move through the body.

The best sources of vitamin E are vegetable oils (including corn, soy, safflower, and cottonseed) and margarine. Whole grains, seeds, nuts, wheat germ, and green leafy vegetables also provide adequate amounts of vitamin E. Processing of these foods may decrease the final vitamin E content.

Deficiency

A primary deficiency of vitamin E is very rare. Secondary deficiencies occur in premature infants and others who are unable to absorb fat normally. Some chronic fat absorption disorders in which deficiencies may occur are **cystic fibrosis, biliary atresia,** other disorders of the hepatobiliary system, and/or liver transport problems.

cystic fibrosis
a genetic disorder in which excessive mucus is produced, primarily affecting respiratory airways; also limits fat-absorption in the digestion system; most common among Caucasian populations

biliary atresia
a congenital condition in which the major bile duct is blocked, limiting the availability of bile for fat digestion

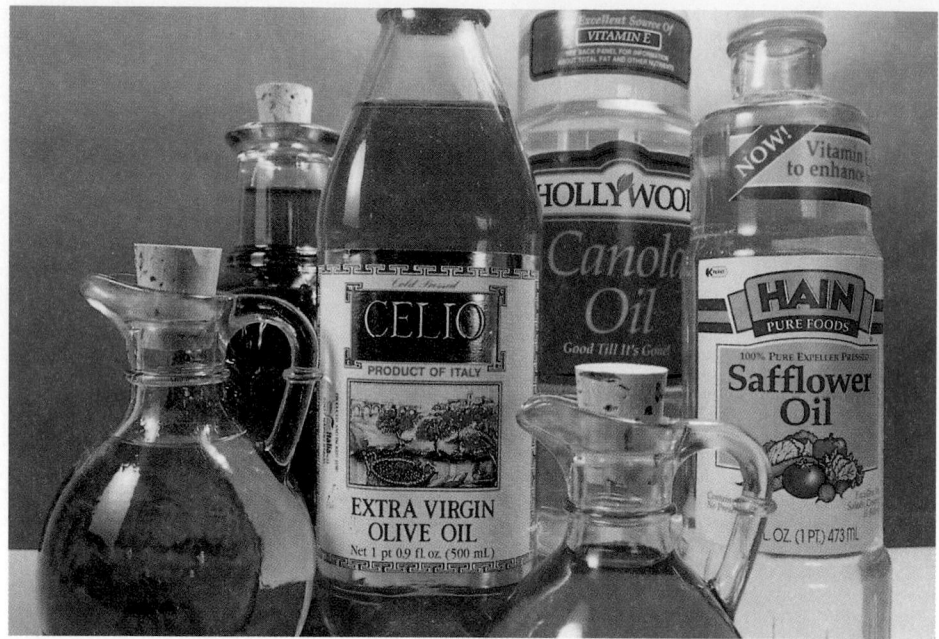

Vegetable oils provide vitamin E.

Symptoms of vitamin E deficiency include neurological disorders resulting from cell damage anemia caused by hemolysis of red blood cells (hemolytic anemia).

Toxicity

There is no evidence of toxicity associated with excessive intake of vitamin E. Intakes of 100 to 800 mg per day appear to be tolerated, but the value of such doses has not been determined (22). Megadoses of vitamin E can exacerbate the anticoagulant effect of drugs taken to reduce blood clotting; vitamin E supplementation is not recommended in persons receiving anticoagulant therapy, with a coagulation disorder, or with a vitamin K deficiency.

Vitamin K

Discovered by a Danish scientist, vitamin K was called *koagulationsvitamin* for its blood clotting properties. Later research revealed that vitamin K is several related compounds with similar functions in the body.

Function

Vitamin K's main function is as a cofactor in the synthesis of blood clotting factors, including prothrombin. Protein formation in bone, kidney, and plasma also depends on the actions of vitamin K.

Recommended intake and sources

The RDA is 70 mcg and 65 mcg for men and women, respectively. This amount provides for sufficient storage of vitamin K in the liver. Vitamin K actually consists of compounds in different forms in plant and animal tissues. All are converted by our livers to the biologically active form of menaquinone called vitamin K.

Vitamin K is available through dietary sources and can also be synthesized by microflora in the jejunum and ileum of the digestive tract. From plants, vitamin K is consumed as phylloquinone; bacterial synthesis produces vitamin K homologues as forms of menaquinones. As noted, phylloquinone and vitamin K homologues are converted to the active form of menaquinone, vitamin K, by the liver.

Vitamin K is still an essential nutrient even though it is synthesized in the body. The key distinction is that bacteria hosted by the human body produce the vitamin. Additionally, not enough vitamin K is produced by the microflora to assure adequate levels for total blood clotting needs; dietary intake is still required (23).

Primary food sources for vitamin K are dark green leafy vegetables. Lesser amounts are found in dairy products, cereals, meats, and fruits.

Deficiency

Deficiency of vitamin K inhibits blood coagulation. Deficiencies may be observed in clinical settings related to malabsorption disorders or drug/medication interactions. Long-term intensive antibiotic therapy destroys the intestinal microflora that produce vitamin K. As with the other fat-soluble vitamins, any barrier to absorption affects the quantity of fat-soluble vitamin absorbed.

Premature infants and newborns are unable to immediately produce vitamin K; their guts are too sterile, free from the microflora necessary to produce vitamin K. Hospitals in the United States routinely give newborns an intramuscular dose of vitamin K to prevent hemorrhagic disease.

Toxicity

Consumption of foods containing vitamin K produces no problems of toxicity. Therapeutic administration of vitamin K in the menadione form has caused reactions in neonates, including hemolytic anemia and **hyperbilirubinemia.** Phylloquinone administration has been acceptable (6).

Table 7-6 provides a summary of fat-soluble vitamins.

hyperbilirubinemia
a neonatal condition of excessively high levels of bilirubin (red bile pigment) leading to jaundice, in which bile is deposited in tissues throughout the body

OVERCOMING BARRIERS

Why do vitamins capture the attention of Americans? We generally do not suffer from vitamin deficiencies, and any problems of vitamin toxicity tend to be self-imposed. Considered through a wellness perspective, vitamins are just one of many factors for achieving optimum health. Yet sales of dietary supplements have significantly increased from $500 million in 1972 to $4 billion in 1993 (5,24). A comprehensive FDA telephone survey of almost 3000 adults indicated that about 36% of the men and 44% of the women (nonpregnant and nonlactating) consumed dietary supplements daily (25). What is the rationale for taking supplements?

Perhaps vitamins are an easier target on which to focus when emphasizing good health. If a person is concerned about vitamin intake, a vitamin pill can always be taken. That's a lot easier than the dietary and behavior modifications required to meet other health factors such as decreasing fat intake or increasing physical activities.

TOWARD A POSITIVE NUTRITION LIFESTYLE: SOCIAL SUPPORT

Social support extends throughout the life span; it goes beyond having friends and family with which to socialize. For families with young children, social support may be cooperative meals when illness strikes (such as during a flu epidemic) and cooking time becomes compromised. The term *cooperative* may mean cooking double portions to feed a friend's family during bouts of chicken pox or childhood ear infections. The kindness would then be reciprocated

Table 7-6   Fat-soluble Vitamins

Vitamin	Function	Clinical Issues Deficiency/Toxicity	Requirements	Food Sources
Vitamin A Precursor: carotenoids Preformed vitamin: retinoids	Maintains epithelial tissues (skin and mucous membranes); rhodopsin formation for vision; bone growth; reproduction	Deficiency: xerophthalmia; night blindness; keratomalcia; degeneration of epithelial tissue; inhibited growth (respiratory and GI disturbances) Toxicity: hypervitaminosis A (from supplements) with blistered skin, weakness, anorexia, vomiting, enlarged spleen and liver	Men: 1000 RE Women: 800 RE	Deep green, yellow, and orange fruits and vegetables; animal fat sources: whole milk, fortified skim, and lowfat milk; butter; liver; egg yolks, fatty fish
Vitamin D Precursor: 7-dehydrocholesterol Active form: cholecalciferol	Calcium and phosphorus absorption; bone mineralization	Deficiency: bone malformation, rickets (children), osteomalacia (adults) Toxicity: hypercalcemia, hypercalciuria	Adults: 10 mcg (< 24 years 5 mcg)	Animal (fat) sources: butter, egg yolks, fatty fish, liver, fortified milk; body synthesis
Vitamin E alpha-tocopherol	Antioxidant for PUFA and vitamin A; antioxidant with selenium and ascorbic acid	Deficiency: primary deficiency rare; secondary deficiency (due to fat absorption) neurological disorders Toxicity: none, but supplements contraindicated with anticoagulation drugs	Men: 10 mg α-TE Women: 8 mg α-TE	Vegetable oil, whole grains, seeds, nuts, green leafy vegetables
Vitamin K Active form: menaquinones	Cofactor in synthesis of blood clotting factors; protein formation	Deficiency: blood coagulation inhibited; hemorrhagic disease (infants) Toxicity: therapeutic vitamin K (menadione form) reactions in neonates causing hemolytic anemia and hyperbilirubinemia	Men: 70 mcg Women: 65 mcg	Green leafy vegetables, intestinal synthesis

RE, Retinol Equivalents; α-*TE,* alpha-tocopheral equivalent.

in the future. Both families gain nutritious meals at times when just thinking about cooking seems overwhelming.

Support for elderly persons, as mentioned earlier in this chapter, may mean assistance with food shopping or having foods delivered. This social support may be provided by neighbors or relatives. In some communities, local Red Cross chapters and other charitable organizations have developed car or bus service specifically to provide transportation so that older residents can safely shop in food stores and have the convenience of being driven to their homes and assisted with carrying groceries into their kitchens. Health care professionals working with older clients can be aware of these services or perhaps help community organizations to initiate similar programs.

SUMMARY

Vitamins are organic molecules that perform specific metabolic functions and are required in very small amounts. As essential nutrients, they must be provided through dietary intake. Vitamins are divided into two categories of water- and fat-soluble vitamins. Solubility of vitamins affects the processes of absorption, transportation, and storage of vitamins in our bodies.

Water-soluble vitamins are vitamin C and the B complex vitamins (thiamin, riboflavin, niacin, folate, pyridoxine (B_6), vitamin B_{12}, pantothenic acid, and biotin). The B vitamins function as coenzymes. Vitamin C serves as an antioxidant in addition to its coenzyme ability. Water-soluble vitamins are easily absorbed into blood circulation. Excesses are excreted so toxicity is less likely but may occur with pyridoxine and vitamin C.

Fat-soluble vitamins are vitamins A, D, E, and K. These vitamins serve structural and regulatory functions throughout the body. Fat-soluble vitamins are absorbed the same as lipids; bile is required, and the nutrients enter the lymphatic system. Since they are retained in fatty substances in the body, toxicity from supplemental intakes is possible.

THE NURSING ROLE
Vitamins and Chronic Alcohol Use: The Nursing Process

As you have read in this chapter, many vitamin deficiencies are seen in people who are chronic excessive alcohol users. In fact, alcoholism is probably the primary cause of vitamin and other nutrient deficiencies in the United States. The nutritional problems arise because the person substitutes alcohol for food and because alcohol is toxic to all cells. Any patient suspected of chronic excessive alcohol use should undergo a thorough nutritional assessment. Following are aspects of the nursing process that should be considered when evaluating vitamin intake status of these individuals.

Continued.

THE NURSING ROLE, cont'd.

Vitamins and Chronic Alcohol Use: The Nursing Process

ASSESSMENT

Factor	Findings of Concern
Objective:	
Intake of foods containing thiamin, niacin, folic acid, vitamins A and C	Underconsumption
Muscle strength	Muscle weakness (especially in the legs), ataxia
Skin	Dermatitis on sun-exposed skin, bruising, poor wound healing
Mouth	Gingivitis, bleeding gums, loose teeth, glossitis
Gastrointestinal function	Anorexia, diarrhea
Mental condition	Irritability, disorientation, depression, paranoia, anxiety
Subjective:	
Pain	Muscular and joint pain
Vision	Diplopia, night blindness

NURSING DIAGNOSIS

Diagnoses are usually based on underconsumption of essential vitamins and other nutrients. The causes are alcohol being consumed instead of food, the toxic effects of ethanol, anorexia, and lack of money for food. An example of the type of diagnosis that may be written is "Altered nutrition, less than body requirements of thiamin, related to alcoholic malnutrition, as evidenced by ataxia and joint pain."

PLANNING

The nurse, nutritionist, primary health provider, and social worker may all need to collaborate on setting goals that are realistic and that address the myriad problems of the person who is a chronic excessive alcohol user. After detoxification, nutritional problems may be the first to be addressed. An example of a goal that may be set is "The client will select, from a choice presented, a daily diet plan which includes adequate vitamins and minerals."

INTERVENTION

The regimen may include:
1. Vitamin supplements
2. Supplements of other nutrients (minerals, protein)
3. Treatment of presenting vitamin deficiency symptoms
4. Weekly weight measurement
5. Recording of daily food diaries
6. Teaching about importance of food variety and Food Pyramid principles

EVALUATION

Each goal should be evaluated to determine whether the outcome has been met as evidenced by such things as:

Decrease in joint pain within 3 months
Improved orientation to time, place, and person within 3 months
Increase in caloric intake to 2000 kcalories daily by 1 month
A daily food diary that reveals food selections adequate in vitamins and minerals

THE NURSING ROLE, cont'd.
Vitamins and Chronic Alcohol Use: The Nursing Process

Because many people who are chronic excessive alcohol users have to make a variety of behavior changes, nurses and other health professionals need patience and understanding when working with them. Goals may have to be modified periodically and new interventions substituted before outcomes are finally reached.

REFERENCES

1. Pagana KD, Pagana JT: *Mosby's diagnostic and laboratory test reference,* St. Louis, 1992, Mosby.
2. Talalay P et al: *The proceedings of the National Academy of Sciences,* April 12, 1994.
3. Tanphaichitr V: Thiamin. In Shils ME, Olson JA, Shike M, eds: *Modern nutrition in health and disease,* ed 8, Philadelphia, 1994, Lea & Febiger.
4. Dreyfus PM, Seyal M: Diet and nutrition in neurological disorders. In Shils ME, Olson JA, Shike M, eds: *Modern nutrition in health and disease,* ed 8, Philadelphia, 1994, Lea & Febiger.
5. National Academy of Science: *Diet and health: Implications for reducing chronic disease risk,* Washington, DC, 1989, National Academy Press.
6. Food and Nutrition Board/National Research Council: *Recommended dietary allowances,* ed 10, Washington, DC, 1989, National Academy Press.
7. McCormick DB: Riboflavin. In Shils ME, Olson JA, Shike M, eds: *Modern nutrition in health and disease,* ed 8, Philadelphia, 1994, Lea & Febiger.
8. Swenseid ME, Jacob RA: Niacin. In Shils ME, Olson JA, Shike M, eds: *Modern nutrition in health and disease,* ed 8, Philadelphia, 1994, Lea & Febiger.
9. Davis J, Sherer K: *Applied nutrition and diet therapy for nurses,* ed 2, Philadelphia, 1994, Saunders.
10. Weinsier RL, Morgan SL: *Fundamentals of clinical nutrition,* St. Louis, 1993, Mosby.
11. Hine RJ: Folic acid: Contemporary clinical perspective, *Persp Appl Nutr* 1(2):1-14, Autumn 1993.
12. Williams RD: FDA proposes folic acid fortification, *FDA Consumer* May 1994:11-14.
13. Herbert V, Das KC: Folic acid and vitamin B_{12}. In Shils ME, Olson JA, Shike M, eds: *Modern nutrition in health and disease,* ed 8, Philadelphia, 1994, Lea & Febiger.
14. Guthrie HA, Picciano MF: *Human Nutrition,* St. Louis, 1995, Mosby.
15. Liddenbaum et al: Neuropsychiatric disorders caused by cobalamin deficiency in the absence of anemia or macrocytosis, *N Engl J Med* 318:1720-1728, 1988.
16. Marshall MW et al: Effect of low and high fat diets varying in ratios of polyunsaturated to saturated fatty acids on biotin intakes and biotin in serum, red cells and urine of adult men, *Nutr Res* 5:801, 1985.
17. Jacob RA: Vitamin C. In Shils ME, Olson JA, Shike M, eds: *Modern nutrition in health and disease,* ed 8, Philadelphia, 1994, Lea & Febiger.
18. Hemila H: Vitamin C and the common cold, *Br Nutr,* 67:3, 1992.
19. Underwood BA: Vitamin A in animal and human nutrition. In Sporn MB, Roberts AB, Goodman DS, eds: *The retinoids,* vol 1, Orlando, Fla, 1984, Academic Press.
20. Olson JA: Vitamin A, retinoids and carotenoids. In Shils ME, Olson JA, Shike M, eds: *Modern nutrition in health and disease,* ed 8, Philadelphia, 1994, Lea & Febiger.
21. Tortorella K: Rickets, a relic shows up again, *New York Times,* sec 13:1, March 12, 1995.
22. Bendich A, Machlin LJ: Safety of oral intake of vitamin E, *Am J Clin Nutr* 48:612-619, 1988.
23. Suttie JW et al: Vitamin K deficiency from dietary vitamin K restriction in humans, *Am J Clin Nutr* 47:475-480, 1988.
24. American Dietetic Association, Positions of the American Dietetic Association: Enrichment and fortification of foods and dietary supplements, *J Am Diet Assoc* 94(6):661-663, June 1994.
25. Stewart ML et al: Vitamin/mineral supplement use: A telephone survey of adults in the United States, *J Am Diet Assoc* 85:1586-1590, December 1985.

Chapter 8

WATER AND MINERALS

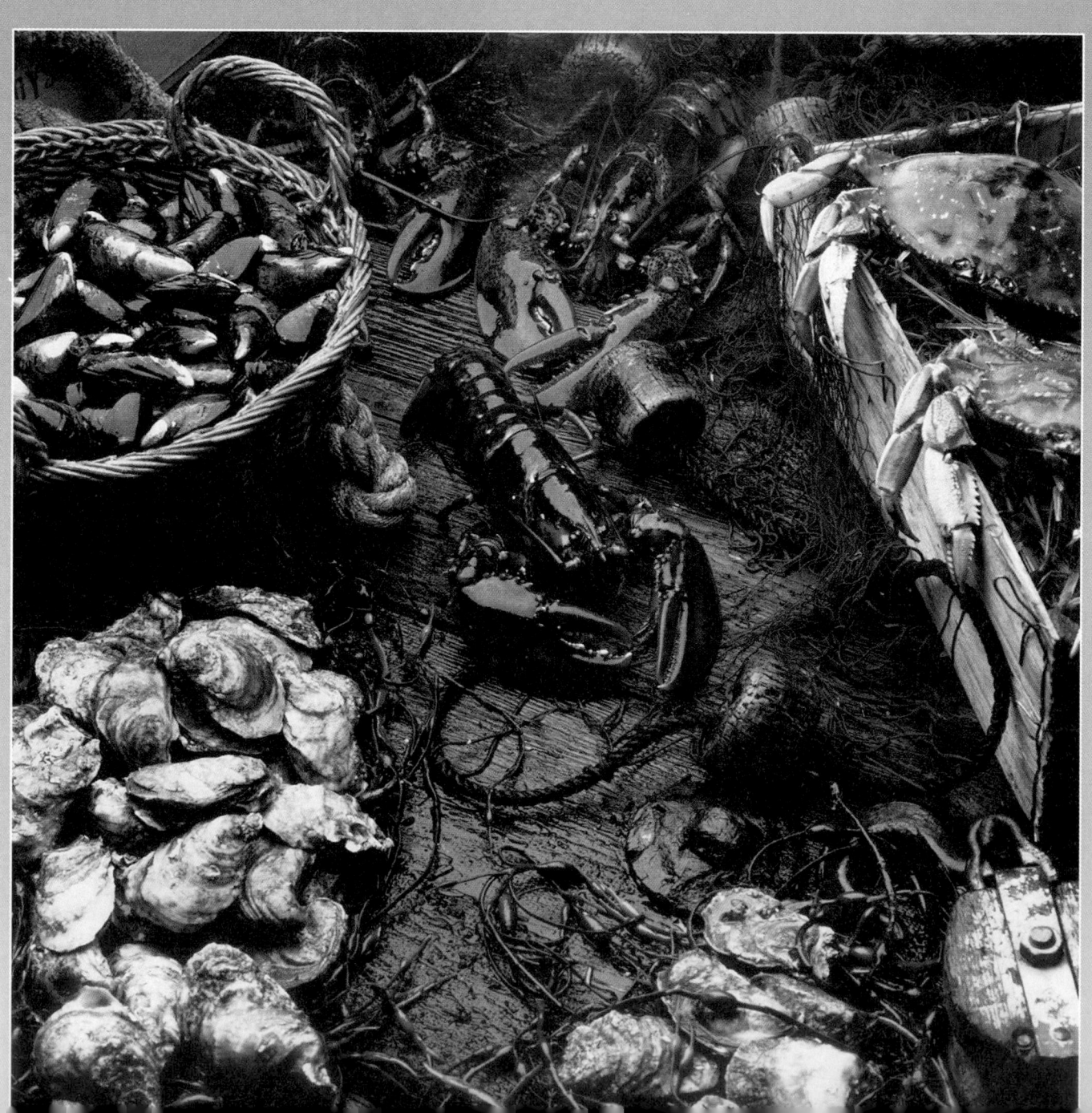

ROLE IN WELLNESS

An ever-circulating ocean of fluid bathes all the cells of our bodies; this fluid allows for chemical reactions, transmission of nerve impulses, and transportation of nutrients and waste products throughout the body. The fluid is not simply *water*, although water is its primary constituent. Some fluid in the body is used to form blood, lymph, and structure for cells. Minerals circulating in our body fluids create the setting for biochemical functions to occur.

Although water and minerals are primary components of body fluids, each performs other functions as well. This chapter explores water and minerals in the context of their nutritional requirements and physiological roles for achieving nutritional wellness.

WATER

We can live several weeks without food, but can survive only a few days without water or fluids. Although our bodies use stored nutrients to fuel energy needs, a minimum intake of water is required for cell function and as a solution through which waste products of the body are excreted in urine.

Food Sources

If we drank only water and no other liquids, we could meet our body's need for fluid. Most of us, however, consume water in addition to other fluids throughout the day. Some fluids also contain other nutrients. Consider the wealth of nutrients found in milk (skim or whole), fruit juices, and soups. Some fruits and vegetables contain as much as 85% to 95% water. Watermelon, grapes, oranges, lettuce, tomatoes, and zucchini have a high water content. Most foods contain water, but some are better sources of fluids than others. Generally, we depend on beverages as our main source of fluids.

Water intake recommendations developed to accompany the RDAs suggest that adults consume 1.0 to 1.5 ml of water for each kcalorie they expend under normal conditions or about 2 l (2 qts) per 2000 kcalories, which equals about 8 glasses of water a day (1). The American Medical Association Health Resolution for 1993 advised 6 to 8 glasses of water daily. Although the minimum amount needed by healthy adults is about 4 glasses, higher amounts may be optimum considering an individual's physiological status and energy output.

Our primary source of water should be the liquids we drink (Table 8-1). Notice that soft drinks, alcohol, coffee, and tea are not listed as primary sources. Although they do contain water, coffee, tea, and alcohol act as diuretics, causing an increase in water loss via the kidneys as urine. Soft drinks add fluid to the body, but they contain solutes (sugar, salt, various chemicals) that must be diluted as they enter the bloodstream. Drinking a soda increases the concentration of these solutes in your blood. Your body responds by pulling fluid from the cells into the bloodstream to dilute the sugar and salt. You lose the increased fluid in your bloodstream when you excrete it as urine. In addition, your body responds to the increased solutes and decreased fluid content by once again triggering your thirst mechanism.

Bottled water has become a mainstay in US beverage selections and an economic force. Sales of bottled water reached almost 3 billion dollars in 1993 (2). Products range from imported sparkling mineral waters to spring waters to waters treated from nearby reservoirs. Although the price range is equally broad, the common

Table 8-1 Sources of Water	
Food	Percent Water
DAIRY PRODUCTS	
Milk	88-91
Cottage cheese	79
Cheddar cheese	37
Ice cream, ice milk	61-66
FRUITS	
Grapefruit (whole or juice)	90
Melons	90
Oranges (whole or juice)	88
Grapes	81
Apples	84
VEGETABLES	
Asparagus	91
Carrots	88
Cucumber	96
Lettuce	96
Potato	75
Spinach	90
Sweet potato	73
Tomatoes	94
MISCELLANEOUS	
Soups	85-98
Gelatin	84
Fruit punch	88
Beans (cooked)	60-70
Meats	50-60
Poultry	65
Oatmeal (cooked)	85
Bread	30-40

From USDA: Nutritive value of foods, *Home and Garden Bulletin* 72, 1991.

denominator is that Americans enjoy the convenience of water as a beverage when available in portable containers and single portions.

Water quality

Minerals found naturally in water vary. **Hard water** refers to water that contains high amounts of minerals such as calcium and magnesium. Drinking this water can provide a significant amount of these nutrients. Nonnutrition-related problems from hard water can develop; appliances and other machinery that interact with water may be damaged by mineral deposits, and soap suds are reduced. To reduce these problems, water can be *softened* by a filtration process that replaces some minerals with sodium chloride (salt). **Soft water** containing sodium, however, can be a problem for sodium-sensitive individuals such as those at risk for hypertension. To prevent health problems, water softeners may be used on only the hot tap in kitchens, leaving the cold tap *unsoftened* for consumption.

Another aspect of water quality is contamination. For example, many older buildings have pipes with lead solder joints that can release lead into the water sitting in or running through them. If the level of lead in water is more than 15 parts per billion (PPB), pregnant women, infants, and children are advised to drink bottled water; even low levels of lead can seriously impair normal development. Your

hard water
water that contains high amounts of minerals such as calcium and magnesium

soft water
water that has been filtered to replace some of the minerals with sodium

local health department can recommend a competent laboratory if you wish to have your water tested.

Some contamination concerns can be remedied by water treatment processes. Others, such as industrial pollution, can be difficult to identify. Complications of bacterial contamination or inadvertent exposure of water to carcinogenic industrial substances can lead to health problems ranging from simple gastroenteritis to cancer. Municipal and regional water processing plants take great care to assure the safest water supply possible. Some water sources (private wells, surface water, springs, and cisterns), however, may exceed the Maximum Contaminant Levels set by the Environmental Protection Agency (3).

The most severe water-related threats such as cholera and typhoid are no longer public health hazards in North America. Other potential industrial and environmental pollutants, however, can enter our water supply and endanger our health. Small suppliers may not have the financial means to improve technological surveillance. A goal of *Healthy People 2000* is to address this need and increase the percentage of Americans receiving the safest water possible (3).

Poorer countries throughout the world continue to struggle with unsafe water supplies. Without the financial and technological knowledge and resources, many people become ill by consuming bacteria-contaminated water. Increased incidence of stomach cancer is associated with exposure to *Helicobacter pylori,* sometimes found in contaminated waters (4).

To reduce the chance of lead leaching into drinking and cooking water:

- Run the water for 2 minutes after it has been standing in the pipes.
- Use only cold water for drinking, cooking, and preparing baby formula (cold water absorbs less lead than hot).

Water as a Nutrient Within the Body

Structure

The structure of water—two hydrogen atoms bonded to one oxygen atom—allows it to provide a base for biochemical reactions in the body and to easily move through the various compartments of cells and body systems. As the basis of body fluids, water can host other substances of different electrical charges and characteristics. **Intracellular fluids** (within the cell) are composed of water plus concentrations of potassium and phosphates. **Interstitial fluids** (between the cells) contain concentrations of sodium and chloride. **Extracellular fluids** include interstitial fluid and encompass all fluids outside cells including plasma and the watery components of body organs and substances (Table 8-2).

Digestion and absorption

Since water is inorganic, it is not digested. It passes quickly to the small intestine. Once there, most water is absorbed; the rest is regulated by the colon and is either absorbed or excreted with feces.

intracellular fluid
fluid within the cells composed of water plus concentrations of potassium and phosphates

interstitial fluid
fluid between the cells containing concentrations of sodium and chloride

extracellular fluid
all fluids outside cells including interstitial fluid, plasma, and watery components of body organs and substances

Table 8-2 Body Fluid Compartments			
Intracellular Fluid (ICF)		**Extracellular Fluid (ECF)**	
PROTEINS	MINERALS	MINERALS	PROTEINS
Enzymes	Potassium	Sodium	Blood proteins
Hemoglobin	Magnesium	Chloride	Antibodies
	Phosphorus	Bicarbonate ions	
		CARBOHYDRATES	LIPIDS
		Glucose	Lipoproteins
65% of body water		35% of body water	

Metabolism

Although not metabolized or broken down by the GI tract processes, water is an integral component of metabolic processes. In some reactions, water of metabolism is water released as a byproduct of oxidative reactions; in others, water may be a part of the process to release energy from adenosine triphosphate (ATP), which is discussed in greater detail in Chapter 9. The released water may be excreted as waste or used elsewhere in the body. Glycogen in muscle and the liver contains water in the structure of glycogen molecules. When glycogen is used for energy, the water becomes available for body functions.

Functions

Water performs a variety of vital functions in the body. It is an important structural component of the body, giving shape and rigidity to cells. It assists in the regulating of body temperature. Water conducts heat, absorbing and distributing it throughout the body, keeping body temperature stable from day to day. Water also helps cool the body by evaporating invisibly from the lungs and the surface of the skin, carrying off excess heat. This type of water loss is called **insensible perspiration.**

Water acts as a lubricant in the form of joint fluid and mucous secretions. It forms a shock-absorbing fluid cushion for body tissues such as the amniotic sac, spinal cord, and eyes.

Water is a major component of blood, lymph, saliva, and urine. As such, it delivers nutrients and removes waste products. Acting as a **solvent,** it enables minerals, vitamins, glucose, and other small molecules to be moved throughout the body. Water also supplies trace minerals such as fluoride, zinc, and copper. Sometimes it is a source of too many minerals, including potentially toxic metals such as lead, cadmium, and incidental substances from pesticides and industrial waste products.

In addition to serving as a medium for biochemical reactions, water also participates as a **reactant.** For example, large molecules such as polysaccharides, fats, and protein are split into smaller molecules by reaction with water.

Ultimately no growth or cell renewal occurs without water; it is part of every cell and is necessary as a medium for reactions and transporter of supplies.

Regulation of Fluid/Water in the Body

Our bodies have delicate but very efficient mechanisms for maintaining appropriate fluid levels. The intake of fluids is balanced with the output through urine, sweat, feces, and insensible perspiration. Regulation of fluid in the body is of physiological importance because most of our body weight is composed of water. Water makes up 50% to 65% of the weight of an average adult; the percentages are even higher for infants whose body weights are 75% water. Fortunately, we just need to take in enough fluids and our body's natural systems take care of the rest.

Homeostasis is maintained by the extracellular distribution of sodium and of potassium intracellularly. Water moves within and between the cells in interstitial fluids in response to the levels of these minerals. An imbalance is corrected by mechanisms that cause thirst and regulate the ability of the kidneys to release or retain fluids.

Thirst, a dryness in the mouth, stimulates the desire to drink liquids. We often ignore our thirst until mealtimes. The thirst mechanism involves several steps. As the water level in the body gets low, the sodium and **solute** level in blood increases. This causes water to be drawn from the salivary glands to provide more fluid for the blood. The mouth then feels dry because less saliva, which keeps the mouth moist, is produced. This sensation, thirst, stimulates the drinking process. If the thirst mechanism is faulty, as it may be during illness or physical exertion, hormonal mechanisms also help conserve water by reducing urine output.

Functions of water

- provides shape and rigidity to cells
- helps to regulate body temperature
- acts as a lubricant
- cushions body tissues
- transports nutrients and waste products
- acts as a solvent
- provides a source of trace minerals
- participates in chemical reactions

insensible perspiration
water lost invisibly through evaporation from the lungs and skin

solvent (H_2O)
the liquid in which another substance (the solute) is dissolved to form a solution

reactant (Mg)
a substance that enters into and is altered during a chemical reaction

homeostasis $(=)$
a state of physiological equilibrium produced by a balance of functions and of chemical composition within an organism

solute
a substance dissolved in another substance

The mechanisms of the kidneys regulate the amounts of water excreted. Obligatory water excretion of at least 500 ml (one pint) must be excreted daily, regardless of the amount ingested, to clear the body of waste products. The mechanism relies on the combined actions of the brain, kidneys, pituitary gland, and adrenal gland. When fluid in the body becomes low, the hypothalamus stimulates the pituitary gland to release the **antidiuretic hormone (ADH)**. ADH is secreted in response to high sodium levels in the body or to low blood pressure or volume. The target organ of the hormone is the kidney. The kidneys then decrease excretion of water; the retained fluid is recycled for use throughout the body.

When the sodium concentration in the kidneys gets high (too much fluid excreted), another process kicks in to counteract the lowered blood volume and pressure. The kidneys release renin, an enzyme that activates the blood protein angiotensin. Angiotensin raises blood pressure by narrowing blood vessels; it is a vasoconstrictor. Angiotensin also prompts the adrenal gland to release the hormone **aldosterone**. The target organ of aldosterone is the kidney. The effect is to decrease excretion of sodium, causing the kidneys to respond by retaining fluid in the body.

Fluid and electrolytes

Dissolved in body fluids are mineral salts required for the regulation of fluid distribution both intracellularly and extracellularly. Fluids follow salt concentrations; this means that cells can control fluid balance by directing the movement of mineral salts.

Electrolytes are minerals that carry electrical charges or ions (particles) when dissolved in water; these minerals separate into positively charged ions called *cations* or negatively charge ions, *anions*. The primary extracellular electrolytes in body fluids are sodium (NA+/cation) and chloride (Cl–/anion), and the primary intracellular electrolyte is potassium (K+/cation). Water will follow electrolyte concentration. To move electrolytes in and out of the cell membrane requires transport proteins. The sodium/potassium pump is a transport protein that works to exchange sodium from within the cells for potassium.

In addition to water regulation, the kidneys also regulate electrolyte levels. If body levels of sodium are low, aldosterone directs the kidneys to reabsorb or retain more sodium. This in turn results in potassium being excreted so the balance of electrolytes is maintained.

Imbalances

What happens when our regulatory mechanisms are unable to maintain the balance? Abnormal shifts in fluid balance may cause fluid volume deficit or fluid volume excess.

Fluid volume deficit

In **fluid volume deficit (FVD)**, a person experiences vascular, cellular, or intracellular dehydration. Severe FVD, when body fluid levels fall 10% of body weight, is a medical emergency (5).

FVD can occur from diarrhea, vomiting, or high fever—symptoms often experienced with stomach and intestinal viral infections or influenza. Other causes of excessive fluid loss may be sweating, diuretics, or **polyuria**. Whenever we lose fluid and have difficulty taking in additional fluids, we are at risk for FVD.

Determining whether symptoms are due to dehydration or illness can be tricky. Characteristics of FVD include infrequent urination, decreased skin elasticity, dry mucous membranes, dry mouth, unusual drowsiness, lightheadedness or disorientation, extreme thirst, nausea, slow or rapid breathing, and sudden weight loss. The person will be less able to maintain blood pressure immediately after rising from a sitting or lying position (called *orthostatic hypotension*). For any illness

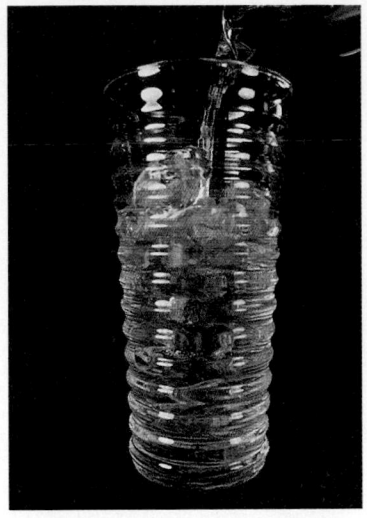

We need water in our diets every day.

antidiuretric hormone (ADH)
a hormone secreted by the pituitary gland in response to low fluid levels; affects kidneys to decrease excretion of water; also called vasopressin

aldosterone
a hormone secreted by the adrenal gland in response to sodium levels in kidneys; affects kidneys to balance fluid levels as needed

fluid volume deficit
the state in which a person experiences vascular, cellular, or intracellular dehydration

polyuria
excessive urination

lasting more than a few days that causes loss of body fluids, a primary health care provider should be consulted. In moderate or severe FVD, intravenous (IV) therapy is indicated to replace fluids.

FVD can also happen when we are not ill. Strenuous physical activity, either athletic or work-related, that causes excessive sweating can lead to FVD. Hot, dry weather also can overwork the body's cooling mechanisms. Drinking fluids throughout the day despite a low level of thirst sensation can alleviate these risks.

Elderly persons and infants are the groups most at risk for FVD. Elderly persons have decreased fluid reserves as well as diminished thirst mechanism acuity. FVD symptoms may be misdiagnosed as senility. Reminding elderly clients to drink even when thirst is not experienced is appropriate to assure adequate intake of fluids. In infants, water makes up a larger percentage of body weight than in adults, and a greater percentage is extracellular fluid; dehydration from fluid loss can occur rapidly. In addition to other signs of FVD, infants may have a depressed fontanel (soft spot) in the skull.

Fluid volume excess

fluid volume excess
the state in which a person experiences increased fluid retention and edema

edema
excess accumulation of fluid in interstitial spaces caused by seepage from the circulatory system

Fluid volume excess is a condition in which a person experiences increased fluid retention and edema. It is associated with a compromised regulatory mechanism, excess fluid intake, or excess sodium intake.

Edema is excess accumulation of fluid in interstitial spaces caused by seepage from the circulatory system or when the body retains about 10% more water than normal amounts. Some of us may notice that if we eat meals that are particularly high in sodium, we may feel *bloated* and our weight may even rise a few pounds the next day. This weight gain is not true weight gain, but simply water retention occurring in response to the excess intake of sodium. Within a few days, weight and water levels in the body return to their usual levels.

Edema can be a symptom of a health risk in certain situations. Sodium-sensitive individuals not only retain fluid when consuming high levels of sodium, but also

CULTURAL CONSIDERATIONS
A Chinese Study: Is it Applicable to Americans?

In Linxian, China the death rate from esophageal cancer is 100 times higher than in the United States; other cancers are high as well. As a joint effort, the National Cancer Institute, Chinese Academy of Medicine Sciences, and Rutgers University conducted a study to assess the effects of vitamin/mineral combinations on decreasing cancer incidence and mortality. Thirty thousand subjects, ages 40 to 69, received supplements daily for 5 years. Doses ranged from one to two times the RDA for various nutrients. Results revealed that the risk of death was lower in groups receiving beta-carotene, vitamin E, and selenium. The effects appeared 1 to 2 years after the start of supplementation and were significant for esophageal and gastric cancers.

Are these results applicable to Americans? Yes and no. This prospective clinical trial supports primary disease prevention in a general population through the use of chemo-prevention (use of drugs to prevent disease).

However, the diets of the Chinese peasants studied were significantly different than the typical American's intake. The Chinese intake is low in fruits, meat, and other animal products. Even their average blood levels of vitamins and minerals are lower than those of Americans. Possible underlying deficiencies, not found in Westerners, may be responsible for the etiology of cancer and mortality rather than the effects of additional quantities of specific nutrients. Nonetheless, these results highlight the potential role of antioxidants in the reduction of disease and mortality.

From Blot WJ et al: Nutrition intervention trials in Linxian, China: Supplementation with specific vitamin/mineral combinations, cancer incidence, and disease-specific mortality in the general population, *J Natl Canc Inst* 85:1483-1492, 1993; and Blumberg JB: Comment: Nutrition intervention trials in Linxian, China: Supplementation with specific vitamin/mineral combinations, cancer incidence, and disease-specific mortality in the general population. In Chernoff R, ed: *Perspectives in Applied Nutrition* 1(3):31-32, Winter 1993.

experience an increase in blood pressure leading to hypertension. Reducing excess water retention through a reduction in sodium consumption is a first step to treating this type of hypertension. A more serious form of edema occurs in victims of kwashiorkor when the protein levels in the body are so low that cellular fluid levels are imbalanced; inappropriate levels of interstitial fluid accumulate in the stomach, face, and extremities.

Water intoxication refers to the consumption of large volumes of water within a short time. It causes muscle cramps, decreased blood pressure, and weakness. Water intoxication is possible if there is extensive loss of electrolytes because of dehydration, and rehydration is accomplished using only water, without the addition of replacement electrolytes. Generally, this condition tends to occur only among psychiatric patients, who have lost the ability to respond to physiological cues to stop drinking.

MINERALS

Minerals serve a variety of functions in our bodies. Structurally minerals provide rigidity and strength to teeth and skeleton; the skeletal mineral components also serve as a storage depot for other needs of the body. Nerve and muscle functions are influenced by minerals, allowing for proper muscle contraction and release. Other functions of minerals include acting as cofactors for enzymes and maintaining proper acid-base balance of body fluids. Minerals are also required for blood clotting and for tissue repair and growth.

Mineral Categories

Based on the amount in our bodies, the 16 essential minerals are divided into two categories: major and trace minerals. To maintain body levels, **major minerals** are needed daily from dietary sources in amounts of 100 mg or higher. In contrast, **trace minerals** are required daily in amounts less than or equal to 20 mg (Table 8-3). Although the required amounts differ greatly between the major and trace minerals, each is absolutely necessary for good health. The RDAs listed in this chapter for minerals are those for young adults. RDAs for other groups are noted when special mention is needed. Keep in mind that since nutrition is a relatively young science, new functions of minerals as nutrients in the human body are still being discovered.

major minerals
essential nutrient minerals required daily in amounts of 100 mg or higher

trace minerals
essential nutrient minerals required daily in amounts less than or equal to 20 mg

Table 8-3 Essential Minerals in the Human Body	
Major	**Trace**
Calcium	Chromium
Chloride	Copper
Magnesium	Fluoride
Phosphorus	Iodine
Potassium	Iron
Sodium	Manganese
Sulfur	Molybdenum
	Selenium
	Zinc

Food Sources

The prime sources of minerals include both plant and animal foods. Valuable sources of plant foods include most fruits, vegetables, legumes, and whole grains. Animal sources consist of beef, chicken, eggs, fish, and milk products. The discussions of individual minerals highlight the best food choices.

In contrast to vitamins, minerals are very stable when foods containing them are cooked. As inorganic substances, they are indestructible. Minerals may leach into cooking fluids but are still able to be absorbed if the fluid is consumed.

Although plants may contain an abundance of various minerals, some minerals in plants are not easily available to the human body. **Bioavailability** is the level of absorption of a consumed nutrient. Bioavailability of minerals is of nutritional concern. Some minerals may be bound to the plant fiber structures by binders such as phytic and oxalic acids. **Binders** are substances in plant foods that combine with minerals to form indigestible compounds, making them unavailable for our use. The amount of plant minerals available for absorption depends on minerals in soils in which the plants are grown.

Minerals from animals foods do not have the same bioavailability issues. In fact, minerals from animal foods can be absorbed more easily than those from plants. Fat content may be an issue for some animal foods, however. Lower fat sources of dairy and meat products are usually available and provide the same levels of minerals. Liver is often cited as a good source of minerals including iron and zinc. Liver is also high in cholesterol and saturated fats and may contain toxins to which the animal's body may have been exposed. These factors, combined with liver's somewhat unusual taste (which many hide by serving liver with high-fat bacon), often leaves the impression that good nutrient intake depends on eating healthy food that tastes bad. Other sources of each nutrient may be more appealing and equally as nutritious.

Food processing may reduce the availability of minerals. Processing oranges into orange juice does not affect potassium levels naturally contained in oranges. But processing whole wheat flour into white flour does cause significant losses of minerals since the whole grain is not used. Iron is the only mineral returned to white flour through enrichment; zinc, selenium, copper, and other minerals are permanently lost.

Since we have difficulty obtaining high enough levels of some minerals naturally, fortification of manufactured foods has become commonplace. It is in this manner that food processing can serve the nutrient needs of consumers while still addressing the issues of convenience and taste appeal. Salt is available fortified with iodine; dry cereals have added minerals such as iron and an assortment of vitamins and other minerals.

Minerals as Nutrients Within the Body

Structure

Minerals are inorganic substances composed of elements from the rock of the earth. Their tendency to gain or lose electrons makes them electrically charged. Thus they have special affinities for water, which itself carries positive and negative charges. As we consume plant and animal foods containing minerals, we can incorporate them into our body structures (bones), organs, and fluids.

Digestion and absorption

During the process of digestion, minerals (as inorganic substances) are separated from the foodstuff in which they entered our bodies. Digestion does change the valence states of some minerals, which changes their ability to be absorbed. Their structure is not changed, however, to prepare them for absorption.

As noted earlier, bioavailability impacts the level of minerals we actually absorb. Generally, consuming a variety of whole foods assures an adequate intake of

bioavailability
the level of absorption of a consumed nutrient

binders
substances occurring in plant foods that combine with minerals to form undigestible compounds which cannot be absorbed

minerals. Mineral deficiencies for which Americans tend to be at risk are iron, calcium, and zinc. Concerns and strategies for consuming appropriate amounts of these nutrients are discussed later in this chapter.

Metabolism

Since minerals are inorganic and do not provide energy, they are not metabolized by the human body. Instead some minerals assist as cofactors of metabolic processes.

MAJOR MINERALS

Calcium

Function

Calcium is the most abundant mineral in the body. Almost all of the calcium in the body, about 99%, is found in our bones, serving structural and storage functions. The other 1% of body calcium is released into body fluids when blood passes through bones; this constant interaction of blood with bone allows calcium to be distributed throughout the body. Other functions that depend on calcium include central nervous system functioning, particularly for nerve impulses; muscle contraction and relaxation when needed; blood clotting; and blood pressure regulation.

Regulation. Our dietary intake of calcium influences the deposition of calcium in our bones. Blood calcium levels, however, do not depend on a daily dietary calcium intake. Instead the skeletal supply of calcium provides the source of calcium to be distributed throughout the body through the circulatory system. If calcium blood levels get too low, three actions can occur to reestablish calcium homeostasis: (1) bones release calcium, (2) intestines absorb more calcium, and (3) kidneys retain more calcium.

The release of calcium from bones is controlled by hormones that regulate the level of calcium in body fluids. Hormones affecting blood levels include **parathormone** (parathyroid hormone), **calcitriol** (active vitamin D hormone) and **calcitonin.** Parathormone is secreted by the parathyroid gland in response to low blood calcium levels. It raises blood calcium levels by stimulating all three ways of providing calcium to body fluids. Vitamin D has a hormone-like effect as calciferol and also increases blood calcium levels by acting on all three systems. The third hormone involved, calcitonin, is released by the Special C cells of the thyroid gland. Calcitonin reacts in response to high blood levels of calcium by lowering both calcium and phosphate in the blood.

Reactions of very low or extremely high blood levels could occur if regulatory mechanisms are hindered by a lack of vitamin D or hormone malfunction. If calcium blood levels get too high, **calcium rigor** (with symptoms of hardness or stiffness of muscles) may occur. Conversely, if levels are too low, a person may experience **calcium tetany**, with spasms caused by muscle and nerve excitability.

Recommended intake and sources

Calcium RDAs for men and women range from 800 mg (ages 1 through 10) to 1200 mg (ages 11 through 24). After age 25, the RDA drops to 800 mg. Higher levels of 1500 mg have been suggested for postmenopausal females to reduce excessive bone loss; this increase however, is not reflected in the RDA recommendations.

Concerns have been raised as to the calcium intake of those most at risk for deficiency—youths age 11 through 24, and pregnant and lactating women. During these times calcium needs are still high, although actual consumption of calcium may decrease. To this end, *Healthy People 2000* proposes that persons in these groups consume at least three or more servings a day of calcium-rich foods. For those over 25, at least two or more servings daily are advised (3). Other issues surrounding calcium intake and children will be discussed in Chapter 12.

parathormone
a hormone that raises blood calcium levels; secreted by the parathyroid gland in response to low blood calcium levels

calcitriol
active vitamin D hormone that raises blood calcium levels

calcitonin
a hormone that reacts in response to high blood levels of calcium; released by the Special C cells of the thyroid gland

calcium rigor
a condition of hardness or stiffness of muscles when blood calcium levels get too high

calcium tetany
a condition of spasms and nerve excitability when blood calcium levels get too low

Primary sources of calcium are dairy products, mainly milk (whole, low-fat, and skim) and milk-based products including ice cream, ice milk, yogurt, frozen yogurt, cheeses, and puddings (Fig. 8-1). Although butter, cream cheese, and cottage cheese are dairy products, they are not good sources of calcium; butter and cream cheese are predominately fat, and cottage cheese loses calcium through processing. Nondairy sources include green leafy vegetables (broccoli, kale, and mustard greens), small fish with bones (sardines and salmon canned with processed edible bones), legumes, and tofu processed with calcium. In addition, a variety of calcium-fortified foods is available, ranging from fortified orange juice to bread products. Table 8-4 gives examples of foods that will boost calcium intake.

Some leafy green vegetables, in particular spinach, collards, Swiss chard, and escarole, contain oxalic acid, a binder reducing the calcium absorbed. Plant foods containing oxalic acid cannot be considered a trustworthy source of calcium. Tea contains oxalic acid as well as tannins (in coffee also), both of which may affect the absorption of calcium in other foods consumed with tea. With the increased consumption of iced tea beverages, this effect should be considered, particularly for female adolescents and young adults.

Some calcium supplements are poorly absorbed because they don't dissolve in the stomach. If a calcium tablet doesn't readily dissolve when stirred into cider vinegar, it probably will not dissolve in the body.

Table 8-4 Suggestions for Boosting Calcium Intake	
DAIRY	**NONDAIRY**
Powdered milk added to baking mixes, soups, puddings, gravies, hamburgers and meat loaves	Bean soups (split pea or lentil soup)
Sliced apples and pears with cheese wedges	Tofu (made with calcium carbonate), fresh or in frozen meals and desserts
Broccoli with melted cheese	Chicken cacciatore (chicken with bones cooked in tomato sauce; acid of tomatoes pulls calcium from bones)
Soups made with lowfat or skim milk	Juices fortified with calcium
Calcium-fortified milk	Bean burritos
Smoothies (fruit drinks made with milk, yogurt, and fruits)	Breads fortified with calcium

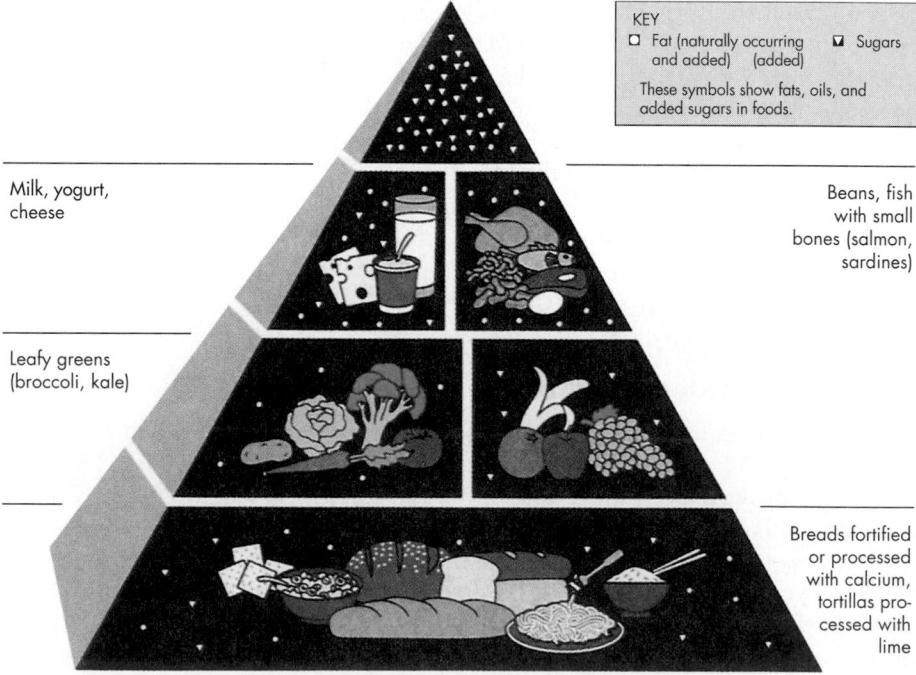

KEY
☐ Fat (naturally occurring and added)   ☑ Sugars (added)
These symbols show fats, oils, and added sugars in foods.

Milk, yogurt, cheese

Beans, fish with small bones (salmon, sardines)

Leafy greens (broccoli, kale)

Breads fortified or processed with calcium, tortillas processed with lime

Fig. 8-1 The Food Guide Pyramid, highlighting calcium-rich foods.

Many adults are lactose intolerant. Lactose intolerance occurs when the body does not produce enough lactase, an enzyme necessary for the digestion of lactose, the carbohydrate found in milk. (Lactose intolerance is detailed in Chapter 4.) Persons experiencing lactose intolerance need to regularly incorporate sources of calcium other than dairy products into their dietary patterns. For some people, calcium supplements may be indicated; a registered dietetian or qualified nutritionist may be consulted.

Absorption factors. Our bodies absorb calcium based on physiological need. During childhood growth phases we may absorb up to 75% of calcium consumed compared with 30% to 60% once we complete our prime growth years. Similarly, during pregnancy and lactation, percentages of absorption are higher based on physiological need (6).

In addition to physiological needs increasing absorption rates, other factors seem to enhance the levels of calcium absorbed. They include the following:

- **Lactose.** Found naturally in milk (an excellent source of calcium), lactose appears to increase calcium absorption.
- **Sufficient vitamin D.** Vitamin D is involved in the synthesis of a protein that allows calcium to pass through the intestinal wall into the blood stream.
- **Acidity of digestive mass.** Calcium is more soluble in acidic substances, so it is better absorbed when ingested as part of a meal. Generally, enough hydrochloric acid passes from the stomach to the intestine for calcium absorption. As we age, the amount of hydrochloric acid in digestive juices may decrease, causing less calcium to be absorbed.

Factors favoring calcium absorption
body's need for higher amounts, as in pregnancy; lactose; sufficient vitamin D; acidity of digestive mass

Factors hindering calcium absorption
binders such as phytic acid and oxalic acid, dietary fat, dietary fiber, laxatives, sedentary lifestyle, drugs

Other factors may decrease calcium absorption. They include the following:

- **Binders.** Naturally occurring substances may bind with calcium in plant foods; two common calcium binders previously mentioned are phytic and oxalic acids (also called phytates and oxalates). Human digestive processes may be unable to separate calcium from the binder; both are then excreted, reducing the calcium available for absorption.
- **Dietary fat.** Dietary fat can form insoluble soaps with calcium; the insoluble soaps are harder to digest, making calcium less accessible for absorption. Moderate and low dietary fat intakes discourage the formation of this insoluble mass.
- **High fiber intake and laxatives.** Excessive fiber consumption or laxative abuse results in foodstuff moving through the gastrointestinal tract too quickly for minerals, particularly calcium, to be absorbed.
- **Sedentary lifestyle.** Being a couch potato has its consequences. A physically inactive lifestyle leads to less bone density. In contrast, weight-bearing exercise that pulls the muscle against the bone enhances calcium deposits in the bone matrix. This action occurs during running, brisk walking, biking, and strength training.
- **Drugs.** Some medications, including anticonvulsants, tetracycline, cortisone, thyroxine, and aluminum-containing antacids, are associated with reduced calcium absorption. Caffeine, the most commonly used drug, can also affect calcium absorption.

Deficiency

Deficiency of calcium primarily affects bone health. During the growing years, inadequate intake of calcium reduces the density of bone mass and if severe can stunt growth.

For adults, long-term calcium deficiency may be one of the risk factors of osteoporosis, a multifactorial disorder. This condition takes many years to develop and overt symptoms appear late in life. Osteoporosis is a condition in which bone density is reduced and the remaining bone is brittle and breaks easily.

One of the most recognizable characteristics of osteoporosis is the *dowager's hump*; as vertebrae in the spine collapse from weakness, the spine is no longer able

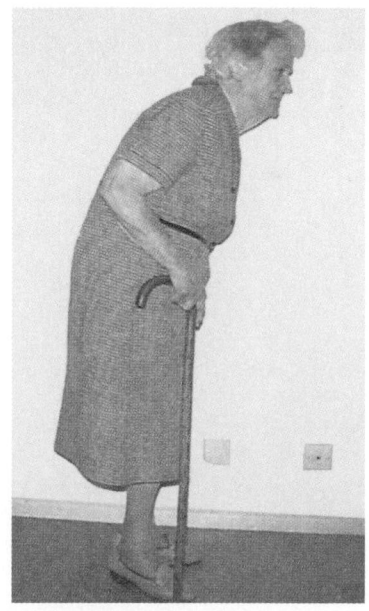

Typical posture in osteoporosis.

to support the weight of the head. The back bows and the head becomes angled down. Most significantly, the internal organs affected by the curvature are unable to function efficiently and other health difficulties develop.

In contrast to osteomalacia, osteoporosis is multifactorial and all the factors are tied to bone mineral density. These factors include genetics, diet, and lifestyle determinants (7). Bone density builds through early adulthood. Peak bone density is reached by about age 20, although some additional bone mineralization continues into the 30s (1). The more density built early in life, the less potential risk encountered.

Factors that affect bone density but cannot be modified include genetic determinants of race and gender (7).

- **Race.** Osteoporosis is more common in Caucasian and Asian women than among African and African-American women. This is due to racial differences in the skeletal density, possibly caused by hormonal differences.

- **Gender.** Men have greater bone density than women. They enter the later years when bone demineralization begins with a larger storage of calcium. The fact that men have more lean body mass or muscularity may cause more calcium to be deposited and retained in comparison with women. Women lose greater amounts of bone calcium during the first few years after menopause. The drop in estrogen levels appears to initiate the calcium loss. To slow the loss and to provide additional protection against heart disease, many primary health care providers prescribe hormone (estrogen) replacement therapy for postmenopausal women.

  Osteoporosis, however, does occur in both men and women. For men, osteoporosis tends to be due to secondary causes that affect peak bone mass development and/or speed loss of bone density. These causes may include steroid therapy, hypogonadism, skeletal metastasis, multiple myeloma, gastric surgery, and anticonvulsant treatment (8).

- **Family history.** A predisposition to lower bone density may be genetically passed between generations, particularly from mother to daughter. If a close family member develops osteoporosis, care should be taken to reduce the effects of other risk factors.

Factors related to development of osteoporosis that can be adjusted include nutrition, particularly calcium intake, and lifestyle determinants.

- **Nutrition/calcium intake.** Dietary calcium intake is of concern throughout the lifespan. In particular, the growth years when calcium is deposited in the bone matrix, and the postmenopause years of bone mineralization loss are the periods when calcium intake appears crucial. Although the RDA for calcium provides sufficient amounts, many individuals consume less than these levels. Adolescent females often consume levels of kcalories and nutrients way below the RDAs while attempting to control body weight. These eating patterns often continue through adulthood. This long-term marginal deficiency of calcium may set the stage for future bone disorders. The issue is even more complicated for older adults. When they consume calcium-containing foods, less calcium may be absorbed because of decreased gastric acidity and reduced levels of available vitamin D.

  For others risk may be related to genes. A specific gene appears to predispose individuals to absorb less calcium. Changes occur in receptor sites for vitamin D, reducing the availability and functioning of vitamin D in relation to maintaining bone density (9). It is not yet known what sets off the changes in the receptor sites.

- **Alcohol.** Long-term excessive intake of alcohol appears to reduce bone density. Alcohol may directly depress bone formation or may take the place of more nutritious foods, producing marginal deficiencies.

- **Smoking.** Cigarette smoking has been associated with a higher risk of osteoporosis. Smokers tend to be of lower weight (less bone density) and appear to lose more bone mineralization after menopause than nonsmokers.

TEACHING TOOLS
Calcium: By Any Means Possible

It's quite simple. The RDA for calcium ranges by age from 800 mg to 1200 mg. The best sources are calcium-rich foods. But what if a client is lactose-intolerant or just doesn't like many calcium-containing foods?

Since the potential ramifications of chronic calcium deficiency are serious—fractures and other complications of osteoporosis—calcium supplementation may be appropriate. Here are some suggestions and cautions for client education:

- Calcium supplementation may increase the dietary intake of calcium, but it does not alleviate other risk factors associated with osteoporosis. Other nutrients and lifestyle behaviors also affect the level of risk. Popping a calcium pill does not mean a person is osteoporosis-free.

- Many people have problems with compliance; the regularity of calcium intake builds dense bones, not an occasional dose. It's better to rely on food sources.

- The source of calcium affects the amount of actual calcium available. Tablets composed of calcium carbonate contain more elemental calcium (often 500 to 600 mg) than those made of calcium citrate or lactate (usually 200 mg per tablet), and it takes fewer pills to achieve the RDA. Calcium citrate, however, is more easily absorbed by the digestive tract, even if more pills are needed.

- Be aware that calcium is always combined with another substance to form the tablet. A tablet may contain 1200 mg of calcium carbonate, but only 500 mg of elemental calcium. The supplements to avoid are those made from dolomite, bone meal, and oyster shell; they may be contaminated with lead and other toxic metals.

- Although the tablets are supplementing dietary intake, it's best to take them with meals. The acid of the digestive process also helps in the breakdown and absorption of the calcium tablet(s), and tying the supplement to meals works as a reminder system. This also helps to spread supplementation throughout the day. One large dose will not be absorbed as well as two or three smaller doses.

- Calcium supplements should not contain vitamin D. Vitamin D should only be taken with the recommendation of primary health care providers; it is too easy to overdose.

- Before supplementing, keep track for several days of sources and amounts of dietary calcium. Intake may be adequate. If not, first contemplate ways to increase intake with foods, then consider supplementation.

- **Caffeine.** Caffeine consumption has been tied to urinary excretion of calcium. Reasonable use of caffeinated beverages, however, may be acceptable (10). More than likely, the relationship of caffeine to lower levels of body calcium concerns caffeinated beverages replacing those containing calcium. A recent study found that although caffeinated coffee consumption affected bone density of postmenopausal women, one glass of skim milk per day overcame the effects of the coffee (11).

- **Sedentary lifestyle.** As noted earlier, a physically active lifestyle not only enhances calcium absorption but also helps to maintain bone matrix mineralization. However, excessive exercise that results in extremely low body fat levels for women may be detrimental to bone density. If amenorrhea (abnormal cessation of menses) occurs because of excessive exercise, the resulting premature drop in estrogen may limit or decrease bone mineralization during the prime growth periods.

Although the risk factors for osteoporosis may seem overwhelming, several can be reduced by following basic recommendations for achieving wellness. By consuming the serving amounts recommended on the Food Guide Pyramid and engaging in regular physical exercise, most of the risk can be minimized. See the box above for tips on educating clients on appropriate calcium intake.

Low levels of calcium intake have also been associated with an increased risk of colon cancer and hypertension.

Toxicity

Calcium toxicity from consuming foods containing calcium is not a concern. Problems may occur when supplements of calcium and other nutrients are used instead of foods. Over-supplementation may cause constipation, urinary stone formation affecting kidney function, and reduced absorption of iron, zinc, and other minerals (12). The general guideline for calcium supplements is that levels should not exceed the RDA for calcium.

Phosphorus

Function

Most of the phosphorus in the body (85%) is in our bones and teeth as a component of **hydroxyapatite**. The other 15% of body phosphorus has functions in energy transfer, as part of the genetic material of DNA and RNA, as a buffer in the form of phosphoric acid balancing body acid-base levels, and as a component of phospholipids used for transportation and structural functions.

hydroxapatite
a natural mineral structure of bones and teeth

Recommended intake and sources

The RDA for phosphorus is the same as for calcium. The RDA for phosphorus is 1200 mg for adolescence to 24 years and 800 mg thereafter.

Phosphorus is widely available in foods. Particularly good sources are protein-rich foods including dairy foods, eggs, meat, fish, poultry, and cereal grains. Because of the processing of convenience foods and soft drinks, both are also sources of phosphorus.

Deficiency

Deficiency of phosphorus is unknown. It is part of the genetic material of every cell of the body.

Toxicity

Excessive amounts of phosphorus, possible only from phosphorus supplements, cause calcium excretion from the body. High phosphorus intakes could affect the calcium/phosphorus ratio, possibly reducing the amount of calcium absorbed. This is a problem only if calcium intake is inadequate. Since phosphorus-containing soft drinks have replaced milk beverages for many American teens and adult women, this may be of dietary concern.

Magnesium

Function

As with calcium and phosphorus, most of the magnesium in the body is found in our bones, providing structural and storage functions. Magnesium assists hundreds of enzymes throughout the body. It also regulates nerve and muscle function including the actions of the heart and has a role in the blood clotting process.

Recommended intake and sources

The RDAs for magnesium are 350 mg for men and 280 mg for women.

Many commonly eaten foods contain magnesium. Particularly good sources are most unprocessed foods including whole grains, legumes, broccoli, leafy green vegetables and other vegetables. Hard water can be a significant source of magnesium.

Deficiency

Magnesium deficiency tends to be related to secondary causes, rather than from a primary lack of magnesium consumption. These secondary causes may include excessive vomiting and diarrhea caused by pathological conditions. A gastrointestinal tract disorder may affect magnesium absorption, or kidney disease may inhibit retention of the mineral. Malnutrition and alcoholism may also impact on magnesium levels in the body. Similarly, drug interference or artificial feeding solutions deficient in magnesium may influence total body levels of magnesium. Whenever body fluids are lost, so is magnesium. Individuals on long-term regimens of diuretics are also potentially at risk for deficiency.

Symptoms of magnesium deficiency include twitching of muscles, muscle weakness, and convulsions.

Toxicity

Toxic effects of magnesium have not been studied or observed.

Sulfur

Function

Sulfur is a component of protein structures. It is present in every cell of the body and is part of several amino acids.

Recommended intake and sources

No RDA has been established for sulfur. Diets adequate in protein provide sufficient amounts of sulfur. Sulfur is found in all protein-containing foods.

Deficiency

Deficiencies of sulfur do not occur; sulfur is so basic to the structure of the human cell that deficiencies cannot develop.

Toxicity

Toxicity to sulfur is not a health issue.

ELECTROLYTES: SODIUM, POTASSIUM, AND CHLORIDE

Sodium, potassium, and chloride are major electrolytes of the body. As electrolytes, these minerals serve very specific functions. The acid-base balance of body fluids depends on regulated distribution of these minerals. Electrolytes also have a role in the normal functioning of nerves and muscles. In addition, each mineral serves other specific functions in the body.

Sodium

Function

Sodium performs a variety of important functions in the body. Blood pressure and volume are maintained by the characteristics of sodium as the major cation in extracellular fluid. Transmission of nerve impulses relies on body sodium levels. As the major extracellular electrolyte, sodium has a role in the regulation of body fluid levels in and out of cells. This movement affects blood volume as well, which is tied to the thirst mechanism and total body fluid levels.

Recommended intake and sources

There is no RDA for sodium. Instead, Estimated Minimum Requirements (EMR) have been set for sodium as well as for the other electrolytes. This dietary recommendation is based on the known minimum intake required for good health. It also acknowledges that it is not possible to determine disadvantages to consumption of large amounts of these nutrients except in particular circumstances discussed under toxicities. The EMR for sodium is 500 mg for adults, or about ¼ teaspoon.

Most sodium enters our diet as sodium chloride (table salt). Sodium occurs naturally in many foods. It is also added to foods as salt during the cooking process and right before consumption. Processing of foods, particularly convenience quick serve foods, often adds substantial amounts of sodium (Table 8-5 and box). Processed foods are *carriers* for other additives that often contain sodium. The sodium adds flavor that may be lost in processing.

Deficiency

Depletion of sodium can develop through dehydration and/or excessive diarrhea. Because of extreme concern over the relationship between sodium and hypertension, some people may overly restrict sodium and be at risk. Typical athletic or physical labor producing excessive sweating may cause dehydration and loss of sodium, but drinking fluids and consuming foods soon restores body levels of sodium. Salt tablets, once a common remedy, are not recommended and may be dangerous.

Symptoms of sodium deficiency include headache, muscle cramps, weakness, reduced ability to concentrate, and memory and appetite loss. It is rare, for sodium deficiency to occur, since we get enough sodium naturally from foods. These symptoms are similar to those of fluid volume deficit, which is more common.

Toxicity

An excess sodium intake is difficult for the body to handle. The kidneys have the primary responsibility to flush out the excess sodium. Some individuals are sodium-sensitive and may develop hypertension and edema in response to high

Table 8-5   Processing Effects on Food Sodium Content

POTATOES	
Baked potato (1)	16 mg
French-fried potatoes (10 strips)	108 mg
Scalloped potatoes from dry mix (1 cup)	835 mg
CHICKEN	
Baked chicken (3 oz)	64 mg
Batter-fried chicken (3 oz)	231 mg
Chicken nuggets (6 pieces)	542 mg
OATS	
Oatmeal prepared with water (1 cup)	2 mg
Oatmeal bread (1 slice)	124 mg
Ready-to-eat oat cereal (1 cup)	307 mg
APPLES	
Apple (1)	Trace
Applesauce (1 cup)	8 mg
Apple pie (1 slice)	476 mg

Data from Pennington *JAT: Bowes & Church's food values of portions commonly used,* ed 16, Philadelphia, 1994, Lippincott; and USDA: Nutritive value of foods, *Home and Garden Bulletin* 72, 1991.

MYTH
Sodium Comes Only From the Salt Shaker

Do you salt your food first, then taste it? Some habits are hard to break, but are worth the effort. However, breaking the salt shaker habit will reduce sodium intake only 15% for most Americans; most of the sodium we eat comes from processed foods.

The more a foodstuff is processed, the higher the sodium content becomes. More nutrients are also lost along the way. Which is saltier, or to be more exact which contains more sodium, a bowl of corn flakes or a large order of fast-food fries? The corn flakes win, containing 290 mg of sodium compared with 200 mg for the fries. Of course, the fries contain a lot more fat and calories.

Consider the potato. A plain baked potato contains only 16 mg of sodium. Fixed up at a local fast-food restaurant, a baked potato with cheese sauce and broccoli skyrockets to over 400 mg of sodium and lots of fat. A cheese or sour cream mix prepared at home is even higher in sodium, close to 600 mg. The sodium in *plain* mashed potatoes from a mix (dehydrated and then reconstituted) jumps from 8 mg in its original whole form to over 300 mg, and that's without butter or gravy. The point is that processing foods adds *invisible* sodium as sodium chloride; in fact it's so invisible that we can no longer taste the saltiness.

Sodium enjoys widespread use in the American diet as a flavoring agent (sodium chloride, monosodium glutamate [MSG], sodium saccharin), dough conditioner (baking powder, baking soda), and preservative (sodium sulfite). Because of consumer demand, lower sodium versions of many products are available. Nutrition labeling information must include sodium content. This is powerful information that allows us to compare the sodium content of similar products.

From Pennington JAT: *Bowes & Church's food values of portions commonly used,* ed 16, Philadelphia, 1994, Lippincott; and Liebman B: The Salt Shake Out, *Nutrition Action Health Letter* 21(2):1, 5-7, 1994.

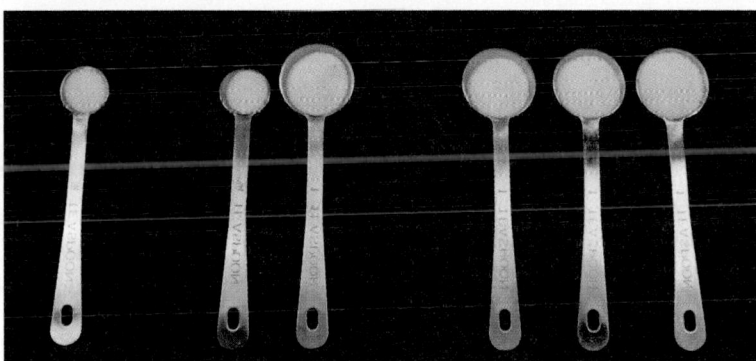

Fig. 8-2 Minimum (¼ tsp. salt: 500 mg sodium), maximum (1¼ tsp. salt: 2400 mg sodium), and typical (3 tsp. salt: 6000 mg sodium) daily salt intake.

intake of sodium. Levels consumed in diets based on highly processed foods and high sodium content foods may be enough to initiate hypertension in the sodium-sensitive. Although others may not experience negative ramifications from high sodium intakes, there are no benefits either. This is one of the few nutrients that we can *overdose* on from foods consumed.

Health-related associations have set guidelines for appropriate and safe levels of sodium. The National Research Council Recommendations suggest limiting daily salt intake to less than 6 g; this equals 2400 mg of sodium (Fig. 8-2). The American Heart Association advises sodium limits of 3 g daily. As a guideline, a teaspoon of salt contains about 2 g or 2000 mg of sodium.

An occasional very salty meal may produce edema, but not hypertension. The best remedy for occasional edema is simply to drink more water to equalize the sodium concentration of body fluids. The kidneys take care of the rest by filtering out the excess sodium.

Potassium

Function

While sodium as a cation maintains the fluid levels extracellularly, potassium, as the primary intercellular cation, maintains fluid levels inside the cells. Potassium is also crucial for normal functioning of nerves and muscles, including the heart.

Recommended intake and sources

The EMR for potassium is 2000 mg.

Whole unprocessed foods, particularly bananas, oranges, and other fruits, vegetables, dairy products, meats, and legumes are good sources of potassium.

Deficiency

Similar to magnesium deficiency, potassium deficiency may be caused by dehydration from vomiting and/or diarrhea, diuretics, and misuse of laxatives. If long-term use of diuretics is warranted to reduce edema associated with hypertension, particular attention should be paid to consuming adequate levels of potassium from foods. Some diuretics are postassium wasting; some are potassium sparing. Supplementation when using a potassium-sparing diuretic could be very dangerous. Potassium supplements should only be taken when prescribed by a primary health care provider.

Symptoms associated with potassium deficiency include muscle weakness, confusion, loss of appetite and, in severe cases, cardiac arrhythmias.

Toxicity

Potassium toxicity occurs only from supplements, not from consuming an excess from foods. Toxicity doesn't usually occur with foods as long as a person has properly functioning kidneys. For individuals with renal disease, high potassium foods are very toxic. Symptoms of toxicity are similar to those of a deficiency. They include muscle weakness, vomiting and, at excessively high levels, cardiac arrest.

Chloride

Function

As the key anion of extracellular fluids, chloride assists in maintaining fluid balance inside and outside cells. In addition, chloride is a component of hydrochloric acid, an indispensable gastric juice produced by the stomach.

Recommended intake and sources

The EMR for chloride is 750 mg for adults. This requirement is easily met by consumption of sodium chloride; foods that provide sodium usually provide chloride as well.

Deficiency

Deficiency of chloride is very rare; adequate amounts are easily consumed. Although deficiency is possible, it would occur from the same circumstances as sodium deficiency.

Toxicity

Chloride toxicity may occur because of dehydration, causing an imbalance of chloride to the other electrolytes; but the other effects of dehydration are more severe.

Table 8-6 provides a summary of the major minerals.

Table 8-6   Major Minerals

Mineral	Function	Clinical Issues Deficiency/Toxicity	Recommended Intakes	Food Sources	Absorption Issues
Calcium (Ca)	Bone and tooth formation; blood clotting; muscle contraction/relaxation; CNS; blood pressure	Deficiency: reduced bone density; osteoporosis Toxicity: constipation; urinary stones; reduced iron and zinc absorption	RDA Adults: 800-1200 mg Pregnancy/lactation: 1200 mg	Milk (whole, lowfat, skim), milk-based products, green leafy vegetables, legumes	Absorption based on need: increased by vitamin D; decreased by binders, inactivity, coffee/tea
Phosphorus (P)	Bone and tooth formation (component of hydroxyapatite); energy metabolism (enzymes); acid-base balance	Deficiency: rare Toxicity: increased calcium excretion	RDA Adults: 800-1200 mg Pregnancy/lactation: 1200 mg	Dairy foods, egg, meat, fish, poultry	Absorbed with calcium
Magnesium (Mg)	Structure/storage; cofactor; nerve and muscle function; blood clotting	Deficiency: secondary with muscle twitching, weakness, convulsions associated with FVD	RDA Men: 350 mg Women: 280 mg Pregnancy/lactation: 320-355 mg	Whole grains, legumes, green leafy vegetables (broccoli), hard water	
Sulfur (S)	Component of protein structures	Deficiency: only if protein malnourished	Protein-adequate diets contain adequate levels	Protein-containing foods	
Sodium (Na)	Major extracellular electrolyte for fluid regulation; body fluid levels; acid-base balance; nerve impulse and contraction; blood pressure/volume	Deficiency: FVD with headache; muscle cramps, weakness, decreased concentration, memory and appetite loss Toxicity: sodium-sensitive hypertension	EMR Adults: 500 mg	Table salt; naturally in many foods; processed foods	
Potassium (K)	Major intracellular electrolyte for fluid regulation; muscle function	Deficiency: muscle weakness, confusion, decreased appetite, cardiac arrhythmias caused by FVD from vomiting/diarrhea or diuretics Toxicity: from diet or supplements if renal disease present	RDA Adults: 2000 mg	Unprocessed foods, fruits, vegetables, dairy products, meats, legumes	
Chloride (Cl)	Acid-base balance; gastric hydrochloric acid for digestion	Deficiency: FVD due to vomiting/diarrhea	EMR Adults: 750 mg	Table salt	

CNS, Central nervous system; FVD, Fluid volume deficit; RDA, Recommended Dietary Allowance; EMR, Estimated Minimum Requirement; ESADDI, Estimated Safe and Adequate Daily Dietary Intake.

TRACE MINERALS

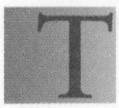race minerals as a group of nutrients function primarily as cofactors, by performing metabolic and transport functions.

Iron

Function

Iron is responsible for distributing oxygen throughout our bodies. Oxygen depends on the iron in **hemoglobin** of red blood cells (erythrocytes) to bring oxygen to all cells. **Myoglobin** holds oxygen in the muscle cells for quick use when needed. Because of its ability to change ionic charges, iron also assists the use of oxygen by enzymes in all cells of the body.

Iron is conserved and recycled by the body. When red blood cells are old or damaged, their iron component is removed by the spleen. Some iron is kept in the spleen for later use, and the rest is sent to the liver for processing. From the liver, iron is transported as transferrin to bone marrow and recycled for use in new red blood cells. Some iron is lost through the shedding of tissue cells in urine and sweat and when bleeding occurs; this lost iron must be replaced by dietary sources.

Recommended intake and sources

The RDA for iron is one of the few that is higher for females than males. When red blood cells break down, the iron in the hemoglobin is recycled to the liver and used to form new red blood cells. Whenever blood is lost from the body, iron is lost as well and cannot be recycled. Internal bleeding such as from acute ulcers can be a deceptive cause of iron loss. More obvious is the loss of blood by women from menstruation. Based on this monthly loss and the increased iron demands of pregnancy, women's overall need for iron is higher than men's. The RDA for men is 10 mg and for women 15 mg. During pregnancy the requirement is 30 mg; the blood supply of a pregnant woman is one and one-half times greater than her normal level.

The RDA allows for the unusual absorption rate of dietary iron. Only about 10% to 15% of dietary iron consumed is absorbed; this amount increases up to 20% if body levels are deficient. Intestinal mucosal cells contain two proteins that assist in absorption of dietary iron. One is mucosal transferrin, which moves iron to a protein carrier in blood transferrin for movement in blood to bone marrow and tissues as needed. The second is mucosal ferritin, which stores iron in the mucosal cells as a reserve if iron is needed. If not used, mucosal cells are replaced every few days so a continuous short-term supply of iron is available. During periods of growth, higher percentages are absorbed.

The RDA is also set to provide adequate storage levels of iron in the liver; iron is also stored in the spleen and bone marrow. In these organs, iron is contained in the proteins ferritin and hemosiderin. Ferritin is always being made and is easily available as an iron source. Hemosiderin is made when iron levels are high; although it is a source of iron, its availability takes longer than ferritin.

Iron is found in both plant and animal sources (Fig. 8-3). **Heme iron,** found in animal sources of meat, fish, and poultry, is more easily absorbed than nonheme iron found in plant foods. Although egg yolks contain iron, the iron is not as well absorbed as other heme sources. **Nonheme iron** sources include vegetables, legumes, dried fruits, whole grain cereals, and enriched grain products especially iron-fortified dry cereals.

Increased absorption of iron occurs when dietary sources are consumed with foods containing ascorbic acid (vitamin C). For example, drinking orange juice or eating slices of cantaloupe with meals increases the amount of nonheme iron absorbed (13). Another way to increase dietary iron intake is to cook foods in cast

---

hemogloblin
oxygen-transporting protein in red blood cells

myoglobin
oxygen-transporting protein in muscle

heme iron
dietary iron found in animal foods of meat, fish, and poultry

nonheme iron
dietary iron found in plant foods

Factors that enhance iron absorption
consuming dietary iron sources with food containing ascorbic acid (vitamin C), such as strawberries or melon or drinking orange or tomato juice; consuming foods containing heme iron from meat, fish, or poultry; combining plant and animal sources of dietary iron; cooking acidic foods in cast iron skillets

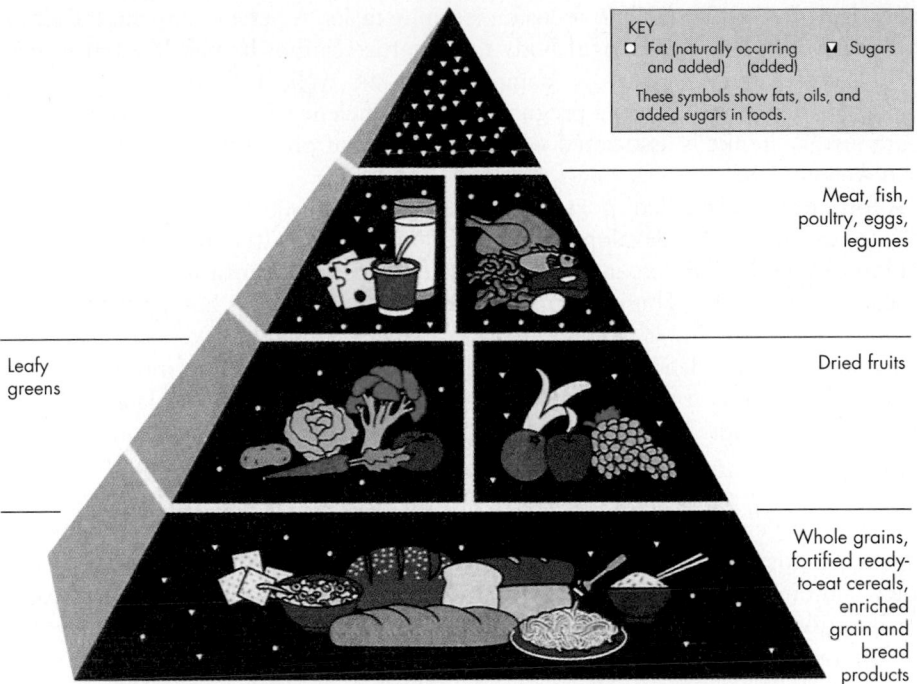

KEY
☐ Fat (naturally occurring   ☑ Sugars
and added)   (added)
These symbols show fats, oils, and
added sugars in foods.

Meat, fish,
poultry, eggs,
legumes

Dried fruits

Leafy
greens

Whole grains,
fortified ready-
to-eat cereals,
enriched
grain and
bread
products

Fig. 8-3 The Food Guide Pyramid, highlighting iron-rich foods.

iron skillets. Iron in the skillet leaches into the foods, providing an easy means for boosting iron intake.

Factors that inhibit iron absorption include consumption of foods that contain binders such as phytates and oxalates that keep the dietary iron from being separated from plant sources. Tannins in plants, most notably in teas and coffee, can also interfere with iron absorption. Continuous use of antacids as well as excessive intake of other minerals competes with the absorption sites for iron. Pica, the consumption of nonnutritive substances, creates health problems by drawing minerals out of the body; pica is discussed in the next section.

Deficiency

Iron deficiency has been a public health problem for many years. Although the incidence has decreased in the United States, most likely because of increased fortification, in other parts of the world it is still the most widespread nutrient deficiency (14). Most at risk are children and women of childbearing age. The effects of iron deficiency can be subtle and may be assigned to other causes. A range of symptoms accompanies different degrees of deficiency. All levels of iron deficiency affect the availability of oxygen throughout the body.

Iron deficiency occurs when there is reduced supply of iron stores available in the liver. If neither the diet nor body stores can supply the iron needed for hemoglobin synthesis, the number of red blood cells decreases in the bloodstream. The blood hemoglobin concentration also falls. When both the percentage of red blood cells (called *hematocrit*) and the hemoglobin level fall, a health care provider should suspect iron deficiency. Appendix E contains the biochemical assessment tests and values to evaluate iron status.

In severe deficiency, the hemoglobin and hematocrit levels fall so low that the amount of oxygen carried in the blood is decreased and the person is pale, tired, and anemic. Iron-deficiency anemia is characterized by microcytes or small, pale red blood cells. Physical activity or work may be difficult to perform because not enough oxygen is available for use by the muscles. Cognitive functioning is compromised. For children, learning problems may develop; an iron-deficient child is

Factors that hinder iron absorption
pica, drinking coffee and tea (tannins) with meals containing iron-containing foods, high-fiber meals, chronic antacid use, excessive intake of other minerals

Paleness can be determined by assessing the lining of the eyelid; it is usually pink, but if iron is deficient it will be without color.

easily distracted and unable to focus on learning tasks. A person may have a sensation of always feeling cold, as if body temperature cannot be regulated appropriately. The immune system is compromised as well, reflected in decreased wound-healing ability. During pregnancy, iron deficiency anemia caused by inadequate dietary intake is associated with greater risk of premature delivery and low birth weight (15).

A form of anemia called *sports anemia* occurs among endurance athletes. As the body adapts to aerobic development from intense exercise, the individual's volume of blood expands. This expansion lowers hemoglobin concentration, producing an appearance of anemia. This condition, however, is not an illness but a positive adaptation of the body.

To alleviate iron deficiency, the cause of the deficiency (either internal loss of blood or lack of dietary intake) needs to be addressed. Children may lack sufficient intake of iron foods. Toddlers may develop iron-deficiency anemia from drinking too much milk, a poor source of iron, which fills them up and keeps them from eating other iron-containing foods. Women tend to be doubly at risk because of dieting habits and female physiology. Chronic dieting may affect the intake of iron-rich foods; loss of blood through menses and the high iron demands of pregnancy combine to greatly increase female iron requirements. The recent increased consumption of iced tea as a popular soft drink may also affect women's iron levels. The tannin in tea reduces iron absorption. For adults iron deficiency is rarely caused by dietary deficiency, but usually results from the blood loss of menstrual bleeding or internal bleeding in the GI tract, perhaps from bleeding ulcers or hemorrhoids.

An unusual behavior associated with iron deficiency is pica. **Pica** is characterized by a hunger and appetite for nonfood substances including ice, corn starch, clay, and even dirt. These substances contain no iron and may even lead to loss of additional minerals, particularly when clay and dirt are consumed. Although *geophagia* (pica of clay or dirt) and *amylophagia* (pica of corn and laundry starch) are primarily recognized among women of rural lower socioeconomic groups, *pagophagia* (excessive ice consumption) has been noted among all socioeconomic levels. Of particular concern is the practice of pica during pregnancy when the risk and implications of iron-deficiency anemia are most severe. A challenge to obstetric nurses is to elicit information about this type of dietary behavior when assessing clients.

If increases in dietary sources of iron-rich foods do not raise hemotocrit levels, supplements may be prescribed. Determination of dose is made based on physiological requirements as assessed by primary health care providers. Long-term compliance is necessary to adequately restore iron storage levels in the body. Client education and support by nurses is advantageous.

Toxicity

Hemosiderosis, storing too much iron in the body, is a health concern. This condition may be caused by either **hemochromatosis,** a genetic disorder that allows more dietary iron to be absorbed than usual, or consumption of very high levels of iron-containing foods, perhaps through iron-fortification. The resulting iron overload can damage tissues cells when storing excess iron. Bacterial microorganisms may thrive on the excessive amounts of iron circulating in the blood. These effects are manifested in vague symptoms of weakness and fatigue. More specific symptoms include liver and heart damage, diabetes, arthritis, and discoloration of skin (14).

Those at risk include men, persons with chronic excessive alcohol consumption, and individuals who are genetically at risk for hemochromatosis. Since men lose no iron through menstruation or childbirth and may consume more foods fortified with iron, their bodies can potentially store more iron than needed. Excessive consumption of alcohol puts people at risk because their livers are affected by alcohol

pica
a condition characterized by a hunger and appetite for nonfood substances

hemosiderosis
a condition in which too much iron is stored in the body

hemochromatosis
a genetic disorder causing excessive dietary iron absorption

Iron supplement tips
- drink a glass of orange juice when taking an iron supplement to maximize iron absorption
- avoid taking iron supplements with milk because the calcium in milk interferes with iron absorption
- Stools will turn black and constipation may result from taking iron supplements

and may malfunction, absorbing too much iron. Treatment for hemochromatosis is blood removal by giving blood regularly and by decreasing dietary intake of iron-containing foods. This disorder is sometimes misdiagnosed as diabetes or as liver disorders. Although they are caused by hemochromatosis, these disorders are treated as individual ailments, rather than addressing the underlying iron overload. However, awareness of hemochromatosis is increasing among primary health care providers and other health professionals.

A final concern about iron toxicity is less a nutritional issue and more of a public health and safety issue. Accidental iron poisoning of children who consume iron supplements and/or vitamin/mineral supplements containing iron is a medical emergency. Only 6 to 12 pills can be lethal depending on the dose and age of the child. All supplements, even the fruit-flavored shapes formulated for children, should be treated as medicinal drugs and kept out of the reach of children.

Zinc

Function

Over 200 enzymes throughout the body depend on zinc. Zinc affects our growth process, taste and smell ability, healing process, immune system, and carbohydrate metabolism by assisting insulin function.

Recommended intake and sources

The RDA is 15 mg and 12 mg for men and women, respectively. During pregnancy and lactation suggested levels for women increase to a range from 15 mg to 19 mg.

Zinc-containing foods include meat, fish, poultry, whole grains, legumes, and eggs. In the United States, a variety of zinc sources are easily available. In parts of the world where animal foods are not regularly consumed and grains are a primary source, deficiencies may develop because of the low bioavailability of zinc from fibrous whole grain plant foods. Grains contain phytic acid that remains bound to zinc in the intestinal tract; human digestive juices cannot break this bond. Use of leavening agents such as yeast to prepare whole grain food products breaks this bond, making zinc available. Zinc deficiency still occurs in parts of the world where food sources may be limited and whole grains are consistently consumed as unleavened breads.

Deficiency

Deficiency symptoms are related to zinc's functions in the body. Symptoms include impaired growth, reduced appetite, and immunological disorders. Severe zinc deficiency during the growth years may result in dwarfism and hypogonadism (reduced function of gonads) leading to delayed sexual development. Reduced appetite is most likely related to reduced ability to taste (hypogeusia) and smell foods (hyposmia). The difficulty is that once appetite is reduced, fewer potential sources of zinc may be consumed and the zinc deficiency may worsen. Marginal deficiencies among children categorized as picky eaters have been noted to negatively affect height status (16). Among older persons, inadequate dietary intake resulting in reduced zinc intake appears to affect wound healing, taste and scent ability, and immune functions (17).

Toxicity

Zinc toxicity from inappropriate supplementation produces gastrointestinal distress leading to vomiting and diarrhea, fever, and exhaustion. The symptoms appear similar to those of the flu. Continual use of supplements decreases iron and copper levels in the body and reduces levels of HDL, thereby increasing risk of coronary artery disease. Intake should be no higher than the RDA unless directed by a primary health care provider; individuals should not self-medicate.

Iodine

Function

Iodine is part of the hormone thyroxin produced by the thyroid gland. Thyroxin is involved with regulating growth and development, basal metabolic rate, and body temperature.

Recommended intake and sources

The RDA for iodine is 150 mcg for both men and women.

Many sources of iodine provide inconsistent amounts. Water may contain some iodine, but the amounts vary. Seafood is a good source, and dairy products and eggs may contain some iodine depending on the feed the animals consumed. Surprisingly, seasalt does not contain iodine; the iodine is lost in processing. The amount of iodine in plant foods depends on the amount in the soil in which the food is grown. Incidental sources of iodine are cleaning products whose residues adhere to cooking and baking equipment and dough conditioners. To assure the population receives adequate amounts of this nutrient, salt in the United States may be purchased fortified with iodine.

Deficiency

Iodine deficiency reduces the amount of thyroxin produced. Symptoms of iodine deficiency then reflect the effects of reduced thyroxin, including sluggishness and weight gain. Severe iodine deficiency during pregnancy causes cretinism of the fetus that results in permanent mental and physical retardation.

Goiter, enlargement of the thyroid gland, occurs during extended iodine deficiency (Fig. 8-4). The thyroid gland works to compensate for the low iodine levels and swells up; most times the goiter remains even after iodine intake is again sufficient.

The incidence of goiter in populations has been endemic or regionally defined. In the past, a *goiter belt* existed in the Midwestern states. Iodine was unavailable in the soil and water of the area since this region is untouched by oceans; oceans provide a natural source of iodine. Since then, fortification of salt with iodine, and the wider availability of seafood because of improved refrigeration and transportation

goiter
enlargement of the thyroid gland
caused by iodine deficiency

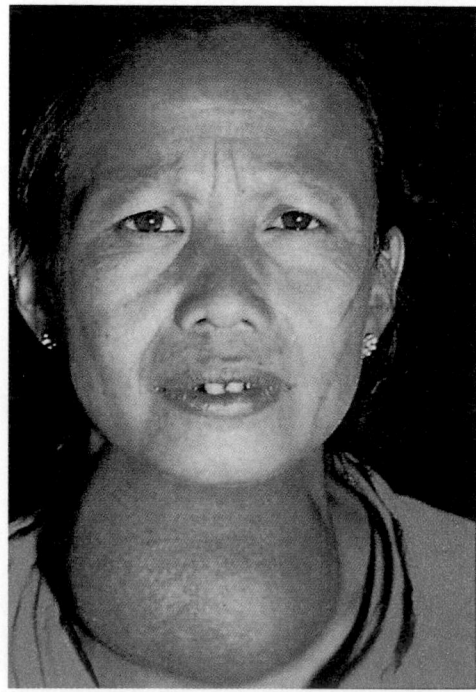

Fig. 8-4 Goiter.

systems has reduced this deficiency. Goiter, while extremely rare in North America, may still occur in parts of Europe, Africa, and South and Central America (18).

Goiter may also be caused by the action of goitrogens. When consumed as a staple component of dietary intake, goitrogens (substances in the root vegetable cassava and in cabbage) suppress the actions of the thyroid gland. Although the thyroid gland swells as in iodine deficiency goiter, the iodine level is not the initiating agent; instead substances in these vegetables suppress the actions of the thyroid gland.

Toxicity

Too much iodine can cause iodine-induced goiter called **thyrotoxicosis.**

thyrotoxicosis
iodine-induced goiter

Fluoride

Function

Fluoride increases resistance to tooth decay and is part of tooth formation. Skeletal health also depends on fluoride for bone mineralization.

Recommended intake and sources

The estimated safe and adequate daily dietary intake (ESADDI) for fluoride is 1.5 to 4.0 mg. Intake should not exceed 4 mg per day regardless of the source.

Sources of fluoride vary. The most consistent is fortified water to which fluoride has been added. Tea, seafood, and seaweed are other reliable sources. Unfortunately, these are not regularly consumed, particularly by children during tooth formation years.

An inadvertent source of fluoride is toothpaste. Most toothpastes have fluoride added as a topical agent to strengthen tooth enamel. However, some fluoride is ingested during the rinsing process, providing a kind of dietary source of fluoride. Children can ingest a lethal dose of fluoride if a tube of toothpaste is consumed.

Deficiency

Low levels of fluoride increase the risk of dental caries. Other factors of hygiene, food choices, and possibly family genes also affect plaque and subsequent dental caries.

Toxicity

Too much fluoride causes **fluorosis.** Fluorosis consists of mottling or brown spotting of the tooth enamel; severe fluorosis may also cause pitting of the teeth.

fluorosis
a condition of mottling or brown spotting of the tooth enamel caused by excessive intake of fluoride

Selenium

Function

Selenium is part of an enzyme that acts as an antioxidant. Vitamin E and selenium work together to prevent cell and lipid membrane damage from oxidizing substances. Selenium is found extensively throughout the body.

Recommended intake and sources

The RDA for selenium ranges from 55 mcg to 70 mcg per day.

Meats, fish, eggs, and whole grains are good sources of selenium. It is a nutrient for which the RDA is easily met.

Deficiency

Deficiency of selenium may predispose individuals to heart disease, particularly Keshan disease. Keshan disease was first noted in China, primarily in children and women of childbearing age with symptoms of cardiomyopathy and other features common to selenium deficiency including muscle pain and tenderness. It is difficult, however, to separate other environmental factors specific to China that may also affect long-term nutritional status. Deficiencies of nutrients other than selenium may have a role in the etiology of Keshan disease. Keshan disease differs from the form of heart disease common in the United States because the myocardium of the heart is affected; in the United States most heart disease is coronary artery disease (19). Therefore selenium deficiency is probably not a factor affecting the American incidence of heart disease.

However, low dietary levels of selenium or reduced blood levels of selenium *are* associated with an increased risk of cancer among Americans (14). The relationship of cancer to selenium consumption is probably caused by selenium's antioxidant functions combined with other antioxidants in the body. This relationship continues to be explored.

Toxicity

Selenium can be toxic at levels as low as five times the RDA of 55 mcg. Effects of toxicity include severe liver damage, vomiting, and diarrhea. Additional symptoms include metallic aftertaste, respiratory distress with lung edema and bronchopneumonia, and garlic-scented breath and sweat (20). The toxicity of selenium highlights the delicate nature of the body's use of trace minerals. Although selenium is proposed as an antioxidant supplement, the amounts suggested are those of the RDA for selenium.

Copper

Function

Although minute amounts are required by the body, copper performs many functions. Some roles of copper include action as a coenzyme involving antioxidant reactions and energy metabolism, a component of wound healing, a constituent of nerve fiber protection, and a required element for iron utilization.

Recommended intake and sources

The ESADDI for copper is 1.5 mg to 3.0 mg.

Good sources include organ meats (liver), seafood, green leafy vegetables, legumes, whole grains, dried fruits, and water if it flows through copper pipes.

Deficiency

Copper deficiency causes bone demineralization and anemia; this form of anemia can also be caused by zinc toxicity reducing body levels of copper. Copper deficiency does not occur in the United States.

Toxicity

Toxicity occurs from supplementation. Common toxic response consists of vomiting and diarrhea. Wilson's disease, an inherited disorder, results in the excessive accumulation of copper in the liver, brain, and cornea of the eye. Eventually the disorder can lead to cirrhosis, liver failure, and neurological disorders. Worldwide, the incidence of copper toxicity appears tied to use of brass and copper pots to prepare and store foods. Nutritional treatment for copper toxicity, whether caused by Wilson's disease or dietary sources, is through dietary restrictions in addition to chelation therapy that initiates excretion of excess copper from the body (21).

OTHER TRACE MINERALS

The amount needed of the following trace minerals is so low that it is easy to meet these amounts through ordinary consumption of foods. All are problematic in large doses; supplements are contraindicated.

Chromium has a role in carbohydrate metabolism as a constituent of the glucose tolerance factor (GTF) that facilitates the reaction of insulin. The ESADDI is 50 to 200 mcg. Found in animal-related foods, eggs, and whole grains, chromium is lost in food processing particularly when wheat is refined to white flour. Nonetheless, outright deficiencies of chromium are unusual. Toxicity has been noted from environmental contaminants in industrial settings rather than from excessive dietary intakes.

Studies are exploring the effects of chromium supplementation on increasing high-density lipoprotein-cholesterol (HDL) and decreasing glucose and insulin levels. The findings may have implications for populations consuming refined foods and those who are exposed to stressors that increase the need for chromium; these may include diets high in simple sugars, infections, and trauma. Inadequate chromium status may be responsible in part for some cases of impaired glucose tolerance, hyperglycemia, hypoglycemia, and unresponsiveness to insulin (22).

Manganese is a component of enzymes involved in metabolic reactions. The ESADDI is 2 to 5 mg. Found in whole grains, green vegetables, legumes, and other foods, manganese deficiency in humans is unknown.

Molybdenum functions as a coenzyme. The ESADDI of 75 to 250 mcg is easily consumed through typical dietary selections. Deficiencies have not been recorded except under medical circumstances in which dietary intake has been greatly altered.

Other trace minerals found in our bodies that may have a role in human health include silicon, boron, nickel, vanadium, lithium, tin, and cadmium. The amounts required are so small we naturally consume enough and are never deficient in these nutrients.

Table 8-7 provides a quick reference to the trace minerals.

OVERCOMING BARRIERS

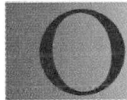O vercoming barriers to wellness pertaining to individual mineral status has been addressed in this chapter. Hypertension appears to be affected by the actions of several minerals and so is explored here.

Hypertension

Continuing research appears to suggest that adequate levels of calcium and magnesium have roles in the maintenance of appropriate blood pressure levels. Population studies point to lower intakes of these nutrients among individuals who are hypertensive (14). Marginal intake of these nutrients, combined with other lifestyle factors such as lack of exercise, excessive weight, cigarette smoking, and sodium sensitivity, sets the stage for hypertension to occur. Sodium sensitivity reflects the need to avoid excesses even if marginally higher intakes than recommended are consumed safely by most of the population.

Consumption levels of calcium, magnesium, and sodium are based on recommendations to consume foods as whole as possible. It is through processing that minerals are lost and sodium levels in foods escalate.

TOWARD A POSITIVE NUTRITION LIFESTYLE: PROJECTING

P rojection is placing responsibility for our own unacceptable feelings or behaviors on others. In relation to health, we may attribute our poor eating patterns to hectic schedules and possibly to roommates or family members who don't want to shop for food or prepare meals. We project our unacceptable behaviors on others, rather than take responsibility for our own health.

Table 8-7   Trace Minerals

Mineral	Function	Clinical Issues Deficiency/Toxicity	Recommended Intakes	Food Sources	Absorption Issues
Iron (Fe)	Distributes oxygen in hemoglobin and myoglobin; growth	Deficiency: microcytic anemia (children and women at risk) Toxicity: hemosiderosis; hemochromatosis	RDA Men: 10 mg Women: 15 mg Pregnancy: 30 mg Lactation: 15 mg	Heme sources: meat, fish, poultry, egg yolks Non-heme sources: vegetables, legumes, whole grains, enriched grains	Conserved and recycled; absorption 10%-15% of dietary iron consumed
Zinc (Zn)	Cofactor for over 200 enzymes; carbohydrate metabolism (insulin function)	Deficiency: decreases wound healing; decreases taste and smell; impaired sexual and physical development; immune disorders Toxicity: similar to flu with vomiting/diarrhea/ fever/exhaustion	RDA Men: 15 mg Women: 12 mg	Meat, fish, poultry, whole grains, legumes, eggs	Binders may decrease absorption in whole grains
Iodine (I)	Thyroxin synthesis (thyroid hormone) regulates growth and development; BMR regulation	Deficiency: decreases thyroxin causing sluggishness and weight gain, goiter, cretinism (if during pregnancy) Toxicity: thyrotoxicosis	RDA Adults: 150 mcg	Iodized salt, seafood	
Fluoride (Fl)	Bone and tooth formation; increases resistance to decay; decreases mineralization	Deficiency: increases dental caries Toxicity: fluorosis	ESADDI Adults: 1.5-4 mg	Fluoridated water, tea, seafood, seaweed	
Selenium (Se)	Antioxidant cofactor with vitamin E; prevents cell and lipid membrane damage	Deficiency: possible Keshan disease/ cancer Toxicity: liver damage, vomiting, diarrhea	RDA Men: 70 mcg Women: 55 mcg	Meat, fish, eggs, whole grains	
Copper (C)	Conenzyme in antioxidant reactions and energy metabolism; wound healing; nerve fiber protection; iron use	Deficiency: bone-demineralization and anemia (not in US) Toxicity: Wilson's disease or with supplements producing vomiting/diarrhea	ESADDI Adults: 1.5-3 mg	Organ meats (liver), seafood, green leafy vegetables	
Chromium (Cr)	Carbohydrate metabolism, part of glucose tolerance factor	Deficiency: possible link with cardio-vascular disorders; hypoglycemia, hyperglycemia, and unresponsive insulin	ESADDI Adults: 50-200 mcg	Animal food, whole grains	

Table 8-7, cont'd Trace Minerals					
Mineral	Function	Clinical Issues Deficiency/Toxicity	Recommended Intakes	Food Sources	Absorption Issues
Manganese (Mn)	Part of metabolic reaction enzymes	Deficiency: unknown	ESADDI Adults: 2-5 mg	Whole grains, green leafy vegetables, legumes	
Molybdenum (Mo)	Coenzyme	Deficiency: unknown	ESADDI Adults: 75-250 mg	Many foods	

CNS, Central nervous system; *FVD*, Fluid volume deficit; *RDA*, Recommended Daily Allowance; *EMR*, Estimated Minimum Requirement; *ESADDI*, Estimated Safe and Adequate Daily Dietary Intake.

One mineral on which projection sometimes occurs is iron. Since iron deficiency is often manifested with tiredness, paleness, and frequent infections, it is frequently self-diagnosed as the pathological cause of poor health. Accurate diagnosis of iron deficiency is based on blood analysis, not on self-reporting. As an aspect of client education, we can help clients clarify the actual cause of their symptoms if they are not clinically iron deficient. Often these symptoms are caused by poor health habits—not enough sleep, irregular meals, and too little exercise. Rather than projecting ill health on the mineral iron, clients can take responsibility and modify their own health behaviors.

WELLNESS AND WATER/MINERALS

Physical Dimension	Water and minerals affect every system of the body; physical health depends on adequate levels of these nutrients.
Intellectual Dimension	Intellectual health is compromised when iron levels are low; iron deficiency affects cognitive abilities, diminishing ability to learn.
Emotional Dimension	Emotional health may rely on our being sufficiently hydrated with fluids; cases of FVD have been mistaken as senility when the thirst acuity of the elderly diminishes.
Social Dimension	Social health may be affected if the elderly become debilitated by bone fractures or osteoporosis caused by chronic calcium deficiencies; social mobility may be limited as their physical movement is inhibited.

SUMMARY

In this chapter water and minerals are explored through their nutritional requirements and physiological roles for achieving nutritional wellness. Although water and minerals are primary components of body fluids, each performs other functions as well.

Water supports a variety of functions including acting as a structural component of the body, a temperature regulator, a lubricant, a fluid cushion, a transportation vehicle, a trace mineral source, and a medium for and participant in biochemical reactions. About 4 to 8 8-oz servings of water per day or 1 to 1.5 ml per kcal of energy expended is required to meet basic physiological needs. Sources may include beverages as well as foods with high water content. The best source is water.

Minerals also fill diverse roles. Structurally, minerals provide rigidity and strength to teeth and skeleton; the skeletal mineral components also serve as a storage depot for other needs of the body. Nerve function is influenced by minerals allowing for proper muscle contraction and release. Minerals also assist enzymes, maintain proper acid-base balance of body fluids, and are required for blood clotting and wound healing.

The 16 essential minerals are divided into two categories: major and trace minerals. Major minerals, needed daily in amounts of 100 mg or higher, include calcium, phosphorus, magnesium, sulfur, and the electrolytes of sodium, potassium, and chloride. Trace minerals, required daily in amounts less than or equal to 20 mg, include iron, zinc, iodine, fluoride, selenium, copper, chromium, manganese, and molybdenum.

Prime food sources of minerals include both plants and animals. Valuable plant sources include most fruits, vegetables, legumes, and whole grains. Animal sources consist of beef, chicken, eggs, fish, and milk products. Although minerals are very stable when cooked, the bioavailability of some minerals may be limited depending on the source. Some plant minerals are not easily available to the human body because of binders inhibiting absorption. Generally, minerals from animals foods are able to be absorbed more easily than those from plants. Whatever the specific food source, dietary patterns consisting primarily of whole foods provide an adequate supply of minerals.

THE NURSING ROLE

Fluid Volume Deficit Case Study: The Nursing Process

Mr. Sales is 82 years old and resides in an extended-care facility. One night he develops nausea, vomiting, and diarrhea from a gastrointestinal virus that has been affecting several other residents also. After 8 hours of repeated vomiting and diarrhea, the RN is concerned that Mr. Sales may be developing fluid volume deficit. The RN uses nursing process skills to investigate and handle the problem as follows.

ASSESSMENT DATA COLLECTED
Objective:
Weight loss from 165 to 161 lb
Dry mucous membranes
Normal filling of hand veins
Pulse rate increase from 80 to 86
Blood pressure in normal range for patient
Temperature 100.6 degrees
Warm extremities
Mentally alert

NURSING DIAGNOSIS
Mild fluid volume deficit related to vomiting and diarrhea as evidenced by weight loss of 4 lb and dry mucous membranes

PLANNING
The RN sets goals in consultation with Mr. Sales to achieve the following outcomes:
No further fluid deficit
Fluid balance restored to normal within 36 hours

INTERVENTION
1. Obtain orders for antiemetic and antidiarrheal drugs
2. Monitor vital signs every 2 hours
3. Try sips of gingerale and broth beginning 1 hour after antiemetic
4. Measure intake and output
5. Weigh patient once a day (OD)

EVALUATION
Goals must be evaluated to see if the outcomes have been met as evidenced by:

THE NURSING ROLE, cont'd.
Fluid Volume Deficit Case Study: The Nursing Process

1. Moist mucous membranes in 36 hours
2. Balanced intake and output in 36 hours
3. Weight of 165 lb within 4 days

REFERENCES

1. Food and Nutrition Board/National Research Council: *Recommended dietary allowances,* ed 10, Washington, DC, 1989, National Academy Press.
2. Prince F, Sfiligo E: Back, back, back, back....(bottled water sales up 8.9% in 1993), *Beverage World* 113(1562):72-76, March 1994.
3. US Department of Health and Human Services, Public Health Service: *Healthy people 2000: National health promotion and disease prevention objectives,* Washington, DC, 1990, US Government Printing Office.
4. Correa P: Is gastric carcinoma an infectious disease? *N Engl J Med* 325(16):1170-71, 1991.
5. Guthrie HA, Picciano MF: *Human nutrition,* St. Louis, 1995, Mosby.
6. Allen LH, Wood RJ: Calcium and phosphorus. In Shils ME, Olson JA, Shike M, eds: *Modern nutrition in health and disease,* ed 8, Philadelphia, 1994, Lea & Febiger.
7. Wardlaw GM: Putting osteoporosis in perspective *J Am Diet Assoc* 93(9):1000-1006, 1993.
8. Scane AC, Sutcliffe AM, Francis RM: Osteoporosis in men, *Baillieres Clin Rheumatol* 7(3):589-601, Oct 1993.
9. Mundy GR: Boning up on genes, *Nature* 367(6460):216-218, Jan 20, 1994.
10. Massey LK: Caffeine, urinary calcium, calcium metabolism and bone, *J Nutr* 123(9):1611-1614, 1993.
11. Barrett-Connor E, Chang JC, Edelstein SL: Coffee-associated osteoporosis onset by daily milk consumption: The Rancho Bernardo Study, *JAMA* 271(4):280-283, Jan 26, 1994.
12. Greger JL: Effect of variations in dietary protein, phosphorus, electrolytes and vitamin D on calcium and zinc metabolism. In Bodwell ED, Erdman Jr. JW, eds: *Nutrient interactions,* New York, 1988, Marcel Dekker.
13. Jacob RA: Vitamin C. In Shils ME, Olson JA, Shike M, eds: *Modern nutrition in health and disease,* ed 8, Philadelphia, 1994, Lea & Febiger.
14. National Academy of Science: *Diet and health: Implications for reducing chronic disease risk,* Washington, DC, 1989, National Academy Press.
15. Scholl IO, Hediger MI: Anemia and iron-deficiency anemia: Compilation of data on pregnancy outcome, *Am J Clin Nutr* 59(2 suppl):429s-500s, Feb 1994.
16. Sanstead HH: Zinc deficiency: a public health problem? *Journal of Disease in Children* 145:853-858, 1991.
17. Greger JL: Potential for trace mineral deficiencies and toxicities in the elderly. In Bales CW, ed: *Mineral homeostasis in the elderly: Current topics in nutrition and disease,* vol 21, New York, 1989, Alan Liss.
18. Dunn H: Iodine deficiency: The next target for elimination, *N Engl J Med* 326(4):267-268, 1992.
19. McLaren D: Clinical manifestations of human vitamin and mineral disorders. In Shils ME, Olson JA, Shike M, eds: *Modern nutrition in health and disease,* ed 8, Philadelphia, 1994, Lea & Febiger.
20. Bedwal RS et al: Selenium—its biological perspectives, *Med Hypotheses* 41(2):150-159, Aug 1993.
21. Turnland JR: Copper. In Shils ME, Olson JA, Shike M, eds: *Modern nutrition in health and disease,* ed 8, Philadelphia, 1994, Lea & Febiger.
22. Nielsen FH: Chromium. In Shils ME, Olson JA, Shike M, eds: *Modern nutrition in health and disease,* ed 8, Philadelphia, 1994, Lea & Febiger.
23. Turnland JR: Copper nutritive bioavailability and the influence of dietary factors, *J Am Diet Assoc* 88 303-308, 1988.
24. American Dietetic Association: Positions of the American Dietetic Association: Enrichment and fortification of foods and dietary supplements, *J Am Diet Assoc* 94(6):661-663, 1994.

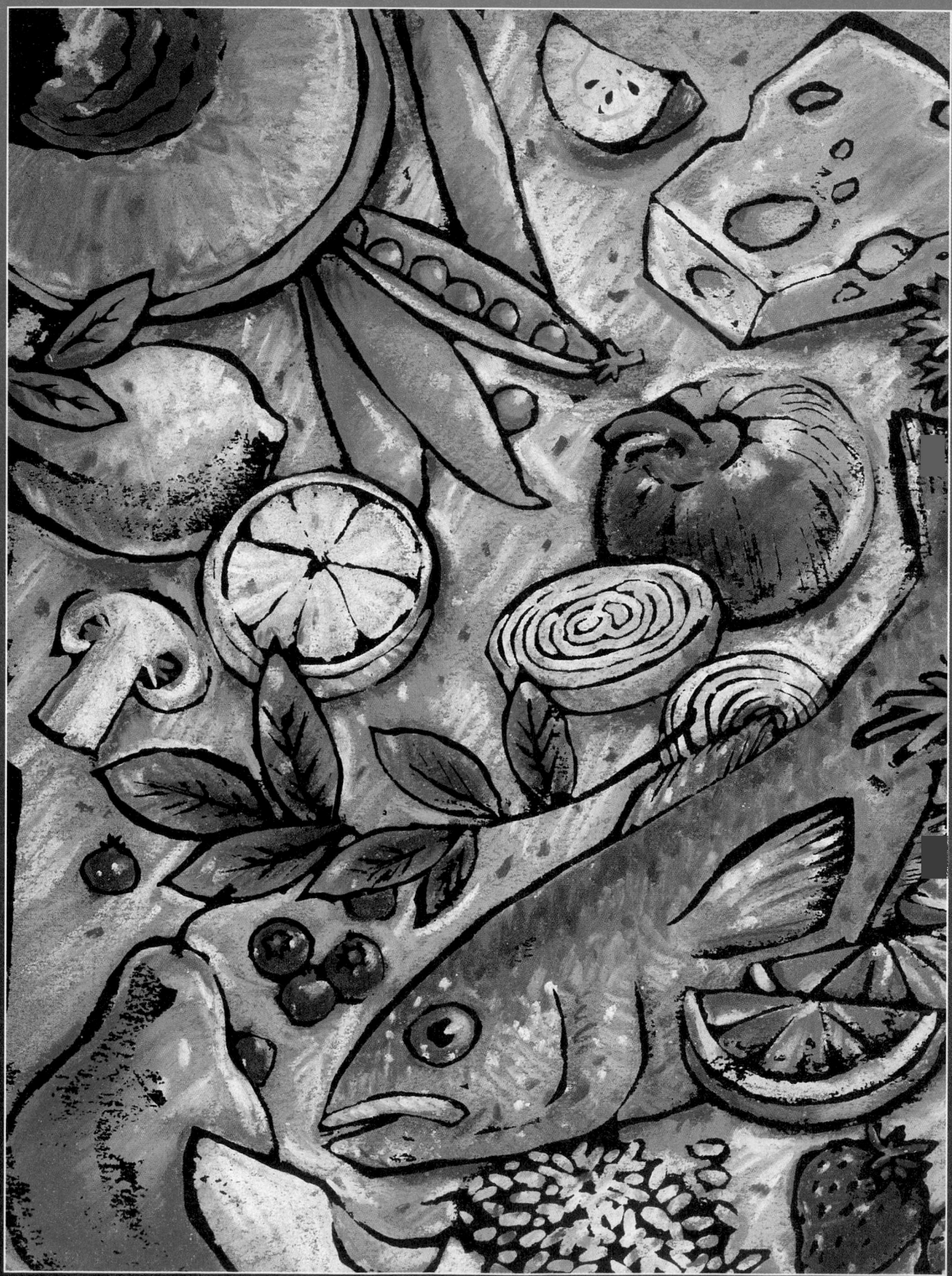

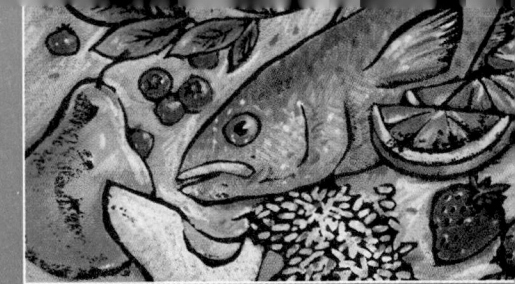

PART THREE

Health Promotion Through Nutrition and Nursing Practice

Chapter 9

ENERGY SUPPLY AND FITNESS

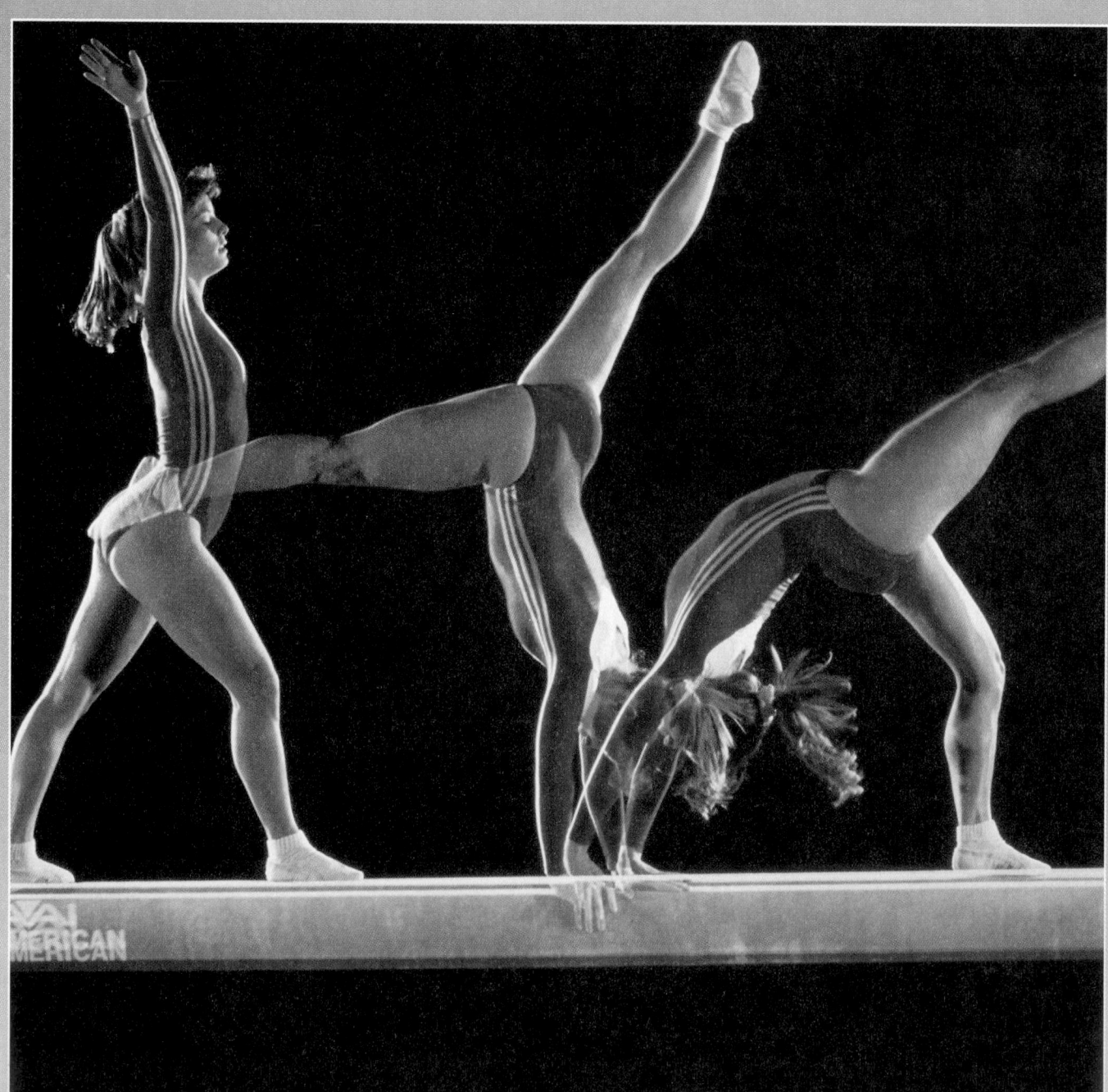

ROLE IN WELLNESS

The abilities to perform work, produce change, and maintain life all require energy. Energy exists in many forms—mechanical, chemical, heat, electrical, light, and nuclear. The laws of thermodynamics tell us that each can be converted from one form to another. As our bodies function, chemical energy from food is converted to mechanical energy and heat.

The ultimate source of energy is the sun. Sunlight is used by plants to produce chemical energy in the form of carbohydrates, proteins, or fats. These foods possess stored energy. People are not capable of doing this. We must convert the chemical energy from the foods we eat into forms useable by the human body.

ENERGY

The energy released from food is measured in kilocalories (thousands of calories) or Calories. Technically a calorie is the amount of heat necessary to raise the temperature of a gram of water 1 degree Celsius. As first noted in Chapter 1, to assure accuracy the term *kilocalories* is used throughout this text, abbreviated as *kcalories* or *kcal*.

Two methods are used to determine the energy a food contains. One is through the use of a bomb calorimeter (Fig. 9-1). This instrument is designed to burn a food while measuring the amount of heat or energy released. This provides an estimate of the energy available to humans. Since the bomb calorimeter method is more efficient than the human body, the kcalorie value assigned to a food item is adjusted to reflect the limitations of the human system. Amounts listed in food tables reflect this adjustment.

The other method of assessing food energy is proximate composition, which determines the grams of carbohydrates, proteins, and fats of a food item. Then the grams are multiplied by the energy value of each (carbohydrates × 4 kcal/g; proteins × 4 kcal/g; fats × 9 kcal/g). The sum of these calculations equals the total energy content of a specific food.

Energy Pathways

The processes of digestion, absorption, and metabolism for each of the three energy nutrient categories of carbohydrates, fats, and protein have been presented in previous chapters. (Alcohol also provides energy, but is not considered a nutrient category.) Carbohydrate digests to glucose, triglycerides (fats) to fatty acids and glycerol, and protein to amino acids. Here we continue to follow their journey as they are used for energy in individual cells.

The nutrients release energy when they are catabolized (broken down), forming carbon dioxide and water. The released energy becomes caught within *adenosine triphosphate* (ATP), the *fuel* for all energy-requiring processes in the body (Fig. 9-2).

Glucose

Glucose releases energy and is converted to carbon dioxide and water through the three processes of glycolysis, citric acid cycle, and oxidative phosphorylation (1). These complicated processes are reviewed in general here; the intricate details are beyond the scope of this text.

Through *glycolysis,* a glucose molecule produces pyruvic acid and ATP. Part of this process depends on niacin, which is a component of the essential coenzyme NAD^+ (nicotinamide adenine dinucleotide). Oxygen is not needed for glycolysis to

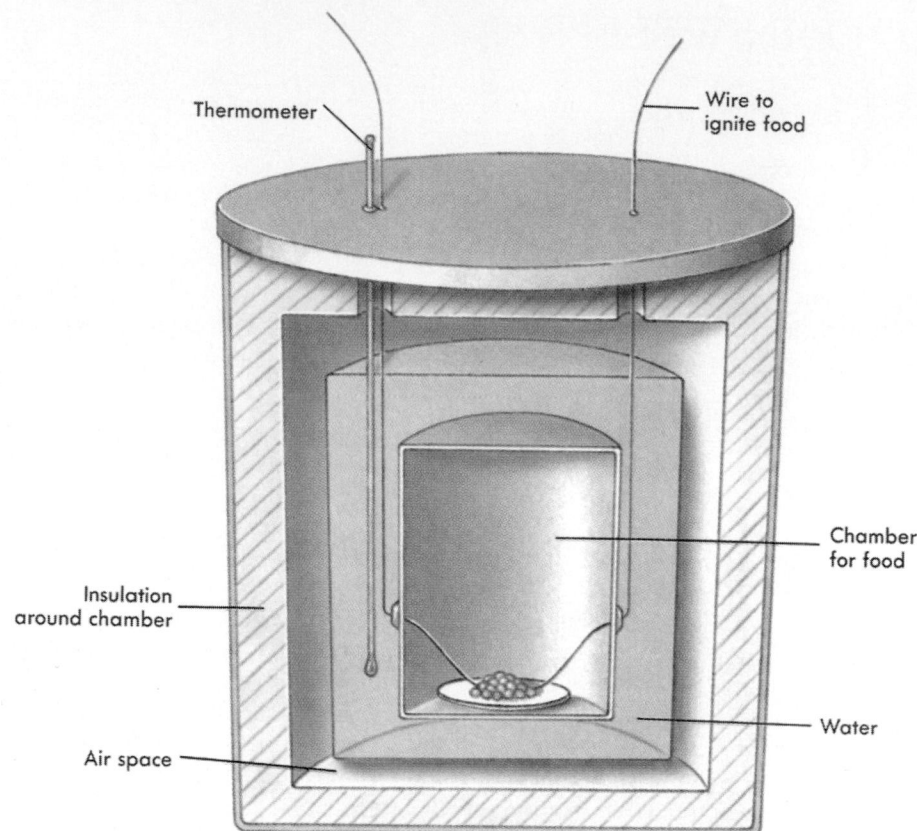

Thermometer

Wire to ignite food

Insulation around chamber

Air space

Chamber for food

Water

Fig. 9-1 Cross-section of a bomb calorimeter. To determine energy, a dried portion of food is burned inside a chamber charged with oxygen that is surrounded by water. As the food is burned, it gives off heat. This raises the temperature of the water surrounding the chamber. The increase in water temperature indicates the number of kcalories contained in the food. One kcalorie equals the amount of heat needed to raise the temperature of 1 kilogram of water by 1 degree Celsius (C).

anaerobic pathway
a form of energy production that does not require oxygen

oxygen debt
the amount of oxygen required to clear lactic acid buildup from the body

anaerobic glycolysis
the conversion of glucose to lactic acid to provide energy in the absence of oxygen

aerobic glycolysis
the conversion of glucose to ATP for energy when oxygen is available

aerobic pathway
a form of energy production that depends on oxygen

occur; it is an **anaerobic pathway.** The anaerobic pathway provides us with energy for short, intense exertion; this exertion is limited because oxygen is not available quickly enough to continue its support. Instead, the incomplete use of glucose causes the pyruvic acid to be converted to lactic acid. As lactic acid builds up, the muscles become sore and stiff. Consequently, the exertion ceases because of pain. Within a few minutes, enough oxygen is available to degrade (break down) the lactic acid, relieving the physical discomfort. This effect is called **oxygen debt.**

The anaerobic pathway provides us with energy for short, intense exercise such as sprinting or a burst of energy in sports such as basketball, soccer, football, golf, and tennis. When we are not involved in athletic pursuits, we still depend on this energy source to run for the train, chase after toddlers, or bound across the room to answer the telephone.

Anaerobic glycolysis takes place in the cell cytoplasm, but oxygen-dependent **aerobic glycolysis** (the **aerobic pathway**) occurs in the mitochondria of the cell. In the mitochondria, pyruvic acid (made without oxygen) reacts with coenzyme A (CoA), creating acetyl CoA. Pantothenic acid (the B vitamin) is required for acetyl CoA conversion. All the energy-producing nutrients are converted into acetyl CoA, revealing the importance of pantothenic acid and acetyl CoA. The energy process continues as acetyl CoA reaches the TCA cycle. The reactions that are part of the cycle lead to the formation of additional ATP and carbon dioxide. One of the coenzymes of this process depends on riboflavin, another of the B vitamins.

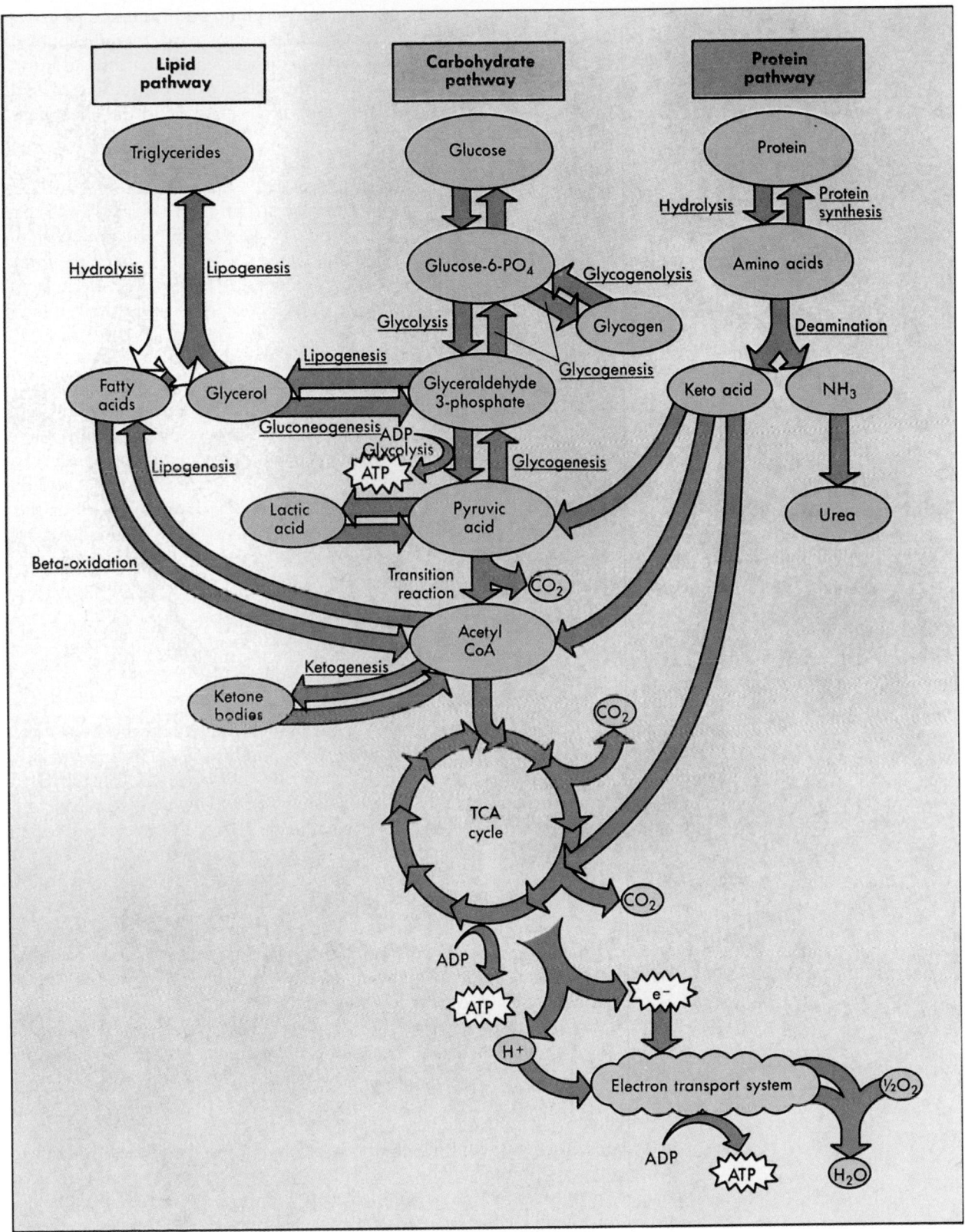

Fig. 9-2 Summary of key steps in the metabolism of glucose, fatty acids, glycerol, and amino acids.

The aerobic pathway is the primary energy source for low-level activities such as walking and most of our daily activities. It is also the primary energy source for endurance-type exercise such as swimming, bicycling, and running.

The last process of glucose conversion to energy is oxidative phosphorylation. A number of actions lead to release of the hydrogens as water and additional energy are captured in ATP. The term *oxidative* reflects the combining of hydrogen with oxygen to form water; *phosphorylation* is the creation of the phosphate bond to form ATP.

Fatty acids and glycerol

Glycerol enters glycolysis by being transformed into pyruvic acid and is used the same way as glucose for energy. Fatty acids, however, enter the glycolysis process at the acetyl unit level and are formed into acetyl CoA. In this form, the fatty acids (now as acetyl CoA) go into the TCA cycle, releasing energy ATP. Because of their structure, many fatty acids are able to form more ATP units than glucose and therefore provide more energy.

Amino acids

Amino acids are first catabolized through deamination as described in Chapter 6. While the nitrogen-containing amino groups are processed by the liver and kidneys, the other amino acid components enter the energy metabolism pathway, with each component entering at a different location. Some of the amino acid components are converted into pyruvic acid; others become intermediaries of the TCA cycle or part of acetyl groups. If sufficient energy is available, amino acids are used for protein functions rather than for energy. If more amino acids are consumed than needed, the extra amino acids are used for energy metabolism.

Alcohol

Alcohol is converted to acetate units that then form acetyl CoA.

Too much energy

If more energy is consumed than is needed for immediate energy needs, extra carbohydrate is stored as glycogen in the liver and muscles. The amount of glycogen able to be stored is only about 1200 to 1800 kcalories (2). Carbohydrate can also continue through glycolysis, with some conversion to glycerol. Eventually triglycerides can be formed and stored in adipose cells (cells specialized for storing fat). Excess triglycerides also continue through the process, but can reverse from acetyl CoA back to fatty acids. These fatty acids can then form triglycerides with glycerol to fill adipose cells.

Amino acids consumed in excess follow a variety of pathways as noted earlier. Some are glucogenic amino acids that can convert into glucose and glycogen. This also means they can be converted into storage triglycerides as well. Other amino acids that form acetyl CoA can also form triglycerides.

The ability of energy nutrients to be converted into triglycerides and stored in adipose cells supports the need to consume adequate energy levels to maintain desirable weight.

Too little energy

Not enough energy entering the body reverses these processes. Energy that is consumed is used immediately, regardless of its source. Stored carbohydrate, glycogen in muscles and liver, adipose energy, and body protein are all potential sources for energy. The first used is glycogen, followed by the energy reserve of body fat in adipose cells. Glucose must be available to the brain. Only a small portion of triglycerides (glycerol) can yield glucose, and continuous use of this source results in a buildup of ketones and the potential imbalance of the body pH (see Chapter 6). Body protein is used as a last resort.

Anaerobic and Aerobic Pathways

How do anaerobic and aerobic energy pathways work together to supply energy? For the first minute or two of exercise, oxygen has not arrived at the muscles and energy must come from anaerobic sources. After several minutes the aerobic pathway takes over. However, as the exertion or exercise continues, there is a constant interchange or use of energy sources.

The energy source that muscles use during exercise depends on the intensity and length of exercise, the person's fitness level, and the foods eaten. Short-term, high-intensity activities such as sprinting rely mostly on the anaerobic pathway for energy, and only carbohydrates (in the form of muscle glycogen) can be used for energy. On the other hand, exercise of low to moderate intensity is supported primarily by the aerobic system, and carbohydrate and fats are the major fuels. Fats are an important energy source during exercise because, unlike carbohydrates, fatty acids are abundant in the body and using them spares muscle glycogen.

The length of activity also determines what type of fuel the muscles will use during exercise. As the duration of exercise increases, glycogen stores become depleted and fat becomes the primary source of energy (Fig. 9-3). A sedentary person breaks down glycogen faster and as a result accumulates more lactic acid in the blood. The lactic acid causes muscle fatigue. A physically fit person has a higher aerobic capacity (the ability of the heart to supply oxygen) so that oxygen is available sooner and in greater quantity; this allows use of the aerobic pathway of energy, avoiding lactic acid buildup. This also means more fat than glycogen can be used for fuel.

If we eat a diet high in carbohydrates, more glycogen is available to be stored as energy. The amount of carbohydrate stored in the body depends on how much carbohydrate we consume and our level of fitness. Endurance training increases the capacity of the muscles to store glycogen, but there is still a limit to the total amount of energy that can be stored. The more glycogen that we store, the more energy we have available for all kinds of activities—not just for marathons.

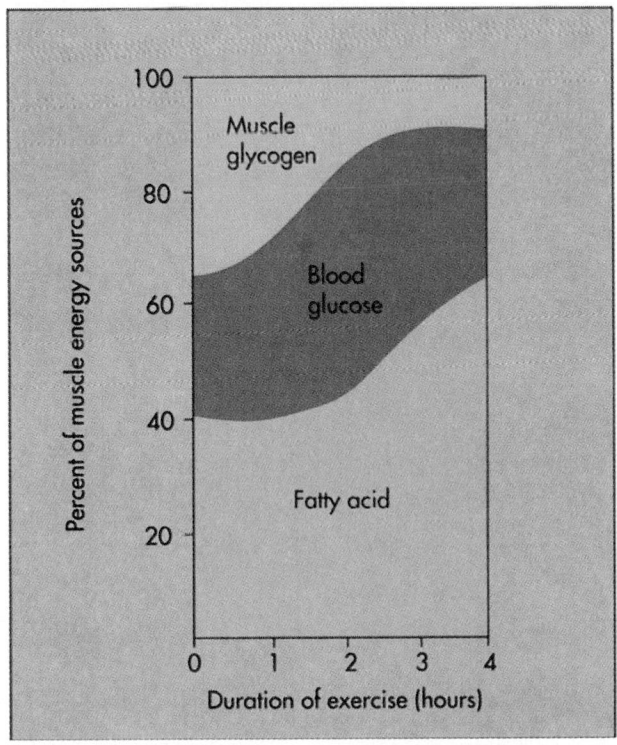

Fig. 9-3 Relative use made of energy sources in the body as exercise continues.

ENERGY EXPENDITURE

To maintain a healthy weight, our energy intake should equal energy expended. Because of our sedentary lifestyles, some of us may need less energy than standard energy requirement charts recommend. In contrast, the serious competitive athlete's energy intake must support a training and competition schedule that allows the athlete to achieve his or her personal best.

Individuals who are acutely ill and hospitalized or adapting to chronic disorders may require individualized levels of energy intake to meet changing physiological needs. Consultation with a registered dietitican may be warranted for patients, their family members, and other caregivers; misconceptions about energy needs can be eliminated by nutrition counseling regardless of the nature of the health disorder.

Estimating Daily Energy Needs

The recommended energy allowances published by the National Research Council appear in Table 9-1. These energy values are based on individuals with a light-to-moderate activity level. The average daily energy intake for the referenced 19-to-24 year-old male is 2900 kcal or 40 kcal/kg. It is 2200 kcal or 38 kcal/kg for the same age referenced female. If a person is more active or of a larger or smaller body size, further adjustments must be made. Most importantly, these levels are simply guidelines; the only accurate recommendation for individuals is one that supports healthy weight levels.

Table 9-1   Median Heights and Weights and Recommended Energy Intake

Category	Age (years) or Condition	Weight (kg)	Weight (lb)	Height (cm)	Height (in)	REE* (kcal/day)	Multiples of REE	Average Energy Allowance (kcal)[†] Per kg	Average Energy Allowance (kcal)[†] Per day[‡]
Infants	0.0–0.5	6	13	60	24	320		108	650
	0.5–1.0	9	20	71	28	500		98	850
Children	1–3	13	29	90	35	740		102	1300
	4–6	20	44	112	44	950		90	1800
	7–10	28	62	132	52	1130		70	2000
Males	11–14	45	99	157	62	1440	1.70	55	2500
	15–18	66	145	176	69	1760	1.67	45	3000
	19–24	72	160	177	70	1780	1.67	40	2900
	25–50	79	174	176	70	1800	1.60	37	2900
	51 +	77	170	173	68	1530	1.50	30	2300
Females	11–14	46	101	157	62	1310	1.67	47	2200
	15–18	55	120	163	64	1370	1.60	40	2200
	19–24	58	128	164	65	1350	1.60	38	2200
	25–50	63	138	163	64	1380	1.55	36	2200
	51 +	65	143	160	63	1280	1.50	30	1900
Pregnant	1st trimester								+ 0
	2nd trimester								+ 300
	3rd trimester								+ 300
Lactating	1st 6 months								+ 500
	2nd 6 months								+ 500

*Resting energy expenditure (REE); calculation based on FAO equations, then rounded.
[†]In the range of light to moderate activity, the coefficient of variation is ± 20%.
[‡]Figure is rounded.

Table 9-2	Factors for Estimating Daily Energy Allowances at Various Levels of Physical Activity for Men and Women (Ages 19 to 50)	
Level of Activity	Activity Factor* (× REE)	Energy Expenditure† (kcal/kg per day)
Very light		
Men	1.3	31
Women	1.3	30
Light		
Men	1.6	38
Women	1.5	35
Moderate		
Men	1.7	41
Women	1.6	37
Heavy		
Men	2.1	50
Women	1.9	44
Exceptional		
Men	2.4	58
Women	2.2	51

*Based on examples presented by WHO (1985).

† REE is the average of values for median weights of persons ages 19 to 24 and 25 to 74 years: males, 24.0 kcal/kg; females, 23.2 kcal/kg.

Many different formulas have been developed for estimating energy expenditure, some of which are very complicated. An easy way of determining kcalorie intake is to multiply weight by one of the numbers in Table 9-2. For example, a 170-lb (77 kg) male who participates in moderate exercise needs about 3060 kcalories a day (77 × 41). Remember that these numbers represent averages. Some people need fewer kcalories; others need more.

Components of Total Energy Expenditure

Our daily energy requirement depends on many variables, including basal metabolism, physical activity, and the thermic effect of food. **Basal metabolism** represents the amount of energy required to maintain life-sustaining activities (breathing, circulation, heart beat, secretion of hormones) for a specific period of time. Basal metabolic rate (BMR) is the rate at which the body spends energy to keep all these life-supporting processes going. Basal metabolic rate is measured in the morning upon awakening, before any physical activity and 12 to 18 hours after the last meal. Two methods are used. One consists of human subjects being placed in a chamber; the body heat given off changes the temperature of the chamber, reflecting the energy used by their bodies for the most basic functions. The second method, indirect calorimetry, uses a calorimeter. The instrument measures the respiratory quotient or exchanges of gases as a person breathes into the mouthpiece of the machine. This determines the amount of oxygen used, which also reflects the energy (as heat) released.

Several factors affect BMR, including age, body size, sex, body temperature, fasting/starvation stress, menstruation, and thyroid function. BMR varies with the amount of lean tissue in the body; higher levels of lean body mass increase BMR. For example, women have lower BMRs than men because of smaller body size and less lean body tissue. The BMR of adults slowly lowers from about age 35 on because of decreases in lean body tissue associated with aging. As a physically fit person ages, the BMR may not slow down as much as that of a person who is physically unfit.

basal metabolism
the amount of energy required to maintain life-sustaining activities for a specific period of time

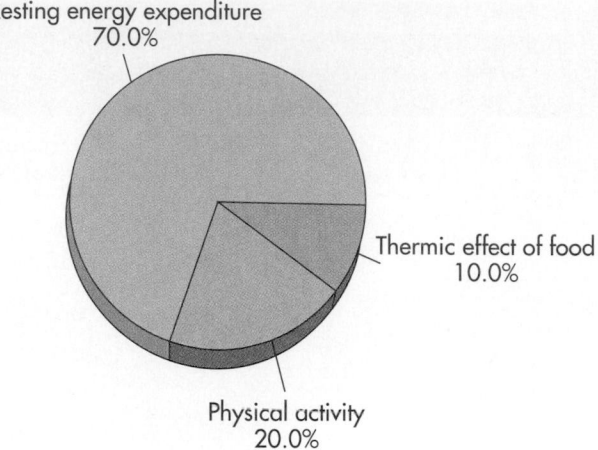

Fig. 9-4 Breakdown of human energy expenditure.

Factors that increase basal metabolism
increase in muscle mass
good physical condition
being a male
hyperthyroidism
pregnancy
puberty
extremes of environmental temperature
smoking

Factors that decrease basal metabolism
increase in body fat
poor physical condition
being a female
hypothyroidism
sleep
aging
undernutrition

resting energy expenditure (REE)
the energy expended in a normal life situation while at rest, and energy used following meals and exercise

thermic effect of food (TEF) or diet-induced thermogenesis
an increase of cellular activity when food is eaten

The process of sustaining fitness maintains the muscle mass of lean body tissue and slows the loss caused by aging. It is never too late to develop fitness; with the approval of a primary health care provider, exercise is appropriate at any age.

BMR also depends on thyroid function. The thyroid hormone *thyroxin* is a key BMR regulator; the more thyroxin produced in the body the higher the BMR. Of course, production of too much thyroxin is not desirable either.

Many scientists, however, prefer to use a more practical measurement called *resting energy expenditure (REE)*. Resting energy expenditure is the energy a person expends in a normal life situation while at rest, and it includes some energy the body uses following meals and exercise. It accounts for approximately 60% to 75% of our total energy needs, similar percentages to those of BMR (Fig. 9-4).

Physical Activity

The second largest component of energy expenditure after REE (or BMR) is physical activity. It demands about 20% to 30% of our total energy needs. Of all the components, it varies the most among people. The amount of energy we expend depends on the intensity and duration of the activity. Walking requires more energy than sitting, and walking for 60 minutes uses more energy than walking for 15 minutes. Thus even a moderate activity can become one of high energy if it is carried on for a long time.

Body size affects energy expenditure more than any other single factor. A heavier person uses more energy to perform a given task than does a lighter person. Table 9-3 shows the number of kcalories burned per hour for two individuals, one weighing 205 lb and the other 125 lb, as they engage in various types of activities.

Thermic Effect of Food

The third component of energy output is the energy required for our body to digest, absorb, metabolize, and store food. When we eat, our body's cells increase their activities. This increase in cellular activity is known as the **thermic effect of food (TEF),** or diet-induced thermogenesis. The thermic effect is relatively small, accounting for approximately 7% to 10% of a person's total energy needs.

Adaptive Thermogenesis

Adaptive thermogenesis is the energy used by our bodies to adjust to changing physical and biological environmental situations. This includes energy used to

Table 9-3   Approximate Calories Used Per Hour

Activity	205 lb Person	125 lb Person
Archery	420	268
Baseball—infield or outfield	382	234
—pitching	488	299
Basketball—moderate	575	352
—vigorous	807	495
Bicycling—on level, 5.5 mph	409	251
13.0 mph	877	537
Canoeing—4 mph	565	352
Dancing—moderate	341	209
—vigorous	464	284
Fencing—moderate	409	251
—vigorous	837	513
Football	678	416
Golf—twosome	443	271
—foursome	332	203
Handball or hardball—vigorous	797	488
Horseback riding—walk	270	165
—trot	551	338
Motorcycling	297	182
Mountain climbing	820	503
Rowing—pleasure	409	251
—rowing machine or sculling 20 strokes/min	1116	684
Running—5.5 mph	887	537
—7 mph	1141	669
—9 mph level	1269	777
—9 mph 2.5% grade	1480	907
—9 mph 4% grade	1564	959
—12 mph	1606	984
—in place 140 count/min.	1993	1222
Skating—moderate	465	285
—vigorous	837	513
Skiing—downhill	789	483
—level, 5 mph	956	586
Soccer	730	447
Squash	849	520
Swimming—backstroke - 20 yds/min	316	194
- 40 yds/min	682	418
—breaststroke - 20 yds/min	392	241
- 40 yds/min	786	482
—butterfly	956	586
—crawl - 20 yds/min	392	241
- 50 yds/min	869	532
—sidestroke	682	418
Tennis—moderate	565	347
—vigorous	797	488
Volleyball—moderate	465	285
—vigorous	797	489
Walking—2 mi/hr	286	176
—110-120 paces/min	425	260
—4.5 mph	540	331
—downstairs	544	333
—upstairs	1417	869
Water skiing	638	391
Wrestling, judo or karate	1049	643

From Grandjean A: *Nutrition for sport success*, Omaha, 1984, Swanson Center for Nutrition.

adapt to coldness, extreme changes in kcalorie intake (of several days duration), and physical and emotional trauma. This category of energy need incorporates additional demands caused by illness and the process of recovery. Since the expenditure depends on individualized variables, it is not calculated into average energy requirements.

FITNESS

Major advances in technology have made our lives more comfortable and simple. We drive instead of walk, take the elevator instead of the stairs, and ride the lawn mower instead of pushing it. The amount of physical activity at work and in the home has declined steadily. How important is physical activity to our health, fitness, and total well-being? Let's take a closer look.

Physical activity is defined as any body movement produced by skeletal muscles that results in energy expenditure. It varies by day, time of year, and stage of life. Physical activity is similar to yet different from physical fitness. Physical activity describes the actions or movements that we make, whereas **physical fitness** describes the limits on the actions that we are capable of making (3).

Being physically fit is more than just being fast or strong. True physical fitness consists of three major components: flexibility, muscular strength and endurance, and cardiovascular endurance. **Flexibility** is the ability to move your muscles to their full extent without injury. **Muscular strength and endurance** describes the ability of the muscles to perform hard and/or prolonged work. **Cardiovascular endurance** is the ability of the body to take in, deliver, and use oxygen for physical work. Although flexibility and muscular strength and endurance are important components of health and well-being, cardiovascular endurance is the best physiological index of total body endurance (4). Life depends on the strength of the heart and lungs to deliver nutrients and oxygen to the cells.

physical activity
any body movement produced by skeletal muscles that results in energy expenditure

physical fitness
the limits on the actions that the body is capable of making

flexibility
the ability to move muscles to their full extent without injury

muscular strength and endurance
the ability of the muscles to perform hard work and/or prolonged work

cardiovascular endurance
the ability of the body to take in, deliver, and obtain oxygen for physical work

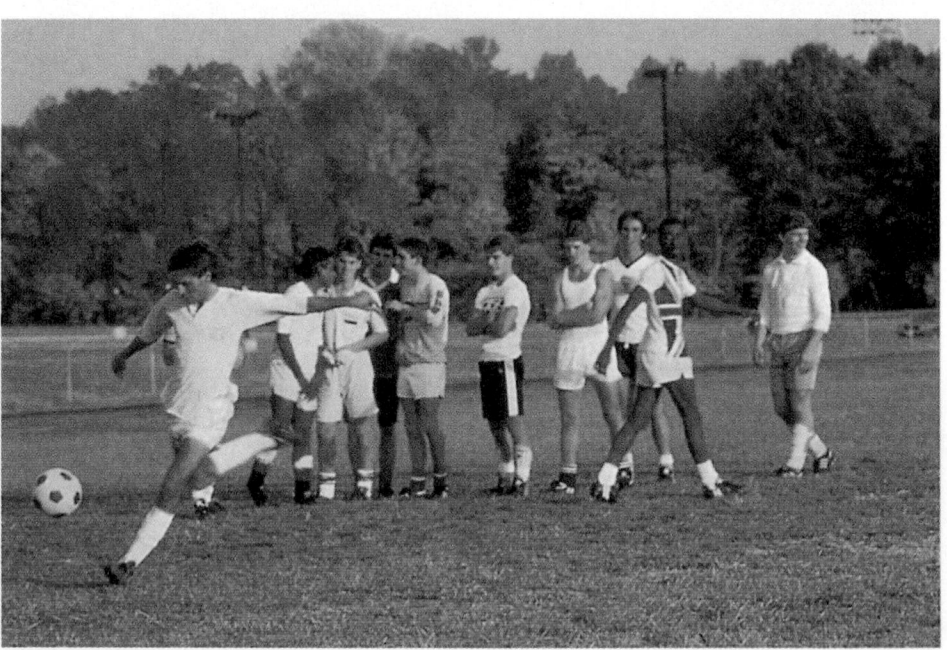

Physical fitness consists of flexibility, muscular strength and endurance, and cardiovascular endurance.

Health Benefits of Physical Exercise

Much of what we do today will affect our future health. In *Fitness and Wellness,* Rosato writes:

> We make choices, both positive and negative, about smoking, wearing seat belts, exercise, weight control, nutrition, alcohol intake, frequency of medical examinations, and so on. These choices and the ensuing behavior patterns profoundly affect the state of our health (4).

Our choices reflect our lifestyles; we are responsible for those choices.

Exercise is one of the many lifestyle factors that we can control. Increased physical activity leads to improved physical fitness and to other physiological changes. It is the combination of these changes that leads to better health. People who exercise regularly often adopt a healthier lifestyle; they may stop smoking, have more energy, handle stress better, and make wise food choices, all of which improve the quality of life.

An inactive person has twice the risk of developing coronary artery disease than one who exercises regularly (5). Studies show that coronary artery disease is 1.9 times more likely to occur in physically inactive people than in those who exercise, independent of other risk factors such as smoking and obesity (6). Those at the lowest fitness level experience the greatest benefits by becoming physically active—even if in very modest activities (7). As we counsel clients and patients in community and acute care settings, we can incorporate suggestions for simple fitness activities into care plans.

There are several ways in which regular exercise can reduce the risk of heart disease. It can improve cardiovascular fitness, decrease blood pressure, aid in losing and maintaining weight, and alter blood lipid and lipoprotein levels. However, individuals with diabetes, coronary artery disease, metabolic disorders, and other conditions should discuss proposed exercise programs with their primary health care providers. Generally, men over age 40 and women over age 50 should check with their primary health care providers before beginning a strenuous fitness program (7).

Well-trained athletes have lower blood triglyceride and higher high density lipoprotein cholesterol (HDL) levels than sedentary individuals. The amount and intensity of exercise needed to produce a beneficial effect on blood levels is not known. However, it is unlikely that exercise alone accounts for the increase in

HEALTH DEBATE
What Kind of Exercise is Best?

Guidelines for physical fitness recommended by the American College of Sports Medicine are 20 to 60 minutes of aerobic activity, 3 to 5 times a week. The lower numbers of 20 minutes, 3 times a week apply to more intense forms of exercise such as running. The higher numbers of 60 minutes, 5 times a week are applicable for less intense activities such as continuous brisk walking.

Some health experts maintain that formal programs may not be necessary. It is possible to be physically fit by doing a variety of tasks throughout the day that produce an adequate level of fitness. For example, if within one day a person takes a 15-minute walk to the store, gardens actively for 30 minutes, and vacuums the house for another 15 minutes, the person has completed the recommended 60 minutes without disrupting or changing his or her lifestyle.

Other health experts believe that a formal fitness program produces more consistent measurable results of improved cardiovascular endurance and overall physical conditioning. The amount of time required is not great and can be individualized to fit a person's lifestyle.

What do you think? Which approach works best? How do you achieve physical fitness—through a variety of tasks or by formal fitness activities?

HDL cholesterol levels. It is the combined effects of a healthy diet, maintenance of ideal body weight, and appropriate exercise that influence lipid and lipoprotein levels (8).

In addition to preventing heart disease, exercise may decrease the risk of colon cancer, stroke, and hypertension. It can also delay the onset of or help treat non–insulin-dependent diabetes (NIDDM), depression, osteoporosis, and obesity. Increasing activity level and consuming a low-fat diet are probably two of the most effective ways to attain a healthy body weight. Physical activity burns kcalories, increases the proportion of lean to fat body tissue, and raises the basal metabolic rate.

One of the major objectives of *Healthy People 2000* is:

> Increase to at least 30 percent the proportion of people aged 6 and older who engage regularly, preferably daily, in light to moderate physical activity for at least 30 minutes per day (9).

Most Americans engage in less physical activity than is proposed in this objective. Only 22% of people ages 18 and older participate in at least 30 minutes of activity 5 or more times a week (9). Health care providers can contribute to meeting this objective by teaching patients about the benefits of exercise and providing information or referrals for exercise programs (Table 9-4).

Table 9-4   Benefits of Moderate Exercise and Possible Adverse Consequences of Excessive Exercise Throughout the Life Span

Benefits of Moderate Exercise During the Life Span	Possible Adverse Consequences of Strenuous Exercise During the Life Span
CHILDHOOD • Establish lifelong exercise and health habits	**CHILDHOOD** • Inability to meet energy needs and compromised growth and development
ADOLESCENCE • Prevent and treat obesity and eating disorders • Establish lifelong exercise and health habits	**ADOLESCENCE** • Inadequate energy intake • Oxidation of dietary protein for energy • Oligomenorrhea or amenorrhea • Negative calcium balance and reduced bone mass • Sports anemia • Anorexia athletica
ADULTHOOD • Control weight • Prevent and treat many diseases • Promote mental health and feelings of well-being	**ADULTHOOD** • Possible increased need for riboflavin and vitamin B_6
PREGNANCY • Control excessive weight gain • More favorable nutrient profile as a result of an increased energy intake • Possibly less constipation and fewer varicose veins	**PREGNANCY** • Low weight gain • Low–birth-weight infant
LACTATION • Promote return to prepregnancy weight • Possibly improve postpartum mental status	**LACTATION** • Excessive rate of weight loss, which compromises milk production and infant growth
ELDERLY • Favorable effects on age-related physiological changes • Prevent and treat osteoporosis • Socialization	**ELDERLY** • Exercise-related injuries leading to disability and other complications

Modified from Kris-Etherton PM: Nutrition and the exercising female, *Nutr Today* 21:2, 1986.

Table 9-5   Target Zone Heart Rate to Achieve Aerobic Physical Effect of Exercise

Age	Maximal Attainable Heart Rate (Pulse: 220 Minus Age)	Target Zone	
		70% Maximal Rate	85% Maximal Rate
20	200	140	170
25	195	136	166
30	190	133	161
35	185	129	157
40	180	126	153
45	175	122	149
50	170	119	144
55	165	115	140
60	160	112	136
65	155	108	132
70	150	105	127
75	145	101	124

Table 9-6   Aerobic Exercises for Physical Fitness*

Type of Exercise	Aerobic Forms
Ball playing	Handball, raquetball, squash
Bicycling	Stationary, touring
Dancing	Aerobic routines, ballet, disco
Jogging or running	Brisk pace
Jumping rope	Brisk pace
Skating	Ice skating, roller skating
Skiing	Cross country
Swimming	Steady pace
Walking	Brisk pace

*Maintained at aerobic level for at least 20 minutes

The American College of Sports Medicine (ACSM) is a medical and scientific organization that provides information on sports medicine and exercise science. ACSM makes the following recommendations regarding the quality and quantity of exercise for developing and maintaining cardiorespiratory fitness and muscular strength and endurance (10):

1. Frequency of exercise—3 to 5 days a week
2. Intensity of exercise—60% to 90% or 50 to 85% of target heart rate (Table 9-5)
3. Duration of exercise—20 to 60 minutes of continuous movement
4. Form of exercise—use of large muscles, continuous, rhythmic, and aerobic in nature (Table 9-6)
5. Strength training—moderate intensity

Strength Training

Strength training has become a popular way to stay in shape. ACSM recommends it as an integral part of an overall exercise program (11). Strength training involves lifting various types of weights to build muscle strength and endurance. It is different from weight lifting. With strength training, improvement is gauged by increased muscle mass. In contrast, weightlifting is a competitive sport in which individuals lift weights in specific body weight divisions.

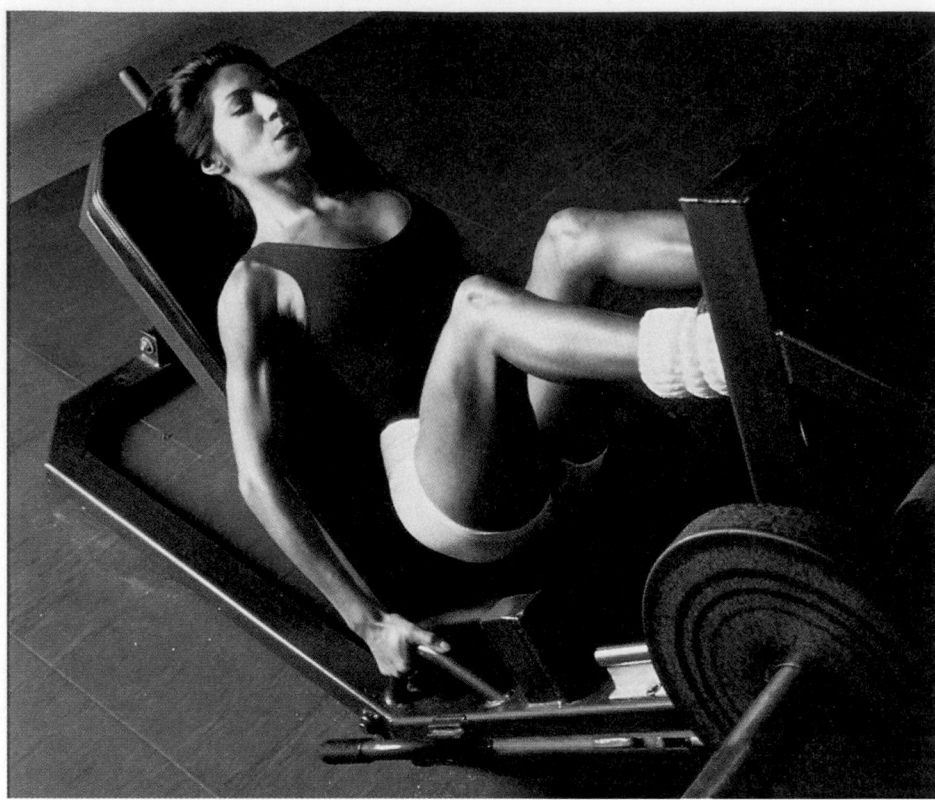

Weight-bearing exercises, including strength training, are beneficial for bone health.

Proper strength training exercise programs can reliably increase muscle size and strength in men and women of all ages. The stimulus for muscle growth is overload—a resistance greater than that to which the muscle has been accustomed must be imposed. Beginners may start with 3 lb weights and progress to higher weights as strength increases.

Most of us know that aerobic exercise, like running and cycling, is good for the heart, making it stronger and more efficient. However, strength training has benefits for cardiovascular health, too. It can help improve blood cholesterol levels, burn fat, and contribute to our well-being. Strength training may also protect against back problems, osteoporosis, and minor injuries. Recent studies show that strength training builds muscle mass of adults in their 80s. Increased muscle mass improves strength and flexibility, both of which reduce the risk of injuries caused by poor muscle coordination and resulting falls (12).

Bone responds to the force of gravity and to muscular contraction. Physical exercise forces bone to adapt to the stresses imposed upon it. When stressed, bones become larger and stronger. Weight-bearing exercises (for example, walking, jogging, weight (strength) training) are beneficial for bone health.

The density and health of bone tissue are of particular concern for women. Being physically fit through aerobic and weight-bearing exercise is a good defense against osteoporosis, for which women are at greater risk. Fortunately, this can be accomplished through daily brisk walking or jogging. Other strategies for reducing the risk of osteoporosis are listed in Chapter 8.

Bodybuilding

In recent years there has been increased interest and participation in bodybuilding among men and women. Bodybuilders work to develop muscle mass, strength, and muscle definition through a combination of dieting, weightlifting, and aerobic exercise (11). Unlike weightlifting and other traditional sports that involve strength, bodybuilders exercise to improve their physique as a form of athletic performance.

To prepare for competition, bodybuilders diet and exercise to reduce their body weight and body fat. Unfortunately, many bodybuilders follow a number of dietary practices that may place them at risk for health problems (13). Bodybuilders are susceptible to misinformation about muscle growth and development because they want quick results and may not understand the dietary requirements of muscle gain. Instead, they may consume protein powders and supplements in the belief that they will provide extra energy and increase muscle mass and strength. These beliefs are reflected in endorsements for a variety of protein and amino acid supplements found in popular fitness and strength magazines. Claims for fast muscle development are made for everything from bee pollen to specific types of exercise equipment.

The composition of muscle is approximately 70% to 75% water, 15% to 22% protein, and 5% to 7% other materials, including inorganic salt, lipids, glycogen, enzymes, and minerals. There is no evidence that extra dietary protein increases muscle mass. Exercise is the single most important factor in increasing the size, strength, and endurance of muscles.

FOOD AND ATHLETIC PERFORMANCE

Physical activity and nutrition have been associated with health since the time of ancient Greece. Hippocrates said, "All parts of the body which have a function, if used in moderation and exercised in labors in which each is accustomed, become thereby healthy, well-developed, and age more slowly, but if unused and left idle they become liable to disease, defective in growth and age quickly." Today, over 2000 years later, this advice is still consistent with our knowledge about nutrition, physical fitness, and health (14).

Physically active people of all ages and levels of competition are seeking information to enhance their training and achieve a competitive edge. They want to know what kinds of foods to eat and specific dietary regimens to follow. Basically, the nutritional needs of athletes are no different from nonathletes, with the exception of kcalories and fluids. A diet that provides a variety of foods supplying 60% to 65% of the kcalories from carbohydrates, 12% to 15% from protein, and no more than 30% from fat is recommended for health and performance (7). However, some forms of heavy training increase the requirement for certain nutrients. For example, carbohydrates are an important source of energy during endurance

TEACHING TOOL
Using Numbers to Guide the Way

For some clients, getting advice to "eat better" and "exercise more" has little effect on their behaviors. For these clients, consider using the charts in this chapter to show clients numerically what their needs are and what benefits will accrue with change.

For example, use Table 9-1 to determine the client's recommended energy allowance and the Table 9-2 factors for estimating daily energy allowances. Use Table 9-5 to teach the client about target heart rates. Also share the list of aerobic activities in Table 9-6. The client may be more interested in exercising if there are goals to be met such as reaching and maintaining the target heart rate during exercise. And, of course, never miss the opportunity to discuss the variety of healthful food choices that support increased physical fitness.

exercise, and therefore runners, cyclists, and swimmers may need more carbohydrates (60% to 70% of their total kcalorie intake) than other individuals.

Nutrition can affect an athlete in many ways. At the most basic level, nutrition is essential for normal growth and development and for maintaining good health. By staying healthy, an athlete will feel better, train harder, and be in better condition. Among comparable athletes, good eating habits can be the factor that determines the winner. However, these good habits do not come from the pregame meal or even what the athlete eats the week before competition. They are built daily over a long period of time.

A number of dietary patterns will provide good nutrition. The Food Guide Pyramid can be a useful outline for athletes of what to eat every day. Each food group provides some but not all of the nutrients an athlete needs. Foods in each of the six food categories in the Food Guide Pyramid provide kcalories from different combinations of carbohydrate, protein, and fat (see Fig. 1-2). For example, fruits provide kcalories from carbohydrates, and milk products contain carbohydrate, protein, and varying amounts of fat.

Athletes should eat at least the minimum number of servings for each group daily to meet energy needs. Depending on their body size and level of training, some athletes may need more than the larger number of servings.

Kcalorie Requirements

As noted earlier in this chapter, kcalorie requirements vary greatly from person to person and are affected by activity level, body size, age, and climate. Body size impacts on kcalorie requirements more than any other single factor. The smaller the athlete, the lower the kcalorie requirement.

Some sports demand high energy expenditure; others do not. A frequently asked question is, "How many kcalories should I consume?" Athletes are consuming enough kcalories if they are maintaining their best competitive yet healthy weight. Ideally, kcalorie intake should balance energy expended. If intake is consistently above or below an athlete's requirement, weight gain or weight loss will occur, both of which can affect performance.

Many athletes are concerned about their appearance and eat less to keep their body weight and percentage of body fat low. However, restricting kcalories can have a negative impact on health and performance. As kcalorie intake decreases, so does nutrient intake. A minimum kcalorie requirement for college athletes is 1800 to 2000 kcalories a day. Eating less than this amount can leave the athlete feeling weak and listless and may lead to iron deficiency, stress fractures, and for women *amenorrhea* (lack of menstruation) and osteoporosis.

Benefits of Snacking

- Helps the athlete get enough kcalories without having to eat large amounts of food at any one meal; this is especially important for staying awake in class and also helps curb hunger pains during practice.
- Helps to replace muscle glycogen stores and fluids that are lost during practice or competition.
- Supplies vitamins and minerals the athlete may not be getting in regular meals.
Whatever kind of snacker you are, ask yourself these questions:
- What nutrients do snacks provide?
- Do I need the extra calories?
- How can these snacks fit into the total day's diet?

Endurance athletes tend to have a higher incidence of iron depletion (15). This so-called *sports anemia* has been attributed to the loss of iron in sweat, the loss of blood as a result of bleeding into the GI tract, or the breakdown of red blood cells as a result of the repeated impact of the athlete's feet on the ground. Although iron supplements can benefit people with evidence of this or any other form of iron deficiency, no benefit is associated with excess iron consumption. African-Americans, 20% of whom suffer from a genetic predisposition for iron overload, should have their iron status checked before supplementing their diet (15).

On the other hand, increasing kcalorie intake to gain weight may also be difficult for athletes. Too much food can cause discomfort, especially if a workout takes place soon after eating. Furthermore, when balancing school, work, and practice, little time is available to eat. Small meals and snacks become an important source of nutrients. How often you snack depends on body size and kcalorie needs.

Water: The Essential Ingredient

Water is the nutrient most critical to athletic preformance. Without adequate water, performance can suffer in less than an hour. Water is necessary for the body's cooling system. It also transports nutrients throughout the tissues and maintains adequate blood volume.

During exercise there is always the risk of becoming dehydrated (fluid volume deficit), especially when the temperature is hot. When athletes sweat, they lose water. Although sweat rates vary among people, losing as little as 2% to 3% of your weight via sweat can impair performance (16). When the water lost via sweat is not replaced, blood volume falls and body temperature rises, causing confusion and loss of coordination. To replace the lost water, athletes must consume extra fluids.

The athlete's sense of thirst is not the best indicator that the body needs water; fluid needs may be greater than thirst can gauge. Adequate water intake before, during, and after an event or practice session is of utmost importance. Athletes should drink 1 to 2 cups of fluid 5 to 10 minutes before exercise and 1 cup of water every 15 to 20 minutes during exercise.

How can athletes be sure they are well-hydrated? One criterion of hydration is that urine should be clear in color throughout most of the day. Athletes should also weigh themselves before and after workouts. For every pound lost, an athlete needs to drink 2 cups of fluid. (See Chapter 8 for effects of fluid volume deficit.)

Sport Drinks

Athletes often wonder which is better for replacing fluids during exercise—water or sport drinks? The number one goal is to remain well hydrated. Whether the athlete drinks water or a sport drink is his or her choice. Cool water is what the body really needs during activities lasting less than 2 hours. However, athletes participating in endurance events requiring more than 90 minutes of continuous moderate to heavy exercise, such as distance running or cycling, may benefit from sport drinks containing carbohydrate and electrolytes (sodium and potassium). Sports drinks provide fluids to keep the athlete well hydrated and extra carbohydrate for energy.

A major consideration in fluid replacement is how quickly the fluid empties from the stomach. To hydrate the total body, the fluid needs to leave the stomach quickly to be distributed throughout the body. Although larger volumes of fluid empty more rapidly from the stomach, many athletes cannot exercise with a full stomach. Cool fluids empty faster from the stomach than warm fluids. Kcalorie content is also important. The greater the kcalorie content of a beverage, the slower the emptying rate.

Stress the importance of adequate fluid intake. Weighing nude before and after exercise is the best way to determine fluid replacement needs. Sweat loss of 1 lb (2.2 kg) of body weight is equal to 2 cups (480 ml) of water.

Carbohydrate: The Energy Food

Carbohydrate stores in the body (glycogen) are limited, and research has shown that low levels of muscle glycogen can impair performance (17). Consuming carbohydrate before and during exercise will delay the onset of fatigue and allow the athlete to compete for a longer period of time.

How much carbohydrate should an athlete eat each day to replace muscle glycogen? It depends a lot on body size. An athlete with more muscle mass will require more carbohydrate. Carbohydrate requirements also depend on intensity and level of training. Athletes participating in high-energy sports requiring short bursts of energy (basketball, tennis, football, soccer) need about 5 grams of carbohydrate per kilogram of body weight daily to maintain muscle glycogen stores. Endurance athletes who train aerobically for more than 90 minutes daily may need up to 10 grams of carbohydrate per kilogram of bodyweight to replace glycogen (17). Individuals who exercise regularly to maintain conditioning do well with general guidelines of high complex carbohydrate diets as represented by the Food Guide Pyramid. The box below shows how to calculate carbohydrate requirements.

Carbohydrate is found in foods in two forms: complex carbohydrates and simple sugars. Both types are effective in replenishing glycogen in the muscles. However, complex carbohydrates provide vitamins, minerals and fiber as well. Examples of complex carbohydrates include bread, potatoes, pasta, cereal, fruits, and fruit juices. Simple sugars include maple syrup, molasses, honey, and table sugar.

Carbohydrate Loading

Carbohydrate loading is the process of changing the type of foods eaten and adjusting the amount of training to increase glycogen stores in the muscle. This concept first became of interest around 1939 when scientists studied the effects of dietary manipulation on the ability to perform prolonged hard work. They found that men consuming a high-carbohydrate diet for 3 days could perform heavy work twice as long as men fed a high-fat diet for the same 3 days (18). Since then, researchers have investigated several techniques for increasing glycogen levels in the muscles.

To achieve maximum muscle glycogen stores through carbohydrate loading athletes should consume a high-carbohydrate diet as part of their regular training program. At least 50% (preferably 60% to 70%) of their total kcalories should come from carbohydrate. For the athlete eating 3000 kcalories a day, this represents a minimum of 375 grams of carbohydrate daily. Three days before competition, exercise should taper off to allow muscles to rest. Dietary carbohydrates should be increased to 60% to 70% of total kcalories. This technique of combining rest and increased carbohydrate intake encourages greater glycogen storage (19,20). Table 9-7 outlines two popular carbohydrate loading methods.

Carbohydrate loading is recommended only for athletes engaged in continuous exercise lasting more than 90 minutes. It is not recommended for athletes participating in short-term events such as sprints, or in sports such as football, baseball,

TEACHING TOOL
How Much Carbohydrate Do You Need?

1. Divide body weight in pounds by 2.2 lb/kg to determine body weight in kilograms. For example:

   154 lbs × 2.2 lbs/kg =
           70 kilograms body weight

2. Multiply each kilogram of body weight by 5 grams to determine the number of grams of carbohydrate needed daily. For example:

   70 kg × 5 g = 350 g of carbohydrate daily.

Table 9-7   Carbohydrate Loading Techniques

	Standard Method		Short Method	
DAY	EXERCISE	DIET	EXERCISE	DIET
1	90 minutes	50% carbohydrate		
2	40 minutes	50% carbohydrate		
3	40 minutes	50% carbohydrate		
4	20 minutes	70% carbohydrate	Normal	70% carbohydrate
5	20 minutes	70% carbohydrate	Normal	70% carbohydrate
6	Rest	70% carbohydrate	Rest	70% carbohydrate
7	4-6 hours before competition	70% carbohydrate meal		
	During event	Carbohydrate-fortified beverages		

Table 9-8   High Carbohydrate Menu for Glycogen Loading*

Meals	Snacks
BREAKFAST	
1 cup orange juice	
1 cup oatmeal, with	
1 banana	
1 cup low-fat milk	
2 slices wheat bread, with	
1 tsp margarine	
LUNCH	**SNACK**
2 slices rye bread	8 graham crackers
3 oz turkey	1 cup low-fat milk
1 oz mozzarella cheese, with	1 apple
lettuce, tomato, mustard	
1 tsp mayonnaise	
1 cup apple juice	
1 orange	
1 cup lemon sherbert	
DINNER	**SNACK**
2 cups spaghetti	6 cups popcorn,
⅔ cup tomato sauce, with	air popped
mushrooms	
2 tbl Parmesan cheese	
4 slices French bread	
2 tsp margarine	
½ cup broccoli	
½ cup ice cream, with	
¾ cup strawberries	

From Coleman E: *Eating for endurance*, Palo Alto, Calif, 1992, Bull Publishing.
*Sample menu contains approximately 3000 calories; 518 grams of carbohydrate.

and wrestling; nor should individuals with diabetes or hypoglycemia consider this dietary pattern that affects carbohydrate metabolism. Furthermore, the degree of benefit from carbohydrate loading varies among individuals.

Therefore athletes should determine before competition the value of this regimen for them. The potential negative side effects of carbohydrate loading include increased water retention and weight gain, stiffness, cramping, and digestive problems (21).

A more practical concern is whether athletes are eating enough carbohydrate on a daily basis to maintain adequate levels of muscle glycogen for training and workouts. Table 9-8 shows an example of a high-carbohydrate diet that will maximize muscle glycogen stores.

Protein

For many years the importance of protein for athletes has been a subject of great controversy. Many athletes and coaches believe that a high-protein diet supplies extra energy, enhances athletic performance, and increases muscle mass. There is no evidence, however, that eating more protein than needed improves athletic ability.

Although carbohydrate and fat are the major fuels used for energy, studies indicate that protein use increases during exercise, and under certain conditions protein may contribute significantly to energy metabolism (22). Two factors that influence the use of protein as an energy source are the length of exercise and the carbohydrate content of the diet. The body may depend on protein for an increased percentage of energy in prolonged exercise (greater than 90 minutes), particularly when carbohydrate intake is low.

The Recommended Dietary Allowance (RDA) for protein for sedentary adults is 0.8 grams per kilogram of body weight per day (23). Current research suggests that athletes need between 1.0 and 1.5 grams of protein per kilogram body weight. (24) For a 150-lb (68 kg) athlete, this amounts to 68 to 102 grams of protein per day. Factors such as kcalorie intake, protein quality, and type and intensity of the sport are important considerations. The higher the kcalorie intake, the lower the protein requirements. When kcalorie intake is adequate, there is enough carbohydrate available for energy use.

The type of protein eaten also affects the amount of protein needed. The 1.0 to 1.5 grams of protein per kilogram of body weight recommendation is based on a diet containing animal foods. Athletes who eat meat, fish, poultry, eggs, milk, or cheese will have little problem meeting their protein needs. Strict vegetarian athletes, however, will need to plan their diets more carefully to ensure that their protein needs are met.

Protein and Amino Acid Supplements

The use of protein and amino acid supplements is common practice among athletes. Various combinations of individual amino acids are sold to athletes with the promise that the acids will stimulate the release of growth hormone and thus increase muscle mass. Promoters claim that amino acids can build muscle, aid fat loss, provide energy, speed up muscle repair, and improve endurance. Others claim that they are more readily digested and absorbed than the protein consumed in foods.

The question is, do athletes need to take these supplements or can they get the protein they need from food alone? Research has not been able to show beneficial effects of protein supplements on performance. Many athletes eat more than the recommended amount of protein (and thus amino acids) from food alone. Amino acids as building blocks of all proteins are found in a wide variety of foods, from pork chops to bread and from beans and peas to milk and tacos. Because the body cannot store extra protein, excess protein and amino acids are broken down and used for energy or stored as fat. If protein or amino acid supplements provide more nutrients than needed for protein functions, the body treats supplements the same as any excess source of protein.

It's safer and cheaper to take amino acids in a glass of milk, a turkey sandwich, or other protein-rich foods. Muscle size and strength increase only after weeks of work. If athletes want to gain muscle mass, they need to become involved in a resistive strength training program and consume a diet rich in carbohydrates.

Fat

In athletic performance, carbohydrate and fat are the major sources of energy. The amount of fat used during exercise depends on the duration and intensity of exercise, degree of prior training, and the composition of the diet. Exercise performed under aerobic conditions will promote fat use as a source of energy. There is a good reason to increase your body's ability to burn fat as fuel; using fat as a source of energy will spare muscle glycogen.

Athletes need a certain amount of fat in their diets and on their bodies for optimal health and performance. The challenge is eating a diet that provides the right amount. The American Heart Association recommends that no more than 30% of total kcalories should come from fat. Because each athlete is different, some may eat less and some slightly more than 30% of their kcalories from fat. Many athletes cannot get the kcalories they need without eating a little extra fat. However, fat intakes greater than 35% of total kcalories have been associated with increased risk of certain diet-related diseases (heart disease, obesity, and cancer). High fat intakes also have been shown to reduce endurance capacity (25).

To lower fat intake, athletes should choose lean meats, fish, poultry, and low-fat dairy products. Fat and oils should be used sparingly in cooking, and fried foods and high-fat snacks should be eaten in moderation. See Chapter 5 for strategies for lowering dietary fat intake.

Ergogenic Aids

In athletics, the term *ergogenic aids* is used to describe drugs and dietary regimens believed by some to increase strength, power, and endurance (Table 9-9). Because winning is often a matter of a split second, it is easy to see why athletes are continuously looking for the competitive edge. The fact that more and more nutritional supplements are being marketed to athletes presents a challenge to coaches, trainers, nutritionists, and health care providers to provide sound nutrition information.

ergogenic aids
drugs and dietary regimens believed by some (but not proven) to increase strength, power, and endurance

The nutritional supplements used by athletes are constantly changing. Often, as athletes find that one doesn't work, they search for another. Today commonly used nutritional aids include amino acid supplements such as arginine and ornithine, vitamins and minerals, L-carnitine, inosine, and herb extracts. Research has shown that these supplements have little effect on performance. Despite a lack of scientific basis for the claims associated with these products, their widespread use continues.

Nutritional supplements are a multimillion-dollar business, and athletes are a prime target for the people who market these products. Athletes make good consumers because, like many Americans, they believe if a little is good, a lot is better. It is not uncommon for an athlete to consume five or six different supplements a day and not know what substances are in them. Many of the supplements athletes purchase from specialty nutrition stores and mail-order catalogs are not subject to the regulations established by the Food and Drug Administration (FDA), and this presents another concern. Athletes have no way of knowing whether these nutritional supplements are safe.

Table 9-9   Ergogenic Aids

Substance	Rationale	Actual Effect
Alcohol	Decreases perception of pain and fatigue	Dehydration Decreases coodination
Antioxidant vitamins	Increases aerobic endurance	No proven benefit
Bee pollen	Benefits linked to its high vitamin and mineral content	No proven benefit
Branched-chain amino acids	Spare glycogen	No proven benefit
Caffeine*	Enhances endurance Increases fat use Spares glycogen	Increases dehydration, anxiety, and stomach acid
Carnitine	Increases fat use and therefore endurance	No evidence of this effect
Coenzyme Q	Increases oxygen use and endurance in patients with cardiovascular disease	No proven benefit in healthy people
Vitamin/mineral supplements, including vitamin B$_{15}$ (a non-vitamin)	Enhance energy use	No proven benefit Potentially toxic

*Proven ergogenic effect at high levels; 1 to 2 cups of coffee are OK before competition, but higher levels are banned by the International Olympic Committee (IOC).

Taking several different supplements at one time, or one that contains a large amount of one nutrient such as vitamin A, can be toxic. There is also the risk of nutrient-nutrient interactions, in which an excess of one nutrient can interfere with the body's ability to use another nutrient. This may occur when excessive amounts of one amino acid are consumed; the body's use of other amino acids may be affected.

In athletes with a high kcalorie intake (>4000 kcal per day), vitamin and mineral intakes greater then 200% of the RDA from food alone are not uncommon. In a study of male triathletes, vitamin D intake from food and supplements was 1065% of the RDA (26). Toxicity and adverse health effects can occur from consuming high doses of vitamins and minerals over a long period of time.

OVERCOMING BARRIERS

American "Couch Potatoes"

The term *couch potatoes* became part of our slang terminology a few years ago. It refers to people who just sit on the couch and vegetate (do nothing) while watching television, viewing movies on a videotape cassette recorder, or playing video games. Those of us who do a lot of sitting, rather than doing, often end up soft and *fluffy* like mashed potatoes. How did this happen?

More than likely, couch potatoes have always existed. Habits that develop during childhood and adolescence may predispose us to lead sedentary lifestyles. If as children our favorite activities involved watching television and sports events rather than playing sports or being physically active, we may end up as couch potato adults. If our parents were also sedentary, we did not have fitness role models.

What has changed is that in the 1980s and 1990s more focus has been placed on the health benefits of physical fitness. We now know that a sedentary lifestyle puts us more at risk for heart disease, some cancers, diabetes, hypertension, and obesity. Even if our body weight is low, we are still at risk for health problems if we are sedentary. These chronic diseases drain the productive and economic resources of our society. Now is a good time for couch potatoes to transform their ways and turn into roadrunners.

Exercise Makes You Hungrier: Myth or Fact?

Does exercise make us hungrier? Do we have a greater physiological need for food when using our bodies more? Or is the hunger psychological?

During and immediately after exercise our digestive system basically slows down. Blood flow through the main digestive organs slows; the blood concentrates on reaching the large muscles that need all the nutrients and oxygen possible to do their work. This means that any foodstuff in the digestive tract takes longer to be processed. When we complete and recover from exercising, the digestive process resumes.

However, we may experience low blood glucose levels depending on how long ago we ate and the amount of exercise we completed. Until the body recovers from the exercise, a glass of juice or other very light snack best serves the needs of the body to raise blood glucose to a comfortable level.

Sustained regular exercise does cause a physiological need for more food. The *work* of exercise uses additional kcalories. Although we may be hungrier and take in more kcalories, we also use more kcalories. The equation of kcalorie input and output can still balance. The bonus is that we will have stronger bodies with more stamina.

TOWARD A POSITIVE NUTRITION LIFESTYLE: MODELING

Want to start a fitness routine but don't know how to get started? Although motivation is essential, sometimes the very basic steps of getting started are the hardest to work out. Should exercise be done in the morning, at lunch, or at night? Every day? Three times per week? How is this done?

A technique to assist in changing behavior is called *modeling*; modeling can be used as an education strategy with patients or may be personally applied to our own lifestyles. Modeling is replicating or imitating the behavior of someone else.

For simplicity, let's apply this technique to you. You are molding your behavior to be similar to that person's behavior. Approaches to modeling include visualization by imagining yourself doing what the other person does or discussion with the person to discover how the desired behavior is performed.

Application to a fitness routine could use both approaches. Perhaps a friend has an established fitness routine, and you would like to begin to work out also. To use visualization, first imagine the friend preparing for the workout, exercising, and resting afterwards. Then substitute yourself for the friend. Imagine getting your exercise clothes ready, setting the alarm clock, getting dressed to exercise, exercising, and then resting afterwards. Do this for several days and then actually exercise.

The other approach is to talk with friends or family members who exercise regularly. Find out how they prepare for workouts. What motivation techniques to maintain a fitness program do they use? How many times per week do they exercise? How do they deal with everyday interruptions to their exercise program such as exams, sick children, or work crises? After adjusting their techniques to your circumstances, actually exercise.

WELLNESS, ENERGY SUPPLY, AND FITNESS

Physical Dimension	Both dietary intake and regular physical activity are essential to achieve physical fitness; exercise affects all muscles, even the muscles of our gastrointestinal tract function better when we regularly exercise.
Intellectual Dimension	The old saying, "a sound body makes for a sound mind" still holds true; by being physically fit, we may be able to devote our full intellectual capacity to our work.
Emotional Dimension	For some persons, depression seems to lift if they regularly engage in sustained aerobic activities. Even if we are not depressed, our general state of mind improves with daily physical exercise.
Social Dimension	Group sports provide an excellent opportunity for social activity while pursuing healthful goals; a sense of belonging and sharing occurs whether the group is a formal organization, such as a running club, or consists of friends who bike together.

SUMMARY

The ability to perform work, produce change, and maintain life all require energy. ATP is the *fuel* for all energy-requiring processes in the body. We convert the energy from the food we eat into ATP energy.

There are two related energy pathways. The aerobic pathway depends on oxygen; the anaerobic pathway functions without oxygen. The physical demands of different sports require specific sources of energy. Carbohydrate in the form of glucose is the only fuel that can be used anaerobically without oxygen to produce ATP. During low to moderate-intensity exercise, muscles cells mainly use fat for fuel.

Our daily energy requirement depends on three major components: basal metabolism, physical activity, and the energy to metabolize food. Each of these components is affected directly or indirectly by many factors including our age, gender, and body size. Physical exercise is important to our long-term health and well-being. Increased physical activity leads to improved fitness and other physiological changes that may reduce the risk of chronic diseases such as heart disease, cancer, diabetes, and obesity. A combination of aerobic exercise and strength training is recommended for overall fitness.

The nutritional needs of athletes are no different from those of nonathletes, with the exception of kcalories and fluids. Many different dietary patterns can meet the athlete's nutrition needs. Carbohydrate is an important nutrient for both health and athletic performance. Athletes should eat enough carbohydrate on a daily basis to maintain adequate levels of muscle glycogen for training and workouts. Protein requirements of athletes may be slightly greater than that of sedentary individuals. Most athletes, however, get enough protein in their diets. There is no need for them to take protein powders or amino acid supplements. For the most part, research has shown that nutritional supplements including vitamins and minerals have little effect on performance in athletes consuming a balanced diet.

THE NURSING ROLE
Nutrition and Athletic Performance

One of your next-door neighbors, Peter, is a high school student who is on the football team. He stops to talk to you one day and says, "Since you're a nurse, I thought I'd ask you. I want to improve my performance on the football team, and people have been telling me all kinds of things about how nutrition can help me." Peter proceeds to ask you the following questions:

1. "Our coach says my weight is OK, but would putting on a little more weight help make me stronger?"
2. "Should I eat more meat and other high-protein foods?"
3. "Someone told me about carbohydrate loading. Is that a good idea?"
4. "Should I be taking extra vitamins?"
5. "How can I know if I am drinking enough when we practice in hot weather, and what should I drink?"

Although you are not working in a professional capacity with Peter, you can certainly answer his questions to the best of your ability. However, you would want to first ask questions about the following areas (your **Assessment**):

1. His present diet
2. His overall knowledge of nutrition
3. Extent of his exercise/training
4. Vitamin or other nutritional supplements being taken

These questions can be asked in a very informal way during the course of the conversation.

Then you could supply Peter with the following information (your **Intervention**):

1. Putting on weight will not make you stronger. Only muscle strength training will do that.
2. Extra protein will probably not make you stronger or more muscular. However, an adequate amount of protein must be eaten (about 10% to 15% of total kcalories). If Peter lacks knowledge about the Food Guide Pyramid or wants to know more about calculating kcalories, offer to get more information for him or refer him to a source of information.
3. Carbohydrate loading is not recommended for football players and other athletes who are not involved in continuous exercise lasting more than 90 minutes.
4. If you are eating a balanced diet, especially if you are eating a high-caloric diet, you are probably getting enough vitamins without a supplement. If you do choose to take supplements, do not exceed 100% of the RDA for each vitamin.
5. You should drink a glass or two of fluid shortly before practice, and probably a few afterward. You can weigh yourself before and after practice. For every pound you lose, drink 2 cups of fluid. Cold water or fruit juice are good fluids to drink.

Because you are not working with Peter in a professional capacity, you may never get to evaluate the results of your interventions. Peter will have to evaluate the advice that he has received from all sources and decide what he wants to do.

REFERENCES

1. Guthrie HA, Picciano MF: *Human nutrition*, St. Louis, 1995, Mosby.
2. Davis J, Sherer K: *Applied nutrition and diet therapy for nurses*, ed 2, Philadelphia, 1994, Saunders.
3. Powell KE et al: Physical activity and chronic disease, *Am J Clin Nutr* 49: 999-1006, 1989.
4. Rosato FD: *Fitness and wellness: The physical connection*, ed 3, St. Paul, Minn, 1995, West Publishing.
5. Powell KE et al: Physical activity and the incidence of coronary heart disease, *Annu Rev Public Health* 8:253-287, 1987.
6. Berlin JA, Colditz GA, A meta-analysis of physical activity in the prevention of coronary heart disease, *Am J Epidemiol* 132:612-628, 1990.
7. American Dietetic Association: Position of the American Dietetic Association and the Canadian Dietetic Association: Nutrition for physical fitness and athletic performance for adults, *J Am Diet Assoc* 93(6):691-697, 1993.
8. Murray TD, Squires WG, Hartung G: Regulation of lipids and lipoproteins by diet and exercise. In Hickson JF, Wolinsky I, eds: *Nutrition in exercise and sport*, Boca Raton, Fla, 1989, CRC Press.
9. US Department of Health and Human Services, Public Health Service: *Healthy people 2000: Health promotion and disease prevention objectives*, Washington, DC, US Government Printing Office.
10. American College of Sports Medicine: The recommended quantity and quality of exercise for developing and maintaining cardiorespiratory and muscular fitness in healthy adults, *Med Sci Sports Exerc* 22:265-274, 1990.
11. Sandoval WM, Heyward VH, Lyons TM: Comparison of body composition, exercise and nutritional profiles of female and male bodybuilders at competition, *J Sports Med Physi Fitness* 29:63-70, 1989.
12. Young A, Skelton DA: Applied physiology of strength and power in old age, *Int J Sports Med* 15(3):149-51, April 1994.

13. Kleiner SM, Bazzarre TL, Litchford MD: Metabolic profiles, diet and health practices of championship male and female bodybuilders, *J Am Diet Assoc* 90:962-967, 1990.
14. Simopoulos AP: Opening address: Nutrition and fitness from the first Olympiad in 776 BC to 393 AD and the concept of positive health, *Am J Clin Nutr* 49:921-926, 1989.
15. Eichner TR: Sports anemia, iron supplements and blood doping, *Med Sci Sports Exerc* 24:S315, 1992.
16. Greenleaf JE: Problem: Thirst, drinking behavior, and involuntary dehydration, *Med Sci Sports Exerc* 24:645-656, 1992.
17. Serman WM, Wimer GS: Insufficient dietary carbohydrate during training: Does it impair performance? *Int J Sports Med* 1:28-44, 1991.
18. Christensen E, Hansen O: Arbeitsfahigkeit and Ernahrung, *Skand Arch Physiol* 81:160, 1939.
19. Sherman WM: Carbohydrates, muscle glycogen, and muscle glycogen supercompensation. In Williams MH, ed: *Ergogenic Aids in Sport*, Champaign, Ill, 1983, Human Kenetics.
20. Hoffman CJ: An eating plan and update on recommended dietary practices for the endurance athlete, *J Am Diet Assoc*, 91:325, 1991.
21. Williams MH: *Nutrition for fitness and sport*, ed 3, Dubuque, Ind, 1992, Brown Publishers.
22. Friedman JE, Lemon PWR: Effect of chronic endurance exercise on retention of dietary protein, *Int J Sports Med* 10:118-123, 1989.
23. Food and Nutrition Board, National Research Council: *Recommended dietary allowances*, ed 10, Washington, DC, 1989, National Academy Press.
24. Ruud J: *Protein*, Omaha, 1990, International Center for Sports Nutrition and the United States Olympic Committee.
25. Bergstrom J et al: Diet, muscle glycogen and physical performance, *Acta Physiol Scand* 71:140-150, 1967.
26. Khoo CS et al: Nutrient intake and eating habits of triathletes, *Annals of Sports Medicine* 3:144-150, 1987.

Chapter 10

MANAGEMENT OF BODY FAT LEVELS

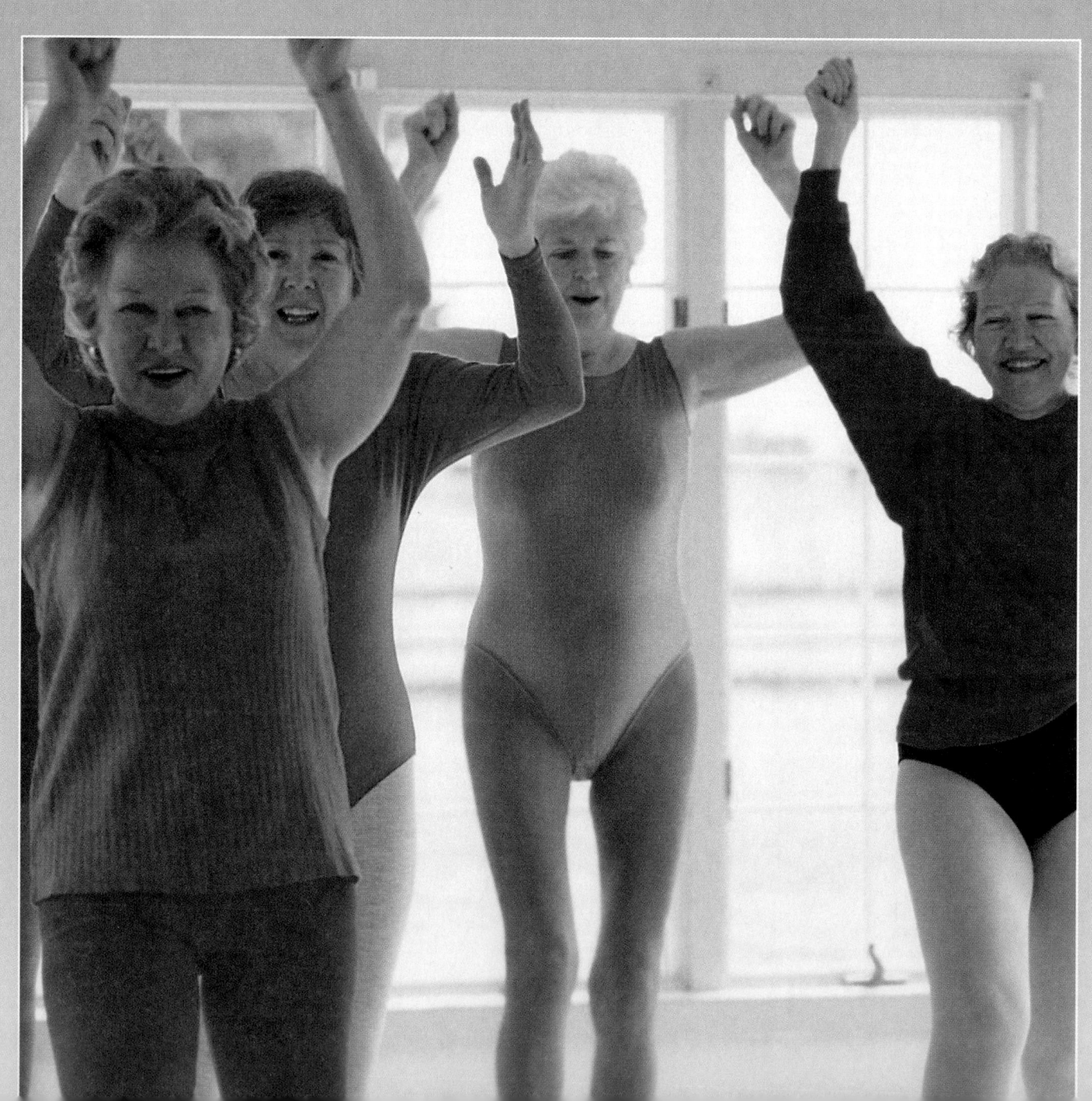

ROLE IN WELLNESS

As members of our contemporary culture, we care a great deal about the size, shape, and composition of our bodies. We understand that body composition is related to emotional and physical health in a number of ways, and we equate slender, youthful bodies with attractiveness, health, power, and control.

Dieting to lose or control weight has become routine, especially for women. Yet in spite of all this effort, most women are largely dissatisfied with their bodies and especially with their fatness levels. Men, usually thought to be relatively free of such fat obsessions, now seem to be following closely on the heels of women in this regard. At the same time, the incidence of disordered eating and of overfat and underfat continues to rise. Clearly, we have a problem with fatness. In this chapter we attempt to cut through the myths, stereotypes, and prejudices and to examine dispassionately the relationship of body fat to our well-being.

Because it is body fat that is really the issue, our focus is on fat rather than on weight. In addition, we use the approach of *management of body composition, specifically body fat levels,* rather than achievement of *ideal* body fatness. In this context *management* is defined as the use of available resources to achieve a predetermined goal. This definition recognizes that individuals differ in the resources available to them and in the goals they set.

BODY COMPOSITION, BODY IMAGE, AND CULTURE

What is Body Image?

The phrase *body image* refers to the perceptions we have of our bodies. Although body image can refer to the functioning of the body, most often it deals with our ideas and feelings about the physical appearance or attractiveness of our bodies. We say that individuals have a distorted body image when their perceptions are inconsistent with reality. For example, most people with anorexia nervosa view their bodies as disgustingly fat when in fact they are emaciated. Body image is important because it affects how we feel about ourselves and how we behave.

This chapter is especially concerned with those aspects of body image that deal with size and shape as they are affected by body composition. We look at how the pursuit of attractiveness affects our health.

Body Perception: What is Attractive?

How do we decide what is attractive? Apparently, biology and culture interact to set the standards (1). Certainly biology plays a role by arranging our genetic inputs so that males and females develop body characteristics that attract the opposite sex and thereby perpetuate the species. It is probably this biological influence that causes us to admire an appearance of strength in males and soft curves in females. Genetics also determine the potential for other characteristics of appearance such as height, color of skin, shape of nose, and texture of hair.

However, within these biologically determined characteristics we make great distinctions as to what is attractive and desirable. At different times and places humans have widely differing notions of what constitutes an attractive male or female.

After the second world war, we entered an era of strong cultural influence. Mass media has created a web of communication of a magnitude and efficiency that was never before possible. Now notions of attractiveness are shared quickly around the globe. Furthermore, sales promotion is a motive underlying much of the communication. The outcome has been a notion of beauty that homogenizes individual differences into a general sameness, decreeing the same size and shape for all. We are pressured both to achieve this ideal appearance and to purchase and consume large quantities of material goods. This creates a dilemma as the ideal person is tall, but curvaceous or well-muscled; youthful, but with ample purchasing power; conforming, but unique; hedonistic, but restrained; and sexually attractive, but safe from disease.

Body Image: Illusions Versus Reality

The effect of these conflicting cultural pressures is bewildering and, for some individuals, overwhelming. Physical attractiveness becomes the expression of personal worth, which translates to thinness and firmness are best. There follows an urgency to be sure one is thin enough. At any given time, about 33% to 40% of American women are dieting to lose weight, even though by objective standards far fewer are overweight (2). The trend is similar for men, though the portion of dieters is somewhat less. Clearly, there is some discrepancy between perception and reality.

Most of us weigh ourselves regularly and have a good idea of our current weight. The figure on the scale, however, does not always agree with how fat we feel. Fig. 10-1 shows the Figure Rating Scale, an instrument that investigators use

How Do You See Yourself?

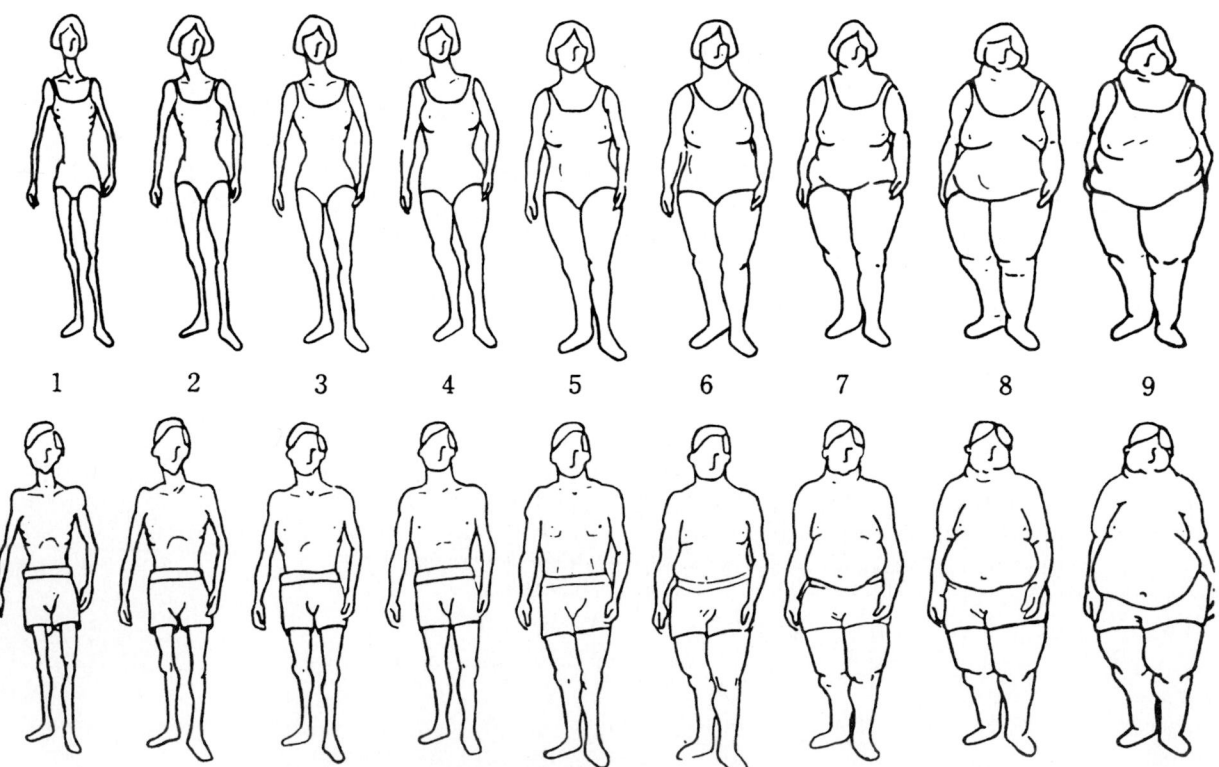

Fig. 10-1 Figure rating scale. (From Stunkard AJ, Sorensen T, Schulsinger: Use of the Danish Adoption Register for the study of obesity and thinness. In *Genetics of neurological and psychiatric disorders*, New York, 1983, Raven Press.)

to assess perceived and preferred body size. The investigator instructs the subjects to mark the figure that is most like the way they feel at that time. When these figures are compared to an objective assessment, the subjects usually have greatly overestimated their size.

Although body image is pretty stable, changes in your feelings of well-being from day to day and from hour to hour may produce small adjustments in your body image. An instrument like the Figure Rating Scale should reflect those changes.

Body preferences: gender concerns

Investigators also use the Figure Rating Scale to determine size preferences; they ask you which figure is most like how you would like to be, which is most like how you currently are, and which you think is most attractive to the opposite sex (3). Ideally, the answers to these three questions would be closely clustered, indicating that you are fairly satisfied with your size. For males, that is the case. Females, however, on average feel much fatter than they think is ideal. Furthermore, the females' personal ideal is thinner than the figure they think males would choose, challenging the assumption that females want to be thin in order to attract males.

Body acceptance: a key to wellness

We may strive mightily to meet the societal standards of attractiveness and thinness, but given our individual genetic makeups we cannot all succeed. Although humans have an awesome potential for growth and development, there are limits (4). Understanding and accepting what we can and cannot expect to achieve in pursuit of the ideal body is a key to wellness (see the box below). Only with this understanding can we establish goals that will guide our behaviors toward health.

SOCIAL ISSUE
Dealing With Our Own Prejudices

We live in a world where fat intolerance or fat phobia is the last socially acceptable prejudice. As a society, we are so committed to self-improvement that it may feel wrong to question the directive that all those who deviate from the *ideal* size and shape should dedicate themselves to rectifying the situation. Our fat intolerance may be motivated by the very best intentions to be helpful to ourselves and to others, but like all prejudices it diminishes the people to whom it is applied.

This prejudice is especially problematic when it exists among health professionals. Obese people often report that they feel degraded by their health care encounters and therefore avoid seeking medical help. The traditional medical model holds the patient responsible for the existence of a health problem; this moralistic philosophy tends to justify blaming the patient for choosing to be fat or thin. Even though this prejudice could be expected to interfere with their effectiveness, health professionals have been found to have high levels of fat intolerance; one study found that among medical students 57% characterized obese individuals as lazy, 52% as sloppy, and 62% as lacking in self control. Encouragingly, the same author found that when medical students participated in a program to increase understanding their negative stereotypes were diminished.

What about you? Have you been successful in questioning and replacing your own prejudices? Are you able to accept yourself and your body? As a future health professional, are you prepared to empower your patients to work toward total wellness, including healthy nondieting habits? Test yourself on the Size Acceptance Scale in Table 10-1 to determine how you rank. If your score indicates you are reflecting society's prejudices, you can take heart from the fact that the authors of the scale have found that negative attitudes can be changed through thoughtful observation, study, and discussion.

From Achterberg C, Trenkner LL: Developing a working philosophy of nutrition education, *J Nutr Ed.* 22:189-193, 1990; Czajka-Narins DM, Parham ES: Fear of fat: Attitudes toward obesity, *Nutrition Today*, Jan/Feb 26-32, 1990; Parham ES: Applying a philosophy of nutrition education in weight control, *J Nutr Ed* 22:194-197, 1990; and Wiese HJC et al: Obesity stigma reduction in medical students, *Int J Obes* 16:859-868, 1992.

Table 10-1   Size Acceptance Scale

Assessing Size Attitudes

This behavior assessment can be used to evaluate your support for the health and well-being of large people. Use the following scale to indicate the frequency of each behavior.

1—never   2—rarely   3—occasionally   4—frequently   5—daily

How often do you:	Never				Daily
1. Make negative comments about your fatness	1	2	3	4	5
2. Make negative comments about someone else's fatness	1	2	3	4	5
3. Directly or indirectly support the assumption that no one should be fat	1	2	3	4	5
4. Disapprove of fatness (in general)	1	2	3	4	5
5. Say or assume that someone is looking good because she or he has lost weight	1	2	3	4	5
6. Say something that presumes that a fat person wants to lose weight	1	2	3	4	5
7. Say something that presumes that fat people should lose weight	1	2	3	4	5
8. Say something that presumes that fat people eat too much	1	2	3	4	5
9. Admire or approve of someone for losing weight	1	2	3	4	5
10. Disapprove of someone for gaining weight	1	2	3	4	5
11. Assume that something is wrong when someone gains weight	1	2	3	4	5
12. Admire weight-loss dieting	1	2	3	4	5
13. Admire rigidly controlled eating	1	2	3	4	5
14. Admire compulsive or excessive exercising	1	2	3	4	5
15. Tease or admonish someone about his/her eating (habits or choices)	1	2	3	4	5
16. Criticize someone's eating to a third person ("so-and-so eats way too much junk")	1	2	3	4	5
17. Discuss food in terms of good/bad	1	2	3	4	5
18. Talk about "being good" and "being bad" in reference to eating behavior	1	2	3	4	5
19. Talk about calories (in the usual dieter's fashion)	1	2	3	4	5
20. Say something that presumes being thin is better (or more attractive) than being fat	1	2	3	4	5
21. Comment that you don't wear a certain style because "it makes you look fat"	1	2	3	4	5
22. Comment that you love certain clothing because "it makes you look thin"	1	2	3	4	5
23. Say something that presumes that fatness is unattractive	1	2	3	4	5
24. Participate in a fat joke by telling one or laughing/smiling at one	1	2	3	4	5
25. Support the diet industry by buying their services and/or products	1	2	3	4	5
26. Undereat and/or exercise obsessively to maintain an unnaturally low weight	1	2	3	4	5
27. Say something that presumes being fat is unhealthy	1	2	3	4	5
28. Say something that presumes being thin is healthy	1	2	3	4	5
29. Encourage someone to let go of guilt	1	2	3	4	5
30. Encourage or admire self-acceptance and self-appreciation/love	1	2	3	4	5
31. Encourage someone to feel good about his/her body as is	1	2	3	4	5
32. Openly admire a fat person's appearance	1	2	3	4	5
33. Openly admire a fat person's character, personality, or actions	1	2	3	4	5
34. Oppose/challenge fattism (intolerance) verbally	1	2	3	4	5
35. Oppose/challenge fattism (intolerance) in writing	1	2	3	4	5
36. Challenge or voice disapproval of a fat joke	1	2	3	4	5
37. Challenge myths about fatness and eating	1	2	3	4	5
38. Compliment ideas, behavior, character, etc. more often than appearance	1	2	3	4	5
39. Support organizations that advance fat acceptance (with your time or money)	1	2	3	4	5

Behaviors 1 to 28 are unhelpful or harmful; look over areas that need improvement and strive to avoid these and similar behaviors in the future. Behaviors 29 to 39 help support size acceptance; reread items you marked "never" (1) or "rarely" (2); make a list of realistic goals for increasing supportive behavior.

From Kano S: Size acceptance scale, *Obesity and Health* Jan/Feb 1994, p. 14.

WHAT IS THE GOAL OF LIFELONG MANAGEMENT OF BODY FATNESS?

If we say that individuals must choose their own values and goals, it is impossible to state one goal for everyone. Nevertheless, we can identify some probable commonalities. Surely most of us would define a goal of maximizing the quality and length of our lives. We probably can go further and say that our goal is to achieve the best possible health, including emotional, social, intellectual, physical, and spiritual aspects of health. This chapter proceeds on the premise that we can agree on some version of this goal. Most of us would also agree that too little and too much fat are likely to compromise physical health; this chapter explores the impact of body fat on health. In addition, we assume that we agree that the relationship between fatness and well-being is limited. That is, being slender does not guarantee happiness and health in all its aspects and vice versa.

What is the Association of Body Fatness With Health?

Physical health

Most of our evidence of the association of fatness and physical health comes from epidemiological studies. Epidemiological research investigates the distribution of disease in a population and seeks to explain associations between causative factors and the disease. This type of research usually involves thousands of subjects and may be longitudinal (involving observations over a number of years). Because it is not practical to measure fatness in these large studies, weight is usually measured instead. If we were to plot the findings of epidemiological studies of the association of weight and risk of certain diseases or mortality from all causes, we would usually produce a J-shaped curve such as in Fig. 10-2 (5).

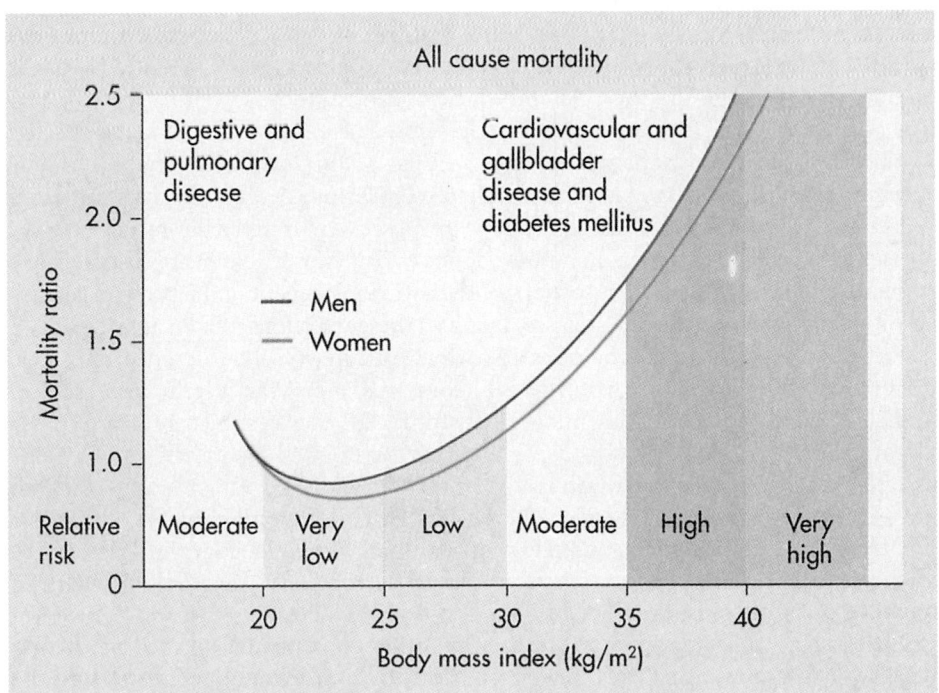

Fig. 10-2 Relationship between body mass index (BMI) and mortality rate. The lowest mortality rates are associated with BMIs between 19 and 27 kg/m^2.

This curve means that individuals at both extremes of fatness, those very thin and those very fat, are at increased risk, whereas those at a more moderate fatness level have the lowest risk. This J-shaped curve is found with four leading causes of death in the United States at this time: heart disease, some types of cancer, stroke, and diabetes. It is a surprise to many people that the low end of the fatness range shows an increased risk, providing strong evidence that you can be too thin. Although the factors contributing to this increased risk of extremely low weight are not completely clear, they are thought to differ from the factors associated with increased risk of heavy individuals.

Because we have far more overfat people in this country than underfat ones, let's consider the impact on physical health of excess fat or obesity.* Higher levels of body fat, especially in the abdominal area, seem to lead to higher blood pressure (hypertension), higher levels of certain blood lipids (LDLs), and more resistance to insulin (6). All of these conditions increase the risk of atherosclerosis, heart disease, and stroke. Diabetes mellitus is characterized by inadequate insulin activity. Some obese persons develop a resistance to their own insulin. Even though they have high levels of this hormone in their blood, it fails to control their blood glucose levels. This type of diabetes, called *non–insulin-dependent diabetes mellitus (NIDDM)*, is the most common type and is highly associated with obesity. Obesity also increases the risk of health conditions that impact well-being but aren't usually life threatening; menstrual irregularities, infertility, gallbladder disease, and some types of arthritis are examples.

In 1985 a group of American scientists was convened by the National Institutes of Health (NIH) to try to reach consensus about obesity's risks to physical health (7). They concluded that there was strong evidence that obesity has adverse effects on health and longevity. The deleterious effect was found to be strongest in young adults.

Some unanswered questions about risks to physical health

Up to this point we have shown some convincing evidence that obesity compromises physical health. However, to get a balanced perspective we must consider some important issues and unanswered questions (8). First, we must recognize that not all well-conducted studies show significant association of risk and fatness. Many other studies do show an increased risk, but do not show that all or even most obese people suffer that risk. For example, it is widely agreed that obesity increases the risk of developing non–insulin-dependent diabetes, but very little consideration is given to the fact that more 90% of obese adults do not develop diabetes. There seems to be wide variability in vulnerability to the risks of greater fatness. What accounts for this variability? Why is obesity more of a risk to young adults than to older ones? How do risks differ between men and women and between ethnic groups? Why is it that in recent decades Americans have gotten fatter, but rates of mortality caused by heart disease have dropped significantly? As scientists sort out the various genetic influences on fatness and on vulnerability to various diseases, many of these questions will be answered.

Does losing weight make the risks go away? Another NIH conference, this time in 1992, concluded that we don't have strong evidence that weight loss reduces risk (2). In fact, numerous epidemiological studies following subjects for a number of years show that weight loss is associated with increased mortality (9). This unexpected finding is a good illustration of the difficulty of interpreting research data—does the increased risk reflect weight lost during terminal illnesses or does it reflect unforeseen, long-term dangers of voluntary weight loss? To determine which was responsible, the investigators would have to have detailed information about the weight losses; this type of data is not yet available.

One issue of contemporary concern is the effect of repeated or chronic dieting on risk (see the box on p. 247). Given our cultural concern about fatness and the

---

* In this chapter, we shall define obesity simply as excessive fatness. More quantitative definitions traditionally used in medicine and the popular press are that weights >110% of desirable weight equals overweight and >120% of desirable weight equals obesity; these definitions imply a precision in interpreting risks of fatness that simply is not available.

HEALTH DEBATE
Balancing the Weight Issue

Which way to go? Recommending that patients lose weight used to seem the only rational option to reduce health risks associated with excessive weight. Recent observations and research reveal that this advice may not be the most risk-reducing or lifesaving approach.

Health factors related to weight-loss dieting may be damaging as well. The success rate of maintaining lost weight is poor; it often leads to cycles of weight gain and loss. Early studies suggested weight *cycling* made weight gain easier and loss even harder. Recent studies show that individuals who weight cycle may have a shorter life span than if they maintain a steady weight, even if the steady weight is higher than their standardized ideal. In-creased deaths from heart disease oc-curred among those whose weight fluctu-ated, although cancer deaths remained the same in all groups.

The question is whether the cure—losing weight by food-restrictive dieting—is more damaging than excessive weight. The ef-fects of weight cycling may cause some of the health risks rather than the weight alone. Are persons who are truly obese (those genetically predisposed to weigh more) less at risk for weight-related health problems than those who are obese as the result of weight cycling caused by chronic unsuccessful dieting? Future research may answer this question; in the meantime the debate continues.

From Bouchard C: Is weight fluctuation a risk factor? (editorial), *N Eng J Med* 324(26):1887-1890, June 27, 1991 and Lee IM, Paffenbarger Jr RS: Change in body weight and longevity, *JAMA* 268(15): 2045-2050, October 21, 1992.

extremely limited success of most weight-loss attempts, there is a high likelihood that a fat adult will have tried to lose weight many times. Is it possible that some of the observed negative effects of obesity are really the outcomes of a lifetime of un-successful dieting? Although the findings to date are not conclusive, animal studies and some limited observations of human beings give support to this hypothesis (9).

Last, we should bear in mind that obesity does not increase all types of health risks. In fact, risks of some types of cancer and of osteoporosis are lower, and risks of other conditions (such as infectious diseases, chronic lung disease, liver disease, and injuries) are no higher among obese people than the general population (8).

Emotional and social health

For many years investigators have searched for a psychopathology that would fit most obese people and would help explain their fatness. Their efforts have failed, for although a minority of fat people suffer from a variety of mental health problems, no set of psychological problems typical of obesity has been identified (10). What these investigators have found is that our culture's extreme stigma against fatness extracts a tremendous toll on people who are obese. Social, eco-nomic, and other types of discrimination against obese persons are widely prac-ticed. This may lead to impaired self-image and feelings of inferiority, which in turn may contribute to social isolation. Some people feel so guilty about their fatness that they hide away and put their lives on hold until they can achieve slenderness.

Other people (both obese and slender) concerned about their weights develop a characteristic known as *restrained eating* (11). Restrained eaters try to use will-power to restrict their eating to a level below their natural **appetites**. Their re-straint is susceptible to disruption by various disinhibitors, especially stress. When disinhibited, restrained eaters usually binge. The binge may be a response to the **hunger** denied for days or weeks. It may be guided by *black/white thinking*, for ex-ample, thinking "if I can't be perfect, I might as well give up." Thus restrained eat-ing makes management of body composition harder.

As is the case with threats to physical health, the psychosocial risks are not uni-form. Many people who are obese feel good about themselves and lead active, pro-ductive lives with a variety of positive relationships with other people.

appetite
desire for food

hunger
a physiological need for food

HOW MUCH BODY FAT IS HEALTHY?

Functions of Fat

Although we tend to think of body fat as something to be avoided, it serves a number of vital functions. In estimating optimal amounts of fat, we must take these functions into consideration. As discussed in Chapter 5, we could not live without some body fat. Although we must always allow for individual differences, **essential fat** in males seems to be 3% to 8% of their body weight; ranges considered healthy are 20% to 22% (12).

In women, the concept of essential fat must be expanded to include gender-specific fat in their breasts, pelvic region, and buttocks that is apparently an evolutionary feature that provides energy during childbearing and lactation. Thus for women the minimum levels of fatness compatible with health are based on the essential fat plus the gender-specific fat and are in the range of 12% to 14%; healthy levels range from 25% to 30% (12).

For most people, the major portion of body fat is **storage fat** (Fig. 10-3). A layer of this fat under our skin provides protection from extremes of environmental temperatures, and cushions of fat defend many internal organs against physical trauma. Storing fat provides an efficient means of storing energy so that we can endure moderate fasts. In fact, this ability is of such importance to our bodies that we have seemingly unlimited capacity to store fat. Some people have set records for the amount of fat they have accumulated in their bodies. Those unfortunate individuals have died young because of the strain of their enormous bodies on the capacity of their vital organs. Even though they weighed more than 500 lbs, there was no evidence that they had lost the ability to gain more fat.

Distribution of Body Fat

From both a health and an appearance perspective, it is not only the amount of fat but its location that is important. Spend a few minutes at a popular swimming pool and notice the diverse patterns of fat distribution. Differences related to gender, age, and stage of development become apparent. Fat patterns may also vary among ethnic groups (6). These distinctions are genetically determined and, although the amount of exercise can affect the tone of the underlying muscle, it cannot change the pattern of distribution.

essential fat
certain components of body fat that are essential for life

storage fat
layers and cushions of fat providing stored energy and protection from extremes of environmental temperatures; also protects internal organs against physical trauma

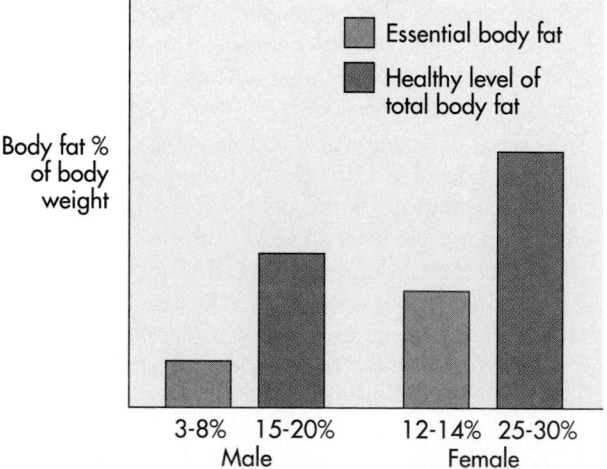

Fig. 10-3 Male and female body fat levels. *Essential body fat*: minimum level of body fat for biological functions. *Total body fat*: range of level of body fat that provides for biological functions but which does not have potential to negatively affect health.

Imagine the various adult shapes seen at the pool; try to classify them as *apples* or *pears*. Apples are biggest around the waist and pears are biggest in their hips, buttocks, and upper thighs. Although some evenly proportioned people will fit neither category, probably most of the *pears* are women and most of the *apples* are men and older women. The upper body fat of apple-shaped people is a far greater health risk than is lower body fat. Although some very sophisticated techniques are used to accurately assess fat distribution patterns, you can make a good estimate by comparing your waist circumference to that of your hips (Fig. 10-4) (6).

Although this exercise may seem frivolous, it focuses attention on the location of fat, which largely determines its effect on health. Fat that is within the abdominal cavity (known as **visceral fat**) is much more involved with the health risks associated with obesity than is the lower body fat or fat under the skin in the abdominal area. Fig. 10-5 shows cross-sectional scans of the bodies of two persons of equal fatness, one having large amounts of visceral fat, the other having lots of subcutaneous abdominal fat. Although male hormones and other genetically determined factors are major influences in fat being deposited primarily in the visceral area, use of alcohol and smoking seem to be involved as well. Thus we see the origin of the term *beer belly*.

The two types of fat distribution also differ in their rate of turnover, with visceral fat being much more easily lost and also more quickly regained than

visceral fat
fat that is within the abdominal cavity

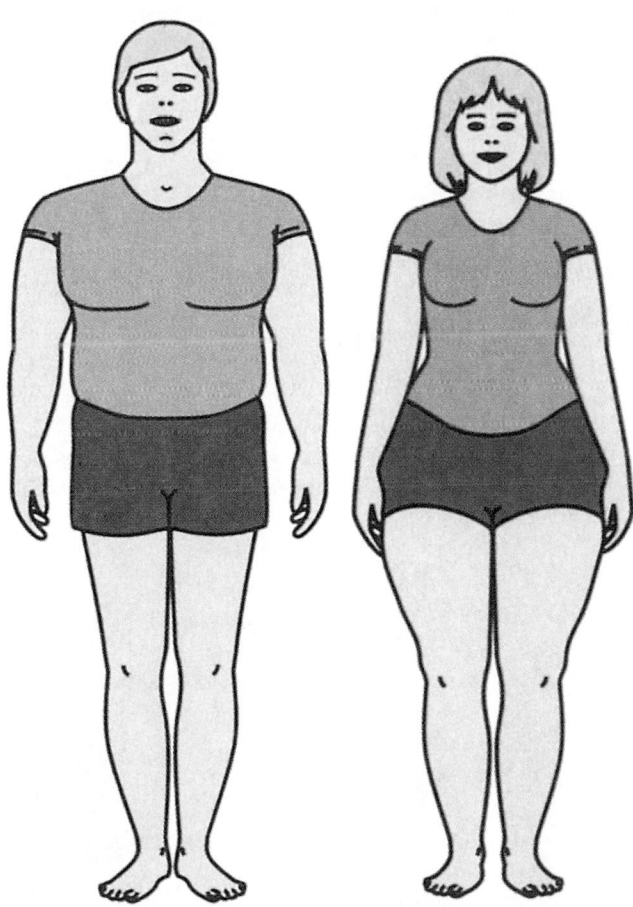

Fig. 10-4 Apple and pear body shapes. To estimate your fat distribution, measure the circumference of your waist and your hips. Divide your waist measurement by your hip measurement. You are an apple if you are a man and your waist to hip ratio is greater than .9, or if you are a woman and your waist to hip ratio is greater than .8. You are a pear if you are a woman and your waist to hip ratio is less than .8.

subcutaneous abdominal fat or lower body fat. This is one of the factors contributing to men's apparent greater ease in losing and regaining fat. It is ironic that although the typical female fat pattern of lower body obesity is more benign, women tend to be more concerned with their fatness than do men (see box).

How Body Fat is Stored

adipocytes
cells specialized for storage of fat

Most of the fat in our bodies is stored in special cells called **adipocytes**. These cells have a nucleus, mitochondria, and other organelles just as other cells do, but as you can see from Fig. 10-6, these features are usually squeezed over to the side to make room for the droplet of stored fat.

The fat in this droplet is in the form of triglycerides, the same type of molecule that makes up most of the fat we eat. These triglycerides are synthesized from glucose, fatty acids, some amino acids, and alcohol that are carried to the adipocyte by the bloodstream. The stored fat is in a constant state of flux, with some triglycerides being broken down while others are being built up. The net effect of this flux—that is, how much fat is in storage—is the result of our energy balance at

CULTURAL CONSIDERATIONS
Valuing Body Sizes

Women's weight has long been a social issue as well as a health issue. Although most conclusions that have been drawn are from studies of white, upper social and economic class women, Allan et al recently studied women of varying socioeconomic status (SES) (31 African-American and 36 Caucasian) to examine their actual weights and their values concerning body size.

African-American women of lower SES were found to be heavier, perceived themselves as heavier, and perceived the heavier body size to be more attractive than did African-American women of higher SES and Caucasian women of all SES groups. Caucasian women and African-American women of higher SES reported feeling pressure to be thin from media images of health and beauty, while African-American women of lower SES are more affected by family and peers.

Although this study is small, it does point out that people of different cultures view issues of size differently. Health care professionals need to remember that just because we might perceive weight reduction as a health benefit, others may not have the same perceptions.

From Allan JD, Mayo K, Michel Y: Body size values of white and black women, *Res Nurs Health* 16:323-333, 1993.

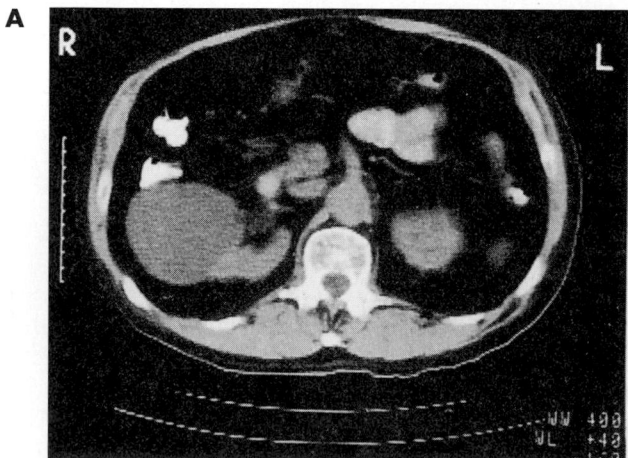
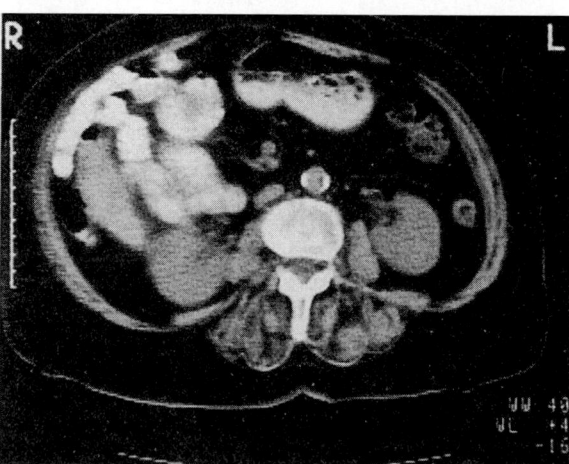

Fig. 10-5 A, Computed tomography (CT) of typical obese male patient shows much fat is contained within the abdomen. **B,** CT of typical obese female shows fat is mainly subcutaneous, with little intraabdominal fat.

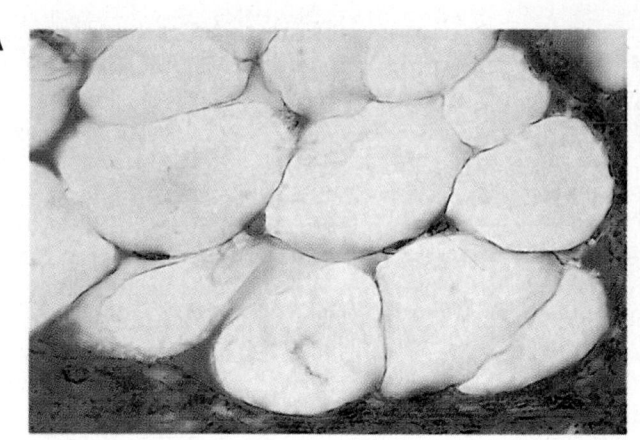
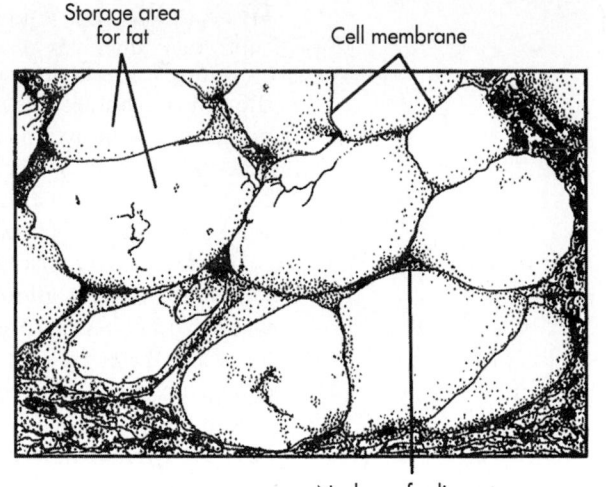

Storage area
for fat

Cell membrane

Nucleus of adipocyte

Fig. 10-6 Filled adipocytes. **A,** Photomicrograph. **B,** Sketch of photomicrograph. Note the large storage spaces for fat inside the adipocytes.

that time. If we need energy, the balance shifts to favor breakdown and release of fatty acids and glycerol to be transported to various cells where they are oxidized or converted to other needed molecules. When we have a ready supply of energy, especially shortly after a meal, the balance tilts toward storage.

At birth, most of us have relatively small numbers of adipocytes, but during the next few years these cells increase in number (a type of growth known as **hyperplasia**) and in size (known as **hypertrophy**). Hypertrophy occurs whenever we continue in positive energy balance for any time. Hyperplasia, however, is more specialized, occurring during the growth spurts accompanying normal development. These growth-related times of hyperplasia occur during infancy, the preschool years, adolescence, and pregnancy. The adolescent increase in numbers of fat cells is much more pronounced among girls and results in the higher level of body fat normal for girls in comparison with boys.

People tend to be very interested in the process of adipocyte hyperplasia because once these cells form there is no natural means of reducing the number. Knowing that there are predictable times of adipocyte hyperplasia, scientists once thought that if we carefully controlled our energy balance during those critical periods, we would have lifetime insurance against becoming too fat. Unfortunately, we now know that this is not true. We can form new adipocytes at any stage of life if the conditions are right (13).

If more energy is consumed than expended, fat storage will go on until the fat droplet reaches its maximum size. If the positive energy balance continues, the body will make new adipocytes, thereby expanding the storage capacity. The stored fat is relatively equally divided so that all cells contain less than their maximum capacity. We are then able to continue to expand our storage capacity as long as the positive energy balance persists.

When fat is lost, whether through reduced intake, increased physical activity, or illness, fat is mobilized from adipocytes to meet energy needs. This reduces the size of the droplet of stored fat, producing a smaller adipocyte. If we have been obese and then lose a lot of fat, our adipocytes may become quite tiny, smaller than the cells of people who were never fat. Our bodies seem to monitor the size of adipocytes, interpreting the shrunken cells as evidence of imminent starvation. We may then feel compelled to eat more. Although the response mechanisms are not fully understood, clearly the effects on metabolism and drive to eat have developed as a means to reverse the threat of further loss. This set of responses is a major part of the theory of *set point*, discussed later in this chapter.

hyperplasia
an increase in the number of cells occurring during the growth spurts accompanying normal development

hypertrophy
an increase in the size of cells

How Body Fatness is Measured

Body weight is the most common way of estimating fatness. Weight is used even though our bodies are made up not only of fat, but also bone, muscle, and other nonfat tissue known as lean body mass. Weighing works fairly well as a means for determining fatness because usually the lean body mass changes only very slowly. Therefore we assume that if the scale says a pound more this week than it did last week, the change is due to a gain of fat.

There are several situations in which weight is not a good measurement of fatness. One involves fluctuations in body fluid; fluid retention premenstrually or during hot weather may be interpreted as fat gain, and losses in a sauna may appear to be fat losses. In these circumstances, normalizing the fluid balance makes the apparent fat change promptly disappear. On the other hand, the scale is also misleading for anyone whose amount of lean body mass deviates from what is expected. A bodybuilder will have a higher portion of lean body mass than the average person and thus will weigh more. Someone who has suffered from a wasting disease will have less lean tissue.

Because weighing is so convenient, it remains a useful assessment. However, if we really need to know how fat we are, we must resort to other means, generally involving other measurements of the size of the body (anthropometric measurements) or assessments distinguishing between fat and other body components on the basis of their physical differences. Of the latter group, underwater weighing (**densitometry**) is the most widely accepted and is often used as a standard to assess the validity of other measures. Unfortunately, densitometry apparatus is bulky and expensive, and not everyone is willing or able to be submerged. There has been a long search for alternative methods. One of these methods, **computed tomography (CT)**, produces the type of images depicted in Fig. 10-5. Although it produces fascinating views of the human body, such imaging is not practical for routine assessments because of the cost. Far more practical is **bioelectric impedance analysis (BIA)**, a method often offered at health fairs and health and fitness centers. This method uses electrodes placed at the wrists and ankles to monitor the ease of passage of a very mild electrical current (14). Fat is a poor conductor of electricity; the conductivity occurs through the nonfat parts of the body. BIA actually estimates the amount of lean body mass, and the amount of fat is calculated from the difference between the lean body mass and the total weight. BIA is safe, inexpensive, easily performed, and reasonably accurate, but it is not considered sensitive enough to detect day-to-day changes experienced by someone trying to gain or lose fat. Other methods of assessing fat level include triceps skinfold and mid-upper arm circumference (see Chapter 15), but again these are unable to detect day-to-day changes.

densitometry
underwater weighing

computed tomography (CT)
an imaging technique for determining body fat composition

bioelectric impedance analysis (BIA)
a method using a very mild electric charge to estimate lean body mass in order to determine body fat composition

Interpreting Body Fatness Measures

In order to interpret fatness measures, we have to agree on some criteria. After all, our interpretation will be far different if our criterion is compatibility with current fashion versus a criterion of lowest mortality rates. Since our focus in this text is achieving wellness, we direct our attention to health-related criteria. Before we consider various measurement systems, let us emphasize the importance of individual interpretations. All systems are based on averages; however, we're all aware that there is no average person. We each must consider our own body configurations, our values, our personal and family health history, the fatness level at which we feel best, and what we find achievable. The standards we review should not be construed as iron-clad laws, but merely guidelines. There are a few numbers that one ought to memorize, but our *ideal* fatness level is not one of them.

Interpreting weight

Weight measurements can be interpreted by consulting a weight for height table such as the one developed by the Metropolitan Life Insurance Company (see inside back cover). This table is based on the weights-for-heights that are associated with the lowest mortality rates. A range of weight is given for each of three sizes of body frame, but this has limited usefulness because a reliable measure of frame size is not readily available. Unless your hands and feet are unusually large or unusually small, it is probably best to assume that you have an average frame. Keep in mind that tables like this are based on insured people, primarily of middle or upper socioeconomic level, and mainly Caucasian. Their applicability to other groups may be limited.

A possibly more convenient way of interpreting weight is to determine our body mass index (BMI). BMI is calculated by dividing the weight in kilograms by the square of the height in meters. This yields a value that can be interpreted without further reference to height. You can determine your BMI and relate it to the associated health risk by consulting Table 10-2. BMIs below 19 to 20 and above 26 to 27 are associated with increased health risks (7,15). Although some controversy exists as to whether the standards should be increased with age, health risk evidence supports increasing the recommended range by one unit for each decade beyond 24 years (15). Thus for people aged 25 to 34 years, the recommended range would be 20 to 25.

Bear in mind that even though BMI is widely used and very convenient, it is still a measure of weight and has all the shortcomings of using weight to estimate fat. When both weight and fat were measured on the same men and women, about 6% of both sexes had weights that were considered normal, but levels of body fat beyond recommended—they were normal weight, but obese. On the other hand, approximately 10% of the men and 8% of the women were overweight, but not overfat (15).

Table 10-2   Relationship Among Height in Inches, Weight in Pounds, and Body Mass Index

Height (in)	Body Mass Index (kg/m²)													
	19	20	21	22	23	24	25	26	27	28	29	30	35	40
	← Body Weight (lb)* →													
58	91	96	100	105	110	115	119	124	129	134	138	143	167	191
59	94	99	104	109	114	119	124	128	133	138	143	148	173	198
60	97	102	107	112	118	123	128	133	138	143	148	153	179	204
61	100	106	111	116	122	127	132	137	143	148	153	158	185	211
62	104	109	115	120	126	131	136	142	147	153	158	164	191	218
63	107	113	118	124	130	135	141	146	152	158	163	169	197	225
64	110	116	122	128	134	140	145	151	157	163	169	174	204	232
65	114	120	126	132	138	144	150	156	162	168	174	180	210	240
66	118	124	130	136	142	148	155	161	167	173	179	186	216	247
67	121	127	134	140	146	153	159	166	172	178	185	191	223	255
68	125	131	138	144	151	158	164	171	177	184	190	197	230	262
69	128	135	142	149	155	162	169	176	182	189	196	203	236	270
70	132	139	146	153	160	167	174	181	188	195	202	207	243	278
71	136	143	150	157	165	172	179	186	193	200	208	215	250	286
72	140	147	154	162	169	177	184	191	199	206	213	221	258	294
73	144	151	159	166	174	182	189	197	204	212	219	227	265	302
74	148	155	163	171	179	186	194	202	210	218	225	233	272	311
75	152	160	168	176	184	192	200	208	216	224	232	240	279	319
76	156	164	172	180	189	197	205	213	221	230	238	246	287	328

From Bray GA, Gray DS: Obesity: Pathogenesis, *West J Med* 149:429, 1988.
*Each entry gives the body weight in pounds (lb) for a person of a given height and body mass index. Pounds have been rounded off. To use the table, find the appropriate height in the left-hand column. Move across the row to a given weight. The number at the top of the column is the body mass index for the height and weight.

Interpreting percent body fat

It is fat that we really care about, not weight. So it is unfortunate that, to date, the evidence to support recommended amounts of fat is relatively scanty. As techniques like BIA are more widely used, this situation will change; in the meantime, we will accept the recommendations that percent body fat be based on the essential fat plus a modest amount of storage fat, yielding a total range of 15% to 20% of body weight for males and 25% to 30% for females (12).

Sometimes athletes and dancers may strive for body fat levels below these ranges. There is concern that low body fat levels may be responsible for the menstrual irregularities experienced by many athletic women (12). Amenorrhea is associated with bone loss and increased risk of fractures. Early work indicated that most girls do not begin menstruation unless their bodies are at least 17% body fat and do not continue regular periods without 22% body fat. Modern methods of assessing body composition do not support these exact fatness levels as predictive of menstrual performance for all physically active women, but body fatness is considered an important factor. The fat level associated with the best athletic performance may not be the level best for all-around long-term health. Working to achieve a lower percent body fat can be very tempting; the desirability of doing this should be carefully assessed, considering the effect on strength, general health, menstruation, and other individual factors.

HOW IS BODY FAT LEVEL REGULATED?

Our bodies form fat as a way of storing energy between eating episodes. When we have excess energy available we synthesize triglycerides and store them in adipose cells. When we have a shortage of energy, we break down those stored triglycerides and use the energy stored in them. Thus the bottom line in adjustment of body fat levels is the status of the body's energy balance: when our energy intake exceeds our expenditure, we gain fat; when it is less than our expenditure, we lose fat. Sounds simple, doesn't it? In fact, it's not simple at all. Our bodies are much more complex than the teeter-totter that is often used to illustrate energy balance. Many factors affect the rate of energy intake and expenditure. We all are familiar with the concept that some cars get good gas mileage and others don't. We humans have many systems that regulate the *mileage* we get from our food energy. The last chapter explored some of these factors. A complete examination is beyond range of this book, but we will strive to convey the scope of the control system.

How Body Fatness Changes

Levels of body fatness change when a disequilibrium in energy balance is established and maintained for a period of time. A pound of body fat is roughly equivalent to 3500 kcalories.* Thus a cumulative positive balance of that magnitude should cause a weight gain of one pound, whereas a negative balance of the same size should result in the loss of a pound of fat. You will recall that energy balance is determined by the relationship of the energy intake to the energy expenditure. The intake side of the equation is simple: it represents the kcaloric value of the food and drink you consume. The expenditure side is more complex, including the energy required to just keep your body going when at rest (basal metabolic rate or BMR),

---

*Although this figure represents the typical energy equivalent of a pound of stored fat, its use implies that the system is much simpler than it really is. In fact, many factors affect the rate of energy utilization and, thereby, the energy equivalent of a given amount of fat varies among individuals and within the same individual from time to time. We should consider the 3500 figure as only a rough estimate.

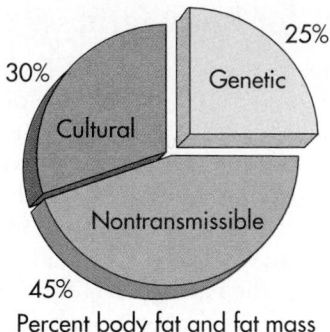

Fig. 10-7 Genetic influence on percent body fat. (Data from Bouchard C et al: *Int J Obs* 12:205, 1988.)

the energy cost of exercise, and the thermic effect of food (TEF). Although there is a lot of interest in factors that affect BMR and TEF, there is not a safe and practical way to alter them.* It would seem simple to manipulate kcalorie intake and kcalorie expenditure from physical activity and to produce desired changes in fatness.

Genetic Influences on Body Size and Shape

During the earlier real or imagined observation at a swimming pool, perhaps it was noticed that families often share tendencies toward certain sizes and shapes. Scientists studying the genetics of fatness examine the fatness (or sometimes weight) of individuals who have identical genetic material (identical twins), who have some genetic material in common (siblings and parents and their children) and individuals who have shared environments but not genetic material (adopted children and their adoptive parents). By comparing various combinations of these groups, scientists are able to estimate heritability, the extent to which certain characteristics are inherited (16,17).

The efforts of these scientists reveal that the role of genetics in the fatness of most people is quite complex. There is no gene for fatness or thinness. True, there are a couple of extremely rare syndromes (Prader-Willi and Bardet-Biedl) where obesity is clearly determined by a genetic factor that also produces mental retardation. Otherwise, fatness must be considered a **multifactorial phenotype**, that is the displayed characteristic (phenotype) is the product of numerous genetic and environmental factors. Regardless of one's genetic makeup, one's fatness is also influenced by nutritional, psychological, economic, and social factors. In addition, there are many different types of obesity and thinness. When a family is characterized by a marked degree of fatness or thinness, we are unable to tell whether we're observing the effect of a shared environment, shared genetics, or both (Fig. 10-7).

How would genes affect the amount and distribution of fat? Research suggests that there is a strong genetic influence on certain components that make up the energy balance equation: basal or resting metabolic rate, thermic effect of food, and the energy cost of light exercise (the previous chapter gives more information about these components). Investigators have also found genetic influences on the ability to use ingested fat for energy, on taste preferences, and on the ability to achieve a high level of physical conditioning. These findings help explain why people differ in their ease of gaining or losing weight. Nevertheless, for almost every component studied there were not only genetic, but also environmental factors involved. Although genetics play a part in the level of body fatness, they are not the only factor. The extent of their influence probably varies from person to person.

multifactorial phenotype
a characteristic that is the product of numerous genetic and environmental factors

---

* There is some evidence that very vigorous physical activity sustained for several hours temporarily raises BMR, but these conditions do not occur often in most people's lives.

Is there a set point for body fatness?

Many of our body characteristics are regulated so that they are maintained at a constant level or within a narrow range. This is true of our body temperature, the level of glucose in our blood, our blood pressure, the acidity of our body fluids, and many other features. Departure from our usual levels of these variables is usually clear indication that something is wrong. Usually when the problem is corrected, the characteristic returns to its usual level. This usual or natural level is referred to as the *set point*. Actually, this term usually indicates not a single point, but a narrow range that defines the natural level for the characteristic. The adjustments our bodies make to return to the set point are referred to as *defending the set point*. Thus we can define **set point** as a natural level (of some characteristic) that the body regulates or defends.

It stands to reason that since energy is a very high priority for the body, the level of energy stores would not be left to chance without regulation. Indeed, as described above, the weight (and body fatness) of most adults is remarkably stable, returning to the usual level after minor gains and losses. In spite of minor gains over the years, this is true of fat people and thin people alike. Let's take a moment to consider just how remarkable this is. On the average it takes an energy surplus of roughly 3500 kcalories to build a pound of fat. Likewise, losing a pound requires an energy deficit of the same magnitude. Now suppose that daily for a year you ate 100 kcalories more than you really needed. This might be a small brownie, a large roll, a fresh pear, or whatever—just a little extra. Over 365 days this little bit would add up to 36,500 kcalories or a little more than 10 lb of fat. In 4 years, the traditional time to get a college degree, this could add up to 40 lb.

Obviously, this doesn't ordinarily happen. True, we do gain and lose weight, but usually this is related to a change in lifestyle or in health status. For the most part, our adult weights are pretty constant. Something is regulating them; there is evidence that we are defending a set point (18). As we will see below, this regulation is skewed toward prevention of weight loss rather than avoidance of weight gain.

Any theory describing set point mechanisms must be able to describe three components: some characteristic that the body monitors, some kind of messenger to carry the information to the central nervous system, and some mechanism of response to exert the control (19). Evidence suggests that fatness, lean body mass, and body mass in general are all monitored. We devote our major attention here to the possible mechanisms of response, the actual regulation. The only options for exerting this control are (1) changing the amount of energy ingested, or (2) changing the efficiency with which we utilize the ingested and stored energy.

The concept of a set point for body weight or composition is still controversial. Some of the controversy involves the question of set point versus set range. Other experts debate *what* characteristic (weight, fat, or lean body mass) is under regulation. Still others resist the concept because they feel it discourages individual responsibility for one's own health behaviors. The importance of these controversies is that they do not refute the basic concept.

Food intake adjustments are part of set point. In discussing the regulation of food intake, one aspect of set point control was identified. When an individual's weight or fatness is below what the body perceives as appropriate, the drive to eat is activated (20). Although the person will experience short-term satiety, this long-term hunger drive apparently is maintained as long as the lower weight exists. Although an individual may learn to ignore this drive, there is no evidence that it goes away, and the ability to ignore or tolerate it is vulnerable to disinhibition. It seems to take effort and attention to resist this hunger drive. People don't always have the psychological energy to devote to this resistance.

Some people come back from a holiday or other situation during which they overate and gained weight, saying "I ate so much then that I'm just not hungry now." Unfortunately, this type of hunger adjustment is rare. It's much more com-

set point
a natural level (of some characteristic) that the body regulates or defends

mon for people to experience their usual degree of hunger and usual intake even after a period of overeating. The regulation system works poorly, if at all, in limiting food intake in this situation. Fortunately, the energy utilization efficiency part of regulation works somewhat better.

Adjustments in energy use as set point regulation. The body can adjust the efficiency of energy use numerous ways; we examine only a few here. We may think first of digestion and absorption as means of regulating how much food energy gets into the body. However, these do not seem to be primary mechanisms of control.

A much better candidate is the rate of energy metabolism. This is implemented primarily in adjustments in the basal metabolic rate (BMR); the level of the thermic effect of food and the energy cost of a given amount of physical activity are probably affected as well. Researchers in numerous laboratories have demonstrated that reduced food intake produces a prompt and significant depression in BMR (21,22). BMR drops promptly and stays depressed throughout the period of lowered intake. If the reduction in intake is not too great, the drop in BMR may be sufficient to prevent weight loss—we would call this a successful defense of set point. With greater dietary restriction, weight is lost, producing a departure from set point (at least temporarily). When weight is lost, there is less body to use energy; this also depresses BMR. Thus these adjustments greatly slow the rate of weight loss. Most often the weight is then regained.

Fig. 10-8 shows the responses of six obese patients who reduced their intake from over 3000 to 450 kcalories for three weeks. BMR has been estimated by measuring the oxygen consumption in liters per hour (this works because the amount

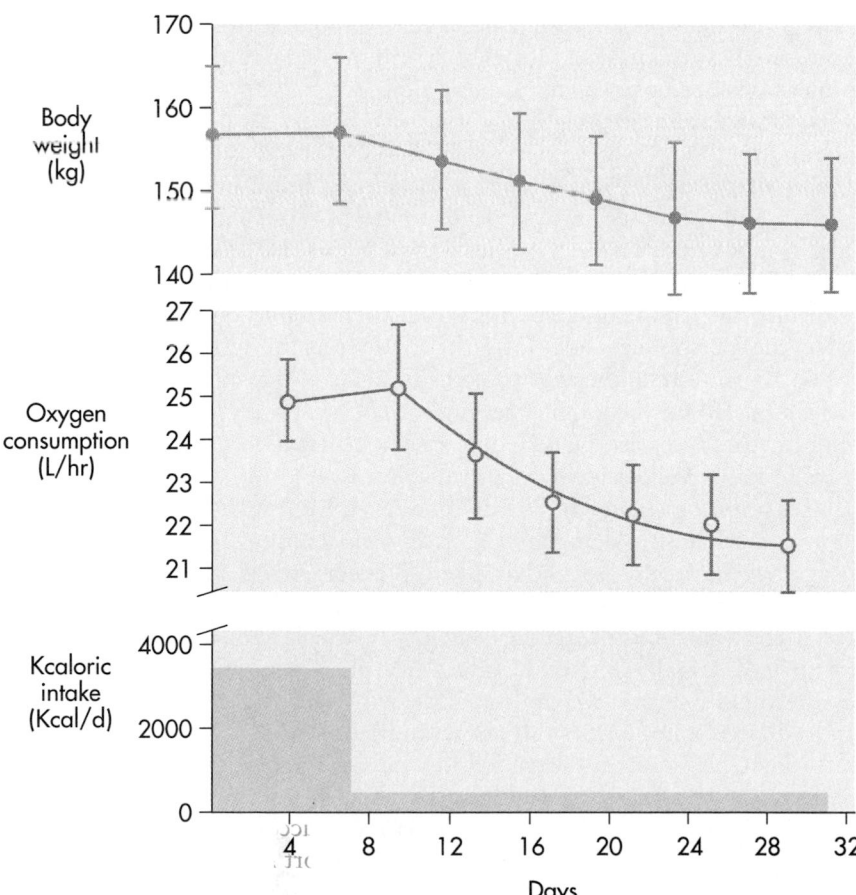

Fig. 10-8 Effect of reduced kcalorie intake on BMR.

of oxygen we use is in direct proportion to the amount of energy being used for basal metabolic activities).

The BMR effect shown in Fig. 10-8 occurs whenever food intake is reduced significantly—in dieters, in victims of disasters, in those suffering from illness, in anyone whose food intake is reduced. Currently there is some concern that yo-yo dieters, persons who repeatedly diet and lose weight only to regain, may lose the ability to raise their BMRs during the regain phase, making it ever harder to lose weight and maintain the loss. At this time there is not good evidence from research to demonstrate that this failure of BMR recovery occurs.

Before leaving Fig. 10-8, note one more point: the vertical lines that extend on either side of each point represent the variability in the response of the six patients. The range from the greatest to least value is usually as great as the overall average effect— a reminder of the high level of individual variability in energy efficiency.

Longer studies have shown that the BMR stays depressed as long as the weight loss is maintained. This means that one's usual amount of food will go further than it did before. One will now gain weight on intakes that previously supported a steady weight. The body is fighting to preserve itself, defending its set point. Although the amount of depression in BMR seems relatively small to have such an effect, we must remember that BMR represents energy expenditure in every second of every day; it adds up fast.

Ordinarily, excursions into overeating trigger an increase in BMR. In many people this increase is sufficient enough that they can overeat periodically without gaining weight. In that case we would say that the set point had been successfully defended. On the other hand, there are limits to the ability to expand BMR, and if overconsumption is sustained, weight gain usually occurs and the set point is reestablished at a higher level.

What determines the set point range? Are we born with our regulatory systems set for slenderness or fatness? Just what determines set point? Definitive answers to these questions are not available at this time but we can explore some probable answers. Observations of weight histories suggest that set point ranges are mainly a matter of the body's adjustment to the maximum size or fatness achieved. The combination of each person's genetic makeup, cultural heritage, environmental experience, and voluntary behavior leads to the development of his/her adult body size and composition. The body seems to assess this size and composition and use it to establish set point. This is easiest to understand in the case of adipocytes. Once formed they are maintained for life. If their size becomes smaller than usual (because the person has lost fat), the body sets in motion the mechanisms described above to refill the cells to their usual size. This means that set point can easily be adjusted upward. One's set point may be at a level of fatness that seems too high or too low. Clearly, set point weight or fatness is not synonymous with what we usually consider ideal or desirable levels.

Can set point be changed? The discussion above has shown that the set point regulatory mechanisms dampen the effects of changes in eating and exercise. However, we have also seen that the set point effects can be overridden by consistent changes in voluntary behaviors of eating and exercise. If these behaviors lead to a consistent positive energy balance, we will gain fat and adjust our set points upward. Usually this seems to be a true change in set point; the new level of fatness becomes one that we can maintain without a great deal of effort and we return to it after minor excursions above and below.

Unfortunately, the situation related to a negative energy balance is not parallel. As we have shown, those rare enduring weight losses seem to be maintained only through continuing effort. True, some people are successful in altering their environment and in changing their habits so that the effort required is manageable, but effort is still required.

Exposure to toxic substances may reduce energy efficiency and/or hunger so that it appears that the set point has been lowered. Cigarette smoking is a prime example. Chronic smokers on the average weigh somewhat less than nonsmokers, and quitting smoking is usually associated with a gain of 6 to 9 lb before the set point becomes reestablished at a new level. It is ironic that, although smoking is usually a far greater health risk than fatness, many smokers report that fear of weight gain prevents them from stopping.

Aerobic exercise is often mentioned as a way of adjusting the set point downward. Although it is true that such exercise increases energy expenditure and may raise BMR, this effect lasts only as long the individual continues to exercise faithfully. So the individual is still having to work hard to maintain the lower status, and it does not seem that set point has really been changed. Nevertheless, exercise is an important factor in fat management and is discussed later in this chapter.

Scientists have looked for factors that would change set point by affecting the rate of breakdown or synthesis of storage fat in adipocytes. Many enzymes and other factors influence these processes, but the search for a factor that could be externally controlled without bodily harm has not been successful to date.

Set point is not the whole story. This discussion of set point has focused on physiological factors regulating fatness. As important as these factors are, we must not lose sight of the fact that one's level of fatness is influenced by environmental and psychosocial influences as well. In fact, because the physiological influences are basically beyond our control, we usually focus on these other factors. Nevertheless, set point often helps us understand what is going on with our weights.

When Body Fatness Deviates From Usual:
Obesity and Eating Disorders

In spite of these various regulatory systems, our population includes many people whose fatness deviates from usual, resulting in obesity or emaciation. Although emaciation may be due to illness or poverty, we are especially concerned with the eating disorder anorexia nervosa, a psychological disorder characterized by extreme voluntarily induced weight loss. One tends to think of obesity and anorexia nervosa as opposites, but in fact they are more appropriately considered as points along a continuum (see Fig. 12-3).

The individuals shown in this continuum differ in their amount of fat, but they tend to have in common a discontent or even anxiety about their size and appearance. At any point along the continuum we may find binge eating or binge/purge behavior. In addition, other than the very low intakes associated with anorexia, the position on the continuum is not predictive of the amount of food eaten. For example, a bulimic individual (midway on the continuum) may be consuming much more than an obese person who does not engage in binge/purge behavior. It is not at all unusual for individuals to occupy various positions all along this continuum at various times in their lives. A preteen girl may become chubby, start a dieting pattern that gets out of control, develop anorexia, move into binge/purge behavior, and under treatment stabilize at a slightly overfat state. Chapter 12 deals more thoroughly with eating disorders, so we focus on obesity here.

Incidence of obesity

If someone asks, "what is the incidence of obesity in the United States?" the answer would depend on the definition of obesity and the age, gender, and ethnicity of those studied. If we use an obesity definition of BMI > 27.5 (a definition that includes not only those frankly obese but also those with mild obesity) and apply that definition to adult Americans in general, we find that roughly 26% meet the criterion (23). Generally, more women than men are overweight, especially for those living in poverty. The incidence usually increases with age, up to about age 55 for men and age 65 for women, and is higher among ethnic minorities, especially

African-American and Hispanic-American women. The higher incidence among ethnic minorities seems to reflect combined genetic and environmental influences. Generally, the incidence of obesity is inversely related to socioeconomic status.

It is especially alarming that the incidence of obesity has increased sharply in recent decades. Currently about 20% of children and adolescents are at least mildly obese—that represents an increase of 39% to 54% in the last 20 years (24). A significant portion of obese young people grow to be obese adults. Add to those early-onset obese persons those who become obese as adults and it appears that the incidence will continue to increase (15,24).

When researchers analyzed data from a large longitudinal study sponsored by the US government to see who was most likely to experience significant weight gains over 10 years, the findings included the following (25):
- Compared with men, women were twice as likely to gain
- The age span from 25 to 34 years was the most likely time for gains
- People already somewhat overfat were most likely to gain more

The *Healthy People 2000* health objectives for our nation include an objective to reduce the incidence of obesity among adults to 20%. Most experts think it is highly unlikely that this objective will be met.

Success of attempts to lose weight

Ironically, during the time reflected in the statistics above, Americans were busily engaged in trying to lose weight. At any one time, about a third of American adults (and even higher percentages of women) are trying to lose weight, primarily through diet and exercise but also through surgery, jaw wiring, pills, hypnosis, acupuncture, sweating devices, and other systems (2). Although many of the commercial programs and products don't release data on the long-term effectiveness of their system, none of those on which data is available produce significant weight losses that are sustained for periods of more than a year in the majority of people trying them. If we ignore for now the downright fraudulent methods and consider only those systems designed to induce a negative calorie balance through reduced intake and/or increased activity, we find that although losing weight is not easy, maintenance is the real pitfall (23,26).

If the members of this class were polled, many would probably report they have dieted to lose weight. Typically, most attempts will have lasted only a few days, but there will be some members who will have stuck with it for some time. They will have worked hard for many weeks, denying their hunger, sticking to their restrictive diet, and increasing their exercise. Usually the losses average about 15 lb. Most of those who lost weight will report that they started regaining almost immediately after leaving the diet (and some will confess that they gained even while continuing to diet). Consistent with the findings of long-term follow-up studies, most will return to their original weights within a few months. Within 5 years, all the weight will have been gained back.

Probably some members of the class will report numerous very short efforts to lose weight—three days on a crash diet and a loss of 3 lb. By the end of the next week the 3 lb were right back. The scale said they lost 3 lb, but if we examined their body composition we would find that the loss was largely water. The typical popular reducing diet is lower in salt and in carbohydrate than the level to which the dieter is accustomed. Both salt and carbohydrate cause the body to retain water, so when we reduce their intake we excrete water and appear to have lost weight. This effect is especially dramatic in the first days of a diet. These fluid losses can be very quickly replaced and the weight returns to the original level.

Table 10-3 summarizes the successfulness of a variety of weight loss efforts. With the exception of stomach surgery, none of the methods has a lasting effect for most people who try them, and all have side effects that cannot be dismissed lightly. Our cure rates for cancer are better than our long-term success with treating obesity.

Table 10-3   Effectiveness of Weight Loss Programs

	All Diets	VLCD*	Fenfluramine & Phentermine†	Diet Pills	Stomach Bypass (Very Obese Only)
Initial Loss	▲▲▲	▲▲▲▲	▲▲▲	▲▲	▲▲▲▲
Dropout Rate	▼▼▼	▼▼▼▼	▼▼	▼▼▼	not applicable
Success Rate	0	0	▲▲	0	▲▲▲
Regain	▼▼▼▼	▼▼▼▼	▼▼	▼▼▼▼	▼▼
Side Effects	▼▼▼	▼▼▼	▼▼	▼▼▼▼	▼▼▼
Cost		inexpensive		inexpensive	expensive
Time Scale For Initial Loss	weeks	months	weeks	weeks	months
Overall	▲	▲	▲▲	0	▲▲▲ ‡

From Seligman MEP: *What you can change and what you can't*, New York, 1993, Alfred A. Knopf.

Initial Loss: ▲▲▲▲ = 80%-100% lose 20 or more pounds
　　　　　　　▲▲▲ = 60%-80% lose 10-20 pounds
　　　　　　　▲▲ = at least 50% lose some weight
　　　　　　　▲ = probably better than nothing
Dropout Rate: ▼▼▼▼ = 55% or more drop out
　　　　　　　▼▼▼ = 40%-55% drop out
　　　　　　　▼▼ = 20%-40% drop out
　　　　　　　▼ = less than 20% drop out
Regain:　　　▼▼▼▼ = 50% or more regain most of their weight
　　　　　　　▼▼▼ = 30%-50% regain most of their weight
　　　　　　　▼▼ = 10%-30% regain most of their weight
　　　　　　　▼ = less than 10% regain
Success Rate: ▲▲▲▲ = 80% remain at the reduced weight 3 years later
　　　　　　　▲▲▲ = 60% remain at the reduced weight 3 years later
　　　　　　　▲▲ = 40% remain at the reduced weight 3 years later
　　　　　　　▲ = 20% remain at the reduced weight 3 years later
　　　　　　　0 = 0%-20% remain at the reduced weight 3 years later
Side Effects　▼▼▼▼ = severe
　　　　　　　▼▼▼ = moderate
　　　　　　　▼▼ = mild
　　　　　　　▼ = none
Overall:　　　▲▲▲▲ = excellent, clearly the therapy of choice
　　　　　　　▲▲▲ = very good
　　　　　　　▲▲ = useful
　　　　　　　▲ = marginal to useless
　　　　　　　0 = useless

*VLCD = very-low-calorie diet
†Insufficient research has been done on the safety and effectiveness of fenfluramine and phentermine. The table is my best guess about their effectiveness. I regard them as for experimental purposes only at this stage of development.
‡NB: Because the surgical patients, unlike patients in the other treatments, come entirely from a superobese group (100% or more of ideal weight), I have allowed "reduced weight" for them to mean a 60% loss in excess weight. On this liberal basis, gastric bypass gets two and a half upward pointers.

You probably know someone who has dieted repeatedly, who never eats without feeling guilty, and yet who remains fat. Dieting changes eating from a simple, enjoyable process into something complicated and laden with guilt and other moral overtones. Hunger is interpreted as temptation, and responding to it becomes evidence of weakness or even sin. After repeatedly denying the call of hunger, most dieters lose touch with the sensations of hunger. Hunger becomes confused with being tired, bored, sad, or other feelings. Dieters rarely eat to satiety; they either force themselves to stop short of satisfaction or they become disinhibited and eat far beyond satiety (27). Their physiological regulatory cues are completely tuned out. They usually develop two lists of foods: *virtuous* ones that they eat when they *are being good* and *forbidden* foods that are constant pitfalls. Rather than increasing the ability to regulate food intake to meet body needs, dieting makes this regulation more precarious.

Certainly one of the harmful aspects of repeated dieting is the sense of personal failure that accompanies the almost inevitable weight gains. Dieters feel pressured by not only those with a commercial interest but also by health care professionals, friends, and family to try every new weight-loss plan that comes along. Most plans do produce initial losses, and dieters are lured into thinking that significant and lasting losses are obtainable. Dieters ignore the powerful and automatic adjustments in metabolism and hunger drive that weight loss triggers. Bodies naturally adjust to restore the lost fat. When the weight comes back, dieters may internalize the failure of their diets and suffer feelings of inadequacy that spread to other areas of their lives.

Gain/loss cycles are not benign; they may lead to nutritional inadequacies, confused food habits, loss of sensitivity to physiological hunger cues, diminished self-confidence and loss of self-esteem, and to greater susceptibility to the health risks associated with obesity.

It's time for some new approaches

This book takes a nontraditional stance regarding attempts to change body composition. The authors, convinced that diets (even the good ones) don't work, have instead chosen to share an approach that emphasizes acceptance of diversity in body size and shape and puts emphasis, not on achieving ideal body composition, but instead upon promotion of wellness, personal satisfaction, and well-being. It is our philosophy that, except for acute medical conditions, it is inappropriate to give weight-loss advice. Instead, the fat, the thin, and the in-between all can benefit by adopting attitudes and behaviors that over time should promote the body composition appropriate to each individual's genetic makeup and contribute to true wellness. To emphasize the lifelong nature of this approach, we will refer to maintenance approaches rather than to efforts to change body composition.

DEVELOPING A PERSONAL APPROACH FOR MAINTAINING AN ACCEPTABLE BODY COMPOSITION

Gain, Lose, or Maintain: a Wellness Approach For Everyone

Although it is untrue that we can mold our bodies to any size or shape we desire, we do have the power to change our attitudes and behaviors if needed so that we can achieve satisfaction and wellness at the body composition most natural for each of us. This section describes some guidelines that are equally applicable to nurses and to their patients who are fat, thin, or just right. We draw on ideas advanced by a number of specialists who support what they call *a non-diet approach* (28-30). All of the behaviors recommended focus on long-term changes. Those who adopt these attitudes and implement these behaviors can expect to feel more comfortable with their bodies and probably better about themselves in general. If we eat well and are physically active, we will look and feel good. Body fatness may or may not change. Although this approach may seem discouraging, the harmful and disheartening effects of diets and other programs that promise a lot but deliver only worse problems will be avoided. Appendix G, kCalorie-Restricted Dietary Patterns, provides dietary procedures for those few people who have a serious health condition justifying the risks of traditional weight-loss efforts.

Establishing Realistic Goals

In setting goals, we must consider two almost opposing factors: (1) our unique and individual values, needs, and characteristics and (2) the limits to the extent of control we have over our bodies and our level of fatness. It is fashionable to deny any limits to this control, but objective observation will reveal the fallacy in that thinking. Aspiring to total control, however, is neither realistic nor healthy for most of us. In goal-setting we need to consider what is practically feasible.

Changing behavior

The most important goals are those related to changes in behavior. By choosing appropriate behaviors for change we can work toward establishing habits that will become almost self-sustaining. The behavioral goals should be related to each person's unique needs. For example, one person in examining his lifestyle may discover that he is always out of food and running out to grab whatever he can find handy, usually pizza and convenience store items. He may try to establish a habit of planning and shopping for the next week every Sunday afternoon. For him this behavior change automatically leads to better food choices; for a different person, this particular goal might be irrelevant.

The Teaching Tool on p. 264 outlines basic principles of behavioral modification applicable to choosing appropriate changes.

In recent decades it has become popular to make superficial use of the principles of behavioral change in weight-loss programs. These techniques have had limited success because they were presented as just a list of handy hints (eat on a smaller plate, put down the fork between bites, etc.) rather than the individualized system described in the box. Don't confuse these principles with those hints having very little to do with the original concepts.

Normalizing Eating

The goal here is to reclaim eating as a comfortable and natural process. It involves being in tune with one's body's needs and its signals about those needs.

Enjoying eating

Normal eating is an enjoyable process. Eating is a very sensual process and has the potential to be highly pleasant. Unfortunately, the ubiquitous dieting mentality dictates a love-hate relationship with food. Those foods we most love, we label sinful and declare off-limits. Then we long for them and feel dissatisfied with the more ordinary foods we allow ourselves.

In normalizing eating we strive to retain the enjoyment of the process. This involves eating with awareness, relaxation, and without guilt, allowing ourselves to eat in appropriate quantities all the foods we enjoy. It also may involve expanding our pleasure by learning to enjoy a wider variety of foods.

TEACHING TOOL
Principles of Behavior Change

1. ***Set a positive, specific, and achievable objective.*** It is helpful to frame a goal in terms of the exact behavior to be practiced. Objectives like "I want to eat better" or "I don't want to be so inactive" fail to give you any guidance about how to achieve them and what constitutes success. On the other hand, an objective such as eating vegetarian meals five times per week can orient you in a helpful direction right from the start. It is easier to replace a behavior with a new one than to just stop doing it. Break major behaviors down into smaller, less daunting parts and try only a few changes at a time.

2. ***Establish a system for monitoring the behavior to be changed.*** This observation helps to assess success in changing the behavior and assists in determining what contributes to and detracts from mastery.

3. ***Modify the environment so that it supports the change.*** If you're trying to eat more vegetarian meals, for instance, it would be helpful if the environment included vegetarian cookbooks and ingredients and opportunities to be with vegetarian friends.

4. ***Set up a plan for rewarding successes.*** Be sure to choose rewards that will be appreciated but are appropriate to the magnitude of the achievement. The reward should be as immediate as possible. Long-range rewards can seem immediate by awarding points toward the reward.

5. ***Recruit support from friends and family.*** These people may want to be helpful but may not be very skilled at it. Tell them of your objectives and how they can help, but do not make them responsible for personal behavior.

6. ***Allow enough time for a new behavior to become habit.*** A simple new behavior, like taking smaller bites, practiced faithfully for 3 weeks should be well on the way to becoming habit. More complex lifestyle behaviors take much longer, usually at least 4 months, to change. Under stress, most of us revert to old habits, so have a plan for how to deal with this.

Enjoyment can be enhanced by keeping meals and snacks simple enough that the true flavors of each item can be tasted. Not only do toppings, sauces, and the like usually involve the addition of extra sugars and fats, but they also obscure flavors.

In spite of all this emphasis on enjoyment, normal eating does not mean depending on food as a major source of pleasure. Just as drinking a long, cool glass of water is a joy when we are thirsty (but is without appeal when we're not thirsty), eating should be a natural source of pleasure and not a preoccupation. We are not advocating that we all live to eat.

Letting hunger and satiety guide eating

As discussed earlier in this chapter, most of us guide our eating not only by physiological cues to hunger and satiety, but also by environmental and cognitive factors. Of these three sets of stimuli, only the physiological cues are triggered by the body's needs. Therefore normalizing eating involves letting hunger and satiety guide eating. It means eating when hungry even if it is not a traditional meal time, and it means stopping with the first signs of satiety even if there is still food on the plate.

Although it would seem that eating this way would be easy, trying to implement this advice is clearly challenging. A person may fear that if the cognitive control that tells us what we *should* be eating is relinquished, all control will be lost and huge amounts eaten. A few people actually do go through such a period—a pretty scary experience. Nevertheless, when they trust that they can eat again as soon as hunger dictates, most find that they are no longer driven to continue eating such large quantities (31).

A great many people actually have a different problem—they have ignored their hunger/satiety cues for so long that they no longer sense them. To reverse this lack of awareness involves relearning how to feel and identify the body's signals for hunger and satiety. An individual can start this process by carefully noting feelings when several hours pass without eating. Then interrupt a meal midway and examine body sensations for satiety cues. A few minutes will be needed to perceive the satiety. If there are no cues to satiety continue eating, stopping again and assessing after a few more bites.

Most people are less aware of their satiety signals than of hunger cues. Eating slowly may enhance awareness of satiety. Keeping meals and snacks simple may help, too. Some research indicates that there is a component of satiety tied to specific tastes: the greater variety, the more food is required to reach satiety because each component is activated by the array of sensations. This may be responsible for eating behaviors at generous buffets.

Sensations of hunger are often confused with those of tiredness, anxiety, relief of anxiety, and other states. Distinguishing the difference may require work. It may be helpful to keep a journal of the various sensations observed.

Minimizing the use of food to meet emotional needs

Probably all humans use food and eating to help them deal with emotions. We use food for expressing positive feelings, celebrating good fortune, rewarding hard work, and creating a sense of companionship. Eating as a means of handling negative emotions such as boredom, frustration, anger, or loneliness is especially problematic for many people. Compared to some other ways of responding to strong emotions, eating may be relatively benign, but when we rely on it as our main means of coping, our consumption patterns may have little or no relationship to our physiological needs. This emotion-driven eating often is followed by feelings of guilt that may feed into the original negative feelings, creating a destructive cycle.

Minimizing emotional eating requires being aware of feelings and any associated eating. For personal understanding or as an adjunct to patient education, a journal or eating record can help achieve this awareness by monitoring feelings, hunger, and eating. Records kept for several weeks catch a range of moods. Examine the records from both the perspectives of what triggered eating and of how the feelings were expressed or coped with.

When we practice eating in response to hunger, we will probably use food less to meet emotional needs. However, if a pattern of eating in response to feelings still occurs rather than in response to hunger, or if we regularly use food to deal with certain emotions, we need to learn some alternative ways to respond to emotions. We can often be our own best resource for discovering alternative responses by using the records to identify coping behaviors that are already working and that can be used more often. The resource list in Appendix C includes several books that deal with making these kind of changes. Counseling can also help.

Since we are probably never going to give up completely using food to meet emotional needs, it's worth considering how to do so effectively. These guidelines may help:

1. Be aware of the reasons behind food use. Verbalize the function intended for the food to serve. Eat food slowly and with concentration.
2. Eat without guilt. If this type of eating occurs only rarely, there is nothing about which to feel guilty.
3. Arrange a *safe* circumstance for eating. If some rich, creamy chocolate is just the thing needed, that's fine. Have some, but make sure there is no danger of overdoing it. Buy just one piece, eat in public, or do whatever is necessary to ensure that a reasonable amount can be enjoyed without feeling at risk of bingeing.

The box on p. 266 describes how the Food Guide Pyramid can be useful in helping clients establish healthy eating habits to manage body composition.

TEACHING TOOL
Making Healthy Food Choices

A major characteristic of normal, nondiet eating is the attention given to making healthy food choices. The Food Guide Pyramid is a helpful guide in making such choices, conveying the idea that some types of food (at the base of the pyramid) should be eaten in much greater quantities than those at the top of the pyramid (see Fig. 2-2). When helping clients toward more healthful management of body composition, consider using the Food Guide Pyramid.

The pyramid emphasizes low-fat foods as the mainstay of dietary intake. Since high-fat foods have such a high energy content, it is difficult to gauge the amount needed to satisfy hunger; minor errors in estimation mount up quickly. Therefore an effective food plan should be relatively low in fat, with about 30% of kcalories coming from fat. If a person has energy needs of 1600 kcalories, that person would limit fat intake to about 50 grams, whereas another person needing 2200 kcalories would aim for no more than 73 grams of fat. Leaf through the food composition table in Appendix A to get an idea of how various foods contribute to the fat content. The nu-trition label also describes fat content in easily used terms.

Low-fat, low-sugar foods should be chosen from each pyramid section. Ideally, hunger should guide decisions as to the number of servings to eat each day.

Many people are surprised that the pyramid contains so many servings of starchy foods and so little meat. This makes sense when considering that carbohydrate and protein are equal in kcaloric value and that, unlike most meats, starchy foods are usually low in fat (unless fat is added). Eating according to the pyramid guidelines means choosing more meatless meals and making sure that vegetables and fruits are available. This takes planning, but it can become a way of life.

No food is excluded from the pyramid, but there are definite distinctions between everyday foods and occasional foods that tend to be lower in nutrient density and higher in sugar and fat. Most of us have our own personal list of occasional foods, ones that we want to continue to enjoy only at infrequent times because of their cost, difficulty to find or prepare, or low nutritive value.

Eating regularly and frequently

Our bodies have evolved so that we function best when we eat several times a day at times spaced throughout our waking hours. Unfortunately, our modern hurried lifestyle often makes eating balanced meals inconvenient. We tend to snack on what is handy early in the day and do most of our eating between 5 PM and bedtime. This pattern has several undesirable effects:

- It puts the greatest food intake at the least active time of day. This means that the energy ingested must be stored as fat to await utilization the next day. Since many individuals do not efficiently mobilize stored fat for energy, they probably feel sluggish and curtail their activity the next day.
- It may mean long stretches of time with very little food. During these times we often find it too inconvenient to eat, and so we deny our hunger or stave it off with inadequate snacks. By late afternoon our hunger, now joined by tiredness and frustrations of school and work, overwhelms us, and we eat frantically, often far more than we need. Thus this pattern runs counter to our goal of hunger-directed eating. Furthermore, with little or nothing to break the overnight fast, it's hard to get a good start in the morning.
- The quick meals or snacks we grab during the day usually are high in sodium and fat with little nutritive value.

There is nothing magical about three meals a day. Five may be better. Whatever pattern works best, it should space food throughout active hours and should not produce overwhelming hunger or the drive to consume excessively. For most of us, how often we eat has to reflect the difficulties of providing ourselves with nourishing options throughout the day. Normalizing eating involves planning ahead to assure that we don't get caught with no alternatives to chips and candy bars.

Adopting an Active Lifestyle

Does physical exercise help maintain a desirable body composition? The conclusions from research are contradictory and confusing. A lot of the confusion disappears when distinguishing between what is possible in a controlled laboratory experiment and what is probable in the reality of most peoples' lives. Bear this distinction in mind as we review the importance of physical activity in a wellness program. Although exercise is not a panacea, it is one of the few factors consistently associated with success in maintaining a healthy body composition.

Exercise increases energy expenditure

Exercise is mechanical work that requires energy—it takes more energy to stand than to sit, to walk than to stand, and so on. Furthermore, vigorous exercise has the potential to increase the rate at which energy is used, even beyond the period of activity. However, for the level of exercise most people are able to accommodate in their lives, the daily effect on energy expenditure is in the range of a few hundred calories (33). Most authorities believe that the beneficial effects of exercise are far greater than can be accounted for by the direct effect on energy balance of these few hundred calories.

Exercise promotes maintenance of lean body mass

Many factors conspire to reduce our levels of lean body mass. These include aging, sedentary lifestyles, wasting caused by illness, and dieting. Exercise reduces the effect of these factors.

Exercise improves many health conditions

Exercise reduces a variety of risk factors for hypertension, coronary artery disease, and diabetes mellitus; these are associated at an increased rate with obesity. Yet even without changes in body fat levels, exercise can decrease heart rate, reduce blood pressure, and improve the blood lipid profile.

Exercise changes our outlook

Practically every investigation that has studied people who are successful in long-term maintenance of a healthy body fatness level has found that exercise was an important factor. Its influence can not be accounted for on the basis of a direct effect on energy balance. Instead, exercise seems to help because it changes how people feel about themselves and about their ability to be in charge on their own lives. Regular, enjoyable exercise increases our awareness and level of comfort with our own body. It provides a good time for thinking and problem solving. It reinforces our commitment to wellness and increases the likelihood that other wellness behaviors will be maintained.

Individuals differ in their response to exercise

Two friends exercise together regularly. Only one of them seems to be changing size. They probably differ in their individual response to exercise. In a recent study of such differences, 31 obese women faithfully exercised for 90 minutes a day 4 or 5 times a week (33). They didn't change their way of eating. After 6 months, two thirds of the women had decreased levels of body fat, whereas the other women had increased levels. Both groups had improved cardiorespiratory fitness, carbohydrate metabolism, and blood lipid profiles. And women in both groups deserved to feel proud of their accomplishments.

Differences in the response to exercise may be related to gender, fat distribution patterns, ability to exercise vigorously, and appetite response to exercise (34). We must remember that our bodies respond differently and that our level of fatness is a poor indicator of the beneficial effects of exercise.

The exercise must suit the individual

Most of the health benefits of exercise are maintained only as long as the exercise is continued regularly. Therefore it is alarming that most people who start an exercise program drop out. Although many factors undoubtedly contribute to this picture, a major one involves attempting exercise that is too difficult for one's physical condition. This is especially true for older or heavier individuals. Driven by sayings such as "it doesn't count if it isn't aerobic" or "no pain, no gain," regimens may be attempted that are initially too demanding. The goal is to do 30 minutes or so of aerobic exercise three or more times a week. Time can be taken to work up to that level. An exercise diary is a good way to monitor one's progress.

We are more likely to exercise if we have access to a variety of activities we enjoy such as walking, swimming, biking, gardening, sports, or even housecleaning—there are lots of options.

OVERCOMING BARRIERS

Prospects for the Future

Will there come a time during our lifetime when no one will have to worry about being too fat, too thin, or too displeasingly shaped? There are several avenues that could lead to such a future—we could learn how to *prevent* deviations from healthy amounts and distributions of fat, we could learn how to effectively *treat* them, or we could become so *accepting* of individual differences that deviations were no longer defined as problems. All avenues will probably be important, but even together they probably will be insufficient to lead to such a future.

MYTH
One Size Fits All

Health professionals may not be aware of ways that their practices fail to meet the needs of their large patients. To assist these professionals, the National Association for the Advancement of Fat Acceptance (NAAFA) has developed the following suggestions:

Office environment
- Provide chairs that are sturdy and armless, with sufficient space between the chairs to accommodate large patients.
- Use wide examining tables bolted to the floor or wall; this prevents tipping when a larger patient sits or gets off the table.
- Offer a solid, secure stool to assist patients getting onto the examining table.

- Have available super-large examining gowns. (One size does not fit all.)

Medical and weight procedures
- Have available blood pressure cuffs in several sizes to prevent false readings.
- Have access to longer needles and tourniquets to draw blood appropriately.
- Provide lavatories with split seats in front to allow large patients to more easily gather urine for specimen collection.
- Weigh patients only if necessary. Do so in a private setting and record weight without commentary. Do not assume that weight is the cause of the patient's condition or the focus of the health visit.

From National Association for the Advancement of Fat Acceptance: *Guidelines for health care providers in dealing with fat patients,* Sacramento, Calif, 1994, NAAFA.

Some Trends are Alarming

Recently we have learned of two alarming trends among the children of this country. Children even in the lowest grades of school are already obsessed with their weight and frequently place themselves on diets, yet there is a significantly increased incidence of obesity among our children. Parents, teachers, and health care professionals usually feel at a loss as to how to deal with this combination. The instinctive response is to restrict the child's intake, but the evidence overwhelmingly indicates that response only creates a terror of not getting enough to eat and contributes to a sense of being ugly and generally unacceptable.

It is not clear what has led to these trends among children, but many suspect that physical inactivity accompanied by a rather generalized passivity may be involved. Furthermore, children are not free of the cultural messages that equate slenderness with happiness—thus the early diets.

Americans want to be physically active, but we are working longer hours and spending more time getting to work or school. When our work days are over, concerns about the safety of our neighborhoods may keep us inside and inactive. It will be interesting to see the impact on physical activity of new communication technologies that allow more people to work at home.

As our country's demographics change, we will have more ethnic diversity. We know that there are major ethnic differences in the incidence of obesity and of eating disorders. However, what causes these differences is unclear, and we certainly are not prepared to deal with them.

Multiple etiologies complicate treatment and prevention

"Coming soon—a drug to cure fatness." This title may appear in the tabloids, but the likelihood of a medication that could reverse all types of obesity (or emaciation) is unlikely because there are too many different causes. One textbook lists about 40 different models of obesity* demonstrated in laboratory animals (32). Humans living in *the real world* are much more complex. Even within a single individual there are numerous factors contributing to fatness level. At one time doctors thought that giving thyroid hormone would reverse all obesity, but experience proved that only a small proportion of individuals were good candidates. Some people lost weight with thyroid treatments, only to regain in response to other factors. The administration of medications may be helpful in some situations, but a pharmaceutical cure-all is unlikely. Likewise, prevention efforts will have to be multifaceted to address all the factors involved.

Prevention efforts may lead to more acceptance

At this time it seems that prevention is our best hope for a better future, fatness-wise. Effective prevention has to encourage behaviors that promote total wellness on a long-term basis. Experience is demonstrating that this requires that people view themselves as valuable and worthy of effort. The Vitality campaign mounted by the Canadian Ministry of National Health and Welfare is a good example of this approach (35). Designed to promote healthy weights, the Vitality program urges Canadians to feel good about themselves, eat well, and be active (see Appendix F). Nutritionists in the state of California have incorporated similar concepts in a statewide cooperative effort to change perspectives about children and weight (36). Thus as more such programs are launched, we may see that good prevention campaigns also lead down the avenue of greater acceptance of individual differences in body size, shape, and fatness.

---

* Although the work demonstrating the multiple etiology of obesity is much more advanced, there is increasing evidence of similar complexity of cause in situations of extreme thinness.

TOWARD A POSITIVE NUTRITION LIFESTYLE: EXPLANATORY STYLE

In his book, *Learned Optimism*, Dr. Seligman, a psychologist and professor, explores applications of explanatory styles to everyday life situations (37). As a component of personal control, explanatory style is the way in which a person regularly explains why events happen. An individual with a pessimistic explanatory style spreads learned helplessness by having a pervasive negative view that no matter what he or she does, nothing will change. In contrast, a person with an optimistic explanatory style feels able to stop the reaction of learned helplessness and understands events in a more positive way. An optimistic person feels competent that he or she can change the course of events.

Explanatory style has been studied in relation to health and wellness. A person's approach to dealing with issues of physical health can be helped or hindered by cognitions about personal control over health conditions and maintenance. As Seligman notes:

- The way we think, especially about health, changes our health.
- Optimists catch fewer infectious diseases than pessimists do.
- Optimists have better health habits than pessimists do.
- Our immune system may work better when we are optimistic.
- Evidence suggests that optimists live longer than pessimists.

How does this apply to body fat management? Having an optimistic explanatory style may mean accepting one's body as it is and acting in ways to improve health by attempting to eat well and exercise regularly. A pessimistic explanatory style would judge one's body negatively and would not attempt behaviors to improve body composition because physical attributes would be understood to be permanent and so unchangeable. Consider other ways that explanatory styles impact on the approach of our patients toward their illnesses and the effect of our explanatory styles on strategies of nursing care.

WELLNESS AND MANAGEMENT OF BODY FAT LEVELS

Physical Dimension	Managing body fat levels by decreasing or increasing, if appropriate, is an aspect of the physical dimension of health. Adequate levels of body fat allow the body to function most efficiently.
Intellectual Dimension	Intellectual dimension of health provides the skills to understand and critique the role of society in molding our attitudes toward the shapes of our bodies.
Emotional Dimension	Regardless of our body size, our emotional health depends on our developing positive self-esteem.
Social Dimension	The social dimension of health may not be affected by body fat levels, although those at either extreme of body size may need to develop a circle of friends and family who are accepting of their size differences.

SUMMARY

Lifelong management of body fat levels provides a more holistic health approach to body size than does body weight. Management is defined as the use of available resources to achieve a predetermined goal. This definition recognizes that individuals differ in the resources available to them and in the goals they set. Goals for body fat levels must take into account an individual's genetic and family factors as well as those of society and health.

Ways of measuring body fat composition include densitometry, computed tomography, and bioelectric impedance analysis. In addition to simple body weight, body mass index provides another way to interpret weight levels. Body weight may be maintained by set point, through which the body regulates its most natural and appropriate weight.

Body size, as an issue of health status, is still a concern among many health professionals. Individuals at both extremes of fatness, those very thin and those very fat, are at increased risk for certain health-related disorders. Obesity, however, does not increase all types of health risks nor are all obese individuals ill. Risks of some types of cancer and of osteoporosis are lower for the obese than for others.

Body acceptance is a key to wellness. Biology and culture interact to set standards of body image, perceptions, and social models of attractiveness. Because of individual genetic makeups, different body types and sizes may not fit the cultural ideals. The goal is to reclaim eating as a comfortable and natural process. This means being in tune with one's body's needs and its signals about those needs. A part of body fat level management is the incorporation of regular exercise. Exercise increases energy expenditure, promotes maintenance of lean body mass, improves many health conditions, and changes one's outlook. Differences in bodies' responses to exercise may be related to gender, fat distribution patterns, ability to exercise vigorously, and appetite response to exercise.

Future considerations of body fat level management include prevention of deviations from healthy levels and distributions of fat, development of effective treatments, and/or the cultivation of acceptance of individual differences.

THE NURSING ROLE
Nursing Diagnosis Related to Body Fat Levels

Has the information in this chapter given you some clues about nursing diagnoses for people who are concerned or not concerned about their body fat levels? Several North American Nursing Diagnosis Association (NANDA) categories could be applicable and an even bigger variety of causative factors. For example, the following nursing diagnoses using NANDA labels could apply:

1. Body image disturbance related to acceptance of society's notion of beauty
2. Body image disturbance related to distorted perception of body size
3. Altered health maintenance related to cyclical dieting and regaining of weight
4. Altered nutrition: less than body requirements, related to fear of being fat

Continued.

THE NURSING ROLE, cont'd.

Nursing Diagnosis Related to Body Fat Levels

5. Altered nutrition: more than body requirements, related to loss of satiety awareness
6. Self-esteem disturbance related to failure of repeated diets

Most NANDA diagnoses are geared toward identifying and labeling patient problems. They do not deal with identification of patient strengths and wellness patterns. Many nurses believe that nursing diagnoses should also include positive aspects of a patient's life that should be supported, encouraged, or enhanced by the nurse.

In the instance of body fat levels, the following are examples of nursing diagnoses that emphasize the positive:

1. Acceptance of body image related to positive self-esteem
2. Good health maintenance related to eating well and exercising adequately
3. Good nutrition related to food intake based on the Food Guide Pyramid
4. Positive self-esteem related to personal acceptance of body fat levels

Nurses, along with other health care professionals and the rest of society, need to become more comfortable with the idea that obese people may not need to diet. If they are healthy, their present weight may be their desirable weight. If they are eating well according to the Pyramid and exercising adequately, the nurse's role may be to support their present behavior. Writing *positive* nursing diagnoses in such cases may help health professionals to throw off prejudices and traditional ways of thinking.

REFERENCES

1. Fallon A: Culture in the mirror: Sociocultural determinator of body image. In Cash TF, Pruzinky T, eds: *Body images: Development, deviance, and change*, New York, 1990, Guilford.
2. National Institutes of Health: *Technology assessment conference statement: Methods for voluntary weight loss and control*, Bethesda, Md, 1992, NIH.
3. Thompson JK: *Body image disturbance: Assessment and treatment*, New York, 1990, Pergamon Press.
4. Brownell KD: Personal responsibility and control over our bodies: When expectation exceeds reality, *Health Psychol* 10:303-310, 1991.
5. VanItallie TB: Body weight, morbidity, and longevity. In Björntorp P, Brodoff BN, eds: *Obesity*, Philadelphia, 1992, Lippincott.
6. Berg FM: *Health risks of obesity*, Hettinger, ND, 1993, Healthy Living Institute.
7. National Institutes of Health Consensus Development Statement: *Health implications of obesity*, Bethesda, Md, 1985, NIH.
8. Ernsberger P, Haskew P: Rethinking obesity: An alternative view of its health implications, *Journal of Obesity and Weight Regulation* 6:57-137, 1987.
9. Berg FM: *Health risks of weight loss*, Hettinger ND, 1993, Healthy Living Institute.
10. Stunkard AJ, Wadden TA: Psychological aspects of human obesity. In *Obesity*, Philadelphia, 1992, Lippincott.
11. Heatherton TF, Polivy J, Herman CP: Restraint, weight loss, and variability of body weight, *J Abnorm Psychol* 100:78-83, 1991.
12. McArdle WD, Katch FD, Katch VL: *Essentials of exercise physiology*, Philadelphia, 1994, Lea and Febiger.
13. Björntorp P: The role of adipose tissue in human obesity. In Greenwood MRC, ed: *Obesity*, New York, 1983, Churchill Livingstone.
14. Lakaski HC: Body composition assessment using impedence methods. In Björntorp P, Brodoff BN, eds: *Obesity*, Philadelphia, 1992, Lippincott.

15. Bray GA: An approach to the classification and evaluation of obesity. In Björntorp P, Brodoff BN, eds: *Obesity*, Philadelphia, 1992, Lippincott.

16. Bourchard C, Pérusse L: Genetics of obesity: Family studies. In Bourchard C, ed: *The genetics of obesity*. Boca Raton, Fla, 1994, CRC Press.

17. Meyer JM, Stunkard AJ: Twin studies of human obesity. In Bourchard C, ed: *The genetics of obesity*, Boca Raton, Fla, 1994, CRC Press.

18. Keesey RE: A set-point analysis of the regulation of body weight. In Stunkard AJ, ed: *Obesity*, Philadelphia, 1980, Saunders.

19. Harris RBS: Role of set-point theory in regulation of body weight, *The FASEB Journal* 4:3310-3318, 1990.

20. Martin RJ, White DB, Hulsey MG: The regulation of body weight, *American Scientist* 79:528-541, 1991.

21. Berdanier CD, McIntosh MK: Weight loss—weight regain a vicious cycle, *Nutrition Today* 6-12, 1991.

22. Jéquier E: Regulation of thermogenesis and nutrient metabolism in the human: Relevance for obesity. In Björntorp P, Brodoff BN, eds: *Obesity*, Philadelphia, 1992, Lippincott.

23. Perri MG, Nezu AM, Viegener BJ: *Improving the long-term management of obesity*, New York, 1992, John Wiley & Sons.

24. Dietz W: Increasing child obesity raises concerns over available treatments, *Obesity & Health* 5:41, 1991.

25. Williamson DF et al: The 10-year incidence of overweight and major weight gain in US adults, *Arch Intern Med* 150:665-672, 1990.

26. Seligman MEP: *What you can change and what you can't*, New York, 1994, Alfred A Knopf.

27. Herman CP, Polivy J: A boundary model for the regulation of eating. In Stunkard AJ, Stellar E, eds: *Eating and its disorders*, New York, 1984, Raven Press.

28. Fanning P: *Lifetime weight control*, Oakland, Calif, 1990, New Harbinger.

29. Foreyt JP, Goodrick GK: *Living without dieting*, Houston, 1992, Harrison Publishing.

30. Omichinski L: *You count, calories don't*, Winnipeg, Manitoba, 1993, Tamos Books.

31. Hirschmann JR, Munter CH: *Overcoming overeating*, Reading, Mass, 1988, Addison-Wesley.

32. Björntorp P, Brodoff BN, eds: *Obesity*, Philadelphia, 1992, Lippincott.

33. Lamarche B et al: Is body fat loss a determinant factor in the improvement of carbohydrate and lipid metabolism following aerobic exercise training in obese women? *Metabolism* 41:1249-1256, 1992.

34. Björntorp P: Physical exercise in the treatment of obesity. In Björntorp P, Brodoff BN, eds: *Obesity*, Philadelphia, 1992, Lippincott.

35. Health and Welfare Canada: *Vitality*, Ottawa, Ontario, 1991.

36. Ikeda JP, Peck EB: California takes action on children and weight concerns, *Obesity and Health* 5:39-41, 1991.

37. Seligman MEP: *Learned optimism*, New York, 1991, Alfred A. Knopf.

Chapter 11

LIFE SPAN HEALTH PROMOTION: PREGNANCY, LACTATION, AND INFANCY

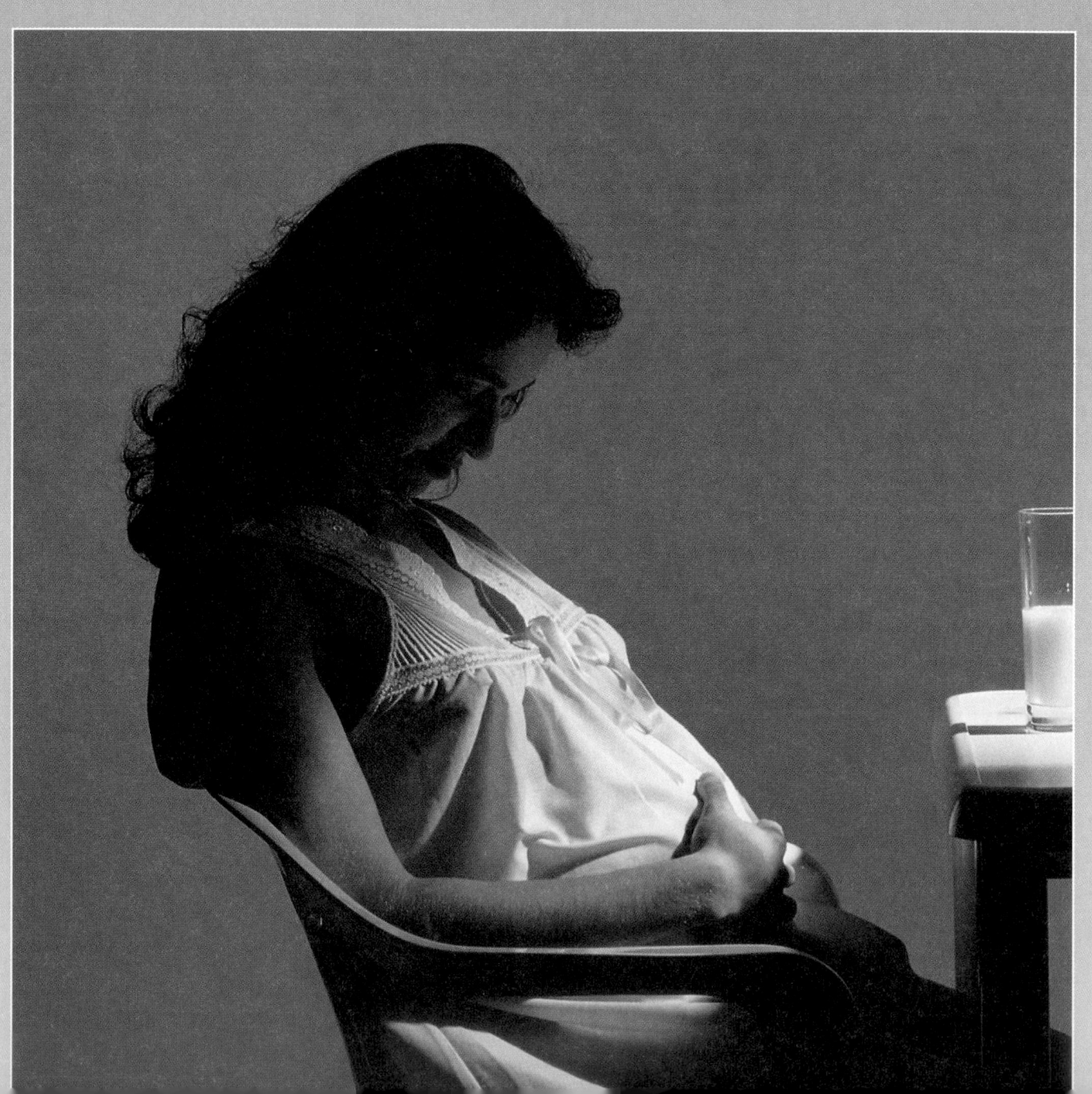

Life span health promotion is the topic of Chapters 11 and 12. These chapters address not only the basic nutrition requirements of pregnancy, infancy, childhood, adolescence, and adulthood through senescence, but also consider the factors affecting health promotion. As presented in Chapter 1, the goal of health promotion is to increase the level of health of individuals, families, and/or communities. Health promotion strategies often focus on lifestyle changes leading to new positive health behaviors.

Development of these behaviors may depend on knowledge, techniques, and community supports. Knowledge is learning new information about the benefits or risks of health-related behaviors. Techniques are strategies for applying new knowledge to everyday activities. By applying our knowledge, we modify lifestyle behaviors. Community supports are available environmental or regulatory measures that support new health promoting behaviors within a social context.

Chapter 11 explores pregnancy, lactation, and infancy through the framework of nutritional requirements and health promotion.

ROLE IN WELLNESS

The prenatal period is characterized by numerous physiological, psychological, and social changes in the mother in preparation for birth and care of the young. It is a time when a woman often expresses interest in and motivation to improve her eating habits, realizing that she is the sole source of nourishment for her developing baby. Following birth, lactation also leads to changes for the mother. Although providing human milk for one's baby is exhilarating, the 24-hour demands of a newborn lead to a reorganization of everyday life that can sometimes be overwhelming. Societal and cultural influences may also affect the acceptability of breastfeeding.

The goal of health promotion is to prepare a woman for these changes by being knowledgeable and taking responsibility for her own health and for the well-being of her infant. Few experience this alone. A spouse, significant others, and family members can be a source of support to further the goals of health promotion. A father-to-be often needs guidance as he grapples with his own expectations of his future responsibilities. Health professionals can use this opportunity to assist individuals to establish healthful habits, such as eating well, being physically active, and avoiding alcohol and drug use.

NUTRITION DURING PREGNANCY

Although the influence of nutrition on the course of pregnancy had been presumed for some time, it was not until this century that research provided a scientific basis to substantiate such assumptions. The most recent, and perhaps the most comprehensive, report outlining recommendations for weight gain, dietary intake, vitamin and mineral supplementation, and substance abuse during pregnancy is *Nutrition During Pregnancy*, published by the Institute of Medicine of the National Academy of Sciences (1).

Body Composition Changes During Pregnancy

Following conception and continuing until *parturition* (childbirth), many metabolic, anatomical, hormonal, psychological, and physiologic changes take place in the mother. This chapter focuses on those most affected by or affecting nutrient intake.

Hormones of pregnancy

The principal hormones of pregnancy are progesterone and estrogen. The action of progesterone promotes development of the **endometrium** and relaxes the smooth muscle cells of the uterus. This relaxation serves both to help the uterus expand as the fetus grows and to prevent any premature contractions of the uterus. The same effect also influences other smooth muscle cells such as the gastrointestinal tract. The resulting slowing of the gastrointestinal tract during pregnancy may increase the absorption of several nutrients, most notably iron and calcium. One perhaps annoying consequence of this decreased gut motility is that it may promote constipation. Progesterone also causes increased renal sodium excretion during pregnancy. The body compensates for this sodium-losing mechanism by increasing aldosterone secretion from the adrenal gland and renin from the kidney. Sodium restriction therefore is not recommended during pregnancy; the body performs its own electrolyte balancing act (2).

Estrogen promotes the growth of the uterus and breasts during pregnancy and renders the connective tissues in the pelvic region more flexible in preparation for birth (2).

Metabolic changes

The basal metabolic rate (BMR) rises during pregnancy by as much as 15% to 20% by term. This increase is due to the increased oxygen needs of the fetus and the maternal support tissues. Interestingly, there are also alterations in maternal metabolism of protein, carbohydrate, and fat. The fetus prefers to use glucose as its primary kcalorie source. Changes occur in maternal metabolism to accommodate this need of the fetus. The adaptation allows the mother to use fat as the primary fuel source, thus permitting glucose to be available to the fetus (2). Increased kcaloric intake by the mother during pregnancy will ensure that these increased metabolic needs are met.

Anatomical and physiological changes

Plasma volume doubles during pregnancy beginning in the second trimester. Failure to achieve this plasma expansion may result in a spontaneous abortion, a stillbirth, or a low birth weight baby. One of the results of this increase in plasma volume is a **hemodilution** effect. In other words, measured components in the plasma such as hemoglobin, serum proteins, and vitamins will appear to be at lower levels during pregnancy because there is a greater volume of *solvent* (the plasma) relative to concentrations of *solute* (the components).

In the kidneys, glomerular filtration rate (GFR) increases to accommodate the increase in maternal blood volume that must be filtered as well as to carry away fetal waste products. As a result of this increase in GFR, small quantities of glucose, amino acids, and water-soluble vitamins may appear in the urine. Although minor losses may be acceptable, a woman who excretes large amounts of protein may be experiencing a more serious problem called pregnancy-induced hypertension, which needs strict medical monitoring. Pregnancy-induced hypertension is described in more detail later in the chapter.

As previously mentioned, progesterone may slow gastrointestinal motility during pregnancy, leading to constipation, heartburn, and delayed gastric emptying. In late pregnancy, these problems may be exacerbated by the weight of the uterus and fetus compressing the abdominal cavity.

Weight gain in pregnancy

The two outcomes that traditionally have been used to evaluate the influence of maternal nutrition on pregnancy outcome are maternal weight gain and infant birth weight. Inadequate weight gain by the mother during pregnancy suggests she may not have received the proper nutrients during pregnancy. Poor weight gain

endometrium
mucous membrane of the uterus

hemodilution
dilution of the blood

Table 11-1   Recommended Total Weight Gain Ranges for Pregnant Women, by Prepregnancy Body Mass Index (BMI)

Weight-for-Height Category	Recommended Total Gain	
	kg	lb
Low (BMI of <19.8)	12.5-18	28-40
Normal (BMI of 19.8-26.0)	11.5-16	25-35
High* (BMI of >26-29)	7-11.5	15-25

Young adolescent and African-American women should strive for gains at the upper end of the recommended range. Short women (<157 cm or 62 in) should strive for gains at the lower end of the range.

*The recommended target weight gain for obese women (BMI of > 29.0) is at least 6 kg (13 lb).

From National Academy of Sciences: *Nutrition during pregnancy: Weight gain and nutrient supplements*, Washington, DC, 1990, National Academy Press.

may then lead to intrauterine growth retardation in the infant. Infants that are born **small for gestational age (SGA)** or **low birth weight** are more likely to require prolonged hospitalization after birth, be ill during the first year of life, or die during the first year of life. Additionally, infant mortality rate is regarded as a measure of a country's health and well-being. Although the 1992 infant mortality rate for the United States declined as a whole (8.5 per 1000 live births, down from 9.1 per 1000 in 1990 (2)), it still remains far greater than other developed countries.

In the 19th century and in the early part of this century a low maternal weight gain was recommended. It was believed that by restricting maternal food intake during pregnancy, babies would be born smaller and easier to deliver. Presently we recognize that women with lower gestational weight gains have smaller babies who are at increased risk for morbidity and mortality. Another consideration is that weight gain should be based on maternal pregravid weight for height (Table 11-1) (3-5). Moreover the Institute of Medicine emphasizes that the pattern of weight gain is as important as the total weight gain (2). It should be a slow, steady gain; any abrupt increases or decreases in weight gain may be a concern.

small for gestational age (SGA)
having a lower birthweight than expected for the length of gestation

low birth weight
weighing less than 5.5 pounds (2500g) at birth

Energy and Nutrient Needs During Pregnancy

The 1989 Recommended Dietary Allowances suggest increases in all of the nutrients during pregnancy except vitamin A (Table 11-2).

Energy

Total energy cost of pregnancy is somewhere between 68,000 kcalories (6) and 80,000 kcalories (7). The increase accomodates the rise in maternal BMR during pregnancy as well as the synthesis and support of the maternal and fetal tissues. The current recommendation is that a woman consume an extra 300 kcalories per day during the second and third trimesters of pregnancy. Although she is *eating for two,* the expectant mother need not and should not double her food intake. An extra sandwich and a glass of milk can easily provide the additional 300 kcalories per day. Personal preference may guide particular food choices to provide the extra kcalories.

What happens if a pregnant woman fails to increase her energy intake during pregnancy? The most well-known example in this century occurred in Holland during World War II. Babies that were born during the famine of 1944-1945 had smaller birth weights and birth lengths when compared with infants born either before or after the famine (7). Recent research shows that when women who begin pregnancy in energy deficit (such as those who are chronically undernourished in

Table 11-2   Recommended Dietary Allowances to Meet Needs of Pregnancy and Lactation: Percentage of Increases Over Those of Nonpregnant Women

	Adult Women (25-49 Years of Age)	Pregnant Women (Third Trimester)	Lactating Mothers*	Percentage of increase in need over that of nonpregnant women	
				Pregnant	Lactation
Energy (kcal)	2200	2500	2700	14	23
Protein (g)	50	60	65	20	30
Vitamin A (RE)	800	800	1300	0	33
Vitamin D (μg)	5	10	10	100	100
Vitamin E (TE, mg)	8	10	12	25	50
Vitamin C (mg)	60	70	95	16	58
Thiamin (mg)	1.1	1.5	1.6	35	45
Riboflavin (mg)	1.3	1.6	1.8	23	38
Niacin (NE, mg)	15	17	20	14	33
Vitamin B_6 (mg)	1.6	2.1	2.1	31	31
Folate (μg)[†]	(180)	400	(280)	†	†
Vitamin B_{12} (μg)	2	2.2	2.6	10	30
Calcium (mg)	800	1200	1200	50	50
Phosphorus (mg)	800	1200	1200	50	50
Iron (mg)[‡]	15	30	15	100	0
Zinc (mg)	12	15	19	25	58
Iodine (μg)	150	175	200	16	33
Selenium (μg)	55	65	75	20	36

NE, Niacin equivalent; RE, retinol equivalent; TE, tocopherol equivalent.

* During the first 6 months of lactation.

† Current recommendation from the US Public Health Service is 400 μg/day for women of childbearing age.

‡ The increases iron requirement for pregnancy cannot be met by the usual American diet or from body stores; thus a supplement of 30 to 60 mg of elemental iron is recommended.

Table 11-3   Changes in the Daily Food Guide Pyramid During Pregnancy and Lactation

Food Group	Nonpregnant	Pregnant or Lactating
Milk, yogurt, and cheese	2-3 servings	3-4 servings*
Meat, poultry, fish, dry beans, eggs, and nuts	2-3 servings	3 servings
Fruit	2-4 servings	2-4 servings (1-2 citrus)
Vegetables	3-5 servings	3-5 servings (1-2 green leafy)
Bread, cereal, rice, and pasta	6-11 servings	7-11 servings

*4-5 servings for pregnant adolescents.

developing countries) are provided with energy supplementation throughout the course of pregnancy, there is a positive effect on maternal weight gain and infant birth weight (8).

Pregnancy is not a time to restrict kcalories or to lose weight, even if the mother begins the pregnancy overweight. This may be particularly important to emphasize to the adolescent population. The mother should be encouraged to eat at least the minimum number of servings from the Food Guide Pyramid (Table 11-3). Sample menus can be helpful in showing the pregnant woman how the pyramid should be used (Table 11-4).

Table 11-4   Sample Menu for Pregnant Women

BREAKFAST Whole grain toast, Banana, Oatmeal, Skim milk or orange juice	**SNACK*** Cereal (ready to eat), Skim milk

LUNCH
Roast beef (lean) sandwich
  with lettuce and tomato,
Green salad,
Orange wedges,
Skim milk[†]
	SNACK
	Apple with cheese,
	  or fruit and yogurt shake

DINNER
Sesame chicken (or fish)
  with broccoli and pasta,
Mixed salad (carrots, tomatoes, spinach, romaine
  lettuce),
Italian bread and butter,
Fruit salad,
Skim milk
	SNACK
	Fig or oatmeal raisin cookies
	  or open-face peanut butter
	  sandwich

*Snacks are all interchangeable.
[†]Assumes water consumed throughout the day as a beverage in addition to skim milk.

Protein

The RDA for protein during pregnancy is 60 grams per day. Women usually can obtain this easily in the American diet; the use of special protein powder supplements is not recommended. Pregnant patients may be counseled to include appropriate sources of protein that also provide vitamins, minerals, and moderate amounts of fat. Patients from low-income populations may need counseling or other assistance to assure that protein intake is sufficient; these clients may qualify for food vouchers through the Special Supplemental Food Program for Women, Infants and Children (see box).

The increase in protein intake over the non-pregnant state is necessary to build and maintain the variety of new tissues of pregnancy. A woman experiencing nausea and vomiting in the first trimester of pregnancy may find it difficult to increase sources of protein in her diet, particularly if meats (which have a strong cooking odor) aggravate the nausea. This is not a cause for concern, as the fetal requirements for increased protein are minimal in the first trimester and increase sharply in the third trimester.

Vitamin and mineral supplementation

The RDAs are increased during pregnancy for all vitamins and minerals except vitamin A. (Excessive intakes of vitamin A during pregnancy can cause birth defects.) Most of these recommendations may be met with a balanced diet, with a few notable exceptions of folate, iron, and possibly calcium. All supplementation, especially during pregnancy, should be prenatal vitamin/mineral supplements as recommended by primary health care providers and/or dietitians.

Folate. Recent research has demonstrated that folate is important for the prevention of neural tube defects (NTDs), which are the most common congenital malformations in the United States (9,10). Approximately 2500 to 3000 infants are born with NTDs each year in the United States, out of a total of 300,000 to 400,000 cases worldwide. The US Public Health Service and the American

Academy of Pediatrics now recommend that all women of childbearing age who are capable of becoming pregnant receive a daily intake of 400 mcg of folate, more than double the nonpregnant allowance (11,12).

Iron. The RDA for iron during pregnancy is 30 mg/day. This level may be difficult to achieve with a normal diet that maintains recommended fat and kcaloric guidelines. Therefore the Institute of Medicine recommends supplementation with 30 mg ferrous iron daily beginning in the second trimester to prevent iron deficiency anemia in pregnancy (1). Iron deficiency anemia is one of the most common complications of pregnancy. The iron requirement increases secondary to the expansion of the maternal red cell volume. Iron deficiency anemia can mean impaired oxygen delivery to the fetus, which may have severe consequences. In addition, during the last trimester, the fetus is storing iron in its liver to use during the first four months of life.

As discussed in Chapter 8, an unusual behavior associated with iron deficiency is pica. Pica is characterized by a hunger and appetite for non-food substances including ice, corn starch, clay, and even dirt. These substances contain no iron and may lead to loss of additional minerals, particularly when clay and dirt are consumed. Intestinal blockages caused by consumption of these substances may be life-threatening. Of particular concern is the practice of pica during pregnancy when the risk and implications of iron-deficiency anemia are most severe. Although more common among African-American women, pica has been diagnosed among all ethnic groups within all socioeconomic levels. A challenge to obstetric nurses is to elicit information about this type of dietary behavior when assessing clients.

Calcium. Calcium needs during pregnancy rise because of the needs of the growing fetus. The RDA increases to 1200 mg/day. Although this level is achievable by following the general pregnancy guidelines of the Food Guide Pyramid, a conscious effort is usually required of a pregnant woman to assure the level is met. The needs of the fetus will be met regardless of the daily calcium intake of the expectant woman. It is the woman's body that loses its store of calcium, which can only be replaced through dietary intake. Women who are unable to consume rich sources of calcium may need to seek advice of a nutrition specialist to determine if supplements are warranted.

Nutrition-Related Concerns

A number of nonnutritive substances that women may be exposed to during pregnancy may have the capability to act as teratogens. A **teratogen** is an agent that is capable of producing a malformation or a defect in the unborn fetus. Some anomalies are apparent at birth or shortly thereafter such as neural tube defects or a cleft lip or palate. Other defects such as delayed growth or learning deficits may not be noticeable for several months or even years. Teratogens include caffeine, drugs, alcohol, and tobacco. Other concerns that may affect the course and outcome of pregnancy include strenuous exercise, maternal age, and medical conditions requiring nutrition intervention such as hypertension, diabetes, phenylketonuria, and AIDS. Although not nutritional in nature, their effect on the course of pregnancy may be so serious as to warrant at least a brief review.

teratogen
an agent that is capable of producing a malformation or a defect in the unborn fetus

Caffeine

The relationship between maternal caffeine consumption and pregnancy outcome is unclear. Caffeine (1, 3, 7-trimethyxanthine) may alter DNA and in some individuals may alter circulating levels of neurotransmitters and increase blood pressure (13-17). It is theorized that any or all of these effects may have direct adverse consequences for the developing fetus. In addition, heavy use of nonnutritive substances such as coffee, tea, and cola may displace needed nutrients in the diet and thus interfere with prenatal development. If a woman chooses to continue consuming caffeine during pregnancy, she might be advised to do so in moderation (<300 mg/day or about 2 cups or less of coffee) providing that she otherwise consumes a well-balanced diet.

Drugs

A pregnant woman should not consume any over the counter or prescription medications unless prescribed by her primary health care provider. The growing fetus, particularly during the period of organogenesis in the first trimester, is highly susceptible to insult.

In the early 1980s the acne medication isotretinoin (Accutane), which contains high levels of retinoic acid in the form of a vitamin A analogue, was found to be the cause of malformations in infants such as craniofacial abnormalities and microcephaly when mothers ingested it in the periconceptional period. The current recommendation is that women of childbearing age not use isotretinoin for the treatment of acne (18). This is consistent with a large body of animal data that show that consumption of large quantities of vitamin A during pregnancy results in an excess of malformations such as anencephaly (defective brain development), cleft palate, spina bifida, webbed fingers or toes, and facial malformations. Vitamin A crosses the placenta by simple diffusion. Since it is fat-soluble, the excess vitamin A can accumulate in the fetal tissues and may cause damage by interfering with cellular growth and differentiation during critical periods of development (19).

Pregnant women should also avoid illicit drugs such as marijuana, cocaine, heroin, and LSD. Drug exposure *in utero* has been reported to result in spontaneous abortion, intrauterine growth retardation, placental insufficiency, premature labor, uterine irritability, placental abruption, congenital infection, and an increased risk of perinatal mortality (2). From a nutritional standpoint, illicit drugs not only replace food, but may also cause changes in metabolism of many nutrients (20).

Alcohol

The use of alcohol during pregnancy may produce **fetal alcohol syndrome** (FAS) or **fetal alcohol effects** (FAE) in the infant. Symptoms include specific anatomical defects such as a low nasal bridge, short nose, flat midface, and short palpebral fissures.

fetal alcohol syndrome (FAS) or fetal alcohol effects (FAE)
a disorder caused by alcohol consumption during pregnancy that may produce a range of specific anatomical and central nervous systems defects

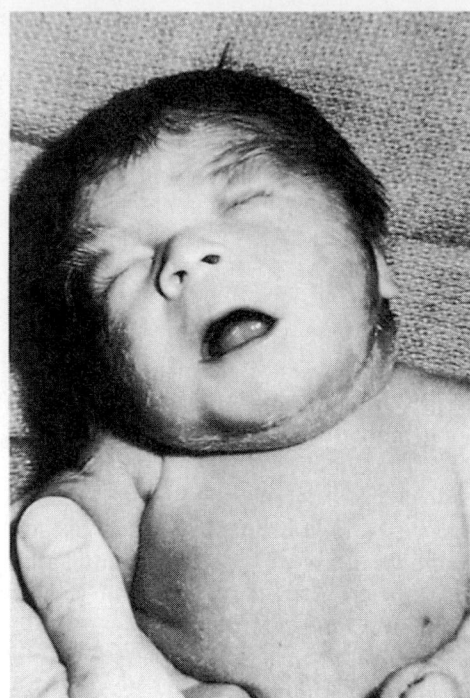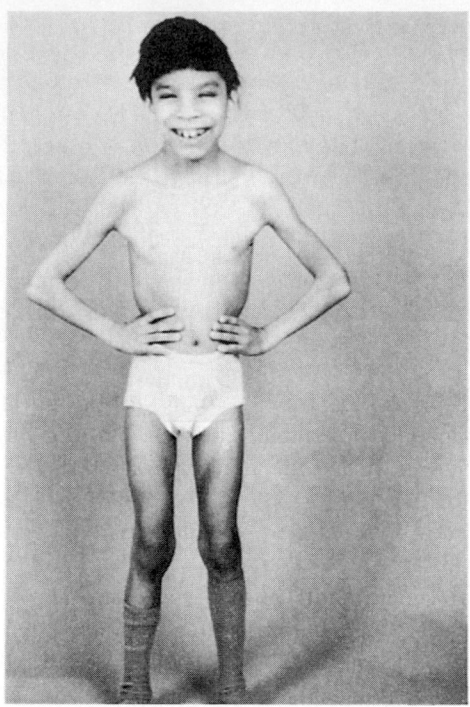

Fig. 11-1 Child with FAS at day 1 and 8 years. This child was diagnosed at birth and has spent all his life in a foster home where his care has been excellent. His IQ has remained stable at 40 to 45.

In addition, infants may be microcephalic, display poor growth patterns, or have central nervous system and mental defects (2) (Fig. 11-1). The children frequently have cognitive or behavioral dysfunctions that can represent substantial economic costs as the children enter school and require special educational services.

There is no safe level of alcohol intake during pregnancy. Fetal alcohol syndrome is not confined to heavy drinkers; anyone who uses alcohol during pregnancy is placing their baby at risk of this very preventable syndrome. Therefore all pregnant women should be urged to cease consumption of all alcoholic beverages.

Tobacco

Considerable research has been conducted on the effects of cigarette smoking during pregnancy. It is well established that women who smoke are at greater risk of giving birth to a growth-retarded infant. Exposure to second-hand smoke also increases the risk. Maternal smoking may lead to an increased risk of prematurity, placenta previa (location in lower uterine area), placentae abruptio (separation from uterine wall), and postnatally, sudden infant death syndrome (SIDS). Furthermore, smoking during pregnancy may cause prolonged effects of impaired intellectual performance and decreased attention span in the offspring.

In spite of the evidence showing the adverse consequences of smoking during pregnancy, many women of childbearing age continue to smoke. Therefore prenatal care should include a smoking cessation component.

Exercise

Women with normal pregnancies should stay active during pregnancy but never exercise to the point of exhaustion. Strenuous exercise should be avoided because the diversion of blood to the exercising muscles can reduce the blood supply to the fetus by as much as 25%. There is also some danger that the rise in the pregnant woman's body temperature during strenuous exercise can cause an undesirable rise in the fetal temperature and heart rate. Some studies have reported an association between low-birth-weight infants and strenuous exercise, but not moderate exercise (21). Recommended activities include walking, swimming, and cycling on a stationary bike.

In addition to having increased energy needs, pregnant women are more susceptible to hypoglycemia and the loss of fluids during exercise. They should be advised to avoid exercising with an empty stomach and to drink fluids before, after and, if necessary, during exercise. General guidelines for exercise during pregnancy are listed in the margin.

Maternal age

Pregnant adolescents represent a special class of high-risk pregnancy. The American Dietetic Association recently issued a Position Statement declaring that teens are in need of special nutrition care during pregnancy because of their "unique biologic, psychologic and developmental vulnerabilities placing them at nutritional risk" (22). Important issues when assessing the nutritional status of the pregnant teen include growth pattern of the mother, poor dietary habits that are typical of many teens, frequency with which meals are eaten away from home each day, psychological maturity of the mother, lack of economic resources to provide for the infant, delay in seeking medical care, and possible preoccupation with weight gain during pregnancy. After the birth of the infant, the teen mother should be counseled about future pregnancy prevention.

Women who become pregnant over the age of 35 years also have distinct nutritional needs, reflecting their longer medical history, their probably long-term use of oral contraceptives and the possibility of a longer history of poor eating habits (23). Careful nutritional evaluation of these patients can be useful in providing guidance to reduce the risk of nutritional deficiencies causing any pregnancy complications.

Pregnancy-induced hypertension

Pregnancy-induced hypertension (PIH), formerly known as toxemia of pregnancy, is characterized by a sudden rise in arterial blood pressure accompanied by rapid weight gain and marked edema. When proteinuria accompanies the other clinical symptoms, it is known as preeclampsia/eclampsia. Onset is generally after 28 weeks gestation.

Pregnancy-induced hypertension (PIH) may occur in as many as 5% to 15% of all pregnancies and is one of the leading causes of prematurity as well as maternal and fetal death (24). Risk factors for PIH are listed in Table 11-5.

Guidelines for exercise during pregnancy
- Limit workouts to 15 minutes.
- Keep pulse rate below 140 beats per minute.
- Drink plenty of fluids before, after, and during exercise.
- Do not exercise lying on your back after the fourth month.
- Avoid exercising in hot, humid weather.
- Consume enough kcalories to meet the extra needs of pregnancy plus the exercise performed.

pregnancy-induced hypertension (PIH)
a sudden rise in arterial blood pressure accompanied by rapid weight gain and marked edema during pregnancy; formerly known as toxemia of pregnancy

Table 11-5 Risk Factors in Pregnancy-Induced Hypertension	
Before Pregnancy	**During Pregnancy**
Never been pregnant	First pregnancy
Diabetes mellitus	Large fetus
Preexisting condition (hypertension, renal, or vascular disease)	Glomerulonephritis
	Fetal hydrops
Family history of hypertension or vascular disease	Hydranmios
Diagnosis of pregnancy-induced hypertension in a previous pregnancy	Multiple gestation
	Hydatidiform mole
Dietary deficiencies	
Age extremes	
20 years or younger	
35 years or older	

From Worthington-Roberts B, ed: *Nutrition throughout the life cycle*, St. Louis, 1996, Mosby.

Nutrition support during PIH includes provision of a well-balanced diet with generous sources of protein to replace losses in proteinuria, adequate vitamins and minerals, plus energy. Energy intake *should not* be limited in an attempt to restrict maternal weight gain. In addition, sodium should not be rigorously restricted; however, moderate sodium use of no more than 2000 mg (about 1 teaspoon) per day is recommended (2).

Diabetes mellitus

Women with preexisting diabetes require specialized care during pregnancy. One of the major concerns is these clients, particularly those with a poorly controlled disease state, are 7 to 10 times more likely than normal pregnant women to bear an infant with a major congenital anomaly (25). Some of the major defects reported include cardiac defects, nervous system defects including neural tube defects, kidney malformations, and skeletal anomalies (26). In addition to these congenital defects, infants born to women with diabetes are more likely to be macrosomic (abnormally large body size), which may be problematic for labor and delivery, possibly requiring a Cesarean section.

Infants born to mothers with diabetes often require immediate monitoring in the neonatal intensive care unit. Accustomed to a high level of glucose in utero since glucose readily crosses the placenta (especially if the diabetes has been poorly controlled), the infants may experience hypoglycemia after birth following withdrawal of the maternal source of glucose. Without quick treatment, this condition can be fatal in neonates.

Fortunately, there may be a decreased prevalence of many of the congenital anomalies associated with diabetes mellitus when diabetic control is achieved before conception and maintained throughout pregnancy. The current recommendation is that women achieve tight glucose control prior to conception in order to maximize the likelihood of a healthy mother and infant. Control includes prudent blood glucose monitoring, adherence to diet, moderate exercise, and strict adherence to the prescribed insulin regimen. Total kcaloric intake, as well as kcalorie distribution, will likely need modification during pregnancy because of the increased kcalorie needs of pregnancy. Insulin dosages may require adjustment, as many of the hormones of pregnancy such as estrogen, progesterone, human chorionic, somatotrophin, and maternal cortisol may act in an antagonistic fashion with insulin.

Oral hypoglycemic agents may have teratogenic effects on the fetus and should be discontinued in women with non–insulin-dependent diabetes mellitus (NIDDM) who previously had used them for glucose control (27). These women should begin using insulin injections before pregnancy when the pregnancy is planned and as soon as pregnancy is diagnosed when pregnancy is unplanned.

gestational diabetes mellitus (GDM)
a form of diabetes occuring during pregnancy, most commonly after the 20th week of gestation

Gestational diabetes mellitus (GDM) is a form of diabetes that occurs during pregnancy, most commonly after the 20th week of gestation. Patients experience abnormal glucose tolerance in a manner similar to other diabetics. Treatment is primarily dietary control combined with moderate exercise that should lead to an appropriate weight gain. These women may receive insulin if they don't achieve glycemic control with these other treatments. Risk factors for GDM include a previous large infant, a prior perinatal death, glycosuria and maternal age greater than 30 years. The majority of women with GDM have normal glucose tolerance following delivery, but they may remain at risk for NIDDM later in life.

Maternal phenylketonuria

Phenylketonuria (PKU) is an inborn error of metabolism characterized by extremely low levels of the enzyme phenylalanine hydroxylase. Absence of this crucial enzyme causes a failure in the metabolism of the amino acid phenylalanine. Successful treatment of this disorder is by adherence to a strict diet that is low in phenylalanine beginning in the first week of life. Failure to detect the disease or a lack of compliance with the dietary therapy results in mental retardation (28,29).

Maternal phenylketonuria, particularly if not well controlled at the time of conception, poses a great risk to the unborn offspring. Mothers with untreated PKU have a high likelihood of spontaneous abortion or having an infant born with microcephaly, mental retardation, congenital heart defects, or intrauterine growth retardation even if the infant does not have the genetic defect (30). Conscientious adherence to a low-phenylalanine diet may lessen but not completely eliminate the risk of an adverse pregnancy outcome (31).

It is recommended that all young women with phenylketonuria continue their low-phenylalanine diets throughout the childbearing years. Family planning is strongly encouraged to establish safe phenylalanine levels before conception and to educate women regarding the high risk of poor pregnancy outcome, even with good dietary control.

AIDS

In 1990 the Centers for Disease Control reported that 11.5% of all cases of acquired immune deficiency syndrome (AIDS) were among women, up from 7% in 1987 (32). Based on these startling figures, clinicians can expect to see a new classification of high-risk pregnancies that require specialized care: AIDS in pregnancy. Pregnancy may put an additional strain on the mother's already fragile immune system because the hormones of pregnancy such as estrogen, progesterone, human chorionic gonadotropin, alfafetoprotein, corticosteroids, prolactin, and alphaglobulin have immunosuppressive effects in vitro (19). Although every effort should be made to help prevent pregnancies in human immuno deficiency virus (HIV) positive women, those women who do become pregnant should be monitored closely for nutrient intake, weight gain, and fetal well-being. Women with AIDS should be counseled about the risks to their unborn fetus, not only concerning the possible vertical transmission of the HIV virus during pregnancy or the birth process, but also the possible teratogenic effects of the medications that the mother may be taking. For example, it is known that drugs such as AZT, trimethoprim, acyclovir sodium, and pentamidine all are able to cross the placenta, but specific effects on the fetus are unknown (19).

The HIV-infected woman who experiences an opportunistic infection during pregnancy will have increased needs for kcalories, protein, vitamins, and minerals. Weight gain must be strictly monitored although there are no current weight gain recommendations for this population.

Overcoming Barriers

Relief from common discomforts during pregnancy

Nausea and vomiting. Nausea and vomiting during the first trimester of pregnancy can be annoying, but it generally begins to subside by the beginning of the second trimester. Symptoms of *morning sickness* may actually occur at any time throughout the day, though vomiting tends to be more common between 6 AM and noon (33). Although the etiology of nausea and vomiting during pregnancy is unknown, it may be caused by hormonal factors such as a rise in estrogen or the placental hormone human chorionic gonadotropin (HCG). Stress or fatigue may exacerbate the condition. There is no cause for alarm unless the mother begins to lose weight or becomes severely dehydrated. If she cannot retain either foods or fluid for 6 hours or longer, a physician should be contacted.

If morning sickness persists into the second trimester or severely interferes with the mother's life, it may be a more serious condition. **Hyperemesis gravidarum** is severe and unrelenting vomiting, and usually requires intravenous replacement of nutrients and fluids. If the mother receives total parenteral nutrition for the treatment of hyperemesis gravidarum, appropriate levels of vitamins and minerals should be included, with careful monitoring and follow-up.

The best dietary advice for a woman plagued with nausea and vomiting of pregnancy is to eat small, frequent, meals; consume liquids between rather than with

hyperemesis gravidarum severe and unrelenting vomiting in the second trimester or that severely interferes with the mother's life; a serious condition usually requiring intravenous replacement of nutrients and fluids

meals; and avoid fried and greasy foods. Some women also find it helpful to reduce coffee intake and to prepare meals near an open window to avoid cooking odors. For women who are employed during pregnancy, snacks to keep in the workplace might include dried fruit, crackers, and small cans of juice.

Heartburn. In late pregnancy, when the fetus is rapidly growing in size, the uterus pushes up against the stomach, which may cause a feeling of fullness in the mother. Additionally, because of the action of progesterone (which can cause relaxation of smooth muscles) a relaxation of the gastroesophageal sphincter may occur, resulting in some reflux of gastric contents into the lower esophagus. This is the cause of the heartburn that is so common during the final weeks of pregnancy. The best dietary remedies include eating small frequent meals, avoiding foods that are high in fat, drinking fluids between rather than with meals, limiting spicy foods, and avoiding lying down for 1 to 2 hours after eating. Many women find relief by wearing clothing that fits loosely around the abdomen. Expectant mothers should not take antacids without primary care provider approval. Heartburn generally disappears after delivery of the baby.

Constipation. Constipation is common during the first and third trimesters of pregnancy. During the first trimester, progesterone (which slows gastrointestinal motility) may be responsible. In the third trimester, the growing fetus crowds the other internal organs, again possibly slowing gastrointestinal motility. Although it may be bothersome, constipation responds well to dietary treatment. A generous intake of fiber as well as inclusion of plenty of fluids in the diet should alleviate constipation. Moderate exercise such as a daily walk may also help. Good sources of fiber include fruits, vegetables, and whole grain cereals (see Chapter 4). Over the counter laxatives or enemas should not be used unless under the direction of a physician.

Enlarged veins in the anus caused by increased pressure from the fetus may contribute to hemorrhoids, which can cause burning and itching. If rupture occurs with bleeding upon defecation, the woman's health care provider should be contacted. The recommendations for alleviating constipation also help prevent hemorrhoids.

NUTRITION DURING LACTATION

All sexually mature female mammals possess milk-producing mammary glands and are able to produce a milk that is specifically formulated to provide optimum growth and development for their offspring. Although there are historical accounts of wet nurses and even artificial feeding implements dating back to Greek and Roman times, breastfeeding (lactation) was the primary mode of infant feeding until this century in the United States and around the world (33). Since World War II, however, there has been a dramatic decline in the incidence and duration of breastfeeding worldwide. In 1989 only slightly more than 50% of the US mothers had chosen breastfeeding at hospital discharge. By 5 to 6 months after birth, only about 20% of the US infants were being breastfed (34). While there is no one isolated cause for this decline in breastfeeding, it can be attributed to a multitude of causes such as advertising of breast-milk substitutes, lack of support for the breastfeeding mother, lack of knowledge of lactation by health care professionals, obstetrical and hospital policies that have promoted mother-baby separation, and the rise in maternal employment without appropriate facilities to nurse babies or pump and store breast milk (35).

A *Healthy People 2000* goal aims to increase the proportion of infants who are breastfeeding at hospital discharge to at least 75%, and to increase the proportion breastfeeding at 5 to 6 months postpartum to 50% (36). Both the American Dietetic Association and the American Academy of Pediatrics have policy statements

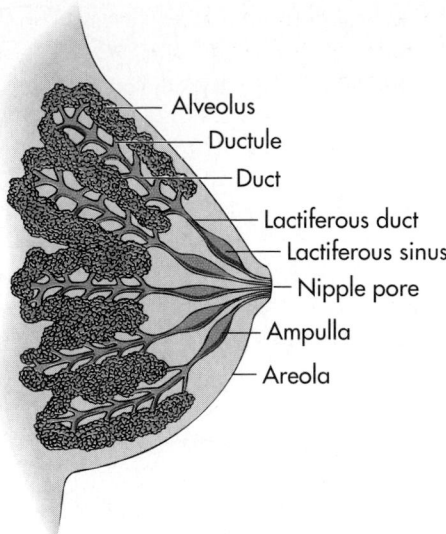

Fig. 11-2 Detailed structural features of human mammary gland.

Table 11-6 Benefits of Breastfeeding
• Confers immunologic protection to the infant against many infections and diseases (especially respiratory and gastrointestinal)
• Offers uniquely suited nutrient composition with high bioavailability
• Reduces risk of food allergy in the infant
• Promotes infant oral motor development
• Offers convenience: always fresh, available, and at the right temperature
• Is generally less expensive than formula feeding
• May protect infant against some chronic diseases such as insulin-dependent diabetes and childhood leukemia
• Promotes mother-infant bonding
• Facilitates uterine contractions and controls postpartum bleeding
• Promotes return to prepregnancy weight

advocating human milk as the preferred feeding choice for infants for at least the first 4 to 6 months of life (37,38). Breastfeeding offers advantages for both infant and mother (Table 11-6).

Anatomy and Physiology of Lactation

The human breast begins its development in utero and goes through two further stages of change after birth: at puberty and during pregnancy. The mature human breast consists of a system of alveoli and ducts. The milk-producing glands, located in the alveoli, are surrounded by myoepithelial cells. The ductules emerge from the alveoli to carry the milk to the lactiferous ducts, which eventually empty into the lactiferous sinuses. The lactiferous sinuses are located behind the areola, or the darkened area of the nipple where the baby latches on during nursing (Fig. 11-2).

Throughout the course of pregnancy, the breast tissue undergoes considerable development. Under the influence of progesterone, the lobules or alveoli increase in size and number, while estrogen stimulates proliferation of the ductal system. Together, these changes render the breast completely capable of milk production after delivery. An extremely uncommon occurrence is a failure of the breasts to undergo development during pregnancy. A women who does not notice any changes

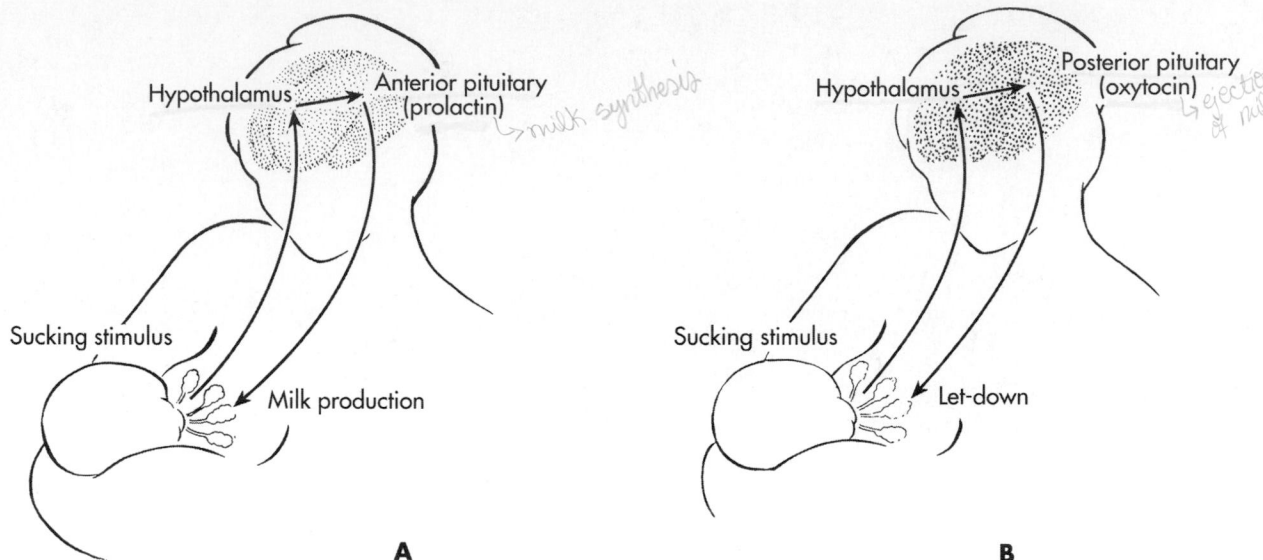

milk synthesis

ejection of milk

Fig. 11-3 Maternal breastfeeding reflexes. **A,** Milk production. **B,** Let-down.

in her breasts during pregnancy, particularly if she is pregnant for the first time, should receive postnatal assistance to determine her ability to fully lactate. Most women, however, are able to fully lactate with no problems. Actual size of breast has no bearing on ability to breastfeed.

Lactation is a normal process that begins via an interplay of various hormones following delivery of the infant. Before the onset of labor, there is a rise in serum levels of **oxytocin.** This hormone is instrumental in initiating the uterine contractions of labor that bring about birth. Oxytocin and another hormone, **prolactin,** instigate the lactation process. Prolactin is primarily responsible for milk synthesis; oxytocin is involved with milk ejection from the breast.

As an infant is allowed to suckle after birth a nerve impulse is sent to the hypothalamus. This stimulates the anterior pituitary to secrete prolactin, which then stimulates milk production in the alveolar cells (Fig 11-3, *A*).

The infant sucking stimulus also initiates the release of oxytocin from the posterior pituitary. The flood of oxytocin into the breast tissue causes the myoepithelial cells around the glands to contract, thereby ejecting the milk into the infant's mouth. This is called the *let-down reflex* or the *milk-ejection reflex* shown in Fig. 11-3, *B*. Many women report that they feel a tingling sensation in their breasts when the let-down occurs. Additionally, if a mother hears her baby's cry or sees another baby, she may also experience a let-down accompanied by a rush of milk ejecting from her breasts. Inhibitors of the let-down reflex may include fatigue, stress, alcohol, smoking, and some prescription medications.

An important point to note here is that milk production is a supply and demand mechanism. The more a baby is allowed to nurse, the more nerve stimulation there will be, resulting in a rise in prolactin levels followed by increased milk production.

Contraindications to Breastfeeding

Although common colds, the flu, and even most illnesses that require short-term antibiotic therapy do not require cessation of breastfeeding, a number of maternal illnesses or conditions are contraindications to breast-feeding (see margin).

Most medications for mild illnesses are safe for the mother to take while breast-feeding; however, mothers should always remind their health care providers that they are nursing an infant should the need for a medication arise. The American

oxytocin
a hormone that initiates uterine contractions of labor and has a role in the ejection of milk in lactation

prolactin
a hormone responsible for milk synthesis

Contraindications to breastfeeding
- Active tuberculosis
- AIDS
- Herpes simplex lesions on the maternal breast
- Maternal alcoholism
- Maternal drug addiction
- Malaria
- Maternal chicken pox (first three weeks postpartum **only)**
- Maternal breast cancer requiring treatment

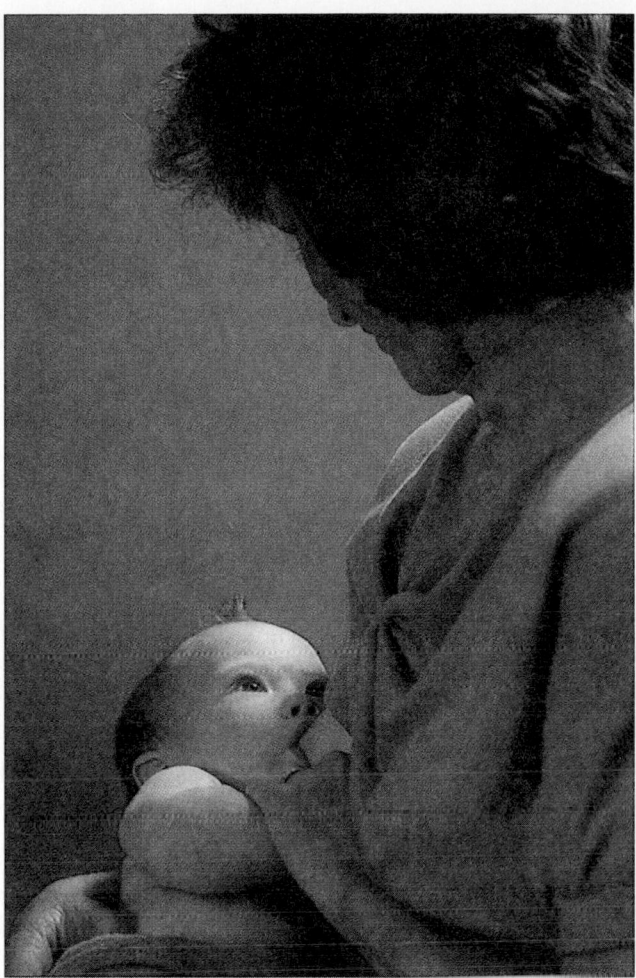

Successful breastfeeding depends on the health and nutritional status of the mother, her attitude toward breastfeeding, and support from health care providers and family.

Academy of Pediatrics has classified medications into five categories based on
safety considerations. For mild illnesses as well as for chronic diseases, a medication that is compatible with breastfeeding can usually be found and substituted for
one that might be contraindicated. The amount of the maternal dose of drug that
is actually secreted into the milk depends on the route of administration, the size of
the molecule, ionization, the pH of the medication, solubility, and protein binding
(39). Health care providers might keep this information in mind as they consider
prescription medications for nursing mothers.

Whether a mother can safely nurse her baby if she is infected with the human
immunodeficiency virus (HIV) has become an important consideration in recent
years. The Centers for Disease Prevention and Control recommend that all women
in the United States who are infected with HIV should not breastfeed their infants.
On the other hand, in developing countries where the risk of death from diarrhea
caused by inappropriate bottle feeding is far greater than the risk of transmission
of HIV via human milk, the World Health Organization recommends that breastfeeding continue in these situations. The woman with active AIDS and opportunistic infections is unlikely to have the physical strength to successfully lactate.

Promoting Breastfeeding

To increase the incidence and duration of breastfeeding in the United States and
around the world, health care professionals must take measures to ensure that

appropriate breastfeeding policies are adopted and practiced in hospitals providing maternity care. In 1991 the World Health Organization and UNICEF launched the *Baby Friendly Hospital Initiative*. The initiative includes *Ten Steps to Successful Breastfeeding* that hospitals must be willing to take to become *baby friendly*. Among the steps are breastfeeding education for all mothers, no separation of mother and baby following birth except for medical reasons, and no supplemental feedings unless medically indicated (40). Nurses play a key role in prenatal counseling and in postpartum support to help mothers successfully establish and maintain lactation.

Another influence on successful lactation is acceptability of lactation within the cultural and ethnic communities of which the mother is a part. Cultures in which breastfeeding is common include Chinese, Finnish, Indian, Saudi Arabian, Muslim, South African, and Swedish. In the following cultures, breastfeeding is common, but infants are not given **colostrum** because it is considered bad or unclean: Cambodian, Filipino, Haitian, Japanese, Korean, Laotian, Mexican, and Vietnamese (26). Socioeconomic and education levels are influences that may also help or hinder a mother's attempt at successful lactation. Organizations such as La Leche League or community-based mothers groups may provide invaluable support to nursing mothers, particularly those nursing for the first time (41).

colostrum
the fluid secreted from the breast during late pregnancy and first few days postpartum; contains immunologically active substances (maternal antibodies) and essential nutrients

Energy and Nutrient Needs During Lactation

A large proportion of the energy stores that are laid down as adipose tissue during pregnancy are mobilized in lactation. The energy cost of milk production is approximately 500 to 800 kcalories per day depending on the volume of milk production. The 1989 RDAs recommend increases for protein (65 g/day for the first 6 months of lactation and 62 g/day for the second 6 months of lactation) and for all the vitamins and minerals over the normal adult levels. The mother can meet most of these increases by consuming a well-balanced diet (see Table 11-3).

A woman need not avoid certain foods while breastfeeding unless a problem occurs. For example, some infants are fussy following the mother's consumption of gas-producing vegetables such as cabbage, onions, and broccoli.

HEALTH DEBATE
Lactation: A Natural Way To Lose Weight?

Considerable controversy has surrounded the role of lactation in postpartum weight loss. It has been generally believed that women who breastfeed their babies return to their prepregnancy weight more easily than those who do not because of the additional energy required for milk production.

Several studies, however, have shown no increase in postpartum weight loss for lactating women when compared with nonlactating women. Some of these studies may have suffered from poor methodological design. Difficulties in quantifying kcaloric intake and levels of physical activity can affect the overall validity of results.

A more recent study shows that when infants are breastfed for at least 6 months, mothers lose significantly more body fat as measured by triceps skinfold thickness and body weight than controls who were matched on age, education, prepregnancy weight, parity, and pregnancy weight gain. Weight loss of lactating women may be slower or equal to nonlactating women who may diet to lose weight. The difference, however, is that the quality of weight lost by lactating women, body fat rather than lean body mass, is better in terms of overall health goals.

What do you think? Should lactation be promoted as a way to lose postpregnancy weight?

From Dugdale AE, Evans JE: The effect of lactation and other factors on postpartum changes in body weight and triceps skinfold thickness, *Br J Nutr* 61:149, 1989; Potter et al: Does infant feeding method influence maternal postpartum weight loss? *J Am Diet Assoc* 91:441,1991 and Dewey KG, Heinig MJ, Mommsen LA: Maternal weight-loss patterns during prolonged lactation, *Am J Clin Nutr* 58:162-166, 1993.

Adequate fluid intake is important during lactation. The average women produces 750 to 1000 ml of milk per day. She can replace this fluid through consumption of water or juice. Coffee or cola drinks should be avoided or used on a minimal basis. They act as diuretics in the mother and caffeine, a stimulant, passes into breast milk in small amounts. The old wive's tale that alcohol helps a mother relax and enhances milk production should not be followed. Alcohol not only passes into milk, becoming available to the tiny infant, but may also inhibit oxytocin, consequently inhibiting the let-down reflex.

Despite the desire of most women to return to their prepregnancy weight quickly, rapid weight loss should not be encouraged while breastfeeding. Recent research shows that women achieve weight loss without compromising nutritional intake when breastfeeding continues for at least 6 months (see box).

The Institute of Medicine's guide to *Nutrition During Lactation* offers a comprehensive review of the nutrient needs of women during lactation (34).

NUTRITION DURING INFANCY

Energy and Nutrient Needs During Infancy

Dramatic changes in growth and development occur during the first 12 months of life. In the first year, a human infant is expected to triple its birth weight and increase its length by 50%. In addition, after birth organs such as the kidney and brain continue to develop and mature. In no other period of life do growth and development occur so rapidly. To support this rapid growth and development, the appropriate balance of all nutrients is essential.

Energy

The World Health Organization suggests that infants receive 108 kcal/kg/day for the first 6 months of life and 98 kcal/kg/day from 6 months until the first birthday (42). Adequate energy intake will be reflected in satisfactory gains in length and weight as plotted on a National Center for Health Statistics (NCHS) growth chart (in Appendix 11).

Protein

Protein needs of infants have been hard to determine because of the difficulty of performing nitrogen balance studies on this population. Requirements therefore are estimated based on the intake and growth rates of normal, healthy infants. Protein requirement is highest during the first four months of life when growth is the most rapid. It is suggested that infants receive 2.2 g/kg/day from birth to 6 months of age and 1.6 g/kg/day for the second half of the first year (43).

An excess of protein in an infant's diet can be problematic. Protein has a large influence on renal solute load. The infant kidney is immature and unable to handle the large renal solute loads that an adult can. Therefore increasing a normal infant's protein intake above the recommended amount should be avoided.

Vitamins and mineral supplementation

The 1989 RDAs may be consulted for appropriate levels of vitamins and minerals for infants. Breast milk or commercial formula should provide infants with all the vitamins and minerals needed for proper growth and development with a few notable exceptions (Table 11-7).

During the third trimester of pregnancy, the fetus stores iron in its liver to be used during the postnatal period. By 4 months of age, this supply of iron is usually depleted. The iron in breast milk, although lower in absolute amounts, is more bioavailable than iron from commercial formula. Many breastfed infants do not

Table 11-7   Recommended Supplementation of Infant Diets

Type of Feeding	Iron	Vitamin D	Fluoride	Vitamin K
Human milk	1 mg/kg/day*	10 µg/day	0.25 mg/day	Single intramuscular dose of 0.5 to 1 mg or oral dose of 1 to 2 mg
Formula	—	—	0.25 mg/day†	Single intramuscular dose of 0.5 to 1 mg or oral dose of 1 to 2 mg

From Guthrie HA, Picciano MF: *Human Nutrition*, St. Louis, 1995, Mosby.
* If an iron-fortified cereal is not used after 6 months of age.
† If fluoride content of water is less than 0.3 parts per million.

need to be supplemented with iron. However, their iron levels should be assessed periodically. Infants who consume commercial formula should use the iron-fortified variety to prevent iron deficiency anemia.

Although humans are able to manufacture vitamin D through exposure to the sun, many young infants may not receive enough sun exposure for adequate synthesis. Although breast milk contains vitamin D, it may not be present in levels sufficient to prevent vitamin D-related rickets. Therefore it is recommended that all breast-fed infants receive a daily oral supplement of vitamin D. It must be recognized that vitamin D can be toxic and therefore the recommended dosage should not be exceeded. Vitamin D is present in commercial infant formula, so formula-fed infants need not receive a supplement.

The water supply of most major cities in the United States may contain fluoride as a preventive measure against tooth decay. It may be particularly important for infants and young children whose teeth are developing to ensure that fluoride is available. Infants who are breast-fed and not receiving water or juice may benefit from a daily oral supplement of fluoride, since fluoride does not readily pass into breast milk even if the lactating mother has fluoride in her diet. Formula-fed infants, on the other hand, only need to receive fluoride if their local water supply is not fluoridated. For example, many rural families who rely on well water would fall into this category. Excess fluoride can result in mottling of tooth enamel; consequently the dosage should be followed precisely.

Newborns are vulnerable to vitamin K deficiency (and thus hemorrhaging) in part because they lack intestinal bacteria to synthesize the vitamin. As a preventative measure, US hospitals routinely give infants 0.5 to 1 mg of vitamin K by injection, or 1 to 2 mg orally, once shortly after birth.

Food for infants

The ideal food for the first 4 to 6 months of life is breast milk. As mentioned previously, breast milk has the correct balance of all the essential nutrients as well as immunological factors that protect the baby from both acute and chronic disease. The breast should be offered at least 10 to 12 times per 24 hours in the first several weeks. As the infant develops a stronger suck, he will be able to extract more milk with each nursing session and thus the frequency of feeding may decline. Although there is no specified time the infant should stay on the breast, between 10 to 15 minutes per breast, offering both breasts per session, is a good recommendation. It is important to realize, however, that this is a *general* guideline because all infants have different nursing styles. It may in fact be more appropriate to *watch the baby not the clock* in an effort to allow the baby to dictate when satiety is reached. The Teaching Tool box offers some suggestions to facilitate successful breastfeeding.

Signs baby is getting enough to eat
- Six or eight wet diapers a day; breast-fed infants often have one or two stools a day for the first few weeks and sometimes as many as one every feeding
- Feeding every 1 1/2 to 3 hours, after which baby seems content
- Adequate weight gain
- Good skin color and tone

TEACHING TOOL

Guidelines for Successful Breastfeeding

Although breastfeeding is the most natural and easiest way to feed infants, our clients who are mothers will welcome these simple suggestions.

- Offer both breasts at each nursing session.
- Baby's mouth should be wide open to latch on correctly.
- At least 1/2 inch–3/4 inch of areola should be in baby's mouth, not just nipple.
- Baby's lips should make a tight seal around the breast.
- Sore nipples are usually caused by incorrect positioning; position baby correctly in a tummy-to-tummy fashion or in a football hold. Support a newborn's head and back with extra pillows on mother's lap or with mother's arm cradling baby.

- Limiting nursing time in the first several days will not prevent sore nipples and it may hinder milk production.
- Remember: milk is produced by supply and demand—the more often the baby nurses, the more milk will be produced.
- Growth spurts can be expected at approximately 10 days, 2 weeks, 6 weeks, and 3 months. Expect a fussy baby who wants to nurse frequently.
- Offer no bottles of formula or water while milk supply is being established. The artificial nipple may confuse baby and substitute feedings that replace breast stimulation may diminish milk production.
- Learn your infant's cues for satiety.

If a mother chooses not to breastfeed, or if she has a medical condition contraindicating breastfeeding, a variety of suitable formulas made from either cow's milk or soy are on the market. In addition, a number of specialty formulas such as protein hydrolysate formulas are available for infants with medical problems. The parents should consult their primary health care provider or nutrition care specialist to identify the most appropriate formula for their infant.

Formulas are either ready-to-feed, where no mixing is required, or they are a powder or liquid concentrate that must be mixed with water. To reduce the chance of lead leaching into water, tap water should be run for 2 minutes after it has been standing in the pipes and only cold water should be used for formula preparation. The formula should be mixed exactly as stated on the package, unless otherwise directed by a primary health care provider. Adding insufficient water can result in a high renal solute load, placing strain on the immature infant kidneys; overdiluting will precipitate undernutrition. For non-English speaking or low-literacy parents or care givers, pictorial mixing instructions may be useful. Alternatively, asking the care giver to demonstrate appropriate formula mixing may be suitable. Formula should never be heated in a microwave oven as microwaves heat food unevenly. Contents of a bottle that appear to be cool on testing may actually have portions that could scald an infant. All unused formula at the end of a feeding should be discarded if not used within two hours because of contamination by saliva enzymes and bacteria. Home-prepared formulas made from evaporated milk are likely to be low in iron, vitamin C, and other essential nutrients and should be avoided (44,32).

Before 1 year of age, cow's milk, regardless of fat content or form (evaporated, liquid, or dried), should not be fed to infants. The fat in cow's milk is less digestible than the fat in breast milk or formula and contains less iron and more sodium and protein. These higher levels of solutes may lead to dehydration caused by increased urine volume to reduce solute levels and deficiencies of other nutrients found in limited amounts such as vitamin C, essential fatty acids, zinc, and possibly other trace minerals (45).

Cow's milk may be introduced after 1 year of age when at least two thirds of energy needs are fulfilled by foods other than milk. Skim milk is generally not recom-

Formula preparation
- Clean all necessary equipment and wash hands before preparing formula
- Read formula label and dilute formula exactly as recommended by the manufacturer
- Use cold tap water for preparation of concentrated or powdered formula, unless directed otherwise by physician or nurse
- Never heat formula in a microwave oven
- Discard unused formula after 2 hours

mended until age 2, when the total fat content of dietary intake is monitored. The delay in cow's milk consumption reduces the risk of developing a milk allergy (45).

Introduction of solid foods. Solid foods may be added to the infant's diet between the ages of 4 and 6 months. Infants who are introduced to solid foods before this time may be prone to excessive kcaloric intake, food allergies, and gastrointestinal upset. Many parents and even some health care professionals believe that offering an infant cereal in the evening will promote sleeping through the night. This notion, however, does not have experimental validity and has not received support in the scientific community (46).

There are two basic issues when considering the introduction of solid foods to the infants diet: *how* to introduce and *what* to introduce.

How to introduce solid foods. Although parents and other care givers may be anxious to introduce foods other than breast milk or formula to their infant's diet, they should be reassured that the baby should be *developmentally ready* for solid foods. The baby should be able to sit with some support; move the jaw, lips, and tongue independently; be able to roll the tongue to the back of the mouth to facilitate a food bolus entering the esophagus; and show interest in what the rest of the family is eating. For example, the baby may try to reach and grab an item off of a family member's plate at meal time. Likewise, parents should become familiar with satiety cues so as not to overfeed the baby. For instance, to indicate satiation the baby may turn her head to the side, refuse to open her mouth, or grimace when the spoon comes close to her mouth. These cues should be respected by the care giver; the baby should never be force fed. If the baby is overtired or is not interested in food, she should be removed from the high chair and the foods offered again later.

When an infant reaches the age of 9 to 12 months, he may enjoy self-feeding. Although this may be a messy process, caregivers should encourage him to develop these skills through food exploration.

Appropriate solid foods during the first year of life. Solid foods should be introduced one at a time with a 4- to 5-day interval between new foods. This timing is crucial because if the infant has any type of allergic reaction such as gastrointestinal upset, upper respiratory distress, or skin reactions such as eczema or hives, the offending food may be easily identified. Families with a documented history of allergies should delay introduction of solid foods until the infant is about 6 months old. If solid foods are introduced too early, the large protein molecules of the offending food may cross the intestinal barrier and elicit an immunological response in the baby. As the gut matures, it is less likely to allow large unhydrolysed proteins to cross the mucosa.

Solid foods offered to baby need not be commercial. Home-prepared foods are a good, practical alternative. Neither salt nor sugar should be added to the baby's food, and there should be strict attention to sanitary food preparation procedures. General guidelines are listed in Table 11-8.

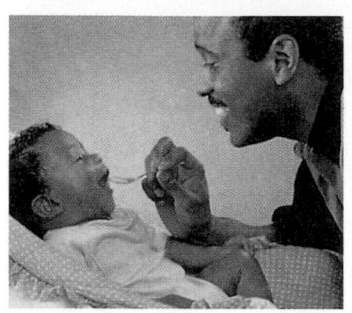

Solid foods should be introduced one at a time.

Table 11-8	Solid Foods During The First Year Of Life	
Age	**Food**	**Foods to Avoid in the First Year of Life**
4-5 months	Iron-fortified infant cereal	Honey (may cause infantile *Clostridium botulinum* poisoning); hot
5-6 months	Strained fruits and vegetables	dogs, grapes, hard candies, raw carrots, popcorn, nuts, peanut
6-8 months	Mashed or chopped fruits and vegetables	butter (choking hazards); skim milk (insufficient calories); cow's milk (potential allergen, may replace breast milk or formula); egg
	Juice from a cup	whites (potential allergen)
9-12 months	Crackers, toast, cottage cheese, plain meats, egg yolk, finger foods	

Baby bottle tooth decay

Baby bottle tooth decay, also known as *nursing bottle caries, nursing bottle mouth,* and *nursing bottle syndrome* is a distinctive pattern of tooth decay in infants and young children that most commonly affects the maxillary incisors, although other teeth may be affected as well (47). From 5% to 15% of all children may be affected, but precise prevalence figures are difficult to obtain (47).

The name *baby bottle tooth decay* has been given to the condition because it commonly occurs in infants who are allowed to sleep with a bottle of milk, juice, or other sweetened liquid. As the infant is falling asleep, the vigorous suck-swallow pattern that normally occurs during feeding diminishes. Moreover, saliva production decreases, resulting in a loss of saliva's buffering action in the mouth. Liquid pools in the infant's mouth, particularly behind the central incisors, becoming a ready source of fermentable carbohydrate for the bacteria that colonize the oral cavity. The acid that is produced by bacterial metabolism, then destroys tooth enamel and initiates caries.

The primary organism thought to be responsible for caries production is *Streptococcus mutans*. There has been considerable research into how *S. mutans* is introduced to the infant mouth because young infants have been found to be free of the bacteria while most adults harbor it (48,49). It now appears that one of the vehicles for colonization of the infant mouth may be the mother. The sharing of cups, spoons, and food between mother and baby provides an easy transport of the bacteria from the mother's mouth to the infant's mouth.

Prevention of baby bottle tooth decay is a *Healthy People 2000* goal (36). Infants should never be put to bed with a bottle of milk, formula, juice, or other sweetened liquid. If a bottle is needed at bedtime, it should be plain water only. Oral hygiene may begin as soon as teeth erupt by a daily gentle cleaning of the tooth surfaces with gauze or a washcloth. Finally, sharing of food and utensils between parents and infants should be discouraged.

Special Nutritional Needs

The nutrition requirements of children with congenital or acquired health problems deserve special attention. These infants often have increased nutrient requirements, increased losses, or malabsorption. Significant drug-nutrient interaction often takes place as well. Although it is beyond the scope of this chapter to describe all of the children's special needs one might encounter in practice, a few of the major disorders are outlined.

The premature infant

An infant is considered to be premature if he or she is born before 37 weeks gestation. As medical technology becomes increasingly sophisticated, infants are surviving at younger and younger ages. Nutrition support of these babies can play a crucial role in their long-term outcome. The major issues of concern in the premature infant are low birth weight, immature lung development, immature gastrointestinal function, inadequate bone mineralization, and minimal energy and mineral reserves (50).

Since the coordinated suck-swallow reflex is not fully developed until an infant reaches 34 weeks gestation, initial feeding of the premature infant may need to be via total parenteral nutrition, tube feeding, or gavage feeding. Many criteria influence the route of nutrient delivery, and thus each infant should receive an individualized nutrition assessment by a Registered Dietitian who specializes in high-risk pediatrics.

Premature infants have increased needs for protein, kcalories, calcium, phosphorus, sodium, iron, zinc, vitamin E, and fluids. If the infant is able to tolerate nipple feeding, a variety of specialized infant formulas are available to meet these additional requirements. Interestingly, milk from mothers who have had premature infants is higher in protein, sodium, and some minerals than term milk (51). Many premature infants are able to successfully breastfeed (52,53). However, the premature infant may tire easily at the breast because of the increased work of breastfeeding, and if the mother and baby are separated for long periods of time because of prolonged hospitalization of the infant, supplementation may be necessary.

Cystic fibrosis

Cystic fibrosis (CF) is an autosomal recessive disorder and is the most common genetic disorder among Caucasian populations, affecting roughly 1 in 2000 live births. Clinical features of the disease include chronic pulmonary disease, pancreatic exocrine insufficiency, and increased sweat chloride (18). The nutrition considerations facing children with CF include growth failure and energy and protein malnutrition. The chronic pulmonary dysfunction leads to malnutrition caused by an increased metabolic rate, increased energy requirement, and frequent use of antibiotics, which can cause anorexia. Steatorrhea, maldigestion, and malabsorption are common because of the lack of lipase secretion in the pancreas. Because of these increased needs as well as increased losses, patients are not always able to meet nutrition needs. To prevent frank protein and energy malnutrition and resulting growth failure, the Consensus Committee of the Cystic Fibrosis Foundation recommends that all CF patients receive a comprehensive nutrition assessment every 3 to 4 months. Further nutrition interventions are discussed in Chapter 14.

Failure to thrive

Failure to thrive (FTT) is defined as a fall of two standard deviations in weight gain over an interval of 2 months or longer for infants less than 6 months of age, or an interval of 3 months or longer for infants greater than 6 months of age (1). An alternative definition is a weight for length measurement that is less than the fifth percentile (1).

Failure to thrive may have organic causes such as an underlying metabolic disorder. For instance, congenital heart disease and AIDS in an infant may cause such an increased kcaloric requirement that oral intake is not able to keep up with metabolic need.

Nonorganic failure to thrive may be diagnosed when no medical reason for poor growth can be recognized. There may be psychosocial causes of the failure to thrive such as inadequate maternal-infant bonding, poverty, child abuse, or neglect. Treatment for nonorganic failure to thrive must include nutrition intervention to promote weight gain as well as therapy to correct any psychosocial problems in the home environment.

Inborn errors of metabolism

Phenylketonuria. All 50 states have newborn screening programs to detect PKU. When discovered early, dietary therapy can commence immediately and long-term prognosis is good. Without treatment phenylalanine and its metabolites reach toxic levels in the blood, resulting in damage to the central nervous system including mental retardation. Treatment consists of a low-phenylalanine diet that must be followed throughout the individual's life. In infancy the use of a special formula such as *Lofenalac* is recommended. As children are introduced to solid foods and make the transition to table foods, meals require careful planning. The use of low-protein breads and pastas may be advised.

Galactosemia. Galactosemia is another autosomal recessive disorder caused by an enzyme deficiency. Absence of the enzyme galactose 1-phosphate uridylyltransferase results in an inability to metabolize galactose. Since the milk sugar *lactose* is a disaccharide of glucose and galactose, these infants are unable to tolerate any milk products containing lactose. Manifestations include diarrhea, growth retardation, and mental retardation. Treatment is dietary therapy that excludes all milk products, including human milk. Soy formulas and casein hydrolysate formulas are acceptable. As with PKU, lifelong diet therapy is required.

Other inborn errors of metabolism that require nutrition therapy include urea cycle disorders, maple syrup urine disease, and homocystinuria.

galactosemia
an autosomal recessive disorder that results in an inability to metabolize galactose and lactose milk products

TOWARD A POSITIVE NUTRITION LIFESTYLE: REFRAMING

Reframing means to change the way a situation or concept is understood to a different *frame* that equally suits and explains the situation (54). Pregnancy and all of the recommendations in this chapter could be viewed as a worrisome burden to the expectant mother. Her body will swell in size, and she may be teased by others for the weight she is gaining. Based on what she hears about pregnancy, it sounds as if every action and every morsel of food consumed will affect the health of her unborn child. Anxiety replaces excitement over the beginning of a new life.

Reframing pregnancy can improve the well-being of the expectant mother physically and emotionally. Nurses can encourage mothers to view the weight gain of pregnancy as a natural feminine process that enhances fetal growth and development. Dietary and lifestyle suggestions can be presented as proactive behaviors to support the nutrient needs of the expectant mother as well as those of the fetus. A more positive frame of pregnancy provides a reassuring gestational period full of anticipatory excitement.

WELLNESS AND PREGNANCY, LACTATION, AND INFANCY

Physical Dimension	The physical health of the newborn depends on the nutrients consumed by the expectant mother and on the teratogens avoided.
Intellectual Dimension	Preparation before conception to take on the responsibilities of pregnancy and future parenting requires application of knowledge.
Emotional Dimension	Emotions may be strained as some women develop postpartum depression after birth; recognition and treatment of this disorder is crucial to the well-being of mother and child.
Social Dimension	The social relationships of mothers and fathers may be altered as lifestyle change occur due to their new social status as parents.

SUMMARY

From before conception through infancy, health promotion concepts are intricate components of wellness. Good nutrition habits form a foundation for proper growth and development. The importance of nutrition during pregnancy, the benefits of breast-feeding, and the establishment and maintenance of positive eating styles during infancy are crucial to overall health goals. Nutrition services should play a role in all health care delivery systems, not only as a vehicle to prevent chronic disease but also as an important part of comprehensive health care for chronic disease such as diabetes mellitus, inborn errors of metabolism, and cystic fibrosis.

Women need to be knowledgeable of dietary patterns that provide the nutritional requirements of pregnancy. They should understand the impact of smoking, drugs, and alcohol on the course of fetal development; health professionals need to review risk factors and never assume that the public is knowledgeable of these dangers. Women whose pregnancies are at high risk, such as those complicated by diabetes mellitus, should have early and regular nutrition services provided during routine prenatal care; specific education may be needed to sensitize them to their special medical and nutritional needs.

298 PART THREE HEALTH PROMOTION THROUGH NUTRITION AND NURSING PRACTICE

Lactation is a natural, physiological process that begins shortly after parturition; it completes the cycle of the female body from pregnancy through motherhood. Human milk is the best health promoter for the neonate. The vast majority of women can successfully breastfeed when given proper instruction, support, and follow-up. The nursing professional is in a unique position to provide such care. Breastfeeding should begin immediately after birth and continue every 2 to 3 hours during the initial weeks postpartum.

Lactating women should continue to consume a diet with adequate sources of protein, energy, vitamins, and minerals. In spite of the desire of most women to return to their prepregnancy weight quickly, rapid weight loss should not be encouraged while breastfeeding.

Health promotion, attending to the needs of the total person, begins as soon as a baby is born. Sound nutrition practices during the first year of life lay the foundation for good health. The ideal food for the first 4 to 6 months of life is breast milk. Supplemental foods may be introduced one at a time at 4 to 6 months of age. Breast milk (or formula) should continue until the infant reaches 1 year of age. Children with medical problems may require specialized nutrition support.

THE NURSING ROLE
Critical Thinking and Problem Solving

Critical thinking and problem-solving are inherent parts of the nursing process. You need to think critically or analytically to arrive at correct assessments and nursing diagnoses. Problem-solving skills are used in the nursing diagnoses to determine how to alleviate or improve the patient's problems or how to reinforce and promote healthy behavior.

Use your problem-solving skills on the following situations. If you are in doubt about approaches that should be taken, look back at the relevant information in the chapter.

1. A woman in the beginning of her third trimester of pregnancy has gained a total of 12 pounds. She has a fear of gaining too much weight. How can you try to convince her of the need to gain more weight? Should she try to play *catch up* on weight gain during the next month? How would you advise her to increase her intake?

2. A teenage new mother responds very positively to nutritional information you give her related to the needs of herself and her baby. But she confides in you that she doesn't think she can afford to buy the types of food and vitamins she and the baby need. To whom could you refer this mother? What advice would you give about low-cost foods?

3. A woman in her first month of pregnancy reports to you that she is very anxious because she has severe morning sickness and cannot keep any food down until around 2 PM. What information would you give her about morning sickness that might alleviate some of her anxiety? What foods or food patterns might help to control her symptoms?

4. A baby in the newborn nursery becomes very fussy about two hours after breastfeeding. The mother is sleeping. What should you do? Rock the infant? Change the diaper? Give a supplemental feeding? Wake the mother to breastfeed again?

5. The mother of a 4-month-old infant would like to start the baby on solid food because her mother advised it. What criteria should you use to determine if the child is ready for solids? How will the mother know how much food to give?

REFERENCES

1. National Academy of Sciences: *Nutrition during pregnancy: Weight gain and nutrient supplements*, Washington, DC, 1990, National Academy Press.
2. Worthington-Roberts B, Williams SW: *Nutrition during pregnancy and lactation,* ed 5, St. Louis, 1993, Mosby.
3. Brown JE: Weight gain during pregnancy: What is "optimal"? *Clin Nutr* 7:181-190, 1988.
4. Niswander KR et al: Weight gain during pregnancy and prepregnancy weight, *Obstet Gynecol* 33:482-491, 1969.
5. Rosso P: A new chart to monitor weight gain during pregnancy, *Am J Clin Nutr* 41:644-652, 1985.
6. van Raaig JMA et al: Body fat mass and basal metabolic rate in Dutch women before, during and after pregnancy: A reappraisal of energy cost of pregnancy, *Am J Clin Nutr* 49:765-772, 1989.
7. Smith C: The effect of wartime starvation in Holland upon pregnancy and its product, *Am J Obstet Gynecol* 53:599, 1947.
8. Task Force on Nutrition: *Guidelines for assessment of maternal nutrition*, Chicago, 1978, American College of Obsetricians and Gynecologists.
9. Medical Research Council, Vitamin Study Research Group: Prevention of neural tube defects: Results of the Medical Council Vitamin Study, *Lancet* 338:131, 1991.
10. Czcizcl AE, Dudas I: Prevention of the first occurrence of neural tube defects by periconceptual vitamin supplementation, *N Engl J Med* 327:1832, 1992.
11. US Centers for Disease Control: *MMWR* 41:1, 1992.
12. Committee on Genetics, American Academy of Pediatrics: Folic acid for the prevention of neural tube defects, *Pediatrics* 92:493, 1993.
13. Tornaletti S et al: Studies on DNA binding of caffeine and derivatives: Evidence of intercalcation by DNA-unwinding experiments, *Biochem Biophys Acta* 1007:112-115, 1989.
14. Shin CG et al: Rapid evaluation of topoisomerase in vivo, *Teratog Carcinog Mutagen* 10:41-52, 1990.
15. Kalow W: Genetics of drug transformation, *Clin Biochem* 19:76-82, 1986.
16. Freestone S, Ramsay LE: Effect of coffee and cigarette smoking on the blood pressure of untreated and diuretic-treated hypertensive patients, *Am J Med* 73:348-353, 1982.
17. Robertson D et al: Tolerance to the humoral and hemodynamic effects of caffeine in man, *J Clin Inves* 67:1111-1117, 1981.
18. Thompson MW, McInnes RR, Willard HF: *Genetics in medicine,* ed 5, Philadelphia, 1991, Saunders.
19. Hurley LS: In *Developmental nutrition*, Englewood Cliffs, NJ, 1980, Prentice-Hall.
20. Mohs ME, Watson RR, Leonard-Green T: Nutritional effects of marijuana, heroin, cocaine, and nicotine, *J Am Diet Assoc* 90:1261, 1990.
21. Guthrie HA, Picciao MF: *Human nutrition*, St. Louis, 1995, Mosby.
22. Position of the American Dietetic Association: Nutrition care for pregnant adolescents, *J Am Diet Assoc* 94:449-450, 1994.
23. Gadsby R, Barnie-Adshead AM, Jagger C: A prospective study of nausea and vomiting during pregnancy, *Br J Gen Pract* 43:245-248, 1993.
24. Imperiale TF, Petrulis AS: A meta-analysis of low-dose aspirin for the prevention of pregnancy-induced hypertensive disease, *JAMA* 266:260-264, 1991.
25. Cousins L: Etiology and prevention of congenital anomalies among infants of overt diabetic women, *Clin Obstet Gynecol* 34:481-493, 1991.
26. Cousins L: Congenital anomalies among infants of diabetic mothers: Etiology, prevention and prenatal diagnosis, *Am J Obstet Gynecol* 147:333, 1983.
27. Bobak IM, Lowdermilk DL, Jensen MD: *Maternity nursing,* ed 4, St. Louis, 1995, Mosby.
28. Platt LD et al: Maternal phenylketonuria collaborative study, obstetrical aspects and outcome: The first 6 years, *Am J Obstet Gynecol* 166:1150-1162, 1992.
29. Rylance G: Outcomes of early detected and early treated phenylketonuria patients, *Postgrad Med J* 65(suppl 2): S7-S9, 1989.
30. Lenke RR, Levy HL: Maternal phenylketonuria and hyperphenylalanemia: An international survey of the outcome of untreated and treated pregnancies, *N Engl J Med* 303:1202-1208, 1980.

31. Kurppa K et al: Coffee consumption during pregnancy and selected congenital malformations: A nationwide case-control study, *Am J Public Health* 14:431-442, 1989.
32. Levin N: HIV disease in pregnancy, *Md Med J* 42:33-36, 1993.
33. Lawrence R: *Breastfeeding: A guide for the medical profession*, ed 4, St. Louis, 1994, Mosby.
34. Institute of Medicine, National Academy of Sciences: *Nutrition during lactation*, Washington DC, 1991, National Academy Press.
35. Mattai J: The Brazilian national breastfeeding programme, *Assignment Children* 61/62:226-247, 1983.
36. US Department of Health and Human Services Public Health Service: *Healthy people 2000: National health promotion and disease prevention objectives*, Washington DC, 1990, US Government Printing Office.
37. Position Statement of the American Dietetic Association: Promotion and support of breastfeeding, *J Am Diet Assoc* 93; 467-469, 1993.
38. Committee on Nutrition, American Academy of Pediatrics: *Pediatric nutrition handbook*, ed 2, Elk Grove Village, Ill, 1985, American Academy of Pediatrics.
39. Trupin S: Personal communication, 1989.
40. Ebrahim GJ: The baby friendly hospital initiative, *J Trop Pediatr* 39:2-3, 1993.
41. LaLeche League International, Inc, 9616 Minneapolis Ave, Franklin Park, IL 60131.
42. World Health Organization: *Energy and protein requirements: Report of a joint FAO/WHO/UNU expert consultation*, Technical Report Series 724, Geneva, 1985, World Health Organization.
43. Williams S, Worthington-Roberts B: *Nutrition throughout the life cycle*, St. Louis, 1996, Mosby.

44. Fomon SJ: *Nutrition of normal infants*, St. Louis, 1993, Mosby.

45. Committee on Nutrition/American Academy of Pediatrics: The use of whole cow's milk in infancy, *Pediatrics* 89:1105,1992.

46. Macknin ML, Medendorp SV, Maier MC: Infant sleep and bedtime cereal, *Am J Dis Child* 143:1066-1068, 1989.

47. Ripa LW: *Baby bottle tooth decay (nursing caries): A comprehensive review, Oral Health Subcommittee of the Healthy Mothers, Healthy Babies Coalition*, Washington DC, 1988, Dental Health Section, American Public Health Association.

48. Catalanotto FA, Shklair IL, Keene HJ: Prevalence and localization of streptococcus mutans in infants and children, *J Am Dent Assoc* 91:606-609, 1975.

49. Carlsson J, Grahnen J, Jonsson G: Lactobacilli and streptococci in the mouth of children, *Caries Res* 9:333-339, 1975.

50. Suskind RM, Lewinter-Suskind L: *Textbook of pediatric nutrition*, ed 2, New York, 1993, Raven Press.

51. Butte NF et al: Longitudinal changes in milk composition of mothers delivering preterm and term infants, *Early Hum Dev* 9:153-162, 1984.

52. Hopkinson JM, Salisbury DM: Milk production by mothers of premature infants, *Pediatrics* 81:815, 1988.

53. Lemons P, Stuart M, Lemons JA: Breastfeeding the premature infant, *Clin Perinatol* 13:111-122, 1986.

54. Watxlawick P, Weakland J, Fisch R: *Principles of problem formation and problem resolution*, New York, 1974, Norton.

Chapter 12

LIFE SPAN HEALTH PROMOTION: CHILDHOOD, ADOLESCENCE, AND ADULTHOOD

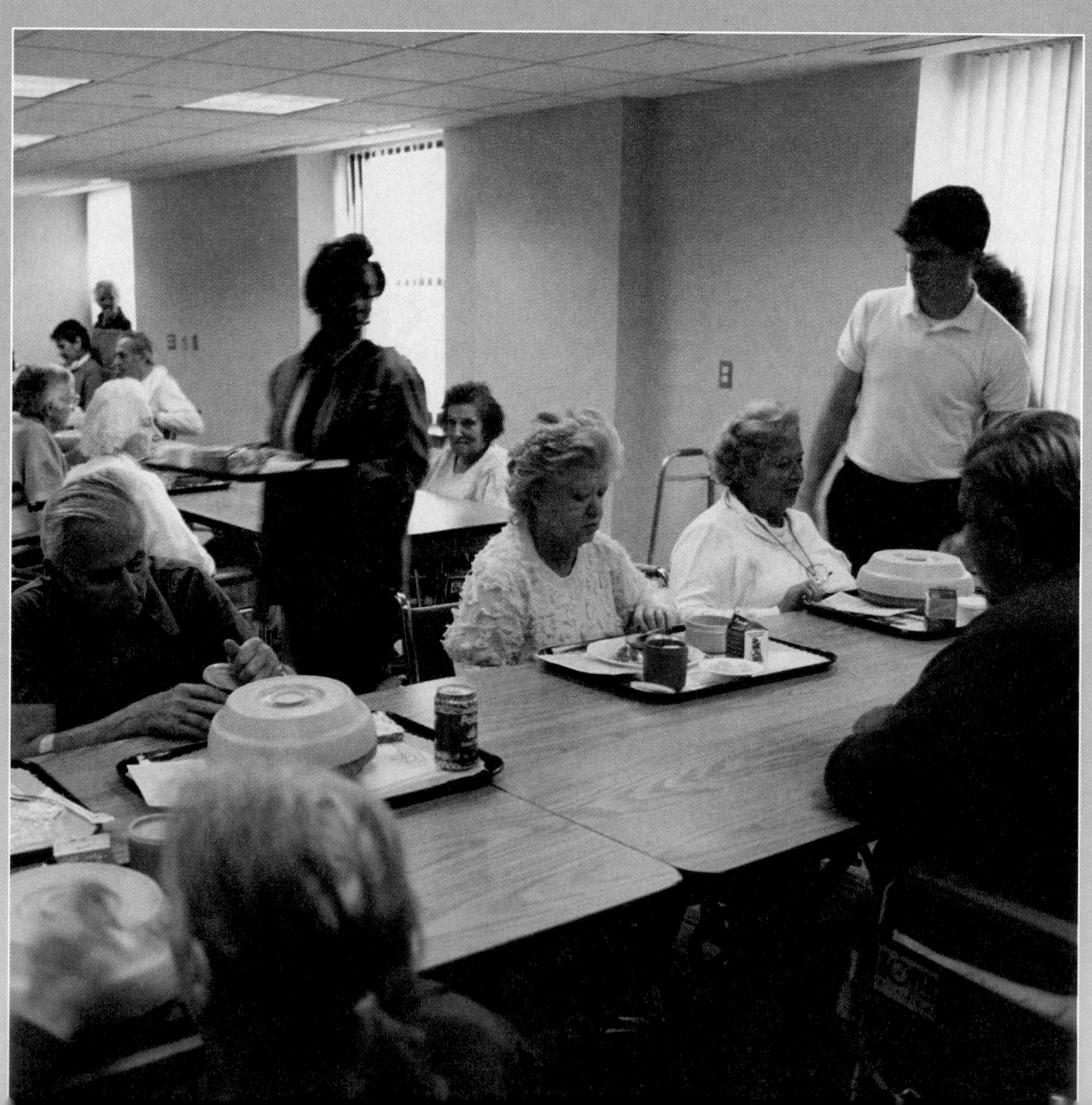

This chapter continues the exploration of the life span. Once past the very specific nutrition and health necessities of pregnancy and infancy, the rest of the life span categories share more similarities than differences regarding nutrient intake and dietary patterns. In striving to increase the level of health of individuals, families, and/or communities, the degree of knowledge appropriate at each stage varies and techniques reflect these limitations. Community supports reveal the commitment of the society regarding health issues.

ROLE IN WELLNESS

The nutrient requirements of humans are basically the same throughout the life span. What differs, depending on age, are the amount of nutrients required and frequency of food consumption (dietary patterns) recommended; these differences are due to physiological and psychosocial needs. For example, consider the amount individuals are able to consume at one time. Toddlers can eat only small amounts at one time. They depend on planned snacks to provide their full assortment of nutrients. Adolescents, however, can eat large quantities, but also need time throughout the day to eat. In contrast, the elderly still have high nutrient needs but require less energy and therefore need more nutrient-dense foods.

LIFE SPAN HEALTH PROMOTION

Stages of Development

The life span stages reflect psychological and physiological maturation. Approaches to health promotion take into account these stages and their impact on nutrient requirements, eating styles, and food choices.

Childhood (1 to 12 Years)

The accelerated growth of infancy slows down by about age 1, marking the transition to childhood. Growth then occurs unevenly until puberty heralds the onset of adolescence. This growth deceleration during childhood results in varying hunger levels that reflect physiological need. Awareness of these fluctuations by parents and caregivers allows children to stay in tune with their internal hunger cues.

Nurses sensitive to normal growth patterns as affected by genetics and environmental influences can assist families in understanding the growth curves of their children. Height, weight, and head circumferences are used with standard growth charts of the National Center for Health Statistics to chart growth (Appendix H). Clinical nutrition assessment procedures are described in detail in Chapter 13.

Childhood categories are based on a combination of psychosocial and physiological developmental stages. Physiological requirements are the basis of the age and gender divisions of the RDAs. There is one set of RDAs for children through age 10. From age 11 on, separate RDAs have been established based on age and gender that reflect differences in physiological requirements. This discussion highlights nutrients of concern (protein, iron, calcium, and zinc); for other specific age-related nutrient recommendations, refer to the RDA table inside the front cover.

Children depend on adults for the provision of food. A discussion of the nutrient needs of the growing body is not complete without a discussion of the role of adults in nourishing children. Children are influenced by and model the behaviors

feeding relationship
the interactions or patterns of behaviors surrounding food preparation and consumption within a family

of adults. The quantity and quality of foods prepared and the environment within which foods are presented for consumption are all controlled by adults. The actual amount consumed, however, is controlled by the children themselves.

Ellen Satter, a Registered Dietitian and therapist, describes the **feeding relationship** as the interactions or patterns of behaviors surrounding food preparation and consumption within a family. This description reveals the contextual nature of food preparation and consumption. Her advice to parents and caregivers is about "the division of responsibility. You are responsible for what your child is offered to eat, but he is responsible for how much of it he eats and even whether he eats" (1).

Adults are also responsible for when meals are offered. Regularity of mealtimes at home—breakfast and dinner—helps to support success at school. Breakfast supplies energy in the morning for school learning (see box); dinner supports the ability to complete homework, study, and relax before bedtime. Most children eat lunch away from home and either brown bag food from home or purchase meals through the School Lunch Program (discussed further in Community Supports).

Snacks boost daily nutrient intake; for children whose energy and general dietary intake are adequate, snacks may sometimes include sweets such as cookies and even an occasional candy bar. A common myth is that sugar makes children hyperactive, yet studies have shown no convincing evidence that consumption of sugar causes attention deficit hyperactivity disorder (2). Sugar, however, can displace more nutritious foods and contribute to nutrient deficiencies. No food should be forbidden; frequency and quantity are the guide.

Children too young for school may attend day care programs if their parents work. The impact on their nutrition may be positive or negative depending on the quality and attitude of the programs toward nutrition and meal times. Most young children, regardless of parental employment, attend some form of preschool; for many, the food and social experiences broaden acceptance to a variety of foods and eating styles.

Although adults may have predominate influence over the eating behaviors of children, another primary influence for some children is television. The influence of television commercials has been studied extensively and is most often con-

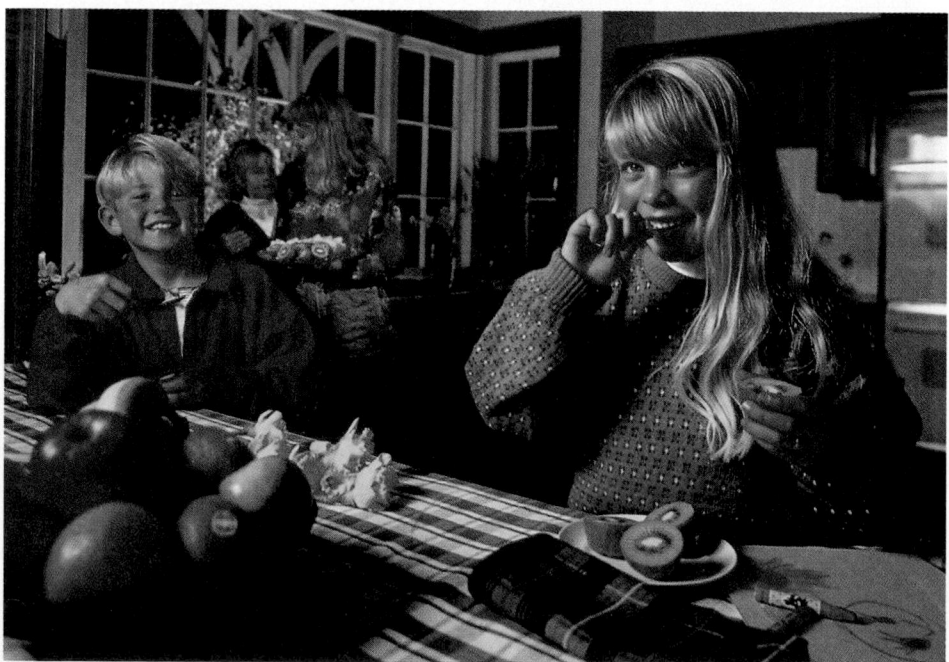

Making low-fat foods a habit throughout childhood is easier than trying to change one's eating style as an adult.

TEACHING TOOL
What's the Best Breakfast?

Foods considered best for breakfast have changed. Although traditional breakfasts consist of eggs, bacon, white toast, and whole milk, this combination is now recognized as being too high in fat and protein. In addition, in the rush of morning preparation few of us have the time to prepare this type of meal. Nonetheless, breakfast, which *breaks* our *fast*, is an important contributor of nutrients and energy.

As we teach clients and their families about nutrition and optimum dietary intake patterns, we can assure them that breakfast can be simple, yet still provide appropriate levels of nutrients. Here are some ideas for parents to use to ignite their children's breakfast appetites.

- For children (and adults) who eat and run, have quick foods available such as fruit, granola bars, muffins, and raisins.
- For older children, offer to prepare a simple breakfast. Although they are able to prepare their own meal, the extra nurturing—and time saved—will be appreciated.
- For creating appetites, toast bread while family members are dressing. The enticing scent will spark their taste buds.
- For picky eaters, create mini smorgasbord plates with several choices such as a small container of yogurt, crackers with cheese, and some pear slices.
- Many of the healthy snacks listed in Table 12-1 can alternate as breakfast foods for everyone.
- Be a role model by also eating breakfast yourself.

demned as negatively influencing children's food choices (3). Parents and caregivers can watch television with their children to assess the type of products advertised and then discuss their nutritional value. As more healthful products are marketed, even if targeted at adults, acceptance by children may increase. Occasional treats of advertised products may lessen their appeal if children are accustomed to high-quality snacks and meals.

The Dietary Guidelines for Americans (see Fig. 2-1) are considered appropriate for ages 1 through 10, particularly in regard to fat intake; 30% or less is the general goal for the population at large. A level of about 30% may also assist with obesity prevention as well by emphasizing fruits, vegetables, and complex carbohydrates. It is easier to enjoy naturally lower dietary fat foods throughout childhood than to try converting one's eating style as an adult. The American Heart Association, the American Health Foundation, and the National Institutes of Health Consensus Development Panel recommend application of the 30% goal to the age group from years 1 to 2 and older. The Committee on Nutrition of the American Academy of Pediatrics, however, has expressed concern that 30% or less of kcalories from dietary fat would overly increase bulky plant foods intake, possibly precluding consumption of enough nutrients by young children. Consequently, the Committee accepts a 30% to 40% dietary fat intake for age 2 and over (4). Levels higher than the 30% to 40% recommendation may actually cause fat to crowd out other nutrients.

Health professionals need to use careful wording when discussing nutrient restriction or reduction for children. Several infants have developed failure to thrive, not because of neglect or lack of food, but because of parental overzealousness about *fat*, both dietary and body fat (5).

Stage I: children 1 to 3 years old

Often referred to as toddlerhood, the age span of 1 to 3 years old is a busy time for young children. They are dealing with issues of autonomy; often food and eating create an arena for asserting newly discovered independence. The eating relationship between parent (or caregiver) and child is forming, and adult reaction to autonomy sets the stage for future encounters (1). Consistency of mealtimes is important. Meals are best accepted when hunger, tiredness, and emotions are still

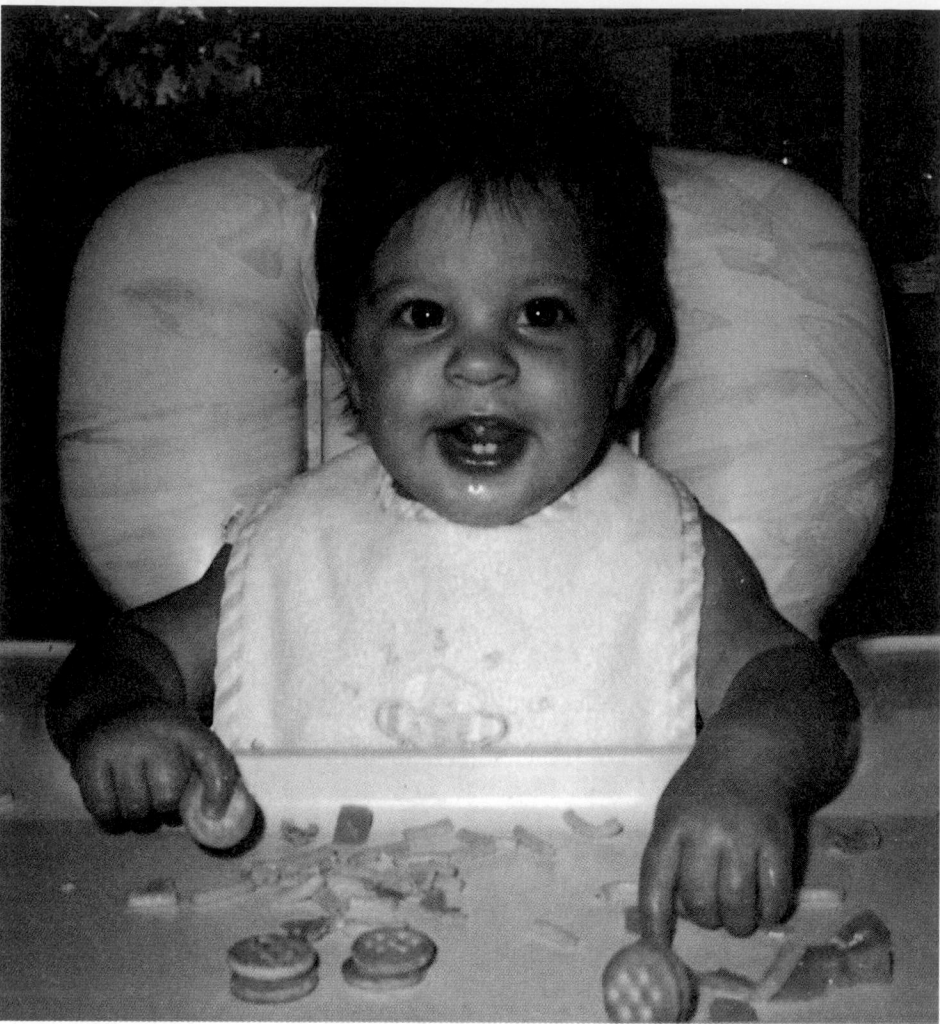

Fig. 12-1 Allowing toddlers to feed themselves promotes physical and psychological development.

controllable; an overly tired child just can't eat. Equally important is fostering self-reliance by allowing young children to feed themselves in a manner most appropriate for their psychomotor abilities. Regardless of the messy results, attempts to self-feed provide the roots of self-empowerment that are crucial to overall physical and psychological development (Fig. 12-1).

Hunger guides the child's perception of *time to eat,* rather than adult meal schedules. Meals for toddlers are based on the same design and food selections as adults, only in smaller portions. (Of course, overly spicy foods may not be acceptable to young taste buds.) Snacks are a necessity in addition to meals. Toddlers are able to eat only small amounts at each meal or food encounter; planned snacks provide required additional nourishment between meals to ensure an adequate dietary intake.

Nutrition requirements. Growth, BMR, and endless activity require an energy supply of 1300 kcal/day for ages 1 to 3. Protein needs increase to 16 grams to meet the demands of growing muscles. For ages 1 through 6, a general guideline is one fruit or vegetable serving equals one tablespoon of fruit or vegetable per year of age. A serving of bread or cereal is equal to about one fourth of an adult's serving. Up to age 3, children should consume two to three cups of milk per day, and meats or meat substitutes can be offered at least twice per day (1).

This age span of 1 to 3 years old is the time to begin introducing lower-fat versions of commonly eaten foods. As mentioned previously, fat-containing foods should not be obsessively restricted; however, high-fat foods are often very filling and may displace other nutrient-containing foods.

This is also a prime time to introduce a variety of foods; toddlers imitate the adults around them. Clever introductions to foods are always helpful. Broccoli is not just a vegetable, but cut up looks like little trees. Peas steamed in their pods are not just peas, but green pearls waiting to be discovered.

Although breast milk or formula is the milk of choice until age 1, toddlers should drink whole milk or formula until age 2, after which low-fat or skim milk is best. Sometimes toddlers consume too much milk or juice, particularly if they are given an unlimited number of bottles. Perhaps drinking from bottles throughout the day simply becomes a habit. Unfortunately, the child fills up on milk or juice, both low sources of iron, and then does not have an appetite for iron-containing foods such as meat, fish, poultry, eggs, or legumes. Iron deficiency anemia may develop. Additionally, apple juice is very sweet-tasting and has few nutrients beyond carbohydrate kcalories; frequent consumption may habituate young children to sweet drinks. Later, apple juice may be replaced with sugar-laden sodas, displacing more nutrient-dense beverages.

Parents and caregivers can view bottles as *cups*. Few of us drink from a cup continuously while watching television, reading, or playing games. Similarly, once past infancy, young children's use of bottles should be viewed as beverages, with the use of cups encouraged.

Stage II: children 4 to 6 years old

The stage of 4 to 6 years old is characterized by independent eating styles although modeling of adults still occurs. Children of this age clearly understand the time frame of meals and can *save* their appetite for meals. Snacks are still an integral part of the child's nutrient intake. Far from the messy eating styles of toddlers, these children accept foods more easily if presented separately, not mixed in a casserole style. Variations of hunger and appetite levels may confuse parents and caregivers. The most practical approach is to be respectful of these vicissitudes of hunger; this diffuses power plays over food consumption.

New foods can continue to be introduced. For some families, back-up meal plans can encourage trying new foods. For instance, if a child does not accept a new dish after a reasonable attempt, the child may be allowed to prepare a meal of a peanut butter sandwich or cereal and fruit. By establishing back-up meals in advance, parents avoid becoming short order cooks preparing three or more individualized meals for dinner.

At this stage children can develop a sense of responsibility for healthful food selections. They can understand that although all foods are okay, some (such as fruits, vegetables, and low-fat foods) can be eaten more often than others. Sometimes children develop food jags, wanting to eat only a narrow range of foods. Parents and teachers can educate the child that each food contains a different assortment of nutrients and offer substitute choices that contain additional nutrients, with the child making the final selections. Eventually food jags diminish and the child consumes a broader selection of foods.

Nutrition requirements. Energy requirements jump to 1800 kcal/day at 4 to 6 years of age, reflecting continued growth and activity levels. Protein needs increase to 24 grams.

Stage III: children 7 to 12 years old

The years from 7 to 12 are tumultuous. Although actual growth may slow down, the body is preparing and seemingly storing up for the puberty growth spurt. Puberty may begin for girls from around age 9 and on; boys may reach puberty in the early teen years. This prepuberty time may be reflected by weight buildup; an increase in chubbiness is not alarming if moderate eating and physical activities are maintained. Adults must be careful not to overreact or they may plant the seeds of eating disorders. To rule out overeating, children can be asked if they are really hungry for food or are they just tired or thirsty. These are very different sensations. By taking time to consider these sensations, children can stay in touch with internal cues of true hunger.

Exposure to other dietary patterns takes place as children spend more time away from home at school and socializing with friends. Peer influence at school lunchtime increases; having the right kind of lunch may be as important as wearing the right kind of clothes. Adults need to be sensitive to these issues. As long as a basic lunch of some protein, complex carbohydrates, and a beverage (preferably milk, juice, or water) is consumed, missing nutrients can be adjusted for later in the day, especially through after school snacks.

It is at this age, when mid-morning school snacks disappear and school lunch scheduling has more to do with numbers of students than with actual lunchtime appetites, that afterschool hunger may intensify. This is the time to provide healthful snacks or at least stock the kitchen shelves with an assortment of nutrient-dense treats (Table 12-1). If children purchase snacks away from home, adults can develop guidelines with children this age to maintain positive eating styles.

Nutrition requirements. Energy needs for 7 to 12 year olds increase to 2000 to 2200 kcal/day. Protein requirements rise to between 28 grams to 46 grams depending on sexual maturity. Sexual maturity leads to an increase of lean body mass, particularly for males. Lean body mass requires more dietary protein for growth and maintenance.

Mineral needs increase as well. Because of increased bone growth and mineralization, calcium recommendations jump from 800 mg/day at age 10 to 1200

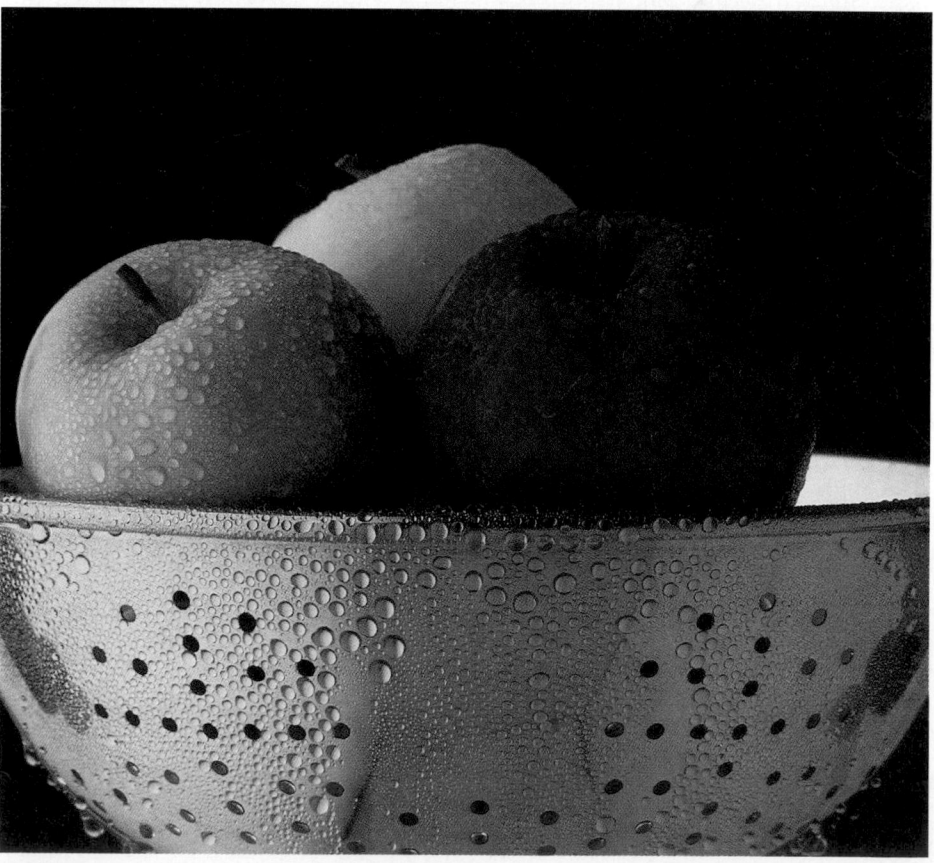

Snacks can play an important role in nutrition.

Table 12-1	Healthy Snacks

- Ready-to-eat cereals: reserve presweetened cereals as special snack treats or mix a sweet cereal with a less sweet cereal—the best of both worlds
- Snack smorgasbord: cut-up apples and oranges, popcorn, cheese, crackers, and cookies
- Fruit juice packs
- Low-fat chocolate milk packs
- Open-face peanut butter sandwich (child-made) with cut fruit, jelly, coconut, and raisins
- Fresh or canned fruit (in fruit juice) with cottage cheese (in 4-oz sizes)
- English muffins (oat bran, raisin, and sourdough)
- Healthier Danish: a slice of toasted bread reheated with low-fat ricotta cheese and preserves
- Bagels with a spread of whipped cream, margarine/butter, or peanut butter; freeze a variety of bagels
- Smoothies or fruit shakes made with skim milk or fruit juice, plain or fruit-flavored yogurt, fresh or frozen fruit—just mix in a blender
- Leftovers from lunch or dinner; a bowl of soup with bread for dipping tops any prepackaged snack

mg/day throughout adolescence. Iron and zinc allowances increase as well. Well-chosen dietary intakes will provide sufficient amounts of these nutrients. Marginal intakes of zinc have been noted among school children who are finicky eaters; low zinc intakes can affect growth rates (6).

Childhood Health Promotion (1 to 12 Years)

Knowledge

The growth cycle of this age span is important for parents and children to understand. Attention to issues related to weight, appropriate appetite, and meal patterning are crucial for the development of positive eating relationships and may prevent the development of eating disorders in the future. By understanding the relationship of nutrients and kcalories to their growth needs, children possess sufficient information to take responsibility for certain aspects of their food choices and dietary patterns. Ultimately, however, adults must provide nourishment for children and guidance as to positive health behaviors.

Techniques

Use of the Food Guide Pyramid to visualize and comprehend the variety and number of servings of foods that constitute a balanced nutrient intake works for both parents and children. The Five-a-Day approach is also ideal for use by children. For young children, however, the five servings would be of smaller sizes.

Keeping a list on the refrigerator door of available nutritious snacks is an excellent reminder for young and old.

Community supports

Community supports for children are presently divided into two categories based on location and services or education offered: school food service and classroom nutrition education.

School food service. The National School Lunch Program was established to protect the health and wellness of American children. Formalized in 1946, the program provides lunches at varying costs depending on family income to all school children at public and nonprofit private schools and residential child care institutions. At the federal level the program is administered by the Food and Nutrition Service (FNS) of the USDA, at the state level by various agencies, and locally by school boards. As an entitlement program, the School Lunch Program provides funds to all schools that apply and meet the criteria of eligibility (7).

Reduced-price meals are offered to children whose household income is below 185% of the federal poverty level; free meals are available to those falling below 130% of poverty.

Specific nutrient guidelines regulate the meals served through this program; at times the definition of these guidelines has been controversial because of their impact nutritionally on children and economically on the farmers and food producers supplying the food. Some foods are available at reduced cost because of federal surplus commodities programs. Although wholesome, these may contain higher fat contents than would otherwise be used in the preparation of school lunches. Fresh fruits and vegetables may be passed over for canned fruits and vegetables that are not as acceptable to children and at times not as nutritious. Whole milk, cheeses, and high-fat meats may be served more often because of economics than health objectives. Meals served may not meet the lower fat and higher fruits and vegetable consumption recommendations of the Dietary Guidelines for Americans. Consequently, a *Healthy People 2000* objective addresses this concern.

> Increase to at least 90 percent the proportion of school lunch and breakfast services and childcare food services with menus that are consistent with the nutrition principles in the Dietary Guidelines for Americans (8).

Basically, lunch must provide approximately one third of the RDA and include the four food groups: dairy; protein; vegetables and/or fruits; and grains, bread, or pasta. For low-income children participating in the program, this provides one third to one half of their daily intake (7).

The School Breakfast Program was created to provide meals to needy children, particularly in economically disadvantaged areas. It is administered through the same governmental offices as the School Lunch Program and is also an entitlement program. Only about half of the schools (53%) that participate in the School Lunch Program also participate in the School Breakfast Program. Of those serving breakfast, over 80% of the participants qualify for free or reduced-priced meals (7).

An assortment of foods can comprise breakfast, but the program requires milk (either as a beverage or with cereal), a serving of fruit (either whole or as juice), and two servings of a bread/cereal product or meat/meat alternative or a combination of bread and meat servings. The breakfast is designed to provide one fourth of the RDA.

During the summer the Summer Food Service Program for Children (SFSP) functions through a range of eligible organizations including schools, summer camps, and community agencies as well as various federal, state, and local government departments. The purpose is to serve meals to school-age children when schools are not in session in communities where children depend on school meals as an essential component of their daily nourishment (7).

School nurses and community health nurses should be aware of these programs as a valuable source of nutrition. Sometimes children do not participate because school payment policies create a stigma associated with participation. Intervention by a health professional may be required to ensure that children's health needs are being meet in a socially-sensitive manner. As health advocates, nurses may be able to highlight the importance of school lunch as well as breakfast programs to educational administrators and to the community at large.

Classroom nutrition education. Health has been taught for many years in most school systems. What varies is the depth of school health curricula and the qualifications of the instructors. Both may affect the quality of the nutrition education. Although basic nutrition facts can be taught within a short-term health course, lifestyle changes that affect dietary patterns take longer to achieve. Unless they have special preparation, instructors may not feel comfortable teaching the intricate and ever-changing discipline of nutrition. This may lead to either poor quality of teaching or the imparting of negative attitudes toward nutrition and food selections.

To address this issue, the Nutrition Education and Training Program (NET) provides nutrition education training for teachers and food service personnel in public and private nonprofit schools and child care centers eligible for other government programs. With training, these professionals can then teach children about food and health through their own specialities, either in the classroom or in the school cafeteria. The program can also provide direct nutrition education to children (7).

To further the goal of increasing the level of nutrition education throughout the country, a *Healthy People 2000* objective addresses this concern.

> Increase to at least 75 percent the proportion of the Nation's schools that provide nutrition education from preschool through 12th grade, preferably as part of quality school health education (8).

Adolescence (13 to 19 Years)

The adolescent years are marked by change. Not only does puberty initiate growth acceleration, but emotional and social developmental struggles also occur as academic and personal responsibilities escalate. Adults often assume the attitude that teenagers can take care of themselves. Although teens need to take responsibility for their behavior and overall health status, they still need the guidance and nurturing of caring adults. There is a fine line between allowing adolescents to be responsible and neglecting their needs. Adult involvement is still necessary to provide physical and emotional support during the stressful years of adolescence.

Part of the physical and emotional support includes creating guidelines for dietary patterns and providing food for consumption. Creating guidelines means maintaining a household in which meals are available, even if family members may not be able to eat together. Knowing that dinner just needs to be reheated means that someone was thinking of the welfare of all family members. Of course, shared responsibility for meal preparation may be an appropriate component of family duties. A kitchen stocked with nourishing snack foods and ingredients for simple meals helps to make stressful, chaotic teenage schedules more manageable.

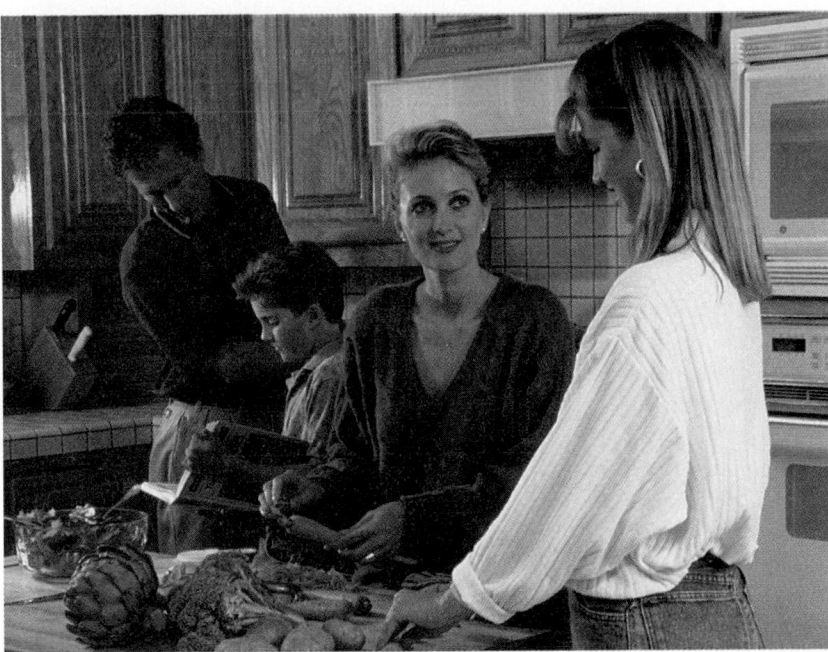

Teens can help plan meals that meet the whole family's nutritional needs while incorporating alternative food styles.

As their sense of social awareness develops, some teens may adopt a vegetarian dietary pattern. Creative planning on the part of the teen and the meal planner can result in meals that meet everyone's nutritional needs without compromising personal convictions.

Discussions of the eating habits of teens tend to be critical of their fast food consumption. Fortunately, most teens can afford the extra kcalories that typically higher-fat foods of hamburgers, fries, and pizza may contain. If teens have grown up accustomed to well-balanced meals, they will more than likely still prefer those meals to high-fat delights. Eating in fast food restaurants, where prices tend to be inexpensive, may have more to do with socializing with peers than with nutrient values.

When fast foods become the mainstay of an individual's diet, regardless of age, then some nutrients such as vitamin A and C may be lacking and overconsumption of dietary fats and kcalories may occur. Although teens may be noticed *hanging out* at such restaurants, most of the other customers consist of families with young children as well as senior citizens; fast foods affect the nutrient intake of all ages.

Nutrition requirements. Because of the natural physiological differences between adolescent males and females, nutrient requirements from age 11 and older are divided by gender. Females need about 2200 kcalories and 45 grams of protein daily. Recommendations for males are 2500-2900 kcalories and 45-59 grams of protein per day. These values for kcalories and protein reflect the increased lean body mass developing in males. They do, however, only represent suggested amounts; physical activity, either work or athletic endeavors, affects the actual nutrient needs for both males and females.

Calcium recommendations are the same for both genders, 1200 mg per day, to allow for skeletal growth (particularly for males) and for bone mineralization, a prime physiological function during adolescence. Bone mineralization for females is a concern as teenage girls often underconsume calcium-rich foods.

As discussed previously in Chapter 10 teenage girls and sometimes teenage boys are at risk for dieting-related disorders and eating disorders. By regularly underconsuming nutrients during a time when the human body is completing maturation, girls are at risk for various deficiencies as they progress toward adulthood and the nutrient requirements of potential pregnancies. In addition to calcium, iron allowances are important to fulfill, particularly for females who begin menstruation; iron is also needed by males, whose accelerated growth necessitates an increased blood volume and lean body mass.

Adolescent Health Promotion (13 to 19 Years)
Knowledge

The adolescent body benefits from a dietary intake most similar to an adult's; however, some nutrient needs are greater. Energy requirements are higher than at any other time of life, especially for adolescents involved in competitive athletics. Calcium recommendations increase to ensure adequate mineralization of bones. Tolerance for alternative food styles enhances overall dietary intake and allows for the acceptance of dietary suggestions to maintain appropriate nutrient consumption.

Teenagers can comprehend the body's physiology and nutrient needs. Ideally this information should be taught within health or science curricula in schools. This knowledge provides a rationale for consumption of *real* food, especially as preparation for sport activities. Although adults may supply provisions for meals and snacks, especially those that can be reheated, ultimately most adolescents take responsibility for their own nutrient intake.

Awareness of the risk factors and symptoms of eating disorders and drug/alcohol abuse should be provided through health classes or interactions with health and educational professionals and parents. Even mild substance abuse in the face

Signs of Substance Abuse		
Appetite loss	Headache	Seizures
Blackouts	Indigestion	Somnolence
Bleeding gums	Insomnia	Sore tongue
Depression	Memory loss	Stomach pain
Diarrhea	Muscle weakness	Taste loss
Dyspnea on exertion	Nausea	Tiredness
Faintness	Nervousness	Vomiting
Hangover	Rash	

From Payne WA, Hahn DB: *Understanding your health,* ed 4, St. Louis, 1995, Mosby.

of the increased nutritional needs of adolescence can compromise nutritional status. For example, alcohol adversely affects absorption of folate and zinc, two nutrients required for normal growth. Nurses need to be aware of the indicators of substance abuse (see box) so they can guide adolescents into treatment. Nutrition assessment, intervention, and support are part of comprehensive physical and psychological rehabilitation of all substance abusers.

Techniques

Similar to techniques for children, the concepts of the Food Guide Pyramid and Five-a-Day can provide a basis for food choices. Often the forces that override good food choices are lack of time and scheduling demands. One strategy that accommodates both is ensuring the availability of simple meals that are easily eaten and/or reheatable. Scheduling of meals can take into account school, sports, work, and recreational agendas.

Community supports

Except for federal government programs that serve children and adults, no food programs are specifically targeted at adolescents. At a time when teens are developmentally ready to be empowered to take care of themselves, society provides few supports. In fact, school, sports, and work schedules often hinder adolescents from taking responsibility for their health behaviors. Television, radio, and print messages rarely promote healthy behaviors. Although the increased interest in physical pursuits of basketball, soccer, biking, skateboarding, rollerblading, and other recreational sports passions enhance fitness, the nutrition component is often overlooked or cloaked in misinformation. This is an area to which all health professionals should be sensitive.

One of the few community supports is comprehensive school health programs. The depth of health issues covered varies and may not include sufficient nutrition guidance, but at the least these programs highlight basic concerns of nutrition and health.

Adulthood

By the time young adults reach about age 24, growth levels off and the body achieves a state of homeostasis. Mental capacity is fully developed as young people begin to assume their roles in adult society. How this transition is experienced depends on cultural views of growing older. Does growing older confer social privileges of respect and authority? Or does it mean the loss of youth and good times? How we accept new responsibilities within family and intimate relationships may affect our overall health status and level of wellness.

Layered on cultural perceptions of aging is the complexity of today's world. Through telecommunications we are exposed to and influenced by numerous world and local events in ways unimaginable to previous generations. Similarly, educational and employment opportunities seem endless; yet some adults are caught in cycles of underemployment and unemployment as the marketplace evolves and others, through economic misfortune, are homeless. Additionally, each stage of adulthood presents particular life stressors. How we cope with these stressors and those of society affects adult nutritional status.

Although previous chapters have addressed nutrition for adults, this section addresses the different influences on nutritional lifestyles through adulthood.

The early years (20s and 30s)

Students tend to imagine that once they finish high school or college and enter the *working world* they will then be able to eat better, sleep more, and generally take better care of themselves than they do during their hectic school years. Unfortunately, that is rarely the experience of young adults. Many find that their lifestyles may be even more time-restricted, and positive health behaviors such as regular meal patterns and exercise may fall by the wayside.

These years mark a transition from one stage of the life span to another; young adults separate from their family of origin, focus on personal and career goals, and often face reproductive decisions (9). As such, it is a prime time to either refine or establish an eating style that promotes health, possibly preventing future development of diet-related diseases. A self-review or assessment by a nutrition professional can assist in creating a personal schedule that allows time for planning and preparation of simple yet high quality meals.

Many women bear children during these years. The nutrition and health requirements of pregnancy are detailed in Chapter 11. Layered on these needs during this life span stage are often employment and other family commitments, all of which affect nutritional and health behaviors. Physically caring for young children, although eminently rewarding, may be exhausting. Throughout the mother's pregnancy and during childbearing, the father's role in terms of health issues is often ignored. While the woman's body is nourishing fetal development, the father is under stress as he prepares to support additional responsibilities. Fathers also need to be at optimum health, especially during the first few years of childrearing when physical stamina is put to the test.

Nutrition requirements. Growth tends to be completed by the late teens for females and early 20s for males, as reflected by the RDAs (inside front cover). For females, the RDA for energy is 2200 kcalories daily; for males it is 2900 kcalories. This reflects the typical differences in body weight and lean body mass of men and women. When this stage includes a departure from high school or college sports training, energy intake should be reduced to meet actual need or weight gain could occur. A teenage boy's serious athletic training may require as much as 5000 to 6000 kcalories a day to maintain weight. Switching to a desk job and exercising for 1 hour per day does not equal previous energy requirements.

The RDA for protein increases for women from 46 grams to 50 grams and for men from 58 grams to 63 grams daily; these ranges reflect lean body mass growth that may still occur in both males and females through about age 24. Vitamin and minerals needs do not significantly change. Calcium and phosphorus needs for men and women decline after age 24 since skeletal growth is complete. Daily recommended calcium and phosphorus levels up to age 24 are 1200 mg, dropping to 800 mg from 25 years on. Because bone development decreases, the need for vitamin D also decreases from 10 mg to 5 mg daily. Maintaining calcium and iron intake continues to be a concern for women because of their often restricted intake of food during dieting.

The middle years (40s and 50s)

The years from 40 to 50 are marked by a continuation of family demands and/or career involvement. Some middle-year adults may be faced with caring for aging parents; the increased stress and responsibility may be offset by the seemingly reduced parenting of their own children. As older children leave for college or move into their own residences, the resultant *empty nest* necessitates rediscovering preparation of dinners for two or, for single parents, dinners for one. With family meals no longer a requirement, many middle-year adults often have the finances and time for restaurant dining; however, making the transition to food preparation styles and dietary patterns that maintain healthful dietary patterns is crucial.

The impact of continued positive dietary patterns coupled with regular exercise provides continued prevention or delay of diet-related diseases such as non–insulin-dependent diabetes mellitus (NIDDM) and coronary artery disease. Increased stamina is an additional benefit from such behaviors.

Nutrition requirements. During the middle years, cell loss rather than replication occurs. Kcaloric needs decline as lean body mass is lost and replaced by body fat that is less metabolically active. Women in particular experience an increase in body fat composition. Body fat increases can be slowed by exercise and strength training to continue maintenance of lean body mass. After age 50 daily energy needs drop from 2200 kcalories to 1920 kcalories for women, and from 2900 kcalories to 2300 kcalories for men. It is a challenge to meet the same nutrient needs with reduced kcaloric intake. Protein needs remain constant for both sexes. Iron requirements for women drop from 15 mg to 10 mg, reflecting reduced iron loss because of menopause.

Overall, dietary patterns that are nutrient-dense and feature lower-fat protein foods coupled with fiber-containing fruits, vegetables, and grains best meet the nutrient needs of middle year adults.

The older years (60s, 70s, and 80s)

The United States has never had a population with as high a percentage of older adults as it will soon have (Fig.12-2). As our life span increases in years, **senescence** or older adulthood is for many a time of life for continued professional or career advancement and recreational enjoyment. Others are in transition, adjusting to retirement and settling into new patterns of activities. **Gerontology,** the study of aging, has provided insights into the emotional, physical, and social aspect of the

senescence
older adulthood

gerontology
the study of aging

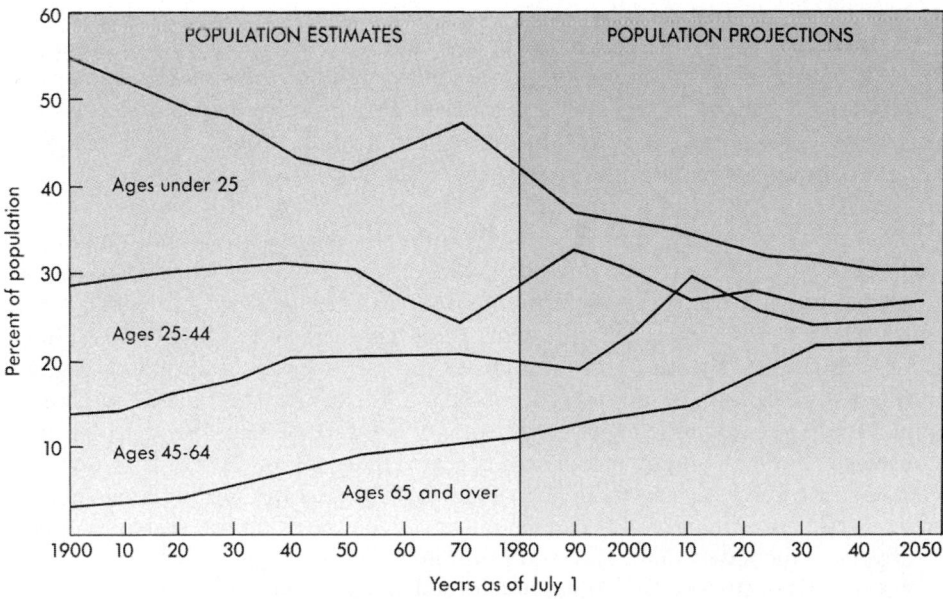

Fig. 12-2 Trend in age distribution of US population (including Armed Forces overseas), 1900-2050. The United States has never had a population with as many elderly people as it will soon have.

Signs of Dehydration in Older Adults
Confusion
Weakness
A hot, dry body
Furrowed tongue
Decreased skin turgor
(may not be valid finding in the elderly)
Rapid pulse
Elevated urinary sodium

later years of life. Preparation for the social and physical transitions of aging actually begins many years earlier, as individual approaches to lifestyle health behaviors, career fulfillment, and leisurely pursuits evolve.

The level of wellness experienced during this stage of life often reflects health behaviors through the several life span stages. A lifetime of physical fitness and good nutrition allows an individual to enter these years with more stamina, cardiovascular conditioning, and solid health-promoting habits that enable him or her to overcome the inevitable slowing down or physical limitation of the later years. Even those who were not always active have been shown to benefit from regular exercise. Strength training has improved muscle tone and stamina of men and women in their 80s (12).

During these later years, individuals may struggle with the deaths of family members and friends and adjusting to retirement. Although some delight in retirement, others view retirement as a loss of social status. This combination of death and loss of status may lead to isolation and depression. The economic realities of retirement without a solid financial base may thrust some elders into unexpected poverty as Social Security and Medicare payments may not be sufficient to cover living and medical expenses adequately. Unless social networking and/or family supports are strong, these conditions may persist. Older adults may abuse alcohol as way to deal with these perceived difficult events.

Disorientation or senility often associated with aging may be caused by improper use of medications or simple dehydration. Elderly clients may intentionally restrict fluids because of incontinence, **nocturia,** or inability to get to the toilet on their own. Some older adults lose their sense of thirst and forget to consume enough fluids. Fluid requirements in the elderly remain the same as in younger adults (about 8 cups a day) unless a medical condition or medication proscribe otherwise. The signs of dehydration are listed in the box above. Medical diagnosis should be sought to determine the specific etiology of such signs.

Nutrition status may be affected by restricted access to food and/or ability to prepare meals. Shopping may be difficult without transportation, and mobility to walk through stores may be limited. Funds for food may be constrained; often food quantities are beyond the amounts that can be used by individuals living alone. Once foods are purchased, preparation may be affected by physical limitations caused by progressive chronic illnesses such as arthritis. Some elderly persons may no longer have an interest in cooking. Others have become so frightened about foods containing too much fat and/or cholesterol that they become malnourished. For individuals in this age bracket, there is not sufficient evidence to warrant restrictive dietary intake; in actuality, malnutrition and underweight are more detrimental than excess dietary fat and cholesterol intake. Table 12-2 lists strategies to increase food intake and promote good nutrition.

Living arrangements also affect nutritional status. A variety of living arrangements exist for the elderly. Although many continue to live in their own homes or with family members, some opt for retirement communities and others, because of health conditions, may reside in long-term care facilities or nursing homes. Living

nocturia
excessive urination at night

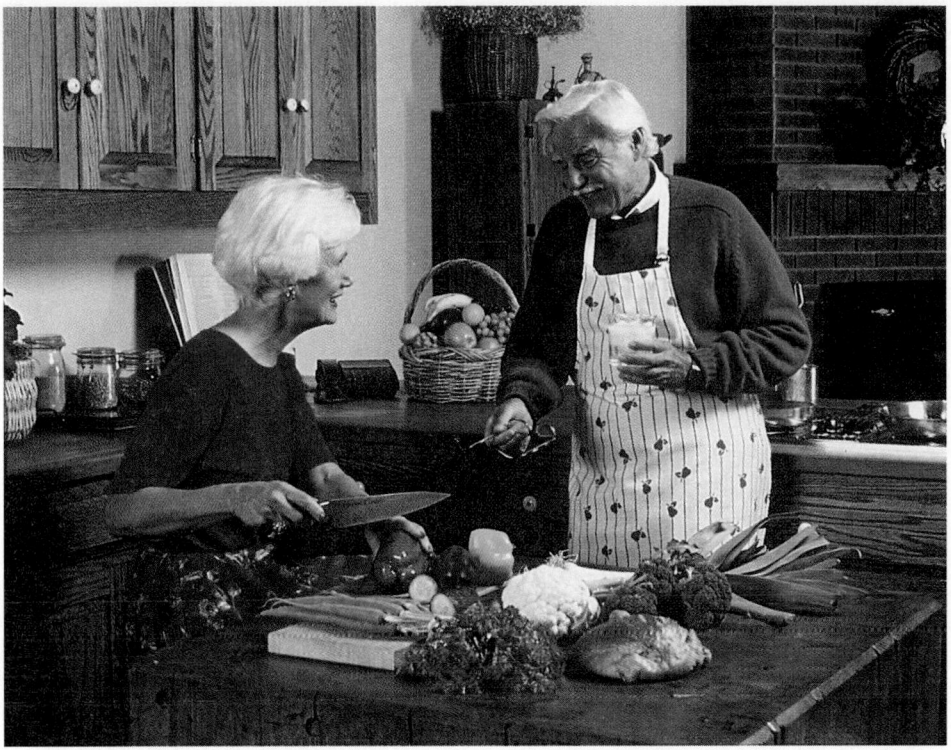

Companionship makes mealtimes more enjoyable for older adults.

in one's own home provides the freedom to prepare and eat foods whenever desired; illness, however, may make shopping for food and preparing it difficult. Retirement communities may provide transportation to foods stores and more social events involving meals, although residents still are responsible for their own food preparation. Long-term care facilities usually provide prepared meals, but the style of cooking may not be as appealing or comforting as home-prepared meals.

A challenge for meeting the nutritional needs of institutionalized elderly is that the RDAs, used to guide nutrient levels, are intended to meet the needs of healthy older adults. Adjustments are necessary for individual circumstances of acute or chronic illness to achieve rehabilitation, recuperation, or maintenance to reduce the risk of further complications (11).

Dietary patterns and preferences of elderly people are the result of long-established habits. When they are ill, lonely, or under stress, older adults may strongly prefer foods they associate with pleasant memories. Ethnic favorites may provide security and comfort. The psychological and social meanings of foods can play an important part in helping an elderly client recover from illness or adjust to changed circumstances (12).

Overall, the elderly may be at nutritional risk because of demographic and lifestyle characteristics. Factors may include gender, smoking, alcohol abuse, dietary patterns, educational level, dental health, chronic illnesses, and living situations (13). Interventions to assist the elderly need to account for these influences.

Nutrition requirements. The RDAs remain constant from age 51 and over for both men and women. What does change is the ability of the body to either process or synthesize certain nutrients. Synthesis of vitamin D is reduced; the elderly either need more exposure to sunlight to produce required amounts or require a supplement if so diagnosed by a physician, qualified nutritionist, or dietitian. Because of decreased production of gastric juices and intestinal enzymes, digestion and absorption may be reduced, further highlighting the need for optimum nutrient intake. The production of the intrinsic factor required for

Table 12-2   Strategies for Overcoming Barriers to Good Nutrition

COUNTERACT DECREASED SENSES OF TASTE AND SMELL
- Recommend smokers refrain from smoking at least 1 hour before meals
- Suggest sipping water before and during the meal to moisten a dry mouth
- Amplify flavors with the use of seasonings other than salt
- Recommend chewing food thoroughly to fully release flavor and aroma
- Vary food textures and flavors

PRESENT FOOD ATTRACTIVELY
- Use colorful foods and table settings
- Provide enough lighting to see food clearly

ENCOURAGE SOCIAL INTERACTION
- Find others who are willing to share food preparation and mealtimes
- Investigate congregate meal programs available through senior citizen centers, religious organizations, and hospital community outreach programs
- Avoid noisy dining areas for clients with hearing aids

PROVIDE OUTSIDE SUPPORT
- Arrange for Meals-on-Wheels for homebound
- Refer eligible clients to the Food Stamp Program, Emergency Food Assistance Program, Child and Adult Care Program, or community food banks or soup kitchens
- Locate grocery stores with delivery service
- Refer to the Expanded Food and Nutrition Education Program (EFNEP) of the Cooperative Extension Service for recipes, meal suggestions, and budgeting assistance
- Refer to home health nurse for routine nutrition screening and appropriate interventions

vitamin B_{12} absorption may also be reduced, increasing the risk of pernicious anemia and necessitating intramuscular injections of the vitamin.

Other factors may affect nutritional status. A marginal deficiency of zinc can alter the sensitivity of taste receptors. This deficiency heightens the ability to taste bitter and sour flavors and reduces sweet and salty sensations; excessive use of sugars and salt to make foods taste appealing may result. Overconsumption of simple sugars and sodium may exacerbate other diet-related disorders such as diabetes and/or hypertension. As the muscularity of the digestive system weakens, constipation may be a problem, especially after a lifetime of low-fiber foods. Constipation may be alleviated by slowly increasing consumption of whole wheat products, fruits, vegetables, and fluids, as well as increasing exercise.

Dental health may also affect the ability of the elderly to be well-nourished. Loss of teeth caused by periodontal disease limits the ability to chew foods such as meats, a prime source of zinc. Chewing ability for some may still be compromised even after dentures have been fitted to replace missing teeth. Dentures may need to be periodically refitted; when old dentures do not fit properly some people do not use them. Instead, they tend to eat foods that can be *gummed* rather than chewed.

The oldest years (80s and 90s)

As life expectancy increases in years, the number of those in the most golden years rises. Although nutrient needs remain basically stable, the effects of aging may continue to reduce the ability of the body to absorb and/or synthesize nutrients. Optimum nutrition continues to be critical. The healthiest of the oldest develop individual patterns of dietary intake that most meet their physical and social needs.

Risk Factors for Malnutrition of the Elderly

Alcoholism
Anorexia
Chewing and swallowing problems
Consuming only one meal a day
Dental difficulties
Depression or dementia
Diabetes
Diminished physical functioning
Feeding problems
Food purchasing/preparation difficulties
Impaired acuity of taste and smell
Living in long-term care institution
Loss of spouse
Multimedications
Nerve disorders
Poverty
Pulmonary disease
Surgery

From Chernoff R: Meeting the nutritional needs of the elderly in the institutional setting, *Nutr Rev* 52(4):132-136, 1994.

Nutrition requirements. Malnutrition and underweight become a concern during this stage (14). Risk factors for malnutrition are listed in the box above. As food preparation becomes more physically difficult to accomplish, kcaloric intake may diminish. Illness and accompanying medications may reduce appetite; malnutrition is associated with increased complications (11). Relatives, friends, and health care professionals can assist in ensuring that adequate meals are available and consumed (see Table 12-2). Although assessment is the responsibility of all health care professionals, home health nurses are particularly able to conduct routine nutrition screening and implement appropriate interventions to prevent or halt malnutrition among this population (14). Government and community meal programs help fill this need and are discussed in Community Supports.

Adult Health Promotion

Knowledge

Health promotion integrates nutrition education and focuses on three areas of knowledge: adequate intake of nutrients found in foods (rather than supplements); the relationship between diet and disease; and moderate kcaloric intake coupled with regular exercise for physical fitness and obesity prevention.

Techniques

Several *Healthy People 2000* objectives address the above key concepts (Table 12-3). Other strategies for adult health promotion include the following.

To promote/maintain positive health status and to reduce risk of diet-related disorders (coronary heart disease, some cancers, NIDDM, and obesity):
- Schedule routine food shopping so staples such as fruits, vegetables, and grains are available for meal preparation.
- When shopping, occasionally compare fat content of commonly purchased foods to similar products; purchase the lower-fat product.
- Aim to limit visible fat-containing foods.
- Reorganize work and personal priorities if necessary to allow time for meal preparation and consumption; for example, get up earlier for breakfast, pack a lunch or afternoon snack, preplan easy-to-prepare dinner menus.

Table 12-3 *Healthy People 2000* Objectives for Adult Health Promotion
• Reduce dietary fat intake to an average of 30% of calories or less and average saturated fat intake to less than 10% of calories among people aged 2 and older • Increase complex carbohydrate and fiber-containing foods in the diets of adults to 5 or more daily servings for vegetables (including legumes) and fruits and to 6 or more daily servings for grain products • Increase calcium intake so at least 50% of youths ages 12 through 24 and 50% of pregnant and lactating women consume 3 or more servings daily of foods rich in calcium and at least 50% of people aged 25 and older consume 2 or more servings daily • Decrease salt and sodium intake so at least 65% of home meal preparers prepare foods without adding salt, at least 80% of people avoid using salt at the table, and at least 40% of adults regularly purchase foods that are modified or lower in sodium • Increase to at least 50% the proportion of overweight people aged 12 and older who have adopted sound dietary practices combined with regular physical activity to attain an appropriate body weight • Increase to at least 85% the proportion of people aged 18 and older who use food labels to make nutritious food selections

From US Department of Health and Human Services, Public Health Service: *Healthy People 2000: National health promotion and disease prevention objectives,* Washington DC, 1990, US Government Printing Office.

- Keep track of dietary intake using the Food Guide Pyramid or 5-a-Day plan. Review Chapter 6 for other dietary fat-lowering techniques and Chapter 5 for approaches that increase use of complex carbohydrates and fiber-containing foods.

For overall bone health and to reduce the risk of osteoporosis:
- Focus on routine dietary habits; for example, drink a glass of milk at lunch each day. A food pattern assessment can assist in creating a practical calcium consumption plan. Review Chapter 8 for other approaches to increasing calcium consumption.

To reduce risk of coronary artery disease and sodium-sensitive hypertension:
- Check food labels to determine sodium content.
- Learn food categories that generally are salty and either consume only occasionally or, if available, purchase low-sodium versions of products. See Chapter 8 for other sodium-reducing strategies.

To attain appropriate body weight and to reduce risk of obesity caused by diet and lifestyle:
- Rather than focusing on food-restricting diets, respond to actual hunger with low-fat, high-fiber foods (with occasional splurges).
- Exercise regularly to increase stamina, strength, and a sense of wellness. Depending on conditioning, incorporate exercise gradually. A 10-minute walk may be comfortable for some; others can begin with more strenuous endeavors. Refer to Chapters 9 and 10 for related strategies.

Community supports

Government, corporate, and social institutions create the environments and structures that can support lifestyle health promotion behaviors. Although the actions of these institutions affect groups of either the public, employees, or communities, it is the individual who can choose to reap the rewards.

Government agencies such as the Food and Drug Administration create regulations that either provide consumers information for decision making (such as nutrition labeling) or that control the quality of foods, which affects the nutrient viability of manufactured products. These issues are addressed by the following objective.

> Achieve useful and informative nutrition labeling for virtually all processed foods and at least 40 percent of fresh meats, poultry, fish, fruits, vegetables, baked goods, and ready-to-eat carry-away foods (8).

Food manufacturers as an institution have been challenged by *Healthy People 2000* to reach the following objective.

> Increase to at least 5,000 brand items the availability of processed food products that are reduced in fat and saturated fat (8).

The intent of this objective is to make it easier for consumers to reduce their intake of fat and saturated fat through manufactured products. Not all health professionals are in favor of this approach. Some suggest that it is better to choose foods that are naturally low in fat than to consume prefabricated foods that may lose other nutritious properties during the manufacturing process.

Although the previous *Healthy People 2000* objectives addressed foods consumed in the home, the next objective concerns eating outside of the home.

> Increase to at least 90 percent the proportion of restaurants and institutional food service operations that offer identifiable low-fat, low-calorie food choices, consistent with the Dietary Guidelines for Americans (8).

This objective may be harder to achieve. The American Heart Association has a program called *Heart Healthy;* its purpose is to help the public identify food choices on restaurant menus that are low in fat, sodium, and cholesterol. Health professionals can request that these food choices be available and highlighted on menus, especially at the food service institutions that serve our patients. Our professional organizations can also request these changes. Many retail and food service institutions already meet the guidelines; specific entrees need to be identified as an educative service for consumers and patients.

Corporations can support health promotion activities. This issue is addressed in the following *Healthy People 2000* objective.

> Increase to at least 85 percent the proportion of workplaces with 50 or more employees that offer health promotion activities for their employees, preferably as part of a comprehensive employee health promotion program (8).

This can be accomplished through wellness centers providing programs about healthy lifestyles. Although most corporations may not be able to provide on-site gyms or similar facilities, some have arranged for corporate discounts at local gym facilities. Perhaps the leader of on-site wellness centers is the NIKE corporate headquarters on the NIKE World Campus in Beaverton, Oregon. Employees are able to use the Bo Jackson Fitness Center, a state of the art health club facility, for a nominal fee and run on an outdoor jogging trail that encircles the NIKE campus. Boats are even available to sail on the lake that is a centerpiece of the corporate headquarters. In addition, employees can take longer lunch breaks, even 2-hour breaks, allowing for complete workouts (15).

Health departments, through their health officers, often provide community programming that meets the next two objectives.

> Establish community health promotion programs that separately or together address at least three of the *Healthy People 2000* priorities and reach at least 40 percent of each State's population (8).
>
> Increase to at least 50 percent the proportion of counties that have established culturally and linguistically appropriate community health promotion programs for racial and ethnic minority populations (8).

Socioeconomic support within the community is provided by government agencies and community groups. Government programs include the Food Stamp

Program, temporary Emergency Food Assistance Program, and community food banks/meals.

The Food Stamp Program provides coupons toward the purchase of foods for people with low incomes. By boosting food purchasing power, overall nutrient intake is improved. This program is administered nationally by the USDA and on the state and local levels by welfare and/or human services agencies. The actual food stamp cost is paid by the federal government; administration costs are divided between the other agencies.

As an entitlement program, it is available to all who are eligible without restriction of age or family size. Financial and nonfinancial factors of households are considered to determine eligibility. Financial factors include income and economic resources such as savings or vehicles; nonfinancial considerations consist of a variety of factors such as social security eligibility, citizenship, and work requirements. Gross incomes must meet certain percentages of the poverty level based on overall factors; the level of support varies based on family membership and net income (7).

The Emergency Food Assistance Program (EMFAP) is administered by the Food and Nutrition Service of the USDA. Various local agencies may administer the program. State agencies determine their own criteria for eligibility based on a household income. The program serves two functions: to reduce government-held surplus dairy commodities and to supplement the dietary intake of low-income households through the distribution of basic commodities. The types of foods distributed vary between actual surplus foods and foods purchased especially for this program. In addition to dairy products of nonfat dry milk and cheese, EMFAP has distributed canned meat, peanut butter, citrus juices, legumes, dried potatoes, and canned and dried fruit. Some of this program's funds are used by states to fund emergency feeding programs such as soup kitchens or food banks (7).

Community food banks and emergency feeding programs may be partially funded by EMFAP in addition to support by foundations and other charitable organizations. Some programs also collect food from the surrounding community and surplus donations from supermarkets and restaurants. Personnel at these facilities are usually volunteers from youth groups, religious organizations, and civic associations. Food banks often provide a bag of food staples to help bridge the gap that may occur when food stamps and monthly welfare support are exhausted before the beginning of the next month. Emergency feeding programs such as soup kitchens may provide hot meals as a safety net to assist individuals to avoid malnutrition among lower socioeconomic populations (7).

Supports specifically for the elderly include the Child and Adult Care Food Program and the Senior Nutrition Program. Community groups may sponsor some of the government programs or may develop their own local programs to meet the following objective.

> Increase to at least 80 percent the receipt of home food services by people aged 65 and older who have difficulty in preparing their own meals or are otherwise in need of home-delivered meals (8).

The Child and Adult Care Food Program provides meals and snacks for children up to age 12 and to senior citizens and specific categories of the handicapped persons participating in day care programs that are nonprofit, licensed, or receive agency approval. Reimbursement rates differ for programs serving children or adults; family income of the participants may be considered. Similar to other programs, it is administered on the federal level by the Food and Nutrition Service of the USDA and on the state level by human services or education departments. Day care programs may be administered locally by a variety of sponsors including adult programs through community groups. For children, eligible programs include Head Start, after-school programs, family day care, and other approved sites (7).

The Senior Nutrition Program serves only the elderly and was created to offer inexpensive meals, education, and socialization. The Congregate Meals Program and Home-Delivered Meals Program (Meals on Wheels) are both part of the Senior Nutrition Program. This program provides for those in financial need as well as for those in social need. Eligibility is open to everyone aged 60 years or older; spouses of participants may also be served regardless of their age. To participate in the Home Delivered Meals Program, individuals must reside in the program service area and be unable to prepare their own meals. Meals are provided Monday through Friday. Those receiving meals at home also are given frozen meals for Saturday and Sunday consumption (7).

OVERCOMING BARRIERS

Food Asphyxiation

Asphyxiation from food is possible at any point along the life span, but toddlers and the elderly tend to be more at risk. As toddlers first become accustomed to a variety of food textures and substances, they sometimes misjudge the size of food being chewed or may be too active when eating and accidentally swallow before sufficient chewing has taken place. Some foods that are potential problems are peanut butter (large clumps can stick in the throat), peanuts, popcorn, hot dogs, hard candies, gum, grapes, and foods containing bones (beef, poultry, and fish). Efforts by parents and caregivers to serve appropriate foods to young children can prevent choking incidents. Children can be reminded to chew food well and sit quietly while eating. The elderly may be at risk because of reduced chewing ability from loss of teeth or poorly fitting dentures. Counseling the elderly about problematic foods may avert asphyxiation occurrences.

Lead Poisoning

Lead poisoning can be an invisible health hazard. Found in old paint dust or chips, enameled porcelain fixtures (bath tubs), and soil or air from industrial and transportation pollution, excessive amounts of lead can be absorbed into the body (16). Children are most at risk; they naturally absorb greater amounts of minerals than adults. Nutritional deficiencies of iron, calcium, and zinc tend to increase the absorption of lead. Lead poisoning and iron deficiency anemia are sometimes diagnosed concurrently. Excessive exposure to lead can permanently affect cognitive and perceptual abilities. These reduced functions affect learning ability (17). School and community nurses in high-risk areas should be sensitive to this risk to both physical and intellectual health. High-risk areas for children include lower socioeconomic areas with poor housing conditions. Once lead poisoning is determined through blood testing, local health departments work with families to ascertain the sources of contamination in the home or school environment while physicians implement lead-reduction therapy.

Overall levels of lead in the environment are lower than in the past because of standards established and enforced by the Environmental Protection Agency. Levels of lead in some communities, however, are still high enough by Centers for Disease Control and Prevention standards, that primary prevention activities to further reduce lead poisoning should remain a community-wide goal (18).

Stress

Stress can affect all aspects of well-being. Although the actual cause of stress may not be related to dietary intake and meal patterns, these may be altered. The *normal* stresses of contemporary life may lead individuals to be so busy that they forget to eat or do not make appropriate food selections, particularly for breakfast and lunch. Some may overeat to soothe their nerves, and others may lose their appetite totally. If these actions become habitual, inappropriate eating patterns reduce the ability to cope with stressors.

Other impediments may occur. Stress may lead the gastrointestinal tract to overfunction, producing excessive gastric juices. The resulting indigestion may lead to the potential development of peptic ulcers. The anxiety of stress could also cause loss of appetite, which further reduces nutrient intake and can affect the absorption of nutrients, including minerals, protein, and vitamin C. Emotional stress increases the release of some hormones such as adrenaline. Adrenaline has a role in the breakdown of bone tissue during bone remodeling. Excess production of adrenaline in response to repetitive stressors affects bone health and is a potential risk factor for osteoporosis (12). The stressors of everyday life may occasionally cause an increase of urinary nitrogen output; however, the amount is not significant. Extreme levels of stress caused by environmental or physiological factors can substantially increase nitrogen loss requiring therapeutic intervention; these interventions are detailed in Chapter 14 (19).

Eating Disorders

eating disorders
a group of behaviors fueled by unresolved emotional conflicts symptomized by altered food consumption

Eating disorders are a group of behaviors fueled by unresolved emotional conflicts, symptomized by altered food consumption. Disorders include anorexia nervosa, bulimia nervosa, and binge eating. These represent a continuum from the starvation of anorexia nervosa to the uncontrollable excessive food intake of binge eating disorder (Fig. 12-3). Most individuals with eating disorders are females; however, males are also susceptible.

Although disordered food consumption is the overt symptom of eating disorders, changed nutrient intake is not the cause. Nourishment becomes a symbolic issue when individuals experiencing eating disorders are not able to deal directly with their emotions and instead *nourish* their psyches by either excessively restricting food or consuming extremely large quantities of foods that may then be purged. Eating disorders cannot be *cured* by eating *properly*. Underlying psychological concerns must first be addressed.

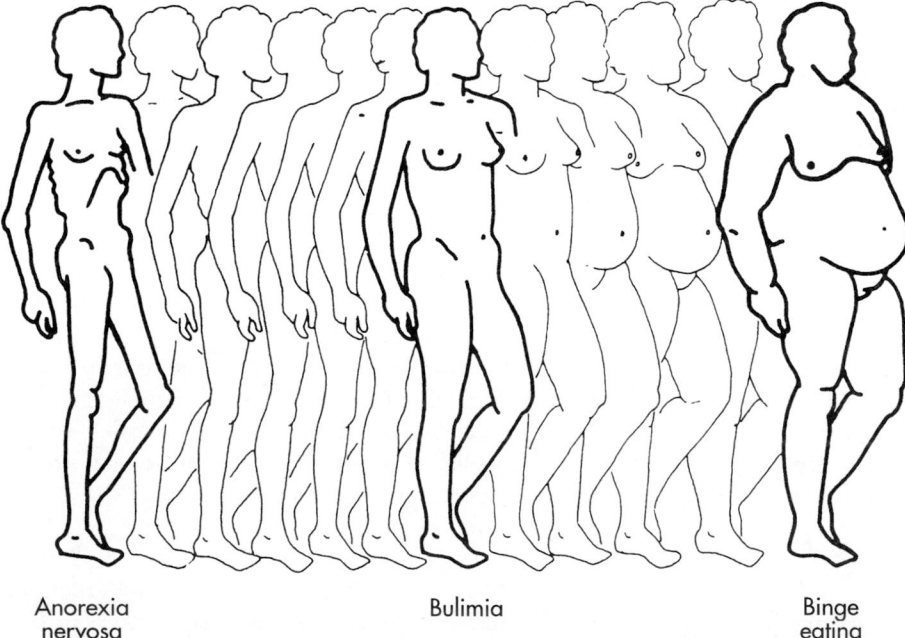

Anorexia   Bulimia   Binge
nervosa   eating

Fig. 12-3 Continuum of eating disorders. Although physical conditions vary, underlying psychological characteristics are held in common across the continuum.

Etiology

The etiology of eating disorders tends to be assigned to our Western obsession with the ideal of thinness. For many American females from early adolescence on, dieting (restrictive food intake) is a way of life. Most who are caught in the web of the culture of thinness experience chronic dieting syndrome. **Chronic dieting syndrome** can be described as a lifestyle inhibited or controlled by a constant concern about food intake, body shape, and/or weight that affects an individual's physical and mental health status (20). Only a small percentage of these chronic dieters manifest eating disorders. Additional risk factors must be present for eating disorders to evolve. Common risk factors include low self-esteem, depression, participation in appearance or endurance sports, history of sex abuse, or self-regulatory difficulties. The influence of risk factors are cumulatively mediated by the context of the individual in relation to societal and familial variables (21).

Diagnosis

Uniform criteria for these psychiatric disorders are established by the American Psychiatric Association and published as the *Diagnostic and Statistical Manual of Mental Disorders, fourth edition, (DSM-IV)*. Periodic revisions allow for updating disorder criteria and for the addition of newly recognized conditions. The DSM-IV criteria for clinical diagnosis of anorexia nervosa, bulimia nervosa, and binge eating disorder are listed in Tables 12-4 through 12-6.

Anorexia nervosa. Anorexia nervosa is characterized as refusal to maintain normal body weight through self-imposed starvation (Fig. 12-4). Because of distorted body images, individuals who experience this disorder do not *see* themselves as underweight and continue to restrict their food intake, often in a ritualistic manner. Some experience binge-eating episodes that are also associated with bulimic behaviors. Psychological characteristics include obsession with body shape and weight and an intense phobia of obesity. Chronic restrictive dieting is coupled with self-imposed limitation of food selection, hoarding, or hiding of food. Although their personal food intake is restricted, anorectics often prepare food for others; otherwise they avoid food-related events. When questioned about their food intake, they deny the disorder and weight loss. Anorectics tend to be overly perfectionist *model children* who are introverted, reserved, or possibly socially insecure. A profile of low self-esteem or a family history of anorexia and/or depression often exists, as well as compulsive behaviors in areas other than food intake. Other areas of compulsion may include excessive exercise, ritualized personal hygiene habits, and intensive study/work behaviors. Bingeing behaviors, if present, are similar to those of bulimia nervosa.

Physical dimensions may include amenorrhea; fatigue yet appearance of hyperactivity; dehydration; electrolyte imbalances including abnormally low levels of magnesium, zinc, phosphorus, and calcium in circulating blood; and metabolic alkalosis or metabolic acidosis caused by laxative abuse. Cardiovascular problems may develop such as hypotension (abnormally low blood pressure), arrhythmias, and sinus bradycardia (unusually slow heartbeat). Also present may be hormonal imbalances of reduced levels of estrogen or testosterone, hypothermia, and hypertension. Lanugo (soft white hair covering the body) is a late-stage effect as is edema not caused by premenstrual conditions or other medical conditions. Other physical conditions may include metabolic changes, constipation, and symptoms associated with starvation including loss of muscular strength, endurance, aerobic capacity, speed, and coordination. Vitamin, mineral, and protein deficiencies may also develop, leading to loss of bone mass and permanent damage to body organs. Mortality for anorexia nervosa is between 5% and 10% (22,23).

Bulimia nervosa. Bulimia nervosa is referred to as the binge and purge syndrome; bulimic behaviors include experiencing repetitive food binges accompanied by purging or compensatory behaviors. **Bingeing** is defined as feeling out of control when eating,

chronic dieting syndrome
a lifestyle inhibited or controlled by a constant concern about food intake, body shape, and/or weight that affects an individual's physical and mental health status

anorexia nervosa
a mental disorder characterized by self-imposed starvation; may include binge eating episodes associated with bulimic behaviors

bulimia nervosa
a mental disorder characterized as the binge and purge syndrome; includes experiencing repetitive food binges accompanied by purging or compensatory behaviors

bingeing
feeling out of control when eating, resulting in the consumption of excessive amounts of food.

CULTURAL CONSIDERATIONS
Is There Sociocultural Protection From Eating Disorders?

Noted in eating disorder literature is the issue of sociocultural protection against eating disorders for women of color. Because of differences in culturally acceptable body shapes, it was theorized that women of color seemed to experience more body satisfaction and self-esteem. This greater acceptance of body shape and size may provide protection against eating disorders.

A concept such as protectionism no longer makes sense within our contemporary society. This view obscures the vast cultural and individual diversity present within American ethnic groups. Eating disorders reflect the illness of the society within which they occur. They can be understood more so as a public health issue, potentially affecting all ethnicities.

For example, sexism is an issue reflecting societal and cultural conditions. Concerns about sexism go beyond those of equal pay. The pressures of the culture of thinness (insecurities about one's body) and career success are touted as sexism concerns. These issues, however, represent the middle/upper socioeconomic class orientation most often researched and are based on feminist analysis.

This perspective, however, is too shallow and underestimates the complexity of being female in Western contemporary society. These issues are superfluous for working and poor women; they deny the experience of working women whose psychological experience is not defined by their bodies nor their careers. Their psychological development is often formed by trauma, sometimes at very early ages, caused by either sexual and/or psychological abuse, racism, or sexual preference. For them, food is not just about thinness and body shape, but functions as a coping mechanism. The resulting eating disorders reflect survival strategies. For these women, just earning a living and caring for one's family are crushing pressures when combined with racism, poverty, and other societal barricades. Others whose sexual orientation differs face discrimination when attempting to live openly as lesbians or increased stress from efforts to keep their sexual identities hidden. Race, sexual orientation, and class are powerful forces in American society.

These same groups would also be underrepresented if prevalence of eating disorders is based on the reports of medical and psychological clinicians and therapists. Knowledge of etiology and treatment are based on the reports and research of therapists, psychologists, and psychiatrists who tend to treat individuals of the upper middle Caucasian socioeconomic group. Criteria based on this information may not represent the experience of all those potentially at risk for or presently experiencing the ravages of eating disorders.

In addition, stereotyping may lead to misdiagnosis. Professionals may not recognize symptoms of eating disorders in individuals from nondominant ethnic groups, since commonly consulted data imply that it is a problem of the dominant group of Caucasian upper socioeconomic females. Symptoms among African-Americans, Latinas, Native Americans, and Asian-Americans may be missed if assumptions are made that they could not possibly have a problem identified with the "white" culture.

Our present view of eating disorder etiology is probably only a piece of the true mosaic of eating disorder causes. The rest of the mosaic needs to be explored to include consideration of the social, economic, and political contexts within which women of color are also at risk.

From Root M: Disordered eating in women of color, *Sex Roles* 22(7/8): 525-536, 1990; and Thompson BW: *A hunger so wide and deep: American women speak out on eating problems,* Minneapolis, 1994, University of Minnesota Press.

Table 12-4   Diagnostic Criteria for Anorexia Nervosa

A. Refusal to maintain body weight at or above a minimally normal weight for age and height (e.g., weight loss leading to maintenance of body weight less than 85% of that expected; or failure to make expected weight gain during period of growth, leading to body weight less than 85% of that expected).

B. Intense fear of gaining weight or becoming fat, even though underweight.

C. Disturbance in the way in which one's body weight or shape is experienced, undue influence of body weight or shape on self-evaluation, or denial of the seriousness of the current low body weight.

D. In postmenarcheal females, amenorrhea, i.e., the absence of at least three consecutive menstrual cycles. (A woman is considered to have amenorrhea if her periods occur only following hormone, e.g., estrogen, administration.)

Specify type:

Restricting Type: during the current episode of Anorexia Nervosa, the person has not regularly engaged in binge-eating or purging behavior (i.e., self-induced vomiting or the misuse of laxatives, diuretics, or enemas)

Binge-Eating/Purging Type: during the current episode of Anorexia Nervosa, the person has regularly engaged in binge-eating or purging behavior (i.e., self-induced vomiting or the misuse of laxatives, diuretics, or enemas)

From American Psychiatric Association: Diagnostic and statistical manual of mental disorders (DSM-IV), ed 4, Washington DC, 1994, American Psychiatric Association.

Table 12-5   Diagnostic Criteria for Bulimia Nervosa

A. Recurrent episodes of binge eating. An episode of binge eating is characterized by both of the following:
(1) eating, in a discrete period of time (e.g., within any 2-hour period), an amount of food that is definitely larger than most people would eat during a similar period of time and under similar circumstances
(2) a sense of lack of control over eating during the episode (e.g., a feeling that one cannot stop eating or control what or how much one is eating)

B. Recurrent inappropriate compensatory behavior in order to prevent weight gain, such as self-induced vomiting; misuse of laxatives, diuretics, enemas, or other medications; fasting; or excessive exercise.

C. The binge eating and inappropriate compensatory behaviors both occur, on average, at least twice a week for 3 months.

D. Self-evaluation is unduly influenced by body shape and weight.

E. The disturbance does not occur exclusively during episodes of Anorexia Nervosa.

Specify type:

Purging Type: during the current episode of Bulimia Nervosa, the person has regularly engaged in self-induced vomiting or the misuse of laxatives, diuretics, or enemas

Nonpurging Type: during the current episode of Bulimia Nervosa, the person has used other inappropriate compensatory behaviors, such as fasting or excessive exercise, but has not regularly engaged in self-induced vomiting or the misuse of laxatives, diuretics, or enemas

From American Psychiatric Association: Diagnostic and statistical manual of mental disorders (DSM-IV), ed 4, Washington DC, 1994, American Psychiatric Association.

Table 12-6   Research Criteria for Binge Eating Disorder

A. Recurrent episodes of binge eating. An episode of binge eating is characterized by both of the following:
   (1) eating, in a discrete period of time (e.g., within any 2-hour period), an amount of food that is definitely larger than most people would eat in a similar period of time and under similar circumstances
   (2) a sense of lack of control over eating during the episode (e.g., a feeling that one cannot stop eating or control what or how much one is eating)

B. The binge-eating episodes are associated with three (or more) of the following:
   (1) eating much more rapidly than normal
   (2) eating until feeling uncomfortably full
   (3) eating large amounts of food when not feeling physically hungry
   (4) eating alone because of being embarrassed by how much one is eating
   (5) feeling disgusted with oneself, depressed, or very guilty after overeating

C. Marked distress regarding binge eating is present.

D. The binge eating occurs, on average, at least 2 days a week for 6 months.
   Note: The method of determining frequency differs from that used for Bulimia Nervosa; future research should address whether the preferred method of setting a frequency threshold is counting the number of days on which binges occur or counting the number of episoded of binge eating.

E. The binge eating is not associated with the regular use of inappropriate compensatory behaviors (e.g., purging, fasting, excessive exercise) and does not occur exclusively during the course of Anorexia Nervosa or Bulimia Nervosa.

From American Psychiatric Association: Diagnostic and statistical manual of mental disorders (DSM-IV), ed 4, Washington DC, 1994, American Psychiatric Association.

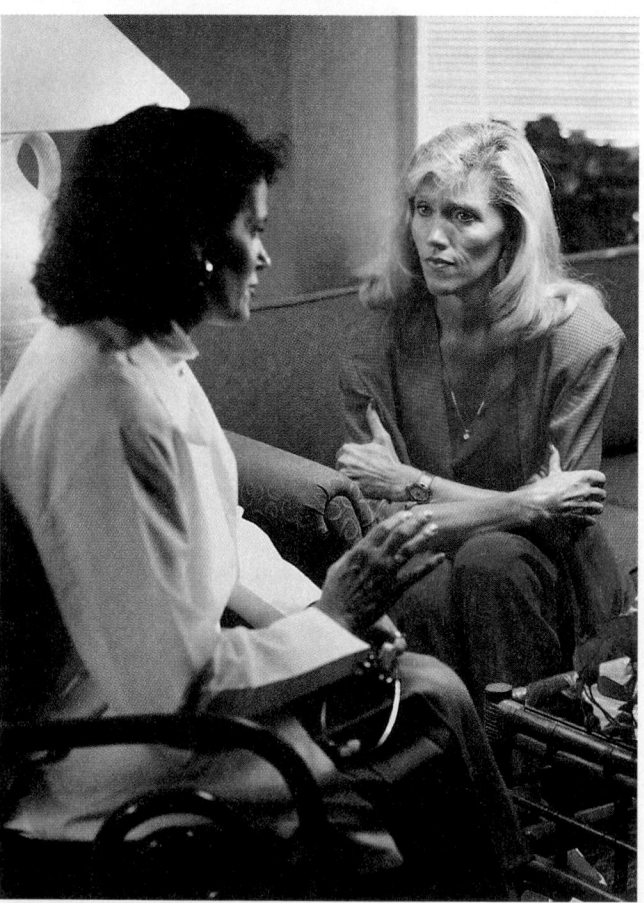

Fig. 12-4 Nurse-client relationships often provide informal opportunities to discuss dietary patterns; if early signs of disordered eating are detected, further assessment or treatment can be initiated.

MYTH
Eating Disorders Affect Only Teens and Young Women

Although most individuals with eating disorders are in their teens and early 20s, these disorders can strike at most any age. Particularly difficult is anorexia nervosa, for which the struggle to recover may be lifelong. Family members may be affected psychologically and physically as their loved ones experience this disorder. Consider the experiences of Mark Stuart Ellison:

Growing Up With An Anorexic Mother

"A hamburger on whole wheat toast and don't cut it." Those words are ineradicably etched in my mind. That's how my mother would order whenever she ate out. Although the hamburger was never to her liking and she would never eat the toast, the order was always the same. I recall the extraordinary patience and compassion of waiters and waitresses trying to please someone who was unpleasable. My mother had anorexia nervosa.

My mother died of anorexia at age 49; I was 17. As an attractive young woman, my mother, at five feet four inches weighed a voluptuous 135 lbs. During the course of her illness, she weighed as little as 60 lbs, while exercising to exhaustion. The circumstances surrounding her illness had caused me to become socially withdrawn years earlier. I am now 34 years old and have only recently begun to emerge from that isolation.

When I was 9, I witnessed a horrifying scene. The bathroom door in my apartment was slightly ajar. My mother was in the bathroom, squirming on the toilet seat, my father struggling to hold her on the bowl. I was terrified. I didn't know what was happening.

A few minutes later, paramedics took her to the hospital on a stretcher. Mom had one too many enemas and suffered the consequences on that day. From then on, my mother was in and out of hospitals for the rest of her life and never lived with me again.

As an anorexic she was ever-present; as a mother, she was absent. I have only begun to fill in the blanks in my own life.

From Ellison MS: Growing up with an anorexic mother, *AABA Newsletter,* Summer 1995.

resulting in the consumption of excessive amounts of food. In response to bingeing, the individual with bulimia purges using laxatives, diuretics, or self-induced vomiting and/or utilizes inappropriate compensatory behaviors of fasting, diet pills, or excessive exercise. Bingeing is one of the primary characteristics of bulimia. A *binge* consists of the consumption of excessively large quantities of food in a short period of time with a feeling of being unable to control the amount consumed. An average of two binges per week for 3 months accompanied by several other psychological and/or physical dimensions constitutes a diagnosis of bulimia nervosa. Binge foods tend to be of high-kcaloric value requiring minimal preparation. The binge is terminated by sleep, abdominal pain, or self-induced or drug-induced vomiting.

Purging and other compensatory behaviors to counteract binges are other characteristics of bulimia. Compensatory behaviors include self-induced vomiting and the use of **emetics,** diuretics, and laxatives as purging agents. Fasting and/or restrictive dieting, appetite suppressants, and excessive exercise may serve as compensatory behaviors. The use of emetics, in particular, to induce vomiting may have serious medical consequences; fatal incidences associated with bulimia have been reported (22).

Psychological dimensions of bulimia encompass obsessions with body shape and weight associated with chronic restrictive dieting. Binge eating and purging are *triggered* by stressful events or initiated as a group activity as part of a social event. Episodes of bingeing are accompanied by a loss of self-control and low self-esteem. Individuals tend to lack the ability to apply appropriate coping skills. Addictive disorders, depression, and family history of obesity, bulimia nervosa, and/or sex abuse may be present.

Physical characteristics may include weight fluctuation, amenorrhea, and fatigue. Dental health is affected as dental caries (from excessive simple-sugar consumption)

emetic
a substance that causes vomiting

develop and dental enamel erosion (from acidic vomitus) occurs. Purging may lead to dehydration and electrolyte imbalances, particularly with abnormally low levels of chloride, sodium, and calcium in circulating blood; laxative abuse may result in metabolic acidosis. Recurrent episodes of vomiting may cause metabolic alkalosis, bruising of the dorsal surface of the hands (from inducing vomiting), sore throats, swollen salivary glands (especially parotid glands), hormonal imbalances, blood-shot eyes (particularly after vomiting), and broken blood vessels on the face. Rare complications may include gastric rupture, esophageal tears, and cardiac arrhythmias. Chronic use of emetics may lead to cardiac and skeletal abnormalities.

Binge eating disorder. The third eating disorder, **binge eating disorder** (BED), is commonly referred to as compulsive overeating. Individuals with this disorder frequently engage in binge eating behavior not accompanied by purging or compensatory behaviors.

Psychological dimensions are reflected by binges *triggered* by stressful events or dysphoric moods including anxiety and depression. The binge eating may occur in secret or private settings and be accompanied by a sense of loss of control. Individuals appear to lack appropriate coping skills. After bingeing episodes, they experience low self esteem, shame, remorse, and/or depression. Other addictive disorders may be present in addition to obsessive behaviors in nonfood areas. A family history of obesity, depression, and/or addictive disorders is likely.

Physical characteristics may include obesity with increased risk of joint pains, breathing difficulties, coronary artery disease, elevated blood cholesterol levels, hypertension, and gastrointestinal tract disturbances. Binge eating disorder, however, is not the only etiological factor of obesity. Obesity may also be caused by excessive kcaloric consumption not associated with emotional turmoil, poor eating habits, sedentary lifestyle, and/or genetic factors. Conversely, binge eating disorder may be present in the absence of obesity, if the criteria of recurrent binges associated with emotional upset and a sense of loss of control occur.

Nutritional Therapy

Dietary patterns in eating disorders may be fractured to a point at which meals are nonexistent or so redefined as to lose all meaning. A challenge in treatment is the relearning of meal patterns.

Medical nutritional therapy is *the use of specific nutrition services to treat an illness, injury, or condition* (24). It involves assessment and treatment that may include diet therapy, counseling, and the use of specialized nutrition supplements. Since medical nutritional therapy is an integral component of eating disorder recovery, knowledge of the process of nutritional care is beneficial for all health care professionals who interact with patients who have eating disorders. As the medical, nursing, and psychological staffs implement their therapeutic approaches, they will be aware of the objectives of the medical nutritional therapy. While underlying psychological issues of eating disorders are worked on through psychological therapy, the registered dietitian works together with the patient to bring about changes in the patient's food-and-weight-related behaviors. This collaborative effort occurs in various phases of outpatient and/or inpatient therapy and constitutes nutrition intervention (24).

Nutrition intervention consists of two phases: the educational phase and the experimental phase. According to the position paper on eating disorders of the American Dietetic Association, all registered dietitians are trained to implement the educational phase, but specialized training and experience in eating disorder counseling is required for the experimental phase (24).

The educational phase provides a knowledge foundation to support the behavioral changes of the experimental phase. The dietitian shares nutrition information about dietary patterns and nutritional adequacy. The interaction is brief and relatively impersonal; the emotional dynamic surrounding food intake as an aspect of eating disorders is not explored in this phase (24).

binge eating disorder (BED)
a mental disorder characterized by frequent binge eating behaviors, not accompanied by purging or compensatory behaviors; commonly referred to as compulsive overeating

medical nutritional therapy
the use of specific nutrition services to treat an illness, injury, or condition

SOCIAL ISSUE
When an Eating Disorder is Suspected: Who is Responsible for Intervention?

Perhaps it is a daughter, sibling, friend, or roommate. An eating disorder is suspected; too much weight is lost, very little is eaten or too much is eaten, and vomiting and other purging is observed. What should you do?

Too often denial occurs, not only by the person with disordered eating but by her family and friends as well. It's easier to ignore what is happening than to risk becoming involved. On the other hand, sometimes overinvolvement happens when family and friends become so embroiled in the battle to eat or not eat that the disorder becomes the center of relationships. Few relationships can survive well based on struggling with eating issues.

When an eating disorder is suspected, the first action is to talk directly to the person about it. She may be waiting for someone to confront her and tell her these behaviors are not okay; such an encounter may be a trigger for her to seek professional help. If that is not sufficient, friends may choose to contact family members who may have more influence and responsibility for the health of the individual. In a college dormitory setting, resident life personnel should be contacted. They are often specially trained to assist students with eating disorders. It is unfair for the eating disorder of a roommate to negatively affect the lives of the others. Roommates can best help the person by intervening, however risky such actions may be to the friendship.

Once intervention has begun, new rules often have to be negotiated. Food and related eating behaviors can no longer be the focus of relationships. Each person becomes responsible for her own intake of nourishment. Although meals may be shared, food policing needs to be curtailed. Parents will need to refrain from pushing food to their child who is anorectic; friends may need to ignore second helpings of a friend who is bulimic. Other rules may evolve; if an individual still binges, she must replace the food she consumes. If the binge is followed by purging, she must completely clean the bathroom after vomiting. The goal is that the person must be responsible for her own actions without interfering with the rights of others. Though friends and family may analyze how their behaviors might have supported this illness, ultimately the struggle to heal is hers alone.

From Siegel M, Brisman J, Weinshel M: *Surviving an eating disorder: Strategies for family and friends,* New York, 1988, Harper Perennial.

The experimental phase does incorporate such issues. Through a long-term counseling relationship, the registered dietitian as a member of a multidisciplinary team works directly with the patient to mediate eating behaviors. The intervention may be a psychonutritional approach through which the dietitian discusses emotional issues of eating with the patient. To do so, the registered dietitian should be supervised by and communicate with the multidisciplinary team since formulating appropriate therapeutic boundaries is crucial.

Based on the position of ADA, there are five objectives of the nutrition education phase: (1) collect relevant information through detailed assessment of the diverse eating disorder population; (2) establish a collaborative relationship between the person with the eating disorder and the registered dietitian; (3) define and discuss relevant principles and concepts of food, nutrition, and weight regulation; (4) present examples of hunger patterns, typical food intake patterns, and the total kcaloric intake of a person who has recovered from an eating disorder; and (5) educate the family.

Primary objectives for the experimental phase have also been established. They include: (1) separate food- and weight-related behaviors from feelings and psychological issues, (2) change food behaviors in an incremental fashion until foods intake patterns are normalized, (3) slowly increase or decrease weight, (4) learn to maintain a weight that is healthful for that individual without using abnormal food- and weight-related behaviors, and (4) learn to be comfortable in social eating situations.

The effectiveness of the multidiscipline approach to treatment is due to the recognition that the complex etiology of eating disorders requires the expertise of various health professionals. With the dietitian addressing the food- and weight-related behaviors, the psychological team members can focus on the psychological issues while the medical and nursing personnel rectify the physical ramifications of the disorder.

Role of nurses. Nurses are members of the therapeutic multidisciplinary team along with physicians, psychiatrists, psychologists, and dietitians or nutritionists. The therapeutic orientation of nursing care depends on the philosophy and clinical modalities of individual treatment programs. Although nurses are central to the staffing of inpatient programs, their participation in outpatient programs may be marginal. If outpatient treatment is within a holistic clinic attending to medical and psychological concerns, the role of nurses is integral. Most outpatient treatment tends to be direct care between the client and a health specialist such as a psychologist or dietitian.

Nurses have an educational role in the prevention of eating disorders. By providing information about nutrition and normal eating patterns to parents, caregivers, and children, healthier feeding relationships can evolve (25). This can help diffuse the behavior of using food as an emotional outlet. Additionally, nurses can be accepting of all body types, taking care to be sensitive to issues of weight and size when providing basic health care. Nurse-client relationships often provide informal opportunities to discuss dietary patterns; if early signs of disordered eating are detected, further assessment or treatment can be initiated before a clinically diagnosable disorder develops.

TOWARD A POSITIVE NUTRITION LIFESTYLE: RATIONALIZING

Rationalization is one of the psychological defense mechanisms used to protect our sense of self when we are under stress. When our behaviors, feelings, or perceptions are irrational or unreasonable, we may use rationalizing to assign reasonable explanations to ourselves as to why we behaved as we did (29).

For example, from adolescents on through the older years, some individuals rationalize their poor eating habits. The list of *reasonable* explanations may include not enough time to prepare *better* meals, lack of knowledge of nutrition or lack of cooking skills. Although these may be *reasonable* explanations, they do not help improve nutritional status. Often these types of rationalizations make it harder to change unproductive behaviors.

Consider the same explanations in a more positive way.

- Not enough time to prepare *better* meals but can reorganize schedule to create time.
- Lack of knowledge of nutrition or of cooking skills but can take a nutrition or cooking course or read books on nutrition and use simple cookbooks to learn basic skills.

Instead of continuing negative rationalization, positive rationalization may provide the means to change.

WELLNESS AND LIFE SPAN

Physical Dimension	Physical health is maintained by beginning health-promoting habits early in life and continuing them through senescence.
Intellectual Dimension	Our intellect provides the ability to change and adapt as circumstances vary according to age and related responsibilities for our health.

WELLNESS AND LIFE SPAN, cont'd.

Emotional Dimension	The symbolic representation and occasions defined by certain foods are often tied to our emotional well-being.
Social Dimension	Food provides a means of communication; customs surrounding eating behaviors vary between cultures and ethnic groups; exposure to these differences is rewarding.

SUMMARY

The nutrient requirements of humans are basically the same throughout the life span. Overall, the issues of health promotion and disease prevention apply regardless of age. This chapter focuses on those issues most tied to nutrition-related concerns such as prevention of diet-related disorders (coronary artery disease, some cancers, NIDDM, and obesity) and emphasizes dietary patterns rather than specific nutrients.

The life span stages reflect psychological and physiological maturation. They include childhood (ages 1 through 12), adolescence (ages 13 through 19) and adulthood. Approaches to health promotion take into account these stages and their impact on nutrient requirements, eating styles, and food choices. Health promotion depends on knowledge, techniques, and community supports. Each stage of development requires different approaches and is supported in various ways by the larger community. Barriers to health promotion across the life span may include food asphyxiation, lead poisoning, stress, and eating disorders.

THE NURSING ROLE
Considering Nutrition Lifestyles

When counseling a patient about normal or therapeutic nutrition and the need to change nutritional habits, a thorough assessment of his or her nutrition lifestyle is first necessary. In addition to assessing nutritional knowledge (see Nursing Process Chapter 2), many of the factors discussed in this chapter could have an impact on the patient's motivation or ability to make needed changes, including the following:

Age
Ethnicity
Income level
Education level
Occupation
Role in household (cooking and/or shopping)
Physical abilities (vision and mobility)
Ability and willingness to read food product labels
Lifestyle factors
  • Use of convenience foods versus home cooking
  • Amount of restaurant eating
  • Use of fresh versus canned or frozen foods
  • Cooking facilities (appliances) and usual cooking methods
  • Amount of time devoted to shopping, cooking, and preparation
Consumption patterns
  • Proportions of food from various levels of the Food Guide Pyramid
  • Food likes and dislikes

An attempt to influence a patient to eat, cook, or shop differently may be in vain if the above factors are unheeded. For example, telling a person

Continued.

THE NURSING ROLE, cont'd.
Considering Nutrition Lifestyles

he should cook all foods from scratch so that ingredients are known and controlled may be a waste of time if he has never cooked very much and has no intention of learning to do so. Encouraging an elderly woman to carefully read product labels may be unrealistic if she has poor eyesight and little stamina for prolonged shopping sessions. Trying to force a 5 year old to eat vegetables when she is on a food jag for spaghetti and peanut butter will be frustrating for everyone. And a busy college student may disregard advice to eliminate fast foods from his diet if they are very important to him.

When suggestions for nutritional changes take lifestyle factors into account, however, there is a greater chance that the patient will comply with the advice. Nurses must develop realistic goals with each individual patient to increase the chances of bringing about necessary and lasting changes.

CASE STUDY

Meg is a senior in high school. Her physical education teacher stopped by the school health office one day to talk to the school nurse about Meg. The teacher has noticed that Meg has lost a lot of weight during the school year, and although she has not missed any time from school, she appears thin, pale, and generally unhealthy. The nurse says she will call Meg in and talk to her.

When Meg arrives in the office, the nurse makes the following assessments by means of observation, Meg's health record, and some information supplied by Meg, although it is difficult to get her to talk about herself.

ASSESSMENT DATA COLLECTED

Subjective:
- Has lost *some weight* because she has been on a diet
- Believes she needs to lose more weight because she is still fat
- Feels tired but has kept up usual activity
- Denies being sick
- Claims she eats *well*
- Has not had her menstrual cycle for a *while*

Objective:
- Height 5'5"
- Weight 1 year ago was 125 lb
- Present weight 100 lb
- Hair dull and straight
- Skin pale

NURSING DIAGNOSIS

Altered nutrition, less than body requirements, related to unwarranted desire to lose weight, as evidenced by undesirable weight loss and intention to lose more weight.

The school nurse does not have enough information to confirm anorexia nervosa as the cause of the problem, but she strongly suspects that it is. She feels she has enough information to make the following plans, which she shares with Meg.

THE NURSING ROLE, cont'd.
Considering Nutrition Lifestyles

PLANNING

The nurse will call Meg's mother and share her concerns about Meg's dieting, and set the following goals. Meg and her mother will:

- Discuss her dieting and weight loss
- Attempt to stop the intentional weight loss
- Consult with their primary care physician

INTERVENTION

1. Call Meg's mother at work and discuss the extent of the problem and possible dangers; find out what the parents' reaction has been thus far
2. Enlist the help of Meg's mother to monitor Meg's diet until she can get professional help for Meg; encourage her to give Meg a balanced diet, even if the portions are small
3. Ask Meg's mother to check her weight twice a week until they see a physician
4. Impress upon Meg's mother the importance of getting professional help immediately, first with the primary care physician, with possible need for a therapist specializing in eating disorders

EVALUATION

The goals will be evaluated in 2 weeks to see if they have been met, as evidenced by:

- Meg's mother stating that she has discussed the dieting behavior with Meg
- No further weight loss (no less than 100 lb) as measured by Meg's mother
- An appointment made with the primary care physician
- The school nurse will continue to follow Meg's case to make sure she is receiving the help she needs

REFERENCES

1. Satter E: *How to get your kid to eat...but not too much*, Palo Alto, Calif, 1987, Bull Publishing.
2. Gans DA: Sucrose and unusual childhood behavior, *Nutrition Today* 26(3):8-14, May/June 1991.
3. Taras HL et al: Television's influences on children's diet and physical activity, *J Dev Behav Pediatr* 10:176-180, 1989.
4. Heird WC: Nutritional requirements during infancy and childhood. In Shils ME, Olson JA, and Shike M, eds: *Modern nutrition in health and disease*, ed 8, Philadelphia, 1994, Lea & Febiger.
5. Parental health beliefs may cause failure to thrive, *Nutr Rev*, 46(6):217-219, 1988.
6. Sanstead HH: Zinc deficiency: A public health problem? *Journal of Disease in Children* 145:853-858, 1991.
7. Food Research & Action Center: Fact sheets on the Federal Food Assistance Programs, February 1993.
8. US Department of Health and Human Services, Public Health Service: *Healthy People 2000: National health promotion and disease prevention objectives,* Washington, DC, 1990, US Government Printing Office.
9. Potter PA, Perry AG: *Fundamentals of nursing*, ed 3, St. Louis, 1993, Mosby.

10. Young A, Skelton DA: Applied physiology of strength and power in old age. *Int J Sports Med*, 15(3):149-51, 1994.
11. Chernoff R: Meeting the nutritional needs of the elderly in the institutional setting, *Nutr Rev* 52(4):132-136, 1994.
12. Guthrie HA, Picciano MF: *Human nutrition*, St. Louis, 1995, Mosby.
13. Posner BM et al: P. Nutritional risk in New England elders, *J Gerontol* 49(3):M123-32, 1994.
14. Cope KA: Nutritional status: A basic 'vital sign,' *Home Healthcare Nurse* 12(2):29-34, 1994.
15. Katz D: *Just do it: The Nike spirit in the corporate world*, New York, 1994, Random House.
16. Revich BA: Lead in hair and urine of children and adults from industrialized areas, *Arch Environ Health* 49(1):59-62, 1994.
17. Brown MJ et al: Lead poisoning in children of different ages, *N Eng J Med* 323(2):135-136, 1990.
18. Gottlieb K, Gottlieb JR: Blood lead levels in children from lower socioeconomic communities in Denver, Colorado, *Arch Environ Health* 49(4):260-265, 1994.

19. Food and Nutrition Board, National Research Council: *Recommended dietary allowances*, 10 ed, Washington, DC, 1989, National Academy Press.
20. Grodner M: Forever dieting: Chronic dieting syndrome, *J Nutr Ed* 24(4):207-210, 1992.
21. Garner DM et al: Psychoeducational principles in the treatment of bulimia and anorexia nervosa. In Garner DM, Garfinkel PE: *Handbook of psychotherapy for anorexia nervosa and bulimia*, New York, 1985, Guilford Press.
22. American Psychiatric Association, *Diagnostic and statistical manual of mental disorders (DSM-IV)*, ed 4, Washington, DC, 1994, American Psychiatric Association.
23. Food and Nutrition Board, National Research Council: *Diet and health: Implications for reducing chronic disease risk*, Washington, DC, 1989, National Academy Press.
24. American Dietetic Association, Position of the American Dietetic Association: Nutrition intervention in the treatment of anorexia nervosa, bulimia nervosa, and binge eating. *J Am Diet Assoc* 94(8):902-907, 1994.
25. Chitty KK: The primary prevention role of the nurse in eating disorders, *Nurs Clin North Am* 26:789-800, 1991.

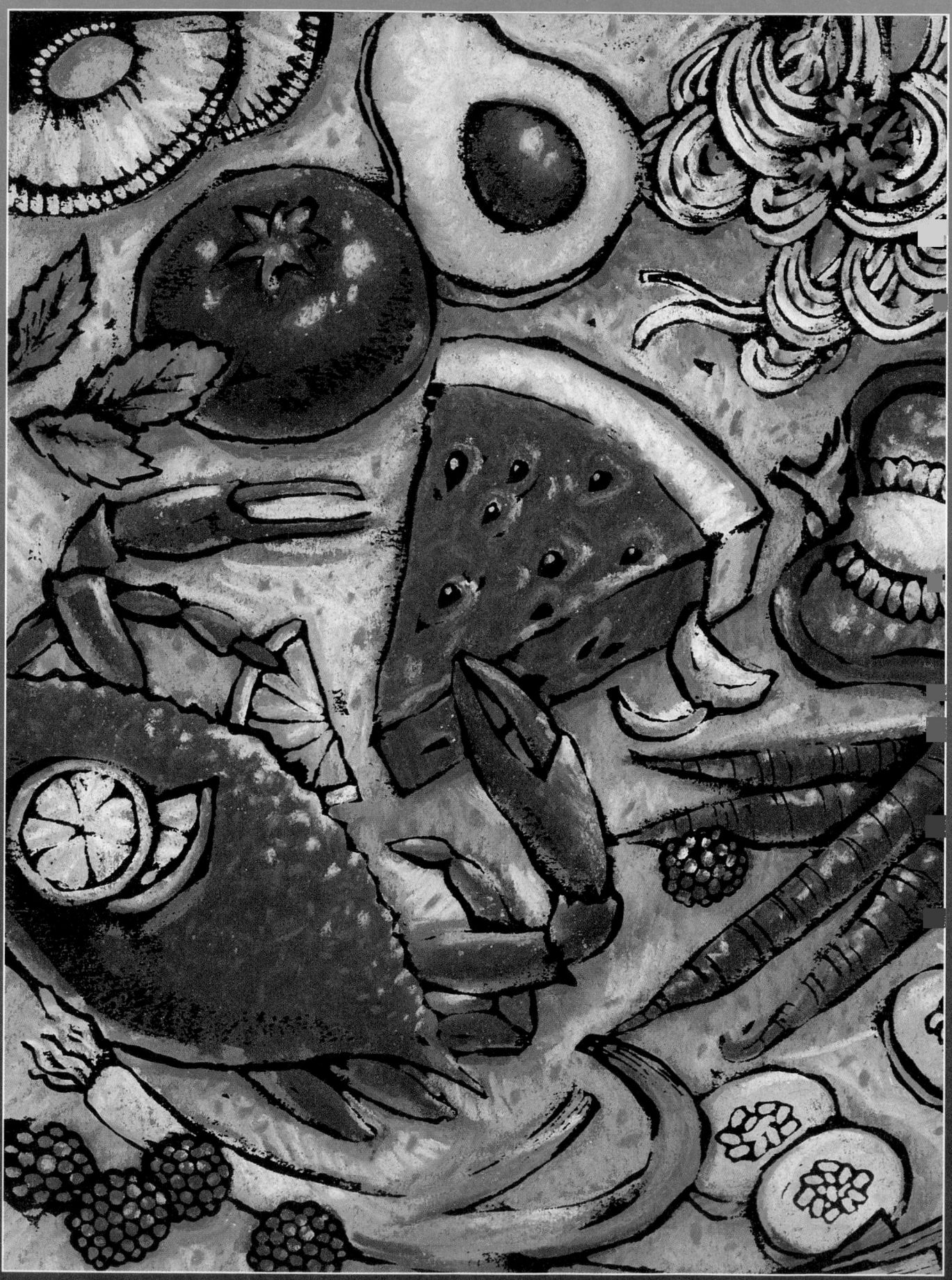

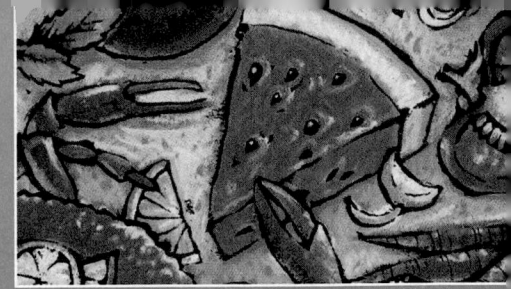

PART FOUR

Overview of Diet Therapy

Chapter 13

NUTRITION IN PATIENT CARE

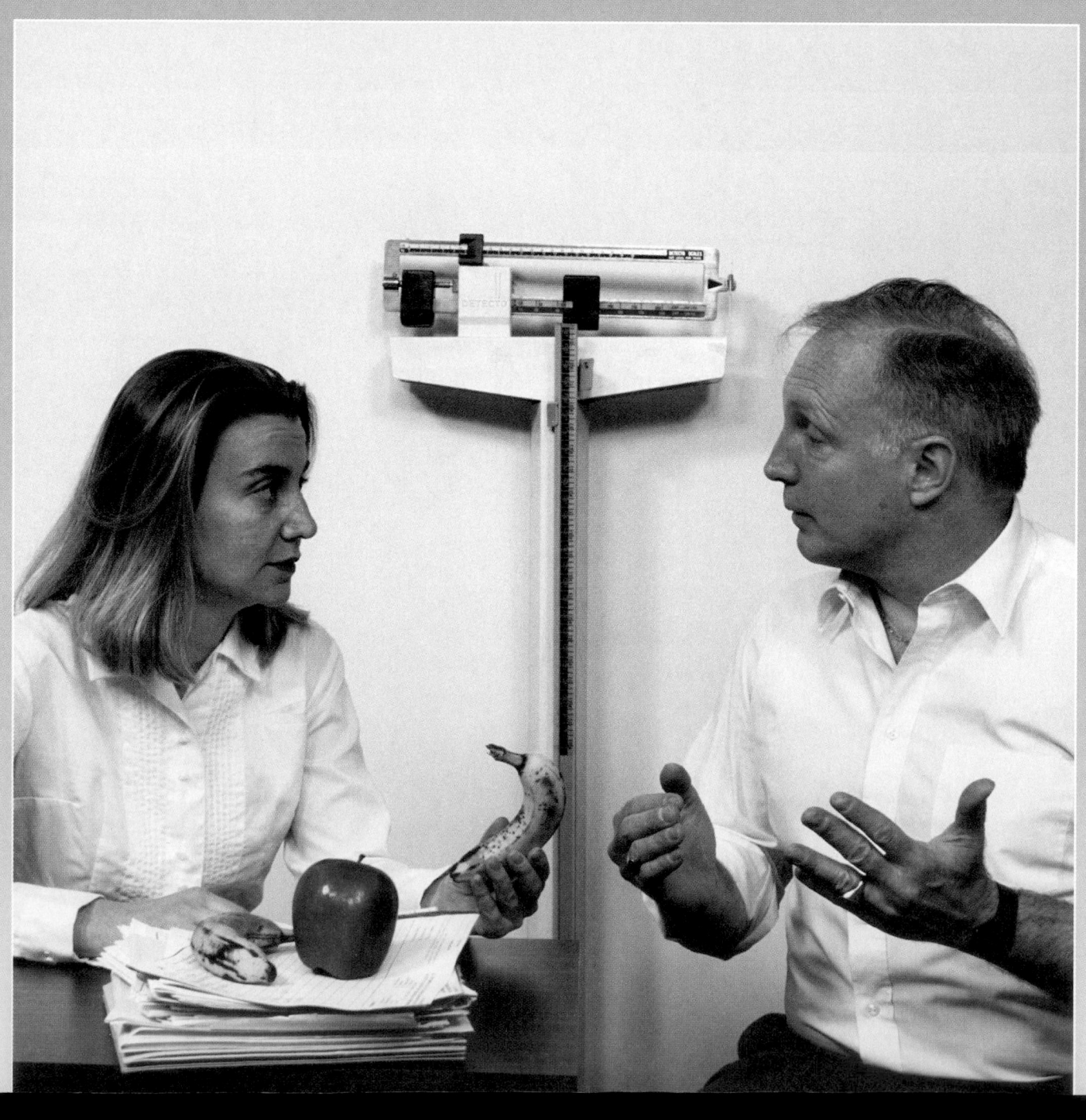

ROLE IN WELLNESS

The first three parts of this text, chapters 1 through 12, discuss basic nutrition as it relates to wellness. This fourth and last part, Overview of Diet Therapy, provides information for nursing professionals on how nutrition pertains to the physiological stresses of disease states.

Nurses are usually the first health care workers with whom the hospitalized patient comes in contact. Hospital size and/or staffing may necessitate that nursing staff perform some basic nutrition assessment and nutrition counseling. This section provides information to enable nurses to perform basic nutrition interventions. Registered dietitians (RDs), however, provide more in-depth knowledge of the aspects of nutritional care beyond basic nutrition interventions. They develop specific dietary patterns to meet therapeutic requirements, consult individually with patients, participate in team meetings, and are a valuable resource for the nursing staff.

NUTRITION AND ILLNESS

Modern health care settings—acute care hospitals—can play havoc with the nutrition status of patients. During their hospitalization, patients who are admitted in good nutritional status encounter several elements, psychological as well as physiological, that have the potential to put them at nutritional risk. If patients are admitted in compromised nutrition status, as many are, the risks are even greater and of more consequence.

Hospital Setting

Imagine that you have been taken to a place where, after answering a multitude of questions about your insurance, financial status, and *durable power of attorney,* you are whisked off to a sterile-looking room that you will share with a stranger. In this room, your clothes are replaced with a thin, flimsy gown and the posterior part of your anatomy is there for all to see, if you can get out of bed. You answer more questions from the nurse who admits you about your medical history. Once he or she finishes, a resident/intern comes into your room to ask many of the same questions in addition to conducting a physical exam.

During your stay in the hospital, your eating habits are open to scrutiny, possibly provoking guilty feelings. You're away from your own refrigerator, and meals are on a schedule that may or may not coincide with your personal meal schedule. Although the food is prepared with the utmost care, it will be different from home cooking (just like any food eaten away from home). Depending on your diagnosis, the food is likely to be modified in texture, consistency, nutrients, or energy. When you're waiting for the meals to be served (you still haven't gotten used to eating in bed), different hospital staff come in and out of your room (usually without knocking) to ask more questions, draw blood, take you elsewhere in the hospital for tests that may or may not be invasive, and ask you about your elimination habits and what you have eliminated, if anything.

Most patients who enter hospitals are miles away from their homes, family, and friends. Although no malfeasance is intended, very little privacy is afforded hospital patients while they are undergoing tests and examinations that may provide them with possibly devastating information regarding their prognosis or life expectancy. During these trying times for patients and staff alike, food becomes very important, both physiologically and psychologically, as it is often one of the few familiar experiences patients encounter in a hospital.

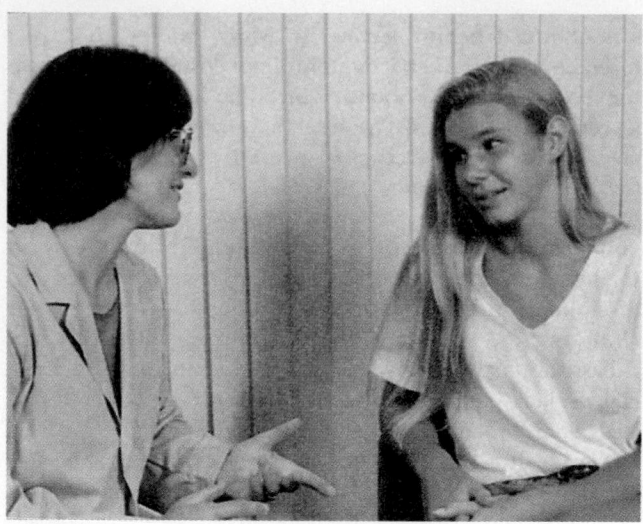

The initial admission procedures allow the nurse to begin knowing the patient and assessing her understanding of the hospital experience.

   Particularly with toddlers and adolescents, food can become a battleground because of all its emotional connotations. As you will see in this chapter and those following, food or alternative nourishment can mean the difference between a good or poor prognosis for many patients' morbidity or mortality.

Bed Rest

Occasionally, bed rest is prescribed as part of patients' medical care, or patients may be unable to ambulate because of the severity of the illness or a multitude of necessary life-saving equipment at bedside. Although it is often necessary or unavoidable, bed rest can cause injurious effects on a patient's body (1). Skin integrity is compromised after just 24 hours of immobilization, and after 3 days of lying supine in bed, muscle tone, bone calcium, plasma volume, and gastric secretions diminish (2). As a result, glucose intolerance and shifts in body fluids and electrolytes may occur. Nursing personnel can provide care that may help prevent the injurious effects of bed rest by turning patients and stimulating the skin and underlying muscles by providing skin care (applying lotion to the skin) and/or passive exercises for the extremities.

Iatrogenic Malnutrition

hypermetabolism
an increase in BMR above expected levels based on age, sex, and body size

Iatrogenic (inadvertently caused by treatment or diagnostic procedures) malnutrition has been likened to a closet skeleton (3). It has been estimated that one third to one half of all patients admitted to hospitals are at nutritional risk. These patients may be experiencing **hypermetabolism** and/or have physiologic stress from injury or illness that increases nutritional needs, further increasing nutritional risk. To add insult to this potential injury, there may be a lack of nutritional screening or monitoring to identify patients at nutritional risk. Additionally, nutritional needs may not be met because of the need for an empty gut for laboratory testing or diagnostic procedures. Nursing personnel can be a fundamental factor in the prevention of iatrogenic malnutrition by paying particular attention to patients' diet orders, recognizing the potential risk when patients have had nothing but clear or full-liquid diets for more than 24 hours, and contacting the registered dietitian to evaluate the patients' nutritional risk (see Myth box).

diagnostic related groups
(DRGs)
classifications used to
determine Medicare payments
for inpatient care, based on
primary and secondary
diagnosis, primary and
secondary procedures, age, and
length of hospitalization

MYTH
Hospitalized, Yet Malnourished? Impossible!

As noted in Butterworth's *Skeleton in the Hospital Closet,* over 20 years ago, more than one third of hospitalized patients are at risk of malnutrition. Sadly, there has not been any data to show this was not just a freak observation. Furthermore, when **Diagnostic Related Groups (DRGs)** became the law of the land, hospitalized patients began leaving the hospitals "quicker and sicker." Obviously, identifying patients who may be at nutritional risk is important. Since nurses are the primary care givers, they can spot potential problems that they can address themselves or refer to the dietitian. Any of the following indicators should alert a nurse to nutritional problems.

INDICATORS OF POTENTIAL NUTRITIONAL PROBLEMS

1. Clear or full-liquid diets for more than 3 days without nutrient supplementation, or with inappropriate or insufficient nutrient supplementation.
2. Intravenous feeding (dextrose or saline) or NPO for more than 3 days without supplementation.
3. Low intakes of prescribed diet or tube feedings.
4. Weight 20% above or 10% below desirable body weight (accounting for edema).
5. Inconsistent growth or weight for height, above or below norms in children.
6. Pregnancy weight gain deviating from normal patterns.
7. Diagnoses that increase nutritional needs or decrease nutrient intake (or both): cancer, malabsorption, diarrhea, hyperthyroidism, excessive inflammation, postoperative status, hemorrhage, wounds (large, draining, or infected wounds), burns, infection, sepsis, major trauma (or multisystem injury).
8. Chronic use of drugs, especially alcohol, that affect nutritional status.
9. Alterations in chewing, swallowing, appetite, taste, smell.
10. Temperature consistently above 37° C (98.6° F) for more than 2 days.
11. Hematocrit: <43% (males), <37% (females)
    Hemoglobin: <14 g/dl (males), <12 g/dl (females)
    Accompanied by mean cell volume <82 cu or >100 cu.
12. Absolute decrease in lymphocyte count (<1500 cells/mm^3).
13. Elevated (>250 mg/dl) or decreased (<130 mg/dl) cholesterol.
14. Serum albumin <3 g/dl in patients without renal disease, liver disease, generalized dermatitis, overhydration

From Butterworth CE: The skeleton in the hospital closet, *Nutrition Today* 9:4, 1974; and Hopkins C: Developing an approach to nutritional assessment. In The American Dietetic Association: *Handbook of clinical dietetics,* ed 2, New Haven, 1992, Yale University Press.

THE STRESS RESPONSE

In its never-ending quest to maintain homeostasis, the human body responds to stress, physiologic or psychologic, with a chain reaction involving the central nervous system and hormones that affect the entire body. The magnitude and duration of the stress determine just how the body will react. It is important for nurses to understand the metabolic changes that take place in reaction to stress, both uncomplicated stress that is present when patients are at nutritional risk and more multifarious variations resulting from severe stress brought about by trauma or disease.

Starvation

If someone must involuntarily go without food, that can be defined as starvation. If we withhold food from ourselves, for instance when we try to lose weight, that can be defined as *dieting* or fasting. Whatever the cause of inadequate food intake and nourishment, the results are the same. After a brief period of going without food (fasting), or an interval of nutrient intake below metabolic needs, the body is able to extract its stored carbohydrate, fat, and protein to meet energy demands.

Liver glycogen is used to maintain normal blood glucose levels to provide energy for cells. Although readily available, this source of energy is limited, and glycogen stores are usually depleted after 8 to 12 hours of fasting. Unlike glycogen stores, fatty acid (triglyceride) stores are ample, and the body also begins to mobilize this energy source. As the amount of liver glycogen decreases, mobilization of free fatty acids from adipose tissue increases to provide the needed energy. After about 24 hours without energy intake (especially carbohydrates), the prime source of glycogen is from gluconeogenesis (4).

Some body cells, brain cells in particular, can only use glucose for energy. During *early* starvation (about 2 to 3 days of starvation), the brain is using glycogen produced from muscle protein. As muscle protein is being broken down for energy, the level of **branched-chain amino acids (BCAA)** in circulation increases even though they are primarily metabolized directly inside the muscle (4). The body does not store any of the amino acids like glucose and triglycerides, so the only sources of amino acids are lean body mass (muscle tissue), vital organ tissues, or other protein-based body constituents such as enzymes, hormones, immune system components, or blood proteins. By the second or third day of starvation, approximately 75 grams of muscle protein is being catabolized daily, which is still not providing enough substrate for glucose utilization by the brain (4). At this point, other sources of energy must be made available. The glycerol portion of adipose tissue triglyceride is hydrolyzed for gluconeogenesis.

As starvation is prolonged, the body tries to preserve proteins by using fat for energy. Ketone production from fatty acids is accelerated, and the body's requirement for glucose decreases. Although some glucose is still vital for brain cells, brain and other body tissues obtain the major proportion of their energy from ketones. Muscle protein is still being catabolized, but at a much lower rate, prolonging survival. During this period of starvation, approximately 60% of the body's energy is being provided by the metabolism of fat to carbon dioxide, 10% from the metabolism of free fatty acids to ketones, and 25% from the metabolism of ketone bodies (5).

An additional *defense* mechanism of the body to conserve energy is to slow its metabolic rate, thereby decreasing energy needs. As a result of declining metabolic rate, body temperature drops, activity decreases, and sleep increases—all to allow the body to preserve energy sources. If starvation continues, the intercostal muscles necessary for respiration are lost, which may lead to pneumonia and respiratory failure (5). Starvation will continue until adipose stores are exhausted.

Severe Stress

Whether stress is accidental (such as from broken bones or burns) or intentional (such as from surgery) the body reacts to these stresses much as it does to the stress of starvation—with a *major* difference. During starvation, the body's metabolic rate slows, becoming hypometabolic. During severe stress, the body's metabolic rate rises profoundly, thus becoming hypermetabolic.

The body's response to stress can be summarized by two phases: ebb phase and flow phase (Table 13-1). The ebb phase, or early phase, begins immediately after the injury and is identified by decreased oxygen consumption, hypothermia (lowered body temperature), and lethargy. The major medical concern during this time is to maintain cardiovascular effectiveness and tissue perfusion. As the body responds to injury, the ebb phase evolves into the flow phase, usually about 36 to 48 hours after injury (6). The flow phase is characterized by increased oxygen consumption, hyperthermia (increased body temperature), and increased nitrogen excretion, as well as expedited catabolism of carbohydrate, protein, and triglycerides

branched-chain amino acids (BCAA)
leucine, isoleucine, and valine

Table 13-1   Metabolic Responses to Severe Stress

Ebb Phase	Flow Phase
↓ Oxygen consumption	↑ Oxygen consumption
↓ Cardiac output	↑ Cardiac output
↓ Plasma volume	↑ Plasma volume
Hypothermia	Hyperthermia
	↑ Nitrogen excretion
↓ Insulin levels	Normal or elevated insulin levels
Hyperglycemia	Hyperglycemia
Hypovolemia	
Hypotension	
↑ Lactate	Normal lactate
↑ Free fatty acids	↑ Free fatty acids
↑ Catecholamines, glucagon, cortisol	↑ Catecholamines, glucagon, cortisol
Insulin resistance	↑ Insulin resistance

to meet the increased metabolic demands (6). The flow stage will last for days, weeks, or months until the injury is healed.

Multiple stresses result in increased catabolism and even greater loss of body proteins. Unfortunately, some of the stresses patients are obliged to endure are iatrogenic. Think of the series of stresses for a patient admitted for elective surgery. Preoperatively, most surgical patients receive only clear liquids or nothing by mouth (NPO). After the surgery, they remain NPO until return of bowel sounds, then progress through clear- and full-liquid diets until they can tolerate food.

If the patient is in poor nutritional status prior to the stress of surgery, he or she is at greater risk to develop pneumonia, or a wound infection accompanied by fever as a result of decreased protein synthesis (Fig. 13-1). As in starvation, energy requirements will be met from **endogenous** sources if **exogenous** sources are not available or adequate (5). Thus intercostal muscles may be depleted, leading to pneumonia, or inadequate amino acids may be available to synthesize antibodies, leading to impaired immune response to infection. Either complication has a negative impact on metabolic demands.

Nutrients affected by hypermetabolic stress include protein, vitamins, and minerals, as well as related nutritional concerns of energy and fluid intake. During moderate metabolic stress, protein requirements increase from .8 gm/kg body weight to 1 to 1.5 gm/kg body weight and for severe stress raises to 1.5 to 2.0 gm/kg body weight (7). These levels are based on sufficient energy consumption to allow for protein synthesis. Requirements of vitamins and minerals all increase during stress. Tissue repair especially depends on adequate intakes of zinc, calcium, magnesium, manganese, and copper. At the least, RDA levels of the nutrients should be consumed, preferably from foods rather than from vitamin/mineral supplements. Achieving requirements through food intake also supports provision of sufficient kcalories to meet increased energy demands during critical illness.

Several formulas can be used to determine the energy needs of patients experiencing hypermetabolic stress. One formula takes into account basal energy expenditure (BEE), activity level, and severity of injury. The activity level considers the energy required if the patient is confined to bed or is ambulatory. The severity of injury is a factor based on whether the injury is due to major or minor surgery, mild to severe infection, skeletal or blunt trauma, or burns (based on percentage of body surface area affected) (8). Another formula is designed to meet energy requirements to maintain body weight of patients while experiencing hypermetabolic stress. It considers normal BMR, tied to age, gender, weight, and height, a stress factor, and energy used within a hospital setting. The stress factor is based on the medical condition of the patient. The formula can also be adjusted to allow for weight gain (9).

endogenous
originating from within the body or produced internally

exogenous
originating outside the body or produced from external sources

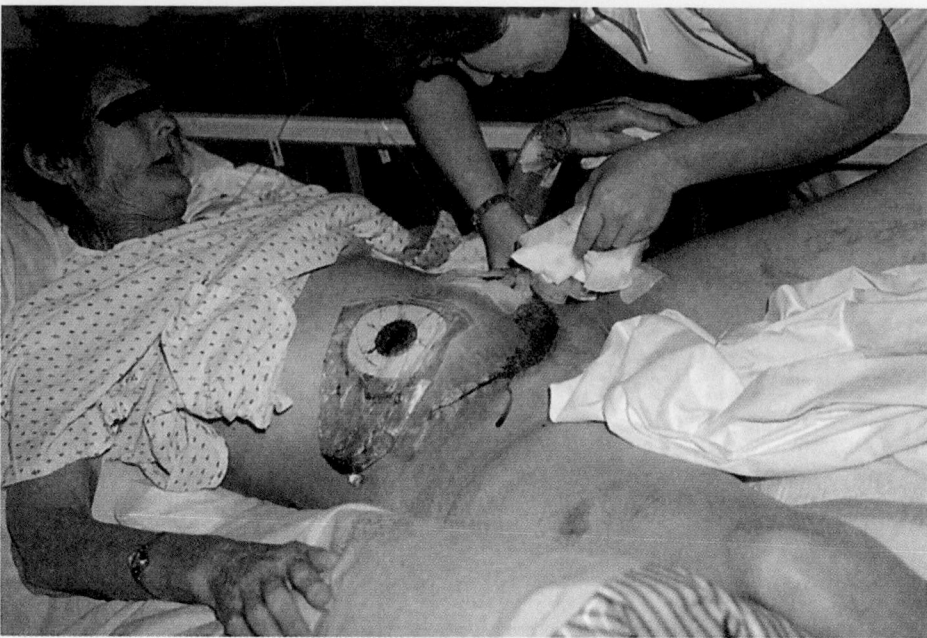

Fig. 13-1 A history of poor protein intake accompanied by surgical stress resulted in poorly healing surgical wounds in this patient.

Registered dieticians, in collaboration with the medical team, use these formulas to determine energy requirements. As factor assessments change, nurses can alert either the registered dietician or other members of the medical team to assure adequate energy provision.

Fluid need during hypermetabolic stress is based on age, reflecting age-related modifications of body composition. For adults younger than 56 years old, fluid intake is 35 to 40 ml/kg body weight. Adults between the ages of 56 to 65 years require a lower amount, 30 ml/kg body weight, and for adults over age 65, 25 ml/kg body weight is recommended (10).

Protein-Energy Malnutrition (PEM)

Inadequate intake of energy, particularly protein, can result in an acute or chronic protein deficiency, or protein-energy malnutrition (PEM). PEM can be primary or secondary. Primary PEM is the result of inadequate intake of nutrients. Secondary PEM is the result of inadequate nutrient consumption as the result of some disease state that impairs food consumption, interferes with nutrient absorption, or increases nutritional requirements (11). PEM, kwashiorkor, and marasmus are presented in detail in Chapter 6 and briefly reviewed here.

Kwashiorkor

The clinical syndrome kwashiorkor is diagnosed largely on the basis of results of laboratory tests on patients in the acute state of poor protein intake and stress. Although etiologic mechanisms are not understood, it appears that the normal adaptive response of protein sparing seen in fasting fails. Kwashiorkor may develop in as little as 2 weeks time (12).

Patients with kwashiorkor appear to be adequately nourished, tending to have normal fat reserves and muscle mass (or even above normal). However, findings such as easily pluckable hair, edema, skin breakdown, and delayed wound healing are telltale signs of kwashiorkor (Fig. 13-2). Characteristic laboratory changes include severely depressed **visceral proteins**: serum albumin (<2.8 g/dl), transferrin

visceral proteins
proteins other than muscle tissue; for example, internal organs and blood

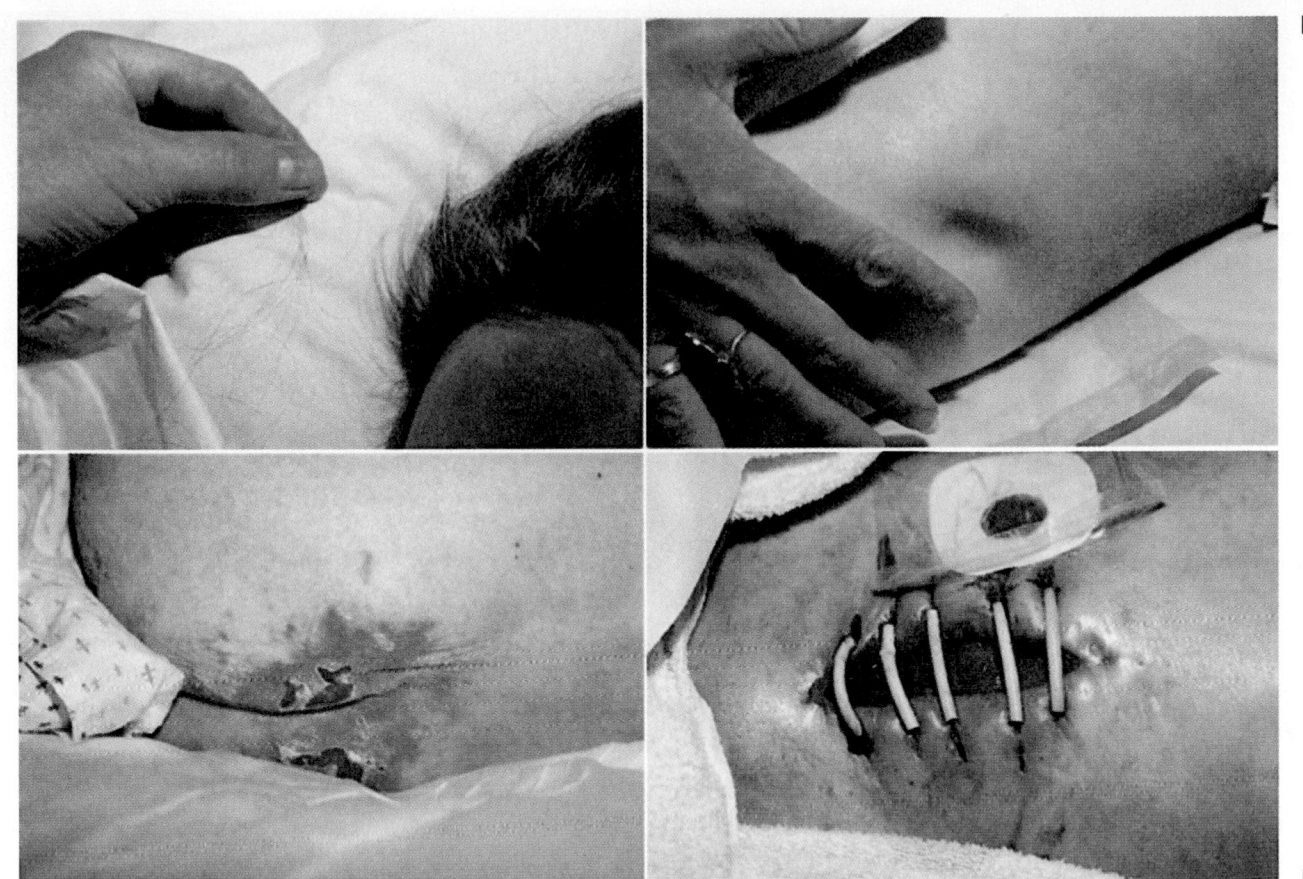

Fig. 13-2 Clinical findings in kwashiorkor include easy painless hair pluckability (**A**), pitting edema (**B**), skin breakdown (**C**), and delayed wound healing (**D**).

(<150 mg/dl), or reduced iron-binding capacity (<200 ug/dl), and depressed cellular immune function (<1500 lymphocytes/mm^3) (12).

Marasmus

Another form of PEM, marasmus, is manifested by severe loss of fat and muscle tissue as a result of chronic energy deficiency. Unlike kwashiorkor, an individual with marasmus will appear thin and is weak and listless. Visceral protein stores are preserved at the expense of **somatic proteins:** skeletal muscle is depleted, but laboratory values are relatively unremarkable (serum albumin is usually within normal range) (12). Immunocompetence and wound healing are fairly well preserved in patients with marasmus.

Marasmus is a chronic condition rather than acute. Treatment is directed toward the gradual reversal of the downward trend. And while medical nutrition therapy or support is necessary, overly aggressive repletion of nutrients can lead to a life-threatening condition referred to as **refeeding syndrome** (see box) (12).

Marasmic kwashiorkor mix

This combined form of protein energy malnutrition develops when acute stress (surgery or trauma) is experienced by a chronically starved or malnourished patient (12). The condition becomes life-threatening because of the high risk of infection and other complications. It is important to determine whether the marasmus or kwashiorkor is predominate so the appropriate medical nutrition therapy can be initiated. The starved, unstressed (hypometabolic) patient is at risk of complications of overfeeding, and the stressed patient at risk for kwashiorkor is more likely to suffer from underfeeding (12).

somatic proteins
skeletal muscle proteins

refeeding syndrome
physiological and metabolic complications associated with reintroducing nutrition (refeeding) too rapidly to a person with PEM; these complications can include malabsorption, cardiac insufficiency, congestive heart failure, respiratory distress, convulsions, coma, and perhaps death

Refeeding Syndrome

Refeeding a patient with protein energy malnutrition can result in many complications if not initiated correctly. In fact, refeeding can be fatal if done too rapidly. The introduction of excess protein and kcalories can overload various enzymatic and physiologic functions that may have adapted during malnutrition. As refeeding is initiated, rapid changes occur in thyroid and endocrine function, causing increased oxygen consumption, cardiac output, insulin secretion, and energy expenditure. Refeeding syndromes are associated more with parenteral nutrition than enteral, but discretion and common sense are of key importance in refeeding semistarved and chronically ill patients. The pathogenesis of refeeding syndrome is as follows:

PHOSPHORUS

hypophosphatemia
low serum phosphorus levels

During starvation total body phosphorus is depleted. During refeeding there is an increase in cellular influx of phosphorus leading to severe extracellular **hypophosphatemia**. This will occur in enteral and parenteral feeding, but can be prevented by a slower rate of nutrient infusion. Hypophosphatemia can also cause **cardiac decompensation.** (Sodium shifts are thought to play a separate, additional role in cardiac overload.) Additionally, hypophosphatemia can lead to tissue **hypoxia** and subsequent altered tissue function.

cardiac decompensation
impaired cardiac output
(reasons not entirely
understood)

hypoxia
lack of oxygen to the cells

POTASSIUM

As potassium is depleted from tissue, it is often not reflected in serum levels because extracellular fluid concentrations are maintained. However, during nutritional repletion potassium is deposited in newly synthesized cells, and serum levels may fall without potassium supplementation.

MAGNESIUM

hyporeflexia
a neurologic condition
characterized by weakened
reflex reactions

Magnesium is also depleted from tissue and under anabolic conditions extracellular fluid levels fall (hypomagnesemia), which in turn can lead to cardiac depression, arrhythmias, neuromuscular weakness, irritability, and **hyporeflexia.**

GLUCOSE METABOLISM

When glucose is reintroduced via high glucose, high volume enteral or parenteral feedings, the starved patient loses the stimulus for gluconeogenesis (an important adaptive mechanism during nutritional depletion). Suppression of gluconeogenic glucose production leads to a corresponding decrease in amino acid utilization and negative nitrogen balance. Additionally, hyperglycemia can precipitate osmotic diuresis, dehydration, hypotension, hyperosmolar nonketotic coma and ketoacidosis (both of these conditions are discussed in Chapter 19), and metabolic acidosis.

FLUID INTOLERANCE

Refeeding with carbohydrate results in sodium and water excretion. With concurrent sodium ingestion, this can lead to a rapid expansion of extracellular fluid volume, which will result in fluid retention and subsequent weight gain. This enhanced fluid retention seen with carbohydrate refeeding may in turn be exacerbated by the loss of tissue mass resulting from starvation.

PREVENTING REFEEDING SYNDROME

Nutrients should be reintroduced slowly to the malnourished patient while medical and metabolic status is monitored closely. Careful estimation of energy requirements should be made through a complete nutritional assessment (see Chapter 14). Care should also be taken to minimize fluid retention (weight gain > 1 kg/wk can be assumed to be fluid retention and should be avoided), and provide adequate repletion of phosphorus, potassium, and magnesium on a daily basis. Weight and fluid balance should be monitored daily to assess the rate of weight regain. Refeeding formulas (whether enteral or parenteral) must also contain adequate amounts of other essential nutrients such as vitamins and minerals. Greater than routine amounts are not necessary, but their absence can be lethal. After one week, intake of kcalories, fluid, and sodium can be liberalized without fear of consequences since the various metabolic equilibrations should have taken place.

From Solomon SM, Kirby DF: The refeeding syndrome: A review, *Journal of Parenteral and Enteral Nutrition*, 14:90-97, 1990; and Apovian CM, McMahon MM, Bistrian BR: Guidelines for refeeding the marasmic patient, *Crit Care Med* 18:1030-1033, 1990.

Nurses can be key players in the recognition and/or prevention of PEM and any of the different forms. By being alert to the clinical symptoms and laboratory values seen in kwashiorkor and marasmus, further deterioration of the patient's nutritional status can be prevented.

THE IMMUNE SYSTEM

One of the first body functions affected by impaired nutritional status is the immune system. When metabolic stress develops, the hormonal and metabolic changes subdue the immune system's ability to protect the body. This activity is further depressed if impaired nutritional status accompanies the metabolic stress. A deadly cycle often develops: impaired immunity leads to increased risk of disease, disease impairs nutritional status, and compromised nutritional status further impairs immunity. Recovery requires that this cycle be broken.

Role of Nutrition

For the immune system to function at its best, adequate nutrients must be available. A well-nourished body will not be ravaged by infections the way a poorly nourished body will. To prove this point, think of the leading causes of death in industrialized countries such as the United States. The majority are chronic diseases associated with lifestyle. In developing countries, however, infections lead morbidity and mortality rates, especially in children, because of the high rate of PEM. The majority of persons in the United States who have serious problems with malnutrition and infections are those with severe medical problems, those who suffer from major metabolic stress, those who suffer from a disease state that causes metabolic stress and/or decreased nutrient intake and/or nutrient malabsorption, or those who have poor nutritional intakes as a result of socioeconomic conditions (poverty, homelessness, and others).

Compromised nutritional status creates a vulnerable immune system by making it difficult to mount both a stress response and an immune response when confronted with a metabolic stress. A number of nutrients affect immune system functioning. It is difficult to determine which specific nutrient factor results in symptoms when the patient is malnourished because of overlapping nutrient deficiencies combined with illness and accompanied by weakness, anorexia, and infection (13).

Immune system components affected by malnutrition include mucous membrane, skin, gastrointestinal tract, T-lymphocytes, macrophages, granulocytes, and antibodies (14). The effects on mucous membrane are flat microvilli, which reduce nutrient absorption and decrease antibody secretions. The integrity of the skin may be compromised as it loses density and wound healing is slowed. Injury to the gastrointestinal tract because of malnutrition may increase the risk of bacteria spreading from inside the tract to outside the intestinal system. T-lymphocytes are affected as the distribution of T-cells is depressed. The effect on macrophages and granulocytes requires that more time be needed for phagocytosis kill time and lymphocyte activation to occur. Antibodies may be less available because of damage to the antibody response. Table 13-2 outlines how specific nutrient deficiencies affect immune system functions; note that the B vitamins and protein are important for adequate functioning of most immune system components (13).

DRUG-NUTRIENT INTERACTIONS

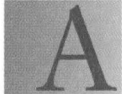All drugs physiologically affect the people who take them, and the use of drugs may involve side effects and risks. The amount and rate of drug absorption can be affected by the composition and timing of the diet.

	Table 13-2	Role of Nutrients and Nutritional Status on Immune System Components	
Immune System Component		**Effects of Malnutrition**	**Vital Nutrients**
Mucus		Flat microvilli, decreased antibody secretions	Vitamin B_{12}, biotin, vitamins B_6 and C
Gastrointestinal tract		Increased risk of bacterial spread to outside GI tract	Arginine, omega-3 fatty acids
Skin		Integrity compromised, density reduced, wound healing slowed	Protein, vitamins A and C, niacin, zinc, copper, linoleic acid, vitamin B_{12}
T-lymphocytes		Depressed T-cell distribution	Protein, arginine, omega-3 fatty acids, vitamins A, B_{12}, B_6, folic acid, thiamin, riboflavin, niacin, pantothenic acid, zinc, iron
Macrophages and granulocytes		Longer time for phagocytosis kill time and lymphocyte activation	Protein, vitamins A, C, B_{12}, B_6, folic acid, thiamin, riboflavin, niacin, zinc, iron
Antibodies		Reduced antibody response	Protein, vitamins A, C, B_{12}, B_6, folic acid, thiamin, biotin, riboflavin, niacin

Conversely, food intake, absorption, and metabolism can be altered by medication. Drug-nutrient reactions have the potential to reduce drug efficacy, interfere with disease control, foster nutritional deficiencies, influence food intake, or provoke a toxic reaction (11,15). The Joint Commission on Accreditation of Healthcare Organizations (JCAHO) strongly recommends evaluation of drug and diet combinations. Documentation of these interactions, which may be done by the registered dietitian or nurse, is essential in complying with JCAHO standards. In addition to medications, use of street drugs also affects nutritional status and nutrient requirements (see box on p. 351).

Risk Factors of Drug-Nutrient Interactions

Determination of risk for drug-nutrient reactions depends on characteristics of the individual including age, physiological status, multiple drug intake, hepatic and renal function, and typical dietary intake (16).

 ### Age

The elderly are more at risk for drug-nutrient reactions because of reduced physiological functioning affecting drug utilization. Older clients often experience several different disorders simultaneously, each with complications and medications that may interact. Nutritional status may be compromised because of physical and social dimensions affecting their ability to procure and prepare nutritious meals. The high rate of drug reactions noted among the elderly may also be due to a combination of these factors, including drug misuse or overuse (16).

Physiological status

Impaired ability to absorb, metabolize, or excrete nutrients and/or medications because of disorders of the gastrointestinal tract and reduced hepatic and renal functioning increases the risk of drug-nutrient reactions. Postoperative trauma or injury may also trigger atypical physiological responses to drug-nutrient interactions.

SOCIAL ISSUE
Nutritional Effects of Street Drugs

References denoting drug-nutrient interactions or a prescription drug's effect on nutritional status are plentiful. Literature on the effects of alcohol on nutritional status is also available. However, nursing personnel may also be faced with caring for patients who use street drugs. Use of nicotine and other addictive drugs can be common, and these drugs also have an impact on nutritional status. Marijuana, heroin, and cocaine can alter food, water, and salt intakes, weight maintenance, and the metabolism and status of other nutrients. The nutritional impact of these drugs can produce unfavorable and sometimes pernicious health effects.

Marijuana

Marijuana increases appetite and food intake in some individuals. This effect occurs also when it is administered orally. This can lead to increased kcaloric intake and increased body weight. Studies have indicated that although kcaloric intake increases with marijuana use, quality of dietary intake may be decreased, especially when marijuana use is coupled with alcohol use.

Heroin

Heroin abuse can alter glucose tolerance and metabolism. In addition, the drug can cause destruction of skeletal muscle (rhabdomyolysis) accompanied by a decrease of myoglobin in the blood to below normal levels and the presence of myoglobin in the urine, which can lead to acute kidney failure. Results of animal studies that have shown depressed water intake, preference for salty solutions, and increased consumption of alcohol could have important implications for humans. These studies also demonstrated a dose-dependent ability of heroin to raise levels of insulin, cortisol, glucagon, and epinephrine, and to induce hypoglycemia and hyperglycemia—findings that could have important consequences for persons with diabetes. Animal subjects also developed hypercholesterolemia (serum cholesterol levels above normal).

Cocaine

Cocaine abuse has been found to lead to diminished intake of meals per day, increased alcohol and coffee consumption, and increased intake of fatty foods. There is also an increased prevalence of anorexia nervosa and bulimia among cocaine users when compared to nonaddicts.

Nicotine

Nicotine, the focal point of smoking research, was designated as an addictive drug in 1988 by the US Surgeon General. Nicotine alone, or in combination with smoking, changes food selections based on taste. Smokers tend to show least preference for sweet foods when offered a choice of bland, salty, and sweet foods; but those who stop smoking show preference for sweet-tasting foods. Smokers also tend to have higher fat intakes than nonsmokers. This effects appears to be dose-dependent; persons smoking more than 20 cigarettes per day consumed more fat than those smoking fewer cigarettes. Women who smoke during pregnancy deliver significantly smaller babies even though maternal weight gain and daily dietary intake during pregnancy is adequate. Research studies have also shown what smokers have been attesting to for years—weight gain occurs after smoking cessation. This phenomenon may be caused by increased consumption of sweet/sugary foods and fatty foods, but there is some indication that nicotine increases metabolism; thus lowered metabolism after smoking cessation may be the reason for weight gain.

Caffeine

Although not really a street drug, caffeine is probably the most widely used drug in the United States. It can be ingested in large enough quantities to alter metabolism. Caffeine is one of the compounds categorized as a **methylxanthine**, along with theophylline and theobromine. These chemicals are found naturally in coffee, tea, cocoa, and cola beverages. Methylxanthines stimulate the central nervous system (keep us awake and alert), produce diuresis, stimulate the cardiac muscle (potential problems for cardiac patients), relax smooth muscle (especially the bronchial muscle, potential benefit for patients with asthma), and increase gastric secretions (potential problems for individuals with gastrointestinal problems). Although moderate amounts of caffeine are probably not harmful in healthy individuals, the safety of its use during pregnancy is inconclusive.

To the extent that these drugs modify or affect nutritional status or food intake, a balanced eating pattern may help renourish individuals and prevent the negative effects of inadequate nutrient intake.

methylxanthines
caffeine, theobromine, and theophylline; found in beverages such as coffee, tea, cocoa, and cola drinks, and have pharmacologic properties that stimulate the central nervous system

From Mohs ME, Watson RR, Leonard-Green T: Nutritional effects of marijuana, heroin, cocaine, and nicotine, *J Am Diet Assoc* 90:1261-1267, 1990; and Gold M: Eating disorders are linked to chemical dependency, *Alcoholism Addiction* 8:13, May-June 1988.

Age alters physiological status as the body matures. Drug doses can vary depending on weight and metabolic function as an aspect of age-related physiological status. Use of medications during pregnancy requires caution because of the multiple effects on the fetus and on the nutritional status of the mother.

Multiple drug intake

Certain types of illness or disease groups tend to require combinations of therapeutic drugs plus medications, including over the counter drugs, for relief of symptoms. The resulting drug-nutrient reactions may be related to the disease itself and/or be a reaction to medications (16). For example, iron deficiency anemia among patients with athritis is often caused by intestinal bleeding. This intestinal bleeding is a common side effect of long-term use of nonsteroidal anti-inflammatory drugs (NSAID), either prescribed or over the counter, taken to reduce the symptoms of athritis. Other chronic conditions such as hypertension and diabetes may result in similar drug-nutrient interactions (16). If other acute disorders develop, the combination of medications may affect nutrient availability and/or function.

Typical dietary intake

The basis of nutritional status depends on foods consumed on a regular basis; it is their nutritional content upon which the body functions. A well-nourished individual is better able to withstand a medical regimen that may affect nutrient functioning. In contrast, individuals who are malnourished or marginally deficient in nutrient intake are more at risk for complications of drug-nutrient reactions as body storage of nutrients are diminished. For example, individuals who excessively consume alcohol tend to be marginally deficient in a number of nutrients either because of inadequate food intake (alcohol is an appetite depressant) or to drug (alcohol)-nutrient interactions. If illness necessitates therapeutic drug intervention, nutritional status may be further compromised, increasing the likelihood of drug-nutrient interactions.

Effects of Drugs on Food and Nutrients

Most drug absorption occurs through the gastrointestinal mucosa, predominately in the small intestine. Before drugs can be absorbed they must first break down and dissolve in gastric juices of the stomach. The speed with which the drug leaves the stomach depends on the gastric emptying time; this affects the rate of drug absorption. The rate of drug absorption may either increase or decrease based on the fed or fast state of the body. In the fasting state, the medication leaves the empty stomach quickly and is absorbed from the small intestine. For some drugs that is too quick because time is needed for disintegration into absorbable particles. For those drugs, it is better to take the medication in the fed state in which the stomach, containing food, empties more slowly, especially after large meals, heated food, and meals containing fat, all of which slow emptying time.

Drugs can alter food intake, nutrient absorption, metabolism, and excretion. If a nutrient binds with a medication, decreased solubility of both the nutrient and drug can result. Drugs used to lower serum cholesterol levels bind with fat-soluble vitamins as well as bile salts. As a result, both the bile salts and vitamins are excreted. Some drugs can decrease the amount of digestive enzymes available and thereby decrease nutrient absorption. Drugs that decrease transit time in the GI tract will also decrease nutrient absorption. The tables in this chapter provide information on selected drug-nutrient interactions.

Mineral status can be affected by drugs, resulting in either depletion or overload. Depletion may occur from the simultaneous use of several medications that each have the side effect of mineral depletion. A common source of mineral depletion is the use of potassium-depleting diuretics in addition to the use of laxatives that may also cause potassium loss. Both are often used by the elderly, whose dietary intake may be marginal in mineral content as well (16). Overload may occur in instances in which renal function is compromised combined with the use of potassium-sparing diuretics (such as Spironolactone) and potassium supplements. Client education is vital regarding the use of potassium supplements. Clear information is essential; clients should be taught about the different kinds of diuretics and potential side effects to reduce inappropriate supplementation.

Medications can also alter food intake by acting as appetite depressants or stimulants (Table 13-3), altering taste sensations (Table 13-4), or producing nausea and vomiting, which further decrease appetite. The Teaching Tool gives suggestions for minimizing drug side effects.

Nutrient absorption may be changed by drugs affecting the motility or pH of the gastrointestinal tract, injury of gastrointestinal mucosa, development of drug-nutrient compounds, decreased bile acid function, and depressed nutrient transport mechanisms (Table 13-5). Nutrient metabolism and excretion may be modified by drug therapy in a mechanism similar to that of nutrient absorption with the addition of effects caused by physical characteristics of solubility and stability of the drug.

The metabolic and excretion rate of the drug itself may also interfere with nutrient metabolism and excretion. Nutrient metabolism can be affected by vitamin analogs that compete metabolically with the vitamin. Certain medications act as

Table 13-3   Selected Drugs That Affect Appetite

APPETITE STIMULANTS	APPETITE DEPRESSANTS

Antidepressants
Amitriptyline (Elavil, Endep)
Clomipramine HCl (Anafranil)
MAOI
  Tranylcypromine sulfate (Parnate)
	Amphetamines
	Benzphetamine HCl (Didrex)
	Fenfluramine HCl (Pondimin)
	Phenylpropanolamine (Dexatrim,
	  Dimetapp, Triaminic)

Antihistamines Astemizole (Hismanal) Cyproheptadine HCl (Periactin)	*Antiarrhythmic* Digitalis Digitoxin (Crystodigin, Digitoxin) Digoxin (Digoxin, Lanoxin)
Bronchodilator Albuterol sulfate (Proventil, Ventolin)	*Antibiotics* Amphotericin B (Fungizone) Gentamicin (Garamycin) Metronidazole (Flagyl) Zidovudine (AZT)

Steroids
Anabolic steroids
  Oxandrolone (Anavar)
Corticosteroids
  Hydrocortisone (Cortef)
Glucocorticoids
  Dexamethasone (Decadron)
  Methylprednisolone (Medrol)
	Antidepressant
	Fluoxetine HCl (Prozac)
	
	Antihistamine
	Azatadine maleate (Optimine)

Tranquilizer
Lithium carbonate (Lithane)
Benzodiazipines
  Chlordiazepoxide HCl (Librium)
  Diazepam (Valium)
  Prazepam (Centrax)
Phenothiazines
  Chlorpromazine HCl (Thorazine)
  Promethazine HCl (Phenergan)
	Antihypertensive
	Amiloride and Hydrochlorothiazide
	  (Moduretic)
	Captopril (Capoten)
	Chlorthalidone (Hygroton)
	
	Muscle relaxant
	Dantrolene sodium (Dantrium)
	
	Stimulant/AntiADD
	Methylphenidate HCl (Ritalin)

From Pronsky AM: *Powers and Moore's food medication interactions,* ed 8, Pottstown, Penn, 1993, Food-Medication Interactions.

Table 13-4   Selected Drugs That Alter Taste

Antiarrhythmic
Amiodarone (Cordarone)

Antiarthritic/chelating agent
Penicillamine (Cuprimine, Depen)

Antibiotics
Ampicillin
Clarithromycin (Biaxin)

Anticonvulsant
Phenytoin (Dilantin)

Antifungal
Griseofulvin (Fulvicin, Grifulvin V,
  Grisactin)

Antigout
Allopurinol (Zyloprim)

Antidepressant
Clomipramine HCl (Anafranil)
Fluoxetine HCl (Prozac)

Antihypertensive
Captopril (Capoten)
Labetalol HCl (Normodyne, Trandate)

Antimanic
Lithium carbonate (Eskalith, Lithane,
Lithobid)
Lithium citrate (Cibalith-S)

Anti-Parkinson
Levodopa (Dopar, Larodopa)

Antiviral/anti-HIV
Didanosine (Videx)

Muscle relaxant
Dantrolene sodium (Dantrium)

Muscle relaxant/antispasmodic
Baclofen (Lioresal)

Stimulant/amphetamine
Dextroamphetamine sulfate (tartrazine,
  Dexedrine)

From Pronsky AM: *Powers and Moore's food medication interactions,* ed 8, Pottstown, Penn, 1993, Food-Medication Interactions.

Table 13-5   Effects of Selected Drugs on Nutrition

DRUG	EFFECT
Antibiotic/sulfonamide	
Trimethoprim/sulfamethoxazole (Bactrim, Cotrim, Septra)	Disrupts folate metabolism
Anticonvulsant	
Primidone (Mysoline)	Decreased calcium absorption
Phenytoin (Dilantin)	Increased metabolism of vitamin D and K; rickets or osteomalacia possible
Antimanic	
Lithium carbonate (Eskalith, Lithane, Lithobid) Lithium citrate (Cibalith-S)	Anorexia, increased thirst, weight changes
Antipsychotic	
Thiothixene (Navane)	Increased need for riboflavin
Antituberculosis	
Isoniazid (Nydrazid)	Osteoporosis, pellagra, increased need for Vitamin D, pyridoxine
Corticosteroid/antiinflammatory/immunosuppressant	
Hydrocortisone (Cortef)	Increased appetite, increased weight, increased folate, calcium lost with osteoporosis/necrosis possible (long-term use)
Diuretic	
Triamterene (Dyrenium)	Decreased use of folate
Stimulant/antiADD	
Methylphenidate HCl (Ritalin)	Anorexia, decreased weight, decreased growth

From Pronsky AM: *Powers and Moore's food medication interactions,* ed 8, Pottstown, Penn, 1993, Food-Medication Interactions.

TEACHING TOOL
Pushing Aside Drug Side Effects

A number of drugs have side effects—symptoms not caused by the illness for which the drugs have been prescribed but as physiological responses of the body to the drug itself. The side effects may be mild or quite bothersome. Some may be serious enough to warrant a change in medication. Before using these strategies as education tools, consult the client's primary health care provider to ascertain if additional medical intervention is required.

SIDE EFFECT: DIMINISHED APPETITE

- Consider eating several small meals or snacks throughout the day.
- Describe a setting and atmosphere for mealtimes that enhances appetite. Assist the client in exploring approaches to encourage an optimum eating environment.
- Discuss client's favorite foods. Brainstorm about how recipes can be adapted to comply with dietary therapeutic plans.

SIDE EFFECT: MODIFIED TASTE SENSATIONS

- Visit a dentist regularly to maintain oral hygiene.
- Mask the taste of medications, if needed, with fruit sauces such as applesauce, crushed pineapple, or milk products. First determine if combinations are acceptable and not contraindicated.

SIDE EFFECT: INCREASED APPETITE

- Alert client to the appetite (and craving sweets) stimulant effect of certain medications.

- Evaluate client's typical dietary intake. Suggest high-fiber foods to provide a quick sense of feeling full.
- Advise limiting availability to high kcalorie foods and drinks to minimize excess kcaloric intake.

SIDE EFFECT: GI TRACT IRRITATION AND DISCOMFORT

- Advise client to sit up or stand after taking medications that have the potential to cause heartburn or indigestion.
- Reduce intake of fat, greasy and/or highly acidic foods, including citrus juices and tomato products.
- Limit food intake in the evening to prevent reflux.
- Control consumption of spicy foods, peppermint, colas, chocolate, alcohol, pepper, decaffeinated coffee, and caffeine if these produce gastric discomfort.

SIDE EFFECT: NAUSEA

- Control liquid intake by serving after meals or drink only small quantities with meals.
- Sustain adequate fluid volume; cold, carbonated, or clear liquids are easier to tolerate.

SIDE EFFECT: DRY OR SORE MOUTH

- Consume softer, moist foods such as applesauce, puddings, pureed foods, and mashed potatoes.
- Include iced and cold foods throughout the day; consider ice pops, frozen yogurt, ice cream, sorbets, and cooled melons.

From Pronsky AM: *Powers and Moore's food medication interactions,* Pottstown, Penn, 1993, Food-Medication Interactions.

vitamin antagonists, preventing vitamins from doing their metabolic function. Coumarin, the anticoagulant, is a vitamin K antagonist that prevents the activation of the the storage form of vitamin K; blood clotting, for which vitamin K is a factor, is then reduced. Other drugs, such as oral contraceptives, may cause marginal deficiencies of B vitamins and vitamin C by causing increased use of these vitamins. Excretion of nutrients may be altered if a medication results in retention of a drug normally excreted. As described in relation to mineral depletion, some diuretics are potassium-saving, causing the body to conserve more potassium than usual; other diuretics are potassium-depleting. Depending on the type of diuretic, dietary support of additional food sources of potassium may be warranted.

Conversely, foods and nutrients may affect drug action, producing uncomfortable side effects. Most noted are the adverse side effects associated with monoamine oxidase (MOA) inhibitors. MOA inhibitors may be prescribed to treat depression. These drugs inhibit the enzyme monoamine oxidase. The function of monoamine oxidase is to inactivate tyramine, a compound found in some foods. Without monoamine oxidase, the level of tyramine increases the release of norepinephrine. Elevated levels of norepinephrine may cause increased blood pressure, headache, pallor, and heart palpitations. Life-threatening severe hypertension can develop. Foods and drugs containing tyramine should be avoided by patients taking MAO inhibitors. Over the counter medications list warnings when appropriate, but foods are not so labeled. An important component of client education is for patients who are taking MOA inhibitors to know which foods contain significant levels of tyramine (Table 13-6).

Effects of Food and Nutrients on Drugs

Teaching patients the best time to take medications in relation to meals allows for optimal absorption.

Medications must be absorbed to have a therapeutic effect. Food intake, or lack thereof, in addition to composition of the food may affect drug absorption. The timing of drug administration and meals also has clinical significance. If absorption is increased by the presence of food, medication should be taken with a meal or a snack. If drug absorption is depressed by the presence of food in the stomach, opti-

Table 13-6   Tyramine-Containing Foods

AVOID: CONTAIN HIGH TYRAMINE LEVELS	USE WITH CAUTION IN SMALL SERVINGS (1/4-1/2 CUP; 2-4 OZ)
Aged foods Hard (aged) cheeses and meats, salami or mortadella, air-dried sausage	*Aged foods* Bologna, pepperoni, aged kielbasa sausage, liverwurst
Pickled/smoked foods Smoked or pickled fish, herring in brine, sauerkraut, kim chee	*Pickled/smoked foods* Smoked meats and fish, Schmaltz herring in oil, pate, lumpfish roe
Beverages Malt beverages (beer and ale), Chianti and vermouth wines, alcohol-free beer	*Beverages* Red and white wines, port wines, distilled spirits, coffee,* cola*
Fermented Fermented bean curd, miso, broad beans, fava beans	*Fermented foods* Soy sauce, yogurt and cream from unpasteurized milk
Extracts Hydrolyzed protein extracts (in many processed foods), concentrated yeast extracts, brewer's yeast	*Fresh foods* Fresh liver, avocado, figs, bananas, raspberries, chocolate,* peanuts

From McCabe BJ: Dietary tyramine and other pressor amines in MAOI regimens: A review, *J Am Diet Assoc* 86:1059, 1986; and Pronsky AM: *Powers and Moore's food medication interactions*, ed 8, Pottstown, Penn, 1993, Food Medication Interactions
*Caffeine in amounts > 500 mg may intensify reactions

mum absorption occurs if medication taken at least 1 hour before or 2 hours after eating or tube feeding. Table 13-7 lists drugs whose absorption is affected by food.

The established drug administration schedules in health care facilities often conflict with the optimal bioavailability of the drug. Absorption response can be altered in 77% to 93% of drugs by the presence of food in the digestive tract (17). Concomitant food intake with drug administration usually delays absorption of the drug, but this may or may not decrease the amount of drug absorbed. As a general guideline, drugs should be given at least 1 hour before or 2 hours after a meal unless the medication causes gastrointestinal distress when taken on an empty stomach. Such timing should enhance drug absorption and decrease hindrance of nutrient absorption.

Table 13-7   Drug Absorption Altered by Food

ABSORPTION ENHANCED	ABSORPTION DIMINISHED
Analgesic Aspirin	*Antibiotic* Amoxicillin (Amoxil) Ampicillin (Polycillin) Penicillin G Penicillin V (K)
Analgesic/narcotic Propoxyphene HCl (Darvon)	
Antiarrhythmic/antianginal/ antihypertensive Propranolol HCl (Inderal)	*Antibiotic/tetracycline* Doxycylcline (Vibramycine) Oxytetracycline HCl (Terramycin) Tetracycline (particularly by dairy)
Antibiotic Nitrofurantoin (Macrodantin)	
Anticonvulsant Carbamazepine (Tegretol)	*Anticonvulsant* Phenytoin (Dilantin)
Antifungal Griseofulvin (Fulvicin)	*Antihistamine* Astemizole (Hismanal)
Antihypertensive Metoprolol tartrate (Lopressor)	*Antineoplastic/antipsoriatric/ antiarthritic* Methotrexate (Methotrexate, Rheumatrex)
Antihypertensive/diuretic Spironolactone (Aldactone)	*Anti-Parkinson* Levodopa (Dopar)
Antihypertensive/vasodilator Hydralazine HCl (Apresoline)	*Platelet aggregation inhibitor* Dipyridamole (Persantine)
	Sedative/hypnotic/anticonvulsant Phenobarbital (Luminal)

Modified from Moore MC: *Pocket guide to nutrition and diet therapy,* ed 2, St. Louis, 1993, Mosby.

WELLNESS, NUTRITION, AND PATIENT CARE

Physical Dimension — The patient's physical dimension of health is considered through nutritional screening and assessment strategies.

Intellectual Dimension — Nurses assist patients to use their intellectual abilities to reduce the impact of psychological stressors of illness, thereby reducing the effects of stress on the immune system.

Emotional Dimension — The emotional effects on patients and their families because of illness and the hospital experience itself can be softened through recognition by the nursing staff of the emotional dimension of health.

Social Dimension — Maintaining the social health dimension is achieved by acknowledging that the social ties of a patient may be an invaluable support for a patient's recovery.

SUMMARY

Although hospital nurses may perform some basic nutrition assessment and nutrition counseling, registered dietitians can provide more indepth knowledge of nutritional care, consult individually with patients, and participate in team meetings. Nurses, however, need to recognize that the nutritional status of patients may be compromised by their stay in acute care hospitals. Psychological and physiological aspects of illness, combined with the effects of bed rest and the potential of iatrogenic malnutrition, emphasize the need for nutritional screening or monitoring to identify patients at nutritional risk.

The stress response of the body also affects nutritional status. Whether the stress response is caused by physiological or psychological determinants, the entire body is affected. Metabolic changes take place in reaction to stress. This includes changes caused by uncomplicated stress that is present when patients are at nutritional risk and severe stress caused by trauma or disease. The functioning of the immune system is also affected by the hormonal and metabolic changes that occur when metabolic stress develops. The immune system's ability to protect the body is further depressed if impaired nutritional status accompanies the metabolic stress.

Drug nutrient reactions have the potential to reduce drug efficacy, interfere with disease control, foster nutritional deficiencies, influence food intake, or provoke a toxic reaction. Medications must be absorbed to have a therapeutic effect. Food intake, or lack thereof, in addition to composition of the food may affect drug absorption. The timing of drug administration and meals also has clinical significance and often the nurse is in a position to influence either or both of these. Awareness of potential drug nutrient reactions enhances the ability of the nursing staff to help the patient maintain nutritional status while enforcing therapeutic drug administration.

THE NURSING ROLE
Health History and Health Assessment

The nurse conducts a health history and health assessment for almost every patient admitted to the health care system. The following routine data are collected on all patients, regardless of medical diagnosis, and are the portions of the health history and assessment that specifically pertain to nutritional status. As you can see, a large portion of the general assessment is devoted to areas related to nutrition.

HEALTH HISTORY
1. Allergies to food or drugs
2. Diet
   - Usual eating patterns
   - Fluid intake
   - Appetite
   - Religious restrictions
3. Food likes and dislikes
4. Current medications
5. Use of alcohol and/or drugs
6. Use of tobacco
7. Weight history
8. Amount of physical activity/exercise

THE NURSING ROLE, cont'd.
Health History and Health Assessment

HEALTH ASSESSMENT
1. Condition of hair
2. Condition of skin
3. Condition of mouth
   Buccal mucosa
   Tongue
   Gums
   Lips
   Teeth/dentures
   Swallowing
4. Height/weight/body fat distribution
5. Muscle tone and strength
6. Gastrointestinal function
   Usual digestion
   Bowel elimination

Additional data such as laboratory tests or physical assessment of other systems would be collected if the medical diagnosis appears to directly affect nutritional status or if the patient is obviously suffering from a nutritional problem.

Critical Thinking | CLINICAL APPLICATIONS

M.G. is a 19-year-old female college student. She is a member of the cheerleading team and was involved in a serious motor vehicle accident when the team was returning from a game. She was admitted through the emergency room of your hospital suffering from multiple fractures and contusions. M.G. is 5'5" tall and weighed 120 lb before the accident. Since she is young, looked healthy, and is somewhat muscular from being a cheerleader, the physician did not request a consult for the dietitian to evaluate M.G.'s nutritional status. After 2 weeks in intensive care, she developed pneumonia. The nurse learned that before the auto accident, M.G. had been using a commercial weight-loss product and was consuming approximately 400 kcal/day for 3 months before the accident in an attempt to "make weight" so that she could remain on the cheerleading team. Answer the following questions:

1. How did the very low calorie diet (VLCD) affect M.G.'s nutritional status?
2. Why did M.G. develop pneunomia?
3. Describe the variety of stresses M.G. was experiencing.
4. Could the pneumonia have been prevented? How?

REFERENCES

1. Rubin M: The physiology of bed rest, *Am J Nurs* 88(1):50, 1988.
2. Williams SR: *Essentials of nutrition and diet therapy*, ed 6, St. Louis, 1994, Mosby.
3. Butterworth CE: The skeleton in the hospital closet, *Nutrition Today*, March/April 1974.
4. Cahill GF: Starvation: Some biological aspects. In Kinney JM et al: *Nutrition and metabolism in patient care*, Philadelphia, 1993, Saunders.
5. Wolfe BM: Nutrition in hypermetabolic conditions. In Zeman FJ: *Clinical nutrition and dietetics*, ed 2, New York, 1991, Macmillan.
6. Bessey PQ, Wilmore DW: The burned patient. In Kinney JM et al: *Nutrition and metabolism in patient care*, Philadelphia, 1988, Saunders.
7. Davis JR, Sherer K: *Applied nutrition and diet therapy for nurses*, ed 2, Philadelphia, 1994, Saunders.
8. Long CL: The energy and protein requirements of the critically ill patient. In Wright RA, Heymsfield SB, McManus CB III: *Nutritional assessment*, Boston, 1984, Blackwell Scientific Publications as published in American Dietetic Association *Handbook of clinical dietetics*, ed 2, New Haven, 1992, Yale University Press.

9. Souba WB, Wilmore DW: Diet and nutrition in the care of the patient with surgery, trauma and sepsis. In Shils ME, Olson JA, Shike M, eds: *Modern nutrition in health and disease*, ed 8, Philadelphia, 1994, Lea & Febiger.

10. Randall HT: Fluid, electrolyte, and fluid base balance. Surgery Clinics in North America. In American Dietetic Association: *Handbook of clinical dietetics*, ed 2, New Haven, 1992, Yale University Press.

11. American Dietetic Association: *Handbook of clinical dietetics*, ed 2, New Haven, 1992, Yale University Press.

12. Weinsier RL, Morgan SL: *Fundamentals of clinical nutrition*, St. Louis, 1993, Mosby.

13. Myrvik QN: Immunology and nutrition. In Shils ME, Olson JA, Shike M, eds: *Modern nutrition in health and disease*, ed 8, 1994, Philadelphia, Lea & Febiger.

14. Cataldo CB, Rolfes SR, Whitney EN: *Understanding clinical nutrition*, St. Paul, 1991, West Publishing.

15. Roe DA: *Handbook on drug and nutrient interactions*, ed 4, Chicago, 1989, American Dietetic Association.

16. Roe DA: Diet, nutrition and drug reactions. In Shils ME, Olson JA, Shike M, eds: *Modern nutrition in health and disease*, ed 8, 1994, Philadelphia, Lea & Febiger.

17. Murray JJ, Healy DM: Drug-mineral interactions: A new responsibility for the hospital dietitian, *J Am Diet Assoc* 91(1):66-70, 1991.

Chapter 14

THE CARE PROCESS: NUTRITION INTERVENTION

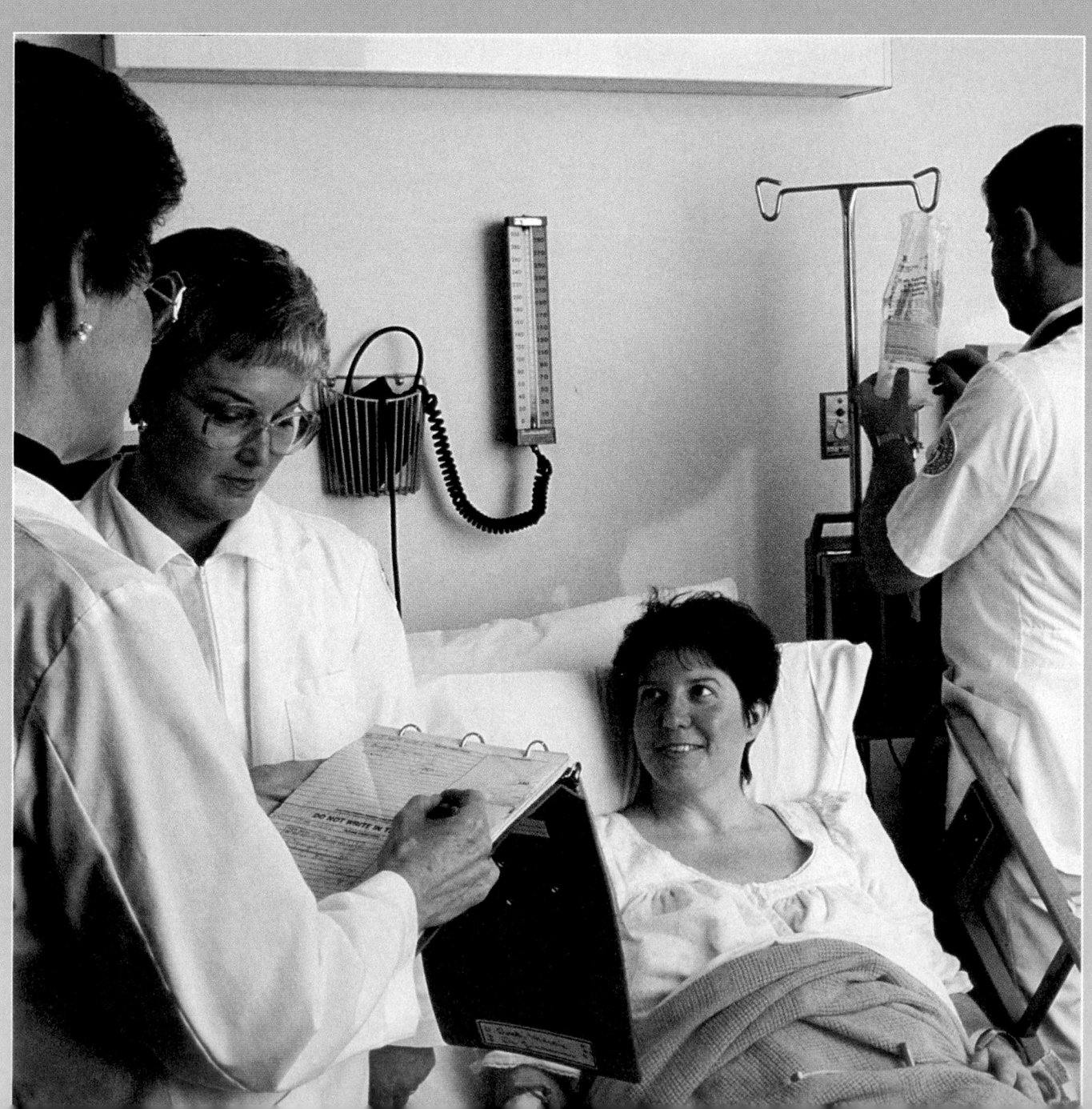

ROLE IN WELLNESS

I t is ironic that the link between nutrition and disease was made almost 3000 years ago by Hippocrates, yet the modern medical community has just recently made the same *discovery.* All the tremendous advances of medical technology are fundamentally impotent if the recipient is malnourished or is at nutritional risk. *Nutritional risk* is the potential to become malnourished because of factors that are primary (inadequate intake of nutrients) or secondary (caused by disease or iatrogenic affects). The capacity for recovery from illness or disease depends on nutritional status. Poor nutritional status delays or prevents recovery, whereas good nutritional status promotes healing and recovery. It is therefore important to determine the nutritional status of those undergoing medical treatment or cure.

NUTRITION CARE PROCESS

E ach patient has unique nutritional needs depending on his or her injury or illness. For nutrition intervention to be efficacious and successful, a systematic, logical strategy is necessary. The nutritional care process provides such an approach. Like the nursing process, this process employs a five-step procedure to identify and solve nutrition-related problems (Fig. 14-1).

Step 1: **Assessment** of patient's nutritional status and needs
Step 2: **Analysis** of assessment data to determine nutritional requirements
Step 3: **Planning** intervention to meet nutritional needs
Step 4: **Implementation** of the plan (steps 1 through 3)
Step 5: **Evaluation** of intervention by ongoing assessment (step 1) and making appropriate changes

Nutritional Assessment

The nutritional care process is often performed during a comprehensive nutritional assessment conducted by dietetic professionals. Dietetic professionals work synergistically with nursing personnel to provide this essential component in medical care. A *comprehensive nutritional assessment* is a procedure conducted by dietetic professionals to determine appropriate medical nutrition therapy based on the identified needs of the patient. This process uses data collected from several different sources to assess patients' nutritional needs, often using the *ABCD* approach: Anthropometrics, Biochemical tests, Clinical observations, and Diet evaluation. Each part of this process is important because there is no one single parameter that directly measures nutritional status, or determines nutritional problems or needs. Thus a combination of these parameters must be used to interpret the overall nutrition picture presented by patients within the context of their personal, social, and economic backgrounds.*

Anthropometric measurements

Anthropometric measurements are determined by simple, noninvasive techniques that measure height, weight, head, arm muscle circumferences, and skinfold thicknesses. The effectiveness of single anthropometric measurements is limited, but serial measurements can be useful in assessing body composition changes or growth over a period of time. Standardized techniques must be used to obtain valid and reliable measurements. Evaluation of anthropometric data involves comparison of

---

*Note that information described in the anthropometric, biochemical, clinical, and dietary assessment data is *not* all-encompassing. In an effort to conserve time and space, only parameters of particular interest to nursing are discussed.

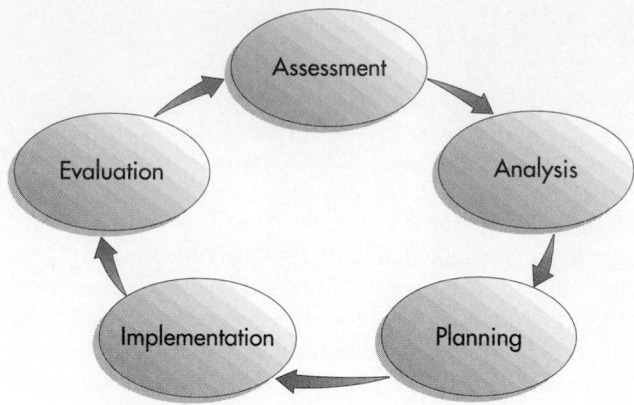

Fig. 14-1 Nutritional Care Process

Measuring Height

1. Have patient stand erect with weight equally distributed on both feet.
   (a) If the legs are of unequal length, place boards under the short limb to make the pelvis level.
   (b) Where possible, make sure the head, shoulder blades, buttocks, and heels all touch the vertical surface.
   (c) Instruct patient to let arms hang free at the sides with palms facing the thighs.
2. Have patient look straight ahead (so the line of vision is perpendicular to the body), take a deep breath, and hold that position while the horizontal headboard is brought down firmly on top of the head. (Measurer's eyes should be level with the headboard to read the measurement.)
3. Read the measurement to the nearest 0.1 cm or 1/8 in.

From Lee RD, Nieman DC: *Nutritional assessment,* ed 2, St. Louis, 1996, Mosby.

data collected with predetermined reference limits or cutoff points that allow classification into one or more risk categories, and in some cases, identification of the type and severity of malnutrition (1). Discussion of various anthropometric measurements follows.

Height. Stature (height) is important in evaluating growth and nutritional status in children. In adults, height is needed for assessment of weight and body size. Height should be measured using a fixed measuring stick or tape on a true vertical, flat surface with no carpeting. If this is not available, the movable measuring arm on platform clinic scales may be used with reasonable accuracy but tends to produce lower measures (2). The patient should be measured standing as straight as possible, without shoes or head coverings, heels together, and looking straight ahead.

Accurate heights are important in nutritional assessment. Many of the calculations used to determine energy requirements and needs are based on height as well as weight. Unfortunately, heights are frequently not available in the medical records of hospitalized patients. When heights are documented, it is often unclear whether they are reported by the patient or measured. Asking patients about their height does not always produce accurate information. On average when asked, people report being slightly taller than they actually are (approximately 0.6 inches or 1.5 cm taller) (3). Men overstate their height more often than women (3,4) and the extent of overstating height increases as people age (3). If the height of a patient recorded in the medical record is not a measured height, it should be documented as a stated height.

 When measuring infants and children (less than 2 to 3 years) who cannot stand, or others unable to stand erect without assistance, a recumbent length table can be

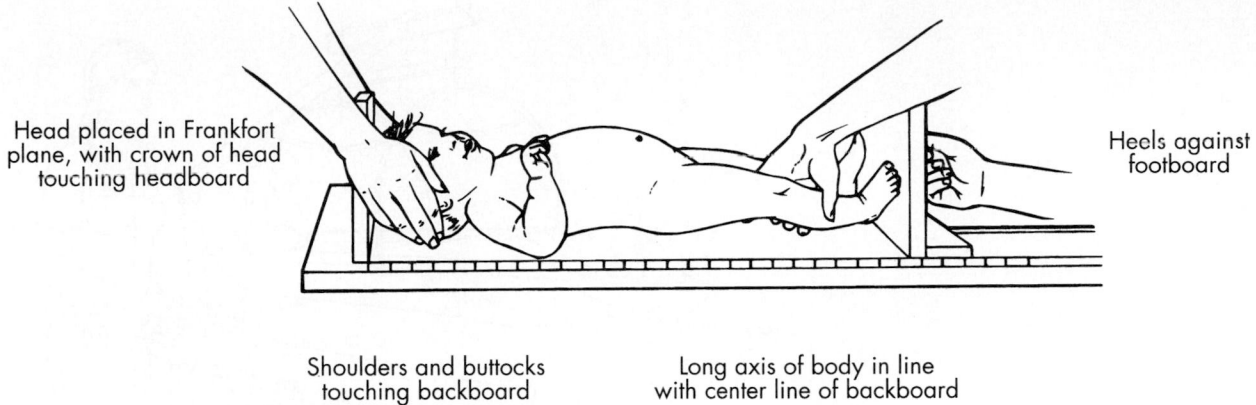

Head placed in Frankfort plane, with crown of head touching headboard

Heels against footboard

Shoulders and buttocks touching backboard

Long axis of body in line with center line of backboard

Fig. 14-2 A recumbent length board.

Measuring Recumbent Bed Height

1. Remove pillows and make bed level.
2. Straighten the patient out in bed, but with the feet flexed.
3. With a clipboard or ruler, extend perpendicular lines from the top of the head and the bottom of the feet out to the side of the bed.
4. Mark the two positions on the bedsheet and measure the distance between them to the nearest 0.5 cm.

From Gray D: Accuracy of recumbent height measurement, *Journal of parenteral and enteral nutrition* 9:712, 1985.

---

used. A recumbent length table or board has a fixed headboard, a moveable footboard, and a permanent measuring tape along the side (Fig. 14-2). To measure a patient, he or she should be placed supine on the board or table with shoulders and legs flat against the measuring board (table) and arms at the sides. The head should firmly touch the headboard while the line of vision is perpendicular to the board or table. Soles of the feet should be vertical, and the footboard should touch the bottom of the feet so that the soft tissue is compressed. Length can be recorded from the measure at the footboard. Two people are often needed to take an accurate measurement (2).

When the patient is comatose, critically ill, or unable to be moved for other reasons, taking a recumbent bed height may be possible (5). Note that when compared to standing height, bed height is significantly greater by at least 2% (5).

A more accurate measurement for patients who cannot stand is knee height. Another plus is that this measurement is minimally affected by aging. Knee height is more accurate when measured in a recumbent rather than sitting position (6). In the elderly, knee height can be measured to estimate height by using the following formulas (7):

Male height (cm) = 64.19 − (0.04 × age) + [2.02 × knee height (cm)]

Female height (cm) = 84.88 − (0.24 × age) + [1.83 × knee height (cm)]

The special calipers necessary for measuring knee height are available from Ross Laboratories in Columbus, Ohio.

Weight. When accurately measured, body weight is a simple, gross estimate of body composition (1). In fact, body weight is one of the most important measurements in assessing nutritional status, and is used to predict energy expenditure (8). Beam scales with moveable but nondetachable weights or accurate electronic scales are recommended for obtaining accurate results (1,2). Spring scales are not recommended (2). If the patient is nonambulatory, wheelchair

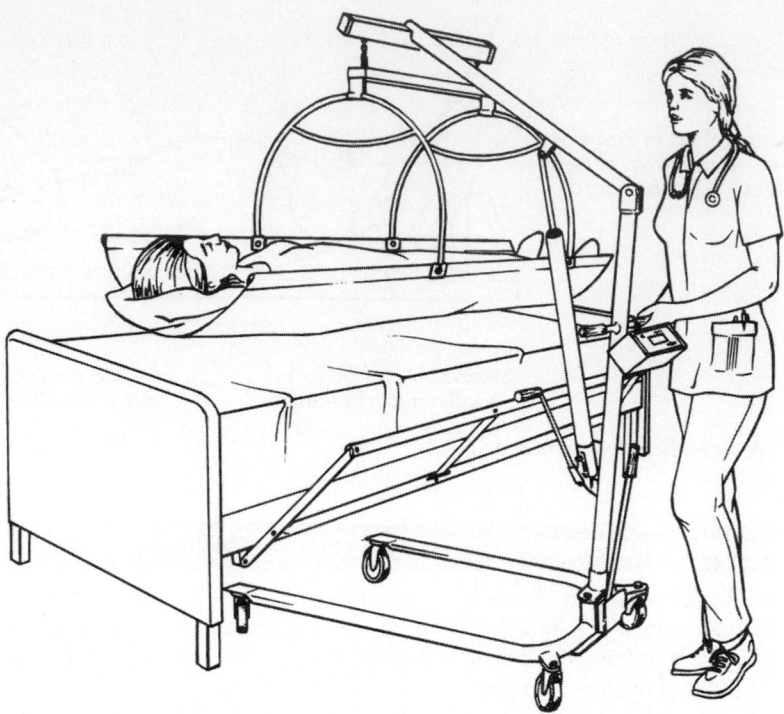

Fig. 14-3 If a patient is nonambulatory, a bed scale can be used.

or bed scales should be used (Fig. 14-3) (1,2). Scales should be checked for accuracy periodically and recalibrated when necessary. Like heights, actual measured weights are more accurate than patients' *guesstimates* because most people report their weight as slightly less than it actually is (by approximately 2.4 lb or 5 kg). Women tend to underestimate their weight more than men, and for both men and women, the extent of underreporting increases as actual weight increases (3).

For accurate weights, patients should be clothed in their underwear or hospital gown. Weights should be measured at the same time of day and after voiding. The patient should stand still with weight evenly distributed on both feet while weight is recorded to the nearest 0.1 kg or ¼ lb (2).

As a nutritional screening tool, weights can be used to recognize changes that may be representative or suggestive of serious health problems. The magnitude and direction of weight change are more meaningful when dealing with sick or debilitated patients than the standardized desirable weight references. Percent weight change is a useful nutrition index and may be computed as follows (1):

$$\% \text{ weight change from usual weight} = \frac{(\text{usual weight} - \text{actual weight})}{\text{usual weight}} \times 100$$

$$\% \text{ weight change from admission weight} = \frac{(\text{admission weight} - \text{actual weight})}{\text{admission weight}} \times 100$$

$$\% \text{ weight change since nutrition intervention} = \frac{(\text{preintervention weight} - \text{actual weight})}{\text{preintervention weight}} \times 100$$

Care should be taken to identify patients with ascites, edema, or dehydration as their weight changes may be more a reflection of their fluid status than actual changes in body composition. If more than 1 lb is gained in a day's time, it may be indicative of excess fluid (1). It is also important to examine any unplanned weight loss the patient might experience: 1% to 2% in usual weight in the past week, 5% over the past month, 7.5% over the previous 3 months, or 10% in the past 6 months indicates significant weight loss, whereas weight losses more than this signify severe weight loss (8). Percent weight losses of these magnitudes could be cause for alarm.

For elderly patients who cannot be weighed because of the severity of their medical condition, or if bed or chair scales are not available, Chumlea et al have developed gender-specific equations for predicting body weight in persons 60 to 90 years of age (9). The estimated weights are based on recumbent measures of arm circumference (AC), calf circumference (CC), subscapular skinfold (SSF), and knee height (KH).

Females: weight (cm) = [0.98 × AC(in cm)] + [1.27 × CC(in cm)] +
                         [0.4 × SSF(in mm)] + [0.87 × KN(in cm)] − 62.35

Males: weight (cm) = [1.73 × AC(in cm)] + [0.98 × CC(in cm)] +
                         [0.37 × SSF(in mm)] + [1.16 × KN(in cm)] − 81.69

Another challenge in obtaining weights is patients who have missing body parts because of amputation. Figure 14-4 shows the approximate percent of body weight contributed by individual body segments so desirable weight can be calculated.

Body mass index. Body mass index (BMI) has been proposed as an alternative to the traditionally used height-weight tables in assessing obesity (1). BMI measures weight corrected for height. You can determine BMI by referring to Table 10-2 (p. 253) or by dividing weight in kilograms by height in square meters using the following steps:

1. Divide weight in pounds by 2.2, to convert it into kilograms
2. Multiply height in inches by 2.54 and divide the result by 100, to convert height to meters; then multiply height in meters by itself (that is, square it).

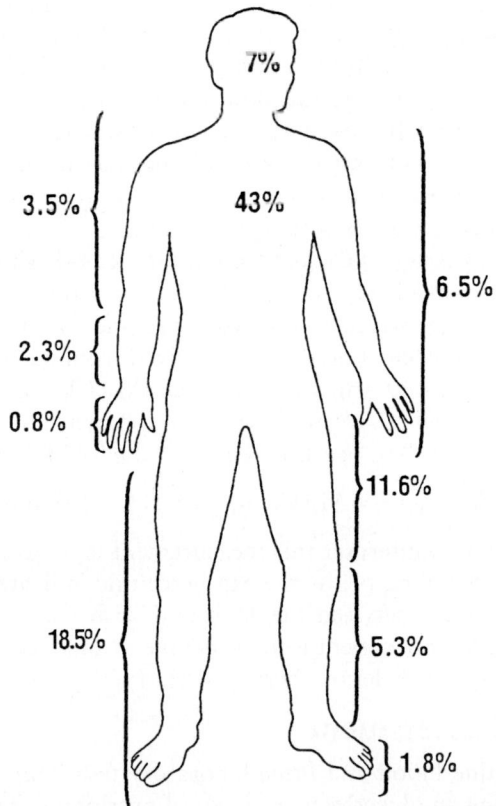

Fig. 14-4 Approximate body weight percentages. Modified from Brunnstrom S: *Clinical kinesiology,* Philadelphia, 1962, FA Davis.

Body Mass Index and Associated Level of Medical Risk	
BMI	**RISK**
<20-25	Very Low
25-30	Low
30-35	Moderate
35-40	High
>40	Very high

3. Divide weight in kilograms (result of step 1) by the square of height in meters (results of step 2). The result is BMI.

$$BMI = Weight (kg)/Height (m) \times Height (m)$$

The desired BMI range for healthy adults is 20 to 25 kg/m^2, which reflects a healthy weight for height. Although at low risk for health problems, persons with BMIs of 25 to 30 kg/m^2 are approximately 20% above desirable levels. Persons with BMIs between 35 to 40 kg/m2 are at high risk, and BMIs greater than 40 indicate very high risk. A BMI of less than 20 for males or 19 for females is classified as underweight and is associated with risk factors such as respiratory disease, tuberculosis, digestive disease, and some cancers (10).

Body measures. Skinfold thicknesses are often used to estimate subcutaneous fat stores or the pattern of fat distribution. This information can then be used to help determine nutritional status. Skinfold measures are taken by measuring a double fold of skin and fat tissue at specific body sites. Although eight sites (chest, triceps, subscapular, midaxillary, suprailiac, abdomen, thigh, and medial calf) can be used, the triceps skinfold (TSF) is the most commonly used single site. The only tools necessary are a tape measure and calipers of acceptable quality. Detailed instructions for measuring various body sites have been published elsewhere and should be studied carefully before undertaking the actual measurement (2). It is important that the person taking the skinfold measures be properly trained and subsequent measurements be taken by the same person (1). As with any other measurement of nutritional status, skinfold measurements should be used in conjunction with other parameters and followed over time to provide an accurate and thorough assessment (1). Skinfold measurements should be compared with percentages of standards (11), be taken from multiple body sites, or be collected as serial measurements to assess changes in fat stores over time (1).

Mid-arm muscle circumference (MAMC) provides an indication of skeletal muscle mass (**somatic protein stores**) and is derived from measurements of the triceps skinfold (TSF) and mid-arm circumference (MAC). Two advantages of this measure are that it takes a relatively short amount of time and the outcome is not affected by edema (1). MAMC is estimated using the following equation:

somatic protein stores
proteins in skeletal muscle

$$MAMC(cm) = MAC(cm) - [0.314 \times TSF(mm)]$$

The most reliable way to interpret this measurement is by using a percentile rank system: measurements falling below the 5th percentile indicate depletion of nutritional reserves, and those between the 15th and 25th percentiles represent marginal reserves (12). This assessment is not sensitive to small changes that can occur during illness or nutrition repletion therapy (13).

Biochemical assessment

Many of the routine blood and urine laboratory tests found in patients' charts are useful in providing an objective assessment of nutritional status. Care should be taken in interpreting test results for a number of reasons. First of all, there is no single available test for evaluating short-term response to medical nutritional therapy.

Biochemical Parameters and How They Are Tested

Visceral protein status
  Serum albumin
  Total iron binding capacity (TIBC)
  Prealbumin (thyroxine-binding prealbumin)
Somatic protein status
  Serum creatinine
  24-hr urinary creatinine
Immune function
  Total lymphocyte count (TLC)
Evaluation of protein intake
  24-hr urea nitrogen (UUN)
Iron status
  Transferrin
  Hemoglobin
  Hematocrit
  Mean corpuscular hemoglobin (MCH)
  Mean corpuscular volume (MCV)

Laboratory tests should be used in conjunction with anthropometric data, clinical data, and dietary intake assessments. Second, some tests may be inappropriate for certain patients, for example, serum albumin cannot be used to evaluate protein status in those patients with liver failure because this test assumes normal liver function. Third, lab tests conducted serially will give more accurate information than a single test (2). Although serial measures can be obtained in long-term care settings, patients in acute care facilities are rarely hospitalized long enough to obtain serial measures. Therefore test results compared to standards should be used.

The most important biochemical parameters are visceral protein status and immune function. Visceral protein status is assessed through tests of serum albumin and prealbumin. Immune function is evaluated based on total lymphocyte count (TLC). The test results of these biochemical assessments provide information to determine the effects of nutritional factors and/or of medical conditions on the health status of patients.

Serum albumin. Serum albumin provides an assessment of visceral protein status. Normal values are within 3.5 to 5.0 g/dl. For nutritional analysis, values between 2.8 and 3.5 g/dl indicate compromised protein status; values less than 2.8 g/dl suggest possible kwashiorkor. This test is most useful when used to monitor long-term nutrition changes since normal values may still be found among patients who are malnourished. If patients are experiencing dehydration (hemoconcentration) or have received infusions of albumin, fresh frozen plasma, or whole blood serum albumin, levels may appear to be normal. As a tool to assess long-term changes, the effects of dehydration and infusions would be dissipated. Alternate causes of abnormally low values may be infection and other stressors (especially with poor protein intake), burns, trauma, congestive heart failure, fluid overload, and severe hepatic insufficiency (1,14,15).

Prealbumin. Prealbumin (thyroxine-binding prealbumin) also provides visceral protein status assessment. Normal values range from 20 to 50 mg/dl. This test is useful in monitoring short-term changes in visceral protein status because of its short half-life of 2 days. Compromised protein status is indicated when levels are between 10 to 15 g/dl. Possible kwashiorkor is a potential diagnosis when levels are less than 10 mg/dl. A nonnutritional cause of normal values despite patient malnutrition is chronic renal failure. Other factors that result in abnormally low levels of prealbumin include surgical trauma, stress, inflammation, infection, and liver dysfunction. (1,14,15)

Total lymphocyte count. Total lymphocyte count (TLC) is a test to assess immune function. A normal TLC is greater than 1500 cells/mm^3. This test should not be used as an absolute indicator of nutritional status, but considered with other diagnostic assessments. A count of less than 1500/mm^3 indicates possible immunocompromise associated with protein-energy malnutrition, especially kwashiorkor. Other causes of abnormal values are not directly related to nutritional status. Abnormally low TLCs may be due to severe stress (such as infections), corticosteroid therapy, renal failure, and cancer. High levels of TLC may indicate infections, leukemia, myeloma, cancer, and adrenal insufficiency (1,14,15).

Other assessment parameters of somatic protein status, nitrogen balance, vitamin and mineral status, and hair analysis are detailed in Appendix E in Routine Laboratory Tests and Values for Nutritional Assessment.

Clinical assessment

Clinical assessment includes collecting data from several sources: medical history, social history, and physical examination. Many environmental factors can influence nutritional status. This information can be obtained by reviewing the patient's medical record or through direct interview. There may be social or family factors that affect nutrient intake or past or present medical conditions that influence nutrient utilization. Many physical signs and symptoms associated with malnutrition are also an integral part of assessing nutritional status (1).

Features associated with nutritional deficiency may be considered through historical and clinical categories (14,16). Historical findings may include alcohol abuse, poverty, avoidance of specific food groups (such as fruits or vegetables), weight loss, drug use (or abuse), family history of inborn errors, and cigarette smoking. Clinical features are extensive; some but not all are surgery or wounds; blood loss; dull, dry, pluckable hair; fever; and bleeding gums. Findings may be organized by symptoms of the eyes, face, skin, muscles, tongue, and central nervous system. Table 14-1 provides additional data about historical and clinical features in relation to nutritional status.

Dietary intake assessment

There are several methods for collecting information regarding actual and habitual dietary intake. Most commonly, data are collected using recall (retrospective) or records (prospective). Each method has its pros and cons, so it is important to chose a method best suited to the type of information needed (1). These data provide information regarding intake of kcalories, protein, carbohydrate, fat, vitamins, minerals, and fluid, which can be calculated manually using food composition tables or analyzed by computer software. There are literally hundreds of programs available to analyze dietary intake. Evaluation of software needs and systems suitable to meet those needs is important when selecting an appropriate software package (2).

24-hour diet recall. In this method, the patient is asked by the interviewer to report all foods and beverages consumed during the past 24 hours. Detailed description of all foods, beverages, cooking methods, brand names, condiments, and supplements, along with portion sizes in common household measures is included. Food models, measuring cups, life-size pictures, or abstract shapes (squares, circles, rectangles) are used to assist the patient in estimating correct portion sizes of foods consumed. This method is useful in screening or during follow-up to evaluate adaptation of dietary recommendations. The advantages of this method are that it is quick (only 15 to 20 minutes are needed) and it can be used with any age group. Since it is retrospective, the patient does not modify his or her actual intake. The information can be obtained by interview, telephone, or patient self-reporting. Some of the drawbacks for this method are that it does rely on the memory, motivation, and awareness of the patient. Since this is only a single day's intake, it may not be representative of the patient's actual diet (1). A sample 24-hour recall form can be found in Appendix I.

Table 14-1   Historical and Clinical Features Associated With Nutritional Deficiency

History or Physical Findings	Nutritional Implication	Possible Deficiency
Alcohol abuse	Inadequate nutrient intake	Kcalories, protein, thiamine, niacin, folate, pyridoxine, riboflavin
	Increased nutrient losses	Magnesium, zinc
Avoidance of fruits, vegetables, grain products	Inadequate nutrient intake	Vitamins A and C, thiamin, niacin, folate
Avoidance of meat, dairy products, eggs	Inadequate nutrient intake	Protein, vitamin B_{12}
Constipation, hemorrhoids, diverticulosis	Inadequate nutrient intake	Dietary fiber
Isolation, poverty, dental disease, food idiosyncrasies	Inadequate nutrient intake	Various nutrients
Weight loss	Inadequate nutrient intake	Kcalories, other nutrients
Drugs (especially antacids, anticonvulsants, cholestyramine, laxatives, neomycin, alcohol)	Inadequate nutrient absorption, decreased nutrient utilization	Various nutrients
Malabsorption (diarrhea, weight loss, steatorrhea)	Inadequate nutrient absorption, increased nutrient losses	Vitamins A, D, K; kcalories; protein; calcium; magnesium; zinc; electrolytes
Parasites	Inadequate nutrient absorption	Iron, vitamin B_{12} (fish tapeworm)
Pernicious anemia	Inadequate nutrient absorption	Vitamin B_{12}
Surgery	Inadequate nutrient absorption	Vitamin B_{12}, iron, folate
gastrectomy		Vitamin B_{12} (if distal ileum),
intestinal resection		iron, others as in malabsorption
Inborn errors of metabolism (by family history)	Decreased nutrient utilization	Various nutrients
Blood loss	Increased nutrient losses	Iron
Centesis (ascitic, pleural taps)	Increased nutrient losses	Protein
Diabetes, uncontrolled	Increased nutrient losses	Kcalories
Draining abscesses, wounds	Increased nutrient losses	Protein, zinc
Nephrotic syndrome	Increased nutrient losses	Protein, zinc
Peritoneal dialysis or hemodialysis	Increased nutrient losses	Protein, water soluble vitamins, zinc
Fever	Increased nutrient requirements	Kcalories
Hyperthyroidism	Increased nutrient requirements	Kcalories
Physiologic demands (infancy, adolescence, pregnancy, lactation)	Increased nutrient requirements	Various nutrients
Surgery, trauma, burns, infection	Increased nutrient requirements	Kcalories, protein, vitamin C, zinc
Tissue hypoxia	Increased nutrient requirements	Kcalories (inefficient utilization)
Cigarette smoking	Increased nutrient requirements	Vitamin C, folic acid
Dull, dry, sparse, easily plucked hair		Protein, energy, zinc
Spoon-shaped, brittle, ridged nails		Iron
Face		
Rotundness, "moon face" appearance		Obesity, protein
Presence of edema or decubiti		Protein
Nasolabial seborrhea		Riboflavin, zinc
Xerosis (dryness of mucous membranes)		Vitamin A
Pallor, listlessness		Iron
Eyes		
Redness or fissures at corners of eyelids		Riboflavin
Dry cornea, Bitot's spots		Vitamin A
Cloudy, pale conjunctiva		Iron
Periorbital numbness		Phosphorus
Angular lesions at corners of the mouth		Riboflavin
Bleeding, spongy gums		Vitamin C
Tongue		
Magenta in color		Riboflavin
Scarlet, raw, swollen, fissures on tongue		Niacin
Thick tongue, difficulty with speaking		Phosphorus

Continued.

Table 14-1 Historical and Clinical Features Associated With Nutritional Deficiency, cont'd.

History or Physical Findings	Nutritional Implication	Possible Deficiency
Goiter		Iodine
Skin		
Scrotal and vulvar dermatosis not accompanied by inflammation		Riboflavin
Swollen skin pigmentation of areas exposed to sun		Niacin
Pinhead size, purplish hemorrhagic spots (petechiae)		Vitamin C
Excessive bruising		Vitamin C or K
Poor wound healing, decubiti		Protein, kcalories
Follicular hyperkeratosis (epidermal hypertrophy causing horny skin formation)		Vitamin A
Muscular system		
Thinness, tissue wasting		Protein, kcalories
Presence of edema		Obesity, protein, sodium
Skeletal system		
Osteoporosis		Calcium, protein
Circumscribed swelling or growth of frontal and parietal areas of skull, bowed legs		Vitamin D
Central nervous system		
Mental irritability		Protein
Hyporeflexia, foot and wrist drop		Thiamine
Psychotic behavior		Niacin
Peripheral neuropathy, forgetfulness		Pyridoxine
Tremor, convulsions, tetany		Magnesium, calcium

From Horne M, Swearingen PL: *Pocket guide to fluids and electrolytes,* St. Louis, 1989, Mosby; and Weinsier RL, Heimburger DC, Butterworth CE: *Handbook of clinical nutrition,* ed 2, St Louis, 1989, Mosby.

nutritional support

although commonly used in reference to enteral and parenteral nutrition delivery systems, it can refer to any nutrition intervention used to minimize patient morbidity, mortality, and complications

Food records. Food records can provide a more realistic picture of a patient's usual intake. All foods, beverages, snacks, and supplements are recorded by the patient, usually over a period of 1 to 7 days using household measures. To assure accuracy, the patient must be trained with food models, measuring cups, or other measuring devices that will help ensure recording of proper or actual portion sizes. Cooking methods, recipe ingredients, and descriptions need to be recorded as completely and accurately as possible. Often, record keeping like this influences the recorder's standard food choices, but in some cases this may be a desirable side effect. In some instances, the recorder is also asked to record locations, times, events, and feelings in addition to foods eaten if information is needed to identify behavioral as well as nutritional patterns. A 7-day food record is considered to be optimal for gathering this kind of information but tends to be rather tedious. Shorter periods are less representative of usual intake, but a 3-day record (including two weekdays and one weekend day) can be acceptable. Obviously for this method of dietary data collection, the patient must be literate, numerate, and well-motivated (1).

Kcalorie counts. In an acute or long-term care setting, one of the most common forms of food records is a kcalorie count. This term is a little misleading because in actual practice, all nutrients can be assessed, but kcalorie and protein intakes are parameters usually quantified. Information gathered in this manner is often used to determine the adequacy of patients' daily oral intake or to document the need for **nutritional support.** Nursing observations are essential to early identification of malnutrition and prevention of iatrogenic weight loss during the hospital stay. Staff who are responsible for recording intake must be accurate in their recordings (1). It is important to record foods and beverages that have been consumed in measurable amounts (such as cups, ounces, teaspoons, tablespoons, cc's) or in percentage of amount eaten (50% baked chicken, 75% bread, 25% green beans).

Table 14-2 Areas of Nutritional Risk		
Data Source	**Moderate Risk**	**High Risk**
Age	65-75 years of age Children over 5 years of age	75 years of age or older Children under 5 years of age
Weight	Evaluation of loss (i.e., self-induced?)	5% weight loss in 1 month 10% loss in 6 months Length/height for age < 5th percentile Weight/height < 5th percentile or < 80th percentile of standard
Lab	Albumin 3.5-3.0 g/dl	Albumin ≤ 3.0 g/dl TLC ≤ 1200 cells/mm^3 Prealbumin ≤ 10 mg

Systems*	Heart, antepartum, pain, orthopedics,
	  selected oncology, short stay,
	  chemotherapy
		Renal, pancreas, GI, liver, diabetes with pregnancy,
		  eating disorders, oncology, transplants, any
		  condition in children associated with
		  development of protein calorie malnutrition

Feeding modalities	Transitional (stable)
	Some selected modified diets with
	  education component
		Parenteral nutrition, tube feeding, NPO, or clear
		  liquids > 3 days

From Grant A, DeHoog S: *Nutritional assessment and support*, ed 4, Seattle, 1991, Anne Grant/Susan DeHoog.
*Systems for risk depend on the individual patient population at risk.

Subjective terms such as *two bites, ate well,* or *three swallows* are virtually useless data and cannot provide objective information needed to calculate protein and kcaloric intake.

Nutritional risk. As mentioned previously, the nutritional care process involves assessing patients' nutritional status, estimating nutritional needs, and planning for nutritional intervention. If done appropriately, it allows for early intervention in both treatment of established malnutrition and prevention of malnutrition among those at high nutritional risk (1). Areas of nutritional risk are age, weight, laboratory test results, (body) systems, and feeding modalities (17) (Table 14-2).

Age: Moderate nutritional risk occurs among adults between ages 65 and 75 and for children over 5 years of age. Age-related high risk is possible for patients ages 75 years or older; for children, high risk most often occurs under the age of 5.

Weight: Weight loss is a potential nutritional risk factor depending on its cause. Based on the percentage of body weight lost combined with the evaluation or cause of the loss determines the possible level of risk (see Table 14-2).

Laboratory: As noted previously, biochemical tests of albumin, TLC, and prealbumin levels provide an assessment of nutritional risk.

Systems: Systems account for conditions of various body systems that present either moderate or high nutritional risk. Moderate nutritional risk may be experienced when a patient is undergoing chemotherapy because of its effects on dietary intake. High risk is incurred among individuals with eating disorders or diabetes when pregnant. (Other conditions are listed in Table 14-2.)

Feeding modalities: Moderate nutritional risk is associated with transition from restrictive therapeutic intervention to a regular dietary intake. Risk may also occur when patients are on modified diets that have the potential to cause nutrient deficiencies. High risk takes place when patients are on parenteral or tube feeding, are NPO, or on clear liquids for more than 3 days.

Nutritional assessment involves examination of (1) anthropometric data, (2) biochemical data, (3) clinical data, and (4) dietary data. It is important to remember that there is no one absolute index for measuring nutritional status. Accurate and meaningful assessment can be made only by incorporating data from several sources.

FOOD SERVICE DELIVERY SYSTEMS

Since nursing personnel are often on the *front line* when food is delivered to patients, it is important to understand how meals are prepared and delivered to patients in hospitals and long-term care facilities. Food service in a health care setting is the responsibility of the director of the food and nutrition services department. This person may be either a management dietitian or a specially trained food service manager. He or she is responsible for hiring, firing, and supervising staff; ordering and purchasing food and supplies; delivery of food to patients and staff; and quality assurance issues. Clinical dietitians may work under the supervision of or alongside the food service director to assess patients' nutritional status, plan appropriate diets and nutrition intervention, and provide nutrition education. Other personnel from the food and nutrition service area include cooks, clerks, dishwashers, aids, and dietetic technicians. Clinical dietitians may also be members of a food service department. Their jobs involve direct patient care. Typically, only registered dietitians (management and clinical) and dietetic technicians have the unique education and training in clinical nutrition and all of its applications, whether that is the delivery of food or assessing nutritional status.

Patients are often able to choose the foods they will be served at meal time. Some institutions provide this service for patients receiving regular and modified

TEACHING TOOL

Assisting Patients With Menu Selections

When we select food items from a restaurant menu while socializing with friends and family, the process is fun. However, choosing foods from the restricted hospital selections, often with little descriptive information, can be a difficult and sometimes intimidating chore when we are ill in a hospital.

As nurses, we are familiar with hospital forms requiring us to choose selections quickly; we cannot assume our patients also share that ability. Patients may need our help. Below are potential menu selection problems and possible solutions.

PROBLEM	SOLUTION
• Patient has a low literacy level, is illiterate, has reduced visual abilities, or is too ill to read or write	Read menu items to patient and mark his/her selections
• Patient does not understand the vocabulary used on menu (we cannot assume dietary terms are common knowledge)	Clarify for patient or ask for clarification from dietetic technician, dietitian, or foodservice personnel
• Patient often must select foods from menu a day in advance, often resulting in choosing too much or too little food (particularly a concern when appetite may be diminished from drug-nutrient interactions or from the effects of the illness)	Remind patients they are selecting food for the next day; if they have not selected enough food, offer them foods kept on the nursing unit for snacks, or order additional foods from foodservice; if they have selected too much food, cover, date, and store appropriate foods for use later in the day
• Patient does not understand why some of his/her favorite foods are not included on the menu, or why smaller amounts are served (when ill, familiar foods are most desired and comforting)	Menus are a great teaching tool for modified diets; discuss dietary concerns of the patient's illness, explaining why specific foods are not included or only limited amounts allowed; contact the registered dietitian to provide education for patient

diets. A menu for a modified diet lists only the foods that are appropriate for each patient to select. This practice allows patients to select foods they like and will eat. A dietitian can plan the most nutritious meals possible, but if patients do not eat the food, then patients are not nourished. A selective menu system also affords patients the feeling of some control over their lives while hospitalized (18).

Some institutions do not offer selective menus. In their place, a standard house diet that is adjusted (or modified) according to special nutritional needs is used. Although a selective menu may not be available, efforts can be made to obtain patient food likes and dislikes. Simple changes or substitutions are common.

Nursing personnel, on behalf of their patients, often interact with the staff of the food service system of their facility. It may be beneficial for nurses to familiarize themselves with the organization and staff of the food service system. Information that is beneficial includes the following (18):

- Procedure and telephone numbers to request a physician-ordered diet, make diet changes, or report problems with a patient's tray
- Procedure and telephone number of the clinical dietitian to request nutrition assessment or education
- Time schedule of meal service so requests or changes can be made *before* meals are delivered to patients
- Location of the **diet manual** on the nursing unit, which is required in each unit by the Medicare Conditions of Participation for Hospitals and the Joint Commission Accreditation for Healthcare Organizations; the diet manual is the reference book (usually in a three-ring binder) that describes the rationale and indications for using a specific diet, lists allowed and restricted foods, and provides sample menus

Most of this information also applies to long-term care facilities, but there are a few additional concerns. Food service provided to residents in long-term care facilities often relies solely upon the food service department for nutritious foods and meals. Repetition and boredom also impact patient acceptance of foods and meals served. Therefore it is of particular importance since these patients are often at high nutritional risk, that patients receive food they can and will eat (18).

diet manual
the reference book (usually in a three-ring binder) that describes the rationale and indications for using a specific diet; lists allowed and restricted foods and sample menus

MEDICAL NUTRITION THERAPY

As discussed in the chapters to follow, specific diseases or conditions require modifications of the nutritional components of a *normal* diet. Each modified diet has a purpose and rationale, and its use is usually determined by the physician and/or dietitian. To appreciate the modified diets described in the following chapters, it will be helpful to have an understanding of the basis for these diets: the regular, general, or house diet.

The general diet is designed to attain or maintain optimal nutritional status in persons who do not require modified or therapeutic diets. Individual requirements for specific nutrients vary and are adjusted depending on gender, age, height, weight, and activity level. This diet is used to promote health and reduce risks for developing chronic diet-related diseases such as cardiovascular diseases or certain cancers (19). Depending on individual food choices, a regular diet is adequate in all nutrients according to the 1989 Recommended Dietary Allowances (20).

Dietary modifications of the regular diet may be made in two ways: quantitative or qualitative. Qualitative diets include modifications in consistency, texture, or nutrients, such as clear liquid or full liquid diets. Quantitative diets include modifications in number of meals served or amounts of specific nutrients, such as six small feedings or kcalorie-controlled diets used in the treatment of diabetes mellitus.

Whatever kind of meals or modified diets patients are receiving, much of their acceptance of the food is influenced by nursing personnel. If a patient's primary care giver expresses criticism about the food service, the patient is likely to do the same. Acceptance of modified diets may also be influenced by whether patients perceive nutrition to be an important part of their medical care and recovery. Patient education can make a difference in patient acceptability of meals. By explaining the rationale of why some foods are allowed and others are to be avoided, the nurse or dietitian may increase patient compliance with modified dietary intake. It is important to remember that food provides the energy and nutrients that aid in the healing process. Food left on the tray does not help.

MYTH
All Hospital Food Is Terrible

Is hospital food as terrible as people think? Or is it just unfamiliar? Or do most people lose their appetite when sick, especially when away from home? Why can't patients just have the same foods they eat at home?

Aside from the fact that patients' illnesses usually dictate what they can eat, medical technology has also influenced what foods are served from the hospital kitchen. Treatments and procedures like chemotherapy, angioplasty, organ transplants, new drugs, and/or diseases such as AIDS have resulted in modifications of meals and foods served to meet patients' special needs. Some hospitals may serve as many as 15 or 20 different menus to patients.

In addition, each hospital food service must conform to federal, state, and professional standards that dictate nutritional content. There are even regulations that impose timing of meals. Added to this are cultural preferences; all of us have a better comfort level when served foods that are familiar to us. Physical mechanical problems that hinder patients from eating *regular* food may require that meat be served cubed or ground. Illness, treatments, or medications may alter patients' ability to taste. Chemotherapy drugs often make meats or high-protein foods taste bitter and metallic. Some other drugs may simply dull all sensation or depress appetite altogether. All of these factors affect perceptions of the quality and taste of hospital meals.

Can anything be done to overcome all these obstacles? The hospital and food service industry *had* to overcome these obstacles. In addition to the desire to improve care, the health care dollar is shrinking, and many hospitals find themselves in competition for paying patients. Once patients were recognized as customers, any service provided by a hospital became a customer service. Food that is appetizing to the palate and the eyes is good advertisement. Many hospital food services have recruited chefs or hired contract food services to provide gourmet menus.

Even without chefs, hospital food services can provide good-tasting, attractively served food. The dietitian or food service director should be notified when patients are having problems with their meals. Without proper nutrition, recovery can be delayed and relapse may only be a matter of time.

From Wielawski I: Is there a cure for hospital food? *Eating Well* May/June:50-57, 1993.

WELLNESS AND NUTRITION INTERVENTION

Physical Dimension Nutrition intervention reduces nutrition risk, allowing healing to occur and thereby promoting the physical health of patients.

Intellectual Dimension Intellectual dimension is tested as nurses are in the tricky position of observing patient's eating patterns and then needing to assess if problems are caused by illness or food availability; nurses need the skill to determine when to alert the clinical dietitian.

Emotional Dimension Emotional health of patients is an issue of nutrition intervention. Are patients upset about food because of their illness or because of other factors?

Social Dimension Social health of patients may be affected since meals are served in their rooms; feelings of isolation deprive meal times of their function of social relatedness.

SUMMARY

The capacity for recovery from illness or disease depends on nutritional status. The nutrition care process provides for the unique nutritional needs of each patient. This is accomplished through nutrition intervention to reduce nutritional risk. The nutritional care process uses a five-step procedure to identify and solve nutrition-related problems. The five steps are assessment, analysis, planning, implementation, and evaluation.

A comprehensive nutritional assessment is a procedure conducted by dietitians to determine appropriate medical nutrition therapy based on the identified needs of the patient. Data is collected from several sources to assess patients' nutritional needs, often using the *ABCD* approach: anthropometrics, biochemical tests, clinical observations, and diet evaluation.

All patient nutrition begins through the food service delivery systems of hospitals and long-term care facilities. Staff includes a director of the food and nutrition services department, clinical dietitians, and also cooks, clerks, dishwashers, aids, and dietetic technicians.

To provide medical nutritional therapy, modified diets are developed to meet the specific needs of patients as determined by the physician and/or dietitian. Dietary modifications of the regular diet may be made in two ways: quantitative or qualitative. Qualitative diets include modifications in consistency, texture, or nutrients. Quantitative diets include modifications in number of meals served or amounts of specific nutrients.

By working together, nurses and dietetic professionals can most efficiently meet the nutritional and medical needs of patients.

THE NURSING ROLE
Working With the Dietitian

In your clinical laboratory practice, you may not yet have had much contact with registered dietitians and may not have a clear understanding of how the roles of dietitians and nurses mesh in patient care. In fact, the roles complement each other very well, and nurses and dietitians enjoy a good professional relationship.

If you are caring for a patient who has a medical or nursing diagnosis unrelated to nutritional status, you may not have any contact with the dietitian on behalf of this patient. However, if your patient has a diagnosis that warrants a special diet, or if the patient has nutritional deficits or very specific food preferences, both you and the dietitian will be working to solve the patient's problems.

As the nurse, you will do a routine assessment that includes nutritional status as indicated in the Nursing Role box in Chapter 13. If this assessment reveals problems, you probably will be in touch with the dietitian who will do a more in-depth assessment as explained in this chapter. You may help collect data for this more thorough assessment, such as measuring height and weight, measuring fluid intake, or recording food or kcalorie intake.

When it comes to setting goals for the patient's nutritional problems, you will either consult with the dietitian or read the information that the dietitian has written in the patient's chart related to anticipated nutritional outcomes.

Planned interventions are also a shared activity. The dietitian calculates the patient's intake and makes sure that the correct food arrives at the correct time; however, the nursing staff is responsible for helping the patient eat,

Continued.

THE NURSING ROLE, cont'd.
Working With the Dietitian

making sure that all needed food is eaten, and recording food intake. Patient requests for different or special foods are usually made to the nurse, who relays the request to the dietary department. If the patient is not able to tolerate the diet or has complaints about it, the nurse contacts the dietitian.

Evaluation of whether goals have been met is done by both professionals. Although the dietitian may visit every few days or even every day if necessary to evaluate the plan, nurses are with the patient 24 hours a day and may pick up changes, problems, or successes even sooner. Consultations between the nurse and the dietitian would take place if the nurse had new information that it was important to share with the dietitian.

It is important to understand the roles of other health professionals, both in theory and practice, so that we can work together to efficiently and expertly meet patient needs.

Critical Thinking CLINICAL APPLICATIONS

R.G. is recovering nicely from surgery to remove his gallbladder. Two days postop, he is not restricted to bed, and is experiencing no complications. He is 6'0" tall and weighed 155 lb on admission. One year ago R.G. weighed 180 lb. Laboratory values are as follows: serum albumin 2.5 mg/dl; TIBC 250 mg/dl; TLC 1350 cells/mm^3; serum creatinine 0.5 mg/dl. Arm muscle circumference and triceps skinfold are decreased. Before admission, his average daily intake was 900 kcalories and 30 grams protein.

1. How would you assess R.G.'s weight status?
2. Are the visceral protein levels low, normal, or high? Why?
3. Are the somatic proteins low, normal, or high? Why?
4. Is the TLC low, normal, or high? Why?
5. What conclusions might you draw from these indices of nutritional status? Will his recovery be affected?

REFERENCES

1. American Dietetic Association: *Handbook of clinical dietetics,* ed 2, New Haven, 1992, Yale University Press.
2. Lee RD, Nieman DC: *Nutritional assessment,* ed 2, St. Louis, 1996, Mosby.
3. Stewart A: The reliability and validity of self-reported weight and heights, *Journal of Chronic Diseases* 35:295-309, 1982.
4. Robinson L, Wright B: Comparison of stated and measured patient heights and weights, *Am J Hosp Pharm* 39:822, 1982.
5. Gray D: Accuracy of recumbent height measurement, *Journal of Parenteral and Enteral Nutrition* 9:712, 1985.
6. Chumlea W, Roche AF, Steinbaugh ML: Estimating stature from knee height for persons 60 to 90 years of age, *J Am Geriatr Soc* 33:116-120, 1985.
7. Chumlea WC, Roche A, Mukherjee D: *Nutritional assessment of the elderly through anthropometry,* Columbus, Ohio, 1984, Ross Laboratories.
8. Blackburn GL, Thornton PA: Nutritional and metabolic assessment of the hospitalized patient, *Journal of Parenteral and Enteral Nutrition* 1:11-22, 1977.
9. Chumlea WC, Shumei G, Roche AF: Prediction of body weight for the nonambulatory elderly from anthropometry, *J Am Diet Assoc* 88:564-568, 1988.

10. Bray GA: An approach to the classification and evaluation of obesity. In Björntorp P, Brodoff BN, eds: *Obesity,* Philadelphia, 1992, Lippincot.

11. Frisancho AR: New standards of weight and body composition by frame size and height for assessment of nutritional status of adults and the elderly, *Am J Clin Nutr* 40:808-819, 1984.

12. Gray GE, Gray LK: Validity of anthropometric norms used in the assessment of hospitalized patients, *Journal of Parenteral and Enteral Nutrition* 3:336, 1979.

13. Swearingen PL: *Manual of nursing therapeutics,* ed 3, St. Louis, 1994, Mosby.

14. Weinsier RL, Heimburger D, Butterworth CE: *Handbook of clinical nutrition,* ed 2, St. Louis, 1989, Mosby.

15. Weinsier RL, Morgan SL: *Fundamentals of clinical nutrition,* St. Louis, 1993, Mosby.

16. Horne M, Swearingen PL: *Pocket guide to fluids and electrolytes,* St. Louis, 1989, Mosby.

17. Grant A, DeHoog S: *Nutritional assessment and support,* ed 4, Seattle, 1991, Anne Grant/Susan DeHoog.

18. Cataldo CB, DeBruyne LK, Whitney EN: *Nutrition and diet therapy: Principles and practice,* ed 3, St. Paul, 1992, West.

19. American Dietetic Association: *Manual of clinical dietetics,* ed 4, Chicago, 1992, The American Dietetic Association.

20. Food and Nutrition Board/National Research Council: *Recommended dietary allowances,* ed 10, Washington, DC, 1989, National Academy Press.

Chapter 15

ENTERAL AND PARENTERAL NUTRITION

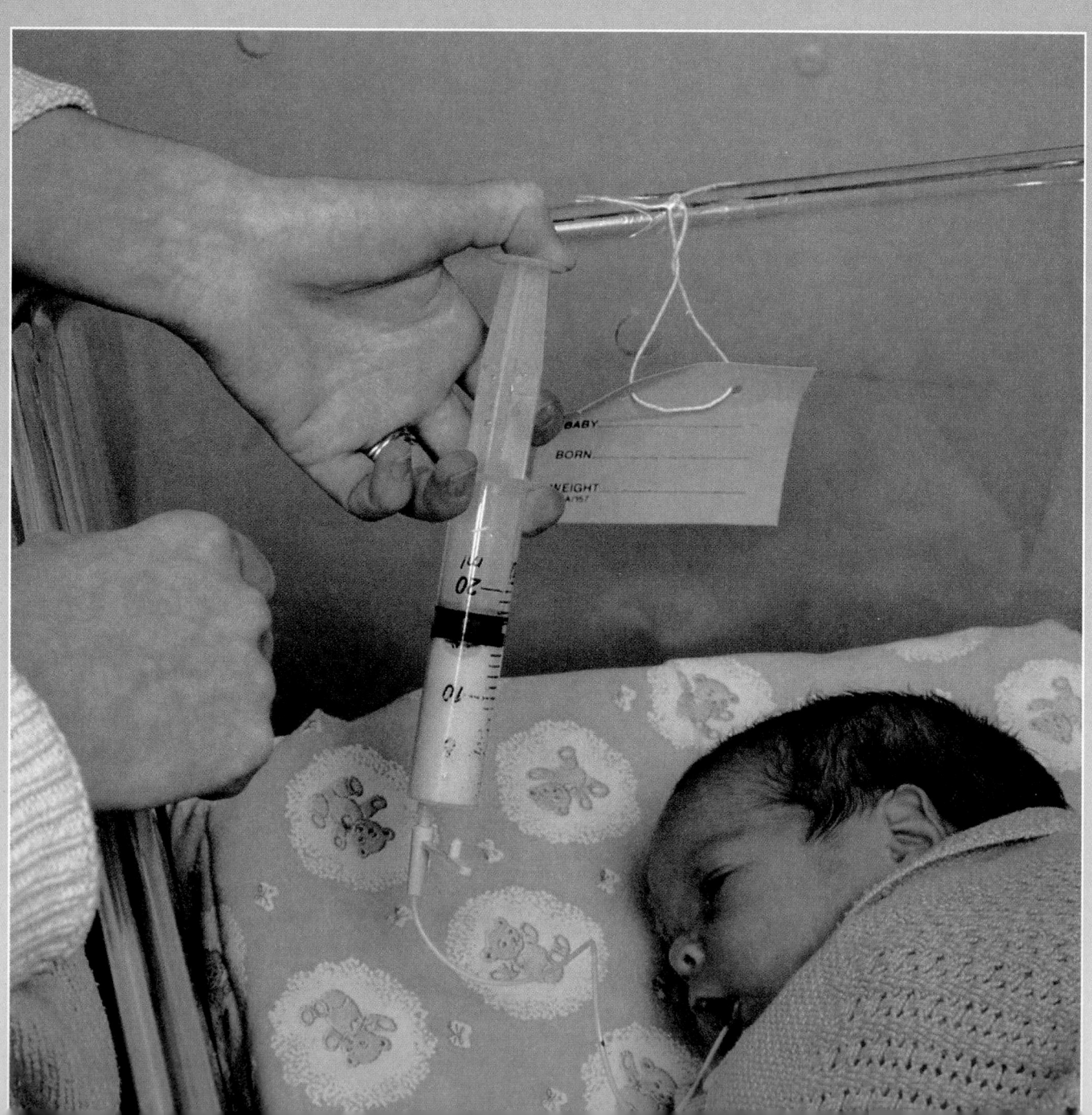

ROLE IN WELLNESS

Sometimes dietary modifications are required to allow the body to heal, to adjust to physical disability, to prepare for diagnostic tests, and/or for surgical procedures. Medical nutrition therapy may involve changes in dietary intake to liquified or pureed foods, tube feeding, or intravenous nourishment. This chapter discusses the promotion of wellness through typical progressive hospital diets, enteral formulas, and parenteral nutrition.

ENTERAL NUTRITION

Anytime the gastrointestinal tract is used to provide nourishment, the feeding can be referred to as enteral nutrition. This includes liquid diets, soft and solid food diets, as well as special nutritionally complete formulas administered orally or via tubes. The consistency of the diet may be modified in progressive steps as discussed below. However, most often when medical personnel talk about *enteral nutrition*, they are referring to the specialized formula feedings.

Basic Hospital Diets

Clear liquid diets

If a patient is scheduled for diagnostic tests or surgery, clear liquid diets are used. A clear liquid diet consists of foods that are clear and liquid at room or body temperature, factors that help prevent dehydration and keep colon contents to a minimum. Although a good source of fluids and water, this modified diet is desolate when it comes to adequate amounts of protein, fat, and energy. In addition, the clear liquid diet is almost devoid of dietary fiber, which is one of the reasons it is used. Whereas this diet can provide adequate amounts of vitamin C, it is nutritionally inadequate for almost all other required nutrients except water. Because of its limited choices, this diet is very boring.

Because a clear liquid diet is inadequate in energy and almost all nutrients except water, *the diet should not be used for more than 24 hours* even when supplemented with low-residue, nutritional products (1). Use of a clear liquid diet for more than 1 day can lead to compromised nutritional status and possible nutrient deficiencies. If the patient is already nutritionally depleted, insult is added to the injury.

Caution also is necessary in regard to the amount of caffeine patients might receive on clear liquid diets. Since food choices are so limited, patients might easily receive and consume excessive amounts of caffeine in the form of coffee, strong tea, or soft drinks containing caffeine. Excess caffeine consumption could lead to increased hydrochloric acid production in the stomach, leading to an upset stomach, and contribute to sleeplessness (2).

Although few conditions contraindicate a clear liquid diet, it is important to reiterate that this diet should not be used as the sole means of nutrition for more than 24 hours in any condition. This diet should also not be used if the patient does not possess adequate gastrointestinal function or has nutrient needs such that **parenteral nutrition** is indicated (3). Clear liquid diets can be adjusted to accommodate other dietary modifications, such as sodium restriction, if necessary.

There is some thought that unsupplemented clear liquid diets are one of the causative factors in the incidence of hospital malnutrition (4). One way to prevent this is quality assurance monitoring by the registered dietitian. This helps identify patients who have been on clear liquid diets too long, as well as those patients with

parenteral nutrition
administration of nutrients by a route other than the gastrointestinal tract, usually intravenously

colonoscopic examination
examination of the mucosal lining of the colon using a colonoscope (an elongated endoscope)

barium enema
rectal infusion of a radiopaque contrast medium to diagnose obstruction, tumors, or other abnormalities (for example, ulcerative colitis)

paralytic ileus
decrease in or absence of intestinal peristalsis

Types of Diets

LIQUID DIETS

Indications for clear liquid diet
Provide oral fluids; before/after surgery; prepare bowel for diagnostic tests (**colonoscopic examination, barium enemas,** and other procedures); minimize stimulation of gastrointestinal tract; promote recovery from partial **paralytic ileus** (early refeeding); minimize residue in the gastrointestinal tract; transition feeding from intravenous feeding to solid foods; acute gastrointestinal disturbances; diarrhea

Contraindications for clear liquid diet
Should not be used more than 24 hours; inadequate gastrointestinal function; nutrient needs requiring parenteral nutrition

Indications for full liquid diet
Provide oral fluids; after surgery; transition between clear liquids and solid food; oral or plastic surgery to the face and neck; mandibular fractures; patients who have chewing or swallowing difficulties; esophageal or gastrointestinal strictures; diarrhea

Contraindications for full liquid diet
Dysphagia

PUREED, MECHANICAL, OR SOFT DIETS

Indications for pureed diet
Neurological changes; inflammation or ulcerations of the oral cavity and/or esophagus; edentulous patients; fractured jaw; head and neck abnormalities; cerebrovascular accident

Contraindications for pureed diet
Situations where ground or chopped foods are appropriate

Indications for mechanical soft diet
Poorly fitting dentures; edentulous patients; limited chewing or swallowing ability; dysphagia; strictures of intestinal tract; radiation treatment to oral cavity; progression from enteral tube feedings or parenteral nutrition to solid foods

Contraindications for mechanical soft diet
Situations where regular foods are appropriate

Indications for soft diet
Debilitated patients unable to consume a regular diet; mild gastrointestinal problems

Contraindications for soft diet
Situations where regular foods are appropriate

any nutritional problems that result from use of the diet. Another way to monitor the use of clear liquid diets would be to establish policy that diet orders for clear liquid diets are valid for only 24 hours (similar to the time-restricted orders for antibiotics), thus allowing physicians to reevaluate the patient and the need for this nutritionally deficient diet. Each day the physician can reorder the diet with documented justification or choose a more appropriate source of nutrition. Along with this method, a mechanism to identify patients who have had clear liquid diets ordered more than three times would be necessary (1).

Full liquid diets

A full liquid diet is one that consists of foods that are liquid at room temperature. It is used to provide oral nourishment for patients that have difficulty chewing or swallowing solid foods. Unlike the clear liquid diet, the full liquid diet offers more variety, and commercial nutritional supplements can be used to supply adequate amounts of energy and nutrients to make it nutritionally complete (1).

There are a few potential hazards associated with full liquid diets. Since all liquids are allowed, lactose-containing (milk-based) foods are included. This is usually not a problem, except for patients who are lactose intolerant. They may experience symptoms of gastrointestinal distress such as nausea, vomiting, distention, or diarrhea when given lactose-rich liquids. Also, temporary lactose intolerance may be experienced by some patients after surgery.

If a patient is to receive a nutritionally complete full liquid diet for an extended period of time, care should be given to reduce the high saturated fat and cholesterol content of the diet from excessive use of whole milk products, ice cream, milk shakes, and eggs as protein sources (custards) (1). Another special concern is for patients with **dysphagia** who cannot swallow thin liquids. Chapter 16 discusses special adaptations that can be used.

Full liquid diets can be nutritionally complete if they are well planned and include between-meal snacks or nourishments of commercially prepared supplements. Amounts of the diet that patients consume should be monitored daily to ensure adequate energy and nutrient consumption. One word of caution about possible problems with food-borne illness: raw eggs should *never* be used in the preparation of any food served to patients, and patients and their families should be educated about possible dangers of food-borne illness.

Pureed diets

When a patient has problems chewing or swallowing, foods can be pureed or strained until they have a smooth consistency. Consistency of the food can be varied according to the patient's ability to chew and swallow. The nurse, dietitian, and patient should work together and evaluate the patient's needs for modifying consistency according to the food preferences.

Some foods such as mashed potatoes and ice cream are already of a smooth consistency. For other foods, small amounts of liquids (such as broth, milk, and gravies) can be added to reach the appropriate consistency needed. Any liquid that is added to pureed foods should complement the food and not conceal the food's original flavor. Care should be taken to add only enough liquid to achieve the desired consistency, yet allow the nutritional quality of the food to be retained.

Butter, margarine, gravies, sugar, or honey may be added to foods to increase kcaloric density. To make pureed foods more attractive, **component pureeing** may be used. For example, a cake decorating tool (icing bag and tips) can be used to make pureed peas look like regular peas.

As mentioned before, the exact composition and consistency of a pureed diet will vary depending on the patient's needs. Pureed diets can be modified for additional needs such as low sodium, kcalorie controlled, or low fat. Care should be taken in evaluating the patient's needs for consistency. Food consistency should be altered only to the degree it is needed. If a patient needs only meats pureed, then only the meats should be pureed. If a patient needs only the foods or meats ground, then they shouldn't be pureed. Sometimes, foods just need to be chopped coarsely or finely. **Edentulous** patients can very often chew solid or soft foods.

Mechanical soft diets

When the texture of foods needs to be modified only slightly, a mechanical soft diet is often used. This diet includes foods that require only minimal chewing before swallowing such as ground meats, canned fruits, and soft-cooked vegetables.

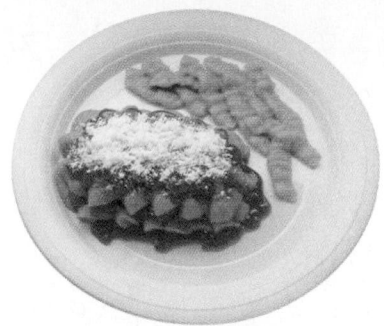

An example of component pureeing: lasagna and green peas, reformed to resemble their original shapes.

dysphagia
the inability to swallow normally or freely or to transfer liquid or solid foods from the oral cavity to the stomach; may be caused by an underlying central neurologic or isolated mechanical dysfunction

component pureeing
each food item is pureed separately (food thickeners may be added to help maintain consistency), then presented in a manner that resembles the original product (for example, a pork chop can be pureed, then molded into a pork-chop shape and served)

edentulous
toothless

Like the pureed diet, the mechanical soft diet can be modified to comply with any other necessary diet modifications.

Soft diets

Soft diets are often used during transition from liquid diets to regular or general diets. Whole foods low in fiber and only lightly seasoned are used. This diet has traditionally been used for patients with mild gastrointestinal problems (5). Food supplements or between-meals snacks may be used if needed to add kcalories.

Regular or general diets

A regular diet is used for patients who do not need dietary restrictions or modifications. Most hospitals offer self-select menus for regular diets, and often for many modified diets. The regular diet serves as the basis for almost all modified diets.

Table 15-1 lists information about each of the basic hospital diets, which progress from a clear liquid to an unrestricted regular diet. Each step or diet of the progression provides appropriate texture and consistency as gastrointestinal function increases. As healing proceeds, dietary restrictions decrease toward a regular diet.

Diet as tolerated

Occasionally when patients are admitted, the physician writes an order for "diet as tolerated." It is also common for this diet to be ordered postoperatively. This permits patients' preferences and situations to be taken into consideration and also allows for postoperative diet progression at the patient's tolerance. Furthermore, this diet order provides an excellent opportunity for collaboration by the nurse, dietitian, and patient to plan and provide food that is eaten, tolerated, and nourishing.

Enteral Feeding by Tube

Often, patients are unable or unwilling to orally consume adequate nutrients and kcalories. When this is the case and the gastrointestinal tract is functioning, nutrients can be provided via feeding tubes placed into the alimentary tract. In fact, when the gastrointestinal tract is functional, accessible, and safe to use, enteral feedings are preferred because they are physiologically beneficial in maintaining the integrity and function of the gut (5). Additionally, enteral tube feedings are much less costly than parenteral nutrition for both the patient and the health care institution.

Enteral tube feeding can be part of routine care when a patient is experiencing protein-calorie malnutrition with 5 days of inadequate oral intake or with a reduced oral intake over the previous 7 to 10 days. Other conditions warranting tube feeding are severe dysphagia, major burns, a short gut from small bowel resection, or when intestinal fistulas (abnormal passages between the intestines) are present. Conditions under which enteral tube feedings are helpful, but not routine, include major trauma, radiation therapy, chemotherapeutic regimens, acute or chronic liver failure, or during severe renal dysfunction. Enteral feeding is of limited or undetermined value if intensive chemotherapy results in gastrointestinal tract dysfunction or if adequate postoperative oral intake is expected to resume within 5 to 7 days. Other conditions for which the benefit is unclear are acute enteritis secondary to radiation, acute infection, active inflammatory bowel disease and if less than 10% of the small intestine is intact after surgery (6,7). Table 15-2 summarizes guidelines and indications for use of enteral tube feedings.

Text continued on p. 388.

Table 15-1   Foods Recommended for Hospital Diet Progressions*

Food Category	Clear Liquid	Full Liquid	Pureed	Mechanical Soft	Soft	Regular
Soups	Broth or bouillon	Broth or bouillon; regular or high-protein consomme; strained vegetable, meat, or cream soups containing finely homogenized meat	Broth or bouillon, consomme, strained or blenderized cream soup	Soups made with allowed foods	Soups made with allowed foods	All
Beverages	Coffee, tea, decaffeinated coffee, carbonated beverages as tolerated	Coffee, tea, decaffeinated coffee, carbonated beverages as tolerated, eggnogs, instant breakfast beverages, yogurt drinks, fruit-flavored drinks	All	All	All	All
Meat and meat substitutes	None	Clean, fresh eggs cooked to a liquid consistency or in custards; egg substitutes; pasteurized eggs used in eggnogs or cooking; salmonella-free frozen eggs	Strained or pureed meat or poultry, cottage cheese, cooked scrambled eggs and egg substitutes pureed as tolerated	Ground or finely diced, moist (gravy or sauces) meats and poultry; flaked fish without bones; eggs; cottage cheese; cheese; creamy peanut butter; soft casseroles	Moist, tender meat, fish, or poultry; eggs; cottage cheese; milk-flavored cheese; creamy peanut butter; soft casseroles	All
Fats	None	Butter, margarine, cream, cream substitute	Butter, margarine, cream, cream substitute, oil, gravy, white sauce, whipped cream, whipped topping	Butter, margarine, cream, cream substitute, oil, gravy, salad dressing, whipped cream, whipped toppings	Butter, margarine, cream, cream substitute, oil, gravy, salad dressing, whipped cream, whipped toppings, crisp bacon	All

Continued.

Table 15-1   Foods Recommended for Hospital Diet Progressions*, cont'd.

Food Category	Clear Liquid	Full Liquid	Pureed	Mechanical Soft	Soft	Regular
Milk	None	Milk and milk beverages; plain or flavored yogurt without seeds, nuts, or fruit pieces; cocoa	Milk and milk beverages; plain or flavored yogurt without seeds, nuts, or fruit pieces; cocoa	Milk and milk beverages, plain or flavored yogurt without seeds or nuts, cocoa	All	All
Starches	None	Refined cooked cereals, strained whole-grain cereals, high-protein cereals; mashed white potato diluted in cream soups	Refined cooked cereals; mashed potatoes; pureed rice or noodles thinned with sauce or gravy; soft, crustless bread pureed with milk or other liquid if tolerated; bread crumbs may be added to soups, casseroles, and vegetables	Cooked or refined ready-to-eat cereals; potatoes; rice; pasta; white, refined wheat, or light rye breads or rolls; graham crackers as tolerated; pancakes; soft waffles; muffins; plain crackers	Cooked or refined ready-to-eat cereals; potatoes; rice; pasta; white, refined wheat, or light rye breads or rolls; graham crackers as tolerated; pancakes; soft waffles; muffins; plain crackers	All
Vegetables	None	Vegetable juice and vegetable purees that are strained and diluted in cream soups	Vegetable juice and strained or pureed vegetables	Soft, cooked vegetables without hulls or tough skin (peas and corn); juices	Soft, cooked vegetables; lettuce and tomatoes; limit gas-forming vegetables and whole kernel corn	All
Fruits	Clear fruit juices (apple, cranberry, grape) or strained fruit juices	Fruit juices, nectars	Strained or pureed fruit, fruit juice, nectars	Cooked or canned fruit without seeds or skins, banana, fruit juice, nectars, citrus fruit without membrane	Cooked or canned fruit, soft fresh fruit, fruit juice, nectars	All

Table 15-1	Foods Recommended for Hospital Diet Progressions*, cont'd.					
Food Category	Clear Liquid	Full Liquid	Pureed	Mechanical Soft	Soft	Regular
Desserts	Flavored gelatin, high-protein gelatin, Popsicles and fruit ices	Flavored gelatin, puddings, high-protein puddings, custard, regular and high-protein gelatin desserts, plain ice cream, frozen yogurt, sherbet, fruit ices, Popsicles	Flavored gelatin; puddings; custard; plain ice cream without seeds, nuts, or fruit pieces; sherbet; frozen yogurt; fruit ices; Popsicles	Flavored gelatin; puddings; custard; plain ice cream without seeds, nuts, or fruit; sherbet; frozen yogurt; fruit ices; Popsicles	Flavored gelatin, puddings, custard, ice cream without nuts, sherbet, frozen yogurt, fruit ices, Popsicles, cake, cookies without nuts or coconut	All
Sweets	Sugar, honey, hard candy, sugar substitute	Sugar, honey, hard candy, sugar substitute, syrup	Sugar, honey, hard candy, sugar substitute, syrup, jelly	Sugar, honey, hard candy, sugar substitute, syrup, jelly	Sugar, honey, candy without nuts or coconut, sugar substitute, syrup, plain chocolate candies, molasses, marshmallows	All
Miscellaneous	Salt	Salt, pepper, flavorings, chocolate syrup, cinnamon, nutmeg, brewer's yeast	Salt, pepper, flavorings, ground spices, smooth condiments	Salt, pepper, flavorings, ground spices, smooth condiments	Salt, pepper, flavorings, mildly seasoned condiments, herbs, spices, catsup, mustard, vinegar in moderation	All
Supplements	High-protein, high-kcalorie, low-residue oral supplements; Polycose	Liquid commercially prepared nutritional supplements, Polycose	Liquid commercially prepared nutritional supplements, Polycose	Liquid commercially prepared nutritional supplements, Polycose	All	All

Modified from Nelson JK et al: *Mayo Clinic diet manual: A handbook of nutrition practices*, ed 7, St. Louis, 1994, Mosby.
*Any foods not listed should be excluded from the diet.

Table 15-2   Guidelines and Indications for Use of Enteral Tube Feedings

Guideline	Indication
Clinical settings where enteral tube feedings should be part of routine care	Existing protein-energy malnutrition* (PEM) with inadequate oral intake for previous 5 days Normal nutritional status with oral intake < 50% or required needs for previous 7-10 days Severe dysphagia caused by strokes, brain tumors, head injuries, multiple sclerosis, amyotrophic lateral sclerosis, or Guillain-Barré syndrome Major, full-thickness burns Short gut because of small bowel resection (given in conjunction with parenteral nutrition when clinically stable to stimulate regeneration of remaining intestine) Low-output (<500 ml/d) enterocutaneous fistulas
Clinical settings where enteral tube feedings would be helpful	Major trauma with functioning GI tract, but may not achieve adequate oral intake for 7-10 days Radiation therapy for cancers of the lungs, head, neck, and cervix, and for lymphomas Recipients of mildly toxic chemotherapeutic regimens who become anorexic Acute or chronic liver failure with severe anorexia and a functioning intestinal tract Severe renal dysfunction (<5% to 10% of normal glomerular filtration) with anorexia and functioning GI tract
Clinical settings where enteral tube feedings are of limited or undetermined value	Recipients of intensive chemotherapy who are experiencing stomatitis, anorexia, nausea, vomiting, diarrhea, and decreased oral intake[†] Immediately postop if it is anticipated that adequate oral intake will be resumed within 5-7 days Acute enteritis secondary to radiation, acute infection, or active inflammatory bowel disease <10% remaining small intestine remaining

From American Dietetic Association: *Manual of clinical dietetics*, ed 4, Chicago, 1992, American Dietetic Association; and ASPEN Board of Directors: Guidelines for the use of enteral nutrition in the adult patient, *Journal of Parenteral and Enteral Nutrition* 11:435-439, 1987.
* PEM is defined as > 10% loss of usual weight or serum albumin < 3.5 g/dl.
[†] Ability to tolerate tube feeding regimen depends on severity of symptoms.

Types of formulas

Enteral nutrition by tube has been used since the late 1800s (8). For years enteral formulas were prepared using foodstuffs, vitamin/mineral preparations, and a blender. Today a wide variety of commercially prepared formulas are available. Some formulas are nutritionally complete, some are formulated for specific diseases or conditions, and others (modular) provide specific nutrients to supplement a diet or other formula. Commercial products are usually preferred over hospital or home-blended concoctions because they provide a known nutrient composition, controlled **osmolality** and consistency, and bacteriological safety. They are also much easier to prepare and store (5). Many are nutritionally complete if consumed in the volumes recommended by the manufacturers.

Polymeric formulas. **Polymeric formulas** are composed of intact nutrients that require a functioning gastrointestinal tract for digestion and absorption of nutrients. There are several categories of polymeric formulas providing 1 to 2 kcalories/ml. Polymeric formulas can be categorized into blenderized

osmolality
concentration of electrically charged particles per kilogram of solution

polymeric formula
a solution that provides intact nutrients (for example, whole proteins and long-chain triglycerides), which require a normally functioning gastrointestinal tract

Classification of Formulas

STANDARD
Polymeric or intact protein

SPECIAL
Predigested or elemental
  Modular
  Specialty formulas

From Swearingen PL: Manual of medical-surgical nursing care, ed 3, St. Louis, 1994, Mosby.

food products, milk-based products, high-kcalorie lactose-free products, and normocaloric lactose-free products. Normocaloric lactose-free products can be categorized into those that are **isotonic, hypertonic,** high-nitrogen, and fiber-containing (5). Blenderized formulas (1 kcal/ml) are a blenderized mixture of ordinary foods that usually contain milk products (lactose). They have a high viscosity and moderate osmolality. Blenderized formulas can be made by dietary staff, at the patient's home, or are available commercially. Noncommercial formulas are very low in cost, but run the risk of bacterial contamination and variation in nutrient composition (9). Commercial formulas provide a sterile product with a fixed nutrient composition (9). Extreme caution should be exercised when using noncommercial (home-made) formulas because of the risk of food-borne illness. For patient safety, commercial formulas should be used.

Normocaloric (1 kcal/ml) lactose-free formulas have low osmolality, which generally makes them well tolerated. **Hypercaloric** (1.5 to 2.0 kcal/ml) formulas are designed to meet kcalorie and protein demands in a reduced volume and have moderate to high osmolality. High-nitrogen lactose-free formulas (1 to 2 kcal/ml) are designed to meet increased protein demands at usual or increased energy needs. They have low to moderate osmolality. Fiber-containing products are low osmolality and are used for patients with abnormal bowel regulation. These formulas contain fiber from natural food sources or soy polysaccharide.

Elemental formulas. **Elemental** or predigested formulas (1.0 to 1.3 kcal/ml) are composed of partially or fully hydrolyzed nutrients that can be used for patients with a partially functioning gastrointestinal tract or those who have impaired capacity to digest foods or absorb nutrients, pancreatic insufficiency, or bile salt deficiency. These products are lactose-free and are usually hyperosmolar. They are not very palatable and are best suited for administration by tube.

Modular formulas. Modular formulas (3.8 to 4.0 kcal/ml) are not nutritionally complete by themselves as they are single macronutrients such as glucose polymers, protein, or lipids. They are added to foods or other enteral products to change composition when nutritional needs cannot otherwise be met.

Specialty formulas. These products (1.0 to 2.0 kcal/ml) are designed to meet specialized nutrient demands for specific disease states such as diabetes, renal failure, liver failure, pulmonary disease, or HIV/AIDS. Some formulas may require supplementation with vitamins, minerals, or trace elements. Some are unpalatable, and most formulas are expensive.

Formula selection

More than 80 enteral feeding formulas are on the market. This fact alone can make product selection a complex process. Choosing an enteral feeding formula includes the following considerations (10):
- What are the patient's digestive and absorptive capabilities?
- Do the patient's fluids need to be restricted?
- Does the patient have high metabolic requirements?

Whether a patient can digest and absorb nutrients indicates whether an elemental or polymeric formula should be used. Individual nutrient requirements determine

isotonic
having the same concentration of solute as another solution, therefore exerting the same amount of osmotic pressure as that solution

hypertonic
having greater concentration of solute than another solution

hypercaloric
more than one kcalorie per ml

elemental formula
a solution that provides ready-to-absorb basic nutrients, requiring minimal digestion

the type and amount of tube-feeding formula. As with previous components of medical nutritional therapy, ongoing assessment of nutritional status and patients' tolerance of the formula is necessary (5).

The successful use of enteral feeding depends on the patient's condition, availability of access for feeding, and the patient's tolerance of the chosen enteral formula (11). Enteral feeding is the feeding route of choice because of the benefits provided. Some of these benefits include improved utilization of nutrients, maintenance of gut mucosa and immunocompetence, decreased catabolic response to injury, administration safety, and lower cost (11). In fact, McClave insists that the only time enteral feedings should not be used is in the absence of a gut (12).

Feeding routes

In addition to choosing an appropriate tube feeding formula, selecting the appropriate feeding tube and feeding route involves consideration of various factors. Patients' medical status and nutritional status often govern the length of the feeding tube (that is, the portion of the GI tract into which the formula is delivered). The anticipated length of time that tube feeding will be required dictates whether the feeding tube should be surgically placed. If the tube feeding will be used for short duration, a nonsurgical placement can be made. If the feeding tube will be long-term or permanent, surgical placement is necessary. Routes for tube feeding include the following (Fig. 15-1):

1. Nasogastric: The tube is passed through the nose to the stomach.
2. Nasoduodenal: The tube is passed from the nose to the duodenum (small intestine).
3. Nasojejunal: The tube is passed through the nose to the jejunum (small intestine).
4. Esophagostomy: The tube is surgically inserted into the neck and extends to the stomach.
5. Gastrostomy: The tube is surgically inserted into the stomach.
6. Jejunostomy: The tube is surgically inserted into the small intestine.

Placing the feeding tube into the stomach, duodenum, or jejunum through the nose are the simplest and most commonly used tube-feeding techniques (5). These techniques are preferred for patients who will resume oral feedings in the near future (5). Placement into the stomach simulates normal gastrointestinal function, but should be reserved for patients who are alert with intact gag and cough reflexes (9). Tube placement into the small intestine has less risk of aspiration, but elemental formulas are often required for easier absorption and continuous feedings are better tolerated (9). Surgical placement of the feeding tube is preferred when long-term use is anticipated or when obstruction makes insertion through the nose impossible. These procedures require surgery with general anesthesia. **Percutaneous endoscopic placement** of a gastrostomy (PEG) can be performed with minimal sedation and has fewer complications than surgical placement (5). Table 15-3 describes the classifications, advantages, and disadvantages of feeding routes.

Method of administration

How enteral tube feedings are administered or given to patients is just as important as formula selection and feeding site. Proper administration safeguards delivery of the desired nutrients, enhances tolerance by the patient, and provides optimal nutrition support (5). Factors affecting decisions about appropriate methods of formula infusion include the patient's medical status, gastrointestinal function, and the feeding route (5). Tube feedings can be administered by three methods: continuous, intermittent, or bolus infusion.

Continuous infusion is generally the preferred method of feeding (13). This method provides controlled delivery of a prescribed volume of formula at a constant rate over a continuous period of time using an infusion pump. Although this method does require the use of special equipment, it is preferred, especially when feeding into the small intestine, because it is similar to typical gastric emptying (5).

percutaneous endoscopic placement
placement of feeding tube into stomach via the esophagus and then drawing it through the abdominal skin using a stab incision

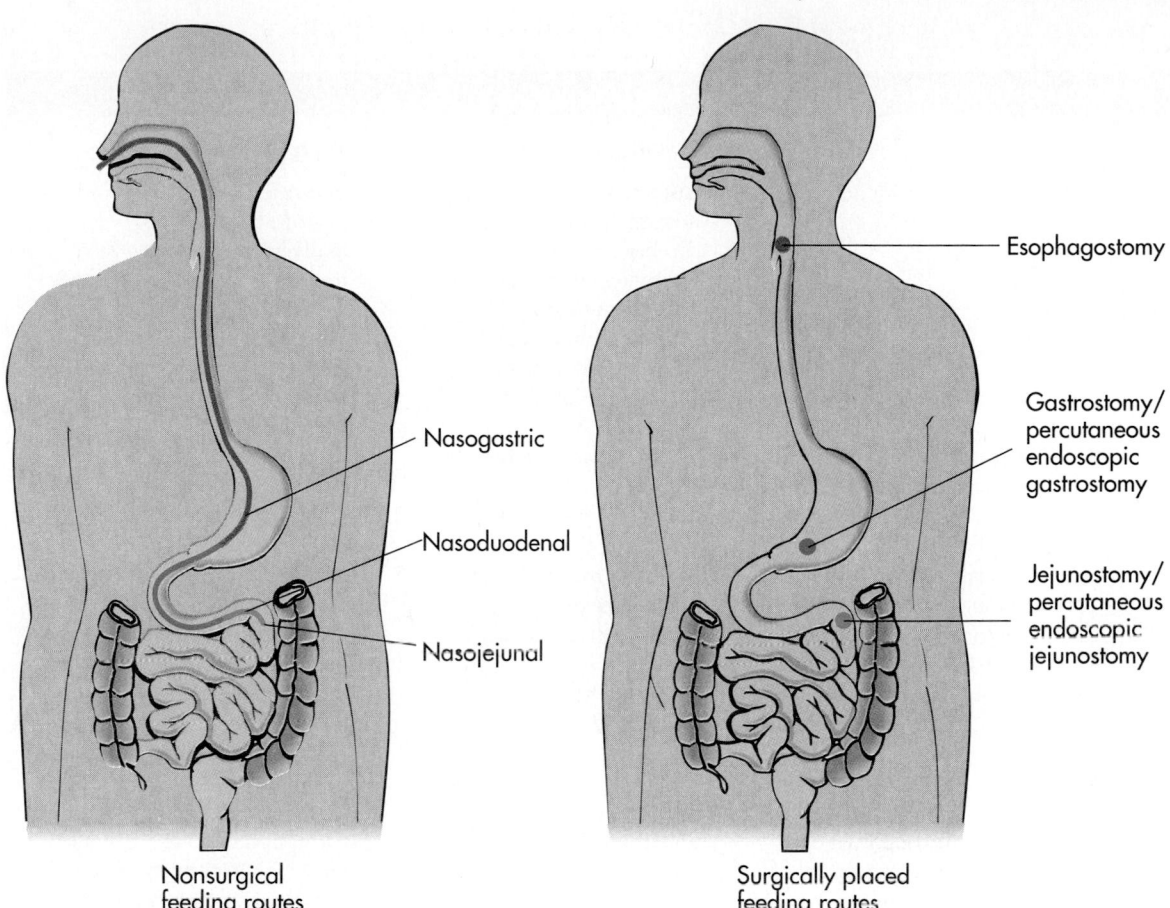

Esophagostomy

Gastrostomy/
percutaneous
endoscopic
gastrostomy

Jejunostomy/
percutaneous
endoscopic
jejunostomy

Nasogastric

Nasoduodenal

Nasojejunal

Nonsurgical
feeding routes

Surgically placed
feeding routes

Fig. 15-1 Types of enteral feeding routes.

Intermittent infusion involves delivering the total quantity of formulas needed for a 24-hour period in 3 to 6 equal feedings. Each feeding is usually delivered by gravity during a 30- to 90-minute period. This method represents a more normal feeding pattern, but patients often do not tolerate this method of feeding if the rate is too rapid. Although equipment needs are minimal, this method is time consuming because feedings must be closely monitored to ensure proper delivery rate (5).

Bolus feedings involve infusing volumes of formula by gravity or syringe over a very short period of time (5,13). This method requires minimal equipment and time, but is associated with increased potential for aspiration, regurgitation, and gastrointestinal side effects (5,9). This method should not be used for intestinal feedings. Table 15-4 summarizes indications for and pros and cons of each feeding method.

Starting the tube feeding

Before initiating enteral tube feedings, placement of the feeding tube must be confirmed and documented. This can be done several ways. Aspiration of gastric contents with a large syringe (60-mL) or radiologic confirmation of placement are the most common. The feeding should then be infused at a rate tolerated by the patient. Isotonic formulas can be administered at a rate of 20 to 50 cc/hr (5,9) and can be advanced every 8 to 12 hours until the desired rate is achieved (9). Most patients will be able to tolerate an advancement of 10 cc every 12 hours (5). Hypertonic formulas can either be given full concentration at a slower rate (15 to 25 cc/hr) or diluted in concentration (5). The high osmolality of a hypertonic formula can lead to GI distress such as intestinal distention and **osmotic diarrhea**. Diluting tube feedings will lengthen the amount of time necessary before nutritional

osmotic diarrhea
diarrhea associated water retention in the large intestine resulting from an accumulation of nonabsorbable water-soluble solutes

Table 15-3   Advantages and Disadvantages of Enteral Feeding Routes

Feeding Route	Characteristics	Advantages	Disadvantages
Nasogastric	Tube extends from nose into stomach	Rapid placement requiring minimal equipment, feedings can begin immediately following confirmation of tube placement and bowel sounds, formula can be delivered by intermittent or continuous infusion	Tube can be easily removed by patient, tube can be inadvertently inserted into trachea, especially in patients with poor gag reflexes, anomalies in nose and neck (deviated septum, esophageal strictures) may prevent tube placement
Nasoduodenal or nasojejunal	Nasoduodenal: Tube extends from nose through the pylorus into duodenum; tube may be advanced by peristalsis or videofluoroscopy Nasojejunal: Tube extends from nose through pylorus into jejunum and is usually placed by videofluoroscopy	Risk for aspiration may be reduced, feedings better tolerated by patients with poor tolerance to gastric feedings (gastric retention or reflux), nasojejunal feedings permit enteral feedings in patients with partial gastric outlet obstruction or duodenal fistula	Dislodgment of tube into stomach by coughing or vomiting is common (will increase risk of aspiration in patients with altered gastric motility, administration usually limited to continuous delivery of formula (small intestine does not tolerate bolus feedings or sudden rate changes well; may require use of pump)
Esophagostomy	Surgical formation of opening into neck through which feeding tube is placed into esophagus and down into the stomach (sometimes used in patients with head and neck cancer)	Procedure can be performed under local anesthesia, does not require opening abdominal wall; feeding can begin immediately	Route requires surgery and formation of a stoma, which must be carefully maintained; skin surrounding stoma may become irritated; wound may become infected; excessive granulation of tissue surrounding stoma may occur; accidental dislodgment of tube common, requires immediate replacement of tube to prevent closure of stoma
Gastrostomy or percutaneous endoscopic gastrostomy (PEG)	Gastrostomy: Tube passed through incision in abdominal wall into stomach PEG: Tube percutaneously placed in stomach under endoscopic guidance, secured by rubber "bumpers" or inflated balloon catheter	Takes advantage of stomach's natural function of adjusting osmolarity, mixing, and serving as a reservoir; ensures provided nutrients are allowed maximal opportunity for absorption; closely simulates natural delivery of nutrients into stomach; eliminates nasal or esophageal irritation gastroesophageal sphincter closed, may reduce risk of aspiration; tube is unobtrusive; PEG placement can be performed under local anesthesia (less expensive); PEG feedings can be started after approximately 24 hrs	Gastric contents may leak around tube with gastrostomy, wound dehiscence may occur, GI bleeding and aspiration may occur; gastrostomy feedings usually not started until up to 72 hrs after surgery; PEG placement often difficult or impossible in severe obesity

Table 15-3   Advantages and Disadvantages of Enteral Feeding Routes, cont'd.

Feeding Route	Characteristics	Advantages	Disadvantages
Jejunostomy or percutaneous endoscopic jejunostomy (PEJ)	Jejunostomy: Types include needle catheter placement, direct tube placement, and creation of jejunal stoma that is catheterized intermittently PEJ: Weighted feeding tube passed endoscopically through gastrostomy tube (from PEG insertion) into duodenum; peristaltic action advances tube into jejunum	Permits feeding in patients with upper GI tract obstruction, esophageal reflux, ulcerative or neoplastic disease of stomach, impaired gastric emptying; reduces risk for aspiration; early postoperative feeding possible (jejunum rapidly resumes its function within 12-24 hrs)	Surgical procedure required, ambulatory patients may find jejunal feeding restrictive because of the need for continuous infusion of formula

Modified from American Dietetic Association: *Handbook of clinical dietetics*, ed 2, New Haven, 1992, Yale University Press; and American Dietetic Association, *Manual of clinical dietetics*, ed 4, Chicago, 1992, American Dietetic Association.

Table 15-4   Administration of Enteral Tube Feedings

Method	Indications	Advantages	Disadvantages
Continuous	Patients who have not eaten for a significant period of time, debilitated patients, those with impaired GI function, patients with uncontrolled IDDM, intestinal feedings	Feedings can be administered at constant rate over 24-hr period, feedings can be cycled (allows formula to be delivered over shorter period, allowing patients freedom of movement and to promote oral intake if appropriate), gastric pooling minimized and fewer GI side effects experienced, continuous feeding into jejunum is very similar to normal gastric emptying	Requires feeding pump if accuracy of volume delivered is required; continuous drip by gravity is possible, but less accurate
Intermittent	Feedings that are infused at specific intervals throughout the day (total volume of feeding divided and given 4-6 times/day)	Requires only simple equipment, can be used in home settings, may be more physiological than continuous infusion, feedings can be administered by gravity over 30-90 minutes	In absence of pumps, feedings must be monitored vigilantly, may become time consuming depending on number of scheduled feedings per day, rate of intermittent infusion (rather than volume) seems to be a major reason for intolerance of tube feedings
Bolus	Appropriate *only* for feeding into the stomach, involves feeding large volumes of formula intermittently over short periods of time, usually by syringe	More manageable for the patient, rate of 30 ml/minute or volume of 500-700 ml per feeding seems to be cutoff of physical tolerance limits	Associated with increased risk of aspiration, regurgitation, and GI side effects; not appropriate for postpyloric feedings

Modified from Nelson JK et al: *Mayo Clinic diet manual: A handbook of nutrition practices*, ed 7, St. Louis, 1994, Mosby; Woolfson AMJ et al: Prolonged nasogastric tube feeding in critically ill and surgical patients, *Postgrad Med J* 52:678-682, 1976; and Heitkemper ME et al: Rate and volume of intermittent enteral feedings, *Journal of Parenteral and Enteral Nutrition* 51:125-129, 1981.

Table 15-5   Criteria for Safe Administration of Enteral Tube Feedings

Criteria	Considerations
Temperature	Administer solutions infused by continuous drip chilled
	Administer intermittent and bolus feedings at room temperature to decrease incidence of GI side effects
Prevention of bacterial contamination	Use closed feeding containers
	Prefilled, ready-to-feed, closed systems are available for some products (less chance of contamination)
	Change extension tubing administration set and bag *daily*. Never add new formula to old formula
	Do *not* hang feedings for longer than 4-8 hours
Prevention of aspiration	Check tube placement prior to administration
	Tubes placed into small bowel are associated with decreased risk for aspiration
	HOB should be elevated 30-45 degrees
	Consider adding vegetable food coloring to formula to allow for detection of aspirated tube feeding from pulmonary secretions (remember, this does not protect against aspiration)
Patency of tubing	Irrigate tubes every 6-8 hours with 40-50 cc of warm water (continuous feeds)
	For intermittent or bolus feedings, irrigate tubes after each feeding with 40-50 cc of warm water
	Flush tube with 40-50 cc of water each time feeding is stopped
	If tubing clogs, flush with 30-50 cc of warm water
	Systems are available that allow for self-flushing of the feeding tube (Ross Laboratories)
Medications	Medications administered through the feeding tube should be in *liquid form*
	Flush tubing before and after giving the medication with 20 cc of water to prevent clogging
	If medication is not available in liquid form, consult the pharmacist *before* crushing or diluting the medication (some medications are pharmacologically altered by mechanical manipulation)
	Never crush time released, liquid-filled capsules or enteric coated medications
	Do *not* give sublingual medications through the tubing
	Because hyperosmolar liquid medications (KCl) may cause gastric irritation or diarrhea, dilute with water before administration
	Supplemental electrolyte preparations (KCl, NaCl, $NaPO_4$) increase the osmolality of the formula and may cause diarrhea
	Bulk-forming agents cause feeding tubes to clog
	Do *not* mix together multiple medications and deliver simultaneously unless the compatibility of the medications is known
	If feeding into the duodenum or jejunum instead of the stomach, check the effect of medication absorption
	Monitor patient response to medications given through the feeding tube and make changes needed
Monitoring	Confirm tube placement before initiation of feeding and before each intermittent feeding
	Record urine glucose every shift until final feeding rate and concentration are established

Table 15-5	Criteria for Safe Administration of Enteral Tube Feedings, cont'd.

Criteria	Considerations
Monitoring, cont'd.	Record gastric residuals every 4 hours (gastric feedings only)
	Record bowel movements and consistency
	Record tolerance to feedings
	Record daily:
	Weight
	Intake and output
	Record weekly:
	Serum electrolytes and blood counts
	Chemistry profile (including liver function tests, phosphorus, calcium, magnesium, total protein, and albumin)
	Nitrogen balance, if appropriate
	Reassess nutrition indexes weekly, adjusting energy and protein as needed

Adapted from American Dietetic Association, *Manual of clinical dietetics*, ed 4, Chicago, 1992, American Dietetic Association; and White WT et al: Contamination of enteral nutrient solution: A preliminary report, *Journal of Parenteral and Enteral Nutrition* 3:459-461, 1979.

requirements can be met by the formula and feeding regimen. Rate of the feedings can be advanced to desired volume, and then concentration can be gradually increased until kcalorie and protein needs are met. Rate and concentration should *never* be advanced at the same time (5). If the feeding is not being tolerated, the rate or concentration can be reduced to the last level of tolerance, then gradually increased again (5).

Other criteria that should be considered to ensure optimal tolerance of the formula and safety of the feedings include solution temperature, prevention of bacterial contamination, prevention of aspiration, patency of tubing, administration of medications, and patient monitoring (Table 15-5).

Possible tube feeding complications

Even though the gastrointestinal tract is being used to nourish the patient, tube feedings are not without problems. Most are preventable; all are correctable. Tube feeding complications can be categorized three ways: gastrointestinal, mechanical, or metabolic problems. Gastrointestinal problems include diarrhea, nausea and vomiting, cramping, distention, and constipation. Mechanical complications consist of tube displacement or obstruction, pulmonary aspiration, and mucosal damage. Metabolic difficulties involve hyperosmolar dehydration, or overhydration; abnormal blood concentration levels of sodium, potassium, phosphorus and magnesium (too high or too low); hyperglycemia; respiratory insufficiency; and rapid weight gain. Table 15-6 summarizes possible complications, probable causes, and suggested corrective actions.

One of the most common complications of enteral feedings, diarrhea, was once thought to be caused by hyperosmolality feeding solutions (13). More recently it has been determined that other factors may contribute to this problem (14). Patients receiving tube feedings are frequently placed on liquid forms of medications, and many of these medications contain sorbitol, which can cause diarrhea. Bacterial dysentery caused by *Clostridium difficile* is also a common cause of diarrhea. Diarrhea should not be attributed to tube-feeding formulas until other causes have definitely been ruled out (13).

Table 15-6 Tube Feeding Complications, Causes, and Corrective Actions

Category	Problem	Possible Cause	Corrective Action
Gastrointestinal	Diarrhea (defined as more than four bowel movements per day or liquid stools greater than 200 g*)	Protein energy malnutrition (PEM)	Switch to isotonic formula and feed at slow rate (will allow intestine to adapt to refeeding)
		Infection, microbial contamination of formula	Confirm with stool, blood, or formula cultures; limit hang time of formula to 8-12 hrs, change bag and tubing every 24 hrs, and rinse after each bolus feeding or before filling bag for continuous feedings
		Malabsorption	Check for pancreatic insufficiency; pancreatic enzymes replacement may be necessary; change to low-fat, lactose-free, or elemental formula; change to continuous feeding
		Bolus feeding, volume overload, rapid administration, dumping syndrome	If infusion rate or concentration was advanced recently, return to previously tolerated rate/concentration; change to continuous feeding; decrease bolus volume and increase frequency of feedings
		Hyperosmolar formula	If started, reduce rate and increase gradually; dilute formula or change to isotonic product; if starting, rate should begin at 25 cc/hr, increasing every 12-24 hours
		Medications	Evaluate types of medications as primary cause (diarrhea has been related to administration of antibiotics and antacids, potassium supplements, cimetidine, and sorbitol-containing meds) and the possibility for change; stool samples should be taken for *Clostridium dificile* culture and toxin; change to fiber-containing formula
		Hypoalbuminemia	Albumin levels < 2.5 g/dL result in decreased colloidal osmotic pressure† with accompanying peripheral edema (which may involve GI tract); try peptide-based, low-fat formula with MCT‡
		Decreased bulk	Fiber-containing formulas may help control diarrhea by normalizing GI transit time and providing bulk
	Nausea and vomiting, cramping, distention	High osmolality	Dilute formula to isotonic concentration if gastric residuals are consistently high; consider changing to isotonic formula
		Patient position	Reposition patient on right side to facilitate passage of gastric contents through pylorus
		Rapid increase in rate, volume, or concentration	Return to slower rate, and advance by smaller increments; advance only when tolerating current rate
		Delayed gastric emptying	Stop feedings for 2 hrs and check residuals; check residuals every 2-4 hrs (continuous feedings) and before administration (bolus feedings); reduce fat content in tube feeding; consider transpyloric feeding; monitor for drugs or disease that may influence gastric or intestinal motility; ambulation may help
		Lactose intolerance	Change to lactose-free formula
		Cold formula	Warm formula to room temperature
		GI tract obstruction	Stop feeding immediately
		Excessive fat in formula	Change to low-fat formula

Table 15-6 Tube Feeding Complications, Causes, and Corrective Actions, cont'd.

Category	Problem	Possible Cause	Corrective Action
Gastrointestinal, cont'd.	Constipation	Dehydration	Monitor intake and output; add free water if intake not greater than output by 500-1000 cc/day
		Decreased fiber	Use formula with fiber; make sure patient gets adequate water
		Medications	Evaluate medication side-effects; suggest stool softener or bulk-forming laxative
		Inactivity	Increase patient activity if possible
		GI tract obstruction	Stop feedings
Mechanical	Tube displacement	Coughing, vomiting	Replace tube, confirm placement before restarting feeding
		Dislodgment by patient	Replace tube; restrain patient if necessary; consider alternate feeding route
		Inadequate taping of tube	Position tube, tape securely
	Tube obstruction	Improperly crushed medications	Use liquid form of medication, medications should not be crushed without first checking with pharmacy; rinse tube with 20 cc warm water before and after giving medications
		Medications mixed with incompatible formula	Review drug/nutrient interaction guidelines; flush tubing before and after adding medications
		Insufficient tube irrigation; failure to irrigate	Flush tubing with 20-50 cc warm water before and after bolus feeding, every 4-8 hours during continuous feedings, and whenever tube is disconnected or feeding is stopped
	Pulmonary aspiration	Patient lying flat	Elevate head of bed 30-45 degrees during continuous feedings and for at least 30-60 minutes after bolus feedings
		Absent or weak gag reflexes	Feed into duodenum or jejunum
		Gastric reflux	May be caused by feeding tube, change to smaller bore tube; feed into duodenum or jejunum
		Delayed gastric emptying	Monitor gastric residual; residual > 200 cc in patients with nasogastric tubes and 100 cc in patients with gastrostomy tubes may indicate intolerance; hold feedings, recheck residual in 1-2 hrs
		Improper tube placement	Confirm tube placement with radiology; reconfirm placement before each feeding and periodically during continuous feeding by injecting air into stomach and listening with a stethoscope
	Mucosal damage	Extended use of large bore tubes	Conscientious mouth and nose care; consider changing to small-bore tubing, or permanent gastrostomy or jejunostomy feeding tubes
		Decreased salivary secretions caused by lack of chewing; mouth breathing	Moisten lips and mouth; let patient chew sugarless gum, gargle, or suck on anaesthetic lozenges if appropriate
Metabolic	Hyperosmolar dehydration	Hypertonic formula used without adequate water	Begin hypertonic feedings at slower rate; dilute with free water; or consider isotonic formula
	Overhydration (fluid overload)	Refeeding patients with PEM; fluid overload	Restrict fluids; use concentrated formula
		Prolonged use of over-diluted formula	Advance concentration as tolerated by patient

Continued.

Table 15-6   Tube Feeding Complications, Causes, and Corrective Actions, cont'd.

Category	Problem	Possible Cause	Corrective Action
Metabolic, cont'd.	Hyponatremia	CHF, cirrhosis, hypoalbuminemia, edema, ascites	Restrict fluids, administer diuretics, use concentrated formulas
		Excess GI losses	Monitor serum Na levels and hydration status, replace Na as needed
	Hypernatremia	Dehydration	Calculate patient's fluid needs: 35 cc/kg can be used unless patient's condition alters fluid needs, <30 cc/kg for the elderly
	Hypokalemia	Refeeding syndrome, insulin administration, diuretics, diarrhea	Monitor electrolytes daily, replete with parenteral potassium
	Hyperkalemia	Renal insufficiency, metabolic acidosis, anabolic metabolism	Reduce potassium intake, consider changing to a lower potassium tube-feeding formula, assess renal function
	Hyperphosphatemia	Renal insufficiency	Use phosphate binder, consider changing formula
	Hypophosphatemia	Refeeding syndrome, insulin administration	Replace phosphorus with parenteral supplement; monitor serum levels daily; once patient is repleted, monitor weekly
	Hypomagnesemia	Refeeding syndrome, alcoholism	Replete with parenteral magnesium sulfate; monitor serum levels daily; once patient is repleted, monitor weekly
	Hyperglycemia	Diabetes mellitus; temporary insulin resistance or insulin deficiency	Monitor blood sugars frequently, adjust insulin dose; reduce rate of tube feeding until blood sugar controlled; avoid formulas high in simple carbohydrates
	Increased respiratory quotient; excess CO_2 production; respiratory insufficiency	Overfeeding (kcalories), especially in form of carbohydrates	Balance kcalories provided from fat, protein, and carbohydrates; consider using a higher-fat formula or adding modular fat
	Rapid, excessive weight gain	Excess kcalories, excess fluids, electrolyte imbalance	Decrease concentration or amount of formula; evaluate electrolyte status

Modified from American Dietetic Association: *Handbook of clinical dietetics*, ed 2, New Haven, 1992, Yale University Press; American Dietetic Association: *Manual of clinical dietetics*, ed 4, Chicago, 1992, American Dietetic Association; Gottschlich MM et al: Diarrhea in tube-fed patients: Incidence, etiology, nutritional impact, and prevention, *Journal of Parenteral and Enteral Nutrition* 12:338-345, 1988; Edes TE, Walk BE, Austin JL: Diarrhea in tube-fed patients: Feeding formula not necessarily the cause, *Am J Med* 88:91-93, 1990.

[*]From Swearingen PL: Manual of medical-surgical nursing care, ed 3, St. Louis, 1994, Mosby.

[†]Pressure difference between the osmotic pressure of blood and that of tissue fluid or lymph; it is an important force in maintaining balance between blood and surrounding tissue, and is usually caused by large particles such as protein molecules that will not pass through a membrane. Also called oncotic pressure.

[‡]Medium chain triglycerides, distinguished from other triglycerides by having 8 to 10 carbon atoms. MCTs are easily digested.

Home enteral nutrition

Because of changing health care reimbursement patterns, the demand for home tube feeding has been growing steadily (5). Although it provides opportunity and convenience for patients, home enteral nutrition (HEN) imparts responsibility that nurses and dietitians must assume and risks that must be planned for (15). In addition to the criteria already discussed regarding selection of appropriate candidates for tube feedings, other criteria that should be considered when sending a patient home on enteral nutritional therapy include the following (15):

• The patient's nutritional needs cannot be met orally
• The appropriate enteral access is in place and functioning, and the patient is tolerating tube feeding regimen

- The patient and/or significant other is (are) able and willing to perform HEN techniques safely and effectively
- Underlying disease state is stable, and the patient is ready for discharge and can be monitored in the home setting
- Affordable HEN supplies are available

Once a patient is considered to be an appropriate candidate for HEN, the nutrition care plan must be modified to an appropriate home plan that includes tailoring the enteral formula, the route and method of administration, and the feeding schedule. The amount or type of formula may need to be adjusted to meet the patient's long-term nutritional requirements. Blenderized formulas are strongly discouraged because of reasons previously discussed. The route of HEN administration should also be examined for its ability to meet the patient's long-term needs and adequacy. If at all possible, the patient should be included in this decision. Keeping the functional level of the gastrointestinal tract and risk of aspiration in mind, the method of administration (continuous, intermittent, or bolus) should be altered if necessary according to patient preference, convenience, and cost (15). Feeding schedules may need to be arranged around family members' schedules or other daily routines. They should be planned to augment patient comfort and convenience and to maximize nutritional benefit (15).

The patient should be stabilized on the home feeding regimen while still hospitalized before patient education is initiated. Education should include oral instructions, written guidelines, staff demonstration, return demonstration by the patient and/or significant other, and their assumption of full responsibility for tube feeding before discharge from the hospital (5,15). Figure 15-2 is an example of a HEN training checklist.

Patients should also be referred to a source for obtaining supplies such as formula and administration equipment prior to discharge (5). Some patients may need help in obtaining financial assistance. Most often, referral to home health agencies provides the necessary supplies, equipment, and staff for home follow-up visits, as well as assistance with third-party payers.

TEACHING TOOL
Tube Feeding the Infant or Child

Parents and caregivers need special support when their infants and children are tube fed. Assure them that the children can still be cuddled and can play without interfering with the tube nourishment. Teach the adults how the process works; they can be allies in helping young children accept and understand these procedures. Be sure to explain the procedures to the children as well. Dolls or stuffed animals can be used to explain how tube feeding helps to speed the healing process.

Every infant and child has individual nutritional requirements based on growth needs and medical conditions. Check with the nurse or dietitian for appropriate rate, concentration, and volume of feedings. Below are some specfic techniques to assure adequate nutrient intake.

- Use additional free water flushes if fluid needs are not met by tube patency flushes.
- Begin feedings with an isotonic formula. Either the strength or the volume of the feeding may be increased every 8 to 12 hours, but not both at the same time.
- Check gastric residual before each feeding if you are feeding the infant every few hours. Hold the feeding if the amount is one-half the volume of the previous feeding.
- Check gastric residual at least every 4 hours if you are feeding with a pump. If residual is equal to the previous hourly rate, hold feedings for 1 hour and recheck. Residual checks are usually not indicated when the tube is placed past the stomach.
- Give medications only in liquid form.
- Elevate the head of the bed 30 to 45 degrees.

From Nelson JK et al: *Mayo Clinic diet manual: A handbook of nutrition practices,* ed 7, St. Louis, 1994, Mosby.

PURPOSE AND INSTRUCTIONS: This checklist will assist in identifying instructional responsibilities and aid in training patients in the skills needed for performing home enteral nutrition (HEN).

   The nurse and dietitian will jointly instruct the patient on tube feeding administration and cares.

   Date and initial section when instruction/demonstration is completed
   RNs: Document training in Nursing Notes.
   RDs: Document training in Progress Notes.

STAGE I: INITIATION OF HEN PROGRAM

_____ Patient assessment   (Dietitian-Nurse)
          Medical-social-nutritional history
_____ Plan of care outlined   (Dietitian-Nurse)
_____ Identification of dismissal date _____   (Nurse)
_____ Home enteral coordinator notified   (Dietitian)

STAGE II: IMPLEMENTATION OF HEN TRAINING   (Dietitian)

INTRODUCTION TO HEN PROGRAM   (Dietitian)

_____ Discuss purpose
_____ Introduce manual *Instructions for Tube Feeding at Home*

EQUIPMENT   (Dietitian-Nurse)
Discuss purpose, assembly, use, care, and cleaning of equipment.

	Discuss	Demonstrate	Patient Demonstrate
Feeding tube	_____	_____	_____
Feeding bag	_____	_____	_____
Gavage syringe	_____	_____	_____
Enteral pump (if needed)	_____	_____	_____

FORMULA—FLUIDS   (Dietitian)
_____ Show formula.
_____ Discuss purpose, type, amount, formula concentrations, fluid needs.
_____ Discuss preparation.
_____ Discuss administration schedule.
_____ Discuss weight expectations.

Fig. 15-2 Home enteral training checklist. (From Nelson JK, Weckwerth JA: Home enteral nutrition. In Skipper A, ed: *Dietitian's handbook of enteral and parenteral nutrition*, Rockville, Md, 1989, Aspen.)

PARENTERAL NUTRITION

Fortunately, there are alternatives for providing nutrients to patients when they can't or won't eat and tube feedings are contraindicated. Parenteral nutrition (PN) affords the provision of energy and nutrients intravenously. When infused into a large-diameter vein, such as the superior vena cava or subclavian (Fig. 15-3), parenteral nutrition is often referred to as central parenteral nutrition (CPN) or total parenteral nutrition (TPN). When a smaller, peripheral vein is used (usually in the forearm), parenteral nutrition is referred to as peripheral parenteral nutrition (PPN). Other terms are also used to characterize parenteral nutrition. These terms include central venous nutrition (CVN), peripheral venous nutrition (PVN), and hyperalimentation (hyperal).

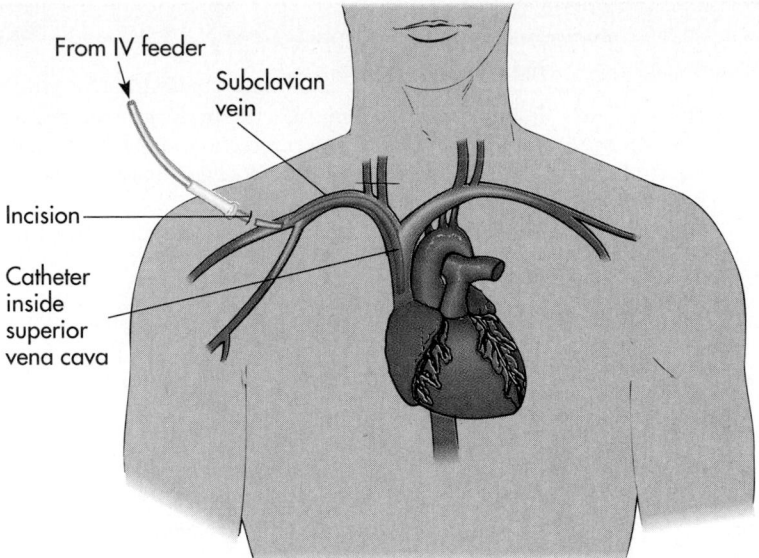

Fig. 15-3 Placement of catheter for cental parenteral nutrition, via the subclavian vein to the superior vena cava.

Parenteral nutrition should be routine when the patient is unable to absorb nutrients or is receiving high-dose cancer chemotherapy, radiation, and bone marrow transplantation. Patients experiencing pancreatitis, severe malnutrition, or catabolism also benefit from parenteral nutrition. Some of the clinical settings in which parenteral nutrition often helps are major surgery, moderate stress/trauma, inflammatory bowel disease, hyperemesis gravidarum (excessive vomiting during pregnancy), and moderate malnutrition. Parenteral nutrition is of limited use in situations of minimal stress or trauma or of untreatable disease. It should not be used when the gastrointestinal tract is functional or when risk of PN exceeds the potential benefits (6,7). Table 15-7 summarizes guidelines and indications for the use of parenteral nutrition.

Components of Parenteral Nutrition Solutions

Parenteral nutrition solutions contain the same nutrients and components you would expect to find in any enteral nutrition source. PN solutions typically contain water, amino acids, dextrose, electrolytes, vitamins, and trace elements. Fat is also included, often by means of *piggyback* administration or by adding it directly to the PN solution (usually referred to as a *3-in-1 solution*, which is discussed later).

Carbohydrate

The most common carbohydrate used in PN is dextrose monohydrate (1,5). Used as an energy source, it yields 3.4 kcal/g because of its hydrated form. Dextrose solutions are available in initial concentrations of 5% through 70%. Higher glucose concentrations are useful when a patient's fluids need to be restricted; lower concentrations are often used to help control hyperglycemia. Concentrations greater than 10% (final concentration) are hypertonic and must be delivered via CPN because the larger central vein can dilute the solution rapidly without damaging the blood vessel. Dextrose solutions are mixed with amino acids and other nutrients to form the final solution. Glucose needs and tolerances are important guidelines. Healthy adults need 2 grams of glucose/kg body weight/day (1).

Amino acids

Protein is provided in PN solutions as a mixture of essential and nonessential crystalline amino acids that are available with or without added electrolytes (1,5).

Table 15-7	Guidelines and Indications for Use of Parenteral Nutrition
Guideline	Indication
Clinical settings where parenteral nutrition should be part of routine care	Inability to absorb nutrients from the gastrointestinal tract (result of massive bowel resection, diseases of small intestine, radiation enteritis, severe diarrhea, or intractable vomiting)
	High-dose cancer chemotherapy, radiation, and bone marrow transplantation
	Moderate to severe pancreatitis
	Severe malnutrition accompanied by a nonfunctional gastrointestinal tract
	Severe catabolism with or without malnutrition when gastrointestinal tract has not been useable within 5-7 days
Clinical settings where parenteral nutrition usually would be helpful	Major surgery—total colectomy, pancreaticoduodenectomy, total pelvic exenteration
	Moderate stress—moderate trauma, 30% to 50% body surface area burns, moderately severe pancreatitis, neurologic trauma
	Enterocutaneous fistulae
	Inflammatory bowel disease
	Hyperemesis gravidarum
	Moderate malnutrition requiring intensive medical or surgical intervention
	Inability to establish adequate enteral nutrition within 7-10 days
	Inflammatory adhesions with small bowel obstruction
	Intensive cancer chemotherapy
Clinical settings where parenteral nutrition is of limited use	Minimal stress or trauma in a well-nourished patient with a usable GI tract (within 10-day period)
	Immediate postoperative or post-stress period
	Proved or suspected untreatable disease
Clinical settings where parenteral nutrition should not be used	When GI tract is functional, useable, and capable of absorbing adequate nutrients
	When PN is needed for less than 5 days
	When aggressive nutrition support is not desired by the patient or legal guardian, and when such action is in accordance with hospital policy and existing law
	When prognosis does not warrant aggressive nutrition support
	When risks of PN exceed potential benefits

From American Dietetic Association: *Manual of clinical dietetics*, ed 4, Chicago, 1992, American Dietetic Association; and ASPEN Board of Directors: Guidelines for use of total parenteral nutrition in the hospitalized adult patient, *Journal of Parenteral and Enteral Nutrition* 10:441-445, 1986.

It is important that the amino acids be used for protein synthesis and not be considered part of the solution's kcalorie source. Some facilities will not include protein kcalories when calculating kcalorie content of PN solutions; others will. Amino acid solutions are available in different concentrations as well as in different compositions of amino acids. Amino acid solutions are available for specialized protein needs such as renal failure, liver failure, stress, and trauma, but their efficacy is controversial (5).

Fats

Intravenous lipid emulsions are used as a concentrated energy source and to prevent the development of essential fatty acid deficiency (1,5,10). Commercial lipid emulsions are formulations of safflower oil, soybean oil, or a combination of the two, with glycerol added for isotonicity, and egg phospholipid added as an emulsifying agent (1,5). The kcaloric density of lipid solutions is useful when volume restriction is necessary. A 10% fat emulsion yields 1.1 kcal/mL or 550 kcal per 500 mL bottle, and a 20% solution yields 2 kcal/mL or 1000 kcal per 500 mL bottle. Another plus for lipid emulsions is that kcalories can be increased without increasing osmolality of PN solutions (5). Traditionally, lipid emulsions have been delivered peripherally using a piggyback system. Even though intravenous (IV) lipids are useful in supplying most of the nonprotein kcalories, care should be taken to not exceed 2.5 grams of lipid/kg (adults) or 60% of nonprotein kcalories (5,16). A baseline serum triglyceride level should be confirmed before administration of IV lipid emulsions, and should be monitored according to institutional policy.

Total nutrient admixtures

When lipid emulsions are added to dextrose and amino acid mixtures, the resulting solution is called a *three-in-one* mixture (Fig. 15-4) or total nutrient admixtures (TNAs) (5). The advantage to this system is that it allows lipid infusion over a 24-hour period, decreasing carbon dioxide production, and reducing hepatic accumulation of fat induced by long-term glucose use (1,17).

Electrolytes

Electrolytes and minerals can be provided by the general amino acid solution, as a combined electrolyte concentrate, or added separately as individual salts (5). Electrolytes and minerals are essential for normal body function and to accommodate excesses and deficiencies of minerals resulting from underlying disease processes. Commercial electrolyte solutions are available. Magnesium, phosphate, and potassium requirements increase in severely malnourished patients during refeeding or when higher levels of dextrose concentrations are used (1).

Vitamins

Adult and pediatric multivitamin formulations for IV use are available commercially. These products have been formulated according to recommendations of the American Medical Association Nutrition Advisory Group (18). In the event of frank vitamin deficiency, multiples of daily doses can be given in accordance with clinical status (5). Vitamin K is not included in adult preparations and must be given either intramuscularly or as an IV injectable added to the PN solution (5).

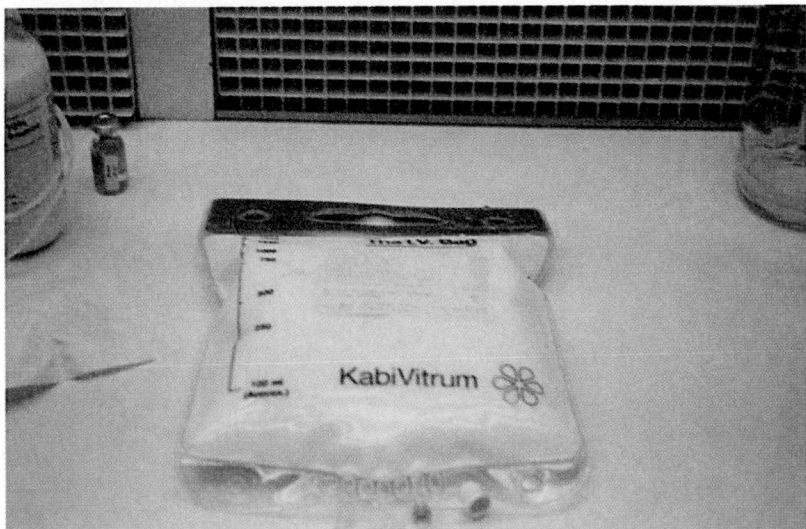

Fig. 15-4 A three-in-one solution includes dextrose, amino acids, and lipids.

Trace elements

Trace elements are another essential component of PN solutions. Their omission from early formulas led to clinical deficiencies and subsequent recommendations by the American Medical Association (19). Formulations that include zinc, copper, manganese, chromium, and selenium are available from commercial sources already combined, or institutional pharmacies may develop their own IV injectable formula.

Peripheral Parenteral Nutrition

PN solutions composed of >10% (final concentration) dextrose and/or >5% (final concentration) amino acids are hypertonic and can be administered only into central veins. PN solutions that are administered via peripheral veins must be isotonic to prevent damage to the vein. Isotonic PN solutions usually contain 5% to 10% dextrose (final concentration) and 3% to 5% amino acids, plus electrolytes, vitamins, minerals, and fat as needed. These nutrient components can only provide a limited amount of kcalories and protein (5). PPN is most often used in situations where only short-term nutrition support is needed in nonhypermetabolic conditions.

Monitoring Guidelines

Monitoring needs and protocols will vary among institutions and patient populations. Frequency of baseline parameter readings range from every 6 hours to a one-time baseline reading. Routine frequencies range from every 6 hours to biweekly or as needed. Specific parameters and recommendations for monitoring patients receiving PN are listed in Table 15-8.

Table 15-8   Recommendations for Monitoring Patients Receiving PN

Parameter	Frequency	
	Baseline	Routine
Glucose (at bedside)	Every 6 hours	Every 6 hours
Vital signs/temperature	Every 6 hours or shift	Every 6 hours or shift
Weight	Daily	Daily
Intake/output	Daily	Daily
Electrolytes	Daily × first 3 days	Biweekly
Creatinine/BUN	Baseline	Biweekly
Magnesium	Baseline	Weekly
Calcium/phosphorus	Baseline	Weekly
Albumin, prealbumin, or transferrin	Baseline	Weekly
Cholesterol	Baseline	As clinically indicated
Liver enzymes	Baseline	Weekly
CBC	Baseline	Weekly
PT/PTT	Baseline	Weekly
Nitrogen balance (24-hr UUN)	Baseline	Weekly
	24-48 hours after full rate achieved	Weekly
Triglyceride	Baseline	
Platelet count*	Baseline	As needed
Serum trace minerals/vitamins	Baseline	As needed
Estimated nutrient needs	Baseline	Weekly
		As needed

From American Dietetic Association: *Handbook of clinical dietetics,* ed 2, New Haven, 1992, Yale University Press; Nelson JK et al: *Mayo Clinic diet manual: A handbook of nutrition practices,* ed 7, St. Louis, 1994, Mosby; and Lenssen P: Monitoring and complications of parenteral nutrition. In Skipper A, ed: *Dietitian's handbook of enteral and parenteral nutrition,* Rockville, Md, 1989, Aspen.
*Needed initially for catheter insertion purposes.

Complications

As with enteral tube feedings, complications can occur with PN. Most can be averted by following the recommendations for monitoring in Table 15-8. Others can be circumvented by adhering to stringent technique. Table 15-9 summarizes possible complications.

Technical complications are related to catheter placement and are not unique to parenteral nutrition. The most common is **pneumothorax** which can be prevented by careful insertion of the central line using proper technique (13). Septic complications, like technical complications, are not unique to parenteral nutrition. Infections can be local or systemic, and usually occur because of poor technique in aseptic catheter care. Metabolic complications are the most common since metabolic requirements (electrolytes and energy) differ from patient to patient. The most common metabolic complication is hyperglycemia, which can be treated by adding insulin to the solution, reducing the dextrose load, and/or ensuring that the total kcaloric load is not excessive (13).

pneumothorax
air introduced into the thorax

Home Parenteral Nutrition

Home parenteral nutrition (HPN) enables selected patients who depend on PN to return to a reasonably normal lifestyle. A specialized catheter is used to reduce the possibility of infection (Fig. 15-5). The catheter is placed through a tunnel under the skin and exits the chest at a place where the patient or caretaker can care for it conveniently (13). As with home enteral nutrition, HPN requires the patient and/or significant other to be willing and able to perform daily procedures involved in administering the PN, which include monitoring laboratory values, temperature, weights, glucose measurements, and fluids (20). Home health care agencies may be utilized to provide equipment, supplies, and services.

Patients may be scheduled to receive HPN at night during sleep (cyclic TPN) to allow freedom to leave home or even work during the day. If the gastrointestinal tract is functional, sometimes HPN is administered only selected nights per week to supplement oral intake. Although expensive, HPN costs less than hospitalization, allows the patient to leave the hospital sooner, and in many cases allows the patient to resume a productive lifestyle (8,20).

Table 15-9 Complications of Parenteral Nutrition
TECHNICAL COMPLICATIONS
Pneumothorax
Malposition of catheter
Subclavian artery puncture
Carotid artery puncture
Catheter embolism
Air embolism
Catheter obstruction
Thrombosis
SEPTIC COMPLICATIONS
Catheter-related sepsis
Septic thrombosis
METABOLIC COMPLICATIONS
Hyperglycemia
Hyperglycemic hyperosmolar nonketotic dehydration
Hypoglycemia
Hyperkalemia
Hypophosphatemia
Hypocalcemia

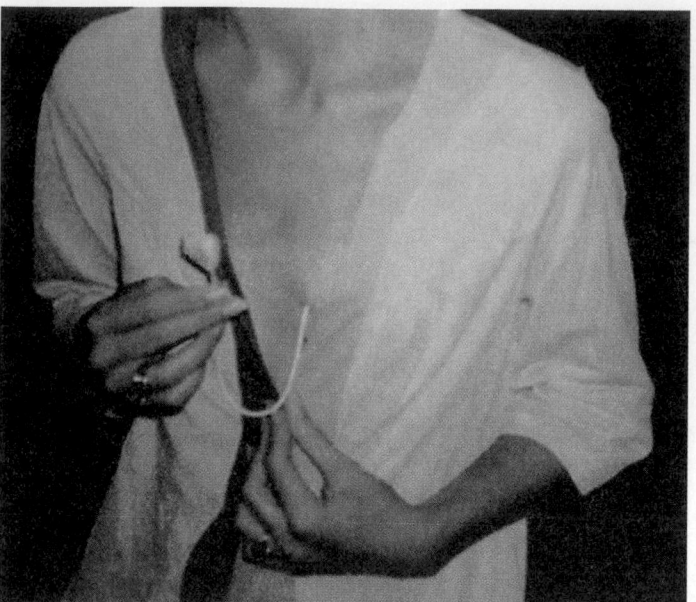

Fig. 15-5 Catheter used for home central venous alimentation.

TRANSITIONAL FEEDINGS

A period of adjustment, or weaning, is necessary before discontinuing nutritional support, or when converting from one form of nutritional support to another. Transition to an adequate oral intake to maintain nutritional status will differ from patient to patient (21). Although the gastrointestinal tract responds quickly to enteral feeding (1), patients who have been receiving TPN usually have decreased appetites and may take 1 to 2 weeks after complete cessation of TPN before they feel hungry and may experience early satiety (21). This necessitates gradual weaning from PN as enteral feeding (oral or tube) progresses to ensure continued adequate intake (1).

Parenteral to Oral or Tube Feeding

As mentioned previously, long periods of PN without enteral feedings result in atrophy of the gastrointestinal tract. If not contraindicated, minimal enteral intake (sips of dilute fruit juice) is encouraged to help maintain normal gastrointestinal tract physiology and gut mucosal immunity (21). Before weaning from PN, judicious assessment of gastrointestinal function is recommended to prevent problems with delayed gastric emptying, nausea, vomiting, or diarrhea (21). As PN is tapered and oral or tube feedings intake increases, it is important to document actual enteral intake, including fluids. This will facilitate the maintenance of nutrient requirements (21). If oral feedings or isotonic formulas are not well tolerated, an elemental formula may be needed.

Tube to Oral Feeding

In addition to documentation of intake per tube and orally, it will be important to assess the patient's swallowing ability before offering oral feedings. Full liquids are usually offered first, followed by pureed or soft foods. Tube feedings should be stopped at least 1 hour before and after meal time to promote appetite. As oral intake increases, tube feeding volume should be decreased. When oral intake consistently exceeds two thirds of energy requirements, the tube feedings can be discontinued.

WELLNESS AND ENTERAL/PARENTERAL NUTRITION

Physical Dimension	Physical health is impacted as these alterations may affect overall nutritional status; careful nursing supervision is necessary to ensure adequate nutrient intake.
Intellectual Dimension	Intellectual health is tested as patients prove their ability to understand, apply, and adapt to these sometimes very different textures of foods.
Emotional Dimension	The loss of symbolic foods, particularly if modifications are to be long-term or permanent, may stress emotional health; nurses can be sensitive to this aspect of dietary modification and assist patients to create new symbols to replace the old.
Social Dimension	Socially, patients will need strategies on how to be active participants at social gatherings and perhaps on how to educate others to be sensitive and comfortable with their special dietary needs.

SUMMARY

Every patient deserves one of the most basic of needs—nourishment. For obvious reasons enteral nutrition (oral or tube feedings) is the preferred method of nutrition support. Feeding patients via the gastrointestinal tract is safer, easier to administer, aids in maintaining gastrointestinal tract integrity, and is as much as five times less expensive. An array of commercial tube feeding products that supply intact nutrients are available. Administered in the appropriate volume, 100% of the RDA for vitamins and minerals can be provided, as well as adequate amounts of energy and protein.

In those instances when patients are unable to obtain nutrition enterally, the use of PN can literally be a life-saving therapy. Peripheral or central infusions of amino acids, dextrose, fat emulsions, vitamins, and minerals can provide the ordinary or extraordinary nutrient needs of patients. Although not without risk, when managed through a team approach and routine monitoring, PN can provide a safe vehicle for meeting patients' nutritional goals.

THE NURSING ROLE

A Stroke Patient: The Nursing Process

Mrs. White suffered a stroke last month that rendered her semicomatose and left her throat muscles partially paralyzed. She is unable to swallow any solid food and aspirates whenever she is given oral fluids. Therefore Mrs. White had a PEG (percutaneous endoscopic gastrostomy) tube inserted two weeks ago. She is now in an extended care facility and is receiving intermittent commercially prepared tube feedings 4 times per day (10 AM-2 PM-6 PM-10 PM). The formula was changed two days ago because she was losing weight. She is now on a full-strength lactose-free formula. She has begun having diarrhea and her respirations are slightly increased.

ASSESSMENT DATA COLLECTED
Objective
Weight: 108 lb
Temperature: 98.4° F
Blood pressure: 130/86, Pulse 84, Respiration 24
Loose or watery stools 3 to 4 times a day
Bowel sounds slightly hyperactive

Continued.

THE NURSING ROLE, cont'd.
A Stroke Patient: The Nursing Process

Skin turgor normal
Mucous membranes moist
Bilateral rhonchi on auscultation

NURSING DIAGNOSIS 1

Diarrhea related to hyperosmolar tube feeding as evidenced by 3 to 4 loose stools per day

PLANNING

Goal: Patient will have normal formed stool within 72 hours.

INTERVENTION

1. Obtain physician's order to reduce concentration or rate of tube feeding.
2. Assess and record consistency and number of stools.
3. After diarrhea subsides, gradually increase concentration or rate as tolerated until desired formula is reached.

EVALUATION

Evaluate whether goal of normal stool has been met as evidenced by one formed stool per day by the end of 72 hours. Continue to evaluate vital signs to rule out infectious process as a contributing factor.

NURSING DIAGNOSIS 2

High risk for aspiration related to tube feedings

PLANNING

Goal: Patient's lungs will sound clear on auscultation

INTERVENTION

1. Before instilling feedings, aspirate stomach contents. If more than 60 ml remain in stomach, reduce feeding by corresponding amount.
2. Elevate head of bed at least 30 degrees during and 1 hour after feedings.
3. Put blue food coloring in feedings for next 48 hours and observe for blue color in pulmonary secretions.
4. Auscultate breath sounds every shift.

EVALUATION

Evaluate whether outcome has been achieved as evidenced by clear lung fields on auscultation.

Critical Thinking ## CLINICAL APPLICATIONS

Advances in medical technology have provided mechanisms to feed or nourish patients that once could not be. However, like most medical advances, it also provides dilemmas and difficult decisions about patient care. Nutrition care dilemmas transpire when this technology will keep the patient alive even when that patient has no hope of ever living a normal life. Often, the dilemma involves legal action for resolution. The Karen Ann Quinlan case (1976) was the first case to go to court to withdraw life-sustaining medical care from a permanently incompetent patient. Most recently (1988), a US Supreme Court decision allowed a feeding tube to be discontinued from Nancy Cruzan, who suffered irreversible

Critical Thinking	**CLINICAL APPLICATIONS, cont'd**

brain damage as the result of a car accident in 1983. What are your thoughts about the following circumstances?

1. An 85-year-old man who suffers from many physical problems but is not terminally ill refuses to be tube fed.
2. A 57-year-old woman is hospitalized as a result of a severe psychiatric disorder that prohibits her from speaking or eating. She is bedridden in a fetal position and has a gastrostomy tube. She repeatedly dislodges the feeding tube and is combative when it is replaced.
3. A 75-year-old woman's husband has requested termination of her nasogastric feedings. She is brain dead and has no living will.

Modified from Edelstein S: *Ethical dilemmas and decisions,* San Marcos, Calif, 1993, Nutrition Dimension.

REFERENCES

1. American Dietetic Association: *Handbook of clinical dietetics,* ed 2, New Haven, 1992, Yale University Press.
2. Mitallo JM: Parenteral therapy. In Lang CE: *Nutritional support in critical care,* Rockville, Md, 1987, Aspen.
3. Philips S: Water and electrolytes in gastrointestinal disease. In Maxwell MH, Klienman CR, eds: *Clinical disorders of fluid and electrolyte metabolism,* New York, 1979, McGraw-Hill.
4. Murray DP et al: Survey: Use of clear and full liquid diets with or without commercially produced formulas, *Journal of Parenteral and Enteral Nutrition* 9:732-734, 1985.
5. Nelson JK et al: *Mayo Clinic diet manual: A handbook of nutrition practices,* ed 7, St. Louis, 1994, Mosby.
6. American Dietetic Association: *Manual of clinical dietetics,* ed 4, Chicago, 1992, American Dietetic Association.
7. ASPEN Board of Directors: Guidelines for the use of enteral nutrition in the adult patient, *Journal of Parenteral and Enteral Nutrition,* 11:435-439, 1987.
8. Rombeau JL, Barot LR: Enteral nutrition therapy, *Surg Clin North Am* 61:605-620, 1981.
9. Swearingen PL: *Manual of medical-surgical nursing care,* ed 3, St. Louis, 1994, Mosby.
10. DeChicco R, Matarese L: Selection of nutrition support regimens, *Nutrition in Clinical Practice* 7:239-245, 1992.
11. Chawla KK, Jeske DJ, Renfro AD: *Assessing and managing nutrition status: A complete guide to meeting complex nutritional needs of acutely ill patients,* St. Louis, 1994, Barnes and Jewish Hospitals.
12. McClave S, Lowen CC, Snider HL: Immunonutrition and enteral hyperalimentation of critically ill patients, *Dig Dis Sci,* 37:1153-1161, 1992.
13. Weinsier RL, Morgan SL: *Fundamentals of clinical nutrition,* St. Louis, 1993, Mosby.
14. Edes TE, Walk BE, Austin JL: Diarrhea in tube-fed patients: Feeding formula not necessarily the cause, *Am J Med* 88:91-93, 1990.
15. Nelson JK, Weckwerth JA: Home enteral nutrition. In Skipper A, ed: *Dietitian's handbook of enteral and parenteral nutrition,* Rockville, Md, 1989, Aspen.
16. Roesner M, Grant JP: Intravenous lipid emulsions, *Nutrition in Clinical Practice* 2:96-107, 1987.
17. Driscoll DF et al: Practical considerations regarding the use of total nutrient admixtures, *Am J Hosp Pharm* 43:416-419, 1986.
18. American Medical Association Department of Foods and Nutrition: Multivitamin preparations for parenteral use: A statement by the nutrition advisory group, *Journal of Parenteral and Enteral Nutrition* 3:258-262, 1979.
19. American Medical Association Department of Foods and Nutrition: Guidelines for essential trace element preparations for parenteral use: A statement by an expert panel, *JAMA* 241:2051-2054, 1979.
20. McCrae JD: Home parenteral nutrition. In Skipper A, ed: *Dietitian's handbook of enteral and parenteral nutrition,* Rockville, Md, 1989, Aspen.
21. Lenssen P: Monitoring and complications of parenteral nutrition. In Skipper A, ed: *Dietitian's handbook of enteral and parenteral nutrition,* Rockville, Md, 1989, Aspen.

Chapter 16

NUTRITION FOR DISORDERS OF THE GASTROINTESTINAL TRACT

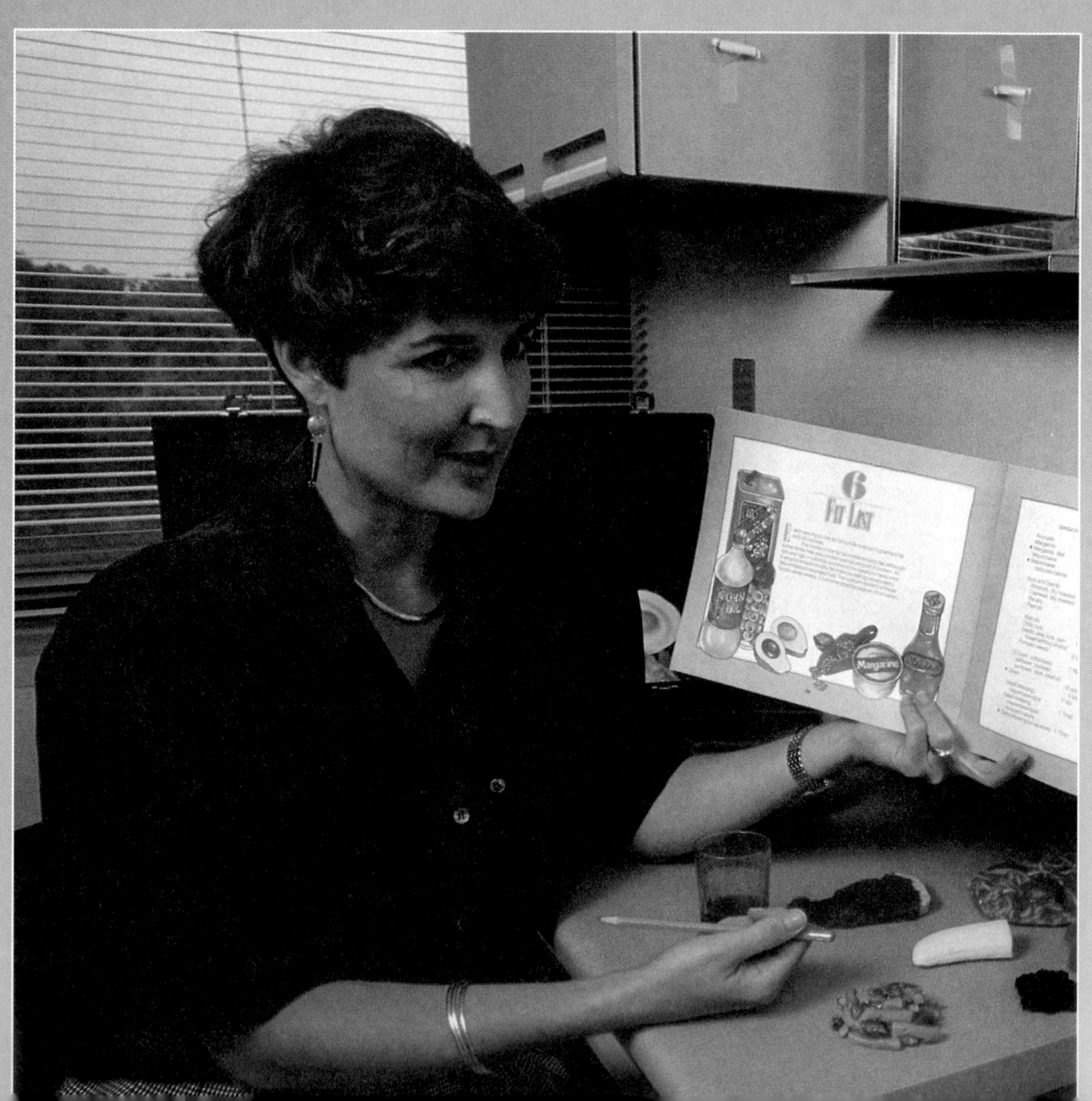

ROLE IN WELLNESS

The simple act of eating an apple is no longer easy when disorders of the gastrointestinal tract occur. The ability to chew, swallow, digest, and absorb nutrients, while passing fiber and other substances on for elimination, may be compromised by disorders of the gastrointestinal tract. These disorders affect the provision of nutrients to all other organs and systems of the body, thereby influencing overall health.

Dysphagia

For patients with chewing or swallowing difficulties, diets must be devised to meet nutritional needs and prevent *aspiration*. Patients may experience changes in consistency tolerance. Thickening agents often are used to provide varying levels of consistency to accommodate individual needs since thin liquids are usually more difficult to swallow. The main focus of dietary management of *dysphagia* is to provide nutrition in a form that fits the specific anatomical and functional needs of the patient while maintaining or improving nutritional status and avoiding aspiration (1).

We rarely think about swallowing, just as we don't think about breathing or our heart beating. Swallowing takes place in three stages, as outlined in Table 16-1: oral preparation and transit, pharyngeal transit, and esophageal transit. A disorder affecting any of these stages may require medical nutrition therapy.

Patients sometimes give *warning signs* that they are at risk for swallowing problems (2). Some of these signs include the following:

- Collecting food under the tongue, in the cheeks, or on the hard palate
- Spitting food out of the mouth, or tongue thrusting
- Poor tongue control
- Excessive tongue movement
- Slow oral transit time
- Delay or absence of elevation of Adam's apple during swallow
- Coughing before or after swallowing
- Choking
- Drooling
- *Gargly* voice after eating or drinking
- Regurgitating food or liquid through nose, mouth, or tracheostomy tube
- Inadequate intake of food or fluids accompanied by weight loss
- Excessive eating time
- Resistance to eating—clenching teeth, pushing food away, clutching throat

Medical nutrition therapy

Diets for patients with dysphagia are individualized based on swallowing ability and personal food preferences (2,3). Successful swallowing depends on several factors regarding the *bolus:* volume (4), viscosity (5), temperature (6), and consistency (7). A nutritionally adequate diet for dysphagia involves taking these characteristics into consideration along with careful planning.

When caring for patients with dysphagia, several aspects are of major concern: bolus consistency, positioning of the patient, rate of feeding, and specific swallowing techniques (1). *Videofluoroscopy* examination is used to determine the level of bolus consistency the patient can tolerate. Different physiological problems dictate different consistencies of food. For example, the most common swallowing disorder in the elderly stroke population is a delayed or absent pharyngeal swallow. Patients with this type of disorder need pureed foods to provide stimulation that provokes the reflex swallow. If the pharyngeal swallow is not delayed or absent, but only reduced, liquids tend to be the most difficult consistency to deal with. The appropriate consistency can usually be acquired by the use of thickening agents (1). For

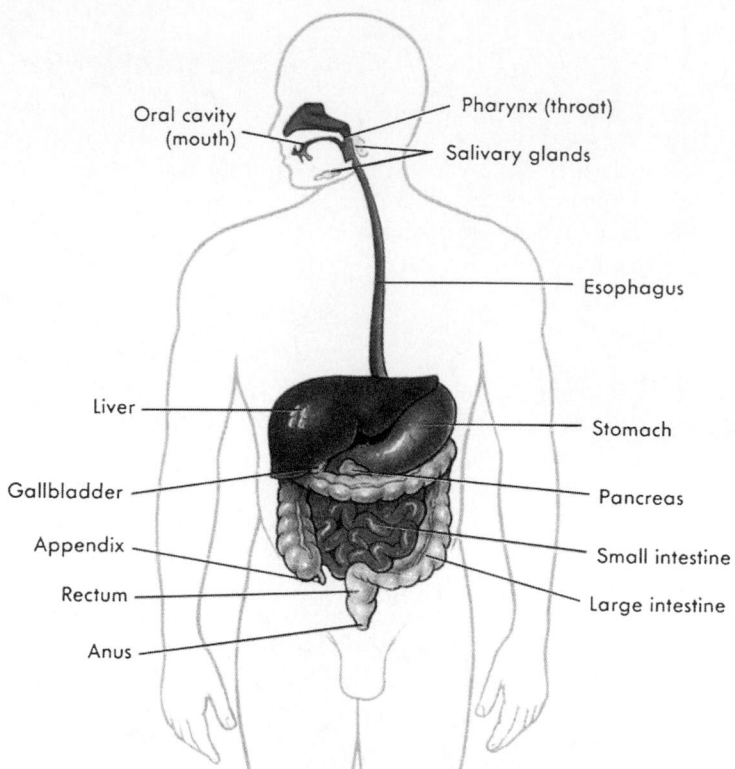

Fig. 16-1 The gastrointestinal tract.

Conditions Causing Dysphagia	
Achalasia	Head or neck cancer or surgery
AIDS, such as from oral or esophageal thrush	Multiple sclerosis (MS)
	Muscular dystrophy (MD)
Alzheimer's disease/dementia	Myotonic dystrophy
Amyotrophic lateral sclerosis (ALS)	Myasthenia gravis
Cerebral palsy (CP)	Parkinson's disease
Cerebrovascular accident (CVA)	Poliomyelitis
Closed head trauma	Reflux esophagitis
Dermatomyositis	Stricture or inflammation of pharynx or esophagus
Dysautonomia	
Huntington's chorea	Tumor or obstruction of throat

From American Dietetic Association: *Handbook of clinical dietetics,* ed 2, New Haven, 1992, Yale University Press; and American Dietetic Association: *Manual of clinical dietetics,* ed 4, Chicago, 1992, American Dietetic Association.

patients who have lost coordination of the upper esophageal sphincter (cricopharyngeal dysfunction), thin liquids are the most appropriate (8).

One of the safest eating positions for patients who have trouble swallowing is the upright position. If patients cannot sit up by themselves, the head of the bed should be raised to provide support, and pillows and wedges should be used to support arms, head, neck, or trunk when necessary. The upright position allows gravity to assist the passage of food along the esophagus and helps prevent choking and aspiration (1,9).

Sometimes patients eat too quickly, stuffing their mouths full of food and then choking when trying to swallow. Staff can observe and supervise the patients while they eat to remind them to complete the swallowing sequence before taking their next bite of food (1).

Table 16-1   Stages of Swallowing

Stage	Action
Oral preparation and transit	Food enters the mouth and is chewed. It is moistened with saliva and pressed against the hard palate to form a bolus. The tongue moves the bolus toward the back of the throat where the involuntary swallowing reflex is triggered.
Pharyngeal transit	The soft palate closes against the pharyngeal wall to prevent nasal regurgitation. The bolus is carried through the pharynx to the sphincter above the esophagus. The larynx closes to prevent food from entering the lungs. Breathing stops momentarily as throat muscles constrict to move the bolus down into the esophagus.
Esophageal transit	The bolus is moved down the esophagus, through the esophageal sphincter into the stomach by esophageal peristalsis and gravity.

From American Dietetic Association: *Manual of clinical dietetics,* Chicago, 1992, American Dietetic Association; and Loustau A, Lee KA: Dealing with the dangers of dysphagia, *Nursing* 15:47, 1985.

Enlisting the aid of a speech therapist is often useful to teach the patient various techniques to compensate for swallowing problems (1). Techniques include the supraglottic swallow and the Mendelson maneuver. The supraglottic swallow is appropriate for patients with reduced laryngeal function. This method requires teaching the patient to take a breath before swallowing, consciously holding the breath during the swallow, exhaling forcefully or coughing gently after the swallow, and reswallowing to clear the mouth. The Mendelson maneuver is helpful for individuals with cricopharyngeal dysfunction. The patient is taught to elevate the larynx voluntarily to the maximum level during a swallow to allow for food to pass (1). Nursing personnel also can use several techniques to assist the patient. Encouraging the patient to think or talk about food before meal time can help stimulate the flow of saliva, which aids in the chewing and swallowing process. Tart or sour foods can stimulate saliva production. Having the patient lick jelly from his lips, pucker them, hum, or whistle helps strengthen mouth muscles, which may help the patient learn to close his lips around a fork or spoon (9). Table 16-2 outlines other considerations for particular features of foods to assist a patient who is dysphagic.

Responsibility for feeding patients with swallowing difficulty usually falls upon nursing personnel. Following safe procedures is important.

1. Position the patient upright.
2. Eliminate distractions so the patient can focus all his attention on the meal at hand.
3. Instruct the patient not to use liquids to clear the mouth of foods; in fact, they should only be used after the patient has cleared the food from his mouth. Encourage frequent dry swallows to help clear food from the mouth between bites.

Table 16-2   Features of Foods to be Considered for Patients With Dysphagia

Feature	Considerations	Possible Solutions
Texture	Texture of foods required depends on patient's degree of control over chewing and swallowing	Texture can be modified by chopping, grinding, or pureeing foods with a food processor (blenders tend to liquify foods); adding coarsely ground food to a smooth, thick puree base; soaking absorbent foods with a gelatin or commercial thickener instead of pureeing them (works especially well with breads, cakes, cookies, and breakfast products)
Cohesiveness	Closely related to texture; describes the ability of the food bolus to stay together; foods modified in texture and assumed easy to chew are not necessarily easy to swallow.	Naturally cohesive foods include custards, hot cereals, and tuna salad; gravies can add cohesiveness to ground meats, rice, and other purees that separate; melted cheese, mashed potato granules, and commercial thickeners also provide cohesiveness
Density	Generally refers to the weight of the bolus; dense foods provide stimulation for patients with reduced swallowing sensation; light foods are more desirable for patients with sensitive mouths and/or flaccid muscles	Heavy or dense foods can be thinned with liquids or combined with lighter foods to make a lighter density food; thickeners can be added to light foods to slow transit time and trigger the swallowing mechanism
Viscosity	Refers to the thickness of a liquid; thin liquids are always contraindicated for patients with delayed swallowing reflex and sometimes for patients with reduced oral coordination	Thickeners can be added to achieve appropriate viscosity; commercial thickeners as well as mashed potato granules and gelatin can be added to fluids
Temperature and seasoning	Temperature extremes and highly seasoned foods can be used to stimulate the swallowing reflex	Acidic vinegar should be avoided because it may cause coughing; food and beverage temperatures should be individualized to patient tolerance and preference

Modified from American Dietetic Association: *Manual of clinical dietetics,* ed 4, Chicago, 1992, American Dietetics Association.

4. Encourage small bites, especially if the patient's ability to manage food is impaired.

5. While the patient is eating, check for voice quality. A wet or *gurgly* voice indicates that food may be resting on the vocal cords (2).

During the early stages of feeding, nursing supervision is necessary at meals to prevent or minimize swallowing problems. Patients should be reevaluated on a regular basis to determine if any changes need to be made in the consistency of fluids or food. Evaluating and documenting the patient's kcaloric and nutrient intake are also prudent to ensure adequate nutritional intake and status. If the patient's nutritional needs are not or cannot be met orally, alternative methods should be considered (1).

For patients with dysphagia, meal time can be made safe and nutritious, but it may be difficult to make eating the pleasure it once was. The one thing nursing personnel can do to make sure meals are as relaxing as possible is to let patients eat at their own pace. Patience may be rewarded with patients who eat with minimal difficulty while maintaining their nutritional status.

Achalasia

Achalasia is a neurogenic disorder of the lower esophagus characterized by ineffective peristalsis in the lower two thirds of the esophagus, a hypertonic lower esophageal sphincter (LES) that does not relax in response to swallowing, and esophageal dilatation (10,11). Achalasia can be divided into two types: classic and vigorous. Classic achalasia is manifested by absent or weak and dysrhythmic esophageal contractions. On the other hand, vigorous achalasia presents with repetitive and hyperactive esophageal contractions, much like in esophageal spasm. In either case, the peristalsis is ineffective and obstruction occurs because of the constricted LES, causing the esophagus to become dilated (10).

The cause of achalasia is unknown, but there is some evidence that it is an impairment in the innervative response of the esophagus to parasympathetic activity (11). It occurs in males and females at any age, but most patients are diagnosed between 20 and 40 years of age (10). Symptoms include dysphagia (both liquid and solid foods), chest pain (particularly in vigorous achalasia), regurgitation (10), and weight loss (11). Complications include esophagitis with edema, possible ulceration and hemorrhage, respiratory complications caused by aspiration of esophageal contents, malnutrition, and a predisposition for esophageal carcinoma (in 3% to 8% of cases) (10,11).

Medical nutrition therapy

Small, frequent meals of semisolid or liquid foods may be best tolerated by patients with achalasia (12). Patients should be taught to eat and drink slowly in a relaxed environment. Drinking fluids with meals may enhance movement of food into the stomach (11). Vitamin and mineral supplements may be necessary. No foods or dietary regimens can prevent achalasia. Guidelines for nutritional care of patients who develop achalasia are outlined in Table 16-3.

Table 16-3 Guidelines for Medical Nutrition Therapy in Achalasia	
Guideline	**Nutritional Treatment**
Texture	Semisolid or liquid foods as tolerated; a low-fiber diet may be used if it is easier to swallow
Meal pattern	Small, frequent meals as tolerated
Nutrients	Moderate carbohydrate and protein and increased fat to reduce LES pressure and gastric secretions
Temperature of food	Avoid extreme temperatures
Irritants	Avoid citrus juices and spiced foods; these can irritate and possibly injure esophageal mucosa if retained

Modified from Zeman FJ: *Clinical nutrition and dietetics,* ed 2, New York, 1991, Macmillan.

Gastroesophageal Reflux, Hiatal Hernia, and Esophagitis

gastroesophageal reflux
return of gastric contents into the esophagus that results in a severe burning sensation under the sternum

esophagitis
inflammation of the lower esophagus

More commonly known as *heartburn*, **gastroesophageal reflux (GER)** is a common experience for some people. In fact, some consider it to be a normal state of being and never report the symptoms to their physicians. The reflux usually takes place within 1 to 4 hours following a meal (11).

Normally, the lower esophageal sphincter (LES) prevents stomach contents from entering the esophagus, but various factors often decrease sphincter pressure. Unlike gastric mucosa, esophageal mucosa can be damaged when exposed to gastric contents. If not treated, GER can result in **esophagitis.** The reflux is thought to be aggravated by reclining after eating, stress, and increased intraabdominal pressure (11). Increased intraabdominal pressure can occur with coughing, straining, bending, vomiting, obesity, pregnancy, trauma, wearing constricting clothing, ascites, and severe physical exertion (11). Older patients often experience respiratory symptoms of pneumonitis (11), chronic bronchitis, or asthma (13,14).

Gastroesophageal reflux is treated medically by reducing intraabdominal pressure and gastric acid production. Patients can do many things to avoid reflux such as limiting activities that increase intraabdominal pressure, elevating the head of the bed at night, avoiding waist-constricting clothing, and not lying down for 2 to 3 hours after meals (11). Table 16-4 summarizes medications that may be used in treating GER as well as their actions.

Medical nutrition therapy

Patients may be able to minimize symptoms of GER by manipulating the way they eat and by avoiding certain foods, especially those high in fat. The Teaching Tool summarizes nutritional recommendations for GER.

TEACHING TOOL
Recommendations for Minimizing Heartburn

Heartburn can be avoided or at least minimized by limiting or avoiding certain foods or manipulating the way meals are eaten. Here are some strategies to share with clients:

1. Avoid large meals. If additional kcalories are needed for weight gain or maintenance, include mid-morning and mid-afternoon snacks.
2. Avoid eating meals or snacks for at least 2 hours before lying down.
3. Avoid or limit foods/beverages that relax the lower esophageal sphincter (allowing stomach contents to back up) such as alcohol, carminatives (oil of peppermint or spearmint, garlic, onion), chocolate, high-fat foods (fried foods, high-fat meats, cream sauces, gravies, margarine/butter, cream, oil, salad dressings).
4. Avoid or limit foods/beverages that can be irritating to damaged esophageal mucosa. These will vary individually and may include carbonated beverages, citrus fruit and juices, coffee (regular and decaffeinated), herbs, pepper, spices, tomato products, and very hot or very cold foods.
5. Increase intake of foods that do not affect the lower esophageal sphincter pressure such as protein foods with low-fat content (lean meats, skim or 1% milk, cheeses and yogurt made from skim milk), carbohydrate foods with low-fat content (breads, cereals, crackers, fruit, noodles, potatoes, rice, and vegetables prepared without added fat).
6. Achieve and maintain a desirable body weight.

From Nelson JK et al: *Mayo Clinic diet manual,* ed 7, St. Louis, 1994, Mosby.

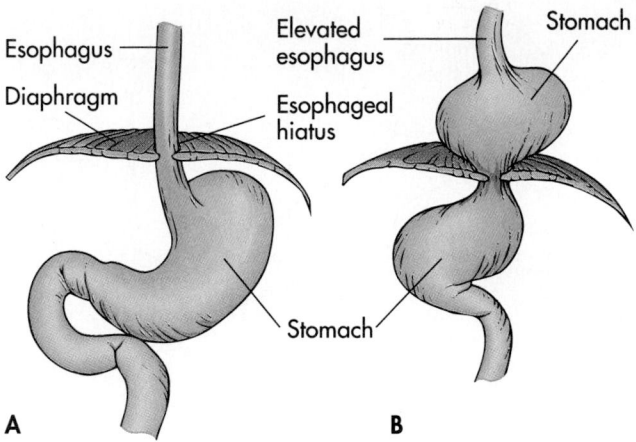

Fig. 16-2 Normal stomach placement compared with hiatal hernia.

Causes of Gastroesophageal Reflux

Increased levels of progesterone caused by pregnancy, oral contraceptives containing progesterone, late stages of the menstrual cycle
Vigorous exercise
Achalasia
Hiatal hernia (Fig. 16-2)

hiatal hernia
herniation of a portion of the stomach into the chest through the esophageal hiatus of the diaphragm

Table 16-4   Medications Used to Treat Gastroesophageal Reflux

Medication	Action
Antacids (Maalox)	Neutralize gastric acid
Histamine H$_2$ receptor blockers (Ranitidine HCI/Zantac)	Suppress gastric acid secretion
Proton pump inhibitor (Omeprazole)	
Alginate antacids (Gaviscon)	Neutralize gastric acid and barrier protection
Gastrointestinal stimulators	Augment gastric emptying and increase LES pressure
Cholinergics (Bethanechol, Urecholine)	Improve LES pressure and esophageal acid clearance
Dopamine antagonists (Metoclopramide, Reglan)	Improve LES and gastric emptying
Antiemetics, cough suppressants, stool softeners	Prevent increased intraabdominal pressure from vomiting, coughing, and straining with bowel movements

From Nelson JK et al: *Mayo Clinic diet manual,* ed 7, St. Louis, 1994, Mosby; and Swearingen PL: *Manual of nursing therapeutics,* ed 4, St. Louis, 1995, Mosby.

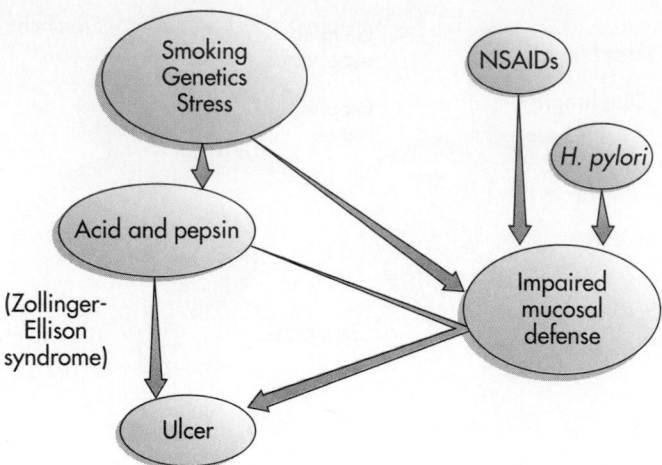

Fig. 16-3 Pathogenesis of peptic ulcer disease.

Peptic Ulcer Disease

Peptic ulcer disease (PUD) is a term for several recurrent chronic diseases characterized by the presence of ulcers in the gastric or duodenum mucosal membrane. Most duodenal ulcers are located within the pylorus, whereas gastric ulcers usually are located at the junction of the antrum and fundus or within 6 cm of the pylorus (15). PUD is caused by a combination of factors: hypersecretion of gastric acid, impaired mucosal defense, and the presence of predisposing factors for peptic ulceration including use of nonsteroidal antiinflammatory drugs (NSAIDs), *Helicobacter pylori (H. pylori),* cigarette smoking, genetic predisposition, and stress (Fig. 16-3) (16). Hypersecretion of gastric acid in the Zollinger-Ellison syndrome is one exception in which ulcers occur in the absence of *H. pylori* infection (16).

Treatment goals are focused largely on relieving symptoms, healing the ulcer, preventing reoccurrence, and avoiding complications (17). The most effective method of treatment appears to be a well-balanced regular diet combined with acid suppression and other medical therapies.

Medical nutrition therapy

Special *bland* diets or *ulcer* diets are no more effective (see box) than a general diet in speeding the healing rate of an ulcer and in reducing gastric acid secretion. Current recommendations are to eliminate foods that increase secretion of stomach acid, worsen symptoms, and damage the lining of the esophagus, stomach, or duodenum. This approach *must* be individualized (17).

Dumping Syndrome

One of the functions of the stomach is to control the rate of gastric emptying of nutrients into the small intestine. This process ensures efficient digestion, absorption, and metabolism (18). In fact, the rate of entry of nutrients into the duodenum is slow enough to allow for about 85% of food to be digested and absorbed by mid-small intestine (19).

When part or all of the stomach (partial or total gastrectomy) is removed (Fig. 16-4) or the pyloric sphincter is removed, **dumping syndrome** may develop. Although almost 40% of patients experience dumping syndrome immediately after surgery, symptoms tend to decrease with time, resulting in 5% or less who sustain chronic symptoms (17). Symptoms are usually related to rapid gastric emptying, which causes distention of the

dumping syndrome
contents from the stomach empty too rapidly into the duodenum, causing symptoms of profuse sweating, nausea, dizziness, and weakness

MYTH
Bland Diets Useful in Treating Peptic Ulcer Disease

For years, bland diets have been used in the treatment of peptic ulcer disease. Starting out as a "white diet" (sometimes called a Sippy diet, after Dr. Sippy, who developed this diet), which allowed the use of only white foods (such as milk, cream, mashed potatoes, cream of wheat), it has experienced waves of liberalization over the years and progressed to what has been called the *liberal bland diet* (which allows all foods except caffeine, alcohol, black pepper, spices, and any other food that could be considered irritating). Foods on the hit list for peptic ulcer disease have always been assumed either to be irritating to intestinal mucosa or to promote gastric acid secretion. However, what makes this interesting is that the efficacy of the bland diet (or any other *ulcer* diet for that matter) has never been scientifically proven.

What has been proven (in the 1950s) is that the traditional bland diet does not decrease gastric acid secretion or increase the rate of healing. Food in the stomach can raise pH, but it does not neutralize gastric acid. This has led the enlightened medical community to prescribe a well-balanced, regular diet combined with antacid or histamine H_2 blocker therapy. Some patients benefit from small, frequent meals—pain relief from the presence of food. General recommendations include the following:

- Eat a well-balanced diet.
- Avoid alcohol, cigarette smoking, and salicylates.
- Avoid eating at bedtime to prevent acid stimulation during sleep.
- Caffeinated and decaffeinated beverages stimulate gastric acid secretion. Use them in moderation. Do not drink them on an empty stomach or before bedtime. Omit coffee if poorly tolerated.
- There is little rationale for completely eliminating a particular food unless it causes repeated discomfort.

Not only has the clinical value of the traditional bland diet never been proven, it may also have several adverse reactions. Ingesting excessive amounts of milk (2 or more quarts) along with antacids (1.4 gram of calcium carbonate) can lead to milk-alkali syndrome, which results in a low to normal serum phosphate level; this responds positively to dietary calcium restrictions. Additionally, the protein and calcium content of milk causes increased gastric acid secretion, which may result in postprandial pain in someone who has an ulcer.

Drug therapy has eliminated the need for restrictive bland diets, and fortunately for patients, medical therapy for peptic ulcer disease is currently based on pharmacological treatment instead of nutritional treatment.

From Alpers D, Crouse R, Stenson W: *Manual of nutritional therapeutics,* ed 2, Boston, 1988, Little, Brown; American Dietetic Association: *Handbook of clinical dietetics,* ed 2, New Haven, 1992, Yale University Press; American Dietetic Association: *Manual of clinical dietetics,* ed 4, Chicago, 1992, American Dietetic Association; Flier J, Underhill L: Pathogenesis of peptic ulcer and implications for therapy, *N Eng J Med* 322:909-915, 1990; Gaska J, Tietze K: Current concepts in the treatment of peptic ulcer disease: A case-oriented approach: Part 1, *Am Pharm* NS29:49-55, 1989; Marotta RB, Floch MH: Diet and nutrition in ulcer disease, *Med Clin North Am* 75:967-979, 1991; Meyer JH: The stomach and nutrition. In Shils ME, Olson JA, Shike M, eds: *Modern nutrition in health and disease,* ed 6, Philadelphia, 1994, Lea & Febiger; Ohning G, Soll A: Medical treatment of peptic ulcer disease, *Am Fam Phys* 39:257, 1989; and Siepler J, Mahakian K, Trudeau W: Current concepts in clinical therapeutics: Peptic ulcer disease, *Clin Pharm* 5:128-142, 1986.

upper small intestine. Additionally, these gastric contents are hypertonic, which will induce a rapid influx of fluid to dilute the **hyperosmolar** contents (17).

Some symptoms occur 15 to 30 minutes **postprandially** (early phase) and are characterized by feelings of epigastric fullness, abdominal cramps, nausea, and/or diarrhea in addition to vasomotor symptoms of tachycardia, postural hypotension, sweating, weakness, flushing, and/or syncope. Some patients experience intestinal symptoms but not vasomotor symptoms, or vice versa. The late phase, which occurs less frequently than the early phase, develops about 2 to 4 hours postprandially and is associated with symptoms similar to hypoglycemia: perspiration, hunger, nausea, anxiety, tremors, and/or weakness (17).

hyperosmolar
abnormally increased osmolarity

postprandial
occurring after a meal

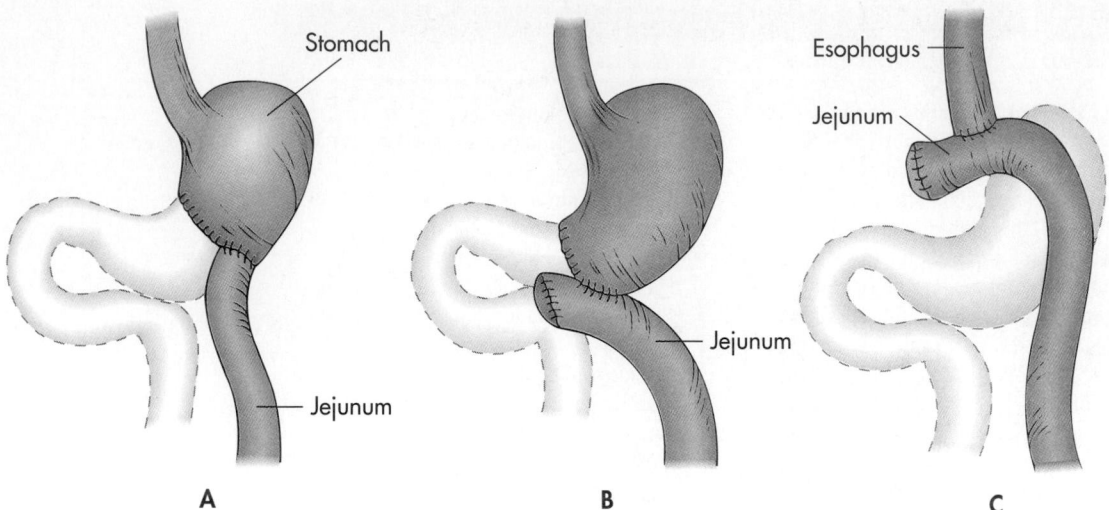

Fig. 16-4 Typical gastric surgery resections. **A,** Partial gastrectomy, Billroth I (gastroduodenostomy). **B,** Partial gastrectomy, Billroth II (gastrojejunostomy). **C,** total gastrectomy.

Medical nutrition therapy

Food and meals can be manipulated and/or restricted to help alleviate patients' symptoms while still providing a nutritionally sound diet. Patients who have dumping syndrome should have their nutritional status evaluated on a regular basis to detect early iron, vitamin B_{12}, protein, and vitamin D deficiencies (17). Basically, the diet should be low in simple carbohydrates, high in complex carbohydrates and protein (1.5 to 2.0 gm/kg), and moderate in fat (1). The Teaching Tool summarizes recommendations for medical nutrition therapy.

Celiac Disease

Celiac disease or sprue is a chronic disease that damages primarily the mucosa of the small intestine, especially the duodenum and proximal jejunum (17). In milder forms of the disease, the microvilli on the villi are destroyed, decreasing the absorptive surface area as much as twofold. In more severe cases, the villi themselves become blunted or disappear altogether, consequently further reducing the absorptive area of the gut (20). Although the exact mechanism remains unknown, this intestinal damage is caused by gliadin, the protein fraction of gluten, which is found only in the grains of wheat, oats, rye, and barley (17). As may be expected, the result of these changes is usually diarrhea and steatorrhea, flatulence, abdominal distention, weight loss, and weakness (17,21).

In the early stages of sprue, fat malabsorption is more typical than other nutrient malabsorption. This condition is often called ***idiopathic steatorrhea.*** In more severe cases of sprue, the absorption of proteins, carbohydrates, calcium, vitamin K, folate, and vitamin B_{12}, as well as other nutrients, becomes impaired. These malabsorptions can result in severe nutritional deficiencies, weight loss, osteomalacia, inadequate blood coagulation caused by lack of vitamin K, and macrocytic anemia of the pernicious anemia type as a result of vitamin B_{12} and folate malabsorption (20).

Medical nutrition therapy

Once gluten is removed from the diet, symptoms gradually improve during the following weeks and months. Intestinal mucosa subsequently returns to a near normal condition. There's only one catch—maintaining an asymptomatic state depends on lifelong avoidance of gluten (17).

Unfortunately, abstaining from wheat, oats, rye, and barley is not as simple as it may sound. Gluten-containing grains and products made from these grains are staples

Alternate terms for celiac disease
Celiac sprue
Nontropical sprue
Gluten-sensitive enteropathy
Gluten-induced enteropathy

idiopathic steatorrhea
fat malabsorption as a result of unknown causes

in the American diet, thanks to the use of emulsifiers, thickeners, and other additives in commercially processed foods (17). Patients must become ardent label readers since unintentional ingestion of gluten is the most common cause of recurrence of symptoms (17). Furthermore, availability of alternatives to wheat breads, crackers, and pasta is limited when eating away from home. And, as might be suspected, a diet that restricts these four grains can become boring (17). Table 16-5 summarizes gluten sources.

Dermatitis Herpetiformis

This is a chronic inflammatory disease of the skin that usually afflicts young or middle-aged adults. It is characterized by an itching, blistering rash that is often accompanied by jejunal lesions similar to those of sprue. The same gastrointestinal symptoms may be present, but often are not. Jejunal and skin lesions usually respond to the elimination of gluten from the diet (17,21).

Lactose Intolerance

The most common disaccharidase disorder is a deficiency of lactase, the enzyme that hydrolyzes lactose into glucose and galactose (see Chapter 4). This lactase deficiency leads to a condition referred to as *lactose intolerance.* More than half of the adults around the world are lactose intolerant (22). Undigested lactose remaining in the intestine will, through osmotic effect, draw water into the digestive tract, resulting in intestinal symptoms such as abdominal cramping, flatulence, and diarrhea. The severity of these symptoms depends on the amount of lactose ingested and the degree of intolerance an individual has (17).

Lactase deficiency sometimes occurs with acute or chronic diseases that damage the intestine such as sprue or Crohn's disease (23), or in persons who have had small bowel or gastric surgery (17). Extended use of central parenteral nutrition may cause atrophy of the small intestine, leading to lactase deficiency (17).

Medical nutrition therapy

Tolerance for lactose varies from person to person (17). For individuals who have or who are suspected of having lactose intolerance, health care professionals

Table 16-5   Sources of Gluten

Foods That Contain Gluten	Foods That May Contain Gluten
MEAT AND MEAT ALTERNATIVES Commercially breaded meats	Meat loaf and patties, cold cuts and other prepared meats, stuffing, cheese foods and other spreads; commercial soufflés, omelets, fondue; soy protein meat substitutes
GRAINS AND GRAIN PRODUCTS Bread, crackers, cereal, and pastas that contain wheat, oats, rye, malt, malt flavoring, graham flour, durum flour, pastry flour, bran, or wheat germ; barley; millet; pretzels; communion wafers	Commercially seasoned rice and potato mixes
VEGETABLES Commercially breaded vegetables or vegetables with a cream or cheese sauce	Commercially seasoned vegetable mixes; canned baked beans
FRUIT None	Commercial pie fillings
FATS AND OILS Commercial gravies, white and cream sauces	Commercial salad dressing, mayonnaise, nondairy creamer
SOUP Most commercial soup and soup mixes; soup that contains barley, wheat pasta; soup thickened with wheat flour or other gluten-containing grains	Broth
SWEETS Commercial cakes, cookies, pastries; commercial desert mixes	Commercial ice cream and sherbet, puddings; commercial candies, especially chocolates
BEVERAGES Milk beverages that contain malt; cereal beverages (Postum), malt, Ovaltine, beer and ale	Commercial chocolate milk; cocoa mixes; other beverage mixes; dietary supplements
MISCELLANEOUS*	Ketchup; prepared mustard; soy sauce; commercially prepared meat sauces and pickles; white vinegar; flavoring syrups (syrups for pancakes or ice cream)

Modified from Nelson JK et al: *Mayo Clinic diet manual,* ed 7, St. Louis, 1994, Mosby.
*Medications may contain trace amounts of gluten. A pharmacist may be able to provide information on the gluten content of medications.

need to establish the patient's tolerance by gradually adding small amounts of lactose-containing foods to a lactose-free diet. Most people can tolerate 5 to 8 grams of lactose at a given time, which is the amount in ½ cup of milk. Small amounts of lactose that are within the patient's tolerance level can generally be consumed on several occasions throughout the day. Individuals generally can tolerate lactose if it is consumed along with other foods, rather than alone as a beverage or a snack. Yogurt may be better tolerated than milk, but this varies with brand and processing method. Lactobacillus acidophilus milk is probably not better tolerated than regular milk. Cocoa and chocolate milk may be better tolerated. Lactase enzyme is available as Lactaid, Lactrase, or Dairy Ease and may be added to milk 24 hours in advance of ingestion. In addition, a tablet form is available that can be ingested just before eating a meal that contains lactose. Depending on the degree of intolerance, patients may use one-half to three tablets (17).

Restricting lactose-containing foods may place a person at risk for calcium, riboflavin, and vitamin D deficiency, depending on the degree of lactose restriction. These nutrients can be provided at the RDA level through the use of lactase enzyme-treated milk and milk products or with supplementation (17). Calcium is of particular importance to children and women. Vitamin D supplementation is necessary only for those individuals who do not obtain adequate exposure to sunlight (17).

Inflammatory Bowel Disease

Inflammatory bowel disease (IBD) refers to two idiopathic chronic inflammatory conditions of the intestines—**chronic ulcerative colitis (CUC)** and **Crohn's disease** (also called **regional enteritis**) (24). The major symptoms in IBD include abdominal pain, diarrhea, intestinal bleeding, protein loss, and fever, all of which result in nutritional depletion (17). Causes of nutritional depletion in IBD include decreased intake, malabsorption, increased nutrient loss, increased nutrient use and thus increased nutrient requirements, and drug-nutrient interactions. Proper management requires persistent attention to nutritional maintenance and/or repletion along with therapies to facilitate healing of the inflamed bowel that may include pharmacotherapy, surgery, and nutritional support (17,24). Surgery is curative in CUC, but Crohn's disease tends to recur following surgical resection of affected sections in the majority of patients (17).

Medical nutrition therapy

The goals of nutrition therapy are to replace nutrients that are lost as a result of the inflammatory process, correct deficits, and provide adequate nutrition to achieve and maintain energy, nitrogen, fluid, and electrolyte balance (17). Attention must be given to intestinal function including previous intestinal resections, site and extent of disease process (Fig. 16-5), and anticipated medical and surgical treatment.

When symptoms are under control in ulcerative colitis, a diet low in fiber (Table 16-6) may be best tolerated. As symptoms lessen, fiber can be introduced as tolerated. In patients with Crohn's disease, different nutrition guidelines are used, depending on the severity of symptoms. Table 16-7 summarizes dietary recommendations.

Colostomies and Ileostomies

Occasionally, when disease or obstruction cannot be resolved, all or a segment of the colon, including the rectum, is removed. Appropriate medical nutrition therapy depends on which procedure is performed. In the case of an **ileostomy**, the effluent is more liquid. Therefore water, sodium, and other minerals are lost, making fluid and electrolyte replacement an important goal. With a **colostomy**, the

chronic ulcerative colitis
an inflammatory process confined to the mucosa of any or all of the large intestine

Crohn's disease
an inflammatory disorder that involves all layers of the intestinal wall and may involve small or large intestine or both; is associated with stricture formation, fistulous tracts, and abscesses

regional enteritis
Crohn's disease

ileostomy
entire colon and rectum removed; surgical formation of an opening of the ileum onto the surface of the abdomen, through which fecal matter is emptied

colostomy
surgical creation of an artificial anus on the abdominal wall by incising the colon and bringing it out to the surface; may be single-barreled (one opening) or double-barreled (distal and proximal loops open onto the abdomen)

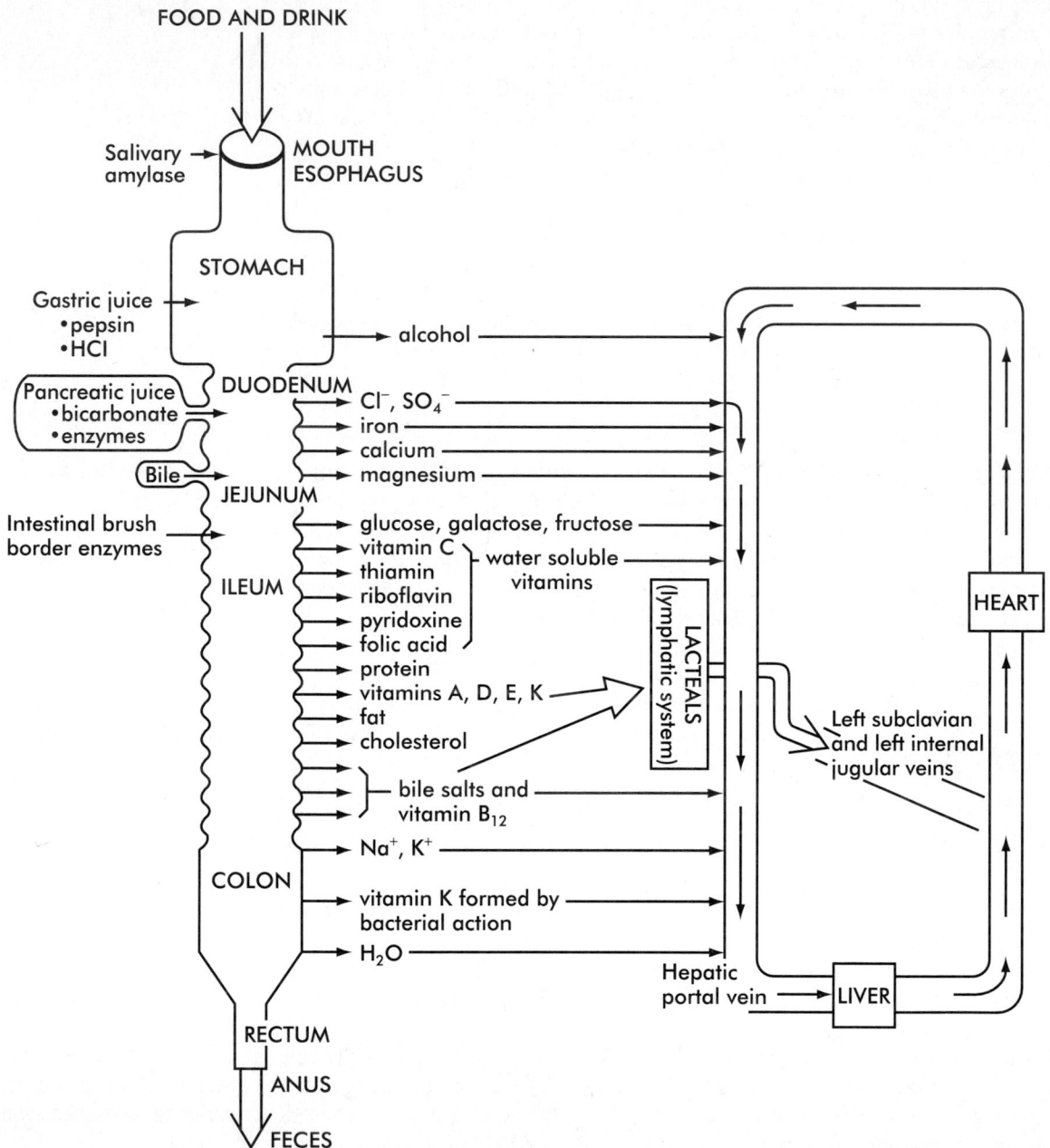

Fig. 16-5 Site and extent of disease process and effect on nutrient absorption.

Table 16-6   Guidelines for Fiber-Restricted Diets

Food Category	Foods Allowed	Foods Not Recommended
Beverages—as desired	Coffee, tea, carbonated beverages, strained or clear fruit juices and drinks, milk	Any containing fruit or vegetable pulp, any containing raw egg
Breads—limit to 3 servings per day	Refined breads, rolls, biscuits, muffins, crackers, pancakes, waffles, plain pastries	Any made with whole grain flour, bran, seeds, nuts, coconut, raw or dried fruits; cornbread, graham crackers
Cereals—limit to 1 serving per day	Refined cooked cereals (grits, farina, Cream of Wheat, Cream of Rice, Malt-O-Meal), refined dry cereals (Cheerios, cornflakes, Rice Krispies, puffed rice, puffed wheat, Special K, Kix, Sugar Smacks)	Oatmeal; any whole grain or bran cereal; granola cereals; any cereal containing seeds, nuts, coconut, or dried fruit
Fruits—limit to 1 serving per day	Canned or cooked fruits, applesauce, fruit cocktail, ripe banana	Dried fruit, all berries, raw fruits except bananas, all fruit not listed as allowed
Vegetables—limit to 2 servings per day	Most well-cooked and canned vegetables without seeds except those listed to avoid, lettuce if tolerated; tomato sauce, paste, and puree	Dried beans, peas, lentils, legumes; sauerkraut; winter squash; vegetables with seeds
Potatoes and potato substitutes—limit to 1 serving per day	Cooked white and sweet potatoes without skin; white rice; refined pasta	All others
Meat and meat substitutes—as desired	Well-cooked, tender meat, fish, poultry, organ meats; eggs, plain cheeses	Meats made with whole-grain ingredients, seeds, or nuts; dried beans, peas, lentils, legumes; peanut butter
Desserts and sweets—as desired	Plain cakes and cookies; pie made with allowed foods; plain sherbet, fruit ice, frozen pops, yogurt, gelatin, custard; jelly, plain hard candy, marshmallows, sugar, honey, ice cream	Any made with whole-grain flour, bran, seeds, nuts, coconut, or dried fruit
Fats—as desired	Margarine, butter, cream, salad oils, mayonnaise, bacon, plain gravies, salad dressings	Any containing whole-grain flour, bran, seeds, nuts, coconut, or dried fruit
Soups—as desired	Bouillon, broth, or cream soups made with allowed vegetables, noodles, rice, or flour; consomme	All others
Miscellaneous	Salt, pepper, sugar, spices, herbs, gravy, vinegar, ketchup, mustard	Nuts, coconut, seeds, popcorn

Modified from American Dietetic Association: *Handbook of clinical dietetics*, ed 2, New Haven, 1992, Yale University Press; and American Dietetic Association: *Manual of clinical dietetics*, ed 4, Chicago, 1992, American Dietetic Association.

Table 16-7   Guidelines for Medical Nutrition Therapy for Inflammatory Bowel Disease

Disease Severity	Nutritional Treatment	Nutritional Recommendations
Mild	Limit foods that are irritating and/or poorly absorbed	Decrease fiber intake, especially popcorn, seeds, nuts, fruit peels, broccoli, dried beans; restrict lactose-containing foods; Limit foods high in fat
Mild to moderate	Correct nutritional deficiencies, increase kcalorie intake	Increase kcalories intake 300-500 kcal/day; increase protein intake to 1.5-3 gm/day; supplement with multivitamin/mineral containing 100%-150% RDA
Moderate to severe	Bowel rest	Use elemental enteral formula orally or via feeding tube; if obstruction is almost total or fistula cannot be bypassed by feeding tube, use parenteral nutrition

Modified from Davis JR, Sherer K: *Applied nutrition and diet therapy for nurses,* ed 2, Philadelphia, 1994, Saunders.

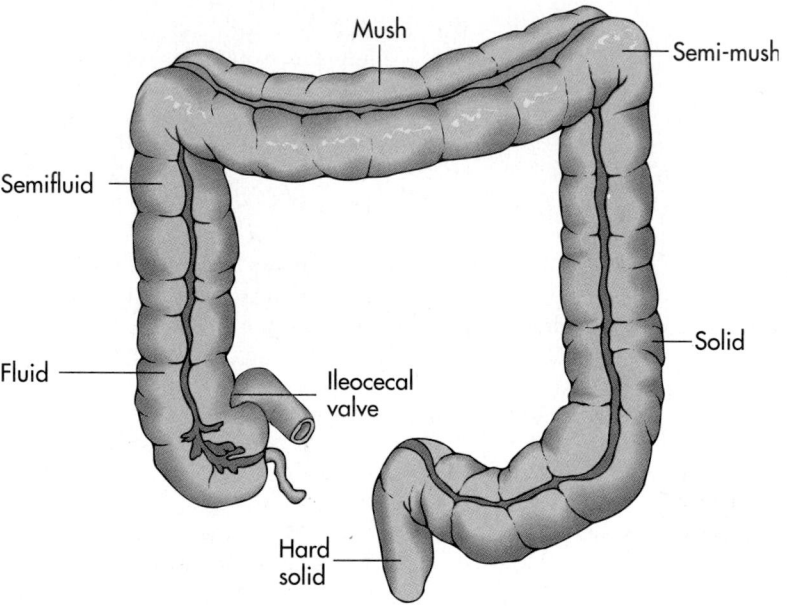

Fig. 16-6 Colostomy site and its effect on output. Excess motility causes less absorption and diarrhea or loose feces. Poor motility causes more absorption, resulting in hard feces and constipation.

effluent is proportional to the length of the remaining bowel (Fig. 16-6) (17). The more liquid the stool, the greater the loss of fluid and electrolytes. Any restrictions placed upon the patient should be based solely on individual tolerance in both cases (17). The Teaching Tool gives nutritional recommendations.

Short Bowel Syndrome

When the small intestine must be resected because of illness or injury, short bowel syndrome (SBS) may occur. Symptoms and resulting consequences of SBS depend on the site of resection, extent of small bowel removed, elapsed time since resection, absence or presence of ileocecal valve, condition of the remaining intestine, and whether or not there is colon continuity (17,25). The most common consequences are malabsorption, steatorrhea, and potential vitamin and mineral deficiencies (17).

TEACHING TOOL
Eating Well With a Colostomy or Ileostomy

Meals can still be an enjoyable experience for patients with colostomies and ileostomies. Individual experimentation works best to determine the most appropriate dietary restrictions. Strategies that may reduce negative symptoms are listed below.

RECOMMENDATION	REASON
Eat meals at regular times, at least 3 times per day.	Bowel pattern may be more regular.
Chew foods thoroughly.	Chewing well assists digestion and reduces the chance of stomal blockages.
Drink 8 to 10 cups of fluids each day.	Adequate fluids prevent constipation and dehydration.
Avoid gaining excessive weight.	Excess weight may affect stomal function.
Limit foods that may produce excessive gas or loose stools or that may not be completely digested (see list below).	*Colostomy:* Foods that have caused problems before surgery may continue to do so as they are digested before they reach the colon. *Ileostomy:* During the first 4 to 6 weeks, limit foods that have caused problems before surgery in order to decrease the chance for stomal blockage and to reduce the amount of gas and stool.
Eat a small evening meal.	This reduces nocturnal stool output.
Try new foods one at a time. Do not eliminate a food from the diet without trying it several times.	This helps determine food tolerance.

Gas-producing foods	Asparagus, beans, broccoli, Brussels sprouts, cabbage, carbonated beverages, cauliflower, onions
Incompletely digested foods	Cabbage, celery, coconut, corn, cucumbers, dried fruit, green peppers, lettuce seeds, mushrooms, nuts, olives, peas, pickles, pineapple, popcorn, spinach, tough skins from fruits and vegetables
Thickening foods	Applesauce, bananas, bread, cheese, pasta, peanut butter (creamy), starchy foods
Thinning foods	Apple juice, grape juice, prune juice, highly seasoned food
Odor-reducing foods	Buttermilk, cranberry juice, parsley, yogurt
Odor-producing foods	Asparagus, eggs, fish, garlic, onions

From Nelson JK et al: *Mayo Clinic diet manual,* ed 7, St. Louis, 1994, Mosby.

Medical nutrition therapy

Nutritional management should take into consideration the individual's digestive and absorptive capabilities. If the patient is unable to consume adequate nutrients or enteral nutrition exacerbates symptoms, then parenteral nutrition support is indicated; however, it is preferable to return to enteral feedings as soon as possible to prevent atrophy of the gastrointestinal tract. Dietary fat restriction and/or the use of **MCT fat** may be beneficial (17). Frequent monitoring of nutritional status, especially fluid and electrolyte balance, is crucial (26).

Diverticular Diseases

When the musculature of the bowel walls weaken, **diverticula** often develop, resulting in the condition **diverticulosis** (see Fig. 4-5). It is thought to develop as the

MCT fat (oil)
specialized modular formulas made of medium chain triglycerides that do not require pancreatic lipase or bile for digestion and absorption; they are absorbed directly into the portal vein (like amino acids and monosaccharides) rather than the lymphatic system like other lipids

diverticula
pouchlike herniations protruding from the muscular layer of the colon

diverticulosis
the presence of diverticula

result of long-term low-fiber eating habits and increased intracolonic pressure such as that created with straining to have a bowel movement (11). Usually, this condition remains undetected unless the diverticula become infected and inflamed from trapped fecal material and colon bacteria. This resulting complication is called **diverticulitis**.

diverticulitis
inflammation of one or more diverticula

Medical nutrition therapy

During periods of inflammation, the medical goal is to rest the bowel, allowing the infection to resolve. Patients are given nothing by mouth, then progress to clear liquids. As inflammation abates, the diet's fiber content is gradually increased to reduce straining during defecation. High fiber diets are planned to increase fiber-rich foods in the general diet such as fruits, vegetables, legumes, whole-grain breads, and cereals. Table 16-8 lists foods that can be used to increase fiber intake.

Although there is no Recommended Dietary Allowance for fiber, several health authorities have made recommendations for fiber intake that are reflected in the Food Guide Pyramid and the Dietary Guidelines for Americans in chapter 5. Translating these recommendations into real food, Americans should consume at least five servings of fruits/vegetables and six servings of breads/cereals/legumes per day.

Fiber should be added to the diet gradually to allow the intestinal tract to adapt (1,2). This minimizes potential adverse side effects such as abdominal distress, bloating, flatulence, cramps, and diarrhea, which are usually temporary and will abate after several days (2). Care should also be taken to consume adequate amounts of fluid, at least 8 to 12 cups per day (1,2).

Intestinal Gas and Flatulence

Excessive gas in the gastrointestinal tract can be the result of several factors. Belching is typically caused by the habit of swallowing air (**aerophagia**) while eating or drinking. Foods that contain high amounts of air, such as carbonated beverages, may also contribute to this problem. Aerophagia does not usually contribute to the formation of colon gas. The presence of *flatus* in the colon is the result of gases formed from food ingestion or fermentation of certain foods by intestinal bacteria. Typically, gas is reabsorbed through the colon wall as it passes through the bowel; but if motility is disturbed, bloating and distention may result, causing abdominal pain (17).

aerophagia
swallowing of air, usually the result of eating with the mouth open, followed by belching, gastric distress, and/or flatulence

Medical nutrition therapy

Since eating habits as well as foods eaten can contribute to excess gas production, a thorough appraisal of the patient's usual eating pattern and habits is necessary. Specific treatment depends on the source of the gas (Table 16-9) (17). Gas-forming foods can be avoided on a trial basis to determine if they are a source of discomfort. Remaining upright for 30 minutes after meals also may be beneficial.

Constipation

There are many causes of *constipation*. Organic causes include intestinal obstruction, spasms of the sigmoid colon, diverticulitis, and tumors. The most common cause of functional constipation is failure to respond to the urge to defecate (28). Other functional causes include lack of fiber and/or fluid, prolonged bed rest or lack of regular exercise, or habitual use of laxatives or enemas. When these conditions are untreated, the colon becomes **atonic** (20). Many women experience constipation during the last trimester of pregnancy as the growing fetus impairs the passage of feces.

atonic
lacking normal muscle tone

Table 16-8 Foods High in Fiber

Food	Serving Size	Approximate Grams of Fiber	Number of Servings
BREADS/STARCHES		2	5 plus ≤ 5 additional servings of refined breads/ starches
Whole grain or rye bread	1 slice		
Whole grain bagel or pita bread	½		
Oat bran muffin	½		
Whole wheat crackers, crisp breads	4		
Whole wheat pasta, corn, peas	½ cup		
Sweet potato, brown rice	⅓ cup		
Potato with skin	1 small		
Popcorn, air popped	3 cups		
Wheat germ	1½ Tbsp		
Corn or flour tortilla	1		
CEREALS		4	1
Whole-grain or bran cereals, cold	1 oz		
Oatmeal, oat bran, grits	⅓ cup dry		
VEGETABLES		2	3 plus ≤ 2 additional servings of other vegetables or juices
Cooked—asparagus, green beans, broccoli, cabbage, carrots, cauliflower, greens, onions, snow peas, spinach, squash, canned tomatoes	½ cup		
Raw—broccoli, cabbage, carrots, cauliflower, tomatoes, celery, green peppers, zucchini	1 cup		
FRUITS		2.5	2 plus ≤ 2 additional servings of other fruits or juices
Apple, nectarine, orange, peach, banana	1 medium		
Grapefruit, pear	½		
Berries	1 cup		
BEANS		5	1
Garbonzo beans, kidney beans, lentils, lima beans, split peas, pinto beans, other beans and peas	½ cup cooked		
NUTS AND SEEDS		1	Optional (high in fat)
Almonds	10 whole		
Walnuts	6 whole		
Peanut butter	1 Tbsp		
Peanuts	15		
Sesame seeds	1 Tbsp		
Sunflower seeds	2 Tbsp		

Modified from American Dietetic Association: *Manual of clinical dietetics,* ed 4, Chicago, 1992, American Dietetic Association; and American Dietetic Association, *Handbook of clinical dietetics,* ed 2, New Haven, 1992, Yale University Press.

Table 16-9 Factors That Contribute to Intestinal Gas and Flatulence	
FOODS THAT MAY CAUSE GAS	Dried beans and peas, baked beans, soybeans, lima beans, lentils, cabbage, radishes, onions, broccoli, Brussels sprouts, cauliflower, cucumbers, sauerkraut, kohlrabi, rutabaga Dried fruit (especially prunes and raisins), apples, bananas Bran cereals, excessive amounts of wheat products, excessive amounts of fruit Lactose-containing foods such as milk, ice cream, ice milk, cream Sorbitol and mannitol (artificial sweeteners found in some *dietetic* candies and sugar-free gums) High-fat foods such as fried foods, fatty meats, rich cream sauces, gravies, pastries
SOURCES OF SWALLOWED AIR	Frequent, repetitive swallowing that may be caused by ill-fitting dentures, chewing gum or tobacco, sucking on hard candy, or sipping beverages Eating rapidly and gulping foods and/or beverages "Drawing" on straws, narrow-mouthed bottles, cigars, cigarettes, pipes Foods containing air such as carbonated beverages, whipped cream Talking (a lot) while eating
OTHER FACTORS	Reclining after meals Inactivity Stress

Modified from Nelson JK et al: *Mayo Clinic diet manual,* ed 7, St. Louis, 1994, Mosby.

megacolon
massive, abnormal dilation of the colon that may be congenital, toxic, or acquired in nature

If constipation becomes severe, bowel movements may diminish in frequency to only once every week or so. This allows tremendous quantities of fecal material to accumulate in the colon, causing its diameter to distend to a diameter as great as 3 to 4 inches. This condition, **megacolon,** can occur because of a number of reasons. Congenital megacolon (also known as Hirschsprung's disease) is the result of lack or deficiency of autonomic ganglion cells in the smooth muscle wall of the colon (20,28). Consequently, neither defecation reflexes or peristaltic motility can occur through this area of the large intestine (20). Toxic megacolon is a complication of ulcerative colitis and may result in perforation of the colon, septicemia, and death. The most common treatment for congenital and toxic megacolon is surgery (28). Acquired megacolon results from chronic refusal to defecate, with the colon becoming dilated by an accumulation of impacted feces. Laxatives and enemas are often the necessary treatment (28).

Medical nutrition therapy

Although laxatives are commonly chosen for self-treatment, diet is usually the treatment of choice for constipation. Recommendations include consuming adequate fluids and a wide variety of foods that contain ample amounts of fiber (see Table 16-8) (17). Fiber is important in providing bulk in the diet, which stimulates peristalsis. Care should be taken to increase fiber in the diet gradually to avoid any potential adverse reactions. Although dietary fiber cannot be digested by humans, it can be broken down by bacteria that live in our intestine. As a consequence, flatulence and **osmotic diarrhea** may result.

osmotic diarrhea
diarrhea associated water retention in the large intestine resulting from an accumulation of nonabsorbable water-soluble solutes

Some foods high in fiber are also high in phytates and oxalate, which decrease the bioavailability of certain vitamins and minerals (29), namely calcium, copper, selenium, zinc, iron, and magnesium (1,2). Nutrient deficiencies are unlikely, however, if an adequate balanced diet from a variety of foods is consumed (30). The body may be able to adjust to the decreased availability of nutrients by increased absorption of those available (1,2).

Corpulent amounts of fiber, particularly wheat bran, may result in the formation of **bezoars** in some persons. This tends to occur more commonly in persons who have diabetes and who suffer from gastroparesis (2). (See Chapter 18 for more information about gastroparesis.)

Diarrhea

Diarrhea (like constipation), is a symptom, not a disease. It is usually categorized in one of two ways: acute or chronic. Treatment is determined by the cause. Acute diarrhea is typically of short duration and is usually the result of **enteritis**. Table 2-4 in chapter 2 lists common food-borne pathogens that may cause diarrhea. Other causes of acute diarrhea include the intended effect or side effects of medications, change in dietary habits or intake, or emotional stress. Diarrhea that lasts longer than 2 weeks is considered to be of a chronic nature. Long-term diarrhea is usually the result of gastrointestinal irritation or malabsorption. Both may necessitate permanent dietary changes (17).

Medical nutrition therapy

Medical nutrition therapy is based on the cause of diarrhea. In severe cases, the patient may be restricted to nothing by mouth to rest the gastrointestinal tract; however, it is usually unnecessary to withhold all feedings (31). Administration of fluids to achieve and/or maintain hydration is a primary concern. This may be done with enteral or parenteral fluids (carbohydrate and electrolytes). Enteral therapy may consist of oral rehydration solutions and/or a clear liquid diet for 1 or 2 days before progressing to a low-fat, low-fiber, and/or low-lactose diet. Small, frequent meals are often better tolerated than three larger meals. After 2 or 3 days, progression to a general or normal diet is usually tolerated (17). It is also important to educate the patient regarding cause and prevention of subsequent incidences of diarrhea (17).

bezoars
physical obstacles created by tangles of fibrous material in the gastrointestinal tract that may cause dangerous gastrointestinal obstructions

enteritis
infection of the small intestine caused by a virus, bacteria, or protozoa

---

WELLNESS AND DISORDERS OF THE GASTROINTESTINAL TRACT

Physical Dimension	The physical dimension of health is most affected if the disorder is chronic and intensifies over time; eventually weight loss and nutrient deficiencies pose other health risks in addition to the primary gastrointestinal tract disorder.
Intellectual Dimension	Intellectual health is tested as the patient, caregivers, and dietetic and nursing staff devise food combinations and textures that are physically and aesthetically acceptable to the patient; other disorders require constant vigilance to restrict inadvertent consumption of problematic substances such as gluten for patients experiencing celiac disease.
Emotional Dimension	Emotional health may be taxed when patients struggle with acceptance of dietary and/or physical limitations; nurses can refer patients to disorder support groups as an additional therapeutic strategy.
Social Dimension	Some disorders may affect social functioning. Nurses can provide patients with social strategies for dealing with the physical ramifications of colostomies, dumping syndrome, and other disorders.

SUMMARY

Disorders of the gastrointestinal tract include those affecting the esophagus, the stomach, small intestine, and large intestine. Some of the disorders affect the muscular action of organs, thereby affecting the flow of sustenance through the gastrointestinal tract; these include dysphagia and hiatal hernia. Other disorders, such as peptic ulcer and diverticulitis, lead to tissue inflammation and pain. Several may be caused by the inability of the body to produce necessary digestive enzymes such as in lactose intolerance, or the inability to metabolize nutrient substances resulting in severe reactions caused by celiac disease. Most of the disorders are additionally influenced by lifestyle behaviors affecting levels of stress and altering dietary patterns. All require medical nutritional therapy individualized to meet the needs of each patient.

THE NURSING ROLE

Impaired Swallowing and Weight Loss: The Nursing Process

Mr. Klein was diagnosed with amyotrophic lateral sclerosis (ALS) 2 years ago. He experienced weakness of the upper arms that progressed to the legs. He is now bed/chair-bound and is beginning to have speech difficulties and dysphagia, with a diminished gag reflex. Mr. Klein is cared for at home by his family and home health aides. Registered nurses visit Mr. Klein at least once a week to evaluate and adjust his care.

ASSESSMENT DATA COLLECTED

Subjective:

Increase in the episodes of choking and regurgitation while being fed (now about one episode every day)

Choking usually precipitated by intake of thin fluids

Amount of time to chew and swallow food has been increasing over the past few months

Objective:

Fluid intake about 800 cc per day

Height 5'10"

Weight 130 lb with weight loss of about 2 lb per month for the last few months

NURSING DIAGNOSIS 1

Impaired swallowing related to weakness of head and neck muscles as evidenced by increased time necessary to chew and swallow and increase in choking episodes.

PLANNING

Goals are set in conjunction with Mr. Klein and his wife:

Patient will experience a decrease in number of choking episodes (less than one per day) within one week

THE NURSING ROLE, cont'd.
Impaired Swallowing and Weight Loss: The Nursing Process

INTERVENTION
1. Test gag reflex every morning
2. Feed only while in upright position
3. Feed slowly in small amounts
4. Avoid thin fluids; thicken juices and water with gelatin, put ice cream in milk
5. Do not use liquids to clear solid food from the mouth, remind patient to swallow food when it remains
6. Have patient take a breath before swallowing, hold breath during swallowing, and exhale forcefully after swallowing

EVALUATION
The achievement of the goal will be evidenced by a fewer number of choking/regurgitation episodes this week compared to last week.

NURSING DIAGNOSIS 2
Altered nutrition, less than body requirements of fluid and kcalories, related to difficulty swallowing, as evidenced by weight loss and fluid intake of only 800 cc per day.

PLANNING
The goals are:
Patient will maintain weight at present level
Patient will increase fluid intake to 1200 cc within 2 weeks

INTERVENTION
1. Use custard, gelatin, and liquid nutritional supplements to increase fluid and kcalorie intake between meals for a total of 3 supplements per day
2. Fluid intake pattern: 300 cc with each meal, the remaining 900 cc between meals and after supper
3. Weigh patient once a week on Mondays at 9 AM on chair scale

EVALUATION
The goals will be evaluated to see if the outcomes have been met as evidenced by:
Record of 1200 cc daily fluid intake after 2 weeks
Weight of 130 lb at each weekly weighing
As Mr. Klein's condition continues to worsen, swallowing and its accompanying problems may get worse, necessitating standby suction, or eventually, gastrostomy tube insertion.

Critical Thinking **CLINICAL APPLICATIONS**

T.E. is a 35-year-old female admitted with microcytic anemia. Her past medical history indicates that she underwent a total gastrectomy 2 years ago for the treatment of bleeding ulcers. Upon admission she weighs 120 lb and she is 5'9" tall. She has lost 30 lb since the surgery. She has been taking ferrous sulfate and monthly injections of vitamin B_{12}. On admission her labs are as follows: hemoglobin 8.0 gm/dl; hematocrit 26%; serum albumin 2.7 gm/dl. Her typical dietary intake is as follows:

Breakfast	10 AM	Lunch
1 egg scrambled in 1 tsp margarine	6 saltine crackers	2 baked chicken wings
½ c cream of wheat with 1 tsp margarine	12-oz can diet cola	1 c cooked carrots
1 slice white toast with 1 tsp margarinee		1 medium boiled red potato
1 c black coffe		1 medium banana
		12 oz diet lemon/lime soda

3 PM	Dinner	9 PM
½ bagel with 1 tbsp cream cheese	1 broiled chicken breast	6 saltine crackers
8 oz chocolate milk	½ c steamed broccoli	1 tbsp peanut butter
	1 c hot tea with artificial sweetener	1 c black coffee

1. What are common nutrition problems found in patients who have gastrectomies?
2. Which of these problems were experienced by T.E.?
3. What factors explain iron deficiency anemia that develops after a gastrectomy? What is used to treat this anemia?
4. How do T.E.'s laboratory values compare with normal values? What do these values indicate?
5. Why is T.E. receiving monthly injections of vitamin B_{12}? Would you advise her to eat more foods high in B_{12}? Explain your rationale.
6. After reviewing T.E.'s usual dietary intake, what food groups and/or nutrients are lacking in her diet?
7. What suggestions would you offer T.E. concerning her dietary habits?
8. Should T.E. continue to consume six smaller meals and snacks? Why or why not?

REFERENCES

1. American Dietetic Association: *Handbook of clinical dietetics,* ed 2, New Haven, 1992, Yale University Press.
2. American Dietetic Association: *Manual of clinical dietetics,* ed 4, Chicago, 1992, American Dietetic Association.
3. Sitzmann JV: Nutritional support of the dysphagic patient: Methods, risks and complications of therapy, *Journal of Parenteral and Enteral Nutrition* 14:60-63, 1990.
4. Vaneck AW, Diamant N: Responses of the human esophagus to paired swallows, *Gastroenterology* 92:643-650, 1987.
5. Dooley CP, Schlossmacher B, Valenzuela JF: Effects of alterations in bolus viscosity on esophageal peristalsis in humans, *Am J Physiol* 254:8-11, 1988.

6. Kaye MD, Kilby AE, Harper PC: Changes in distal esophageal function in response to cooling, *Dig Dis Sci* 32:22-27, 1987.

7. Dooley CP, Schlossmacher B, Valenzuela JF: Modulation of esophageal peristalsis by alterations of body position: Effect of bolus viscosity, *Dig Dis Sci* 34:1662-1667, 1989.

8. Milazzo LS, Buchard J, Lund DA: The swallowing process: Effects of aging and stroke. In Erickson RV: Medical management of the elderly stroke patient, *Phys Med Rehab* 3:489-499, 1989.

9. Loustau A, Lee KA: Dealing with the dangers of dysphagia, *Nursing* 15:47-50, 1985.

10. Hill JW, Deluca SA: Achalasia, *Am Fam Phys* 37:201-203, 1988.

11. Swearingen PL: *Manual of nursing therapeutics,* ed 4, St. Louis, 1995, Mosby.

12. Zeman FJ: *Clinical nutrition and dietetics,* ed 2, New York, 1991, Macmillan.

13. Sontag SJ et al: Effect of positions, eating and bronchodilators on gastroesophageal reflux in asthmatics, *Dig Dis Sci* 35:849-856, 1990.

14. Mansfield LE: Gastroesophageal reflux and respiratory disorders: A review, *Ann Allergy* 62:158-163, 1989.

15. Gaska J, Tietze K: Current concepts in the treatment of peptic ulcer disease: A case-oriented approach. Part 1, *Am Pharmacol* NS29:49-55, 1989.

16. Flier JS, Underhill LH: Pathogenesis of peptic ulcer and implications for therapy, *N Eng J Med* 322:909-915, 1990.

17. Nelson JK et al: *Mayo Clinic diet manual* ed 7, St. Louis, 1994, Mosby.

18. Meyer JH: The stomach and nutrition. In Shils ME, Olson JA, Shike M, eds: *Modern nutrition in health and disease,* ed 8, Philadelphia, 1994, Lea & Febiger.

19. Borgström B et al: Studies of intestinal digestion and absorption in the human, *J Clin Invest* 36:1521-1536, 1957.

20. Guyton AC: *Textbook of medical physiology,* ed 8, Philadelphia, 1991, Saunders.

21. Kelly CP et al: Diagnosis and treatment of gluten-sensitive enteropathy, *Avd Intern Med* 35:341-363, 1990.

22. Macdonald I: Carbohydrates. In Shils ME, Olson JA, Shike M, eds: *Modern nutrition in health and disease,* ed 8, Philadelphia, 1994, Lea & Febiger.

23. Pironi L et al: Lactose malabsorption in adult patients with Crohn's disease, *Am J Gastroenterol* 83:1267-1271, 1988.

24. Rosenberg IH, Mason JB: Inflammatory bowel disease. In Shils ME, Olson JA, Shike M, eds: *Modern nutrition in health and disease,* ed 8, Philadelphia,1994, Lea & Febiger.

25. Purdum PP, Kirby DF: Short bowel syndrome: A review of the role of nutritional support, *Journal of Parenteral and Enteral Nutrition* 15:93-101, 1991.

26. Williams SR: *Essentials of nutrition and diet therapy,* ed 6, St. Louis, 1994, Mosby.

27. Slavin JL: Dietary fiber: Classification, chemical analyses, and food sources, *J Am Diet Assoc* 87:1162, 1987.

28. *Mosby's medical, nursing, and allied health dictionary,* ed 3, St. Louis, 1990, Mosby.

29. Position of the American Dietetic Association: Health implications of dietary fiber, *J Am Diet Assoc* 93:1446-1447, 1993.

30. Federation of American Societies for Experimental Biology, Council on Scientific Affairs: Dietary fiber and health, *JAMA* 262:542-546, 1989.

31. Davis JR, Sherer K: *Applied nutrition and diet therapy for nurses,* ed 2, Philadelphia, 1994, Saunders.

Chapter 17

NUTRITION FOR DISORDERS OF THE LIVER, GALLBLADDER, AND PANCREAS

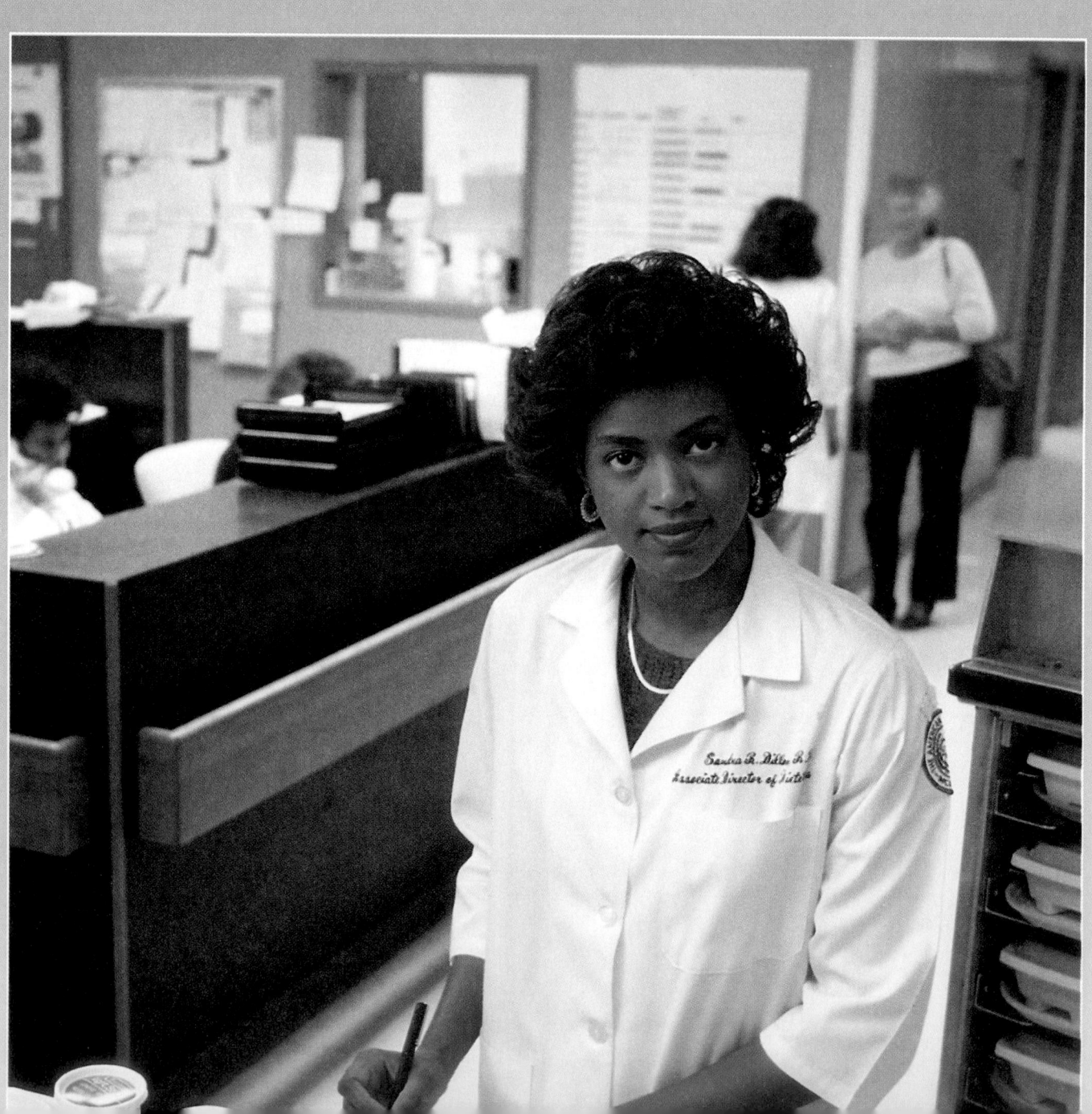

ROLE IN WELLNESS

Although they are not part of the digestive tract proper, little digestion, absorption, or metabolism would take place without the liver, gallbladder, and pancreas. Disease or injury to these ancillary digestive organs can have a devastating effect on nutritional status. Medical nutrition therapy is part of the treatment for disorders of the liver, gallbladder, and pancreas; it is also necessary to prevent nutritional deficiencies because of the role of these organs on digestive functioning.

LIVER DISORDERS

The liver, the largest organ in the body, lies beneath the diaphragm in the right upper quadrant of the abdomen (see Fig. 3-6, p. 67) and is responsible for the majority of biochemical functions that take place in the body. Nutritional status is influenced by the liver's management of bile production and its role in intermediary metabolism of carbohydrates, protein, lipids, and vitamins (1). Thus it is easy to understand that impaired liver function can result in major imbalances of metabolic and nutritional status. And, as you will see in so many diseases, progressive decline of nutritional status can further impair liver function (2). Fig. 17-1 summarizes the role of the liver in metabolism and nutritional status.

Fatty Liver

Fatty liver (also called *hepatic steatosis*) is typically a symptom of an underlying problem. It is the earliest form of alcoholic liver disease, but can also be caused by excessive kcaloric intake, obesity, complications of drug therapy (corticosteroids, tetracyclines), total parenteral nutrition (TPN), pregnancy (3), inadequate intake of protein (as seen in kwashiorkor), infection, or malignancy. Fatty infiltration of the liver develops when triglycerides build up in the liver tissue, which will eventually produce an enlarged liver. This infiltration is a function of improper fat metabolism. It can be reversed if the causative agent is removed (3). Therefore if alcohol abuse is the culprit, then abstinence from alcohol is necessary to reverse the infiltration and prevent further fibrosis or necrosis. Whatever the cause, proper nutrition in the form of a well-balanced diet is important in reversing fatty infiltration.

Hepatitis

Defined as inflammation of the liver, acute hepatitis can occur as the result of infectious mononucleosis, cirrhosis, toxic chemicals, or viral infection. There are six types of hepatitis, and although symptomatology is similar, immunological and epidemiological characteristics are different.

Type A hepatitis is usually transmitted through the fecal-oral route, and large scale outbreaks caused by food and drinking water contamination can occur (4). It is most often the result of poor hand washing and/or stool precautions, and is common in overcrowded areas with poor sanitation. Onset is rapid, usually within 2 to 6 weeks (5). Type B and type C (previously called non-A, non-B) hepatitis are transmitted through contaminated blood, saliva, or semen, although type C is predominately associated with blood exposure, for example, transfusion or IV drug use (4). Type C hepatitis is diagnosed only when types A and B have been ruled out (5). Onset for Types B and C is usually slow, anywhere from 6 weeks to 6 months, and can develop into some form of chronic liver disease (5,6). Type D hepatitis

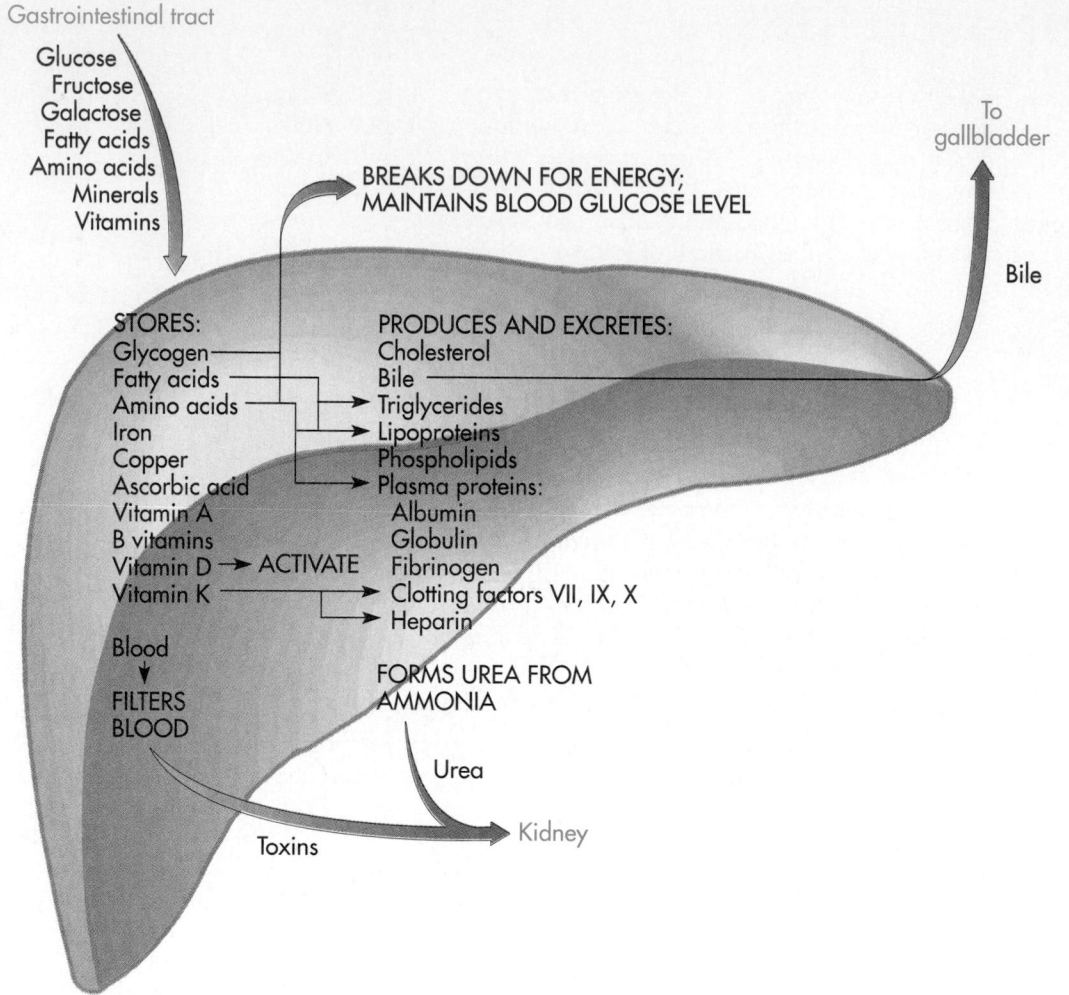

Fig. 17-1 Role of the liver in metabolism and nutrition. Any damage to the liver may affect nutritional status.

jaundice
yellow discoloration of the skin, mucous membranes, and sclerae of the eyes caused by greater than normal amounts of bilirubin in the blood

fatty infiltration
accumulation of fat (triglycerides) in the liver

necrosis
localized tissue death that occurs in response to disease or injury

hepatic coma
neuropsychiatric symptom of extensive liver damage caused by chronic or acute liver disease

infection can only occur if an individual with chronic hepatitis type B is subsequently exposed to hepatitis type D (superinfection), or if an individual is simultaneously infected with both hepatitis types B and D (coinfection) (4). Hepatitis D is found throughout the world but is endemic to the Mediterranean basin, the Middle East, and portions of South America.

Outside these areas, infections occur predominately in persons who have received multiple transfusions and, in the United States, in IV drug users (4). Transmission of hepatitis E closely resembles that of hepatitis A and has been implicated in epidemics in areas of the world such as India, Southeast Asia, Africa, and Mexico (4). Non-A, non-B hepatitis is the exclusionary classification of hepatitis viruses that remain when serologic tests for other viruses are negative. As noted above, previously hepatitis C constituted a significant portion of this group. Non-A, Non-B occurs sporadically, usually following blood exposure (4).

Regardless of the cause, symptomatology of hepatitis viruses is similar: nausea, fever, liver tenderness and enlargement, **jaundice,** pale stools, and anorexia. Normally, hepatitis is reversible after recovery from the acute phase; however, in some instances, expanded liver damage (**fatty infiltration** and/or **necrosis**) can lead to **hepatic coma,** liver failure, or death (5,6).

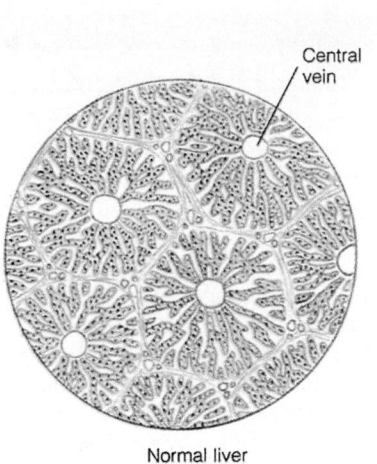
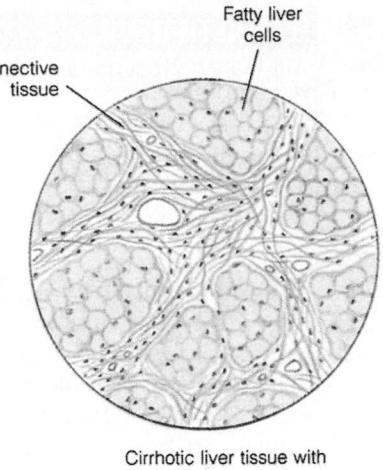

Normal liver
tissue structure

Cirrhotic liver tissue with
scarring and fatty infiltration

Fig. 17-2 Comparison of normal liver tissue structure with cirrhotic liver tissue changes.

Medical nutrition therapy

Treatment for all types of hepatitis is the same. Since there are no medications to treat hepatitis, bed rest and proper nutrition are the major constituents of therapy. During periods of nausea and vomiting, hydration via intravenous fluids is necessary.

Oral feedings should be initiated as soon as possible, beginning with a liquid diet then progressing to small, frequent feedings that are high in kcalories (3000 to 4000 kcal) and high quality protein (100 grams to 150 grams or 1.5 to 2.0 g/kg body weight) as tolerated. Carbohydrates should provide at least 40% of the kcalories to promote glycogen synthesis and spare protein. Dietary fats should not be limited unless they are not well tolerated (as in steatorrhea). Fat plays an important role in providing concentrated kcalories and making food taste better, which is very important when trying to get a lot of kcalories into a patient who probably doesn't have much of an appetite. Fluid intake should be high (2500 to 3000 ml/day) to accommodate the high protein intake unless otherwise contraindicated. Supplementation with a multivitamin that includes vitamin B complex (especially thiamine and vitamin B_{12} because of decreased absorption and/or hepatic uptake of these vitamins), vitamin K (to normalize bleeding tendency), vitamin C, and zinc for poor appetite is recommended (6).

Cirrhosis

Cirrhosis is a chronic degenerative disease in which liver cells are replaced by the buildup of fibrous connective tissue and fat infiltration (Fig. 17-2). This damage can be the result of several insults: **alcohol** (see Health Debate box), hepatitis (**postnecrotic**), **biliary** disorders, chronic autoimmune disease, metabolic disorders (**Wilson's disease** or **hemochromatosis**), or chronic use of **hepatotoxic** drugs (Table 17-1). These insults cause liver cells to die, and the formation of new cells results in scarring that can cause congestion of hepatic circulation (blood backing up in the portal vein), which results in further decline of liver function, **portal hypertension, and esophageal varices.**

Esophageal varices are the result of collateral circulation that develops around the esophagus when normal blood flow through the liver is blocked. The blood vessels tend to be large and bulge into the lumen of the esophagus where they may

alcoholic cirrhosis
associated with chronic alcohol abuse, accounts for 50% of all cases, also called Laennec's cirrhosis

postnecrotic cirrhosis
associated with history of viral hepatitis, improperly treated hepatitis, or hepatic damage from toxic chemicals; accounts for about 20% of all cases

biliary cirrhosis
associated with obstruction of biliary drainage or biliary disorders, accounts for 15% of all cases

Wilson's disease
a rare, inherited disorder of copper metabolism in which copper accumulates slowly in the liver and is then released and taken up in other parts of the body; as copper accumulates in RBCs, hemolysis, then hemolytic anemia occur

hemochromatosis
a rare disease of iron metabolism characterized by excess iron deposits throughout the body

hepatotoxic
potentially destructive to liver cells

portal hypertension
increased blood pressure in the portal circulation caused by compression or occlusion in the portal or hepatic vascular system

esophageal varices
large and swollen veins at the lower end of the esophagus that are especially vulnerable to ulceration and hemorrhage, usually the result of portal hypertension

HEALTH DEBATE
Alcohol: Proscribe or Prescribe?

Alcohol is probably the most commonly used hepatotoxic drug. Next to caffeine, it is probably the most socially acceptable drug in the United States. It is legal, but sales are regulated by state-controlled establishments, and anything stronger than beer or wine cannot be advertised on television. The advertisements we do see give us the message that if we would just drink a specific brand of beer or wine we would: (1) be more athletic, (2) become very good pool players, (3) become irresistible to a gorgeous male/female, (4) hike through the Rocky Mountains, (5) fulfill a deep desire to become an English bulldog with an attitude, and/or (6) pretend we're jet-setters by drinking imported beer.

However, we get negative messages too, and rightly so. Alcohol's link to birth defects and traffic accidents is well accepted. Heavy alcohol intake (three or more drinks* daily) causes damage to the liver (such as fatty liver and cirrhosis), brain, and heart and increases the risk of cancer. Could any possible good come from such a drug? Well, it seems so. Present research indicates that alcohol *may* decrease the risk of heart disease.

Several population studies have found a lower coronary artery disease mortality risk among moderate drinkers (defined as one to two drinks daily) as compared to non-drinkers. At first it looked as if red wine was the magic elixir, but white wine, beer, and hard liquor seem to be just as beneficial. On the other hand, it appears the more one drinks, the greater the risk of developing certain cancers. Chronic, heavy drinking is associated with cancers of the mouth, throat, larynx, and liver. Moderate alcohol consumption has been linked to cancers of the breast, colon, and rectum.

So what's a person to do? Don't drink if: you do not currently drink, you're pregnant or trying to conceive, you're taking medication, you'll be driving, or you're unable to control your drinking. The dangers outweigh any possible benefits. If you're concerned about heart disease and drink small quantities of alcohol every day or every other day, you're probably OK. Remember that *alcohol is a drug.* And like any drug, it is most effective when administered at the appropriate dosage. It may be beneficial to discuss this matter with your personal physician.

From Forman A: Tapping the benefits of alcohol: A drink a day? *Environmental Nutrition,* 17:1,6, Mar 1994; Klatsky AL, Armstrong MA: Alcoholic beverage choice and risk of coronary artery disease mortality: Do red wine drinkers fare best? *Am J Cardiol* 71:467-469, 1993; and Kris-Etherton PM: Abstract, *Perspectives in Applied Nutrition,* 1:34-35, 1993.
*One drink equals 12 oz of beer, 5 oz of wine, or 1½ oz of hard liquor.

Table 17-1   Hepatotoxic Drugs

Acetaminophen*	Isoniazid (INH)
Alcohol*	Ketoconazole
Allopurinol	Mercaptopurine (6-MP)
Amiodarone	Methotrexate (MTX)
Androgenic steroids	Methyldopa
Aspirin and other salicylates*	Mitomycin
Carbamazepine	Monoamine oxidase (MAO) inhibitors
Carmustine (BiCNU)	NSAIDs
Chlorpromazine (CPZ)	Oral contraceptives
Cyclosporine	Oxacillin
Dantrolene	Phenindione
Diazepam	Phenylbutazone
Erythromycin	Phenytoin sodium
Glucocorticoids	Rifampin
Haloperidol	Sulfonamides
Halothane and related anesthetics	Vitamin A*

From Swearingen PL: *Manual of nursing therapeutics,* ed 3, St. Louis, 1994, Mosby.
*Available without prescription

rupture. This bleeding tends to recur and can eventually be fatal. Patients with esophageal varices should be given soft, low-fiber foods. Another complication of cirrhosis, **ascites,** is the result of increased pressure in the portal vein (portal hypertension), which forces plasma out of the blood vessels into the abdominal cavity (7). This causes the characteristic swollen or distended abdomen so often seen in patients with cirrhosis. Ascites disappears if the causes are eliminated (8). To treat patients with ascites, a dietary sodium restriction (500 to 1000 mg) is used, sometimes along with a fluid restriction of 1000 to 1500 ml per day (6). If diuretics are used, attention should be given to whether the drug depletes or spares potassium. If a potassium-depleting diuretic is used, potassium levels should be monitored.

As liver disease continues to progress, blood is shunted from the portal circulation to the systemic circulation. This causes blood to bypass the liver, resulting in **hepatic encephalopathy,** which if left untreated can lead to hepatic coma. As a result, toxins are not eliminated from the body and nutrient metabolism is compromised (especially amino acids), which has been causally linked to the development of hepatic encephalopathy (3). Patients with hepatic encephalopathy will experience changes in consciousness, behavior, loss of concentration and memory, confusion, apathy, personality changes, and other psychiatric symptoms (3,9). Neurological changes include spasticity, muscle spasms, asterixis or *flapping* (involuntary jerky movements, especially of the hands), **athetoid** postures, and rigidity of the limbs with flexion withdrawal of the lower limbs (3,6).

Although the exact cause of hepatic encephalopathy is unknown, several factors have been implicated (9). Excessive ammonia and nitrogenous waste, accumulation of false neurotransmitters, and a deficiency in branched-chain amino acids (BCAA) are proposed mechanisms that are related to protein metabolism (3). Increased blood ammonia levels can be caused by decreased production of urea (result of impaired liver function), increased bacterial production of ammonia in the intestine from available nitrogen substrates (dietary protein, gastrointestinal bleeding), enterohepatic circulation of urea, renal failure (increased availability of urea for enterohepatic circulation), and constipation (increased ammonia production and prolonged transit time, which allows increased absorption) (9). Several methods are used to lower ammonia levels, but each has potential side effects. Neomycin is an antibiotic used to reduce the numbers of bacteria in the gastrointestinal tract thus decreasing the amount of urea that can be converted to ammonia (6). Neomycin treatment allows more protein to be included in the diet for tissue regeneration. One disadvantage of neomycin use is that it contributes to malabsorption of most nutrients and can cause nausea, vomiting, and diarrhea (6). Another method is use of Lactulose, a nonabsorbable disaccharide that is metabolized by intestinal bacteria. This decreases ammonia and aromatic amino acid formation and improves tolerance to dietary protein (6). It has a laxative action and diarrhea is common.

In a healthy liver, aromatic amino acids (AAAs) are catabolized and BCAAs pass through the portal circulation into the systemic circulation. In chronic liver failure, catabolism of AAAs is impaired, causing serum levels to rise (8). Since muscles can metabolize BCAA, they are used for energy, thereby decreasing plasma concentrations of BCAA (deficiency in BCAAs) (7). Aromatic amino acids are precursors of neurotransmitters; high levels of these amino acids interfere with certain neurotransmitters (dopamine and norepinephrine), and instead cause the production of substances that act like neurotransmitters (accumulation of false neurotransmitters) (3). These *false* neurotransmitters are believed to contribute to hepatic coma (9).

Medical nutrition therapy

The most important aspect of medical nutrition therapy to keep in mind is that each patient has individual nutritional needs that must be addressed. In the presence of hepatic encephalopathy, dietary protein is often restricted to reduce ammonia

ascites
abnormal intraperitoneal accumulation of fluid containing large amounts of protein and electrolytes, usually resulting in abdominal swelling, hemodilution, edema, or a decreased urinary output

hepatic encephalopathy
a type of brain damage caused by liver disease and consequent ammonia intoxication

athetoid
purposeless weaving motions of the body or extremities

Sample 50 Gram Protein/Sodium-Restricted Diet Menu

(Exchanges adjusted for 30 gram and 40 gram diets)

BREAKFAST
Apple juice
Low-sodium white toast
Scrambled egg
Low-sodium margarine and jelly
Low-fat yogurt
Decaffeinated coffee (½ cup)

LUNCH
Lemonade (½ cup)
Sirloin tips (1 oz)
Noodles
Green beans
Cinnamon applesauce
Low-sodium margarine
Ice tea

DINNER
Fruit punch (½ cup)
Low-sodium turkey breast (2 oz)
Small baked potato
Garden salad with Italian dressing
Pear halves
Hot tea

From Memorial Hospital, Carbondale, Ill.

dry body weight

an estimate of actual weight without the weight of ascites fluid

levels. Protein should be given in the highest amount that will not induce or worsen encephalopathy, with a goal of 1.0 to 1.5 g/kg of **dry** (or desirable) **body weight** (10,11) (see Sample Menu). If this level of protein causes exacerbation of symptoms, further restriction to 0.75 or 0.5 g/kg of dry (or desirable) body weight may be used (10,11). If symptoms do not improve, dietary protein should be decreased to 10 to 20 g/day while an adequate energy intake is maintained (11). As symptoms improve, the patient's tolerance to protein can be tested by adding 10 to 20 gram of dietary protein every 2 to 3 days until reaching the highest tolerance level (10,11). If signs of encephalopathy occur, dietary protein should be reduced to the previous restriction where the patient was asymptomatic (11). Some patients may tolerate higher levels of protein if the majority comes from dairy, starch, and vegetable sources of protein and animal sources are limited to 20 to 40 g/day (≤0.5 g/kg) (10). One word of caution: diets containing 50 gram or less of protein may be deficient in thiamin, riboflavin, calcium, niacin, phosphorus, and iron based on the 1989 Recommended Dietary Allowances (11).

Energy intake should be high enough to prevent protein (muscle) catabolism and spare dietary protein for anabolism. Most patients' protein requirements will be met by 30 to 35 kcal/kg (dry or desirable) body weight (10,11). However, adjustments must be made for catabolic stress factors such as infection, trauma, surgery, or loss of nutrients (steatorrhea) (11). Furthermore, patients with cirrhosis may be anorexic, drowsy, or confused and usually have early satiety. They may have problems consuming adequate kcalories at meal times, so supplements and/or between-meal feedings may be required to increase kcalorie intake (10).

Sodium may need to be restricted to 2000 mg or less if edema or ascites are present (10,11). Sometimes it is necessary to restrict sodium to as little as 500 mg to

1000 mg of sodium per day for patients whose edema and ascites are resistant to diuretic therapy. Diets this low in sodium are very restrictive, unpalatable, difficult to comply with and can be deficient in calcium (10,11). Potassium may need to be restricted if renal function is inadequate, or it may need to be supplemented if potassium-wasting diuretics are used (11).

Fluids should be given in relation to input/output records, daily weights, and electrolyte values (10,11). Fluid restrictions are often necessary to prevent or decrease ascites formation (11). Fluid restrictions usually begin at 1500 ml/day and may decrease to 1000 to 1200 ml/day depending on the patient's response. The nurse may provide suggestions on how to cope with thirst in an effort to improve compliance with these kind of fluid restrictions (9). Sample suggestions are listed in the following Teaching Tool.

It is not uncommon to find vitamin deficiencies in patients with cirrhosis, and chances are that nutrition intake was poor before the onset of liver disorders. If deficiencies are present, water-soluble supplements with emphasis on folate, B_{12}, and thiamin may be necessary. Fat-soluble vitamins should be given in water-soluble form if steatorrhea is present (11). Prophylactic supplementation of minerals is not recommended unless they are recognized as being deficient. If conditions such as hemochromatosis and/or Wilson's disease are present, mineral toxicity is possible (11).

Liver Transplantation

Once considered experimental, liver transplantation is regarded as an appropriate treatment for end stage liver disease. Most patients in this condition show some indications of compromised nutritional status and therefore require special

TEACHING TOOL
Suggestions for Coping With Fluid Restriction

These simple yet effective suggestions may help patients cope with fluid restrictions while maintaining personal comfort.

1. Drink to quench thirst only. Avoiding high-sodium foods will result in less thirst. (See Table 8-5, p. 194, for a list of high-sodium foods.)
2. Try to avoid drinking from habit or to be sociable.
3. Eat ice-cold fruit between meals.
4. Sliced lemon wedges can stimulate saliva and moisten a dry mouth.
5. Keep the mouth clean by brushing teeth frequently and rinsing mouth with water (do not swallow rinse water).
6. Chew gum, suck hard candy (tart or sour is best), or use mints to stimulate saliva flow.
7. Try sucking on ice; most people find it more satisfying than the same amount of water since it stays in the mouth longer.
8. Limit fluids at meal time; when appropriate, take medications with meal time liquids or soft foods like applesauce.
9. Take medications at one time to decrease amount of total fluid needed.
10. Add lemon juice to ice cubes to suck on; you will use fewer since the tartness of the lemon will make your mouth water. Use about half of a lemon per tray of water. Or freeze lemonade into small, individualized popsicles in an ice cube tray.
11. Take small amounts of fluid at one time.
12. If allowable, use high-fat foods to help decrease the desire for fluid with a meal. (Gravies and margarine will moisten foods and make them easier to swallow.)

Modified from Davis JR, Sherer K: *Applied nutrition and diet therapy for nurses*, ed 2, Philadelphia,1994, Saunders; and Dunning S: *Ideas to Control Fluid*, Bio-Medical Applications of Carbondale, Dialysis Services Division, National Medical Care Inc, Carbondale, Ill.

attention to nutritional needs (12-15). In addition, dietary restrictions used in treatment of liver disease before liver failure often contribute to the decline of nutritional status (13). It is often difficult to assess nutritional status in patients with liver disorders/because many assessment parameters (body weight, nitrogen balance studies, total lymphocyte count, and serum protein levels) are affected by edema, ascites, and hepatic necrosis seen in end stage liver failure (11-13,15). Therefore it may be more appropriate to use subjective parameters such as weight changes, appetite, satiety level, taste changes, diet history, and gastrointestinal symptoms (11,16).

Medical nutrition therapy

Each phase of the transplant procedure dictates specific nutritional requirements. The primary objective in pretransplant medical nutrition therapy is to provide enough kcalories and protein to decrease protein catabolism and correct any nutritional deficiencies.

The 4 to 8 weeks following surgery, the immediate posttransplant period, requires individualization of medical nutrition therapy according to the needs of the patient (11). Ascites, edema, or excess fluid makes using the patient's actual weight unreliable for determining kcalories and protein needs. Ideal (desirable) weight is a better reference point. Adequate kcalories and protein are necessary for the hypercatabolic (but not necessarily hypermetabolic) stresses resulting from surgery and high doses of glucocorticoids (10,11). Total parenteral nutrition may be necessary if nutritional needs cannot be met enterally (feeding by mouth and/or with nasoenteric feeding) (10,11). When oral intake is initiated, early satiety and altered tastes may prevent adequate intake. Between-meal feedings and/or supplements should be used to meet kcalorie and protein goals (10,11).

For the long-term posttransplant patient, a healthy, well-balanced diet is the nutrition goal (10). Because of common posttransplantation complications such as excessive weight gain, hypertension, hyperlipidemia, and diabetes, adjustments in kcalories, fat, and concentrated carbohydrates may be necessary (10,17-19).

In some institutions, while the patient is waiting for transplant surgery a low-bacteria diet is used in combination with an oral selective bowel decontamination solution (OSBD) (10). Foods that should be avoided on a low-bacteria diet are listed in Table 17-2.

Table 17-2   Foods to Avoid on a Low-Bacteria Diet for Liver Transplantation

Food Groups	Foods to Avoid
Meats and eggs	Any undercooked; all cheese and cottage cheese products
Fat	None
Milk	Unpasteurized milk and milk products
Starch	None
Vegetables	All raw vegetables (including salads and garnishes)
Fruit	Fresh fruit with peels that are consumed (grapes, cherries, berries*)
Beverages	None
Condiments/Seasonings	None

Modified from Nelson JK et al: *Mayo Clinic diet manual,* ed 7, St. Louis, 1994, Mosby.
*Fresh fruit that can reasonably be peeled and rinsed is allowed (apples, oranges, bananas, grapefruit, pears, melon, pineapple, peaches, nectarines, kiwi).

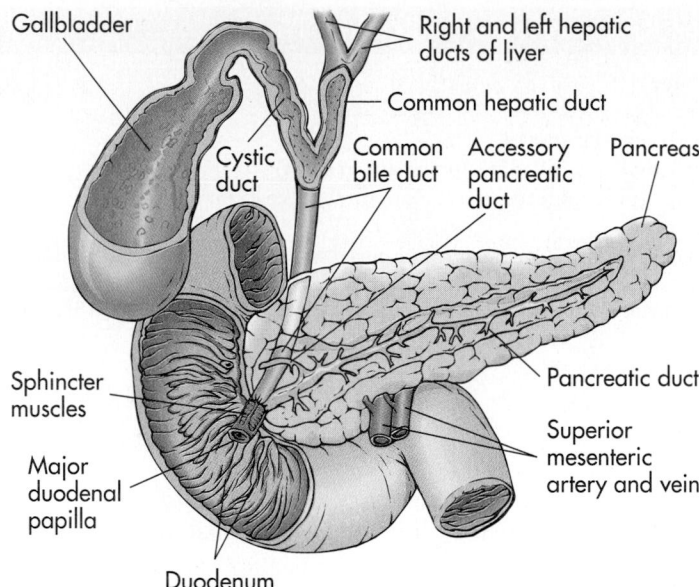

Fig. 17-3 Gallbladder and bile ducts. Obstruction of either the hepatic or the common bile duct by stone or spasm prevents bile from being ejected into the duodenum.

GALLBLADDER DISORDERS

The gallbladder lies directly beneath the right lobe of the liver, and along with the hepatic, cystic, and common bile ducts composes the biliary system (Fig. 17-3). Bile is transported from the liver to the gallbladder via the biliary duct system where it is concentrated and stored until released into the duodenum to expedite absorption of fats, fat-soluble vitamins, and certain minerals, and activate the release of pancreatic enzymes (5). The most common disorders of the gallbladder include **cholelithiasis, choledocholithiasis,** and **chole-cystitis.**

One of the main constituents of bile is cholesterol, which is also a major constituent of gallstones. The amount of cholesterol in bile is determined somewhat by the amount of dietary fat consumed (3,20). As might be expected, chronic intake of high-fat foods increases the risk of developing cholelithiasis (Fig. 17-4). Gallstones are commonly found in women who are multiparous, on estrogen therapy, or who use oral contraceptives; obese individuals; those with sedentary lifestyles; and the aged (5). Approximately 70% of Native American women over the age of 30 have gallstones (6). Other predisposing conditions to the development of gallstones are diabetes mellitus, regional enteritis, and familial tendencies (5).

An interesting phenomenon is that people who lose a great deal of weight rapidly, as found with the use of **very low calorie diets (VLCDs)** and some commercial weight-loss programs, are at a greater risk for developing gallstones than obese persons. In fact, gallstones are one of the most medically significant complications of voluntary weight loss (21). Although no studies have directly linked a diet's nutrient composition to the risk of gallstones, it is believed that VLCDs may not contain enough fat to cause the gallbladder to contract enough to empty the stored bile, thus causing gallstones to form (21). Approximately 10 grams of fat is necessary for normal contraction of the gallbladder (21). Persons who are

cholelithiasis
presence of stones in the gallbladder

choledocholithiasis
gallstones in the common bile duct

cholecystitis
acute inflammation of the gallbladder associated with pain, tenderness, and fever

very low calorie diets (VLCD)
usually defined as diets containing 800 kcalories per day or less

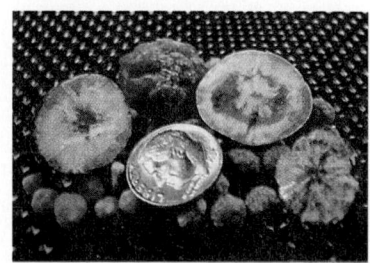

Fig. 17-4 Gallstones.

Suggested Risk Factors in Gallbladder Disease
Advanced age
Gender (female)
Obesity with high-fat intake
Hormonal imbalance (estrogen, progestin, insulin)
Certain drugs (oral contraceptives, clofibrate, cholestyramine)
Enzyme defects
Very low kcalorie diets (medically supervised VLCDs used for weight loss)

From Escott-Stump S: *Nutrition and diagnosis-related care,* ed 3, Philadelphia, 1992, Lea & Febiger.

colic
sharp visceral pain

cholecystectomy
surgical removal of the
gallbladder, performed to treat
cholelithiasis and cholecystitis

considering losing a significant amount of weight should see a physician to evaluate their past medical history, individual circumstances, and the proposed method of weight loss.

If cholelithiasis is asymptomatic, no specific therapy is necessary (22). Symptoms usually manifest after eating, especially a high-fat meal, and include a mild, aching pain in the midepigastrium that may increase in intensity during a **colic** attack. The pain may radiate to the right upper quadrant and right subscapular region. Nausea, vomiting, tachycardia, and diaphoresis may also be present (5).

Cholecystitis occurs when gallstones block the cystic duct or as the result of stasis, bacterial infection, or ischemia of the gallbladder. This inflammation is associated with pain, tenderness, and fever. Fat intolerance may manifest as regurgitation, flatulence, belching, epigastric heaviness, indigestion, heartburn, chronic upper abdominal pain, and nausea. Jaundice and steatorrhea may also be present (5). The recommended therapy for symptomatic cholelithiasis and cholecystitis is surgical removal of the gallbladder (**cholecystectomy**).

Medical nutrition therapy

Since cholelithiasis and cholecystitis usually produce rather painful symptoms, the main objective of nutritional care is to decrease the patient's discomfort. Most patients become acutely aware of foods that cause discomfort and they avoid these foods. Low-fat diets are traditionally used to treat cholecystitis, but some recount that fat content of meals has little influence on the action of the gallbladder (7). During an acute attack, the patient receives IV fluids with nothing orally. The diet can progress to the patient's tolerances, and a low-fat diet excluding gas-forming vegetables is recommended (see Table 16-9) (5,6).

Chronic cholecystitis with inflammation is usually treated with a fat and kcalories controlled diet until surgery can be performed. Adequate amounts of carbohydrates are important, especially fiber (such as pectin), which binds excess bile acids (6). If the patient is obese, weight loss is usually advised before surgery. Foods that should be avoided to reduce dietary fat are fried foods, fatty meats, and rich desserts. Any other foods known to cause gastrointestinal discomfort should also be avoided.

Following cholecystectomy, bile enters the small intestine continually rather than in response to food in the gastrointestinal tract. Immediately postoperatively, patients receive clear liquids until they can tolerate a regular diet. Some patients need to follow a low-fat diet for several weeks after surgery, but other than individual patient tolerance there is little need to restrict the diet (7). A low-fat diet is outlined in Table 17-3.

Table 17-3   Recommended Diet Modifications to Decrease Dietary Fat (25 grams or 50 grams of fat)

Food Groups	Choose	Decrease
BEVERAGES 2 or more servings of milk and dairy products per day are recommended	Skim milk (liquid, powdered, and evaporated), skim buttermilk, skim chocolate milk, coffee, tea, soft drinks, other nondairy products	1%, 2%, whole milks; buttermilk made from whole milk; chocolate milk; evaporated milk; cream
BREADS AND CEREALS 6 to 11 servings per day are recommended	Whole-grain breads, enriched breads, saltines, soda crackers, English muffins, whole-grain or enriched bagels, flour tortillas	Biscuits, breads containing egg or cheese, sweet rolls, pancakes, French toast, doughnuts, waffles, fritters, muffins, egg bagels, popovers, snack crackers with added fat, snack chips, stuffing, fried tortillas
	Whole-grain cereals except regular granola-type cereals, low-fat granola cereals, unbuttered popcorn	Granola-type cereals, buttered popcorn
FRUITS 2 to 4 servings per day are recommended	Fresh, frozen, canned, or dried fruit; fruit juices	Avocado
VEGETABLES 3 to 5 servings per day are recommended	All fresh, frozen, or canned vegetables prepared without fats, oils, or fat-containing sauces	Buttered, au gratin, creamed, or fried vegetables unless made with allowed fat allowance
POTATOES	Potatoes; rice; barley; noodles; spaghetti, macaroni, and other pastas	Fried potatoes, fried rice, potato chips, chow mein noodles
MEATS AND MEAT SUBSTITUTES For 50 g fat diet—6 oz For 25 g fat diet—5 oz Recommended preparation methods are broiling, roasting (on rack), grilling, or boiling; weigh meat after cooking	Poultry: breast meat without skin Veal: all cuts Lean beef: USDA good or choice cuts (round, sirloin, flank steak, tenderloin, and chopped beef); roast (rib, chuck, rump); steak (cube, Porterhouse, T-bone); meatloaf made with ground beef (95% lean) Lean pork: fresh, canned, cured, or boiled ham; Canadian bacon; tenderloin; chops; loin roast; Boston butt; cutlets Lean lamb: chops, leg, or roast Fish: all fresh, frozen, or canned in water; crab, lobster, scallops, shrimp, clams, oysters, tuna; herring (uncreamed or smoked), sardines (canned, drained), salmon (canned in water) Luncheon meats: 95% fat-free; lean ham, turkey, or beef	Any fried, fatty, or heavily marbled meat, fish, or poultry Poultry: duck, goose Beef: most USDA prime cuts of beef, ribs, corned beef Pork: spareribs, ground pork sausage (patty or link), ham hocks, pigs' feet, chitterlings Lamb: patties (ground lamb) Fish: tuna (packed in oil), salmon (packed in oil) Most luncheon meats including bologna, salami, pimento loaf Sausage: Polish, Italian, knockwurst, smoked bratwurst, frankfurter Legumes cooked with added fat

Continued.

Table 17-3 Recommended Diet Modifications to Decrease Dietary Fat (25 grams or 50 grams of fat), cont'd.

Food Groups	Choose	Decrease
DESSERTS AND SWEETS In moderation	Sherbet, fruit ice, gelatin, angel food cake, vanilla wafers, graham crackers, meringues, pudding made with skim milk, fat-free commercial baked products, nonfat ice cream, frozen yogurt, sugar, honey, jelly, jam, marmalade; molasses, maple syrup, sourballs, gumdrops, jelly beans, marshmallows, hard candy, cocoa powder	All other cakes, cookies, pies, pastries; puddings made with whole milk or eggs; cream puffs Butter, coconut, chocolate and cream candies
FATS Amounts equal 1 fat equivalent 3 to 5 equivalents per day of unsaturated fats are recommended	*Unsaturated* Margarine (1 tsp); diet margarine 1 tbsp); mayonnaise (regular = 1 tsp; reduced-calorie = 1 tbsp); creamy salad dressings (regular = 2 tsp; reduced-calorie = 1 tbsp); other salad dressings (regular = 1 tbsp; reduced-calorie = 2 tbsp); vegetable oils (1 tsp); nuts: almonds (6 whole), cashews (2 whole), peanuts (20 small or 10 large), peanut butter (2 tsp), cashew butter (2 tsp), walnuts (2 whole), pistachios (18 whole), other nuts (1 tbsp); seeds: sesame (1 tbsp), sunflower (1 tbsp), pumpkin (2 tsp); olives: 10 large or 5 small *Saturated* Bacon (1 slice), bacon fat (1 tsp); butter (1 tsp); whipped butter (2 tsp); chitterlings (1/2 oz); shredded coconut (2 tbsp); cream: light, coffee, table (2 tbsp); heavy whipping (1 tbsp); sour cream (2 tbsp); cream cheese (1 tbsp); coffee whitener: liquid (2 tbsp), powder (4 tsp); lard (1 tsp); oil: coconut (1 tsp), palm (1 tsp); shortening (1 tsp); sour cream (2 tbsp); salt pork (1/4 oz)	Any in excess of amounts recommended on diet and all others
SOUPS	Fat-free broth, fat-free vegetable soup, cream soup made with skim milk and allowed fat, packaged dehydrated soups	All others
MISCELLANEOUS	Catsup, chili sauce, vinegar, pickles, vanilla, unbuttered popcorn, white sauce made with skim milk and allowed fat, mustard, all herbs and seasonings, apple butter	Olives and nuts in excess of specified portions, cream sauces, gravies, buttered popcorn

Modified from American Dietetic Association: *Manual of clinical dietetics,* ed 4, Chicago, 1992, American Dietetic Association; and American Dietetic Association: *Handbook of clinical dietetics,* ed 2, New Haven, 1992, Yale University Press.

PANCREATITIS

In addition to hormonal functions, the pancreas secretes enzymes necessary for protein, carbohydrate, and fat digestion. The pancreas also secretes sodium bicarbonate to neutralize acidic gastric contents as they enter the duodenum, which provides the optimal pH for the activation of these enzymes (5).

Pancreatitis is an inflammatory process characterized by decreased production of digestive enzymes and bicarbonate, and malabsorption of fats and proteins. This acute inflammation causes the blood vessels that supply the pancreas to become exceptionally permeable and leak fluid and plasma proteins into the spaces between the pancreatic cells, causing localized edema and damage. Pancreatic enzymes are ordinarily secreted into the intestinal lumen where they are activated (8). But if the pancreas is damaged, however, the enzymes are retained and activated within the pancreas, resulting in autodigestion and severe pain (5). When the enzymes amylase and lipase cannot be secreted into the intestine, they enter the bloodstream and levels can become quite high. In fact, elevated levels of serum amylase are an indication of pancreatitis. In addition to severe pain, patients with pancreatitis often experience nausea and vomiting (5).

Acute pancreatitis is most commonly caused by excessive alcohol consumption and gallbladder disease (8,24) combined with a genetic predisposition to damage (8). Chronic pancreatitis is usually associated with chronic alcohol consumption and is characterized by chronic pain and exocrine and endocrine insufficiency (22). Diabetes mellitus can occur as the result of chronic pancreatitis if **beta cells** are damaged thus decreasing insulin production (5).

Medical nutrition therapy

The primary goal is to provide for the patient's nutritional needs while minimizing pancreatic secretions (23,25). This may be accomplished with either enteral or parenteral nutrition, although enteral nutrition is generally not used until pain is controlled, gastrointestinal symptoms have abated, and inflammation resolved (23,25). Because malabsorption of fats and protein and severe weight loss are benchmarks of chronic pancreatitis, most patients are malnourished when diagnosed. This factor is the cause for concern to initiate nutritional support as soon as possible.

When enteral feeding is appropriate, low-fat, elemental formulas are recommended because they tend to reduce pancreatic stimulation (23). Feeding into the lower small bowel, in the jejunum distal to the ligament of Treitz, allows for the areas associated with pancreatic stimulation to be bypassed (22). Patients receiving enteral feedings should be monitored for increases in pancreatic enzymes, abdominal pain, or discomfort. Enteral feedings should be terminated if any of these symptoms occur (23).

The American Society of Parenteral and Enteral Nutrition (ASPEN) guidelines recommend use of parenteral support when enteral feedings exacerbate abdominal pain (26). Peripheral parenteral nutrition can be used for nonstressed patients who are expected to be NPO for less than 10 days. Central parenteral nutrition may be necessary if the patient will be NPO for longer than 5 to 7 days (23).

Whatever feeding route is chosen, the patient must receive adequate energy and nutrients based on the severity of the pancreatitis. Restricting fat to less than 50 grams per day typically prevents symptoms of steatorrhea. A medium-chain triglyceride product such as MCT oil may be used to increase kcalories if needed. The rest of the kcalories should come from protein (at least 120 grams per day) and carbohydrates ($\geq$450 gram). Since patients are usually anorectic, providing meals in six feedings daily may facilitate adequate nutritional intake (7). Replacement pancreatic enzymes are taken orally with meals to control maldigestion and malabsorption. Complete abstinence from alcohol is essential but often difficult to achieve (8).

pancreatitis
inflammation of the pancreas, may be acute or chronic

beta cells
insulin-producing cells situated in the islets of Langerhans of the pancreas

CYSTIC FIBROSIS

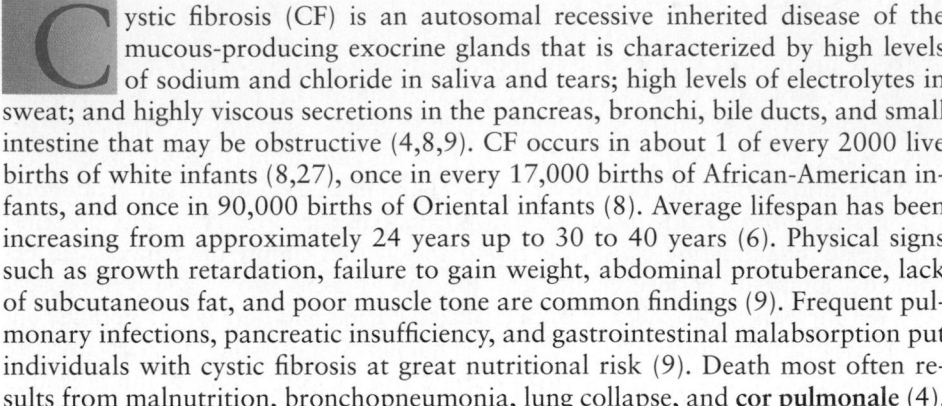

Cystic fibrosis (CF) is an autosomal recessive inherited disease of the mucous-producing exocrine glands that is characterized by high levels of sodium and chloride in saliva and tears; high levels of electrolytes in sweat; and highly viscous secretions in the pancreas, bronchi, bile ducts, and small intestine that may be obstructive (4,8,9). CF occurs in about 1 of every 2000 live births of white infants (8,27), once in every 17,000 births of African-American infants, and once in 90,000 births of Oriental infants (8). Average lifespan has been increasing from approximately 24 years up to 30 to 40 years (6). Physical signs such as growth retardation, failure to gain weight, abdominal protuberance, lack of subcutaneous fat, and poor muscle tone are common findings (9). Frequent pulmonary infections, pancreatic insufficiency, and gastrointestinal malabsorption put individuals with cystic fibrosis at great nutritional risk (9). Death most often results from malnutrition, bronchopneumonia, lung collapse, and **cor pulmonale** (4).

Medical nutrition therapy

Nutrition is of prime importance in the treatment of cystic fibrosis (9). Poor nutritional status because of undernutrition contributes to poor growth, pulmonary complications, and susceptibility to infection (9). The primary goal of nutritional therapy for patients with cystic fibrosis is to exceed the Recommended Daily Allowance (RDA) for kcalories and all other nutrients (9). Dietitians estimate individual energy requirements based on basal metabolic rate, activity level, lung function, and fat absorption. Improvement in pancreatic enzyme replacement therapy allows higher amounts of dietary fats that previously were prohibited (28). Since fat provides such a concentrated source of energy, it does not need to be restricted below 30% to 40% of total kcalories, and pancreatic enzyme replacement therapy can be individualized according to the patient's intake (9). Additional salt is usually necessary, especially during periods of hot weather, febrile illness, and strenuous physical exertion (9). Multivitamin supplements should be prescribed for all patients with cystic fibrosis (9,29). Additional fat-soluble vitamins may be prescribed as well, in a water-miscible form if fat malabsorption is severe.

Infants. Pancreatic enzyme replacement therapy should be used along with all types of milk products, including breast milk (27). Supplemental fat or carbohydrate may be necessary for some infants to increase kcaloric density to over 20 kcal/oz (9). Introduction of **beikost** is not different for infants with cystic fibrosis (25).

Children and adolescents. Nutritional adequacy of the diet, compliance with pancreatic enzymes, and growth patterns should be monitored because as the child becomes older and more independent, compliance may become questionable (9,28).

Reevaluation of the patient's diet is important to ascertain whether recommendations are adequate to support growth and maintain nutritional status. As changes occur in the disease process and growth occurs, nutritional needs will also change. Weight gain, linear growth, and level of pancreatic enzyme replacement therapy should be assessed also during this time (9).

cor pulmonale
an abnormal cardiac condition characterized by hypertrophy of the right ventricle as a result of hypertension of the pulmonary circulation

beikost
(BYE-cost), supplemental or weaning foods

WELLNESS AND LIVER, GALLBLADDER, AND PANCREAS DISORDERS	
Physical Dimension	As ancillary digestive organs, their malfunctioning can devastate nutritional status.
Intellectual Dimension	Reasoning skills are required to make lifestyle decisions related to levels of alcohol consumption and fat intake if at risk for cirrhosis or pancreatic disorders.
Emotional Dimension	The strain in dealing with chronic life-threatening illness such as CF challenges emotional health.
Social Dimension	Because of the relationship of these disorders to digestive functioning, restrictive dietary guidelines may inhibit ability to easily socialize with others.

SUMMARY

The liver, gallbladder, and pancreas are important ancillary digestive organs. Disorders of the liver include hepatitis, an inflammation of the liver, and cirrhosis, a chronic degenerative disease causing fibrous connective tissue and fat infiltration of the liver. Medical nutrition therapy includes bed rest and proper nutrition for hepatitis, and individual nutrition plans for cirrhosis that often restrict protein to ease liver function. Meeting medical nutrition therapy needs while still providing for adequate RDA nutrient levels is challenging. Liver transplants occur as treatment for end stage liver disease. Medical nutrition therapy involves a variety of dietary plans specific to each phase of the procedure.

Gallbladder disorders include cholelithiasis, choledocholithiasis, and cholecystitis; these disorders are characterized by the formation of gallstones within the gallbladder. Medical nutrition therapy often requires low-fat diets, but individuals may not all respond. Chronic cholecystitis with inflammation is usually treated with fat- and kcalorie-controlled diets until surgery. Moderation of fat is often indicated postoperatively.

Pancreatitis affects production of digestive secretions, resulting in malabsorption of fats and protein. Medical nutritional therapy tends to require enteral or parenteral nutrition. Regardless of the feeding route, fat intake is restricted.

Cystic fibrosis is an inherited disease of the mucous-producing exocrine glands. Medical nutrition therapy is of prime importance with the goal to exceed the RDA for kcalories and all other nutrients necessitating use of vitamin supplementation.

THE NURSING ROLE
A Patient With Cirrhosis: The Nursing Process

Mr. Ashaad is seriously ill with cirrhosis of the liver related to chronic hepatitis. He has developed severe ascites and mild encephalopathy. He is being treated with diuretics (spironolactone) and lactulose to reduce ammonia levels. His fluids are restricted to 1200 cc per day, and he is to receive 2000 calories, 20 grams of protein, and 1 gram of sodium. However, it is becoming more difficult to get Mr. Ashaad to eat all of his food.

ASSESSMENT DATA COLLECTED
Objective:
Abdominal distention; ascites
Peripheral edema, ankles and lower legs
Jaundice of skin and sclera
Muscle wasting of upper extremities and thighs
Body weight 210 lbs
Dark amber urine
Confusion and disorientation most of the time
Laboratory results:
   BUN 7 (norm 8-25 mg/dL)
   Hematocrit 40 (norm 45%-52%)
   Albumin 3.0 (norm 3.5-5.0 gm/dL)
   Total Bilirubin 2.4 (norm 0.4-1.0 mg/dL)

Subjective:
Anorexia, occasional nausea
Premorbid weight 205 lb
Thirst

Continued.

THE NURSING ROLE, cont'd.

A Patient With Cirrhosis: The Nursing Process

NURSING DIAGNOSIS 1

Altered nutrition, less than body requirements, related to anorexia, nausea, and necessary protein restriction, as evidenced by muscle wasting, and apparent loss of true body weight.

PLANNING

The RN sets goals, consulting Mr. Ashaad when possible, to achieve the following outcomes:

Consumption of prescribed diet

No further weight loss other than that accounted for by fluid loss.
  Note: Every 500 cc of excess fluid loss should account for 1 lb of weight loss.

INTERVENTION

1. Contact dietitian about decreasing size of main meals and increasing between-meal snacks
2. Determine past and present food likes and encourage them
3. Administer prescribed antiemetics as indicated
4. Weigh once a day at 8 AM
5. Record fluid intake and output and food intake

EVALUATION

Evaluate whether outcomes have been met as evidenced by adequate food consumption recorded in chart and maintenance of body weight.

NURSING DIAGNOSIS 2

Fluid volume excess related to increased intrahepatic pressure and decreased colloidal osmotic pressure as evidenced by ascites and peripheral edema.

PLANNING

The RN sets the goal of reducing fluid excess and reducing its harmful effects as seen in the following outcomes:

Decrease in fluid weight of 1 lb in 1 week

Intact skin over edematous areas

INTERVENTION

1. Maintain sodium restriction
2. Restrict fluids to 1200 cc per day, 300 cc with each meal and 300 cc total between meals
3. To deal with thirst, give ice, hard candy, and lemon wedges as tolerated
4. Weigh and measure intake and outtake as above
5. Administer diuretics as prescribed and monitor for side effects
6. Measure abdominal girth in supine position daily at 10 AM
7. Reposition every 2 hours and keep heels off mattress

EVALUATION

Evaluate whether outcomes have been achieved as evidenced by loss of excess 1000 cc fluid (1 lb) in 1 week and no skin breakdown over sacrum, ankles or heels.

Critical Thinking **CLINICAL APPLICATIONS**

Chronic alcohol abuse is usually the cause of chronic liver disease (cirrhosis and hepatic encephalopathy) and chronic pancreatitis. One way to evaluate the risk of alcoholic-related liver disease is to assess the pattern, quantity, and duration of alcohol intake; usual dietary intake; and socioeconomic factors affecting eating habits. Data can be collected from the patient or reliable friend or family member, and evaluated to determine amount (grams) and the kcaloric value of alcohol consumed. When consumed in large quantities, alcohol can provide the majority of the day's kcaloric intake.

To assess this information, we should review a few basics. Alcohol provides 7 kcalories per gram. The average percent alcohol content (based on weight per volume) of various forms of alcoholic beverages is as follows:

Beer = 4% to 6%
Wine = 9% to 12%
Distilled alcohol (whiskey, rum, gin, or brandy) = 35% to 50%

The concentration of alcohol in distilled beverages (hard liquor) is usually referred to as *proof*. One proof equals 0.5% alcohol, which means that 80-proof tequila contains 40% alcohol. Hard liquor is routinely measured in a jigger or shot, which is 1½ oz or 45 ml.

1. How many grams of alcohol and kcalories would 2 shots of 80-proof tequila provide?
2. What is the best way to obtain information from an individual about his/her alcohol consumption?
3. You obtain the following information from the alcohol intake questionnaire and diet history: Alcohol is consumed 7 days/week at home, work, and at bars. A typical day's intake consists of a Bloody Mary (1 cup tomato juice, 2 shots 80-proof vodka) first thing in the morning, followed by 5 cups of black coffee (some at home, some at work). Three more shots of 80-proof vodka are consumed at work. Lunch is usually fast food double cheeseburger, small fries, and a cup of black coffee. After work 4 12-oz bottles of beer (4% alcohol) and pretzels (about 30) are consumed at the local pub with friends. Dinner at home consists of a lunchmeat sandwich (usually 2 slices white bread, 2 oz bologna, 1 tsp mustard), 10 potato chips, and 2 more 12-oz beers. Total kcalorie intake for the day is approximately 3200 kcal.

How many grams of alcohol are consumed? _____ grams alcohol
How many kcalories are provided by the alcohol? _____ kcal from alcohol
What percent of the kcalories are provided by alcohol? _____ % energy from alcohol

ALCOHOL INTAKE ASSESSMENT TOOL

1. How many days a week do you drink alcoholic beverages?   Circle number of days:
   0 <1 1 2 3 4 5 6 7
2. Where do you drink?   Circle all that apply:
   a. at home
   b. at a friend's
   c. at a bar
   d. at work
   e. in the car
   f. other (specify)

Continued.

Critical Thinking   **CLINICAL APPLICATIONS, cont'd.**

3. Which alcoholic beverages do you consume?

Circle all that apply:
a. beer
b. white, red, or rose wine
c. sherry or port
d. gin
e. whiskey
f. vodka
g. rum
h. other (specify)

4. How do you determine how much you drink?

Circle all that apply:
a. Count the number of beer cans
b. Count the number of wine glasses
c. Count the number of shots poured
d. Count the number of bottles of wine
e. Count the number of bottles of liquor used a day or week
f. I don't know exactly how much I drink
g. Other method of deciding alcohol intake (specify)

5. On any drinking day, how many drinks do you usually have?

Circle letter(s) indicating drinks consumed and number within each category consumed to indicate number of drinks per day:
a. beer   1 2 3 4 >5
b. white, red, or
   rose wine   1 2 3 4 >5
c. sherry or port   1 2 3 4 >5
d. gin   1 2 3 4 >5
e. whiskey   1 2 3 4 >5
f. vodka   1 2 3 4 >5
g. rum   1 2 3 4 >5
h. other (specify)   1 2 3 4 >5

6. For how long have you been drinking this quantity?
7. Do you drink this amount on a regular basis?

Professionals working with individuals who consume excessive amounts of alcohol advise that self-reported intakes may constitute about half of what is actually consumed. Therefore double-checking any information obtained from a patient about alcohol intake with a reliable family member or friend is recommended.

From Zeman FJ, Ney DM: *Applications of clinical nutrition*, Englewood Cliffs, 1988, Prentice Hall.
*Any beverages used as mixers should be included in the estimated kcalorie intake.

REFERENCES

1. Korsten MA, Lieber CS: Nutrition in pancreatic and liver disorders. In Shils ME, Olson JA, Shike M, eds: *Modern nutrition in health and disease,* ed 8, Philadelphia, 1994, Lea & Febiger.

2. Weinsier RL, Morgan SL: *Fundamentals of clinical nutrition,* St. Louis, 1993, Mosby.

3. Lee SP: Diseases of the liver and biliary tract. In Kinney JM, JeeJeebhoy KN, Hill GL, and Owen OE, eds: *Nutrition and metabolism in patient care,* Philadelphia, 1988, Saunders.

4. White HM: Hepatic diseases. In Woodley M, Whelan A, eds: *Manual of medical therapeutics,* ed 27, Boston, 1992, Little, Brown.

5. Swearingen PL: *Manual of nursing therapeutics,* ed 3, St. Louis, 1994, Mosby.

6. Escott-Stump S: *Nutrition and diagnosis-related care,* ed 3, Philadelphia, 1992, Lea & Febiger.

7. Davis JR, Sherer K: *Applied nutrition and diet therapy for nurses,* ed 2, Philadelphia, 1994, Saunders.

8. Zeman FJ: *Clinical nutrition and dietetics,* ed 2, New York, 1991, Macmillan.

9. Fischer JE, Baldesarini RJ: False neurotransmitters and hepatic failure, *Lancet* 2:75-80, 1971.

10. Nelson JK et al: *Mayo Clinic diet manual,* ed 7, St. Louis, 1994, Mosby.

11. American Dietetic Association: *Manual of clinical dietetics,* ed 4, Chicago, 1992, American Dietetic Association.

12. DiCecco SR et al: Assessment of nutritional status of patients with end-stage liver disease undergoing liver transplantation, *Mayo Clinic Proc* 64:95-102, 1989.

13. Hehir DJ et al: Nutrition in patients undergoing orthotopic liver transplant, *Journal of Enteral and Parenteral Nutrition* 9:695-700, 1985.

14. Porayko MK, DiCecco SR, O'Keefe SJD: Impact of malnutrition and its therapy on liver transplantation, *Seminars in Liver Disease* 11:305-314, 1991.

15. Hasse JM: Nutritional implications of liver transplantation, *Henry Ford Hospital Medical Journal* 38:235-240, 1990.

16. Hasse JM: Role of the dietitian in the nutrition management of adults after liver transplantation, *J Am Diet Assoc* 91:473-476, 1991.

17. Munoz SJ et al: Hyperlipidemia and obesity after orthotopic liver transplantation, *Transplantation Proceedings* 23:1480-1483, 1991.

18. Palmer M, Schaffner R, Thung SN: Excessive weight gain after liver transplantation, *Transplantation* 51:797-800, 1991.

19. Eid A et al: Beyond one year after liver transplantation, *Mayo Clinic Proc* 64:446-450, 1989.

20. Guyton AC: *Textbook of medical physiology,* ed 8, Philadelphia, 1991, Saunders.

21. Public Health Service, National Institutes of Health, and National Institute of Diabetes and Digestive and Kidney Diseases: *Dieting and gallstones,* Washington, DC, 1993, US DHHS.

22. Rubin DC: Gastroenterologic diseases. In Woodley M, Whelan A, eds: *Manual of medical therapeutics,* ed 27, Boston, 1992, Little, Brown.

23. Hurst J, Gallagher AL: Pathophysiology and nutritional management in acute pancreatitis, *Support Line* 16:6-11, 1994.

24. Ranson JNC: Etiological and prognostic factors in human acute pancreatitis: A review, *Am J Gastroenterol* 77:633-638, 1982.

25. Havala T, Shronts E, Cerra F: Nutritional support in acute pancreatitis, *Gastroenterol Clin North Am* 18:525-542, 1989.

26. ASPEN Board of Directors: Nutrition support for adults with specific diseases and conditions, *Journal of Parenteral and Enteral Nutrition* 17(suppl):16SA, 1993.

27. Ramsey BS, Farrel PM, Pincharz P: Nutritional assessment and management in cystic fibrosis: a consensus report, *Am J Clin Nutr* 55:108-116, 1992.

28. Wilson-Goodman V et al: Factors affecting the dietary habits of adolescents with cystic fibrosis, *J Am Diet Assoc* 90:429-431, 1990.

29. Gerson WT, Swan P, Walker WA: Nutrition support in cystic fibrosis, *Nutr Rev* 45:353-360, 1987.

Chapter 18

NUTRITION FOR DIABETES MELLITUS

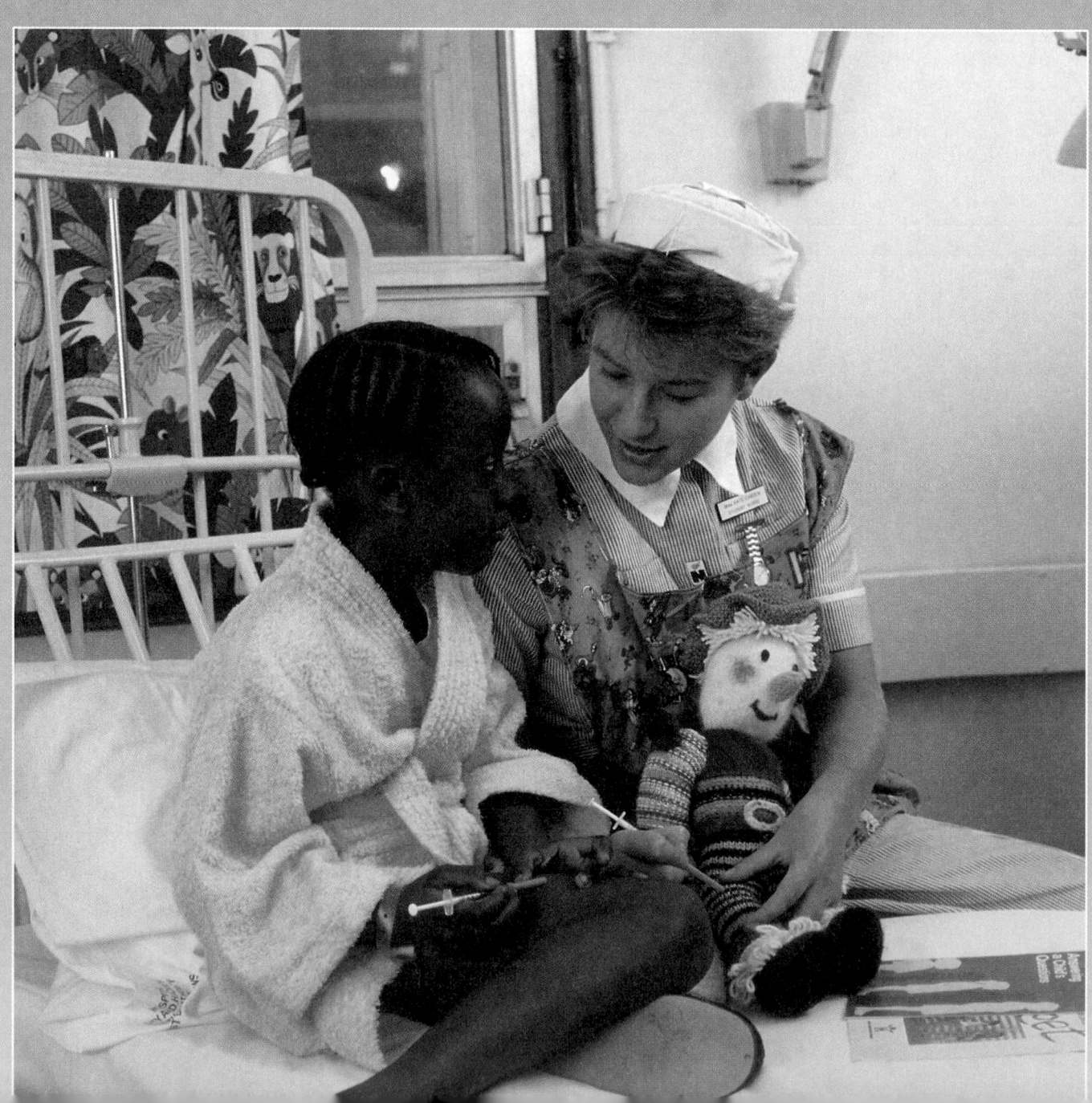

ROLE IN WELLNESS

As a chronic disorder, diabetes mellitus requires long-term lifestyle changes of both dietary intake and physical activity. Approaching this disorder in a proactive manner can lessen the negative impact of diabetes and achieve a higher level of wellness.

DIABETES MELLITUS

Diabetes mellitus is a group of conditions characterized by either a relative or complete lack of insulin secretion by the beta cells of the pancreas or by defects of cell insulin receptors, which result in disturbances of carbohydrate, protein, and lipid metabolism (1,2). Diabetes is usually diagnosed and characterized by elevated blood sugar (>120 mg/dl) or *hyperglycemia.* The main goal of treatment is maintenance of insulin/glucose homeostasis.

In addition to the everyday maintenance necessary to control blood sugar levels, diabetes mellitus is associated with disability and premature death because of the disease's effect on structural and functional alterations in many body systems, especially *macrovascular* and *microvascular* damage (Table 18-1) (2). Macrovascular complications increase the risk of coronary artery disease, peripheral vascular disease, and cerebrovascular accidents. Microvascular effects include nephropathy (kidney disorder) and retinopathy (eye disorder from blood vessel changes). Because of nephropathy, approximately half of all individuals with insulin-dependent diabetes mellitus develop chronic renal failure and end stage renal disease. Retinopathy is the leading cause of blindness in North America. In addition, neuropathy complications affect peripheral circulation, causing decreased sensations in extremities that may result in injury without the patient's knowledge. Healing is impaired because of the effects of diabetes on the circulatory system; gangrene may develop, and amputation may be necessary. Autonomic effects of diabetes may include orthostatic hypotension, persistent tachycardia, *gastroparesis,* neurogenic bladder (urinary bladder dysfunction from neurological damage), impotence, and impaired visceral pain sensation that can obscure symptoms of angina pectoris or myocardial infarction.

The development of these long-term complications is believed to be correlated to the level and frequency of hyperglycemia experiences throughout the life span of a person who has diabetes (3). These are considered *long-term complications* because individuals generally do not suffer these until they have lived with diabetes for more than 15 to 20 years. Genetic and environmental factors also play a role in the development of these complications (4).

Glucose intolerance can be classified into two primary categories: non–insulin-dependent diabetes (NIDDM) and insulin-dependent diabetes (IDDM). Other types include gestational diabetes, impaired glucose tolerance, and other forms of diabetes (5). These classifications, based on etiology, treatment needs, and their symptoms, are summarized in Table 18-2. The majority (over 90%) of persons with diabetes have NIDDM, whereas 5% to 10% have IDDM (4).

Insulin-Dependent Diabetes Mellitus

The onset of IDDM is usually very sudden. Cells use glucose for energy, and without *endogenous* insulin, cells literally start starving. The body responds by sending signals to eat because the cells are *hungry,* but since the end product of digestion (glucose) cannot enter the cells, the glucose builds up in the bloodstream. It is common for the person to experience weight loss while consuming large quantities of

Symptoms of IDDM
sudden onset of polyphagia, polyuria, polydipsia, weight loss

polyphagia
excessive hunger and eating

polyuria
excessive urination

polydipsia
excessive thirst

Symptoms of NIDDM
gradual onset of polyuria,
polydipsia, easily fatigued,
frequent infections (especially
urinary tract)

food (**polyphagia**). Since glucose cannot enter the cells and builds up in the blood-stream, the blood becomes hypertonic and the body tries to *get rid* of the excess glucose by increasing urine output (**polyuria**). In reaction to the increased excretion of urine, the body again responds by increasing thirst (**polydipsia**) to replace lost fluids.

By the time IDDM is diagnosed, approximately 80% to 90% of beta cell function has been lost (4). The destruction of the insulin-producing beta cells is thought to result from a progressive autoimmune response believed to be caused by a combination of genetic predisposition, viral infections, and environmental or unknown stimuli (6).

Non–Insulin-Dependent Diabetes Mellitus

Non–insulin-dependent diabetes mellitus is an insidious disease. Persons with NIDDM rarely present with the *classic* symptoms of diabetes (polyuria, polyphagia, polydipsia). In fact, some of the first symptoms that cause persons to seek medical attention are the complications (heart attack, stroke, neuropathic problems) associated with diabetes. It is not uncommon for a person to have NIDDM years before diagnosis (4). Unlike IDDM, the primary metabolic problem in NIDDM is insulin resistance or the failure of the cells to respond to insulin being produced by the body. Family history and obesity are the two strongest risk factors for NIDDM. In fact, obesity by itself produces an insulin-resistant state that causes beta cells to produce excessive amounts of insulin. Since not all obese persons develop diabetes, there seems to be a genetic tendency for diabetes that leads to beta

Table 18-1	Clinical Complications of Diabetes Mellitus	
Complication	**Target Site**	**Incidence/Manifestations**
Macrovascular*	Coronary artery disease	13 times greater than general population
	Peripheral vascular disease	5 times greater
	Cerebrovascular accident	3 times greater
Microvascular†	Nephropathy	Approximately half of all individuals with IDDM develop chronic renal failure and end stage renal disease; one third requiring dialysis or renal transplantation have diabetes
	Retinopathy	Leading cause of blindness in North America
Neuropathy	Peripheral	Decreased sensation in extremities; resulting injury may lead to gangrene and amputation
	Autonomic	Orthostatic hypotension; persistent tachycardia; gastroparesis; neurogenic bladder; impotence; impaired visceral pain sensation

From American Dietetic Association: *Handbook of clinical nutrition,* ed 2, New Haven, 1992, Yale University Press; Kenshole AB: Diabetes. In Jeejeebhoy KN, ed: *Current therapy in nutrition,* Toronto, 1988, Decker; Swearingen PL: *Manual of nursing therapeutics: Applying nursing diagnoses to medical disorders,* ed 2, St. Louis, 1990, Mosby; and Orland MJ: Diabetes mellitus. In Woodley M, Whelan A, eds: *Manual of medical therapeutics,* ed 27, Boston, 1992, Little, Brown.
*Exacerbated by concurrent of hypertension, hypercholesterolemia, smoking, aging.
†Compounds the effects of macrovascular problems.

cell exhaustion and hyperglycemia in some obese persons (4). Additionally, upper body obesity has been recognized as being an even greater risk factor for diabetes than degree of obesity (7). Upper body obesity, defined as a waist-to-hip ratio greater than 0.8, is a risk factor not only for diabetes but also for heart disease and hypertension (4).

Insulin

As the name implies, all persons with IDDM require *exogenous* insulin to maintain normal blood glucose levels. Some individuals with NIDDM may require insulin to optimize blood glucose control. Regardless of the type of diabetes, the goal of insulin therapy is to mimic physiologic insulin delivery (4,8). This is usually accomplished by a variety of methods: split-dose regimen, multidose therapy, or insulin pumps.

For the most part, insulin is not recommended for obese patients because of the large doses required to normalize blood glucose levels. Since obesity promotes insulin resistance and large doses of insulin can stimulate appetite, insulin therapy can result in increased food intake, weight gain, and the need for more insulin. Furthermore, insulin is an anabolic hormone, which may increase fat deposits and fluid retention (9).

Oral Hypoglycemic Agents

Oral hypoglycemic agents (sulfonylureas) are used to treat NIDDM when diet and physical activity cannot control hyperglycemia. Their primary action is to increase insulin production from the beta cells to overcome insulin resistance at the peripheral level. Patients taking oral hypoglycemic agents can experience hypoglycemia, which can be caused by not eating enough food or interactions with other medications (prescription or over-the-counter).

Table 18-2   Classifications of Glucose Intolerance

Classification	Former Terms	Symptoms or Indicators
Insulin-dependent diabetes mellitus (IDDM)	Type I diabetes, juvenile-onset diabetes, ketosis-prone diabetes, brittle diabetes	*Early:* fatigue, weakness, polyuria, polydipsia, nocturnal incontinence, polyphagia, weight loss *Late:* dehydration, electrolyte imbalance, possible hypovolemic shock, possible coma, Kussmaul's respirations, acetone breath, weak and rapid pulse, hypotension, hyperglycemia
Non–insulin-dependent diabetes mellitus (NIDDM)	Type II diabetes, adult-onset diabetes, maturity-onset diabetes, ketosis-resistant diabetes, stable diabetes	*Early:* fatigue, polyuria, polydipsia *Late:* retinopathy (some are diagnosed with NIDDM after seeking medical care for blurred vision), marked dehydration, hypovolemic shock, shallow respirations, gross hyperglycemia, absence of ketosis
Diabetes associated with certain conditions or syndromes	Secondary diabetes	
Gestational diabetes mellitus (GDM)	Gestational diabetes, Type III diabetes	Does not include those with known diabetes mellitus who become pregnant; if glucose intolerance remains after delivery, patient is reclassified (IDDM or NIDDM)
Impaired glucose tolerance (IGT)	Borderline diabetes, chemical diabetes	Diabetes mellitus may develop if dietary and exercise habits not modified

From American Dietetic Association: *Handbook of clinical dietetics,* ed 2, New Haven, 1992, Yale University Press; *Mosby's medical, nursing, and allied health dictionary,* ed 4, St. Louis, 1990, Mosby; Swearingen PL: *Manual of nursing therapeutics: Applying nursing diagnoses to medical disorders,* ed 3, St. Louis, 1990, Mosby; Weinsier RL, Heimburger DC, and Butterworth CE: *Handbook of clinical nutrition,* ed 2, St. Louis, 1989, Mosby; Orland MJ: Diabetes mellitus. In Woodley M, Whelan A, eds: *Manual of medical therapeutics,* ed 27, Boston, 1992, Little, Brown.

Exercise

Along with medical nutrition therapy (discussed later in this chapter) and insulin, exercise is the third component of treatment of diabetes. Exercise, like insulin, lowers blood glucose levels, assists in maintaining normal lipid levels, and increases circulation. For most individuals, consistent and individualized exercise helps reduce the therapeutic dose of insulin (10). Patients should be instructed not to perform exercise at the time insulin is at its peak. Ideally, they should exercise when blood glucose levels are between 100 and 200 mg/dl or about 30 to 60 minutes after meals. They should avoid exercising when blood glucose is above 250 mg/dl and ketones are present in the urine (9). Fig. 18-1 describes metabolic effects of exercise on IDDM and NIDDM. In the case of IDDM, glucose control can be compromised if proper adjustments are not made in food intake or insulin administration. Patients with NIDDM who are taking oral hypoglycemic agents may be at risk of post-exercise hypoglycemia (11).

Exercise can increase the risk for hypoglycemia in persons with IDDM. Hypoglycemia during exercise of 40 minutes or less is rare. The onset is more likely to occur after exercise, often between 4 and 10 hours after (9). Blood glucose levels should be monitored at 1 or 2-hour intervals after exercise to assess response to the exercise and allow for adjustments in insulin and food intake (9).

The best time to eat a small snack is after exercising, rather than before. Guidelines for adjusting or increasing food intake should be based on blood glucose levels before and after exercise, how close exercise is to scheduled meals/snacks, and how often the exercise is performed. Persons who exercise regularly (same time each day) usually require less additional food than someone who exercises intermittently (9).

Persons with diabetes should schedule exercise 1 to 3 hours after meals, with the starting blood glucose above 100 mg/dl. In addition to the regularly planned meals, patients should consume extra food following moderate exercise. A general rule is 10 to 15 gm of carbohydrate (one fruit or starch/bread exchange) should be eaten for one hour of moderate exercise. Moderate exercise is defined as tennis,

IDDM

Insulin	Hepatic Glucose Output	Peripheral Glucose Use	Counter-regulatory Hormones		Blood Glucose
Adequate	⇓	⇓	⇓	➡	⇓
Inadequate	⇑	⇑	⇑	➡	⇑

NIDDM

Hepatic Glucose Output	Peripheral Glucose Use	Counter-regulatory Hormones	Insulin Sensitivity		Blood Glucose Control
⇓	⇑	⇓	⇑	➡	Improved

Figure 18-1 Metabolic effects of exercise in IDDM and NIDDM.

swimming, jogging, or cycling. Mild exercise, such as walking less than a mile, generally does not require additional food. Strenuous activity (football, hockey, soccer, racquetball, basketball, strenuous cycling or swimming, and shoveling heavy snow) may require 30 to 50 gm of carbohydrate (one-half meat sandwich with one milk or fruit exchange) (9).

Blood Glucose Monitoring

Blood glucose levels are the cornerstone of diabetes management (11). Blood glucose levels can be monitored several ways: (1) **fasting blood glucose,** (2) **glycosylated hemoglobin,** and (3) self-monitoring.

Fasting blood glucose, also called fasting blood sugar, is the level of glucose in the blood after an 8-hour fast. Normal values range from 70 to 110 mg/dl depending on the standards set by individual laboratories. Fasting levels of blood glucose are elevated in uncontrolled diabetes.

Glycosylated hemoglobin ($HgbA_{1c}$) is formed through an irreversible process. As the red blood cells (RBC) circulate in the bloodstream, hemoglobin combines with glucose, forming glycohemoglobin. The amount of glycohemoglobin formed depends on the amount of glucose in bloodstream circulation over the RBCs 120-day life span. Therefore the amount of $HgbA_{1c}$ is a reflection of the average blood glucose level for the 100- to 120-day period before the test; the more glucose the RBC was exposed to, the greater the value. This value is not affected by factors such as food intake, exercise, or stress so the blood sample can be drawn at any time; this is an easier sample to obtain than the fasting blood glucose test.

Self-monitoring can be performed in the patient's home with blood glucose meters (sometimes called glucometers) that can be purchased at pharmacies. A droplet of blood is obtained by finger prick on a regular basis to monitor glucose levels before and after meals and at bedtime (10). Self-monitoring is particularly useful in evaluating glycemic control and effectiveness of the meal plan in meeting the goals of medical nutrition therapy.

Records should be kept of self-monitored blood glucose levels for review by the health care team to determine food, insulin, and exercise needs. This allows for individualized treatment, especially with meal plans, making indiscriminate, general dietary advice or tear-off diet sheets unjustified. The frequency of monitoring depends on the type of diabetes and therapy. For some, monitoring up to seven times a day may be appropriate: before and after (1 to 2 hours after) breakfast, lunch, and dinner; and at bedtime (11).

Hypoglycemia

Hypoglycemia (below normal values of blood glucose levels) usually results from too much insulin, skipping meals, or too much exercise without a concomitant increase in food intake. The onset is sudden and can be fatal if left untreated. Most often, hypoglycemia occurs during the peak time of insulin (or oral hypoglycemic agents) or during the night when the patient is sleeping (fasting) (10).

Symptoms usually occur when blood glucose drops below 50 mg/dl or there is a relatively significant drop in blood glucose. For example, if a patient is in a consistent state of hyperglycemia (may be 180 to 200 mg/dl) and blood glucose levels are brought down to 90 mg/dl, he may experience hypoglycemia even though the blood glucose level is in the normal range. The key is, the *normal blood glucose* is low for that patient (10).

Diabetic Ketoacidosis

Diabetic ketoacidosis (DKA) is a life-threatening condition caused by insulin deficiency. When glucose cannot be used by cells, the body breaks down fats and

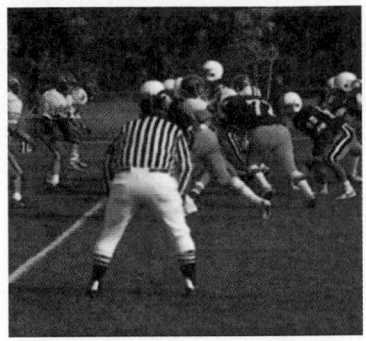

Exercise, like insulin, lowers blood glucose levels, helps to maintain normal lipid levels, and increases circulation.

fasting blood glucose
level of glucose circulating in blood serum after an 8-hr fast; also called fasting blood sugar

glycosylated hemoglobin ($HgbA_{1c}$)
a substance (glycohemoglobin) formed when hemoglobin combines with some of the glucose in the bloodstream

Symptoms of hypoglycemia
hunger; erratic behavior; confusion; trembling, shaking; cool, clammy, pale skin

Symptoms of DKA
polyuria; polyphagia; weight loss; nausea; dry, flushed skin and mucous membranes; dehydration and metabolic acidosis; polydipsia; *fruity* (acetone) breath; generalized weakness; vomiting; weakness, fatigue

proteins for energy that can cause ketosis. Ketosis is an abnormal accumulation of ketones caused by the metabolism of fatty acids for energy with little carbohydrate metabolism occurring; ketoacidosis may then occur. This condition results in hyperglycemia that causes osmotic diuresis, leads to dehydration, and precipitates lactic acidosis. Lowered pH, resulting from the acidosis, stimulates the respiratory center and produces deep, rapid respirations known as *Kussmaul respirations*. Large amounts of ketones in the body also produce a *fruity* or acetone odor on the breath (a person suffering from DKA could be mistaken for someone who is inebriated). If this condition is not recognized and treated promptly, the acidosis and dehydration lead to loss of consciousness, and possibly coma and death (10). Common conditions that precipitate DKA include insufficient or interrupted insulin therapy, too much food, infection, or other stresses (trauma, surgery, emotional stress, myocardial infarction) (8).

Symptoms of HHNK
polyuria; polyphagia; weight loss; nausea; dry, flushed skin and mucous membranes; dehydration secondary to osmotic diuresis; polydipsia; possible seizures and tremors; generalized weakness; vomiting; weakness, fatigue

Hyperosmolar Hyperglycemic Nonketotic Coma

Hyperosmolar hyperglycemic nonketotic coma (HHNC), like DKA, is a life-threatening emergency caused by a relative or actual insulin deficiency resulting in severe hyperglycemia. Most often HHNC is triggered by stress (trauma, infection) that increases the body's demand for insulin. Although enough insulin may be present to prevent the formation of ketones, thus preventing acidosis, there may not be enough to prevent hyperglycemia. If hyperglycemia is left untreated, the serum becomes hyperosmolar and produces osmotic diuresis and simultaneous loss of electrolytes. Mortality for HHNC is 10% to 25% (10).

MEDICAL NUTRITION THERAPY

In 1994 the American Diabetes Association published its fifth set of recommendations since 1950 (Table 18-3). These new recommendations introduce two major changes in the philosophy of nutrition care for diabetes. First, the calculated kcaloric prescription tailored to meet individual needs has been replaced by individually developed dietary prescriptions based on metabolic, nutrition, and lifestyle requirements. This change was guided by the appreciation that diabetes encompasses a variety of metabolic abnormalities and that a single formula for planning diets is not adequate to treat all types of diabetes (12).

The second change deals with the approach to nutrition management of NIDDM. Although weight loss continues to be a focus of therapy for overweight persons, blood glucose and lipid goals have also been included. A variety of methods to achieve these metabolic goals are advocated, only one of which is weight loss (12). In the words of the Diabetes Care and Education Practice Group (of The American Dietetic Association):

> Overall, the 1994 recommendations make obsolete the concept of one diet for diabetes and physician orders for an 'ADA diet.' They mandate a comprehensive approach to nutrition management of diabetes that demands more resources than the mathematical methods but also has the potential to be more effective (12).

Adherence to nutrition and meal planning principles has always been one of the most challenging facets of diabetes care (13). Medical nutritional therapy is an essential component of successful diabetes management and the complexity involved requires a team approach to enhance the ability of the patient to obtain good metabolic control (12). The diabetes management team should include a registered nurse, a physician or primary health care provider, the person with diabetes, and a registered dietitian knowledgeable and skilled in implementing current principles and recommendations for diabetes (12,13).

Year	Percent of Carbohydrates	Percent of Protein	Percent of Fat
pre-1921		Starvation diets	
1921	20	10	70
1950	40	20	40
1971	45	20	35
1986	≤60	12-20	<30
1994	Based on nutrition assessment and treatment goals	10-20	Based on nutrition assessment and treatment goals; less than 10% of energy from saturated fats

Table 18-3   Historical Perspective of Nutrition Recommendations for Diabetes Mellitus

Modified from American Dietetic Association: Nutrition recommendations and principles for people with diabetes mellitus, *J Am Diet Assoc* 94:504-506, 1994.

What's Out/What's In

PRIMARY GOAL
Out: Weight loss as the primary goal for management
In: Aim for near normal blood sugar levels and optimal lipid levels (cholesterol, LDLs, HDLs, triglycerides)

DIET PLAN
Out: Preprinted diet plans
In: Individualized diet plans based on food preferences, lifestyle, and medication

WEIGHT
Out: Striving to reach an *ideal* or *desirable* weight, which may be unattainable or frustrating
In: Focus on reaching a *reasonable* weight that can be maintained; even a 10-20 lb weight loss can improve blood glucose control

SUGAR
Out: The idea that simple sugar should be avoided and replaced with complex carbohydrates (starches)
In: Some sugar, and foods that contain sugar, can be substituted for other carbohydrate foods, but not simply added to the meal plan

Modified from *Environmental Nutrition,* 17:3, 1994.

Goals of Medical Nutrition Therapy

Whereas the overall goal of nutrition therapy is to facilitate changes in nutrition and exercise habits leading to improved metabolic control, there are additional specific goals (13):

- Maintain as near normal blood glucose levels as possible by balancing food intake with insulin (either endogenous or exogenous) or oral hypoglycemic agents and activity levels
- Achieve optimal serum lipid levels
- Provide adequate energy for maintaining or attaining reasonable weights for adults, normal growth and development rates in children and adolescents, increased metabolic needs during pregnancy and lactation, or recovery from catabolic illnesses (reasonable weight is defined as the weight an individual

and health care provider acknowledge as achievable and maintainable, both short- and long-term; this weight may not be the same as the traditionally defined *desirable* or *ideal* body weight)
- Prevent and treat acute complications of insulin-treated diabetes (hypoglycemia, short-term illnesses, and exercise-related problems) and long-term complications of diabetes (renal disease, autonomic neuropathy, hypertension, and cardiovascular disease)
- Improve overall health through optimal nutrition

Successful medical nutrition therapy involves the diabetes management team conducting a thorough assessment, encouraging patient participation in goal setting, selecting an appropriate nutrition intervention, and evaluating the effectiveness of the nutrition care plan (12).

Assessment

Assessment helps identify goals and determines the types of nutrition intervention to be used. It includes the collection of clinical data, dietary history, and nutrient intake. With this information, nutrition problems are identified and misinformation corrected.

Goal setting

The goal setting step uses information gathered from the assessment to guide the patient to identify his needs in relation to overall diabetes management. A number of questions are asked of the patient about the types of behavior changes the patient is willing to make. The outcome is for the patient to develop personal, realistic, and specific goals regarding positive changes in eating and exercise behaviors. The goals, however, are not permanent and are adjusted for a variety of reasons.

Nutrition intervention

The third step, nutrition intervention, considers any metabolic abnormalities experienced by the patient. The patient acquires knowledge and skills to change or maintain eating habits. The dietitian considers the literacy level of the patient and determines the appropriate amount and format of information to present. Basic nutrition intervention provides an overview of nutrition and nutrient requirements, diabetes nutrition management, and other related information. In-depth nutrition intervention details meal planning with a more structured approach regarding menu content, portion size, and carbohydrate (intake) to insulin ratio(s).

Evaluation

The fourth step, evaluation, involves the dietitian and the patient deciding the effect of the intervention. Part of the evaluation includes analysis of the clinical data to assess effectiveness. Follow-up interventions may be needed as changes occur in the patient's life; these may be related to lifestyle or to modifications in diabetes management recommendations. For adults, additional interventions may occur every 6 to 12 months. Because of their growth patterns, follow-ups for children are recommended every 3 to 6 months (12).

These four steps are outlined in Table 18-4.

Exchange Lists for Meal Planning

One of the most widely used methods of creating individualized meal plans for persons with diabetes is the Exchange Lists for Meal Planning (14). Food exchange lists provide one of the easiest ways to allow flexibility in meal planning while preserving consistency in carbohydrate, protein, and fat intake. No special or *diet* foods are necessary when using this system as the exchange lists divide foods into three different groupings. Each group of foods, or exchange, is similar in kcalorie, carbohydrate, protein, and fat content (unlike the Basic Four Food Groups or

Table 18-4   Steps Involved in Medical Nutrition Therapy for Diabetes

Step	Purpose	Information Needed	Desired Outcome
Assessment	Helps identify goal, determines types of nutrition intervention to be used, establishes rapport with patient	*Clinical data:* Height/weight; body frame; reasonable weight; blood pressure; results of patient's self-monitoring of blood glucose levels, blood lipid levels, and glycosylated hemoglobin; daily medications (insulin or oral hypoglycemic agents); daily energy needs *Dietary history:* Usual food intake, attitudes toward nutrition and health, previous nutrition education and outcomes *Nutrient intake:* Overall nutritional adequacy, kcalorie intake, nutrient distribution (type of carbohydrate, protein, and fat)	*Dietitian will:* Identify nutrition problems and misinformation, provide positive feedback on patient's current eating habits and lifestyle activities
Goal Setting	Enables patient to use assessment information to identify his needs in relation to overall diabetes management	The following questions may help negotiate goals and obtain information about patient's understanding and about his willingness and interest in making changes: What would you like from nutrition counseling? What is the most important goal for you in managing your diabetes and the way you eat? Regarding your present plan of eating, what are some changes you are willing to make? What would you do to make these changes? Of the changes we've discussed, what could you do first?	*Patient will:* Establish realistic and specific goals to make positive changes in eating and exercise behaviors, goals are *not* permanent and change for a variety of reasons
Nutrition intervention	Provides the patient with knowledge and skills necessary to change or maintain eating habits	Information on metabolic abnormalities of patient, literacy level of patient, type of audiovisual materials to use (handouts, videos, audiotapes, flip charts, or food models)	After basic nutrition intervention, patient will be able to state overview of nutrition and nutrient requirements, diabetes nutrition management guidelines, and other appropriate information (label reading, sick-day management, travel tips) After in-depth nutrition intervention, patient will be able to plan meals with more structure (menus, calorie counting, fat counting, exchange lists, and carbohydrate to insulin ratio)

Continued.

Table 18-4   Steps Involved in Medical Nutrition Therapy for Diabetes, cont'd.

Step	Purpose	Information Needed	Desired Outcome
Evaluation	Determines effect of medical nutrition therapy intervention	Clinical data	If effective, patient continues adhering to guidelines and follow-up sessions to revise diet because of lifestyle and life span changes or to modification of diabetes management guidelines; follow-up for children should occur every 3-6 months; adults every 6-12 months

Modified from Tinker LF, Heins JM, Holler HJ: Commentary and translation: 1994 nutrition recommendations for diabetes, *J Am Diet Assoc* 94:507-511, 1994.

Table 18-5   Summary of Exchange Lists for Meal Planning

Groups/Lists	Carbohydrate (gm)	Protein (gm)	Fat (gm)	Kcal
Carbohydrate group				
Starch	15	3	1 or less	80
Fruit	15	—	—	60
Milk				
Skim	12	8	0–3	90
Low-fat	12	8	5	120
Whole	12	8	8	150
Other carbohydrates	15	varies	varies	varies
Vegetables	5	2	—	25
Meat and meat substitute group				
Very lean	—	7	0–1	35
Lean	—	7	3	55
Medium-fat	—	7	5	75
High-fat	—	7	8	100
Fat group	—	—	5	45

Food Guide Pyramid, which categorize foods according to their source). Portion sizes vary from food to food, which allows each food (in its proper portion) to be kcalorically equivalent. The Carbohydrate group is subdivided into lists of starch, fruit, milk (skim, low fat, or whole), other carbohydrates, and vegetables. The Meat and Meat Substitutes group is sorted by fat content into categories of very lean, lean, medium fat, and high fat. Accordingly, foods *within* any one group can be exchanged (traded) for another food *within* the same group. Generally, it is a good idea not to trade food from one group for food in another group. Table 18-5 outlines the exchange groups and distribution of nutrients. A listing of foods included on each exchange list can be found in Appendix B.

To help clarify the exchange concept, consider this analogy. Meal planning with exchange lists is like having different bank accounts that are designated for the *purchase* of different products. A certain amount of *money* (number of exchanges allowed per day) can be spent from each account (the exchange lists) each day. The only stipulation is that the money from each account can only be used to purchase products designated for that account. Let's say that you have bank accounts set up for your home. There is a utilities account, clothing account, mortgage/rent account, groceries account, entertainment account, and savings account. You can take money out of your utilities account to pay for electricity, water, or gas, but money from this account cannot be used to by a new dress. Likewise, money from the clothing account cannot be used to make rent payments.

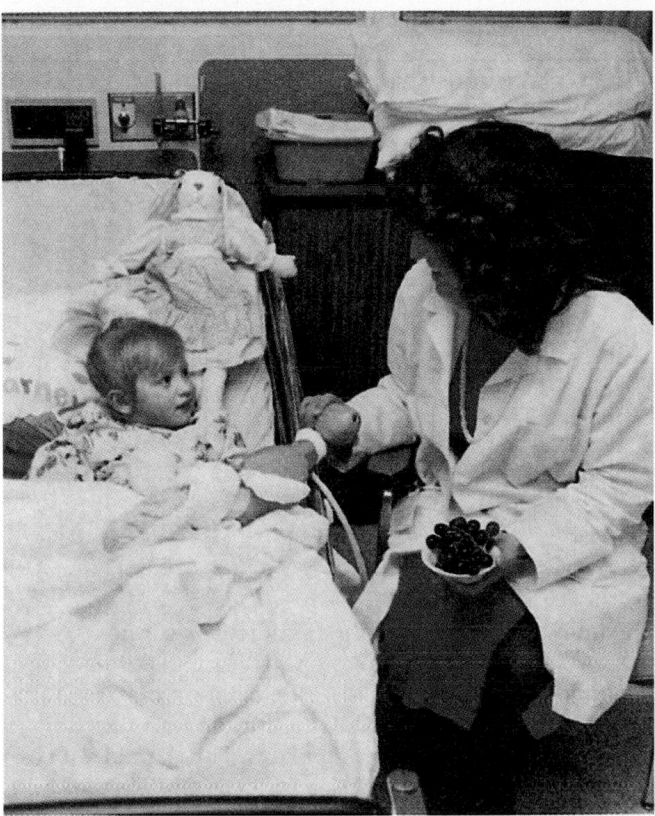

Educating children to make healthy food choices is an ongoing task.

When reviewing the exchange lists, pay particular attention to the foods included in each list. Although we're used to using the Food Guide Pyramid, which groups foods from the same or similar sources together (for example, all milks and milk products are grouped in the milk group), we cannot use the Exchange Lists in a similar manner. The only dairy products listed in the Milk Exchange are milk and yogurt. Cheeses are in the Meat Exchange. Starchy vegetables (such as corn and potatoes) are listed in the Starch List instead of the Vegetable List.

The total amount of food allowed for each day is divided into a specific number of exchanges from each group depending on the patient's preferences obtained from the diet history. Diet instruction is usually conducted by the registered dietician, with reinforcement and guidance from the nurse. Educational needs of patients with diabetes in addition to basic meal planning include exercise guidelines, hypoglycemic treatment, nutrition planning in the event of short-term illnesses such as flu, blood glucose monitoring, and plans for continuing care (11). Once the meal plan has been developed, it should be reviewed, reinforced, and possibly adjusted on a regular basis, at least every 3 to 6 months. The sample menu (see box) reflects a 1500 kcalorie controlled meal plan.

Additional education topics that can enhance nutrition *survival* skills include label reading, foods for sick days, alcohol use, adjusting meal times, healthy snack choices, eating at fast-food restaurants, brown bag lunches, and making meal plans more flexible (11). These topics are usually taught by registered dietitians after clients master basic education and skills.

Nutrition Therapy and IDDM

Meal plans should be based on an individual's usual food intake and used as a foundation for integrating insulin therapy into the usual eating and exercise patterns. Patients should also be taught to eat at consistent times synchronized with the time/action of the insulin preparation used. Insulin doses need to be adjusted according to blood glucose levels and the amount of food usually eaten. Insulin pumps and

Sample 1500 Kcalorie-Controlled Diet Menu for Diabetes Management

BREAKFAST
Orange juice
Corn flakes
Whole wheat toast
Margarine
Skim milk
Coffee

LUNCH
Beef sirloin tips (2 oz)*
Sweet potatoes with green beans
Tossed salad with Italian salad dressing
Applesauce with cinnamon
Margarine (1-2 exchanges)*
Diet soda

DINNER
Turkey breast (2 oz) with peas and parsley carrots*
Tomato soup with whole wheat crackers
Baked custard
Pear halves
Sugar-free lemonade

From Memorial Hospital, Carbondale, Ill.
*Quantities not exact; for representation only.

multiple daily injections allow for considerable flexibility in when and what individuals eat. When appropriate, insulin regimens should be integrated with the patient's lifestyle and adjusted for departures from usual eating and exercise habits (9).

Nutrition Therapy for NIDDM

Traditional therapy has incorporated weight loss and hypokcaloric diets to improve short-term, and hopefully long-term, glycemic levels. Because these traditional dietary strategies have usually not been effective in achieving long-term weight loss, emphasis should be placed on achieving glucose, lipid, and blood pressure goals. Although weight loss is desirable, and some individuals are able to lose and maintain weight lost, further strategies can be realized to improve metabolic control. There is no one proven strategy or method that is uniformly recommended (13). Table 18-6 suggests approaches that may be successful.

Individualized Recommendations

Medical nutrition therapy for diabetes is complex. Physicians and nurses can no longer depend on preprinted diet sheets or formulated meal patterns to provide nutrition care to patients with diabetes (12). There is no **one** *diabetic* or *ADA* diet. The recommended diet can only be defined as a dietary prescription based on nutrition assessment and treatment goals. Medical nutrition therapy should be individualized, taking into consideration a person's usual eating habits and other lifestyle factors (13). Consistency within an eating pattern will result in lower glycosylated hemoglobin levels than following an arbitrary eating style (15).

Nutrition recommendations for total fat, saturated fat, cholesterol, fiber, vitamins, and minerals are the same for individuals with diabetes as for the general population. Recommendations are modified for protein, carbohydrates, sucrose, and alcohol because of the nature of diabetes in relation to carbohydrate metabolism or

Table 18-6   Strategies for Metabolic Control (NIDDM)

- Nutritionally adequate meal plan with a reduction of total fat, especially saturated fats
- Meals spaced throughout the day
- Mild to moderate weight loss (5-10 kg [10-20 lb]) even if desirable body weight is not achieved (moderate decrease in energy intake + increase in kcalorie expenditure)
- Regular exercise
- Monitoring of blood glucose levels, glycosylated hemoglobin, lipids, and blood pressure
- Oral hypoglycemic or insulin may be required if above does not work
- Serotonergic appetite suppressants (long-term safety and efficacy unknown)
- Gastric reduction surgery for individuals with BMI [kg/m^2] > 35 (long-term safety and efficacy unknown)

the effects of diabetic complications. Protein intake can range from 10% to 20% of daily kcalories from animal and vegetable protein sources. If the patient has nephropathy, lower intakes of protein (about 10% of daily energy intake) may be warranted. Carbohydrate recommendations are individualized based on the person's eating habits and blood glucose and lipid goals. Blood glucose control is not impaired by the use of sucrose in the meal plan, but sucrose-containing foods are substituted for other carbohydrates and foods and are not eaten in addition to a meal plan. Blood glucose levels are not affected by moderate alcohol use if diabetes is well controlled. For individuals using insulin, ≤2 alcoholic beverages can be consumed as an addition to a meal plan. Alcohol is best consumed with meals to reduce the risk of hypoglycemia for those using insulin or on sulfonylureas. Alcohol kcalories, if figured as part of the meal plan, are substituted for fat exchanges or fat kcalories.

Other related nutrient issues include the use of fructose, other nutritive and nonnutritive sweeteners, and mineral intake of chromium, magnesium, and potassium. Although fructose creates a smaller rise in plasma glucose than sucrose and other carbohydrates, large amounts of fructose (up to 20% of daily kcalorie intake) provide no advantage as a sweetener based on its negative effects on serum cholesterol and LDL-cholesterol levels. Other nutritive sweeteners such as corn sweeteners, fruit juice or juice concentrate, honey, molasses, dextrose, and maltose affect glycemic response and caloric content in a manner similar to that of sucrose. The sugar alcohols (sorbitol, mannitol, and xylitol) result in lower glycemic responses than other simple and complex carbohydrates, and ingesting large amounts may have a laxative effect. Nonnutritive sweeteners approved for use by the FDA, including saccharin, aspartame, and acesulfame K, are considered safe for consumption by individuals with diabetes. Additional supplementation with vitamins and minerals is not required if dietary intake is adequate. Deficiencies of chromium and magnesium affect carbohydrate metabolism and cause insulin resistance. However, most individuals with diabetes are not deficient in these minerals; therefore supplementation would not reduce their hyperglycemia. Potassium supplementation may be harmful. For persons with renal insufficiency caused by diabetic complications, dietary potassium restriction may be necessary. Table 18-7 summarizes nutrition therapy recommendations.

Role of the Nurse

The role of the nurse in caring for the nutritional needs of patients with diabetes varies depending on the setting and age of the client. However, the general approach is to assess the patient's knowledge and understanding and adherence with the prescribed diet. When possible, observing meals and food choices as well as monitoring glucose levels can give important clues to the level of compliance.

When compliance is faulty, the nurse needs to determine whether knowledge or motivation is the problem. Knowledge deficits can be remedied by the nurse or dietitian; lack of motivation may be harder to deal with. For example, adolescents with diabetes may not believe that long-term complications are related to diet and may be more motivated by the need to eat like their peers. The elderly with diabetes may be very set in long-time food intake patterns and may not want to change them as long as they are taking medication for hyperglycemia.

When a trusting relationship exists between the nurse and the patient, discussions about motivations and concerns can take place. The nurse may then influence the patient to be more concerned about his long-term welfare. A care plan that meets the patient's social, psychological, and physical needs can be developed as a result of collaboration among the nurse, the physician or primary health care provider, the dietitian, and the patient. An additional form of support may be pro-

Table 18-7 Summary of 1994 Medical Nutrition Therapy Recommendations for Diabetes Mellitus	
Nutrient	**Recommendation**
Protein	Animal and vegetable protein sources: 10%-20% of daily kcalorie intake; if nephropathy develops, consider lower intakes of protein: 0.8 g/kg body weight/day (approximately 10% of daily energy intake)
Total Fat	Percentage of energy from fat depends on desired glucose, lipid, and weight goals; for individuals with normal lipid levels and who maintain a reasonable weight (and for normal growth and development in children and adolescents) recommend 30% or less of energy intake from total fat, and < 10% from saturated fat
Saturated fat and cholesterol	Saturated fat intake: <10% of daily energy intake Dietary cholesterol: limit to ≤ 300 mg daily
Carbohydrates	Percentage of daily energy intake individualized based on eating habits and glucose and lipid goals
Sucrose	Use as part of the meal plan does not impair blood glucose control; substitute sucrose and sucrose-containing foods for other carbohydrates and foods; do not add to the meal plan
Fructose	Produces a smaller rise in plasma glucose than sucrose and most starchy carbohydrates; fructose may have no overall advantage as a sweetening agent based on possible adverse effects of large amounts of fructose (20% of energy) on serum cholesterol and LDL-cholesterol levels
Other nutritive sweeteners	Corn sweeteners, corn syrup, fruit juice or fruit juice concentrate, honey, molasses, dextrose, and maltose do not have any significant advantage or disadvantage over sucrose in terms of improvement in caloric content or glycemic response; sugar alcohols (sorbitol, mannitol, and xylitol) create lower glycemic response than sucrose and other carbohydrates, but excessive amounts may have a laxative effect
Nonnutritive sweeteners	Saccharin, aspartame, and acesulfame K are approved for use by the FDA and are considered safe to consume by all people with diabetes
Fiber	20 to 35 g dietary fiber daily from a wide variety of food sources (same as for the general population); dietary fiber effect on glycemic control is probably insignificant
Sodium	2400-3000 mg/day; for those with mild to moderate hypertension: ≤ 2400 mg/day (same as for the general population)
Alcohol	When diabetes is well controlled, blood glucose levels are not affected by moderate alcohol use; if using insulin: ≤ 2 alcoholic beverages (1 alcoholic beverage = 12 oz beer, 5 oz wine, or 1½ oz distilled spirits) ingested with and in addition to the usual meal plan; alcohol may increase the risk for hypoglycemia if taking insulin or sulfonylureas so alcohol should be ingested with meals; when kcaloric intake from alcohol is calculated as part of the total kcaloric intake, substitute alcohol for fat exchanges or fat kcalories (1 alcoholic beverage = 2 fat exchanges)
Vitamins and minerals	Additional supplementation when dietary intake is adequate **Chromium:** Although chromium deficiency may affect glucose metabolism, most people with diabetes are not chromium deficient and chromium supplementation has no known benefit **Magnesium:** Although magnesium deficiency may result in insulin resistance and carbohydrate intolerance, very few are at risk for hypomagnesium **Potassium:** Dietary potassium restriction may be necessary in those with renal insufficiency and hyperkalemia

Modified from Tinker LF, Heins JM, Holler HJ: Commentary and translation: 1994 nutrition recommendations for diabetes, *J Am Diet Asssoc* 94:507-511, 1994; and American Dietetics Association: Nutrition recommendations and principles for people with diabetes mellitus, *J Am Diet Assoc* 94:504-506, 1994.

vided by community agencies and associations. These resources, such as the American Diabetes Association, are listed in Appendix C: Nutrition and Health Organizations.

As mentioned previously, nutrition and diet are considered, both by patients and health professionals, to be the most difficult problem in the management of diabetes. Every day we are faced with changes in our environments that require some adaptation to the situation. We're late for work, so maybe we skip breakfast or grab something quick along the way. The kids have ball practice tonight, so dinner becomes sandwiches and fruit instead of a full-course meal. Most of us make the required changes in stride, not thinking too much about it. Why should we think life for persons with diabetes is any different? Historically, those with diabetes have been taught consistency in every thing they do: eat at the same time every day, eat the same number of kcalories every day, take the same amount of insulin every day, and on and on. The new recommendations for medical nutritional therapy take these perpetual lifestyle changes into consideration.

But wouldn't it also be practical when encouraging dietary adherence with a person who has diabetes, to discuss situations that cause the individual problems in maintaining control over his eating? Schlundt et al (16) have identified 12 situations that provide obstacles to adhering to a prescribed diet (Table 18-8). Complete education for persons with diabetes should include assessment of these obstacles and situational problem-solving (16).

Table 18-8   Obstacles to Dietary Adherence in Diabetes Mellitus

Obstacle	Assessment
Extent to which social, career, recreational, and personal goals create situations in which the person must choose between making appropriate food choices and furthering another important life goal	Does the patient see this as a problem? To what extent? Does he feel frustrated about it? How has he dealt with it in the past? Does the patient make compromises, or does he give in to the competing goals? Is the conflict planned for, or simply handled when they arise? Does time pressure have any effect on the patient's ability to make appropriate choices?
Tempted to overeat to cope with stress and negative emotions	How stressful is the patient's life? How does he respond to frustration, stress, anxiety, and depression? Any conflicts with friends, family, supervisors, or other authorities? Is food used as an escape or avoidance strategy? If so, how much and what kinds of foods are eaten? How is boredom handled?
Ability to resist temptation when confronted with inappropriate foods or when experiencing specific food cravings?	Does the patient encounter inappropriate foods in his everyday environment? If so, how often? How does the patient react to seeing other people eat these foods? Does the patient experience specific food cravings? If so, what foods, how often, and how strong are the cravings? Is there family support to reduce the availability of inappropriate foods?
Reaction to eating in restaurants, social events, parties, special occasions, and holiday	What are family food traditions? How often does the patient eat socially with his peers? Do friends and/or family eat in moderation, or do they overeat at holidays and social events? How does the patient make food choices when faced with a large array of foods? Can the patient order an appropriate meal from a menu? Does the patient even try to stick to the meal plan, or does he simply give up?
Social support	Do family and friends make it easier or harder to eat appropriately? What behaviors from family and friends create obstacles? Do others deliberately sabotage the patient? Are there any supportive behaviors that friends or family could do?
Assessment of patient's history of dietary adherence	Does the patient get discouraged and give up altogether? Is there a history of taking *vacations* from appropriate diabetes care? Does the patient work out compromises or give up entirely?
Assessment of whether the patient can respond assertively when being pressured to deviate from an appropriate eating pattern	Can the patient say no clearly and firmly? How worried is the patient about being different from others?

Modified from Schlundt DG et al: Situational obstacles to dietary adherence for adults with diabetes, *J Am Diet Assoc* 94:874-879, 1994.

SPECIAL CONSIDERATIONS

Illness

During periods of illness, blood glucose levels become elevated and diabetes control may worsen. This is caused by an increase in hepatic production of glucose that has been stimulated by infection, illness, injury, or stress (specifically, by the release of epinephrine, norepinephrine, glucagon, and cortisol). This hyperglycemia increases insulin requirements (4).

Often, while illness causes an increased need for insulin, there is also a decreased appetite and food intake. Liquids and soft foods are usually better tolerated and also help provide some kcaloric intake while preventing dehydration. The following guidelines can be used on an emergency basis for a maximum of 3 days (4,17):

1. Monitor blood glucose at least 4 times per day (before each meal and at bedtime).
2. Test urine for ketones (if blood glucose is > 240 mg/dl).
3. If regular foods are not tolerated, carbohydrates in the meal plan should be replaced with liquid, semiliquid, or soft foods. The source of the carbohydrate is not of major concern. Sugar-containing liquids may be the only food source tolerated. More important is what the patient can tolerate. A general rule of thumb: Every 1 to 2 hours, approximately 15 grams carbohydrate (½ cup juice or ½ cup applesauce) should be consumed, or every 3 to 4 hours, 50 grams (1 cup juice and ¾ cup applesauce or 10 saltine crackers, 1 cup soup, and ½ cup juice) should be consumed. If blood glucose is > 240 mg/dl, the entire amount may not need to be consumed.
4. Each hour, 8 to 12 oz of fluid (water, broth, tea) should be taken. A carbohydrate source may also be the fluid source.
5. If vomiting, diarrhea, or fever are present, small amounts of salted foods and liquids should be taken more frequently to replace lost electrolytes.

Gastroparesis

Approximately 20% to 30% of individuals with diabetes develop gastroparesis with delayed gastric emptying that can manifest with heartburn, nausea, abdominal pain, vomiting, early satiety, and weight loss for some persons. Gastroparesis occurs as a result of vagal autonomic neuropathy, and occurs more often in IDDM than in NIDDM (18).

Dietary treatment of gastroparesis involves monitoring intake carefully. Carbohydrates should be replaced with tolerated foods. Six small meals may be better tolerated than three large meals. If constipation or diarrhea are present, fiber intake is altered according to patient needs. If the patient complains of dry mouth, fluids can be increased and food moistened with broth. A low-fat (40 grams) soft or liquid diet may be useful to prevent delay in gastric emptying. If metoclopramide (Reglan) is used to increase gastric contractions and relax the pyloric sphincter, the patient may experience side effects of dry mouth or nausea. Insulin should be matched with meals to regulate delayed absorption and glucose changes. Bezoar formation is common with oranges, coconuts, green beans, apples, figs, potato skins, Brussels sprouts, and sauerkraut. If problems are severe, a jejunostomy tube feeding may be indicated (18).

Diabetes Management Through the Life Span

The role of medical nutrition therapy is crucial for optimal blood glucose control. In various life stages, pregnancy outcome, growth and development of children, and quality of life of older persons can be influenced by nutritional intake (Table 18-9).

TEACHING TOOL
Sick Day Guidelines

Colds, fever, flu, nausea, vomiting, and diarrhea can cause special problems for individuals with diabetes. Teach these guidelines to clients to help them manage common illnesses *and* maintain control of their diabetes.

1. If you take insulin, you must continue to take your usual dose to prevent ketoacidosis. Your need for insulin continues or may increase during illness. **Never omit your insulin.**

2. If you take oral hypoglycemic agents (tablets), continue to take your usual dose unless you are vomiting. Resume your medication when you are able to tolerate fluids and food again. If vomiting continues, contact your physician.

3. Monitor your blood glucose and test urine for ketones at least four times per day—before each meal and at bedtime. If your blood glucose reading is > 240 mg/dl and there are moderate to large ketones in the urine, call your physician.

4. If you can't eat your regular food, replace it with carbohydrates in the form of liquids or soft foods. Eat at least 50 grams of carbohydrates every 3 to 4 hours, especially if your blood sugar is < 240 mg/dl. If your blood sugar is > 240 mg/dl, continue to drink liquids, especially those that don't contain kcalories (water, broth, diet soft drinks, and tea).

Foods containing 10 grams carbohydrates
½ cup regular soft drink (ginger ale, cola)
½ Popsicle (twin bar)
2 tsp corn syrup or honey
2½ tsp granulated sugar
¼ cup regularly sweetened gelatin

Foods containing 15 grams carbohydrates
½ cup orange or grapefruit juice
⅓ cup grape or apple juice
½ cup ice cream
½ cup cooked cereal
¼ cup sherbet
⅓ cup regularly sweetened gelatin
1 cup broth-based soups (reconstituted with water)
1 cup cream soups
¾ cup regular soft drink (ginger ale, cola)
¼ cup milkshake
1½ cups milk
½ cup eggnog (commercial)
⅓ cup tapioca pudding
½ cup custard
1 cup plain yogurt
1 slice toast
6 saltine crackers

5. Drink a large glass of kcalorie-free liquid every hour to replace fluids. If you feel nauseated or are vomiting, take small sips (1 to 2 tablespoons) every 15 to 30 minutes. Call your physician.

6. These guidelines apply only to mild, short-term, 1-day illnesses. Call your physician if:
   - You can't keep *any* liquids or carbohydrates down for more than 8 hours.
   - You are vomiting or have diarrhea.
   - You are spilling ketones in your urine.
   - You begin to breathe rapidly, become drowsy, or lose unconsciousness.
   - You have questions or concerns.

7. When illness subsides, return to your regular meal plan and usual insulin schedule.

Franz MJ, Mooynes JO: *Diabetes and brief illness,* Minneapolis, 1993, International Diabetes Center.

Pregnancy

Women with preexisting diabetes who become pregnant are vulnerable to fetal complications, and maternal health can be compromised when complications of diabetes occur (8). Occasionally, the stress of pregnancy may induce gestational diabetes mellitus, which is a form of glucose intolerance that has its onset during pregnancy and is resolved on parturition (4). Whether the mother has preexisting diabetes or gestational diabetes, the risk of fetal abnormalities and mortality are increased in the presence of hyperglycemia, so every effort should be made to control blood glucose levels (4,11).

Changes that take place during pregnancy greatly affect diabetes control and insulin utilization. Hormones and enzymes produced by the placenta are antagonistic to insulin, thus reducing its effectiveness. Maternal insulin does not cross the placenta, but glucose does. This will cause the fetus's pancreas to increase insulin

Table 18-9   Diabetes Management Through the Life Span

PREGNANCY

- Individualize meal plan on the basis of diet history, prepregnancy weight, and activity level; the meal plan should meet nutritional needs for pregnancy *and* allow normal blood glucose levels
- Plot weight gain; the pattern of weight gain should be appropriate for pregnancy
- Use food and blood glucose monitoring records to meet glycemic control goals and prevent or correct ketosis
- Ideal blood glucose monitoring schedule: 8 tests/day (before each meal, 1-2 hours after each meal, bedtime, in the middle of the night)
- Minimum blood glucose monitoring schedule: 4 tests/day (before each meal and at bedtime)
- Test urine ketones during illness (morning sickness, flu), when blood glucose is greater than 200 mg/dl, when meals are delayed or missed, and before breakfast every day

CHILDHOOD AND ADOLESCENCE

- Individualize meal plan to provide adequate energy for normal growth and development; energy requirements vary with age, sex, height, weight, stage of development, and level of physical activity

Estimating energy needs:

Method 1: NAS/RDA Guidelines

Method 2: 1000 kcalories for 1st year

- Add 100 kcal per year up to age 11
- For girls 11-15 years, add 100 kcal or less/year after age 10
- For girls > 15 years, calculate as an adult
- For boys 11-15 years, add 200 kcal/year after age 10
- For boys >15 years, add 23 kcal/lb if very active, 18 kcal/lb for usual activity, 16 kcal/lb if sedentary

Method 3: 1000 for 1st year

- For boys add 125 kcal × age
- For girls add 100 kcal × age
- Add up to 20% more kcal for activity

(For toddlers between 1-3 years, add 40 kcal/inch of length)

- During dietary assessment, include the role of parents, older siblings, grandparents, day-care workers, and teachers
- Assess previous nutrition education of client, parent, and/or caregivers to determine accuracy of information
- Include in the nutrition history any factors in a child's life that influence eating:

School routine: including class schedule, when/where lunch is eaten, how birthday parties/special events are handled

Weekday routine: including after-school activities, after-school snacks, how this differs from weekend routine

Relationships with siblings and friends: including role of food in social activities, how the child reacts to peer pressure when eating (if everyone goes to McDonald's and orders fries and a milk shake, what does the child choose?)

Factors that influence food choices: including family food preferences and traditions, the small child's self-feeding skills, does the child consume a variety of foods

Self-care skills: including responsibility for any/all of the diabetes management, including preparing any of his/her own meals

OLDER AGE

Considerations for home care

- Routine weights
- Diet history or 3-day recall
- Alcohol intake
- Ability to perform self-monitored blood glucose

Table 18-9   Diabetes Management Through the Life Span, cont'd.

Considerations for home care, cont'd.
- Chewing and swallowing ability
- Ability to feed self, and assistance available
- Activity level
- Assessment of kitchen and storage abilities
- Financial and community resources

Considerations for care at long-term facilities
- Monthly weights
- Percent intake of daily meals or kcalorie counts
- Fasting blood glucose
- Glycosylated hemoglobin
- Chewing and swallowing ability
- Ability to feed self
- Activity level

From American Diabetes Association: *Maximizing the role of nutrition in diabetes management,* A clinical education program of American Diabetes Association in cooperation with Diabetes Care and Education, a practice group of The American Dietetic Association, Alexandria, Va, 1994, American Diabetes Association; Davis M: Application of the 1994 nutrition recommendations to the elderly population and long-term care facilities, *On the Cutting Edge* (Newsletter of the Diabetes Care and Education Practice Group) 16:29-30, 1995; Holzmeister LA: Application of the 1994 nutrition recommendations to children and adolescents, *On the Cutting Edge* (Newsletter of the Diabetes Care and Education Practice Group) 16:31, 1995; and King J: Medical nutrition therapy in diabetes and pregnancy, *On the Cutting Edge* (Newsletter of the Diabetes Care and Education Practice Group) 16:32-34, 1995.

production if blood glucose levels get too high. The increased production of insulin causes the most typical characteristic of babies born to women with diabetes—macrosomia. Newborns may also have other problems such as respiratory difficulties, hypocalcemia, hypoglycemia, hypokalemia, and/or jaundice (9).

macrosomia
larger body size

Desired weight gains and nutrient requirements are the same as for established pregnancy guidelines: 0.9 kg to 1.8 kg (2 to 4 lb) for the first trimester and 1 lb per week for the second and third trimesters based on prepregnancy BMI. No kcalorie adjustments are needed for the first trimester (11). During the second and third trimesters, an increased energy intake of approximately 100 to 300 kcalories per day is recommended (11). Protein (high quality) should be increased by 10 grams per day and can be met easily be one or two extra glasses of low-fat or skim milk and/or 1 to 2 ounces of meat or meat substitute (11). As with any pregnancy, alcohol consumption is not recommended in any amount.

Pregnancy in overt diabetes. A successful pregnancy for a woman who has diabetes requires planning and commitment (19). Since most fetal malformations occur during the first trimester of pregnancy, achieving and maintaining excellent glycemic control prior to conception and during early pregnancy is a must (19).

Pregnancy will require greater attention to medical nutrition therapy on a day-to-day basis. Guidance during early pregnancy should include special consideration for food cravings and nausea. The meal plan should be individualized and should evolve throughout the pregnancy to meet changing nutritional needs and insulin requirements. Three meals and three snacks are usually recommended. The use of frequent home blood glucose monitoring can help the patient maintain normal fasting and postprandial glucose levels and avoid frequent or severe hypoglycemic reactions (11,19).

Gestational Diabetes. Gestational diabetes (GDM) will develop in nearly 2% of all pregnancies (5). Women who develop GDM are often obese, but weight reduction should not be attempted at this time (19). Although the specific components of an *ideal diet* for GDM have not been determined, good glucose control must be maintained and is usually accomplished by individualization of intake and graphing of weight gain (11). Often, insulin may be prescribed in addition to medical nutrition therapy to reduce the risks of fetal macrosomia, neonatal hyperglycemia, and perinatal mortality (19). Oral hypoglycemic agents are not recommended. Glucose levels usually revert to normal following delivery, but there is an increased risk for later development of IDDM or NIDDM. Nearly 30% of women with GDM eventually develop NIDDM (5).

WELLNESS AND DIABETES MELLITUS

Physical Dimension Long-term serious physical health complications may be avoided if hyperglycemia is controlled through dietary and lifestyle modifications.

Intellectual Dimension The ability of the individual to understand his condition, to be compliant on a regular basis regarding insulin injections, if required, and to follow dietary and exercise recommendations may depend on the intellectual dimension of health.

Emotional Dimension Emotional health may be tested. Not only is the individual dealing with a chronic lifelong condition, but changes in dietary intake may necessitate the loss of symbolic foods, which may be emotionally upsetting. Support, especially by family members and friends, is crucial.

Social Dimension Social health may be pivotal in adjustment to this disorder. If secure in social relationships, adaptations in social situations will be easier and more acceptable.

SUMMARY

Diabetes mellitus is a group of conditions characterized by either a relative or complete lack of insulin secretion by the beta cells of the pancreas or defects of cell insulin receptors, which results in disturbances of carbohydrate, protein, and lipid metabolism and hyperglycemia. Long-term complications develop, often leading to disability and premature death. The complications may be related to the level and frequency of hyperglycemia experiences throughout the life span, in addition to genetic and environmental factors.

The two primary categories of glucose intolerance are non–insulin-dependent diabetes (NIDDM) and insulin-dependent diabetes (IDDM). IDDM symptoms appear suddenly and include polyphagia, polyuria, polydipsia, and weight loss. All persons with IDDM require exogenous insulin to maintain normal blood glucose levels. The primary metabolic problem in NIDDM is insulin resistance. Family history and obesity are the two strongest risk factors for NIDDM. The gradually occurring symptoms of NIDDM are polyuria, polydipsia, fatigue, and frequent infections. Some individuals with NIDDM may require insulin to optimize blood glucose control. Additional types of diabetes include gestational diabetes, impaired glucose tolerance, and other less common forms of diabetes. Related conditions that may occur are hypoglycemia, diabetic ketoacidosis (DKA), and hyperosmolar hyperglycemic nonketotic coma (HHNC).

The main goal of treatment is maintenance of insulin/glucose homeostasis.

Treatment includes the use of insulin, medical nutrition therapy, and exercise. Blood glucose levels are the cornerstone of diabetes management and can be monitored several ways: (1) fasting blood glucose, (2) glycosylated hemoglobin, and (3) self-monitoring.

Medical nutritional therapy is an essential component of successful diabetes management, and the complexity involved requires a team approach to enhance the ability of the patient to obtain good metabolic control. The diabetes management team should include a registered nurse, a physician or primary health care provider, the person with diabetes, and a registered dietician. Successful medical nutrition therapy involves the diabetes management team conducting a thorough assessment, encouraging the patient's role in goal setting, implementing nutrition intervention, and evaluating the nutrition care plan.

The present guidelines for medical nutrition therapy for diabetes management include: aim for near normal blood sugar levels and optimal lipid levels; individualize diet plans; reach a reasonable weight; and, if desired, consume some sugar and foods that contain sugar if substituted for other carbohydrate foods. Nutrition recommendations for total fat, saturated fat, cholesterol, fiber, vitamins, and minerals are the same for individuals with diabetes as for the general population. Recommendations are modified for protein, carbohydrates, sucrose, and alcohol because of the nature of diabetes in relation to carbohydrate metabolism or the effects of diabetic complications.

THE NURSING ROLE
Non–Insulin-Dependent Diabetes Mellitus: The Nursing Process

Mrs. Alvarez is 72 years old, lives alone, and has had a medical diagnosis of NIDDM for the past year. She comes to the physician's office for fingerstick glucose testing every 2 weeks because she has resisted learning how to do home glucose monitoring. She is presently taking Glyburide, an oral hypoglycemic agent, every morning.

ASSESSMENT DATA COLLECTED

In talking to Mrs. Alvarez, the office nurse finds out that the client *treats herself* to foods that are not on her diabetic diet, such as chocolate bars, potato chips, and rich cake, several times a week. When asked questions about her diabetic diet, she does not seem to have a good grasp of the principles, and finds it difficult to understand her printed diet plan. She does take her Glyburide regularly, but seems to view medication as the only therapy she really has to be concerned with. Although previous blood sugar levels have been under 170 mg/dl, they have been steadily increasing. Her fingerstick blood sugar today, before lunch, is 200 mg/dl. Mrs. Alvarez had little formal schooling and does not read very well.

NURSING DIAGNOSIS

Noncompliance with diabetic diet related to complexity and lack of understanding of diet as evidenced by intake of high-sugar and high-fat foods and blood sugar of 200.

PLANNING

The office nurse sets the following goals with Mrs. Alvarez. The client will:
Attend two sessions with a dietitian at a local clinic
Limit foods not on the diet to one portion per week until meeting with the dietitian
Reduce blood sugar to 150 mg/dl by next office visit

INTERVENTION

1. Discuss with Mrs. Alvarez the importance of keeping blood sugar within normal limits to prevent complications

Continued.

THE NURSING ROLE, cont'd.

Non–Insulin-Dependent Diabetes Mellitus: The Nursing Process

2. Teach about foods that are high in sugar and fat and should be avoided
3. Assure Mrs. Alvarez of her ability to follow the diabetic diet with help
4. Make an appointment with dietitian for teaching and reinforcement of diabetic diet
5. Provide dietitian with assessment data and ask dietitian for simplification of written diet plan for Mrs. Alvarez

EVALUATION

The goals will be evaluated in 2 weeks to see if outcomes have been achieved as evidenced by:

Mrs. Alvarez saying she has met with the dietitian

Mrs. Alvarez's report of her dietary intake revealing her avoidance of foods high in sugar and fat

Blood sugar at or below 150 mg/dl

Critical Thinking   ## CLINICAL APPLICATIONS

D.E. is a 75-year-old white male admitted to the hospital following a cerebrovascular accident. He has a history of NIDDM, hypertension, moderate obesity, and possible alcohol abuse. Medications upon admission include Lasix (furosemide), hydrochlorothiazide, propranolol hydrochloride (Inderal), and Diabinese 500 mg BID. D.E. comes to the clinic regularly and at his last visit complained of blurred vision, polydipsia, polyuria, and a weight loss of 8 lb in the past 2 weeks. He was admitted to the hospital with a diagnosis of urinary tract infection and hyperglycemic hyperosmolar nonketotic (HHNK) syndrome. Physical examination revealed the following: Ht - 5'11", Wt - 215 lb, BP 160/82, chol 380 mg/dl, TG 300 mg/dl, BS 750 mg/dl. Family history: sister has had NIDDM for 10 years.

1. Explain how D.E.'s blood glucose level could become so high without producing ketones.
2. If this patient's HHNK was not treated, how would you expect his disease to progress?
3. What are D.E.'s blood glucose and lipid goals?
4. What is the purpose of the prescribed medications? Are there any possible drug-nutrient interactions?
5. How frequently should blood sugars be monitored?
6. What are possible complications?

REFERENCES

1. *Mosby's medical, nursing, and allied health dictionary,* ed 4, St. Louis, 1995, Mosby.
2. Kenshole AB: Diabetes. In Jeejeebhoy KN, ed: *Current therapy in nutrition,* Toronto, 1988, Decker.
3. Raskin P, Rosenstock J: Blood glucose control and diabetic complications, *Ann Intern Med* 105:254, 1986.
4. American Dietetic Association: *Handbook of clinical dietetics,* ed 2, New Haven, 1992, Yale University Press.

5. National Institutes of Health, National Diabetes Data Group: Classification and diagnosis of diabetes mellitus and other categories of glucose intolerance, *Diabetes* 28:1039, 1979.

6. American Diabetes Association: *Physician's guide to insulin dependent (Type I) diabetes: Diagnosis and treatment,* Alexandria, Va, 1988, American Diabetes Association.

7. Kissebah AH et al: Relation of body fat distribution to metabolic complications of obesity, *J Clin Endocrinol Metab* 54:254-260, 1982.

8. Orland MJ: Diabetes mellitus. In Woodley M, Whelan A, eds: *Manual of medical therapeutics,* ed 27, Boston, 1992, Little, Brown.

9. Franz MJ, Norstrom J: *Diabetes actively staying healthy: Your game plan for diabetes and exercise,* Wayzata, Minn, 1990, International Diabetes Center/DCI Publishing.

10. Swearingen PL: *Manual of nursing therapeutics,* ed 3, St. Louis, 1992, Mosby.

11. *Maximizing the role of nutrition in diabetes management,* A clinical education program of American Diabetes Association in cooperation with Diabetes Care and Education, a practice group of The American Dietetic Association, Alexandria, Va, 1994, American Diabetes Association.

12. Tinker LF, Heins JM, Holler HJ: Commentary and translation: 1994 nutrition recommendations for diabetes, *J Am Diet Assoc* 94:507-511, 1994.

13. American Dietetic Association: Nutrition recommendations and principles for people with diabetes mellitus, *J Am Diet Assoc* 94:504-506, 1994.

14. American Diabetes Association: *Exchange lists for meal planning,* Alexandria, Va, 1995, The American Dietetic Association.

15. Delahanty LM, Halford BN: The role of diet behaviors in achieving improved glycemic control in intensively treated patients in the Diabetes Control and Complications Trial, *Diabetes Care* 16:1453-1458, 1993.

16. Schlundt DG et al: Situational obstacles to dietary adherence for adults with diabetes, *J Am Diet Assoc* 94:874-879, 1994.

17. Franz MJ, Joynes JO: *Diabetes and brief illness,* Minneapolis, 1993, International Diabetes Center.

18. Escott-Stump S: *Nutrition and diagnosis-related care,* ed 3, Philadelphia, 1992, Lea & Febiger.

19. Anderson JW, Geil PB: Nutritional management of diabetes mellitus. In Shils ME, Olson JA, Shike M, eds: *Modern nutrition in health and disease,* ed 8, Philadelphia, 1994, Lea & Febiger.

Chapter 19

NUTRITION FOR CARDIOVASCULAR DISEASES

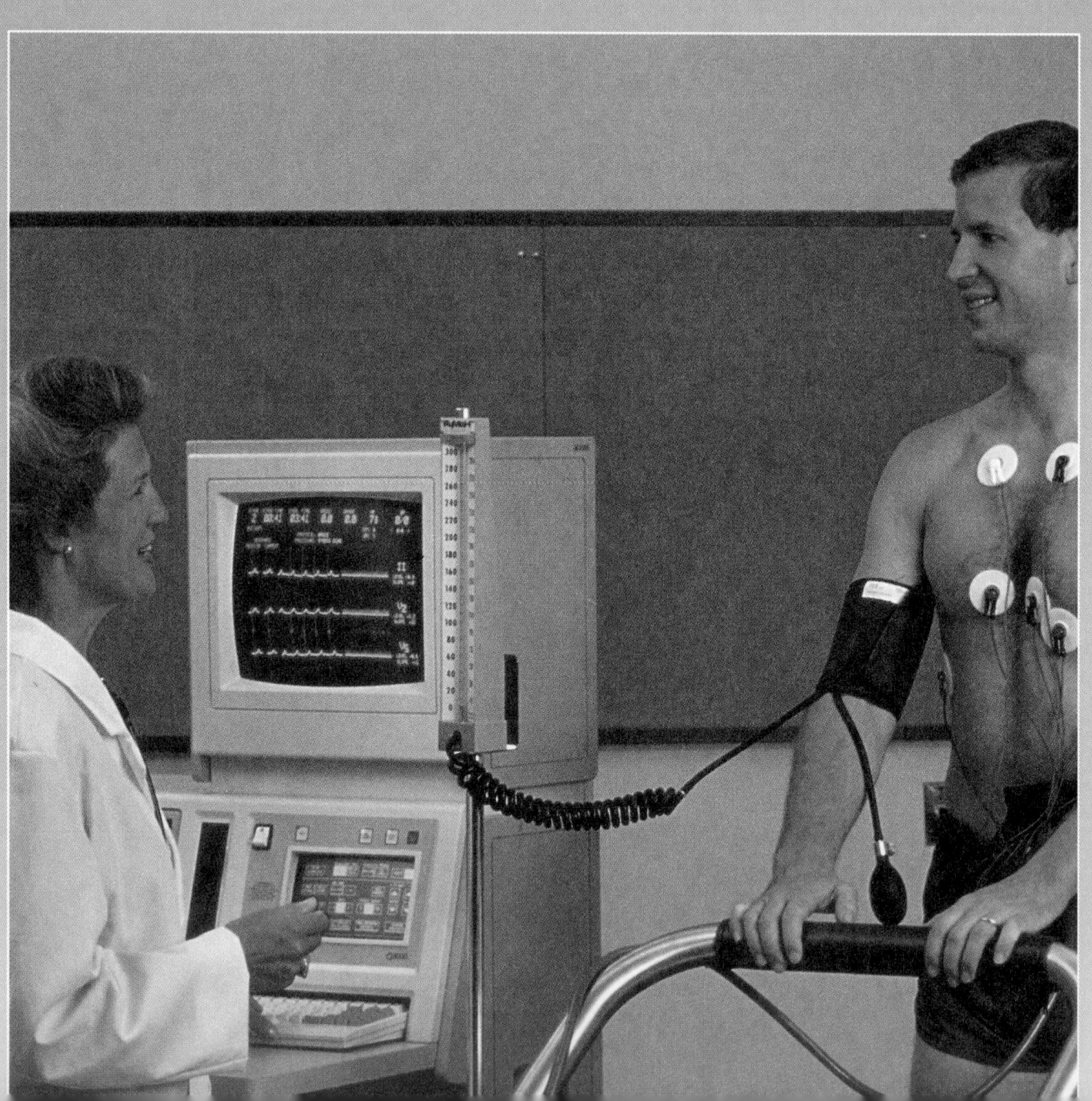

ROLE IN WELLNESS

Nurses working in varied settings play a major role in teaching people how to reduce cardiovascular risk factors through lifestyle changes that include dietary modifications. Education about dietary factors can be performed by both nurses and dietitians. Even though dietitians are responsible for developing the medical nutrition plan and for the majority of diet education instruction, nurses reinforce that teaching and answer any additional questions of patients and their families. Therefore familiarity with diet as it affects cardiovascular disease is essential.

The term *cardiovascular disease* encompasses a group of diseases and conditions affecting the heart and blood vessels (1): coronary artery disease (also referred to as coronary heart disease), hypertension, peripheral vascular disease, congestive heart failure, and congenital heart diseases. Cardiovascular disease has been a public health issue since 1920 and is currently the leading cause of death in the United States (2) for both men and women and in all ethnic and racial groups (3). Over 58 million Americans have some form of cardiovascular disease, including hypertension. Approximately 11 million Americans have coronary artery disease (CAD), and over 3 million have cerebrovascular disease (4). It has been estimated that 2.5 million Americans are diagnosed with CAD or stroke each year (5,6). More than 1.25 million Americans suffer heart attacks yearly because of CAD, and approximately 500,000 die as a result (5). Most people who have heart attacks die before they ever reach a hospital for treatment, a situation that emphasizes the need for preventing heart disease (7).

Although CAD has been a public health concern for decades, as health professionals we cannot assume that our newly diagnosed CAD patients, regardless of education or socioeconomic level, are knowledgeable of the disorder and treatment approaches. These approaches often include implementing secondary and tertiary preventive strategies. Secondary prevention behaviors reduce the effects of a disease or illness. For CAD, reducing risk factors can minimize negative health effects. The purpose of tertiary prevention is to minimize further complications or to assist in the restoration of health. For CAD, these efforts may involve significant lifestyle changes combined with continued medication and medical care. Learning more about the disorder is often helpful for patients and their families.

Several of the risk factors for cardiovascular disease are modifiable or altogether preventable; nonetheless, more than 80% of Americans have at least one major risk factor (8). The risk factors are categorized into three groups: controllable, noncontrollable, and predisposing. Controllable or lifestyle factors include tobacco use and physical inactivity. Noncontrollable factors are gender, age, and family history. Predisposing conditions may be diabetes mellitus, hypertension, obesity, and hypercholesterolemia (total blood cholesterol levels over 200 mg/dl).

CORONARY ARTERY DISEASE

The underlying pathological process responsible for coronary artery disease (CAD) is **atherosclerosis** (Fig. 19-1). Beginning in childhood, atherosclerosis may gradually lead to **arteriosclerosis** (1). The most common and serious manifestation of atherosclerosis is the development of lesions in the coronary arteries that can cause **angina pectoris** if blood flow is partially occluded by a **thrombus,** or **myocardial infarction** if blood flow to the heart is completely occluded. If **thrombosis** occurs in a cerebral artery, a cerebrovascular accident (CVA) or stroke occurs. Peripheral vascular disease (PVD) occurs when atherosclerosis in the abdominal aorta, iliac arteries, and femoral arteries produces temporary arterial

atherosclerosis

development of lesions (also called fatty streaks) in the intima of arteries; during aging, the lesions develop into fibrous plaques that project into the vessel lumen and begin to disturb blood flow

arteriosclerosis

thickening, loss of elasticity, and calcification of arterial walls, resulting in decreased blood supply

angina pectoris

chest pain that often radiates down the left arm and is frequently accompanied by a feeling of suffocation and impending death

thrombus

blood clot

myocardial infarction

occlusion of a coronary artery; sometimes called heart attack

thrombosis

thrombus (blood clot) development within a blood vessel of the body

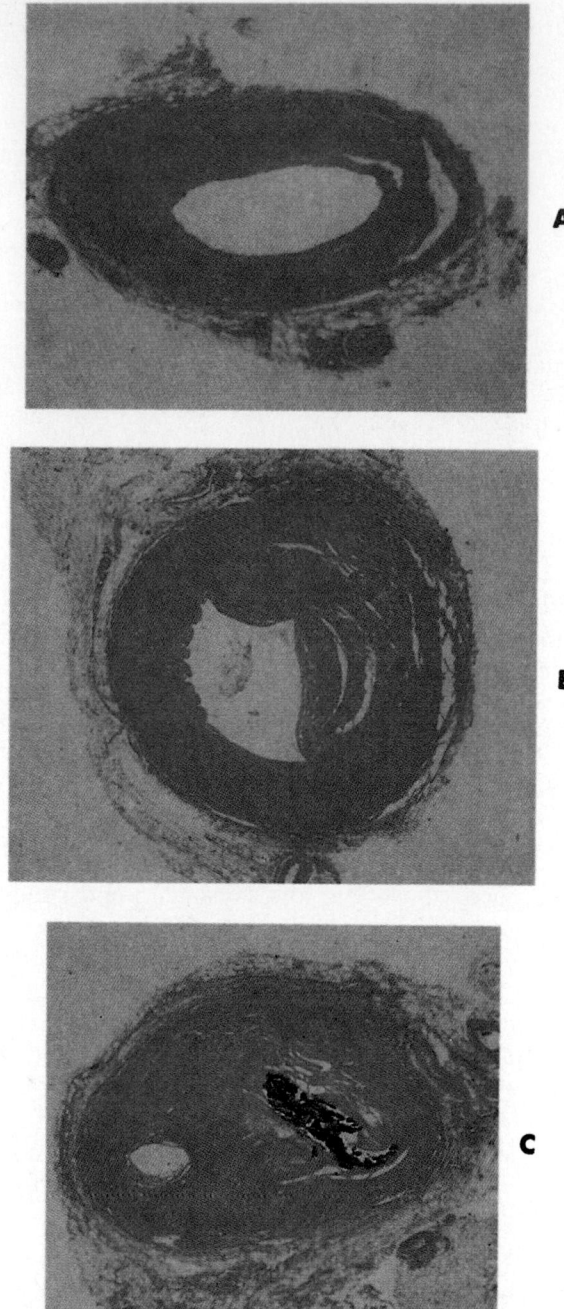

Fig. 19-1 The path to a heart attack. **A,** The coronary artery shows only minor blockage. **B,** The artery exhibits severe atherosclerosis; much of the passage is blocked by buildup of cholesterol and other lipids on the interior walls of the artery. **C,** The coronary artery is almost completely blocked.

ischemia

decreased blood supply to a body organ or part

insufficiency upon exertion (intermittent claudication) or **ischemic** necrosis of the extremities (gangrene) (1).

The most frequent approach in assessing coronary artery disease risk is to measure total blood cholesterol (TC), as well as the proportions of the different types of lipoproteins that carry cholesterol in the blood. Cholesterol is an essential component of cell membranes and a precursor of bile acids and steroid hormones. Cholesterol is a not actually a lipid, but travels in the bloodstream in spherical particles containing lipids and proteins called lipoproteins. Cholesterol levels in the

Table 19-1 CAD Risk Classifications		
Risk Classification	Total Cholesterol	LDL-Cholesterol
Desirable	<200 mg/dl	<130 mg/dl
Borderline-high	200-239 mg/dl	130-159 mg/dl
High	≥ 240 mg/dl	≥ 160 mg/dl

Modified from National Cholesterol Education Program: *Report of the expert panel on detection, evaluation, and treatment of high blood cholesterol in adults,* NIH Pub No 89-2925, Washington, DC, 1989, US Dept of Health and Human Services, Public Health Services, National Institutes of Health.

blood are determined by genetic factors, fat and cholesterol content of the diet, and other factors such as obesity and physical inactivity (9).

Three major classes of lipoproteins can be measured in blood from a fasting individual: very low density lipoproteins (VLDL), low density lipoproteins (LDL), and high density lipoproteins (HDL) (9). The LDL-cholesterol contains approximately 60% to 70% of the total serum cholesterol, and high serum levels are causally related to increased risk of CAD. The HDLs usually contain 20% to 30% of the total cholesterol, and serum levels are inversely correlated with risk for CAD. The VLDLs are largely composed of triglyceride, containing 10% to 15% of the total serum cholesterol (9).

Because most of the cholesterol in the blood is found in the LDLs, the concentration of TC is closely correlated with the concentration of LDL-cholesterol (9). This means that although LDL-cholesterol is a more precise and preferable risk factor measure, testing TC levels (which is more available and less expensive) can be used in the initial stages of evaluating CAD risk (9). As cholesterol (TC) levels rise, so does coronary risk, particularly when cholesterol levels rise above 200 mg/dl. Table 19-1 summarizes the CAD risk classifications based on TC and LDL-cholesterol.

Risk factors for cardiovascular diseases
Controllable (lifestyle)
 tobacco use
 physical inactivity
Noncontrollable
 gender
 age
 family history
Predisposing conditions
 diabetes mellitus
 hypertension
 obesity
 hypercholesterolemia

Medical Nutrition Therapy

For many, lowering cholesterol and LDL-cholesterol can be achieved by dietary intervention, including weight loss (if necessary) and exercise (9,10). Approximate intake of cholesterol, total fat, saturated fat, unsaturated fat, alcohol, and simple and complex carbohydrates should be assessed by diet history before a meal plan is developed. For patients who are overweight, the assessment should include review of weight history, any previous weight-reduction efforts, eating-related behaviors, exercise history, and current medications (11).

The goals of medical nutrition therapy are to reduce total fat, saturated fat, and cholesterol intake in an attempt to reduce total cholesterol, LDL-cholesterol, and triglyceride levels. The National Cholesterol Education Program (NCEP) recommends a two-step approach to accomplish these goals (Table 19-2) (10).

Currently, Americans consume approximately 37% of total kcalories from fat, with 15% to 20% of the fat derived from saturated fat sources (animal fats, tropical oils, cocoa butter, hydrogenated vegetable fats), only 7% from polyunsaturated fats (vegetable oils), and the rest from monounsaturated fats (olive, canola, and peanut oils). The NCEP guidelines to reduce total fat intake to 30% of total kcalories (<10% saturated fats, no more than 10% polyunsaturated fat, the remainder monounsaturated fat) creates a corresponding need to increase carbohydrate intake to meet kcalorie demands (11). This increased carbohydrate intake should come in the form of complex carbohydrates: whole-grain breads and cereals, fruits, and vegetables. Protein intake is commonly 12% to 15% of the total kcalories. The average cholesterol intake per day in the United States is approximately 450 mg. Although reducing dietary cholesterol is not as effective in lowering serum cholesterol as reducing total fat and saturated fat levels, the NCEP guidelines (Step 1) recommend that less than 300 mg of cholesterol

Table 19-2   Medical Nutrition Therapy for High Blood Cholesterol

Nutrient	Recommended Intake*	
	STEP 1	STEP 2
Total fat	≤30% of total kcalories	≤30% of total kcalories
Saturated fats	8% to 10% of total kcalories	<7% of total kcalories
Polyunsaturated fats	≤10% of total kcalories	≤10% of total kcalories
Monounsaturated fats	≤15% of total kcalories	≤15% of total kcalories
Carbohydrates	≥55% of total kcalories	≥55% of total kcalories
Protein	Approximately 15% total kcalories	Approximately 15% total kcalories
Cholesterol	<300 mg/day	<200 mg/day
Total kcalories	To achieve and maintain desirable weight	To achieve and maintain desirable weight

From National Cholesterol Education Program: *Second report of the expert panel on detection, evaluation, and treatment of high blood cholesterol in adults (adult treatment panel II)*, NIH Pub No 93-3093, Washington, DC, 1993, US Dept of Health and Human Services, National Institutes of Health.
*Kcalories from alcohol not included.

Sample Fat and Cholesterol-Controlled Diet Menu

BREAKFAST
Citrus sections (or juice)
Cheerios with skim milk
Scrambled eggs (from egg substitute)
Toasted English muffin
Coffee or sugar-free hot cocoa

LUNCH
Fruit punch
Sirloin tips (2 oz) with a bed of noodles and green beans*
Garden salad with dressing (low-fat or regular)
Fruit cocktail
White or whole wheat bread with whipped spread and honey
Iced tea

DINNER
Tomato soup
Turkey breast (2 oz) and gravy with dinner roll and carrot/pea medley*
Gelatin with applesauce
Whole wheat bread with margarine
Low-fat baked custard
Coffee

From Memorial Hospital, Carbondale, Ill.
*Quantities not exact; for representation only.

Cholesterol can usually be decreased by:
• decreasing total fat intake
• decreasing saturated fat intake
• using unsaturated fats in recommended amounts
• decreasing high-cholesterol food intake, and
• reducing weight or maintaining a desirable body weight

hyperlipidemic
excess lipids in the blood

should be consumed per day. In patients remaining **hyperlipidemic** after using this plan for 3 months, the Step 2 diet is then recommended: 30% of total kcalories from fat (less that 7% saturated fat) and cholesterol less than 200 mg per day.

Obviously, these guidelines must be translated into foods and directions for quantities to consume for them to be useful to patients. A dietitian's individualized meal plan with specific recommendations for portion sizes is integral for practical medical nutrition therapy intervention. See Table 19-3 for general guidelines for the Step 1 and Step 2 diets. Chapter 5 also contains strategies for reducing dietary fat and cholesterol consumption, including discussion on hydrogenated fats and transfatty acids. The Cultural Considerations box discusses aspects of selected European dietary lifestyles that have recently received attention.

Table 19-3   Medical Nutrition Therapy to Lower Blood Cholesterol: Guidelines for the Step 1 and Step 2 Diets

Food Group and Servings per Day/Week	Avoid	Decrease	Use Instead
MILK AND DAIRY PRODUCTS Step 1: 3 servings/day Step 2: 2 servings/day	Whole milk (regular, evaporated, condensed), cheese, yogurt made from whole milk, custard-style yogurt, cream, half-and-half, most nondairy substitutes, whole milk ricotta, neufchatel, brie, hard cheeses (Swiss, American, mozzarella, feta, cheddar, Muenster), cream cheese, sour cream	2% milk, ice milk, creamed cottage cheese (4%), part skim milk cheeses, low-fat yogurt (1%-2%)	Skim or 1% milk, nonfat yogurt, no-fat or fat-free cheese*, low-fat cottage cheese (1%-2%)*, pot cheese
MEAT, POULTRY, FISH, AND SHELLFISH Step 1: 6 oz/day (cooked) Step 2: 6 oz/day (cooked)	Organ meats, fatty and heavily marbled meats (corned beef, brisket, regular ground beef, short ribs, pork spareribs, blade roll), goose, domestic duck, regular cold cuts, frankfurters, sausage, bacon, fried meats, canned meats or meat mixes	*Prime* grade meats, peanut butter, nuts, fish canned in oil, oysters, shrimp	Lean meats with fat trimmed (beef round, sirloin, chuck, loin; pork tenderloin, leg, shoulder; lamb leg, arm, loin, rib; all cuts of veal except ground), poultry without the skin, fish, water-packed tuna or salmon, low-fat cold cuts*, and low-fat frankfurters*
EGGS Step 1: 3 yolks/week Step 2: 1 yolk/week	None	Egg yolks	Egg whites or egg substitutes
BREADS, CEREALS, PASTA, RICE, DRIED PEAS, AND BEANS Step 1: 4-7 servings/day† Step 2: 5-8 servings/day†	Egg noodles	Crackers, cakes, cookies, muffins, and other bakery products made with unsaturated fat and less than 3 g fat per serving (check the label)	Whole-grain breads and cereals, English muffins, bagels, bread sticks, rice, pasta, macaroni, potatoes, low-fat crackers (such as matzo, zwieback, soda, graham, rye, plain)*, dried beans and peas (split peas, blackeyed peas, chick peas, kidney beans, navy beans, lentils, soybeans, soybean curd [tofu])
FRUITS AND VEGETABLES Step 1: 3 fruit/4 vegetable servings/day Step 2: 3 fruit/4 vegetable servings/day	Coconut, fruits and vegetables in cream or cream sauces, butter, and dips	Avocado, olives	Fresh, frozen, canned, or dried fruits and vegetables

Continued.

Table 19-3   Medical Nutrition Therapy to Lower Blood Cholesterol: Guidelines for the Step 1 and Step 2 Diets, cont'd.

Food Group and Servings per Day/Week	Avoid	Decrease	Use Instead
SWEETS AND SNACKS Step 1: 2 servings/day Step 2: 2 servings/day	Ice cream; frozen tofu; commercially prepared pies, cakes, cookies, donuts, sweet rolls, pastries, and muffins; potato and corn chips prepared with saturated fat; buttered popcorn; frappes; milk-shakes; floats; and eggnogs	Crackers, cakes, cookies, muffins, and other bakery products made with unsaturated fat and less than 3 g fat per serving (check the label); chocolate; most candy	Sherbet, sorbet, Italian ice, frozen yogurt, Popsicles, angel food cake, fig bars, gingersnaps, jelly beans, hard candy, plain popcorn, pretzels; carbonated drinks, juices, tea, coffee
FATS AND OILS Step 1: 5-7 servings/day[†] Step 2: 4-6 servings/day[†]	All fats, especially saturated fats (butter, lard, bacon, bacon fat, gravy and cream sauces, hydrogenated margarine and shortening, cocoa butter, coconut oil, palm oil, palm kernel oil, most nondairy creamers); dressings made with egg yolks	Mayonnaise, creamy salad dressings, reduced-calorie sour cream or cream cheese (not fat-free)	Polyunsaturated oils (safflower, corn, sunflower, soybean, sesame, or cottonseed); monounsaturated oils (olive, canola, peanut oil); salad dressings made with unsaturated oils listed above; margarine from polyunsaturated oil or margarine where the first ingredient listed is *liquid* oil; no-fat or fat-free spreads, dressings, cream cheeses and sour creams[†]

Modified from Nelson JK et al: *Mayo Clinic diet manual,* ed 7, St. Louis, 1994, Mosby; Davis JR, Sherer K: *Applied nutrition and diet therapy for nurses,* ed 2, Philadelphia, 1994, Saunders; and National Cholesterol Education Program: *Eating to lower your high blood cholesterol,* NIH Pub No 89-2920, Washington, DC, 1989, US Dept of Health and Human Services, Public Health Services, National Institutes of Health.
*Low-fat is defined as less than or equal to 3 g fat per serving. No-fat or fat-free products are defined as 0 to 0.5 g fat per serving. Check the label.
†Variations in quantity reflect different kilocalorie intake—1600 or 2000 kcal/day.

CULTURAL CONSIDERATIONS
Do the French, Greeks, and Italians Know Something We Don't?

THE FRENCH PARADOX

Even if you didn't watch the *60 Minutes* program (1993) to learn that the French eat about as much fat as Americans, yet are much less likely to die from heart disease, you probably heard about it the following day. One aspect of the French diet that gained plenty of media attention is the widespread practice of moderate wine consumption with meals. Research leaves little doubt that light to moderate alcohol consumption is protective of heart disease (moderate amounts raise HDL-cholesterol, but no one agrees on the specific mechanism). But are there other reasons? Other dramatic differences in French and American dietary habits have been brought to light:

• The French eat their largest meal at lunchtime, consuming over half (about 57%) of their total energy intake before 2 PM and work until

CULTURAL CONSIDERATIONS, cont'd.
Do the French, Greeks, and Italians Know Something We Don't? cont'd.

evening (a practice thought to help fat metabolize more efficiently and synthesize less LDL-cholesterol); Americans consume less than 40% of their total energy intake by 2 PM, eating their largest meal in the evening and engaging in predominantly sedentary activities before going to bed

- The French eat less red meat and other flesh foods and larger amounts of vegetables and fiber-rich whole grain breads at their meals (these foods are high in fiber, which helps keep blood cholesterol levels down)
- The French include fresh fruits (more fiber) in their meals as desserts (eating less shortening, oil, eggs, and sugar—common ingredients in rich desserts)

There is no clear evidence that shows *how* these differences account for the differences in rate of heart disease between France and the United States, or even *whether* they have an impact. Yet read ahead, there may be some clues.

A MEDITERRANEAN ODYSSEY

Residents of Greece and southern Italy not only consume wine comparable to the French, but they also use a lot more olive oil than Americans and they, too, have less risk from heart disease. What are they doing right? What are we doing wrong? One thing people in the Mediterranean region learn to do is drink wine as an integral part of meals in a family setting, not as alcohol is often used in the United States—away from the table as a recreational drug. Residents of Greece and Italy average about 2 to 3 tablespoons of olive oil per day. Americans average about 3 tablespoons of olive oil per person every 4 to 5 months. Olive oil is a monounsaturated oil that doesn't elevate levels of LDL-cholesterol and helps maintain blood levels of HDL-cholesterol. Although olive oil is probably the most expensive cooking oil, it is very flavorful. A little goes a long way.

However, as in the case of the French

paradox, the Mediterranean diet (based on studies done during the 1950s and 1960s) entails some other dietary and lifestyle habits that may affect risk for heart disease:

- In the Mediterranean, saturated fat contributed only 7% to 8 % of total energy intake; intake of red meat and flesh foods (combined) averaged less than 1 lb per week; nuts, seeds, and legumes were used as alternatives to meat
- People in the Mediterranean region consumed very little transfatty acids (formed when liquid vegetable oils are hardened by hydrogenation to make margarines, and which like saturated fats can raise blood cholesterol)
- Residents of the region ate about twice as many fruits and vegetables as Americans do (back to the fiber thing again); additionally, fruits and vegetables are high in antioxidant nutrients (vitamin C and beta-carotene) and contain a number of biologically active nonnutrient substances that may exert health-promoting influence
- Whole grain-based foods (bread and pastas) were consumed at a volume of around 1 lb a day; Americans eat about ½ lb of grain products a day
- People of the Mediterranean region enjoyed a greater level of physical activity and ate their meals at a more leisurely pace than Americans in general, which may play some role in the complex association between stress and heart disease

The Harvard School of Public Health, the World Health Organization, and the nonprofit Oldways Preservation & Exchange Trust have developed a Mediterranean Diet Pyramid to capture the diets of Greeks and southern Italians during the 50s and 60s (Fig. 19-2). It does not offer specific recommendations for amounts of foods to be eaten daily, but makes weekly and monthly recommendations. Exercise and wine consumption are considered important lifestyle benefits.

From Bellizzi MC et al: Vitamin E and coronary heart disease: The European paradox, *Eur J Clin Nutr* 48:822-831, 1994; Broihier CA: How you can borrow from the global pantry and come up healthy, *Environmental Nutrition,* 16:1,4, April, 1993; Shields D: Healthy eating heads full-speed for the Mediterranean Sea, *Environmental Nutrition* 17:1,4, Sep 1994; *Tufts University diet and nutrition letter,* Better to eat ze main meal earlier? 11:1, June 1993; and *Tufts University diet and nutrition letter,* In search of a better diet: A Mediterranean odyssey 11:3-6, Aug 1993.

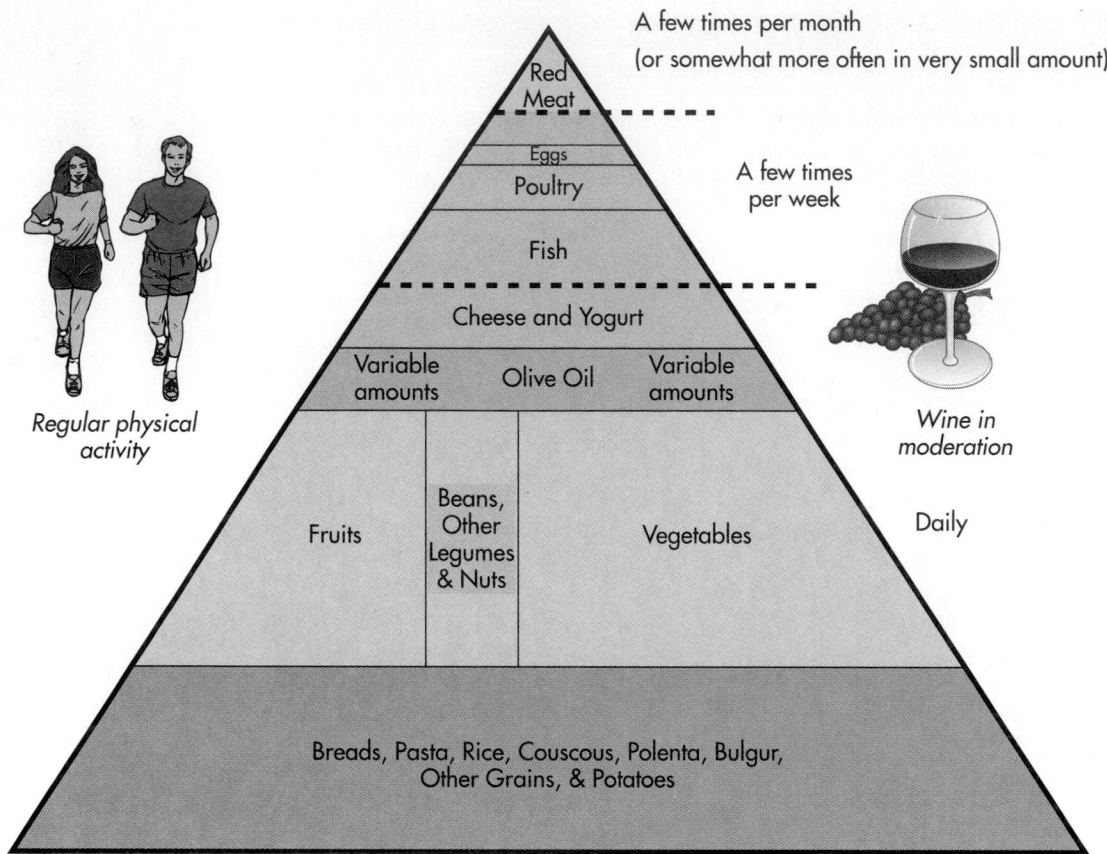

Fig. 19-2 The traditional healthy Mediterranean diet pyramid.

HYPERTENSION

As many as 50 million Americans age 6 and older have **hypertension** (one in every four adults) (4). Not only is it a cardiovascular disease itself, but hypertension is also a risk factor for coronary artery disease. According to the American Heart Association, the incidence of hypertension is higher in the following groups (4):

- Men <55 years old have greater risk than women
- Women >75 years old have greater risk than men
- African-Americans, Puerto Ricans, Cuban-Americans, and Mexican-Americans are more likely to have hypertension than Anglo-Americans
- People with lower educational and income levels tend to have higher levels of blood pressure
- African-Americans and Anglo-Americans living in the southeastern United States have a greater prevalence of hypertension than those from other regions of the country

In about 95% of cases of hypertension, the cause is not known and is referred to as **primary** or **essential hypertension** (4). **Secondary hypertension** is the term used when a cause for the elevated blood pressure can be identified. Conditions that are possible causes of secondary hypertension include renal insufficiency, renovascular diseases, Cushing's syndrome, and primary aldosteronism (12). Although sometimes called a *silent killer*, hypertension is easily detected and usually controllable.

Medical Nutrition Therapy

Prescribed treatment regimens for hypertension are individualized and vary because the disease differs in its degree of severity. The first line of treatment is usually nonpharmacological or focused on lifestyle modifications. These include possible beneficial effects of reducing weight if overweight, decreasing alcohol consumption, increasing physical activity if sedentary, terminating cigarette smoking, decreasing sodium intake, and dietary increases of other minerals such as potassium, magnesium, and calcium. Table 19-4 summarizes these lifestyle modifications that help reduce high blood pressure and/or overall cardiovascular risk. Modifying dietary intake is a predominate element of the nonpharmacological treatment of existing hypertension (11). The Health Debate box discusses research into the use of garlic to reduce hypertension and blood cholesterol.

In addition to being primary treatments for hypertension, weight reduction and sodium restriction augment antihypertensive medications. Weight loss is *the* most effective means of lowering blood pressure. Weight reduction facilitates lowered blood pressure even when it is only a 10 lb to 15 lb loss (11). The diet for weight loss and control should include a specific kcalorie restriction and exercise (aerobic) prescription. Weight loss cannot be maintained without a subsequent increase in physical activity. (See Appendix G on kcalorie-controlled diets.)

The average daily sodium intake in America has been estimated to be approximately 4 to 6 grams (175 to 265 mEq) (13). Most of this comes from sodium added during processing and manufacturing (11) (see Table 8-5, p. 194). The other main source of dietary sodium is table salt (sodium chloride). A small portion of dietary sodium comes from the natural sodium content of foods. The level of sodium restriction should be determined by the patient's physical condition and ability to comply with dietary restrictions. For example, for someone with a high intake of sodium (over 6 g/d) and mild hypertension, a diet order of "no added salt" (approximately 4 g or 174 mEq/d) may represent a significant decrease in sodium intake. Table 19-5 lists sodium-restricted dietary guidelines. A salt substitute may be prescribed (see MYTH box). The Teaching Tool gives tips on helping patients recognize foods potentially high in sodium.

Sodium intake affects the level of urinary sodium output. Showing patients the level of sodium in urine output is a way to help them become more sensitized to their intake. Sodium restriction combined with sodium loss caused by use of diuretics, extreme sweating from high fevers or prolonged exercise, or loss of fluid from vomiting and diarrhea may be problematic. Clients need to be aware of symptoms of **hyponatremia** (sodium depletion) such as muscle cramps and weakness, tiredness, low blood pressure (hypotension), disorientation, and decreased urination (oliguria).

Older patients require additional supervision on antihypertensive and reduced-sodium diets. The elderly are more at risk for dehydration and for **orthostatic hypertension** caused by reduced cardiovascular reflexes and hypertensive medications. Dietary modifications may be interpreted as restricting total food intake rather than just sodium intake. Adapting to restriction may necessitate careful food pattern development geared to the specific taste preferences of individuals.

Sodium makes up about 40% of salt, one teaspoon of salt contains about 2000 mg of sodium, 1 g sodium = 1000 mg sodium, 2300 mg sodium = 100 mEq sodium, 1 mEq sodium = 23 mg sodium

hyponatremia
abnormally low concentrations of sodium in circulating blood

orthostatic hypotension
a sudden drop in blood pressure when changing from a lying to a sitting or a sitting to a standing position; also referred to as postural hypotension

HEALTH DEBATE
Sure, Garlic Keeps Vampires Away, but What About Heart Disease?

Worldwide, garlic is considered one of the most popular herbal cure-alls, used as everything from a treatment for athletes' foot to an aphrodisiac. Today its role in prevention of chronic diseases is topping the research lists. Evidence suggests that one half to one clove of garlic daily reduces blood cholesterol by about 9%, a significant reduction in total cholesterol levels. This indicates that two cloves of garlic per day might be as efficacious as some cholesterol-lowering drugs. Another bonus: some research suggests that garlic also prevents formation of blood clots that can block arteries, whereas other research implies that it may help lower blood pressure.

What, then, is keeping the medical community from prescribing this *wonder herb* as a panacea for heart disease? Most of the research that has been done on garlic is lacking in overall quality: dietary habits and unintended interventions were not monitored rigorously enough, and most of the studies lasted only weeks or months, nothing long-term. Although the jury is still out on making actual dietary recommendations based on garlic intake, there's nothing wrong with continuing to use garlic as a flavorful seasoning. Just don't rely on garlic to prevent heart disease. As with most food-based factors, incorporating garlic into a well-balanced diet is more beneficial than relying on garlic pills or supplements. No one can say for certain which of the many substances in garlic produces the beneficial effects, not to mention that no long-term studies have been conducted on garlic supplements to rule out any possible negative effects. The studies that have produced positive results were all based on real garlic consumption.

From Pressing garlic for possible health benefits, *Tufts University diet and nutrition letter* 12:3-6, Sep 1994; and Warshafsky S, Kamer RS, Sivak SL: Effect of garlic on total serum cholesterol, *Ann Intern Med* 119:599-605, 1993.

Table 19-4 Lifestyle Modifications That Help Reduce Hypertension and/or Overall Cardiovascular Risk

Modification	Reason
Reduce weight if overweight	Although not all obese individuals have hypertension, obesity and blood pressure are closely associated; as weight decreases, so does blood pressure; excess abdominal fat, especially, increases risk
Limit alcohol consumption	Alcohol (specifically ethanol) intake of > 2 oz/day is associated with hypertension; the effect is independent of age, obesity, exercise, smoking status, and gender
Increase physical activity	Less active and less physically fit persons have a 30% to 50% greater risk of developing hypertension; regular aerobic exercise is recommended
Decrease sodium intake	Blood pressure response to dietary sodium varies from person to person; it has been estimated that about one third of those with hypertension are *sodium-sensitive* (blood pressure will decrease with a decrease in dietary sodium); for persons receiving diuretic therapy, sodium restriction may reduce the dosage needed for blood pressure control
Increase intake of potassium, calcium, magnesium	Higher intakes of potassium, calcium, and magnesium are connected with lower risk of hypertension; good sources of these minerals are fruits, vegetables, and dairy products
Stop smoking	Nicotine increases CAD risk
Decrease fat intake	Decreasing saturated fat intake decreases CAD risk; decreasing total fat intake is an important factor in weight control

Modified from *Environmental Nutrition*, 15:7, Nov 1992; National Institutes of Health: *The fifth report of the Joint National Committee on Detection, Evaluation, and Treatment of High Blood Pressure*, NIH Pub No. 93-1088, Washington, DC, Oct 1992; Nelson JK et al: *Mayo Clinic diet manual*, ed 7, St. Louis, 1994, Mosby; and Nowlan MH, Hiser E, Hudnall M: Remember when? Salt, sugar, and cholesterol used to be major nutrition concerns, Are they still? *Eating Well*, March/April 28-36, 1995.

Table 19-5   Levels of Dietary Sodium Restriction

Food Groups	Serving Size	Number of Servings Allowed				Foods Allowed	Foods to Avoid	Average Natural Sodium Content per Serving (mg)
		3 gm* (3000 mg or 130 mEq)	2 gm (2000 mg or 87 mEq)	1 gm (1000 mg or 43 mEq)	500mg† (22 mEq)			
Milk and other beverages	8 oz	2	2	2	2	8 oz buttermilk/day allowed on 3 gm Na diet; milk; tea; coffee; lemonade; carbonated beverages (limit to 16 oz/day)	Buttermilk, evaporated milk, condensed sweetened milk, malted milk, and milkshakes	120
Low-sodium milk‡	8 oz	Unlimited	Unlimited	Unlimited	Unlimited			7
Meats, fish, poultry, or low-sodium cheeses	1 oz	6–8	6	4	4	Fresh or frozen meats (beef, lamb, pork, veal, game, poultry); eggs; unbreaded fish and shellfish; low-sodium canned tuna, salmon, or sardines; low-sodium cottage cheese and peanut butter; dried beans and peas	Smoked, salted, or canned meats such as bacon, chipped beef, corned beef, luncheon meats or cold cuts, ham, hot dogs, sausage, sardines, anchovies, marinated herring, pickled meats; regular hard or processed cheeses	25
Regular breads and cereals	1 slice, ¾ oz, ½ cup	5 or more	5	2	0	Regular whole grain or enriched bread; regular biscuits; pancakes, cornbread, waffles; graham crackers, unsalted crackers, yeast doughnuts		200
Low-sodium breads and cereals	1 slice, ¾ oz, ½ cup	Unlimited	4 or more	7	7	Puffed rice, puffed wheat, shredded wheat, low-sodium cornflakes, unsalted popcorn, matzo; cooked cereals, rice, macaroni, noodles, pastas cooked without salt; melba toast, low-sodium crackers		5

Continued.

Table 19-5   Levels of Dietary Sodium Restriction, cont'd.

Food Groups	Serving Size	Number of Servings Allowed				Foods Allowed	Foods to Avoid	Average Natural Sodium Content per Serving (mg)
		3 gm* (3000 mg or 130 mEq)	2 gm (2000 mg or 87 mEq)	1 gm (1000 mg or 43 mEq)	500 mg† (22 mEq)			
High-sodium vegetables	½ cup	Unlimited	Unlimited	1	0	Artichoke, beets, carrots, celery, dark leafy greens (mustard, turnip, dandelion, kale, spinach), black-eyed peas, sweet potato	Regular canned vegetables and vegetable juices, frozen peas, lima beans, mixed vegetables, and corn; frozen vegetables in sauce; sauerkraut, pickles, and other vegetables prepared in brine	50
Low-sodium vegetables	½ cup	Unlimited	Unlimited	2-4	2	Fresh, frozen, or canned without salt: asparagus, bean sprouts, broccoli, Brussels sprouts, cabbage, cauliflower, cucumbers, eggplant, green beans, green pepper, lettuce, mushrooms, okra, onions, potatoes, radishes		9
Fruits	Varies	Unlimited	Unlimited	Unlimited	2	All but those to avoid	Dried fruit with sodium sulfite added, crystallized or glazeits, and maraschino cherries	2
Salted butter or margarine	1 tsp	6 or more	6	2	0	Cream cheese, salted butter, regular margarine, and mayonnaise-type salad dressing		50
Unsalted fats	1 tsp	Unlimited	Unlimited	Unlimited	5	Vegetables oils, unsalted butter and margarine, nondairy coffee creamer, low-sodium mayonnaise, cream, and sour cream		5

Table 19-5   Levels of Dietary Sodium Restriction, cont'd.

| Food Groups | Serving Size | Number of Servings Allowed | | | Foods Allowed | Foods to Avoid | Average Natural Sodium Content per Serving (mg) |
		3 gm* (3000 mg or 130 mEq)	2 gm (2000 mg or 87 mEq)	1 gm (1000 mg or 43 mEq)	500mg† (22 mEq)			
Sweets	Varies	Unlimited	Unlimited	Unlimited	2	Sugar, syrup, honey, jelly, marmalade, jam, hard candy and other sugar candies, molasses, marshmallows		
Desserts	Varies	Unlimited	Unlimited	1	0	Plain gelatin and fruit juice or dietetic gelatin with no sodium added, unsalted bakery goods, ice cream, pudding and custard (made from milk and/or egg allowance), sherbet, water ice, flavored gelatin (limit to <1 cup/day)		20
Seasonings	Varies						Sauces and seasonings such as bouillon cubes, barbecue sauce, catsup; celery salt, seeds, or leaves; chili sauce; garlic salt; horseradish made with salt; meat extracts, sauces, and tenderizers; monosodium glutamate, prepared mustard; olives	

*May use up to ¼ tsp salt per day in cooking and at the table.
†500 mg sodium diet is not recommended for longer than 2–3 days.
‡ Low-sodium milk may be unpalatable for certain patients.

MYTH
Any Salt Substitute Will Do

All salt substitutes are not created equal; some substitutes reduce total sodium content through the use of fillers or replace sodium with potassium, whereas others completely replace sodium with a combination of spices. Use of salt substitutes should be discussed with the patient's primary health care provider because they may be medically contraindicated (for example, individuals with renal disease whose kidneys may not be able to handle additional minerals). Some health care facilities may require primary health care providers to systematically prescribe salt substitutes when ordering sodium-restricted diets. Listed below are common types of salt substitutes and manufacturers' information to assist in locating substitutes for patients.

Type of Salt Substitute	Brand Name	Sodium Content	Manufacturer/Phone Number
Herb-spice	Mrs. Dash	Sodium free	Alberto-Culver Co, 800/622-DASH
Potassium chloride	Adolph's	Salt free	Chesebrough-Pond's Inc, 800/243-5804
Reduced sodium	Morton's Lite Salt	50% sodium (still contains salt)	Morton Salt Division, Morton Thiokol Inc, 312/807-2695
	Papa Dash	Low sodium	Alberto-Culver Co, 800/622-DASH

Modified from *Manual of clinical dietetics,* ed 4, Chicago, 1992, The American Dietetic Association.

Sample Sodium-Controlled Diet Menu

BREAKFAST
Orange juice
Oatmeal with 2% milk
Low-sodium French toast with syrup
Blueberry muffin with low-sodium margarine and jelly
Coffee or tea

LUNCH
Low-sodium chicken broth
Fresh ham (2 oz) with sweet potatoes and green beans
Garden salad with low-sodium or regular dressing
Fruit cocktail
Whole wheat or white bread with whipped spread and honey
Sugar-free hot cocoa or iced tea

DINNER
Cranberry juice cocktail
Turkey breast and low-sodium gravy
 with dinner roll and carrot/pea medley
Whole wheat bread with low-sodium margarine
Baked custard
Skim milk or coffee

From Memorial Hospital, Carbondale, Ill.

MYOCARDIAL INFARCTION

Myocardial infarctions (MI) or heart attacks are the single largest killer of males and females in the United States. An American will suffer a heart attack every 20 seconds and someone dies from one every minute. Disability or death can result after an MI, depending on how much heart muscle is damaged (4).

Medical Nutrition Therapy

The purpose of medical nutrition therapy for patients suffering from an MI is to reduce the workload of the heart. This is also a good time to initiate education about modification of diet-related cardiac risk factors.

The patient may receive a liquid diet initially (for approximately 24 hours) and progress as tolerated to foods of regular consistency. Smaller, frequent meals are usually better tolerated than large meals that can increase myocardial oxygen demand by increasing splanchnic (visceral) blood flow (11). Caffeine-containing beverages are restricted to avoid myocardial stimulation (11). Foods and beverages served should be of moderate temperatures, neither very hot nor very cold. Sodium, cholesterol, fat, and kcalories (if weight loss is indicated) are controlled according to the patient's needs.

Consuming omega-3 fatty acids appears to reduce the risk of blood clots that may cause a myocardial infarction, as discussed in Chapter 5. Sources of omega-3 fatty acids include fish such as tuna, salmon, halibut, sardines, and lake trout.

CONGESTIVE HEART FAILURE

Almost one half million new cases of **congestive heart failure** (CHF) occur each year (4). CHF can be caused by CAD, lung disease, hypothyroidism, or damage to the myocardial or cardiac muscle. Congestion and edema develop in the lungs, liver, bowel, and legs. The condition is characterized by decreased blood flow to the kidneys and retention of sodium and fluid. Patients with congestive heart failure often experience edema of the feet and ankles and shortness of breath.

congestive heart failure
circulatory congestion resulting in the heart's inability to maintain adequate blood supply to meet oxygen demands

TEACHING TOOL
Heart Healthy Changes

Advising patients to start eating *heart healthy* is vague; instead, give specific, yet simple, dietary changes such as the following:

Stock your refrigerator and pantry with foods low in saturated fat. It will be much easier to adjust your eating habits if heart-healthy foods are readily available.

General:

Eat a variety of foods every day. Choose foods from the different groups (see Food Guide Pyramid, Chapter 2).

Meats:

Substitute dried beans or legumes as a main dish to reduce fat, cholesterol, kcalories, and add variety. Trim fat from meats before grilling, broiling, or baking. Remove the skin from poultry before cooking. Most fish is lower in fat than meat and poultry. Substitute baked, broiled, or grilled fish for meats and poultry. Buy tuna or other canned fish packed in water. If you buy oil-packed, rinse it in a strainer before making your recipe. Baste meats with fat-free ingredients such as wine, tomato juice, or lemon juice instead of fatty drippings. Self-basting turkeys can be high in saturated fat. Use meats as flavorings or seasonings in dishes rather than as the main ingredient.

Milk:

Ease your way from whole milk to skim milk gradually. Drink 2% milk for a few weeks, then 1%, and finally skim milk. Each step will decrease saturated fat, cholesterol, and kcalories.

Cheeses:

Many cheeses are higher in saturated fats than meat. Read the label and choose low-fat cheeses that have 2-6 grams of fat per ounce. Choose low-fat cottage cheese, farmer cheese made with skim milk, or pot cheese.

Ice Cream:

Try frozen desserts such as ice milk, yogurt, sorbets, and the new low-fat or fat-free frozen desserts.

Eggs:

Limit yolks to three per week. Two egg whites can be substituted for one whole egg in recipes.

Fats & oils:

Substitute soft or liquid margarine or liquid oils in recipes. 1 tablespoon margarine or ¾ tablespoon oil will substitute for 1 tablespoon of butter. One cup of plain yogurt will substitute for one cup of sour cream. Limit butter, lard, fatback, and solid vegetable shortenings in your cooking.

Fruits and vegetables:

Keep plenty of fresh or frozen fruits and vegetables handy for meals and snacks. Make your own *convenience* foods or *fast food* by storing the fruits or vegetables after any needed preparation (for example, store broccoli after it's been cut into bite-sized pieces). This will make for quick snacks.

Breads, cereals, and pastas:

Try pasta, rice, and dried peas and beans (split peas, lentils, kidney beans, and navy beans) as main dishes, casseroles, soups, or other one-dish meals without high-fat sauces. Most granola-type cereals are high in fat. Look for the low-fat versions. Commercial baked goods will be high in saturated fat. However, breads and most rolls are low in fat (plus, whole-grain types will be higher in fiber).

From Public Health Service, National Institutes of Health, National Cholesterol Education Program, National Heart, Lung, and Blood Institute: *Eating to lower your high blood cholesterol,* NIH Pub No 89-2920, Washington, DC, 1989, US DHHS.

Medical Nutrition Therapy

To lessen the workload of the heart, medical nutrition therapy focuses on restricting dietary sodium. The more severe the heart failure, the more severe the sodium restriction to reduce extracellular fluids. Patients in severe failure may receive a diet that contains 1000 mg (45 mEq) or less of sodium per day, whereas patients in moderate failure may receive a diet containing 2000 mg (90 mEq) or less of sodium (11). Fluid may also be restricted if hyponatremia occurs. Restrictions of 1.5 to 2.0 liters/day are common, but patients in severe failure may require fluids to be restricted to less than 1 liter/day (11).

Energy requirements may be 30% to 50% above basal needs because of increased cardiac and pulmonary energy demands (11). If the patient has cardiac

Small feedings supplied throughout the day—as many as 5 or 6—reduce the risk of stomach distention and associated diaphragm pressure that could increase cardiac stress.

cachexia, additional kcalories are needed to prevent further catabolism. Caution must be used when increasing energy, however, so as not to overfeed the patient. Kcalorie dense (1.5 to 2.0 kcal/ml) nutritional supplements may be helpful to increase kcalories and protein intake. Enteral or parenteral nutrition may be necessary for patients who cannot meet their nutritional needs through oral intake.

cachexia
general ill health and malnutrition, marked by weakness and emaciation

LIFE SPAN IMPLICATIONS

Cardiovascular disease often seems to be the realm of our older patients, but the illness may strike in the middle years of 40s and 50s. With later marriages and/or delayed childbearing, the middle years may often still be a time of parenting young children as well as teens. Dietary modifications are easier to follow when the whole family is supportive and compliant.

Dietary education should include the individuals who buy and prepare meals (and snacks, too) for the patient. Lists of health associations, community hospitals and other organizations that offer cooking courses, and bookstores or public libraries with available heart healthy cookbooks are excellent adjuncts to dietary prescriptions. By including all family members in the educative process, not only is the health of the individual with CAD enhanced, but primary risk factors for the younger members are also decreased. Although children may not need to follow the sometimes extreme restrictions of CAD patients, it still is easier for a 10 year old to understand that it is heart healthy to have popcorn with little or no salt than to simply blame restrictions on "Daddy's sickness." Lifelong health promotion habits develop early and benefit everyone.

OVERCOMING BARRIERS

Demystifying Labels

Label reading is an important skill for all of us, but is especially so for someone with hypertension or cardiovascular disease. Educating patients about the use of food label information demystifies the process of consuming recommended levels of dietary fat and sodium (14,15). Food labels may display two types of messages about the packaged food: nutrient content claim and health claims. Federal regulations formulated by the Food and Drug Administration (FDA) control how certain terms can be used in labeling. Below are terms related to sodium, dietary cholesterol, and fat—nutrients of concern for cardiovascular diseases.

Nutrient content claims

Free: a product contains virtually none of one or more of these: fat, saturated fat, cholesterol, sodium, sugars, and kcalories

Low: a product has a low enough amount of a nutrient (fat, saturated fat, cholesterol, sodium, and kcalories) to allow frequent intake without concern of getting too much:

  low fat—≤3 grams per serving
  low saturated fat—≤1 gram per serving
  low sodium—≤140 mg per serving
  very low sodium—≤35 mg per serving
  low cholesterol—≤20 mg per serving
  low calorie—≤40 kcal per serving

Lean and extra lean: used to describe the fat content of meat, poultry, seafood, and game meats lean—<10 grams fat, 4 grams saturated fat, and <95 mg of cholesterol per serving and per 100 grams

extra lean—<5 grams fat, <2 grams saturated fat, and <95 mg of cholesterol per serving and per 100 grams

Good source: one serving of a food contains 10% to 19% of the Daily Value for a particular nutrient

Reduced: a nutritionally altered product that contains 25% less of a nutrient or kcalories than the regular product (this claim cannot be made on a product if the regular food already meets the requirement for *low*)

Less: contains 25% less of a nutrient than a comparable food (example: pretzels can have 25% less fat than potato chips)

Light or lite: a product has one third fewer kcalories than a comparable product or 50% of the fat found in a comparable product, or the sodium content of a low-kcalorie, low-fat food has been reduced by 50% (*light* may still be used to describe properties of foods such as texture and color)

Healthy: by January 1, 1996, *healthy* individual foods must have no more than 480 mg of sodium per serving (meals and main dishes can't exceed 600 mg); by January 1, 1998, *healthy* foods must have no more than 360 mg of sodium (meals and main dishes can't exceed 480 mg)

Health claims

Relationships between nutrients or foods and the risk of a disease or health-related condition are allowed if the claim meets FDA requirements. The following nutrient-CAD relationship claims are allowed to appear on food labels:

saturated fat and cholesterol and CAD

fiber-containing fruits, vegetables, and grain products and risk of CAD

sodium and hypertension

WELLNESS AND LIPIDS

Physical Dimension	CAD affects the heart, an essential organ; this disease impairs functioning of many body systems.
Intellectual Dimension	Determining one's own risk factors and devising a program to reduce their effects depends on intellectual skills.
Emotional Dimension	Patient denial may occur; some individuals view heart problems as only happening to others. Mortality caused by CAD, as well as the many lifestyle modifications necessary, may be very frightening; how can we reassure patients, yet still assist them to change behaviors?
Social Dimension	Because of increased education through the work of health associations and health departments, many restaurants and resorts serve *Heart Healthy* entrees; with careful selections, socializing can continue unaffected.

SUMMARY

C ardiovascular disease consists of a group of diseases and conditions affecting the heart and blood vessels; they are coronary artery disease, hypertension, peripheral vascular disease, congestive heart failure, and congenital heart diseases. Cardiovascular disease risk factors are categorized into three groups: controllable, noncontrollable, and predisposing. Controllable or lifestyle factors include tobacco use and physical inactivity. Noncontrollable factors are gender, age, and family history. Predisposing conditions may be diabetes mellitus, hypertension, obesity, and hypercholesterolemia.

Coronary artery disease (CAD) begins with atherosclerosis. Atherosclerosis is the development of lesions in the coronary arteries that can lead to arteriosclerosis and cause angina pectoris or myocardial infarction. If thrombosis occurs in a cerebral artery, a cerebrovascular accident or stroke occurs. CAD risk is assessed by measuring total blood cholesterol, as well as the proportions of the different types of lipoproteins that carry cholesterol in the blood. Lowering total cholesterol and LDL-cholesterol can be achieved by dietary intervention, including weight loss and exercise. The goals of medical nutrition therapy are to reduce total fat, saturated fat, and cholesterol intake in an attempt to reduce total cholesterol, LDL-cholesterol, and triglyceride levels.

Hypertension for which the cause is not known is referred to as primary or essential hypertension. Secondary hypertension occurs when the cause of elevated blood pressure can be identified. Prescribed treatment regimens for hypertension are individualized and vary because the disease differs in its degree of severity. The first line of treatment is usually nonpharmacological or focused on lifestyle modifications. Weight reduction and sodium restriction augment antihypertensive medications as well.

Myocardial infarctions are the single largest killer in the United States. The purpose of medical nutrition therapy is to reduce the workload of the heart. The patient may receive a liquid diet initially and progress as tolerated to foods of regular consistency. Smaller, frequent meals are usually better tolerated than large meals.

Congestive heart failure can be caused by CAD, lung disease, hypothyroidism, or damage to the myocardial or cardiac muscle. Congestion and edema develop in the lungs, liver, bowel, and legs. The condition is characterized by decreased blood flow to the kidneys and retention of sodium and fluid (11). Patients with congestive heart failure often experience edema of the feet and ankles and shortness of breath. To lessen the workload of the heart, medical nutrition therapy focuses on restricting dietary sodium.

THE NURSING ROLE
Reducing Fat and Cholesterol: The Nursing Process

Mr. Stanton is a 56-year-old with a family history of heart disease and a personal history of high cholesterol levels (260 and above) and high low-density lipoprotein levels (180 and above). He has an appointment in the health maintenance organization (HMO) where you are a cardiovascular clinical nurse specialist.

ASSESSMENT DATA COLLECTED
The newest lab results reveal a total cholesterol (TC) of 256 mg/dl and LDL level of 170 mg/dl. You ask Mr. Stanton if he has been limiting fat and cholesterol in his diet as previously instructed and he says "yes." However, when you ask him to describe some of his typical meals, you find that he is eating a lot of fried foods, some bakery pastries, and several portions of lean beef each week. He states that he is careful to buy low-cholesterol foods when available. You arrive at the following diagnosis.

NURSING DIAGNOSIS
Knowledge deficit related to lack of understanding of relationship between fat and cholesterol as evidenced by purposeful use of some low-cholesterol foods but intake of high-fat foods.

Continued.

THE NURSING ROLE, cont'd.

Reducing Fat and Cholesterol: The Nursing Process

PLANNING

Together you set the following goals. Mr. Stanton will:

Express understanding that controlling total fat intake is as important as controlling cholesterol

Limit fried foods and beef to one portion per week and eat only low-cholesterol, low-fat pastry in small amounts

Increase intake of whole-grain breads and cereals, fruits, and vegetables

By next clinic visit in 3 months, reduce total cholesterol level to 220 and LDLs to 160.

INTERVENTION

1. Review the physiological differences between fat and cholesterol
2. Give Mr. Stanton another copy of a handout on fat and cholesterol that included foods to be limited and avoided in each category
3. Assess Mr. Stanton's understanding of the effects of high TC and LDL levels on the body
4. Schedule appointments for Mr. Stanton with the laboratory and yourself in 3 months
5. Ask Mr. Stanton to call the dietitian he originally worked with if he is having difficulty with the diet during the next 3 months.

EVALUATION

The goals will be evaluated in 3 months to see if outcomes have been achieved as evidenced by:

Mr. Stanton giving a simple explanation of the difference between fat and cholesterol

Total cholesterol of 220 mg/dl or lower and LDL of 160 or lower

---

Critical Thinking   ## CLINICAL APPLICATIONS

I.C. is 69-year-old male admitted to the coronary care unit of your hospital. He is 5'11" tall, of medium frame, and weighs 210 lb. He has gained 30 lb since he retired 4 years ago, which he attributes to boredom and lack of exercise. Three months prior to admission, I.C. began to experience chest pain that radiated up his neck and down to his stomach. He has a history of hypertension and elevated serum cholesterol levels. After admission to the hospital, I.C. was diagnosed with an acute MI.

Test results for serum lips were as follows: Chol 300 mg/dL, LDL-cholesterol 190 mg/dL, HDL-cholesterol 30 mg/dL, TG 600 mg/dL

Meds prescribed after admission: tenormin, cardizem, nitroglycerin

Diet order: NCEP Step 1 diet and no added salt

1. Define the term *myocardial infarction* and describe what happens when a myocardial infarction occurs.
2. What are the risk factors for cardiovascular disease?
3. What are I.C.'s risk factors?
4. What specific guidelines are included in the NCEP's Step 1 recommendations?

Critical Thinking   **CLINICAL APPLICATIONS, cont'd.**

5. While caring for I.C., you learn that he snacks on high-fat cheeses, ice cream, potato chips, corn chips, peanuts, and crackers. He also drinks whole milk and eats a lot of butter on his bread at every meal. What characteristics of I.C.'s intake contradict the NCEP Step 1 recommendations?
6. What are some alternative foods I.C. could use for snacks?

REFERENCES

1. National Center for Health Statistics, CDC: Advance report of final mortality statistics, 1990, *Month Vital Stat Rep* 41(7)(suppl) DHHS publication 93-1120, 1993.
2. Food and Nutrition Board, National Research Council: *Diet and health: Implications for reducing chronic disease risk,* Washington, DC, 1989, National Academy Press.
3. US Department of Health and Human Services: *Report of the Secretary's Task Force on Black and Minority Health, Volume 1: Executive summary,* Washington, DC, 1985.
4. American Heart Association: *Heart and stroke facts: 1995 statistical supplement,* Dallas, 1994, American Heart Association.
5. Centers for Disease Control and Prevention: *Cardiovascular disease surveillance: Ischemic heart disease, 1980-1989,* Issued 1993.
6. Centers for Disease Control and Prevention: *Cardiovascular disease surveillance: Stroke, 1980-1989,* Issued 1994.
7. CVD Plan Steering Committee: *Preventing death and disability from cardiovascular diseases: A state-based plan for action,* Washington, DC, 1994, Association of State and Territorial Health Officials.
8. Centers for Disease Control and Prevention: Prevalence of adults with no known major risk factors for coronary heart diseases—behavioral risk factor surveillance system, *MMWR* 43:61-63, 69, 1994.
9. National Cholesterol Education Program: *Report of the Expert Panel on Detection, Evaluation, and Treatment of High Blood Cholesterol in Adults,* NIH Publication No. 89-2925, Washington, DC, 1989, US Dept of Health and Human Services, Public Health Services, National Institutes of Health.
10. National Cholesterol Education Program: *Second Report of the Expert Panel on Detection, Evaluation, and Treatment of High Blood Cholesterol in Adults (Adult Treatment Panel II),* NIH Publication No 93-3093, Washington, DC, 1993, US Dept of Health and Human Services, National Institutes of Health.
11. Nelson JK et al: *Mayo Clinic diet manual,* ed 7, St. Louis, 1994, Mosby.
12. National Institutes of Health: *Fifth report on the Joint National Committee on Detection, Evaluation, and Treatment of High Blood Pressure,* NIH Pub No 93-1088, Washington, DC, 1992, NIH.
13. US Department of Health and Human Services: *Surgeon General's report on nutrition and health,* DHHSA (PHS) Pub No 88-50210, Washington, DC, 1988, US Dept of Health and Human Services.
14. Legislative Highlights: Final food labeling regulations, *J Am Diet Assoc* 93:146-148, 1993.
15. Liebman B: Label loopholes, *Nutrition Action Newsletter* 21:10-11, 1994.

Chapter 20

NUTRITION FOR DISEASES OF THE KIDNEYS

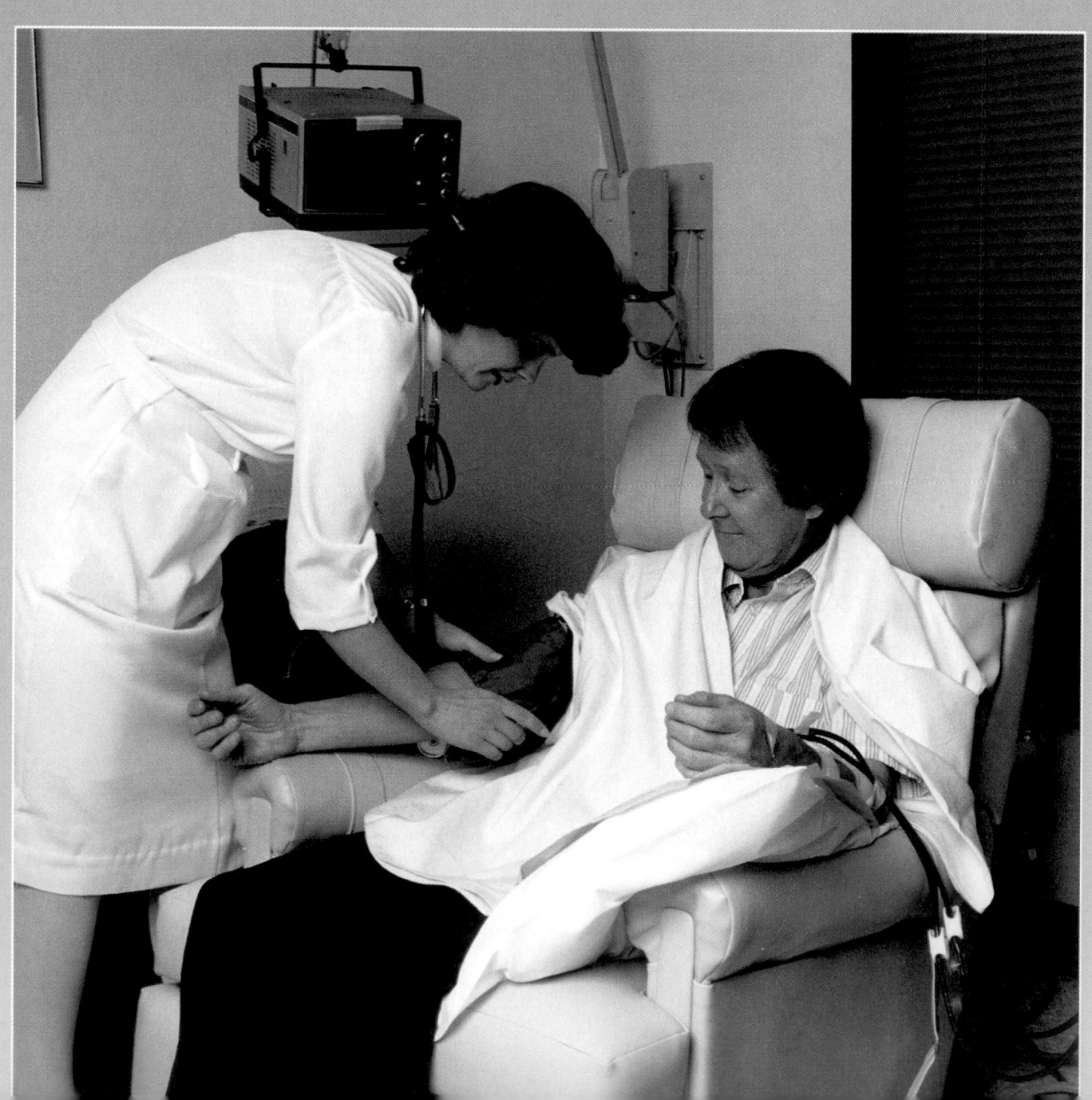

ROLE IN WELLNESS

Often taken for granted, the kidneys filter approximately one liter of blood per minute to remove excess fluid and over 200 waste products from the body. In addition, the kidneys perform vital metabolic and hormonal functions. Because the kidneys play so many roles in wellness, kidney disease has serious consequences. Nutritional needs of these patients are complex and ever-changing. The constant assessment, monitoring, and counseling required provide an ongoing challenge to nursing personnel.

KIDNEY FUNCTION

The chief, life-preserving function of the kidneys is to maintain chemical homeostasis in the body. They do this by processing blood plasma to maintain fluid, electrolyte, and acid-base balance, and by eliminating wastes in the urine. Within each kidney there are approximately 1 million microscopic workhorses called nephrons (Fig. 20-1). Each nephron filters and resorbs essential blood constituents, secretes ions as needed for maintaining acid-base balance, and excretes unwanted substances as urine. Other important functions of the kidneys include manufacturing hormones to regulate blood pressure (renin), stimulating production of red blood cells (erythropoietin), and regulating calcium and phosphorus metabolism (vitamin D). The kidneys also detoxify some drugs and poisons.

Various inflammatory, obstructive, and degenerative diseases affect the kidneys in different ways. These disorders interfere with the normal functioning of the nephrons to regulate products of body metabolism. In short, kidney failure means homeostatic failure and, if not relieved, death.

NEPHROTIC SYNDROME

Nephrotic syndrome is a term used to describe a complex of symptoms that can occur as a result of damage to the capillary walls of the glomerulus. Glomerular damage results in increased urinary excretion of protein (*proteinuria*), decreased serum levels of albumin (*hypoalbuminemia*), *hyperlipidemia,* and edema [1,2]. Nephrotic syndrome is often the result of secondary disease processes: primary glomerular disease (*glomerulonephritis*), nephropathy secondary to diabetes mellitus, *lupus erythematosus,* or infectious disease. It may be treated with corticosteroid or immunosuppressive medications, but in some patients nephrotic syndrome is resistant to treatment and may progress to chronic renal failure (CRF) [1].

It is essential for nursing personnel to monitor patients' weight and intake and output closely. Intake and output should be documented in the medical record every shift [1]. The nurse and dietitian play important roles in developing a nutrition care plan for patients with CRF and in educating them regarding foods high in sodium. Table 20-1 lists foods high in sodium. For the specific sodium content of foods, refer to Appendix A.

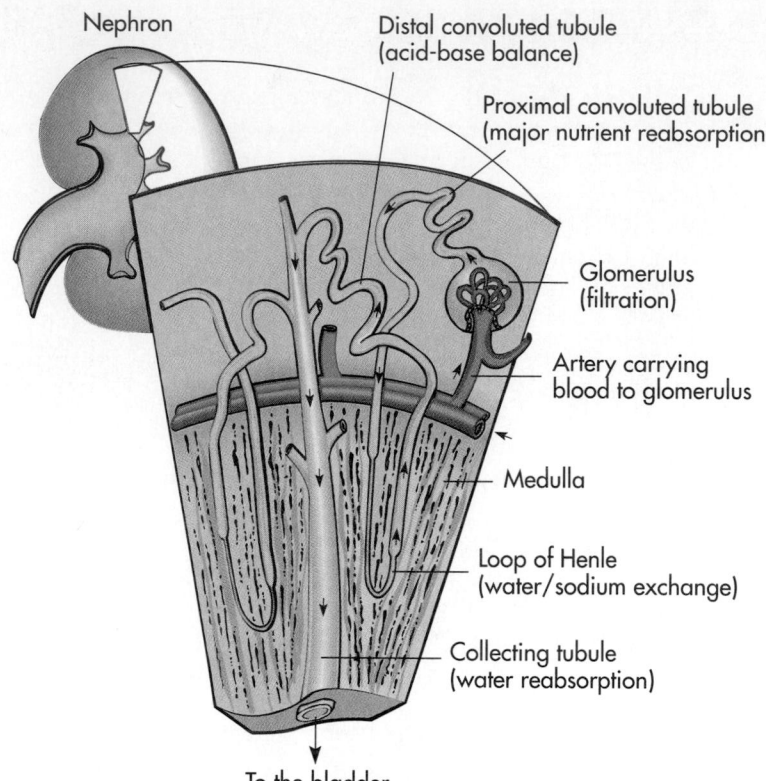

Fig. 20-1 The nephron. Blood flows into the glomerulus and some of its fluid is absorbed into the tubule. Waste products are filtered and passed through the tubule into the bladder. The fluid and dissolved substances needed by the body are resorbed in vessels alongside the tubule.

Table 20-1	Foods High in Sodium				
Condiments	**Breads/Starches**	**Meats/Meat Substitutes**	**Beverages**	**Soups**	**Vegetables**
Pickles, olives (black and green), salted nuts, meat tenderizers, commercial salad dressings, monosodium glutamate (MSG, Accent), steak sauce, ketchup, soy sauce, Worcestershire sauce, horseradish sauce, chili sauce, commercial mustard, salt, seasoned salts (onion, garlic, celery), butter salt	Salted crackers, potato chips, corn chips, popcorn, pretzels; dehydrated potatoes	Cured, smoked, and processed meats (ham, bacon, corned beef, chipped beef, hot dogs, luncheon meats, bologna, salt pork, canned salmon and tuna); all cheeses except low-sodium and cottage cheese; convenience foods (microwave and TV dinners); peanut butter	Commercial buttermilk, instant hot cocoa mixes	Canned soups, dehydrated soups, bouillon	Sauerkraut, hominy, pork and beans, canned tomato and vegetable juices

Kidney Functions
• Maintain fluid, electrolyte, and acid-base balance • Eliminate waste products • Regulate blood pressure • Stimulate red blood cell production • Regulate calcium and phosphorus metabolism • Eliminate many drugs

Hidden Sources of Sodium

Baking powder
Drinking and cooking water
Medications
    Antacids
    Antibiotics
    Cough medicines
    Laxatives
    Pain relievers
    Sedatives
Mouthwash
Toothpaste

MEDICAL NUTRITION THERAPY

The primary goals of medical nutrition therapy are to control hypertension, minimize edema, decrease urinary albumin losses, prevent protein malnutrition and muscle catabolism, supply adequate energy, and slow the progression of renal disease (3). Patients need to consume adequate amounts of protein (0.8 to 1.0 g/kg/day) and kcalories (≥35 kcal/kg/day) to prevent catabolism of lean body tissue and avoid malnutrition. The majority of the patient's kcalories should be provided by carbohydrates (50% to 60% of total kcal) and monounsaturated and polyunsaturated fats (approximately 30% to 40% total kcal). Monounsaturated and polyunsaturated fats are recommended because of the increased risk of hyperlipidemia (4).

Limiting dietary sodium can help control hypertension and edema. (Appendix A lists sodium content of foods.) Processing of foods, especially convenience foods, often adds substantial amounts of sodium (discussed in Chapter 8). Patients should also be mindful of possible hidden sources of salt such as their water supply and medications. Toothpaste and mouthwash often contain a significant amount of sodium, and patients should be instructed not to swallow these products.

ACUTE RENAL FAILURE

Acute renal failure (ARF) is characterized by an abrupt loss of renal function that may or may not be accompanied by **oliguria** or **anuria** (1,5). The most common causes of ARF are trauma, hemorrhage, shock, nephrotoxic chemicals or drugs, **septicemia**, and streptococcal infection (2,3). Although a few patients do not experience any reduction in urine output, two thirds experience the following three stages (1,3,6):

oliguria
<400 ml urine excretion/24 hr

anuria
<250 ml urine excretion/24 hr

septicemia
systemic infection in the circulating bloodstream

Foods High in Potassium	
Apricots	Oranges, orange juice
Avocado	Peanuts (also high in sodium)
Banana	Potatoes, white and sweet
Cantaloupe	Prune juice
Carrots, raw	Spinach
Dried beans, peas	Swiss chard
Dried fruits	Tomatoes, tomato juice, tomato sauce
Melons	Winter squash

azotemia
retention of excessive amounts of nitrogenous compounds in the blood caused by the kidney's failure to remove urea from the blood; characterized by uremia

1. Oliguric (usually lasting approximately 7 to 21 days)—manifested by **azotemia**, acidosis, high serum potassium, high serum phosphorus, hypertension, anorexia, edema, and risk of water intoxication (indicated by low sodium levels)
2. Diuretic (usually lasting approximately 7 to 14 days)—output of urine is gradually increased
3. Recovery (usually 3 to 12 months)—kidney function gradually improves, but there may be some residual permanent damage

It is important to monitor intake and output closely and document each shift. Weight should also be taken and recorded daily. When patients do not eat, they may lose approximately 0.5 kg/day (1). Conversely, any sudden weight gains suggest excessive fluid retention. Monitoring intake, output, and weight will help differentiate whether weight loss or gain is from fluid versus lean body mass or adipose tissue. Fluid retention can mask loss of lean body mass.

Nurses are the health care professionals who will assist patients in adhering to prescribed fluid restrictions. See the Teaching Tool, Chapter 17, for a list of hints for helping patients with fluid restrictions. Nurses work closely with renal dietitians to coordinate meal planning and nutrition education with patients and their significant others (1). Nutrition education may involve reduced protein, sodium, potassium, and fluid intake. Appendix A lists protein, sodium, and potassium content of foods. Nurses should be watchful for constipation as a result of restricted intake of fluids and fresh fruits (most are high in potassium), bed rest, and medication side effects (1).

dialysis
a procedure that involves diffusion of particles from an area of high to lower concentration, osmosis of fluid across the membrane from an area of lesser to greater concentration of particles, and the ultrafiltration or movement of fluid across the membrane as a result of an artificially created pressure differential

Medical Nutrition Therapy

Nutritional needs are partially determined by whether or not **dialysis** is used for treatment. Another determinant of nutrient needs is the underlying cause of the ARF. Patients may be hypermetabolic if the renal failure was caused by trauma, burns, septicemia, or infection. These conditions, other underlying medical problems, and the renal failure will more than likely have a negative impact on the patient's appetite, thus increasing concern for nutritional status (3).

Energy should be provided in sufficient amounts for weight maintenance or to meet the demands of stress accompanying the ARF, usually 30 to 50 kcal/kg (3,6). Nonprotein kcalories should be provided by fats, oils, simple carbohydrates, and low-protein starches. If dialysis is not used for treatment, 0.6 grams of protein per kg body weight (but not less than 40 grams per day) is recommended (3,4). This amount can be increased as kidney function improves. When dialysis is used as part of the medical treatment, protein intake can be liberalized to 1.0 to 1.5 g/kg (3,4). In either situation, the use of high **biological value** or **high quality proteins** is recommended (3). Diets containing less than 60 gm of protein may be deficient in niacin, riboflavin, thiamin, calcium, iron, vitamin B_{12}, and zinc (4), and these nutrients may need to be supplemented.

biological value
a measurement of nitrogen balance determining the protein availability of a particular food

high quality protein
a food containing the best balance and assortment of essential and nonessential amino acids for protein synthesis

During the oliguric stage, sodium may be restricted to 1000 to 2000 mg and potassium to 1000 mg per day. (The Teaching Tool gives tips on reducing potassium.) Both electrolytes may be lost during the diuretic phase or during dialysis.

TEACHING TOOL
Reducing Potassium Content of Foods

Many commonly consumed vegetables are good sources of potassium. Unfortunately, renal disorders often require restricting vegetables that are high in potassium. Clients may become frustrated by the limited selection of vegetables available that are naturally low in potassium.

By using the same principle of dialysis on food preparation, the potassium content of vegetables that are usually restricted can be reduced. This method, sometimes called *leaching*, **does not** eliminate potassium, it just reduces the amount of potassium in the food item so it can be used more often in the meal plan. Clients can then choose from an expanded selection of vegetables, while still limiting potassium intake.

Leaching potatoes, carrots, beets, and rutabagas
1. Peel and slice ⅛ in thick

2. Place vegetables in a volume of warm water that is 10 times the amount of vegetables (example: 1 cup of potatoes should be placed in 10 cups water); soak for at least 2 hours
3. Rinse and cook for 5 minutes in five times the amount of water
4. Cooked vegetables can be frozen in individual portions and prepared later in a variety of ways

Leaching greens (kale, mustard, or spinach), lima beans, squash, mushrooms, and cauliflower
1. Place frozen greens in a strainer (or sieve) and allow to thaw at room temperature
2. Drain and rinse fresh or frozen vegetables in warm water
3. Soak and cook as above

Therefore losses should be replaced as needed depending on urinary volume, serum levels, and frequency of dialysis (4). Fluids are usually restricted to the patient's output (urine, vomitus, and diarrhea) plus 500 ml during the oliguric phase (3,4,6). During the diuretic phase, large amounts of fluid may be needed to replace losses.

CHRONIC RENAL FAILURE

Chronic renal failure (CRF) is the result of progressive, irreversible loss of kidney function (1). It can develop over days, months, or years and progress to end stage renal disease (ESRD) (1,2). CRF has many causes; some of the most common are glomerulonephritis, **nephrosclerosis,** obstructive diseases (kidney stones, tumors, congenital birth defects of kidneys and urinary tract), diabetes mellitus, lupus erythematosus, and illicit use of analgesic or *street* drugs. Regardless of the cause, results will be the same: retention of nitrogenous waste products and fluid and electrolyte imbalances that can affect all body systems (1).

Before ESRD, management focuses on slowing the progression of CRF and avoiding complications (1). Once CRF progresses to ESRD, management centers on reducing **uremia** by the use of various treatment modalities: conservative management, **hemodialysis, peritoneal dialysis,** and **renal transplantation** (1,3).

Medical Nutrition Therapy

Planning diets for CRF, ESRD, hemodialysis, and peritoneal dialysis patients requires calibrating intakes of energy, protein, lipids, phosphorus, potassium, sodium, vitamins and other minerals, and fluids. It is not only important to design food combinations that include the necessary nutrients, but the foods must be ones that the patient will accept and enjoy. This task can be overwhelming, but there are specialists—renal dietitians—who do this on a daily basis. Most often, a system similar to the exchange system, called the National Renal Diet, is used to develop diet guidelines and meal plans (Appendix K).

nephrosclerosis
necrosis of the renal arterioles, associated with hypertension

uremia
excessive amounts of urea and other nitrogenous waste products in the blood

hemodialysis
a procedure to remove impurities or wastes from the blood in treating renal insufficiency by shunting the blood from the body through a machine for diffusion and ultrafiltration and then returning it to the patient's circulation

peritoneal dialysis
a dialysis procedure performed to correct an imbalance of fluid or electrolytes in the blood or other wastes by using the peritoneum as the diffusible membrane

renal transplantation
the transfer of a kidney from one person to another

Table 20-2   Treatments and Major Concerns for Pre-ESRD, Hemodialysis, and Peritoneal Dialysis

	Pre-ESRD	Hemodialysis	Peritoneal Dialysis*
Treatment	Diet + medications	Diet + medications + hemodialysis	Diet + medications + peritoneal dialysis
Modality		Dialysis using vascular access for waste product and fluid removal	Dialysis using peritoneal membrane for waste product and fluid removal
Duration	Indefinite	3-5 hours 2-3 days/week	3-5 exchanges 7 days/week
Concerns	Hypertension, glycemic control in patients with diabetes mellitus	Bone disease, hypertension	Bone disease, weight gain, hyperlipidemia, glycemic control in patients with diabetes mellitus
	Glomerular hyperfiltration, rise in BUN, bone disease	Amino acid loss, interdialytic electrolyte and fluid changes	Protein loss into dialysate, glucose absorption from dialysate

From American Dietetic Association: *National renal diet: Professional guide,* Chicago, 1993, American Dietetic Association.
*Includes continuous ambulatory peritoneal dialysis (CAPD) and continuous cyclic peritoneal dialysis (CCPD).

uremic toxicity
buildup of toxic waste products (urea and other nitrogenous waste products) in the blood; symptoms include anorexia, nausea, metallic taste in the mouth, irritability, confusion, lethargy, restlessness, and pruritus (itching)

Nurses play a very important role in helping patients maintain good nutritional status, weight, morale, and appetite by working with renal dietitians to reinforce medical nutrition therapy and nutrition education. Through formal and informal teaching, nurses can help patients appreciate the need for the stringent diet and help them recognize the direct relationship between adherence to the diet and progression or lack of progression of symptoms that reduce their quality of life.

Nutritional management depends on the method of treatment in addition to medical and nutritional status of the patient (7). Table 20-2 compares treatment methods and primary concerns associated with each.

No clear guidelines define the exact point when medical nutrition therapy should begin, but conventional wisdom indicates that dietary modifications (Table 20-3) should be initiated as early as possible to minimize **uremic toxicity,** delay the progression of renal disease, and prevent wasting and malnutrition (2). This can be accomplished by limiting foods whose metabolic byproducts add to the buildup of toxic substances and providing adequate kcalories to prevent body tissue catabolism (2). Patients often find this diet difficult to follow for a long period of time, so motivation and encouragement from nursing and other health professionals are crucial.

Reducing protein and phosphorus to minimum requirements can slow the progression of renal insufficiency (2). Phosphorus content of foods is listed in Appendix A. Continuing to assess the nutritional status and dietary compliance of patients with CRF is very important. Because patients may find that foods "don't taste like they used to," encouraging the uses of spices such as garlic, onions, and oregano to enhance the flavor of allowed foods can be helpful (1).

The National Renal Diet was developed by the Renal Dietitians Practice Group and the National Kidney Foundation Council on Renal Nutrition to provide a renal diet with nationwide applicability. Diet prescription guidelines for pre-ESRD, hemodialysis, and peritoneal dialysis patients were developed over a 5-year period. Because of the national focus of these guidelines, ethnic and geographically unique foods are not included but can be incorporated as part of the individualized diet plan. Vegetarian choices are also not included because high biologic value proteins are the preferred protein sources for renal patients, and vegan diets usually are of low biologic value. Ovovegetarian and lacto-ovovegetarian diets include high biological value protein sources, but they tend to be high in phosphorus. One point that requires emphasis is that the National Renal Diet guidelines and food lists are only a starting point for individualized meal plans and education. Patient compliance is enhanced by designing meal plans to meet the specific needs of each patient (7). The accompanying box provides a sample menu for a patient with chronic renal failure.

Table 20-3 Nutrition Guidelines for Pre-ESRD, Hemodialysis, and Peritoneal Dialysis

Nutrient	Pre-ESRD	Hemodialysis	Peritoneal Dialysis	Comments
Energy	35-40 kcal/kg	30-35 kcal/kg	25-35 kcal/kg	Based on ideal body weight
Protein	0.6-0.8 g/kg	1.1-1.4 g/kg	1.2-1.5 g/kg	Based on ideal body weight
Sodium	1-3 g if necessary	2-3 g	2-4 g	
Potassium	Usually unrestricted	Approximately 40 mg/kg	Usually unrestricted	Based on ideal body weight
Phosphorus	8-12 mg/kg	≤17 mg/kg	≤17 mg/kg	Based on ideal body weight; 5-10 mg/kg, but 8-12 mg/kg is a more practical restriction; a diet high in protein may make it impossible to meet the optimum phosphorus prescription
Calcium	1200-1600 mg	Depends on serum levels	Depends on serum levels	
Fluid	Usually unrestricted	500-750 plus daily urine output or 1000 ml if anuric	>2000 ml	

From American Dietetic Association: *A clinical guide to nutrition care in end-stage renal disease,* ed 2, Chicago, 1994, American Dietetic Association; and American Dietetic Association: *National renal diet: Professional guide,* Chicago, 1993, American Dietetic Association.

Sample Renal Diet Menu

85 mg protein; 2000 mg sodium; 2000 mg potassium; 1000 mg phosphorus; 1000 ml fluid

BREAKFAST
Apple juice
Oatmeal
Blueberry muffin
Scrambled egg
Low-sodium margarine (2 exchanges)*
2% milk (½ cup)*
Decaffeinated coffee (½ cup)*

LUNCH
Lemonade (½ cup)*
Sirloin tips (3 oz) with noodles*
Salad with Italian dressing
Fruit cocktail

DINNER
Fruit punch (½ cup)*
Low-sodium turkey (3 oz) with parsley carrots*
White bread with margarine (2 exchanges)*
Cinnamon applesauce
Hot tea (½ cup)*

From Memorial Hospital, Carbondale, Ill.
*Quantities not exact; for representation only.

HEMODIALYSIS

During hemodialysis, blood is removed by way of a special vascular access or shunt (usually in the nondominant forearm), **heparinized,** cleansed of excess fluid and waste products through a semipermeable membrane, and then returned to the patient's circulation (Fig. 20-2, *A*) (1,7). The **dialysate** is an electrolyte solution similar to the composition of normal plasma. Each of the constituents may be varied according to the patient's needs, the most common being potassium (1). The average treatment lasts 2 to 4 hours and is usually performed three times per week (2). Hemodialysis can be performed in a dialysis unit by staff or patients who have received special training, or it can be performed at the patient's home where a significant other or paid aide is required to assist in the procedure.

Medical Nutrition Therapy

Individual diet prescriptions (see Table 20-3) are determined by residual kidney function, dialysate components, duration of dialysis, and rate of blood flow through the artificial kidney (2). The meal plan is designed, monitored, and reevaluated by the dietitian. Nurses and others on the medical team are crucial for providing positive reinforcement and encouragement to the patient and family members on an ongoing basis (2). Objectives for medical nutrition therapy are to attain or maintain good nutritional status, prevent excessive accumulation of waste products and fluid between treatments, and minimize the effects of metabolic disorders that occur as a result of ESRD (7).

Phosphorus is routinely restricted in patients receiving hemodialysis because high levels of serum phosphorus contribute to secondary hyperparathyroidism and raise the calcium-phosphorus product in the plasma (2,4). Although an intake of 12 mg/kg/day is the usual recommendation, it is often necessary to liberalize this restriction to meet protein needs (2,7). Foods high in phosphorus, such as milk, milk products, cheese, beef liver, chocolate, nuts, and legumes, are usually limited or avoided (2). Medications are also used to control serum phosphorus levels. The medications of choice are calcium carbonate or calcium acetate (2,3,7). They are given at meal times to bind the phosphate in the food.

Calcium carbonate or calcium acetate also provide a much needed source of calcium in the diet of hemodialysis patients. Calcium supplements are necessary because of impaired calcium absorption caused by the lack of the active form of vitamin D (calcitriol) (2,3). Additionally, diets used to treat hemodialysis patients are low in calcium as a result of the restriction of dairy products (which are also high in phosphorus). Serum calcium levels should be monitored for hypercalcemia (2-4,7).

In renal failure, the kidneys also lose their endocrine function of producing calcitriol (the active form of vitamin D). Although many forms of vitamin D are available for supplementation, it is the active form that helps prevent bone disease (2,3). The active form of vitamin D is available in oral form (Rocaltrol) and IV form (Calcijex), which is given during hemodialysis (2,4).

Anemia results from another endocrine function affected by CRF—decreased production of the hormone erythropoietin, a hormone that stimulates bone marrow to produce red blood cells and blood loss. An adequate available iron supply is necessary for erythropoiesis to take place. **Recombinant erythropoietin (EPO)** (Epogen) can be given during dialysis (by IV) or subcutaneously just after dialysis treatment. Oral or IV iron supplementation is often necessary before administration of recombinant EPO to replenish iron stores (2-4).

Patients treated with hemodialysis are at risk for deficiencies of water-soluble vitamins, particularly vitamin B_6 and folic acid. The reason is two-fold: poor intake or loss of the nutrients during dialysis (3,7). Supplementation of the fat-soluble

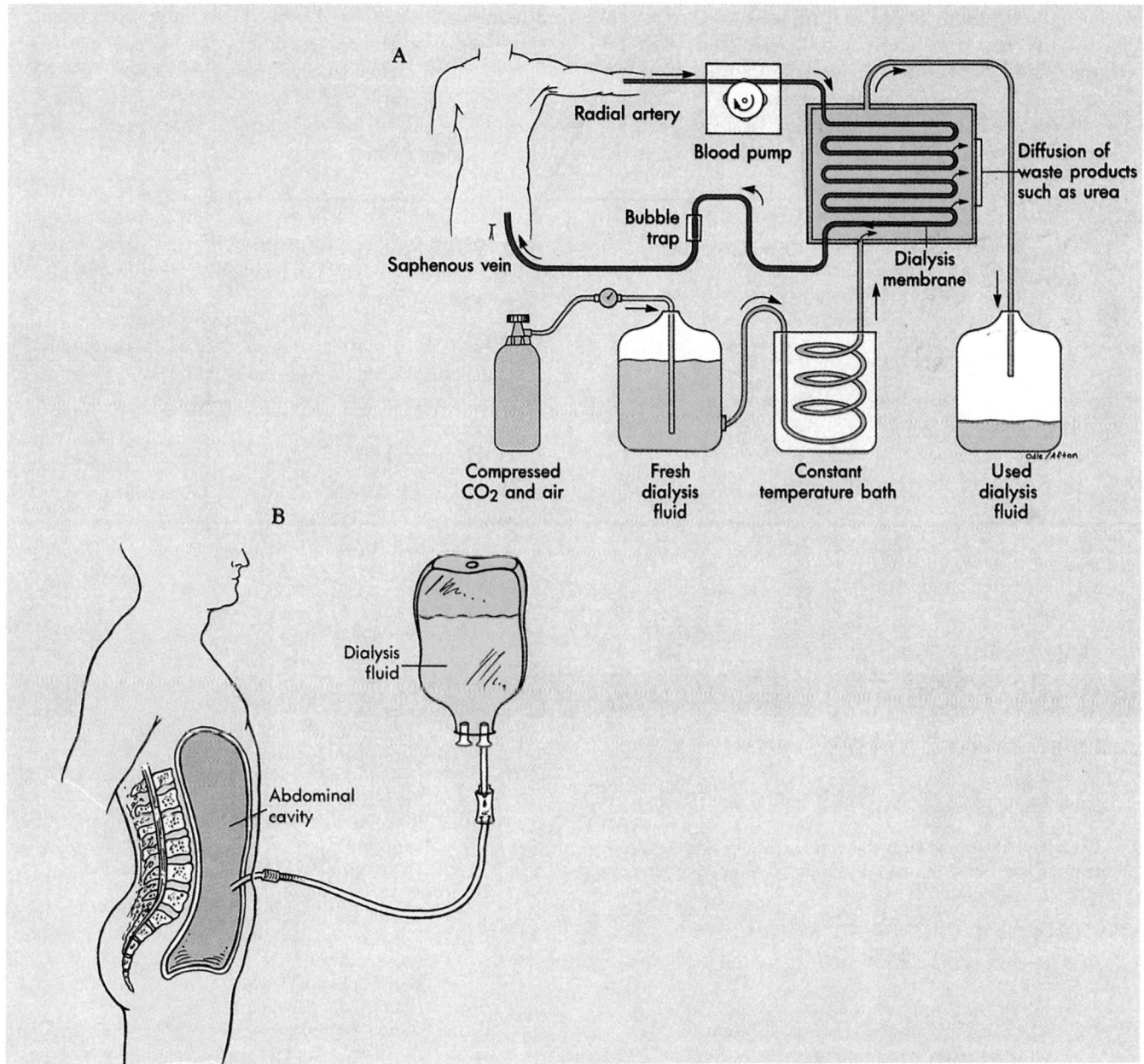

Fig. 20-2 Kidney dialysis. **A,** During hemodialysis, blood usually is taken from an artery, passed through tubes composed of a selectively permeable membrane and then returned to a leg or wrist vein. In the dialysis tank the tube is surrounded by a bath, or dialysis fluid, containing varying concentrations of electrolytes and other chemicals. The membrane allows only very small molecules, such as urea and other waste products, to escape into the surrounding fluid. **B,** in continuous ambulatory peritoneal dialysis (CAPD), 1 to 3 liters of dialysis fluid is introduced directly into the peritoneal cavity through an opening in the abdominal wall. Peritoneal membranes in the abdominal cavity transfer waste products from the blood into the dialysis fluid, which is then drained back into a plastic container. This technique is less expensive than hemodialysis and does not require the use of complex equipment.

Suggestions for Patients With Altered Taste
Brush teeth 6 to 8 times per day
Rinse mouth with a chilled mouthwash (commercial product or water mixed with lemon juice or vinegar)
Eat sour-ball candy
Chew gum
Before meals drink water with lemon or eat a small amount of sherbet or fruit sorbet

From American Dietetic Association: *National renal diet: Professional guide,* 1993, American Dietetic Association.

vitamins A, E, and K is usually not necessary. In fact, patients treated with hemodialysis have been reported to experience vitamin A toxicity. Supplementation of trace minerals is not necessary unless a deficiency is suspected or documented (3).

Obviously, patients who have a poor dietary intake are at increased risk of nutrient deficiencies and poor nutritional status. Intake can be the result of poor appetite, changes in taste acuity and in food preferences (especially red meat and sweets), nausea and vomiting, or diet limitations (3). When patients develop changes in taste, foods with sharp, distinct flavors may be useful in stimulating appetite (6).

Approximately one third of patients requiring hemodialysis each year have diabetes mellitus. Diets for these patients should incorporate nutritional modifications necessary for ESRD as well as providing consistent content and timing of meals and snacks to facilitate glycemic control (7).

PERITONEAL DIALYSIS

Peritoneal dialysis (PD) removes excess fluid and waste products from the blood using the peritoneal membrane as a filter. Dialysate is instilled and removed through a catheter that has been surgically placed into the peritoneal cavity. The peritoneum, the lining of the abdominal cavity, is used as the dialysis membrane (Fig. 20-2, *B*). The waste products cross the membrane by passive movement from the peritoneal capillaries into the dialysate in the peritoneal cavity. The dialysate contains dextrose, which increases the osmolality of the solution and facilitates removal of the excess fluid. As the fluid moves from the vascular space into the peritoneal cavity, the osmolality of the solutions becomes equal. The toxins and excess fluids collected in the peritoneal cavity are then drained from the body through the catheter and discarded (8). The advantage of peritoneal dialysis is that it is usually performed in the home. All forms of peritoneal dialysis require special training of the patient, caregiver, or both.

Intermittent Peritoneal Dialysis

Intermittent peritoneal dialysis (IPD) involves infusion of approximately two liters of dialysate instilled over a 20- to 30-minute period. The dialysate is then drained by gravity, and the process is repeated over an 8- to 10-hour period 4 to 5 times per week. IPD can be performed manually or mechanically. During the time of dialysis, patients are restricted to a chair or bed (1). This method is not commonly used as a long-term treatment modality because of the time involvement (2).

Continuous Ambulatory Peritoneal Dialysis

Continuous ambulatory peritoneal dialysis (CAPD) entails the infusion of dialysate for a 4- to 6-hour intraperitoneal dwell time during the day and an

8-hour dwell time overnight (7). At the end of the designated time, the dialysate is drained by gravity and a new exchange begins. Dialysis exchanges are done continuously, 7 days a week (1).

Continuous Cycling Peritoneal Dialysis

Continuous cycling peritoneal dialysis (CCPD) is a combination of IPD and CAPD. At night, a cycler (mechanical) performs three dialysate exchanges. During the day, a fourth exchange is infused for the entire day (1,7). At bedtime, the fourth exchange is drained and the process is started again. Although restricted to bed during night-time infusions, patients are ambulatory during the day (1).

Medical Nutrition Therapy

The objectives of nutrition therapy (see Table 20-3) are to maintain good nutritional status while replacing albumin lost in the dialysate, minimize complications of fluid imbalance, minimize symptoms of uremic toxicity, and minimize metabolic disorders secondary to ESRD and peritoneal dialysis (7). As with hemodialysis, patients treated with PD are at risk for deficiencies of water-soluble vitamins and minerals. A daily multivitamin supplement that includes folic acid is recommended (3). Some patients may receive recombinant EPO for correction of anemia and need iron supplementation to maximize the effectiveness of the drug (3).

Energy needs for patients treated with PD are usually lower than for those receiving hemodialysis. Dextrose is used as an osmotic agent in PD dialysate and must be considered when energy needs are calculated (2,3,7). Approximately 75% to 80% of the dialysate is absorbed (3,7) and needs to be calculated as part of the patient's energy source.

Protein losses during PD range from 5 grams to 15 grams per day (2,7) and are reflected in higher dietary protein recommendations (see Table 20-2). Hemoglobin, serum albumin, urea, and total serum protein can be used as indicators of sufficient protein intake (3). Values will decline suddenly when protein intake decreases or when there are excessive losses during peritonitis (3). At least 50% of dietary protein should be high biological value (complete sources of essential amino acids) (7).

During PD, sodium, potassium, and fluid are continually being removed, making severe dietary restrictions unnecessary (2,3,7). However, it is important to remember that nutrient needs vary among patients; individualized recommendations are necessary. Restriction of dietary phosphorus is critical to prevent development of **osteodystrophy**. Unfortunately, the higher protein requirements for PD consequently provide high amounts of phosphorus. Therefore severely restricting or eliminating dairy products is necessary to control phosphorus intake, which may result in the need for calcium supplementation (2,3,7).

The absorption of glucose from PD dialysate presents unique challenges in patients with diabetes. Blood glucose levels and hyperlipidemia are more difficult to control (2,7). Weight gain caused by the kcalorie load of the dialysate is another common problem with peritoneal dialysis (3). Another condition to watch for is dehydration, which is caused by excessive fluid removal and extracellular fluid volume deficits (3). Careful monitoring of blood glucose, intake and output, and weight are preventive measures.

osteodystrophy
defective bone development associated with disturbances in calcium and phosphorus metabolism and renal insufficiency

RENAL TRANSPLANTATION

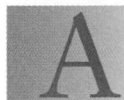
pproximately 10,000 patients with ESRD receive kidney transplants each year, and more than 13,000 are on waiting lists (1,2). Recipients have decreased hospitalization rates with increased survival rates compared with

those receiving dialytic therapy (2). Nutritional care of renal transplant recipients involves continual reassessment of nutritional goals and efficacy of therapy during the different phases of care (2).

Pretransplant

Nutritional status is evaluated to identify and correct deficits before surgery (2). Medical nutrition therapy usually involves a protein- and sodium-controlled diet (3). As the recipient progresses toward ESRD, potassium and/or phosphorus may need to be restricted (see Table 20-3) (3).

Immediate and Long-Term Posttransplant

Kcalorie needs in the immediate posttransplant period are high (30 to 35 kcal/kg) because of stress from surgery and catabolism. Energy requirements decline approximately 6 to 8 weeks after transplant, and kcalories should then be provided at a level to achieve and maintain a desirable body weight (3). Restriction of dietary protein is not necessary. In fact, protein catabolism is increased as the result of surgery and the administration of corticosteroids for immunosuppression (2,3).

Steroid therapy may cause glucose intolerance and therefore necessitate restriction of simple carbohydrates (2,3). Fats are used to supply energy, but may need to be limited if hypercholesterolemia and/or hypertriglyceridemia occur (2,3). Recommendations regarding sodium and potassium should be individualized for each patient (3). Fluids are generally unrestricted and limited only by graft function. Many of the drugs used postoperatively and posttransplant have the potential to influence nutritional needs and status. Careful observation of the patient may prevent potential problems.

RENAL CALCULI

Renal calculi (kidney stones or urolithiasis) are a common and often recurrent urologic condition (1,2). Most calculi are composed of calcium, oxalate, or phosphorus, with a small proportion formed from cystine or uric acid (2,3). Formation of kidney stones depends on the simultaneous occurrence of the following factors: (1) low urine volume (usually the result of low or inadequate fluid intake), (2) high urine pH, (3) excessive urinary excretion of calcium, oxalate, uric acid, or a combination, and (4) decreased levels of substances in the urine that normally inhibit stone formation. Dietary habits can increase the risk of stone formation in susceptible persons. The following advice may be beneficial in preventing kidney stones.

Fluid

Fluid intake has the most significant impact on reducing the risk of stone formation. An increased fluid intake increases urine output, thereby diluting the concentration of minerals in the urine. Advise the patient to maintain a urine output of over 2 liters per day by maintaining adequate hydration. Two to three liters of fluid intake per day is recommended to obtain this level of output (1).

Uric Acid Stones

Uric acid is a metabolic product of purines (a nitrogen-containing compound). Although the efficacy of limiting foods high in purines (lean meats, organ meats, legumes, and whole grains) has not been proven, restriction of dietary protein may

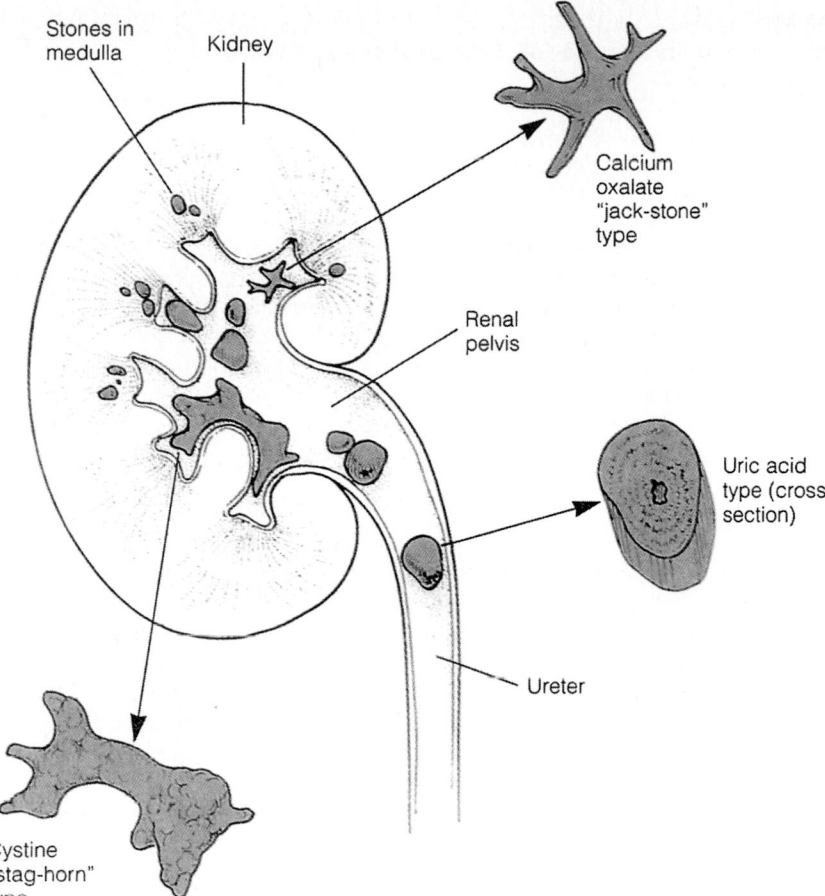

Fig. 20-3 Renal calculi.

be effective. Dietary protein intake should not exceed 100 grams per day since excessive animal protein may increase urinary uric acid and lower the pH of the urine (3). A more complete listing of purine content of foods can be found in Appendix L.

Calcium Stones

Conventional wisdom regarding calcium stones has been to limit foods high in calcium (milk, cheeses, yogurt, and green leafy vegetables) and sodium (2000 to 3000 mg/day). But research indicates that there is no need to restrict dietary calcium, and in fact a high-calcium diet appears to protect against calcium stone development (9). Kidney stone formation is more influenced by the amount of oxalate in the urinary tract, not calcium. Restricting calcium seems to allow more oxalate to be absorbed and then excreted through the urinary tract. Higher levels of dietary calcium bind with the oxalate so that it cannot be absorbed, leading to less oxalate in the urinary tract. Research also confirms that a high-protein diet contributes to stone formation, whereas potassium and fluid intake protect against stones forming. High sodium still appears to increase the potential risk for kidney stones (10,11).

Oxalate is found primarily in foods of plant origin and is the end product of ascorbic acid metabolism. Restriction of dietary oxalate intake has been used to reduce the risk of recurrence of calcium oxalate kidney stones. (See Appendix M for

CULTURAL CONSIDERATIONS
Cranberry Juice: A Folk Remedy That May Really Work

For years, cranberry juice has been touted as a means to prevent urinary tract infections (UTI), the theory being that drinking cranberry juice makes urine more acidic and consequently a less friendly environment for bacteria that cause UTIs. But research dating back to the 1920s has never proven this theory. Until now.

Recent research doesn't prove the more-acid-urine theory, but it does show that elderly women who were given 10 oz of cranberry juice cocktail each day had lower levels of bacteria in their urine than women consuming the same amount of a placebo beverage. However, the lower levels of bacteria were not the result of acidic urine. In fact, the cranberry juice drinker's urine was less acidic than the placebo drinker's. The new theory is that a compound in cranberry juice keeps the UTI-causing bacteria from clinging to the wall of the urinary tract where they multiply and cause symptoms. This reinforces an earlier study that identified a substance found only in cranberry and blueberry juice that seemed to interfere with bacteria's ability to adhere to tract cells.

These findings don't mean that people with urinary tract infections should forego seeking medical advice and drink cranberry juice instead. What they do mean is that further research should be conducted on younger women and women with recurring UTIs to determine the efficacy of cranberry juice. In addition, follow-up studies should be conducted to identify the active agent in cranberry juice.

And by the way, cranberry juice is a very bitter drink. The cranberry beverage sold in stores is cranberry juice *cocktail,* which is a mixture of cranberry juice, water, and sweetener. Regular cranberry juice cocktail provides approximately 150 kcalories per cup and low-kcalorie cranberry juice cocktail provides about 50 kcalories per cup.

From Avorn J et al: Reduction of bacteriuria and pyuria after ingestion of cranberry juice, *JAMA* 271:751-754, 1994; Fleet JC: New support for a folk remedy: Cranberry juice reduces bacteriuria and pyuria in elderly women, *Nutr Rev* 52:168-170, 1994; Ofek I et al: Anti-*Escherichia coli* adhesion activity of cranberry and blueberry juices, *N Eng J Med* 324:1599-1602, 1991; and On cranberry juice and urinary tract infections, *Tufts University diet and nutrition letter* 12:1, 1994.

Best Current Advice for Avoiding Kidney Stones

Do not restrict dietary calcium
Increase intake of fruits and vegetables (rich sources of potassium)
Keep meat intake at a moderate level
Increase intake of complex carbohydrates (whole-grains, fresh fruits and vegetables)
Limit foods high in oxalate
Drink plenty of water and other fluids (3 L/day)

From No need for kidney stone sufferers to curb calcium, *Environmental Nutrition*, 16:7, 1993.

---

a more complete list of oxalate content of foods.) Studies indicate that although oxalate-rich foods enhance excretion of urinary oxalate, the increase is not always proportional to the oxalate content of the food (2-4). Only eight foods—spinach, rhubarb, beets, nuts, chocolate, tea, wheat bran, and strawberries—caused a significant increase in urinary oxalate excretion. Therefore initial medical nutrition therapy for stone-forming individuals can be limited to the restriction of foods definitely shown to increase urinary oxalate (15). It may also be prudent to instruct patients that vitamin C supplements (≥1000 mg/day) should be avoided since they may increase urinary oxalate excretion.

WELLNESS AND DISEASES OF THE KIDNEYS

Physical Dimension	Functions of the kidneys affect total physical well-being; implementing medical nutrition therapy to aid treatment is essential.
Intellectual Dimension	Clients need to know (or be taught) anatomy and physiology to fully understand the dysfunction processes leading to kidney disorders.
Emotional Dimension	The chronic nature and potentially life-threatening aspects of kidney disorders may be emotionally devastating; clients may benefit from psychological counseling to deal with these illnesses.
Social Dimension	Significant others may become worn down by the responsibility of caring for loved ones with renal disorders; the ever present need for dialysis, once initiated, disrupts normal social relationships unless new ways of coping are established.

SUMMARY

The chief, life-preserving function of the kidneys is to maintain chemical homeostasis in the body. Various inflammatory, obstructive, and degenerative diseases affect the kidneys in different ways. These disorders interfere with the normal functioning of the nephrons to regulate products of body metabolism.

Because of glomerular damage, nephrotic syndrome results in increased urinary excretion of protein, decreased serum levels of albumin, hyperlipidemia, and edema. Although treated with corticosteroid or immunosuppressive medications, nephrotic syndrome may resist treatment and progress to chronic renal failure. The primary goals of medical nutrition therapy are to control hypertension, minimize edema, decrease urinary albumin losses, prevent protein malnutrition and muscle catabolism, supply adequate energy, and slow the progression of renal disease.

Acute renal failure is characterized by an abrupt loss of renal function that may or may not be accompanied by oliguria or anuria. The most common causes are trauma, hemorrhage, shock, nephrotoxic chemicals or drugs, septicemia, and streptococcal infection. Nutritional needs are determined by the underlying cause of the condition and whether dialysis is used for treatment. Patients may be hypermetabolic if the renal failure was caused by trauma, burns, septicemia, or infection.

Chronic renal failure (CRF) is the result of progressive, irreversible loss of kidney function. It can develop over days, months, or years and progress to end stage renal disease (ESRD). Regardless of the cause, the results are the same: retention of nitrogenous waste products and fluid and electrolyte imbalances affecting all body systems. Before ESRD, management focuses on slowing the progression of CRF and avoiding complications. Once CRF progresses to ESRD, management centers on reducing uremia by various treatment modalities: conservative management, hemodialysis, peritoneal dialysis, and renal transplantation.

Planning diets for CRF, ESRD, hemodialysis, and peritoneal dialysis patients requires calibrating intakes of energy, protein, lipids, phosphorus, potassium, sodium, vitamins and other minerals, and fluids. Often, the National Renal Diet is used to develop diet guidelines and meal plans. Individual diet prescriptions are based on residual kidney function, dialysate components, duration of dialysis, and rate of blood flow through the artificial kidney. Medical nutrition therapy objectives are to attain or maintain good nutritional status, prevent or minimize symptoms of uremic toxicity and fluid imbalance between treatments, and minimize the effects of metabolic disorders caused by ESRD, hemodialysis, and peritoneal dialysis. Nutritional care of renal transplant recipients involves continual reassessment of nutritional goals and efficacy of therapy during the different phases of care.

Renal calculi are a common, recurrent urologic condition. Most are composed of calcium, oxalate, or phosphorus, with a small proportion from cystine or uric acid.

Fluid intake has the most significant impact on reducing the risk of stone formation. Uric acid is a metabolic product of purines. Although limiting foods high in purines has not been proven effective, restriction of dietary protein may be effective. Kidney stone formation is more influenced by the amount of oxalate in the urinary tract than the amount of calcium. Oxalate is found primarily in plant foods and is the end product of ascorbic acid metabolism. Restriction of dietary oxalate intake is used to reduce the risk of recurrence of calcium oxalate kidney stones.

THE NURSING ROLE
Renal Calculi

Mrs. Tajian is a 55-year-old secretary who recently suffered an attack of severe flank pain that was found to be caused by renal calculi. The calculi were passed without surgical intervention, and Mrs. Tajian is now being treated with a preventive regimen since recurrence of stones occurs in the majority of cases. Based on a chemical analysis of the stones, which revealed calcium oxalate composition, the physician prescribed a low-calcium and low-oxalate diet. As the physician's office nurse, you are to teach Mrs. Tajian about her dietary restrictions. You develop the following teaching plan.

Objectives	Content	Strategy	Evaluation
Client will state the etiology of stone formation	Influence of diet, climate (heat leading to possible dehydration), genetics, sedentary occupation	Discuss factors with client, emphasizing which ones put her at high risk	Client will verbalize her risk factors
Client will identify dietary sources of calcium and oxalate	*Foods high in calcium:* dairy products, green leafy vegetables *Foods high in oxalate:* chocolate, coffee, tea, nuts, green leafy vegetables	Supply a list of foods to be reduced or eliminated in the diet, discuss list and client's usual dietary intake of these foods	Client will accurately list five or more foods that she must limit in her diet
Client will explain the importance of high fluid intake and physical exercise	Approximately 3000 cc (3 qts) of fluid should be ingested per day to ensure at least 2000 cc of urine output, more fluid may be needed in hot weather or during exercise, prolonged sitting should be avoided to prevent pooling of urine	Discussion of such factors that can help prevent future stones	When questioned, the client will correctly explain the importance of 3000 cc fluid intake and exercise
Client will express fears regarding diagnosis or uncertainties regarding diet	Any topic the client raises	Discussion with validation of feelings	Client will state that any anxiety has been addressed

K.D. is a 40-year-old female who works full time in an office and has a sedentary lifestyle. She is 5'6" tall, has a medium frame, and weighs 125 lb (dry weight). Her usual body weight is 132 lb. Her appetite has not been good for the past 3 months, but it is improving. She is on hemodialysis for 3 hours, three times per week. Her urine output is approximately 500 ml/24 hours.

Her predialysis labs include: BUN 57 mg/dL, Na 133 mEq/L, K^+ 4.7 mEq/L, PO_4 6.3 mg/dL, Ca 9.5 mg/dL, serum albumin 3.0 g/dL, and ferritin 7 ug/L. Her diet prescription is 2200 kcalories, 70 to 80 grams protein, 2000 mg Na, 2000 mg K, 1000 mg PO_4, and 1500 ml fluid.

K.D.'s diet history indicates that she doesn't like meat very much, but does like cheese and orange juice and will occasionally overindulge on these foods. She admits to having too much cheese and orange juice when she came in for her last dialysis. The patient is taking Nephro-Vites.

1. What is the purpose of hemodialysis?
2. How are metabolic waste products removed during dialysis?
3. Give two explanations why K.D.'s serum albumin levels are decreased?
4. Why is the serum ferritin often low in renal patients?
5. Why are high biological value proteins recommended for patients with renal disease?
6. Why are water-soluble vitamins supplements (Nephro-Vites) usually prescribed for patients with renal disease?

K.D. is considering trying a type of peritoneal dialysis so she won't have to go to the kidney dialysis center three times each week.

7. Explain to K.D. how peritoneal dialysis works.
8. What dietary changes might need to be made if K.D. switches to peritoneal dialysis?

Information courtesy of Kim Dittus, PhD, RD.

REFERENCES

1. Swearingen PL: *Manual of medical-surgical nursing care,* ed 3, St. Louis, 1994, Mosby.
2. American Dietetic Association: *A clinical guide to nutrition care in end-stage renal disease,* ed 2, Chicago, 1994, American Dietetic Association.
3. Nelson JK et al: *Mayo Clinic diet manual,* ed 7, St. Louis, 1994, Mosby.
4. American Dietetic Association: *Manual of clinical dietetics,* ed 4, Chicago, 1992, American Dietetic Association.
5. Weinsier RL, Morgan SL: *Fundamentals of clinical nutrition,* St. Louis, 1993, Mosby.
6. Escott-Stump S: *Nutrition and diagnosis-related care,* ed 3, Philadelphia, 1992, Lea and Febiger.
7. American Dietetic Association: *National renal diet: Professional guide,* Chicago, 1993, American Dietetic Association.
8. Popovich RP et al: Continuous peritoneal dialysis, *Ann Intern Med* 88:449-456, 1978.
9. Curhan GC et al: A prospective study of dietary calcium and other nutrients and the risk of symptomatic kidney stones, *N Eng J Med* 328:833-838, 1993.
10. Sakhaee K et al: The potential role of salt abuse on the risk for kidney stone formation, *J Urol* 150:310-312, 1993.
11. Burtis WJ et al: Dietary hypercalciuria in patients with calcium oxalate kidney stones, *Am J Clin Nutr* 60:424-429, 1994.
12. Brinkley L et al: Bioavailability of oxalate in foods, *J Urol* 17:534-538, 1981.
13. Brinkley LJ, Gregory J, Pak CYC: A further study of oxalate bioavailability in foods, *J Urol* 144:94-96, 1990.
14. Finch AM, Kasidas GP, Rose GA: Urine composition in normal subjects after oral ingestion of oxalate-rich foods, *Clin Sci* 60:411-418, 1981.
15. Massey LK, Roman-Smith H, Sutton RA: Effect of dietary calcium oxalate and calcium on urinary oxalate and risk of formation of calcium and oxalate kidney stones, *J Am Diet Assoc* 93:901-906, 1993.

Chapter 21

NUTRITION IN CANCER, AIDS, AND OTHER SPECIAL PROBLEMS

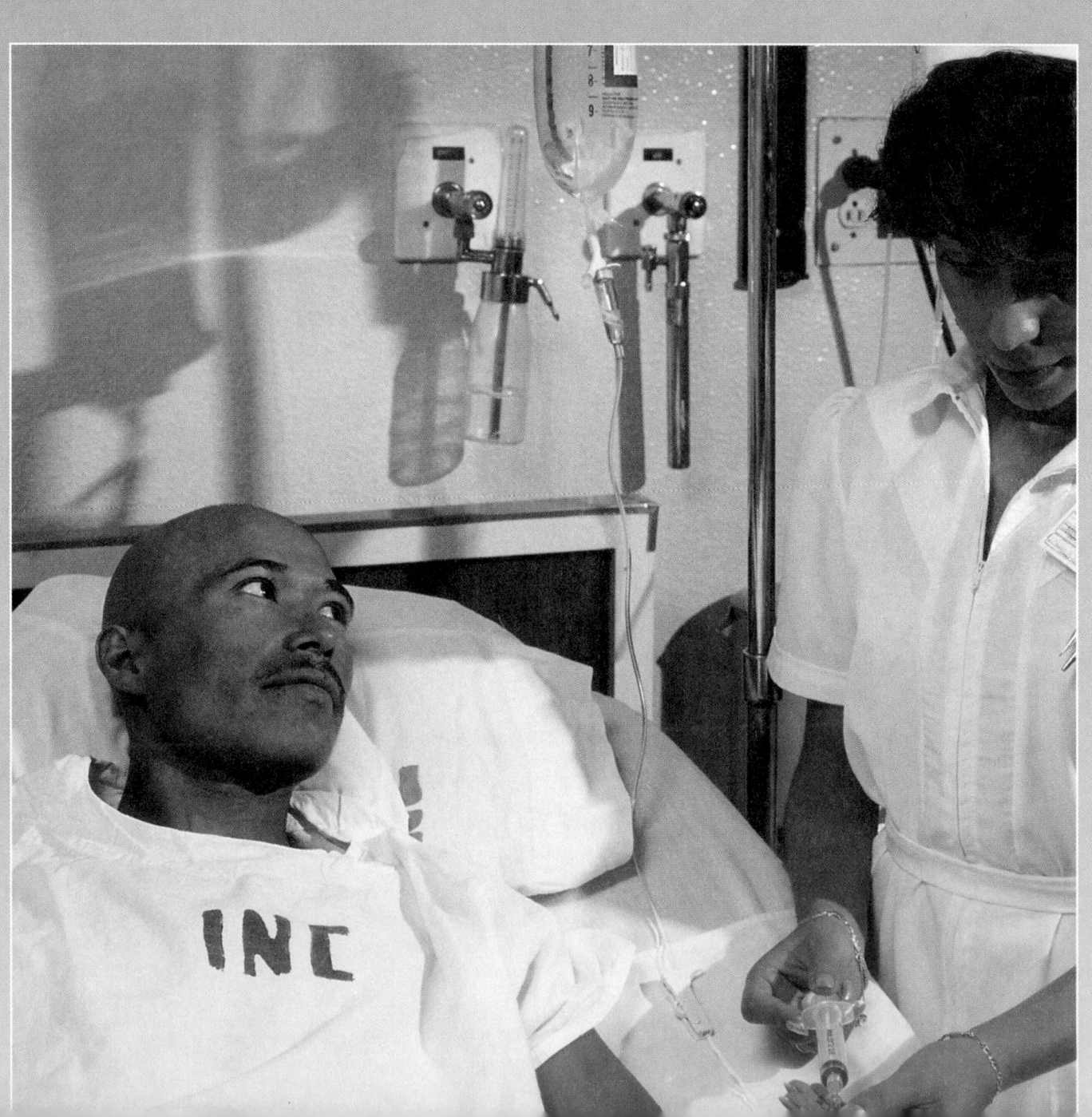

ROLE IN WELLNESS

The disorders of this chapter are characterized by wasting and malnutrition, largely because of the effect of the disease itself or the secondary consequences of treatment on the gastrointestinal tract. Consequently, the nutritional status of patients with cancer, acquired immune deficiency syndrome, and/or pulmonary disease is challenged by manifestations not only of the disease, but by the ramifications of treatment as well.

Most of the medical nutrition therapy prescribed focuses on reducing these effects and supporting patients through the potentially debilitating side-effects of treatment. Since these disorders are chronic, nursing care often continues after the patient leaves the hospital setting and returns home. The role of home health care nurses is crucial for providing not only medical care, but nutritional support and food consumption strategies as patients recover and/or become acclimated to their conditions (see box). Maintaining good nutritional status may improve survival rates, reduce treatment side effects, and increase the quality of life.

CANCER

Like all cells, **cancer** cells originate from preexisting cells. The process of carcinogenesis is thought to occur in two stages: initiation and promotion. During initiation, a *mutation* (spontaneous change) takes place in a normal cell and in turn forms a *neoplasm* (abnormal growth). Neoplasms are either *benign* or *malignant* in nature. During the promotion phase, neoplastic cells are activated (1). Although the exact causes of cancer are not fully known, initiators and promoters are believed to be environmental and lifestyle factors, which would indicate that most cancers are preventable (1,2).

Diet is considered to be one of the important environmental/lifestyle factors in the etiology and prevention of cancer in the United States. Although the contribution of diet to total incidence of and mortality from cancer cannot be specified, it is believed to be related to approximately one third of all cancer mortality (3). Whereas evidence of a diet/cancer connection does not establish a cause-and-effect relationship, epidemiological and laboratory animal research suggests that some specific dietary components may increase the risk of developing some types of cancer and other components may be protective (4) (see box). It is important to remember that no one food causes cancer, and no one food can prevent it. The National Cancer Institute and the American Cancer Society have issued the following guidelines for cancer prevention based on current available information:

- Eat a variety of foods
- Maintain a desirable body weight
- Eat a variety of both fruits and vegetables every day
- Eat more high-fiber foods such as whole-grain breads and cereals, legumes, vegetables, and fruits
- Reduce fat intake to $\leq$ 30% of total kcalories
- If you drink alcohol, use in moderation
- Limit consumption of salt-cured, smoked, and nitrite-preserved foods

You'll notice that these guidelines are consistent with good nutrition practices. The use of nutritional supplements is not recommended because most of the desired effects are assumed to be acquired through eating a variety of foods.

With over 100 variations, cancer is the second leading cause of death in the United States, following heart disease. Local or systemic effects of the cancer combined with **antineoplastic therapy** place the patient with cancer at increased risk of developing malnutrition or the wasting syndrome of *cancer cachexia* (5). Protein-

cancer
uncontrolled growth of cells that tend to invade surrounding tissue and metastasize to distant body sites

carcinogenesis
the process of cancer production

antineoplastic therapy
substance, procedure, or measure that prevents the proliferation of malignant cells; usually chemotherapy, radiation therapy, surgery, biologic response modifiers, bone marrow transplantation

Home Health Care: Expansion of Nursing Practice

Images of the old-fashioned visiting nurse come to mind when the topic of home health care comes up. In the past, visiting nurses working for charitable organizations bridged the gap for the poor who could not afford care in a hospital or clinic. Today, however, nurses from home health care agencies provide a wide range of specialized services in the homes of patients of all socioeconomic levels who have varying physical and psychological conditions. Several factors account for this change.

Hospitals, because of changes in medical reimbursements, are discharging patients more quickly than in the past. Patients arrive home while just beginning the process of recuperation; complications of their illness or surgery may not yet be evident. Chronic long-term illnesses may require consistent nursing care, but not require as intense a health care setting as a hospital. Pro-

viding health care services at home, even if daily, tends to be more cost effective than a prolonged hospital stay. As described in this chapter, recovery from cancer or an invasive AIDS-related disorder necessitates a well-devised home health care plan; patients and their significant others benefit from the education nurses provide in their homes. Nurses tailor medication schedules and medical nutrition therapy to the overall needs of the family. Reinforcing strategies of prescribed medical nutrition therapy while in the patient's kitchen provides a powerful teaching setting.

Home health care nurses are an important link between the other members of the health care team and the patient. The nurse's daily assessments and care plan records provide a wealth of information and document the patient's progress towards the goal of self-care.

HEALTH DEBATE
Fact or Fantasy? Food as Pharmaceuticals?

They're touted as being able to prevent cancer, heart disease, and depression. Some say they can even boost our immune system. There's some opinion that they can even slow down the aging process. They're the foods our mothers tried to make us eat when we were kids. They're *fruits* and *vegetables*.

What a surprise. Over the past 20 years, epidemiological researchers have consistently found that people who eat greater amounts of fruits and vegetables have lower rates of cancer. Fruits and vegetables contain hundreds of compounds such as antioxidants (beta-carotene and vitamins C and E), folic acid, fiber, and at least a dozen groups of chemicals that are not strictly nutrients called phytochemicals (specific chemicals found in plants, primar-

ily in fruits and vegetables). Some families of plants have more than others, but none of the phytochemicals are found in animal foods. The list below lists known phytochemicals, their action in the body, and common food sources.

Most health professionals believe that the whole plant is probably more important than the sum of its nutrients and chemical components. More benefits (some we don't even know yet) are derived from nutrients and phytochemicals by eating foods rather than swallowing supplements. Clients may question why they shouldn't just take specialized supplements of phytochemicals if we know their actions. What do you think? How will you explain your view to clients? Was Mom right? Should we all eat our vegetables?

PHYTOCHEMICAL	ACTION	FOOD SOURCE
Limonene	Speeds up enzyme production that may dispose of potential carcinogens	Citrus fruits
Allyl sulfides	Aids potential carcinogen excretion	Garlic, onions, leeks, chives
Allium compounds	May decrease tumor cell reproduction	Garlic, onions, leeks, chives
Dithiolthiones	May block damage to cell DNA by carcinogens	Broccoli

HEALTH DEBATE, cont'd.
Fact or Fantasy? Food as Pharmaceuticals?

PHYTOCHEMICAL	ACTION	FOOD SOURCE
Ellagic acid	Scavenges carcinogens, may prevent their altering cell's DNA	Grapes
Protease inhibitors	Suppresses enzyme production in cancer cells, slows tumor growth	Soybeans, dried beans
Phytosterols	Slows cell reproduction in large intestine, possibly prevents colon cancer	Soybeans, dried beans
Isoflavones	Blocks estrogen entry into cells, possibly reduces risk of breast or ovarian cancer	Soybeans, dried beans
Saponins	May prevent cancer cell multiplication	Soybeans, dried beans
Genistein	Inhibits cancer cell growth	Soybeans
Caffeic acid	May ease disposal of carcinogens from body	Fruits
Ferulic acid	May prevent nitrate conversion to carcinogenic nitrosamines, binds nitrates in stomach	Fruits
Indoles	Stimulates enzymes that make estrogen less effective, may reduce breast cancer risk	Cruciferous vegetables (bok choy, broccoli, Brussels sprouts, cabbage, cauliflower, collards, kale, kohl-rabi, mustard greens, rutabaga, turnip greens, turnips
Isothiocyanates	May block carcinogen damage to a cell's DNA	Cruciferous vegetables

From Meisler JG: Soy: The bean most likely to succeed in fending off cancer, heart disease, *Environmental Nutrition*, 17(5):1, 4, 1994; Schardt D: Phytochemicals: Plants against cancer, *Nutrition Action Health Letter*, 21(3):1, 9-11, 1994; and To take antioxidant pills or not? The debate heats up, *Tufts University diet and nutrition letter*, 12(3):3-6, 1994.

energy malnutrition (PEM) is the single most common problem in patients with cancer (6). The presence of malnutrition adversely affects tissue function and repair and immunocompetence, leading to a poor prognosis for recovery. Furthermore, patients who are malnourished do not tolerate treatment as well, and each form of cancer treatment is associated with adverse nutritional consequences (5,7,8). A vicious cycle is propagated: malnutrition caused by treatment in patients already debilitated as a result of disease process.

Nutritional Effects of Cancer Therapy
Chemotherapy
The activities of chemotherapeutic agents are not specific only to cancer cells. Normal or noncancerous host cells are frequently common targets of chemotherapy side effects (6,9). The severity and manifestation of the side effects depend on the particular chemotherapy agent, dosage, duration of treatment, rates of metabolism, accompanying drugs, and individual susceptibility (5,6,9). Chemotherapy agents include alkylating drugs, antibiotics, antimetabolites, hormones, enzymes, plant alkaloids, and biological response modifiers. These agents act by inhibiting one or more steps of DNA synthesis in rapidly proliferating cells; bone marrow

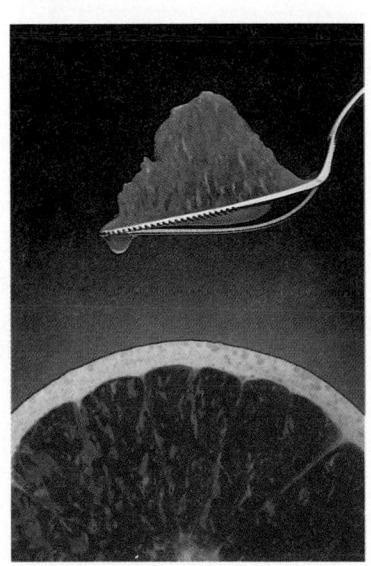

Dietary fiber may play a role in preventing cancer.

mucositis
inflammation of mucous membranes

stomatitis
inflammation of mucous membranes of the mouth

fractionation
administration of radiation in smaller doses over time rather than in a single large dose; minimizes tissue damage

and cells lining the gastrointestinal tract tend to be susceptible to damage as well (5,6,9). This damage can lead to malnutrition through a variety of mechanisms: anorexia, nausea, vomiting, **mucositis**, **stomatitis**, organ injury (toxicity), and learned food aversions (6). Nutritional implications of chemotherapeutic agents are summarized in Table 21-1.

Radiation therapy

Radiation is used to treat tumors sensitive to radiation exposure or tumors that cannot be surgically resected. Nutritional problems vary according to the region or area of the body radiated, dose, **fractionation**, and whether radiation is being used as combination therapy with surgery or chemotherapy (6). Complications may develop just during radiation treatment or become chronic and progress even after treatment is completed (6). As with chemotherapy, radiation therapy damages rapidly replicating normal host cells along with cancerous cells.

Primary radiation sites affected are the head and neck, the abdomen and pelvis (gastrointestinal tract), and the central nervous system (5). All three radiation sites may cause anorexia, nausea, and vomiting. In the head and neck, these common effects create problems of food ingestion as stomatitis, esophageal mucositis, loss of taste sensation, and dry mouth may also occur. Side effects to the abdomen and pelvis alter the gastrointestinal tract, reducing digestion and absorption of nutrients because of diarrhea and steatorrhea, malabsorption, ulceration, and bowel damage or obstruction.

Table 21-1   Nutritional Implications of Chemotherapeutic Agents

Drug Classification	Selected Examples	Actions	Nutritional Implications
Alkylating agents	Cisplatin Hexamethylmelamine Dacarbazine	React with susceptible DNA sites	Anorexia, nausea, vomiting, mucositis/stomatitis
Antibiotics	Bleomycin Doxorubicin Dactinomycin	Bind to DNA and inhibit cell division, interfere with RNA transcription	Anorexia, nausea, mucositis/stomatitis, diarrhea; some may cause decreased calcium and iron absorption
Antimetabolites	Methotrexate 5-Fluorodeoxyuridine 5-Fluorouracil	Inhibit a stage of DNA synthesis	Anorexia, nausea, vomiting, diarrhea, mucositis, abdominal pain, intestinal ulceration; some may cause decreased absorption of vitamin B_{12}, fat, and xylose
Hormones	Prednisone Tamoxifen Diethylstilbestrol	Alter cell metabolism to cause unfavorable tumor growth	*Corticosteroids:* sodium and fluid retention, hyperglycemia, gastrointestinal upset, osteoporosis (calcium losses), negative nitrogen balance *Estrogens:* nausea, vomiting, anorexia, hypercalcemia
Enzymes	Asparaginase	Delay DNA and RNA synthesis by inhibiting protein synthesis (deprive cells of asparagine)	Anorexia, nausea, hyperglycemia, pancreatitis, azotemia (uremia), weight loss
Plant alkaloids	Vinblastine Vincristine	Inhibits mitosis	Nausea, vomiting, constipation, diarrhea, abdominal pain
Biologic response modifiers	Interferon Interleukin	Modify host biologic response to tumor	Nausea, vomiting, anorexia, weight change (increase or decrease)

From Charuhas PM: Dietary management during antitumor therapy of cancer patients, *Topics in Clinical Nutrition*, 9:42-53, 1993; and Shils ME: Nutrition and diet in cancer management. In Shils ME, Olson JA, Shike M, eds: *Modern nutrition in health and disease*, ed 8, Philadelphia, 1994, Lea and Febiger.

Table 21-2   Nutrition Side Effects of Cancer Surgery

Site of Surgery	Side Effect
Head and neck	Impaired chewing and swallowing
Esophagectomy	Diarrhea, steatorrhea, esophageal stenosis
Vagotomy	Gastric stasis, diarrhea, fat malabsorption
Gastrectomy	Dumping syndrome; hypoglycemia; malabsorption; possible deficiencies of iron, calcium, vitamin B_{12}, and fat-soluble vitamins
Pancreatectomy	Insulin-dependent diabetes mellitus (IDDM); possible malabsorption of fats, protein, fat-soluble vitamins, minerals
Small bowel resection	Possible malabsorption of many nutrients; depends on extent and site of surgery
Ileostomy	Sodium and water losses, vitamin B_{12} malabsorption, fat malabsorption, bile salt diarrhea

From Charuhas PM: Dietary management during antitumor therapy of cancer patients, *Topics in Clinical Nutrition* 9:42-53, 1993.

Surgery

Surgery is the preferred treatment for solid tumors and tumors in the gastrointestinal tract (9). Radical resections of any portion of the gastrointestinal tract often cause alterations in nutrition intake and may lead to significant nutritional problems (5,6). Although some of the changes are temporary, many patients endure permanent complications (6). Malabsorption tends to be the primary nutritional problem with surgery; yet unless small bowel resection is extensive, the adaptability of the small intestine may prevent major clinical problems from occurring (6). Pancreatic enzymes, histamine H_2 receptor blockers, and insulin ease the nutritional problems associated with pancreatectomy. To ensure adequate energy intake, traditional dietary modifications for diabetes may not be necessary (6).

Any problems associated with surgery (Table 21-2) will be further complicated if the patient receives subsequent radiation and chemotherapy (5).

Bone marrow transplantation

Bone marrow transplantation (BMT) is used to treat certain hematologic malignancies (acute and chronic leukemia and some forms of lymphoma) and, more recently, solid tumors such as in breast cancer (5,6). Before the transplant, patients receive several days of high-dose chemotherapy and possible total body irradiation to eradicate the cancer (6). The development of protein-energy malnutrition is almost inevitable because of the nutrition sequelae associated with these treatments (6). Glutamine-supplemented parenteral nutrition improves nitrogen balance, shortens the length of hospital stays, and lowers the incidence of positive microbial cultures and clinical infections in BMT patients (10).

BMT also impairs immune function and leaves patients susceptible to bacterial and fungal pathogens found in fresh fruits and vegetables that are ordinarily no hazard to healthy persons; therefore a low-bacteria diet is indicated whenever the neutrophil (white blood cell) count is less than 0.5×10^9 per liter (6). A low-bacteria diet requires restrictions to avoid undercooked meats and eggs, raw vegetables (including salads and garnishes), and all fresh fruits. Frequent monitoring of nutritional intake and encouragement to take in adequate amounts of energy and protein are essential in the care of these patients (6).

Although it is not recommended that food be brought in by family members or others while the patient is experiencing **neutropenia,** the physician may approve food from outside the hospital when the patient has been engrafted and oral intake remains inadequate (6). The low-bacteria diet is used from the time the patient is

To destroy tap-water contaminants that may cause illness, the Centers for Disease Control and Prevention recommends boiling tap water before consumption by individuals with weakened immune systems. Immune system functioning may be diminished because of the effects of HIV/AIDS, chemotherapy drugs, and immunosuppressive drugs (to prevent organ-transplant rejection).

neutropenia
abnormally low levels of circulating white blood cells (neutrophils) that remove bacteria

admitted until discharge. The patient may eat carefully washed fruits and vegetables if the neutrophil (white blood cell) count is greater than 0.5×10^9 per liter (6).

A major complication that may occur with BMT is graft versus host disease (GVHD), which is best described as *reverse rejection*. The grafted tissue or organ recognizes the host's cells as foreign. GVHD may involve multiple organ damage, but the skin, gastrointestinal tract, and liver are particularly involved. Dietary management of gastrointestinal GVHD is documented elsewhere (6).

It may take patients up to 1 year to regain lost weight after BMT. Common problems influencing oral intake include sore mouth (stomatitis), taste changes, xerostomia, and anorexia. Patients should be encouraged to eat whatever is tolerated, including nutritional supplements. Weight should be monitored monthly, and patients should be referred to a dietitian in the event of inappropriate weight loss and/or eating problems (6).

Medical Nutrition Therapy

As with any other disease, nutrition support of cancer patients must be individualized. Staff and patients alike should realize that nutrition is an essential component of the total management of the disease. Prognosis should be considered to appropriately adjust the aggressiveness of the nutritional intervention (supportive, adjunctive, definitive) (6). As previously mentioned, nutritional problems arise as a result of the cancer itself and the treatment method. One of the most important medical interventions to increase nutrient intake is pain control (11); reducing pain discomfort improves the success of nutrition intervention. Nutritional interventions include the following (6):

1. Obtain diet history. Determine past weight changes, food preferences and eating habits, use of food/nutritional supplements, present kcalorie and protein intake, food intolerances, taste abnormalities, distribution of meals throughout the day, who does the cooking, and whether the patient eats alone. Consider nutritional side effects from past or current treatment (chemotherapy, radiation, surgery).
2. Monitor kcalorie and protein intake daily and adjust according to individual patient response.
3. Prevent further weight loss. Megestrol acetate (Megace) is a hormone (progestin) used to decrease gastrointestinal distress and stimulate appetite.
4. For nausea, use antiemetic drugs 30 to 60 minutes before meals.
5. For pain, use analgesics 30 to 60 minutes before meals.
6. Assess meals patterns and snacks. Previous dietary restrictions (for example, cholesterol, fat, and total kcalories) may need to be liberalized. Patients may hesitate to eat between meals or eat high-kcalorie foods. Inform patients and significant others that this is no longer necessary.
7. Consider patient's strength and ability to prepare food. Suggestions for easily obtainable food may be appropriate if patient is alone during the day.
8. Give patients and significant others written nutrition guidelines. Although encouragement to eat recommended foods is important, advise significant others not to place excessive pressure on the patient to eat as this may become counterproductive.
9. Encourage patients to eat food whenever possible, but sometimes nutritional supplements (high-kcalorie, high-protein liquid feedings) are necessary.
10. Multiple vitamin/mineral supplements are required for patients unable to ingest well-balanced meals or who have specific nutrient deficiencies.

Table 21-3 lists recommendations for specific nutrition-related problems. The most commonly encountered nutrition-related problems in cancer patients are loss of appetite and early satiety, diarrhea, nausea and vomiting, chewing and swallowing difficulties, constipation, abdominal gas and bloating, dry mouth, and taste or smell alterations.

Table 21-3 Nutritional Approaches to Nutrition-Related Problems in Cancer and Cancer Therapy	
Problem	**Recommendations**
Loss of appetite/early satiety	Eat frequent small meals, increase kcal/protein content of foods, use high-protein/high-kcalorie supplements, serve foods cool or at room temperature, avoid excess fat, exercise regularly if tolerated, limit liquids at meal time; appetite may be best in the morning
Diarrhea*	Eat frequent small meals, serve foods cool or at room temperature, increase fluid intake, eat and drink slowly, decrease fiber intake, avoid excess fat, avoid gas-forming foods, limit liquids at meal time, avoid highly seasoned foods, limit beverages containing caffeine and alcohol; trial avoidance of lactose may be helpful; take antidiarrheal medication per MD
Nausea and vomiting	Eat frequent small meals, avoid strong odors, serve foods cool or room temperature, increase fluid intake, eat and drink slowly, avoid excess fat, limit liquids at meal time, avoid highly seasoned foods, rest after meals with head elevated, take antiemetic per MD
Chewing and swallowing difficulties	Eat frequent small meals; increase kcal/protein content of foods; use high-protein/high-kcal supplements; serve food cool or at room temperature; increase fluid intake; eat and drink slowly; add sauces and gravy to soften and moisten foods; avoid highly seasoned foods; avoid alcohol, tobacco, and commercial mouthwashes; coarse-textured and acidic foods may irritate
Constipation	Increase fluid intake, increase fiber intake, exercise regularly if tolerated; stool softener and/or laxative may be necessary
Abdominal gas	Eat and drink slowly, decrease fiber intake, avoid excess fat, avoid gas-forming foods, exercise regularly if tolerated, limit lactose if not tolerated
Dry mouth	Increase fluid intake; add sauces and gravy to soften and moisten foods; tart foods or sugar-free hard candy may be used to stimulate saliva; avoid alcohol, tobacco, and commercial mouthwash
Taste/smell alterations	Serve food cool or at room temperature, increase fluid intake, use seasonings to enhance flavors, avoid cooking odors, try alternative protein sources for meat aversion

From Nelson JK et al: *Mayo Clinic diet manual*, ed 7, St. Louis, 1994, Mosby.
*Diarrhea secondary to malabsorption, dumping syndrome, or other causes may require different treatment modalities.

ACQUIRED IMMUNODEFICIENCY SYNDROME (AIDS)

Acquired immunodeficiency syndrome is a life-threatening disease that surfaced in the United States in the early 1980s. It is caused by the **retrovirus** human immunodeficiency virus (HIV), which attacks **T cells** and **monocytes/macrophages** and results in severe depression of immune functions. HIV is transmitted through sexual contact that involves exchange of body fluids, contaminated blood or blood products, or sharing needles with IV drug users. The hallmark of AIDS is the breakdown of the immune system that is manifested by neoplasms, opportunistic infections, and/or enteropathy (Table 21-4). These disorders also negatively affect the overall health and nutritional status of those infected.

Because of these complications, malnutrition is a common problem of HIV infection and plays an important role in the morbidity and mortality of the disease (12). Occurring in 80% or more of people with HIV/AIDS, the development of malnutrition is multifactorial, ranging from decreased nutrient (food) intake, malabsorption, and altered metabolism (12-15). Decreased nutrient intake occurs because of physical symptoms, psychosocial determinants, and economic considerations. Physical symptoms include anorexia, nausea, vomiting, and diarrhea. Psychosocial determinants encompass depression, dementia, food beliefs, or restrictive regimens that may alter appetite and limit the variety of foods viewed as selectable. Economic considerations may limit access to food availability. Malabsorption among individuals with HIV/AIDS occurs because of infections damaging the gastrointestinal tract or causing surface area blockage. Digestive changes such as pancreatic and/or enterocyte dysfunction further reduce absorption of nutrients. Altered metabolism, caused by infection, fever, and changes in organ function,

retrovirus
an RNA virus that becomes integrated into the DNA of a host cell during replication; HIV is a retrovirus

T cells
a small circulating lymphocyte produced in the bone marrow that mediates cellular immune responses

monocytes
white blood cells (large leukocytes)

macrophages
cells that are able to surround, engulf, and digest microorganisms and cellular debris

Table 21-4 Clinical and Nutritional Complications of AIDS

	Manifestation	Clinical/Nutrition Complications
Neoplasms	Kaposi's sarcoma (KS)	Oral and esophageal lesions, lesions along small and large intestine, diarrhea and malabsorption
Opportunistic infections	**Fungi**	
	Candida albicans	Thrush, stomatitis, esophagitis, pneumonia
	Cryptococcus neoformans	Meningitis, pneumonitis
	Aspergillus	Fungemia, pneumonia
	Coccidioides immitis	Pneumonitis
	Histoplasma capsulatum	Pneumonitis, skin lesions
	Viruses	
	Cytomegalovirus (CMV)	Esophagitis, pneumonitis, diarrhea
	Herpes simplex	Ulcerative lesions of the mucous membranes, stomatitis, esophagitis, pneumonia
	Epstein-Barr (EBV)	EBV-positive non-Hodgkin's lymphomas, oral hairy leukoplakia
	Hepatitis B	Nausea, vomiting, fever, antigenemia
	Herpes zoster	Multiple dermatomal zoster
	Papilomavirus	Oral hairy leukoplakia
	Bacteria	
	Mycobacterium avium-intracellulare	Tuberculosis, diarrhea, other mycobacteria
	Legionella	Pneumonia
	Salmonella	Diarrhea, bacteremia
	Listeria monocytogenes	Meningitis, bacteremia
	Brucella	Fever, anorexia, pneumonia, meningitis
	Shigella	Diarrhea, bacteremia
	Campylobacter	Diarrhea, bacteremia
	Staphylococcus aureus	Pneumonia
	Streptococcus pneumoniae	Pneumonia
	Haemophilus influenzae	Pneumonia
	Protozoa/parasites	
	Pneumocystis carinii (PCP)	Pneumonia
	Toxoplasma gondii	
	Cryptosporidium	Focal encephalitis, pneumonia
	Isospora belli	Malabsorption, diarrhea
	Microspora	Diarrhea
	Entamoeba histolytica	Malabsorption, diarrhea
	Entamoeba coli	Diarrhea
	Giardia lamblia	Diarrhea
	Acanthamoeba	Diarrhea
		Meningoencephalitis
Direct HIV infection	Enteropathy	Malabsorption, diarrhea

From Collins CL: Nutrition care in AIDS, *Dietetic Currents* 15:11-16, 1988; Resler SS: Nutrition care of AIDS patients, *J Am Diet Assoc* 88:828-832, 1988; Gold JWM: HIV-1 infection: Diagnosis and management, *Med Clin North Am* 76:1-10, 1992; Bernard EM et al: Pneumocystosis, *Med Clin North Am* 76:107-119, 1992; and Ralten DJ: Nutrition and HIV infection: A review and evaluation of the extent knowledge of the relationship between nutrition and HIV infection, *Nutrition in Clinical Practice* 6:1S, 1991.

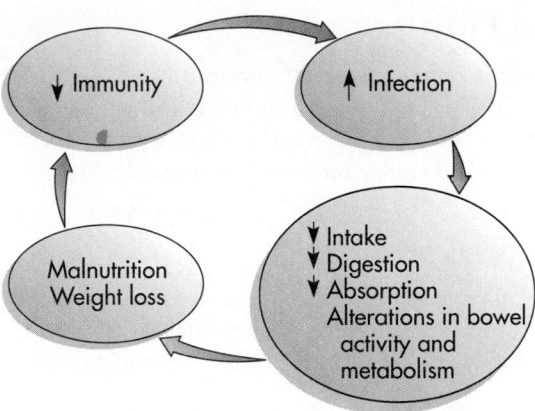

Fig. 21-1 Vicious cycle of malnutrition and AIDS.

Table 21-5   Nutritional Warning Signs in HIV/AIDS Patients

Warning Sign	Parameters	Possible Causes
Rapid weight loss	Any unintentional weight loss, 20-lb weight loss over 6 months	Decreased nutrient intake, decreased absorption or malabsorption, increased nutrient needs
Gastrointestinal problems	Losses of fluids and nutrients through vomiting and diarrhea	Oral/intestinal infection or malignancies, medication interactions, malnutrition, malabsorption
Inadequate intake	Decreased intake of energy: protein, fat, carbohydrates	Anorexia, dysphagia, fear of diarrhea or pain, drug-nutrient interaction
Increased nutrient needs	Increase in established energy/protein requirements	Hypermetabolism during infection
Food aversions	Diarrhea with specific foods Nausea/vomiting	Lactose/fat intolerance Alterations in taste/smell
Fad diets/supplements	Use of fad diets Self-prescription of diet supplements	Nutrient inadequacy Nutrient-nutrient competition

From Cameron AM, ed: Nutrition in HIV/AIDS, *Dietetic Currents* 21:11-16, 1994.

results in a state of hypermetabolism that requires elevated levels of nutrients for individuals already struggling with meeting basic nutrient requirements.

The malnutrition and wasting in patients with HIV creates a vicious cycle (Fig. 21-1) that can be fatal (16). Decreased immunity increases the development of infections, which then lowers nutrient intake, digestion, and absorption, further affecting bowel functions and metabolism. These factors combine to cause malnutrition and weight loss, which continue the decreased immune functions of the physiological systems. In particular, the weight loss appears to be particularly prognostic of negative clinical outcomes (17).

Assessment of Nutritional Status

To help identify HIV/AIDS patients who are at risk for malnutrition and wasting, nurses can be familiar with factors that determine nutritional status in this population. All patients in this population undergo standard nutritional assessment (18,19). It is important to remember that, as mentioned in Chapter 14, no one nutrition assessment parameter stands alone as an assessment tool. Parameters are evaluated to determine a patient's nutritional profile and appropriateness of interventions to support nutritional status (18,20).

Awareness of the following *warning signs* that are detrimental to nutritional status provides nurses with potential factors to discuss with patients (13) (Table 21-5).

Rapid weight loss

Rapid weight loss is defined as any unintentional weight loss or a 20-lb weight loss over 6 months. This type of weight loss may indicate decreased nutrient intake or alterations with the body's ability to absorb nutrients. The nutrient needs of the individual may have significantly increased because of infection-induced hypermetabolism.

Gastrointestinal problems

Gastrointestinal problems may lead to extensive loss of fluids and nutrients through vomiting and diarrhea. These losses may be caused by oral/intestinal infections or malignancies, medical interaction, or malnutiriton.

Inadequate intake

Decreased intake of energy (protein, fat, or carbohydrates) may not provide sufficient nutrients. Anorexia, dysphagia, or a drug-nutrient interaction may cause the reduced-energy intake. A patient may also be fearful of developing diarrhea or pain from eating and may knowingly restrict food intake.

Increased nutrient needs

Because of hypermetabolism during infections, an increase in established energy/protein requirements may be warranted.

Food aversions

Based on past experiences when eating specific foods that caused diarrhea or nausea and vomiting, patients may develop food aversions. This may decrease the overall intake of important nutrients. The actual cause of the physical reaction may be lactose or fat intolerance or alterations in taste and smell sensations.

Fad diets/supplements

The use of fad diets may lead to nutrient inadequacy if the fad diet does not provide sufficient quantities of nutrients, particularly important when the body is defending itself against the invasive infections common to AIDS. Self-prescribed supplements may be problematic by providing an imbalance of nutrients that may lead to nutrients being in competition with each other for absorption sites.

Medical Nutrition Therapy

Medical nutrition therapy is as important as drug therapy in the management of HIV disease. It may extend and improve the quality of life of people with HIV/AIDS, and improve efficacy of other medical therapies by maintaining lean body mass stores. Nutrition therapy should be considered as an integral part of the care planning process and not as an alternative or adjunctive therapy (20).

Goals of medical nutrition therapy need to be realistic and individualized for each patient. The bases of interventions are nutritional status, causes of malnutrition, complications that impact nutritional status, and feasibility of rehabilitation (14,15). The overall goals of nutrition management are as follows (13,15):
- Preserve lean body mass and gut function
- Prevent development of malnutrition
- Provide adequate levels of all nutrients to maintain daily physical and mental functioning
- Minimize symptoms of malabsorption
- Present nutrition-related immune suppression
- Improve sense of well-being and quality of life

TEACHING TOOL
Maximizing Food Intake in HIV/AIDS

Clients dealing with the chronic effects of HIV/AIDS may have difficulty consuming enough to meet physiological requirements. Home health care nurses can teach the following strategies that increase kcalories and protein without necessarily expanding the volume of food.

- Substitute kcalorie-containing and nutrient-dense foods and beverages for low or no-kcal foods and beverages (milk or shakes instead of coffee or tea; regular soft drinks for sugar-free drinks)
- Increase the number and/or size of feedings daily (Offer 5 to 6 small meals/snacks)
- Fortify foods with kcalories and protein-containing ingredients (add skim milk powder to milk, shakes, gravies, hot cereals)
- Use kcalorie-containing condiments (add butter/margarine to hot cereals, vegetables, starches)
- Modify diet according to tolerances (cold or room temperature foods, bland or salty foods; avoid greasy and sweet foods, liquids between meals)
- Add kcalorie-containing supplements as needed (commercial nutritional supplements)

From Newman CF: The role of nutritional supplements and nutritional plans in the management of HIV/AIDS: An overview of the PAAC Nutrition Initiative, *Nutrition and HIV//AIDS* 1:57-106, 1992.

Fluid, energy, protein, and vitamin/mineral requirements are based on nutritional evaluation and assessment. Depending on the clinical profile, a patient may require anywhere from 25 to 60 kcalories per kilogram of weight (15). Protein needs should be approximately 20% of total kcalories (15). Patients are monitored on a daily basis to evaluate the efficacy of the prescribed diet. Nutritional supplements are encouraged when additional energy and nutrients are needed. See the Teaching Tool for ideas to help patients increase energy and nutrients in their diets.

Fluid loss because of malabsorption and diarrhea may be considerable. Urine and/or diarrheal losses may be as high as 2 to 4 liters per day. Sources and volume of losses are considered when providing fluids to patients. Medications to minimize symptoms and IV fluids to maintain fluid and electrolyte balance may be necessary (14). Determining the cause of the diarrhea and/or fluid loss makes treatment more effective (15).

The use of enteral and parenteral nutrition is not regarded as a last-ditch effort but rather as a maintenance therapy or as a means to prevent nutritional problems (15). Many enteral products available are tailored to the requirements of HIV/AIDS patients. Patient preferences, cost, availability, and nutritional requirements are determining factors in selecting enteral products and their route of delivery. Parenteral nutrition is appropriate in patients who have severe underlying malabsorptive disorders. As in any patient under consideration for nutrition support, patient quality of life and preservation of gut function are considered. The risk of infection that accompanies parenteral nutrition in an immunosupressed patient is another important factor. Some suggest the use of combination therapy: high-kcalorie oral nutrition supplements during waking hours and cyclic parenteral nutrition while sleeping (15).

The malnutrition and wasting in HIV/AIDS patients may be slowed at times and possibly reversed or delayed. It requires a multidisciplinary approach, including collaboration between the nurse and an HIV-specialist dietitian. Early recognition and intervention for nutritional risk factors and indicators are the keys to successful nutrition support and related medical therapies (15). Probably the most important factor in care of HIV/AIDS patients is the provision of supportive and nonjudgmental care in clinical and home health care settings (14).

Because no cure for AIDS is known, patients with this disease are potential victims for unproven or fraudulent health and nutrition therapies. These alternative or unconventional therapies may not only be extremely costly, but may interfere with traditional medical methods, putting the patient at even more risk. Patients with AIDS may adopt macrobiotic diets or ingest supplements of lecithin mixtures, glandulars (desiccated glands such as pancreas, liver, thyroid), or megavitamins. The macrobiotic diet is a strict vegetarian diet that is very low in kcalories and high in fiber. It is deficient in niacin, riboflavin, vitamin B_{12}, and vitamin D and may be low in bioavailable iron, calcium, zinc, and protein.

Research on the efficacy of vitamin/mineral megadoses is still inconclusive. Alternative health and nutrition practices should be evaluated for harmful effects. If dangerous, they should be discouraged. If the practice is not harmful, however, a placebo effect may be beneficial for the patient's mental and physical well-being. Following is a list of contacts where persons can get advice or report questionable practices or products:

False advertising	FTC Bureau of Consumer Protection; regional FTC office; Chief Postal Inspector, US Postal Service; editor or station manager of media outlet where ad appeared
Product marketed with false or misleading claims	Regional FDA office, state attorney general, state health department, local Better Business Bureau, Congressional representative
Bogus mail-order promotion	Chief Postal Inspector, US Postal Service; editor or station manager of media outlet where ad appeared
Improper treatment by licensed practitioner	Local or state professional society, local hospital (if practitioner is a staff member), state licensing board
Improper treatment by unlicensed individual	Local district attorney, state attorney general
Advice needed about questionable product or service	National Council Against Health Fraud (PO Box 1276, Loma Linda, CA 92340); Consumer Health Information Research Institute; local, state, or national professional or voluntary health groups

From Nelson JK et al: *Mayo Clinic diet manual,* ed 7, St. Louis, 1994, Mosby; Resler SS: Nutrition care of AIDS patients, *J Am Diet Assoc* 88:828-832, 1988; and Collins CL: Nutrition care in AIDS, *Dietetic Currents,* 15:11-16, 1988.

---

chronic obstructive pulmonary disease (COPD)
a progressive and irreversible condition identified by obstruction of air flow; chronic bronchitis, asthma, and emphysema (also called chronic obstructive lung disease)

respiratory distress syndrome
a respiratory disorder identified by insufficient respiration and abnormally low levels of circulating oxygen in the blood

acute respiratory failure
sudden absence of respirations, with confusion or unresponsiveness caused by obstructed air flow or failure of the pulmonary gas exchange mechanism

OTHER SPECIAL PROBLEMS

Disorders of the pulmonary system are classified into two categories. One category is disorders that result in chronic long-term changes in respiratory function such as **chronic obstructive pulmonary disease (COPD).** COPD is a collective phrase for chronic bronchitis, asthma, and emphysema and is the second leading cause of disability in the United States (18,21). The goal of medical nutrition therapy is to maintain respiratory muscle strength and function. The second category is disorders that cause acute changes in respiratory function such as **respiratory distress syndrome (RDS)** and **acute respiratory failure (ARF).** Patients who are critically ill, in shock, severely injured, or who have sepsis can develop these disorders (22). For ARF and RDS, the function of medical nutrition therapy is to inhibit tissue destruction by providing the extra nutrients required for hypermetabolic conditions.

Similar to cancer and HIV/AIDS, as these pulmonary disorders progress nutritional status tends to decline and malnutrition exacerbates declining respiratory muscle function and ventilatory drive. In addition, the specific energy nutrient content (fat versus carbohydrate versus protein) of a patient's diet has the ability to influence ventilation and gas exchange (23).

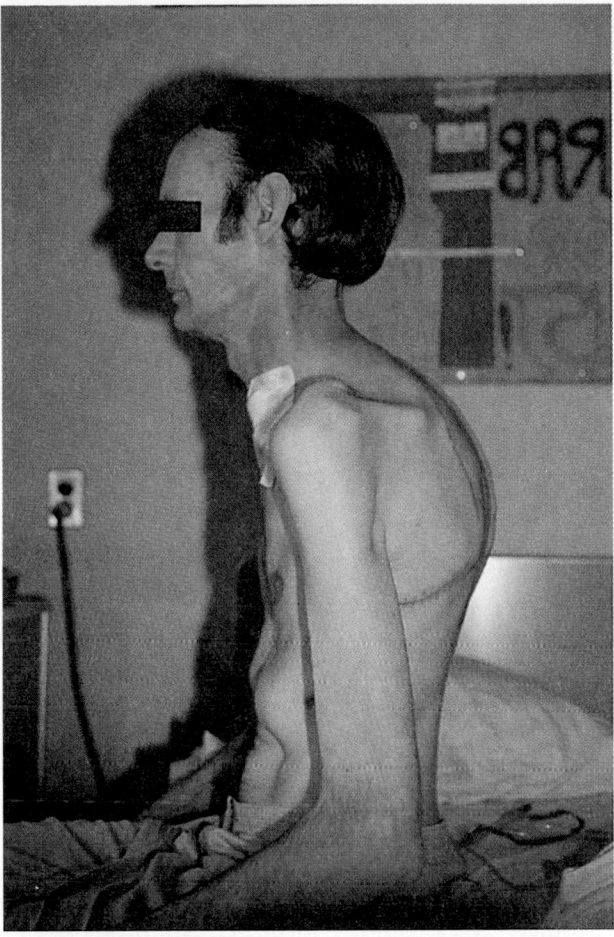

Fig. 21-2 Patient with chronic obstructive pulmonary disease.

Chronic Obstructive Pulmonary Disease

The energy required for breathing is something most of us often take for granted. Energy needs, however, become quite evident in patients with respiratory problems. Because of their weakened respiratory system, patients with COPD expend a great deal of energy just breathing; therefore they have an increased likelihood of malnutrition. It is common to see weight loss and loss of fat reserves and muscle mass, including the diaphragm and other respiratory muscles (Fig. 21-2) (23). The more severe the COPD, the greater the associated malnutrition and weight loss; the more weight that is lost, the greater the loss of respiratory muscles and diaphragm (1,23). Assessment of the patient's nutritional status is an important consideration in the management of COPD (1).

Medical nutrition therapy

Of major importance is providing adequate nutrition to counter the nutritional manifestations produced by COPD. Sufficient energy and protein is necessary to maintain the integrity of the immune system. Patients may require a range of 25 to 45 kcal/kg depending on whether they require maintenance kcalories or repletion (< 90% ideal body weight) kcalories. Adequate protein stimulates the ventilatory drive (1). Patients may require 1.2 to 1.9 gm protein/kg for maintenance and 1.6 to 2.5 gm/kg for repletion (24).

Providing nutrients in the proper mixture is also important to reduce production of carbon dioxide and maintain respiratory function (1). The **respiratory quotient (RQ)** indicates that carbohydrate metabolism produces the greatest amount

respiratory quotient (RQ) ratio of CO_2 exhaled to O_2 inhaled; depending on the net metabolic needs of the body, the ratio ranges from 0.7 to 1.0, and averages around 0.8; carbohydrate metabolism produces an RQ = 1; protein metabolism RQ = 0.8; and fat metabolism RQ = 0.7

TEACHING TOOL
Maximizing Food Intake in COPD

Even though well-balanced, nutritionally sound meals are provided, it is sometimes difficult for patients with COPD to consume adequate amounts of nutrients, particularly in the home setting. Here are ideas to make meal times easier and more nutritious by increasing kcalorie and protein without increasing the amount of food eaten.

IN CLINICAL AND HOME HEALTH CARE SETTINGS
- Eat high-kcalorie foods first
- More frequent meals and snacks may be helpful
- Increase kcalories by adding margarine, butter, mayonnaise, sauces, gravies, and peanut butter to foods
- Limit liquids at meal times
- Cold foods can give a lesser sense of fullness than hot foods
- Rest before meals

IN A HOME HEALTH CARE SETTING
- Have favorite foods and snacks on hand
- Have ready-prepared meals available for periods of increased shortness of breath
- Eat larger meals when you are not as tired
- Avoid foods that you know cause gas
- Skim milk powder (2 tablespoons) can be added to regular milk (8 oz) to add protein and kcalories
- Use milk or half-and-half instead of water when making soups, cereals, instant puddings, cocoa, or canned soups
- Add grated cheese to sauces, vegetables, soups, and casseroles
- Choose dessert recipes that contain egg, such as sponge cake, angel food cake, egg custard, bread pudding, or rice pudding

of carbon dioxide and fat metabolism produces the least amount. An RQ greater than 1.0 is evidence of accumulating carbon dioxide, which will make respiration that much more difficult for a COPD patient (1). Nonprotein kcalories should be divided evenly between fat and carbohydrate (24). The important issue is to provide adequate nutrition without overfeeding the patient.

Acute Respiratory Failure and Respiratory Distress Syndrome

Almost half of all patients with acute respiratory failure suffer from malnutrition that impairs recovery and prolongs weaning from mechanical ventilation (23). A diet that minimizes carbon dioxide production while maintaining good nutrition is recommended (1,18,23). Since patients in acute respiratory failure or respiratory distress syndrome may require mechanical ventilation, nutritional needs may be provided via enteral or parenteral nutrition.

Medical nutrition therapy

Nutrition support should be initiated as soon as possible to help wean the patient from the ventilator, since 2 to 3 weeks are required to refeed patients (22). (See Chapter 13, Refeeding box.) Nutritional recommendations are similar to those for patients with COPD: high-kcalorie, high-protein, moderate to high (50% nonprotein kcalories) fat, with moderate (≤50% nonprotein kcalories) carbohydrate.

Care must be taken to provide adequate kcalories and protein without overfeeding the patient. Excess kcalories and protein can result in shortness of breath in patients with limited respiratory function (21,25). **Hypophosphatemia** can also adversely affect respiratory muscle function (21,23). Low serum levels of phosphorus decrease oxygen delivery to tissues and decrease energy production, thereby impairing respiratory muscle function (23). Phosphorus levels should be monitored in patients in respiratory failure.

hypophosphatemia
abnormally low phosphate levels in circulating blood

Enteral nutrition (tube feedings). Commercial formulas that provide 40% to 50% of total kcalories from fat are available. Low osmolality feedings are started slowly to avoid gastric retention or diarrhea. Continuous administration is recommended unless otherwise contraindicated (22). Since these patients are at risk for aspiration, special precautions such as elevating the head of the bed and/or using a tube placed into the duodenum or jejunum, are necessary (1). Blue food coloring can be added to the formula so that aspiration can be easily detected if it occurs (1,22).

Parenteral nutrition. Although total (or central) parenteral nutrition may be more useful for extended support, some limitations exist. High glucose concentrations can lead to excess carbon dioxide production, making weaning more difficult (1,22). Since phosphate depletion occurs frequently with glucose infusions (which reduces respiratory drive), serum phosphorus is monitored (1,23). If depleted, phosphorus is provided at 2.5 to 5 mg/kg body weight (22).

Daily kcalorie counts are functional for assessing the patient's response to nutrition support. If fluid retention is not evident, daily weights and biochemical parameters are also useful. In the event of edema or fluid overload, these parameters are not accurate and indirect calorimetry provides more useful information to monitor the effects of nutrition support (1). Collaboration with clinical dietitians is best to monitor transition from parenteral to enteral feedings to conventional feeding.

Malnutrition and the method of refeeding unquestionably influence the outcome in respiratory disease or respiratory failure (23). Medical nutrition therapy is important to maintain or replenish nutritional status and can positively or negatively influence weaning from mechanical ventilation. Since a significant number of patients with respiratory disease or failure have clinically relevant malnutrition, nurses and other health care professionals should always be alert to alterations in nutritional status.

WELLNESS AND CANCER, AIDS, AND OTHER PROBLEMS

Physical Dimension	The physical health challenge of these disorders is to halt or minimize malnutrition often associated with the symptoms or treatments.
Intellectual Dimension	These disorders are marked by either their chronic and/or potentially life-threatening outcomes; maintaining optimal nutrient intake while dealing with serious illness requires intellectual abilities to comprehend the different aspects of treatment and rehabilitation.
Emotional Dimension	Facing death with AIDS or cancer or dealing with the chronic pulmonary diseases stresses our emotional ability to cope; nurses need to be sensitive to the emotional burden patients and families are experiencing.
Social Dimension	Social health may be compromised as prejudice against (and fear of) clients with HIV/AIDS and/or cancer affects the ability of individuals to continue their social and work relations as they did in the past. Dealing with societal and emotional issues may warrant counseling support for clients and their families.

SUMMARY

The disorders of cancer, acquired immune deficiency syndrome, and pulmonary disease are characterized by wasting and malnutrition, largely caused by the effect of the disorders or the secondary consequences of treatment on the gastrointestinal tract. Medical nutrition therapy focuses on reducing these effects.

Local or systemic effects of the cancer combined with antineoplastic therapy place the patient with cancer at increased risk of developing malnutrition or cancer cachexia through a variety of mechanisms: anorexia, nausea, vomiting, mucositis, organ injury (toxicity), and learned food aversions. Chemotherapy and radiation therapy damage rapidly replicating normal host cells along with cancerous cells. Surgery is the preferred treatment for solid tumors and tumors in the gastrointestinal tract, but often causes alterations in nutrition intake and may lead to significant nutritional problems. Malabsorption tends to be the primary nutritional problem with surgery. Bone marrow transplantation is used to treat certain hematologic malignancies and some solid tumors. The development of protein-energy malnutrition often develops because of the affects associated with these treatments. Nutrition support must be individualized and is an essential component of the total management of cancer. Common nutrition-related problems are loss of appetite, early satiety, diarrhea, nausea and vomiting, chewing and swallowing difficulties, constipation, abdominal gas and bloating, dry mouth, and taste or smell alterations.

Acquired immunodeficiency syndrome (AIDS), caused by the retrovirus human immunodeficiency virus (HIV), leads to the breakdown of the immune system, resulting in neoplasms, opportunistic infections, and/ or enteropathy. Malnutrition, a common complication of HIV/AIDS, is multifactorial and includes decreased nutrient (food) intake, malabsorption, and altered metabolism. Goals of medical nutrition therapy are individualized, and interventions are based on nutritional status, causes of malnutrition, complications that impact nutritional status, and feasibility of rehabilitation. Medications to minimize symptoms and IV fluids to maintain fluid and electrolyte balance may be necessary. Patient preferences, cost, availability, and nutritional requirements are determining factors in selecting enteral products and their route of delivery. Early recognition and intervention for nutritional risk factors and indicators are the keys to successful nutrition support and related medical therapies.

The two categories of pulmonary disorders cause either chronic long-term changes in respiratory function, such as chronic obstructive pulmonary disease (COPD), or acute changes in respiratory function, such as respiratory distress syndrome (RDS) and acute respiratory failure (ARF). The goal of medical nutrition therapy for COPD is to maintain respiratory muscle strength and function. ARF and RDS may develop in patients who are critically ill, in shock, severely injured, or who have sepsis. For ARF and RDS, the function of medical nutrition therapy is to inhibit tissue destruction by providing the extra nutrients required for hypermetabolic conditions. As all pulmonary disorders progress, nutritional status tends to decline and malnutrition exacerbates declining respiratory muscle function and ventilatory drive. Sufficient energy and protein is necessary to maintain the integrity of the immune system, but without overfeeding. Malnutrition and the method of refeeding influence the outcome in respiratory disease or respiratory failure.

THE NURSING ROLE
Acquired Immunodeficiency Syndrome: The Nursing Process

Joe McCoy is a 28-year-old former IV drug abuser who is now suffering from AIDS. He has had multiple episodes of opportunistic infections and is presently being treated for oral and esophageal candidiasis, diarrhea, and wasting. You see Joe in an HMO clinic every 2 weeks. He has previously been seen by the nutritionist. On this visit, you complete the following assessment:

THE NURSING ROLE, cont'd.
Acquired Immunodeficiency Syndrome: The Nursing Process

ASSESSMENT DATA COLLECTED
Objective
Body weight 110 lb (Baseline weight 148 lb; last visit 111 lb)
Lower abdominal tenderness
Oral and pharyngeal whitish/yellow lesions
Generalized muscle wasting
Laboratory results
  Total serum protein 5.1 (norm 6.6 to 7.9 gm/dl)
  Serum albumin 2.7 (norm 3.5 to 5.5 gm/dl)

Subjective
Fatigue
Periodic lower abdominal pain
Discomfort when chewing and swallowing

NURSING DIAGNOSIS 1
Pain in mouth and throat related to disruption of mucous membranes as evidenced by plaques and discomfort when eating.

PLANNING
The following goal was set with Joe's input:
Decrease in pain when chewing and swallowing

INTERVENTION
1. Eat cool or room temperature foods
2. Increase fluid intake from approximately 1200 cc to about 1800 cc
3. Eat mechanically soft foods or foods with sauces
4. Avoid highly seasoned foods

EVALUATION
Evaluate whether outcome of subjective decrease in pain has been met by next visit.

NURSING DIAGNOSIS 2
Altered nutrition, less than body requirements, related to diarrhea and HIV wasting, as evidenced by weight loss and protein depletion.

PLANNING
You plan to achieve the following outcome:
Weight gain of 1 lb by next visit

INTERVENTION
1. Eat frequent, small meals
2. Eat favorite foods, especially those high in fat and sugar
3. Drink a total of 200 cc of commercial nutritional supplement between meals
4. Use high-calorie condiments such as butter and mayonnaise

EVALUATION
Weigh Joe at next visit in 2 weeks in same amount of clothing to see if he has gained 1 lb. If he has not, consult again with the nutritionist.

Critical
Thinking   **CLINICAL APPLICATIONS**

M.N. is a 20-year-old female college student with an uneventful medical history with no significant illness. After finals, she came down with the flu and has felt run-down ever since. She has also had a persistent low-grade fever and cough since the flu. With much insistence by her parents, she went to see her doctor for a physical. She was admitted to the hospital after her chest x-ray indicated a possible malignancy. Following a bone marrow biopsy, chest CT, MRI, and biopsy of suspect lymph nodes, a diagnosis of non-Hodgkins lymphoma with positive lymph nodes was made. Bone marrow, as well as other organs, indicated no presence of the disease. M.N.'s physicians have determined a chemotherapy regimen using a combination of drugs to be given over 5 days every 4 weeks. M.N. complains of an overall lack of appetite, but no nausea, vomiting, constipation, or diarrhea. She is 5'6" tall and weighs 120 lb upon admission. Her usual weight is 130 pounds.

1. What are the possible causes of her decreased appetite?
2. What side effects from her chemotherapy might she encounter?
3. How will this affect her nutritional status?

From Marcia Nahikian-Nelms, PhD, RD.

REFERENCES

1. Zeman FJ: *Clinical nutrition and dietetics,* ed 2, New York, 1991, Macmillan.
2. Cotugna N et al: Nutrition and cancer prevention knowledge, beliefs, attitudes, and practices: The 1987 National Health Interview Survey, *J Am Diet Assoc* 92:963-968, 1992.
3. Committee on Diet and Health, Food and Nutrition Board, Commission on Life Sciences, National Research Council, *Diet and health: Implications for reducing chronic disease risk,* Washington, DC, 1989, National Academy Press.
4. Krenkel J, St Jeor S: Nutrition interventions for cancer prevention, *Topics in Clinical Nutrition* 9:1-9, 1993.
5. Charuhas PM: Dietary management during antitumor therapy of cancer patients, *Topics in Clinical Nutrition* 9:42-53, 1993.
6. Nelson JK et al: *Mayo Clinic diet manual,* ed 7, St. Louis, 1994, Mosby.
7. DeWys WD et al: Prognostic effect of weight loss prior to chemotherapy in cancer patients, *Am J Med* 69:491-497, 1980.
8. Dreizen S et al: Nutritional deficiencies in patients receiving cancer chemotherapy, *Postgrad Med* 87:163-167, 1990.
9. Shils ME: Nutrition and diet in cancer management. In Shils ME, Olson JA, Shike M, eds: *Modern nutrition in health and disease,* ed 8, Philadelphia, 1994, Lea & Febiger.
10. MacBurney M et al: A cost-evaluation of glutamine-supplemented parenteral nutrition in adult bone marrow transplant patients, *J Am Diet Assoc* 94:1263-1266, 1994.
11. Feuz A, Rapin CH: An observational study of the role of pain control and food adaptation of elderly patients with terminal cancer, *J Am Diet Assoc* 94:767-770, 1994.
12. Kotler DP: Causes and consequences of malnutrition in HIV/AIDS, *Nutrition and HIV/AIDS,* 1:5-8, 1992.
13. Cameron AM, ed: Nutrition in HIV/AIDS, *Dietetic Currents,* 21:11-16, 1994.
14. Resler SS: Nutrition care of AIDS patients, *J Am Diet Assoc* 88:828-832, 1988.
15. Cohan GR, Fields-Gardner C: Malnutrition and wasting in HIV disease: A review, *Perspectives in Applied Nutrition* 2:10-19, 1994.

16. Wong G: *HIV disease nutrition guidelines: Practical steps for a healthier life*, Chicago, 1993, The Physicians Association for AIDS Care.
17. Chlebowski RT et al: Dietary intake and counseling, weight maintenance, and the course of HIV infection, *J Am Diet Assoc* 95:428-432, 435, 1995.
18. Swearingen PL: *Manual of medical-surgical nursing care*, ed 3, St. Louis, 1994, Mosby.
19. Cerda JJ: AIDS and nutrition issues, *Clinics in Applied Nutrition* 63-68, Jan 1991.
20. Newman CF: The role of nutritional assessments and nutritional plans in the management of HIV/AIDS: An overview of the PAAC Nutrition Initiative, *Nutrition and HIV/AIDS* 1:57-106, 1992.
21. Chin R, Haponik EF: Nutrition, respiratory function, and disease. In Shils ME, Olson JA, Shike M, eds: *Modern nutrition in health and disease*, ed 8, Philadelphia, 1994, Lea & Febiger.
22. Escott-Stump S: *Nutrition and diagnosis-related care*, ed 3, Philadelphia, 1992, Lea and Febiger.
23. Weinsier RL, Morgan SL: *Fundamentals of clinical nutrition*, St. Louis, 1993, Mosby.
24. Menashian L, ed: *Standards of practice: Guidelines for the practice of clinical dietetics*, Fresno, Calif: 1991, Servicemaster.
25. Askanazi J et al: Respiratory diseases. In Kinney JM et al, eds: *Nutrition and metabolism in patient care*, Philadelphia, 1988, Saunders.

Appendices

A   Food Composition Table

B   Exchange Lists

C   Nutrition and Health Organizations: Sources of Nutrition Information

D   Lactose Content of Foods

E   Values for Common Laboratory Tests

F   Recommended Nutrient Intakes for Canadians Vitality—A Fresh Approach

G   Kcalorie-Restricted Dietary Patterns

H   Physical Growth NCHS Percentiles

I   Dietary Intake Assessment: Sample 24-hour Recall Form

J   National Renal Diet

K   Foods High in Purines

L   Foods High in Oxalates

M   Cultural Dietary Patterns

USING THE FOOD COMPOSITION TABLE

The following Food Composition Table was developed by Positive Input Corp. and includes a majority of the foods listed in *Mosby's NutriTrac* software, which is available as a supplement to this text. As we go to press with this textbook, we are still adding foods to *Mosby's NutriTrac* so that it will be as complete as possible. Thus you will be able to find foods in *Mosby's NutriTrac* that are not in the Food Composition Table.

The easiest way to look for a food is to use the "Search For" feature in *Mosby's NutriTrac* software. However, if you do not have access to a computer or your computer time is limited, you can easily look for a food using this Food Composition Table. The foods in the table are arranged alphabetically. Note, however, in some cases foods are arranged alphabetically in groups such as Baby Food, Beef, Bread, etc., rather than by name alone.

Code	Food Name	Amount	Unit	Grams	kCalories	Carbohydrate (gm)	Protein (gm)	Fat (gm)	Saturated Fat (gm)	Monounsaturated Fat (gm)
11001	Alfalfa Seeds, Sprouted, Fresh	½	Cup	16.5	5	1	1	0	0	0
19065	Almond Joy Candy Bar	1	Bar	50	232	29	2	14	8	3
12067	Almonds, Toasted, Unblanched	½	Cup	71	418	16	14	36	3	23
19066	Alpine White Bar w/ Almonds	1	Bar	35	197	18	4	13	7	5
15002	Anchovy, European, Cnd In Oil	3	Ounce	85.1	179	0	25	8	2	3
55188	Angel Hair Pasta, Lean Cuisine-Stouffer's	1	Each	283.5	240	38	10	5	1	-
18150	Animal Crackers	1	Each	2.5	11	2	0	0	0	0
19294	Apple Butter	1	Tbsp.	18	33	9	0	0	-	-
19186	Apple Crisp	1	Cup	282	460	91	5	10	2	4
9400	Apple Juice, Unsweetened	¾	Cup	185.8	87	22	0	0	0	0
18302	Apple Pie	1	Slice	155	411	58	4	19	5	8
9007	Apples, Cnd, Sweetened	½	Cup	102	68	17	0	0	0	0
9009	Apples, Dehydrated, Sulfured	¼	Cup	15	52	14	0	0	0	0
9003	Apples, Fresh, w/ Skin	1	Medium	138	81	21	0	0	0	0
9004	Apples, Fresh, w/o Skin	1	Medium	128	73	19	0	0	0	0
9020	Applesauce, Sweetened	½	Cup	127.5	97	25	0	0	0	0
9019	Applesauce, Unsweetened	½	Cup	122	52	14	0	0	0	0
9403	Apricot Nectar, Cnd, w/ Added Vit C	¾	Cup	188.2	105	27	1	0	0	0
9036	Apricot Nectar, Cnd, w/o Added Vit C	¾	Cup	188.2	105	27	1	0	0	0
9028	Apricots, Cnd, Heavy Syrup Pack	½	Cup	129	107	28	1	0	0	0
9024	Apricots, Cnd, Juice Pack	½	Cup	124	60	15	1	0	0	0
9026	Apricots, Cnd, Light Syrup Pack	½	Cup	126.5	80	21	1	0	0	0
9022	Apricots, Cnd, Water Pack	½	Cup	121.5	33	8	1	0	0	0
9030	Apricots, Dehydrated, Sulfured	¼	Cup	29.8	95	25	1	0	0	0
9032	Apricots, Dried, Sulfured	¼	Cup	32.5	77	20	1	0	0	0
9021	Apricots, Fresh	3	Medium	106	51	12	1	0	0	0
9035	Apricots, Frozen, Sweetened	½	Cup	121	119	30	1	0	0	0
11705	Asparagus, Ckd	½	Cup	90	23	4	2	0	0	0
11015	Asparagus, Cnd	½	Cup	121	23	3	3	1	0	0
11011	Asparagus, Fresh	½	Cup	67	15	3	2	0	0	0

Restaurant foods, including fast foods (quick service), are listed separately, starting on p. A-62. These foods are listed alphabetically by restaurant name. If the fast food/quick service restaurant where you ate is not listed, use the generic "Fast Food" category within the Restaurant list.

The code number before each food listing corresponds to the food data bank in *Mosby's NutriTrac* software. When you input your dietary intake into the software program, you may choose to use code numbers. Alternatively, you may choose to enter your dietary intake into *Mosby's NutriTrac* by typing a food's name or partial name and using the "Search For" option.

Polyunsaturated Fat (gm)	Fiber (gm)	Cholesterol (mg)	Folate (µg)	Vitamin A (re)	Vitamin B6 (mg)	Vitamin B12 (µg)	Vitamin C (mg)	Vitamin E (mg)	Riboflavin (mg)	Thiamin (mg)	Calcium (mg)	Iron (mg)	Magnesium (mg)	Niacin (mg)	Phosphorus (mg)	Potassium (mg)	Sodium (mg)	Zinc (mg)
0	0	0	6	3	0	0	1	-	0	0	5	0.2	4	0.1	12	13	1	0.2
1	-	1	4	2	0	0.1	0	-	0.1	0	40	0.6	33	0.2	70	186	67	0.4
8	8	0	45	0	0.1	0	0	-	0.4	0.1	201	3.5	216	2	390	549	8	3.5
1	2	4	5	9	0	0.3	0	-	0.1	0	81	0.2	13	0	82	146	26	0.4
2	0	72	11	18	0.2	0.7	0	-	0.3	0.1	197	3.9	59	16.9	214	463	3120	2.1
1	-	10	-	250	-	-	6	-	0.3	0.3	80	1.5	-	2.9	-	500	410	-
0	-	0	0	0	0	0	0	-	0	0	1	0.1	0	0.1	3	3	10	0
-	0	0	0	0	0	0	0	-	0	0	1	0	1	0	1	16	0	0
3	-	0	14	87	0.1	-	6	-	0.2	0.2	79	2.1	20	2.2	71	274	513	0.5
0	-	0	0	0	0.1	0	77	0	0	0	13	0.7	6	-	13	221	6	0.1
.5	-	0	6	19	0	0	3	-	0.2	0.2	11	1.7	11	1.9	43	122	327	0.3
0	2	0	0	5	0	0	0	-	0	0	4	0.2	2	0.1	5	69	3	0
0	2	0	0	1	0	0	0	-	0	0	3	0.3	3	0.1	8	96	19	0
0	4	0	4	7	0.1	0	8	0.8	0	0	10	0.2	7	0.1	10	159	0	0.1
0	2	0	1	5	0.1	0	5	0.3	0	0	5	0.1	4	0.1	9	145	0	0.1
0	2	0	1	1	0	0	2	-	0	0	5	0.4	4	0.2	9	78	4	0.1
0	1	0	1	4	0	0	1	-	0	0	4	0.1	4	0.2	9	92	2	0
0	-	0	2	248	0	0	102	-	0	0	13	0.7	9	0.5	17	215	6	0.2
0	1	0	2	248	0	0	1	-	0	0	13	0.7	9	0.5	17	215	6	0.2
0	-	0	2	160	0.1	0	4	-	0	0	12	0.6	10	0.5	17	173	14	0.1
0	2	0	2	210	0.1	0	6	-	0	0	15	0.4	12	0.4	25	205	5	0.1
0	2	0	2	167	0.1	0	3	-	0	0	14	0.5	10	0.4	16	175	5	0.1
0	2	0	2	157	0.1	0	4	-	0	0	10	0.4	9	0.5	16	233	4	0.1
0	-	0	1	377	0.2	0	3	-	0	0	18	1.9	19	1.1	47	550	4	0.3
0	3	0	3	235	0.1	0	1	-	0	0	15	1.5	15	1	38	448	3	0.2
0	3	0	9	277	0.1	0	11	-	0	0	15	0.6	8	0.6	20	314	1	0.3
0	2	0	2	203	0.1	0	11	-	0	0	12	1.1	11	1	23	277	5	0.1
0	-	0	88	75	0.1	0	24	-	0.1	0.1	22	0.6	17	0.9	55	279	216	0.4
0	2	0	116	64	0.1	0	22	-	0.1	0.1	19	2.2	12	1.2	52	208	472	0.5
0	1	0	86	39	0.1	0	9	-	0.1	0.1	14	0.6	12	0.8	38	183	1	0.3

Code	Food Name	Amount	Unit	Grams	kCalories	Carbohydrate (gm)	Protein (gm)	Fat (gm)	Saturated Fat (gm)	Monounsaturated Fat (gm)
11019	Asparagus, Frz, Ckd	½	Cup	100	28	5	3	0	0	0
9037	Avocados, Fresh	1	Medium	201	324	15	4	31	5	19
3117	Babyfood, Applesauce	1	Ounce	28.4	10	3	0	0	-	-
3280	Babyfood, Bananas w/ Tapioca	1	Ounce	28.4	19	5	0	0	-	-
3681	Babyfood, Barley, Ppd w/ Whole Milk	1	Ounce	28.4	31	5	1	1	-	-
3003	Babyfood, Beef	1	Ounce	28.4	30	0	4	1	1	1
3049	Babyfood, Beef and Rice	1	Ounce	28.4	23	2	1	1	-	-
3043	Babyfood, Beef Lasagna	1	Ounce	28.4	22	3	1	1	-	-
3287	Babyfood, Beef Noodle	1	Ounce	28.4	16	2	1	1	-	-
3052	Babyfood, Beef Stew	1	Ounce	28.4	14	2	1	0	0	0
3098	Babyfood, Beets	1	Ounce	28.4	10	2	0	0	-	-
3100	Babyfood, Carrots	1	Ounce	28.4	9	2	0	0	-	-
3013	Babyfood, Chicken	1	Ounce	28.4	42	0	4	3	1	1
3069	Babyfood, Chicken Noodle	1	Ounce	28.4	14	2	1	0	-	-
3070	Babyfood, Chicken Soup	1	Ounce	28.4	14	2	0	0	-	-
3014	Babyfood, Chicken Sticks	1	Stick	10	19	0	1	1	-	-
3214	Babyfood, Cookies, Arrowroot	1	Ounce	28.4	125	20	2	4	1	3
3120	Babyfood, Corn, Creamed	1	Ounce	28.4	18	5	0	0	-	-
3028	Babyfood, Cottage Cheese w/ Fruit	1	Ounce	28.4	22	5	1	0	-	-
3018	Babyfood, Egg Yolks	1	Ounce	28.4	58	0	3	5	1	2
3201	Babyfood, Egg Yolks and Bacon	1	Ounce	28.4	22	2	1	1	-	-
3236	Babyfood, Fruit Dessert	1	Ounce	28.4	18	5	0	0	-	-
3092	Babyfood, Green Beans	1	Ounce	28.4	7	2	0	0	-	-
3009	Babyfood, Ham	1	Ounce	28.4	35	0	4	2	1	1
3166	Babyfood, Juice, Apple	¾	Cup	185.8	87	22	0	0	-	-
3179	Babyfood, Juice, Mixed Fruit	¾	Cup	185.8	87	22	0	0	-	-
3172	Babyfood, Juice, Orange	¾	Cup	185.8	82	19	1	1	-	-
3090	Babyfood, Macaroni and Cheese	1	Ounce	28.4	17	2	1	1	-	-
3045	Babyfood, Macaroni and Tomato and Beef	1	Ounce	28.4	17	3	1	0	-	-
3021	Babyfood, Meat Sticks	1	Stick	10	18	0	1	1	1	1
3279	Babyfood, Mixed Vegetable	1	Ounce	28.4	9	2	0	0	-	-
3076	Babyfood, Noodles and Chicken	1	Ounce	28.4	18	3	0	1	-	-
3228	Babyfood, Peach Cobbler	1	Ounce	28.4	19	5	0	0	-	-
3230	Babyfood, Peach Melba	1	Ounce	28.4	17	5	0	0	-	-
3131	Babyfood, Peaches w/ Sugar	1	Ounce	28.4	20	5	0	0	-	-
3133	Babyfood, Pears	1	Ounce	28.4	12	3	0	0	-	-
3124	Babyfood, Peas, Buttered	1	Ounce	28.4	17	3	1	0	-	-
3135	Babyfood, Plums w/ Tapioca	1	Ounce	28.4	21	6	0	0	-	-
3694	Babyfood, Rice, Ppd w/ Whole Milk	1	Ounce	28.4	33	5	1	1	-	-
3210	Babyfood, Rice, w/ Mixed Fruit	1	Ounce	28.4	24	5	0	0	-	-
3050	Babyfood, Spaghetti and Tomato and Meat	1	Ounce	28.4	18	3	1	0	-	-
3103	Babyfood, Spinach, Creamed	1	Ounce	28.4	12	2	1	0	-	-
3058	Babyfood, Split Pea and Ham	1	Ounce	28.4	20	3	1	0	-	-
3105	Babyfood, Squash	1	Ounce	28.4	7	2	0	0	-	-
3109	Babyfood, Sweetpotatoes	1	Ounce	28.4	17	4	0	0	-	-
3216	Babyfood, Teething Biscuits	1	Biscuit	11	43	8	1	0	-	-
3238	Babyfood, Tropical Fruit	1	Ounce	28.4	17	5	0	0	-	-
3016	Babyfood, Turkey	1	Ounce	28.4	37	0	4	2	1	1
3083	Babyfood, Turkey and Rice	1	Ounce	28.4	14	2	1	0	0	0
3017	Babyfood, Turkey Sticks	1	Stick	10	18	0	1	1	-	-
10124	Bacon	1	Slice	6	35	0	2	3	1	1
10131	Bacon, Canadian-style Bacon, Grilled	1	Slice	21	39	0	5	2	1	1
62528	Bacon, Turkey	1	Slice	14	25	0	3	2	1	-
18005	Bagels, Cinnamon-raisin	1	3-1/2 In.	71	195	39	7	1	0	0
18006	Bagels, Cinnamon-raisin, Toasted	1	3-1/2 In.	66	194	39	7	1	0	0
18003	Bagels, Egg	1	3-1/2 In.	71	197	38	8	1	0	0
18004	Bagels, Egg, Toasted	1	3-1/2 In.	66	197	38	8	1	0	0
18007	Bagels, Oat Bran	1	3-1/2 In.	71	181	38	8	1	0	0
18008	Bagels, Oat Bran, Toasted	1	3-1/2 In.	66	181	38	8	1	0	0
18001	Bagels, Plain	1	3-1/2 In.	71	195	38	7	1	0	0

Polyunsaturated Fat (gm)	Fiber (gm)	Cholesterol (mg)	Folate (μg)	Vitamin A (re)	Vitamin B6 (mg)	Vitamin B12 (μg)	Vitamin C (mg)	Vitamin E (mg)	Riboflavin (mg)	Thiamin (mg)	Calcium (mg)	Iron (mg)	Magnesium (mg)	Niacin (mg)	Phosphorus (mg)	Potassium (mg)	Sodium (mg)	Zinc (mg)
0	-	0	135	82	0	0	24	-	0.1	0.1	23	0.6	13	1	55	218	4	0.6
4	12	0	124	123	0.6	0	16	-	0.2	0.2	22	2.1	78	3.9	82	1204	20	0.8
-	0	-	0	0	0	0	11	-	0	0	1	0.1	1	0	2	22	1	0
-	0	-	2	1	0	0	7	-	0	0	2	0.1	3	0.1	3	31	3	0
-	-	-	3	-	0	0.1	-	-	0.2	0.1	65	3.5	9	1.7	43	54	14	0.2
0	0	-	2	9	0	0.4	1	-	0	0	2	0.5	3	0.9	20	54	19	0.6
-	-	-	2	22	0	0.1	1	-	0	0	3	0.2	2	0.4	10	34	101	0.3
-	-	-	2	44	0	0.1	1	-	0	0	5	0.2	3	0.4	11	35	129	0.2
-	0	-	2	25	0	0	0	-	0	0	2	0.1	2	0.2	9	13	5	0.1
0	0	4	2	65	0	0.1	1	-	0	0	3	0.2	3	0.4	12	40	98	0.2
-	1	-	9	1	0	0	1	-	0	0	4	0.1	4	0	4	52	24	0
-	0	-	5	335	0	0	2	-	0	0	7	0.1	3	0.1	6	57	14	0
1	0	-	3	16	0.1	0.1	0	-	0	0	16	0.3	3	1	26	35	14	0.3
-	0	-	2	30	0	0	0	-	0	0	5	0.1	3	0.1	7	10	5	0.1
-	0	-	1	63	0	0	0	-	0	0	10	0.1	1	0.1	7	19	5	0.1
-	0	-	1	95	0	0	0	-	0	0	7	0.2	1	0.2	12	11	48	0.1
0	0	0	3	-	0	0	2	-	0.1	0.1	9	0.9	6	1.6	33	44	105	0.2
-	1	-	4	2	0	0	1	-	0	0	5	0.1	2	0.1	9	23	15	0.1
-	0	-	1	1	0	0	7	-	0	0	9	0	1	0	11	12	14	0
1	0	208	26	107	0	0.4	0	-	0.1	0	22	0.8	2	0	81	22	11	0.5
-	0	-	1	8	0	0	0	-	0	0	8	0.1	1	0.1	14	10	14	0.1
-	0	-	1	7	0	0	1	-	0	0	3	0.1	1	0	2	27	4	0
-	1	-	9	12	0	0	2	-	0	0	18	0.3	6	0.1	5	36	1	0.1
0	0	-	1	3	0.1	0	1	-	0.1	0	1	0.3	3	0.8	25	60	19	0.5
-	0	-	0	4	0.1	0	108	-	0	0	7	1.1	6	0.2	9	169	6	0.1
-	0	-	12	7	0.1	0	118	-	0	0	15	0.6	9	0.2	9	188	7	0.1
-	0	-	49	11	0.1	0	116	-	0.1	0.1	22	0.3	17	0.4	20	342	2	0.1
-	0	-	0	1	0	0	0	-	0	0	14	0.1	2	0.2	17	12	22	0.1
-	0	-	2	31	0	0.1	0	-	0	0	4	0.1	2	0.2	12	20	5	0.1
0	0	-	1	2	0	0	0	-	0	0	3	0.1	1	0.1	10	11	55	0.2
-	-	-	2	69	0	0	1	-	0	0	5	0.1	3	0.1	6	32	3	0.1
-	0	-	1	37	0	0	0	-	0	0	7	0.1	3	0.2	9	17	7	0.1
-	0	-	0	4	0	0	6	-	0	0	1	0	1	0.1	2	16	3	0
-	-	-	1	6	0	0	7	-	0	0	3	0.1	1	0.1	1	26	3	0.1
-	0	-	1	5	0	0	5	-	0	0	1	0.1	1	0.2	3	44	1	0
-	1	-	1	1	0	0	6	-	0	0	2	0.1	3	0.1	3	33	1	0
-	-	-	10	12	-	-	4	-	0	0	13	0.3	-	0.4	-	33	1	-
-	0	-	0	3	0	0	0	-	0	0	2	0.1	1	0.2	2	24	2	0
-	-	-	2	-	0	0.1	-	-	0.1	0.1	68	3.5	13	1.5	50	54	13	0.2
-	0	-	1	1	0.1	0	6	-	0.2	0.1	6	1.3	1	0.8	7	9	3	0.1
-	0	-	2	38	0	0	1	-	0	0	5	0.2	2	0.3	10	31	6	0.1
-	1	-	20	104	0	0	1	-	0	0	32	0.4	18	0.1	14	63	16	0.1
-	0	-	4	23	0	0	1	-	0	0	7	0.1	-	0.1	14	39	4	0.2
-	1	-	4	57	0	0	2	-	0	0	7	0.1	3	0.1	5	52	0	0
-	0	-	3	188	0	0	3	-	0	0	5	0.1	3	0.1	7	69	6	0
-	0	-	2	1	0	0	1	-	0.1	0	29	0.4	4	0.5	18	36	40	0.1
-	-	-	1	1	0	0	5	-	0	0	3	0.1	1	0	2	16	2	0
0	0	-	3	48	0	0.3	1	-	0.1	0	8	0.4	3	1	27	51	20	0.5
0	0	-	1	42	0	0	0	-	0	0	7	0.1	2	0.1	5	10	4	0.1
-	0	-	1	7	0	0.1	0	-	0	0	7	0.1	2	0.2	10	9	48	0.2
0	0	5	0	0	0	0.1	2	-	0	0	1	0.1	1	0.4	20	29	96	0.2
0	0	12	1	0	0.1	0.2	5	-	0	0.2	2	0.2	4	1.5	62	82	325	0.4
-	-	10	-	0	-	-	0	-	-	-	0	0	-	-	-	-	170	-
0	-	0	15	6	0	0	0	-	0.2	0.3	13	2.7	15	2.2	55	108	229	0.5
0	-	0	11	5	0	0	0	-	0.2	0.2	13	2.7	15	2	55	108	228	0.5
0	-	17	16	23	0.1	0.1	0	-	0.2	0.4	9	2.8	18	2.4	60	48	359	0.5
0	-	17	11	21	0.1	0.1	0	-	0.1	0.3	9	2.8	18	2.2	59	48	358	0.5
0	-	0	33	0	0.1	0	0	-	0.2	0.2	9	2.2	40	2.1	117	145	360	1.5
0	-	0	23	0	0.1	0	0	-	0.2	0.2	9	2.2	41	1.9	117	145	360	1.5
0	1	0	16	0	0	0	0	-	0.2	0.4	53	2.5	12	3.2	68	72	379	0.6

Code	Food Name	Amount	Unit	Grams	kCalories	Carbohydrate (gm)	Protein (gm)	Fat (gm)	Saturated Fat (gm)	Monounsaturated Fat (gm)
18409	Bagels, Plain, Toasted	1	3-1/2 In.	66	195	38	7	1	0	0
55189	Baked Cheese Ravioli, Lean Cuisine-Stouffer's	1	Each	241	240	30	13	8	3	-
41297	Baked Cheese Ravioli-Healthy Choice	1	Each	255.1	250	44	14	2	1	-
55190	Baked Potato w/ Sour Cream, Lean Cuisine-Stouffer's	1	Each	294.1	230	38	9	5	2	-
11028	Bamboo Shoots, Cnd	½	Cup	65.5	12	2	1	0	0	0
11026	Bamboo Shoots, Fresh	½	Cup	75.5	20	4	2	0	0	0
19400	Banana Chips	1	Ounce	28.4	147	17	1	10	8	1
18304	Banana Cream Pie	1	Slice	148	398	49	7	20	6	8
41240	Banana Nut Muffin-Healthy Choice	1	Each	70.9	180	32	3	6	-	-
19311	Banana Pudding	1	Cup	298.1	379	63	7	11	2	5
9040	Bananas, Fresh	1	Medium	114	105	27	1	1	0	0
6150	Barbecue Sauce	½	Cup	125	94	16	2	2	0	1
7001	Barbeque Loaf, Lunch Meat	1	Slice	23	40	1	4	2	1	1
15187	Bass, Freshwater, Ckd, Dry Heat	3	Ounce	85.1	124	0	21	4	1	2
15188	Bass, Striped, Ckd, Dry Heat	3	Ounce	85.1	105	0	19	3	1	1
41276	Bean and Ham Soup-Healthy Choice	1	Each	212.6	220	35	12	4	1	-
16006	Beans, Baked, Cnd, Vegetarian	½	Cup	127	118	26	6	1	0	0
16007	Beans, Baked, Cnd, w/ Beef	½	Cup	133	161	22	8	5	2	2
16008	Beans, Baked, Cnd, w/ Franks	½	Cup	128.5	182	20	9	8	3	4
16009	Beans, Baked, Cnd, w/ Pork	½	Cup	126.5	134	25	7	2	1	1
16005	Beans, Baked, Home Prepared	½	Cup	126.5	191	27	7	7	2	3
16315	Beans, Black, Ckd	½	Cup	86	114	20	8	0	0	0
11056	Beans, Green, Cnd	½	Cup	68	14	3	1	0	0	0
11052	Beans, Green, Fresh	½	Cup	55	17	4	1	0	0	0
11061	Beans, Green, Fzn	½	Cup	67.5	18	4	1	0	0	0
16029	Beans, Kidney, Cnd	½	Cup	128	104	19	7	0	0	0
16073	Beans, Lima, Cnd	½	Cup	120.5	95	18	6	0	0	0
11040	Beans, Lima, Fzn	½	Cup	90	95	18	6	0	0	0
16039	Beans, Navy, Cnd	½	Cup	131	148	27	10	1	0	0
16044	Beans, Pinto, Cnd	½	Cup	120	94	17	5	0	0	0
16103	Beans, Refried, Cnd	½	Cup	126.5	135	23	8	1	1	1
11932	Beans, Yellow, Cnd	½	Cup	68	14	3	1	0	0	0
11722	Beans, Yellow, Fresh	½	Cup	55	17	4	1	0	0	0
41335	Beef and Bean Burritos (medium)-Healthy Choice	1	Each	148.8	270	42	12	7	3	0
41334	Beef and Bean Burritos (mild)-Healthy Choice	1	Each	148.8	250	45	11	5	1	-
55191	Beef and Bean Enchiladas, Lean Cuisine-Stouffer's	1	Each	262.2	240	32	15	6	3	-
41270	Beef and Potato Soup-Healthy Choice	1	Each	212.6	110	17	9	1	-	-
14114	Beef Broth and Tomato Juice, Cnd	¾	Cup	183	68	16	1	0	0	0
55192	Beef Cannelloni w/ Sauce, Lean Cuisine-Stouffer's	1	Each	272.9	200	28	14	3	1	-
41249	Beef Enchilada-Healthy Choice	1	Each	379.2	370	66	15	5	2	-
19002	Beef Jerky, Chopped and Formed	3	Ounce	85.1	287	12	34	11	5	5
55149	Beef Pie-Stouffer's	1	Each	283.5	460	37	18	27	-	-
57806	Beef Pot Pie-Swanson	1	Pie	198.5	370	36	12	19	-	-
43405	Beef Ravioli, Micro Cup-Hormel	1	Each	212.6	270	34	9	11	4	5
41251	Beef Sirloin Tips-Healthy Choice	1	Each	318.9	270	29	22	7	3	-
43413	Beef Stew, Micro Cup-Hormel	1	Each	212.6	230	11	13	15	5	4
55158	Beef Stroganoff w/ Parsley Noodles-Stouffer's	1	Each	276.4	390	28	24	20	-	-
13347	Beef, Corned, Brisket, Ckd	3	Ounce	85.1	213	0	15	16	5	8
13353	Beef, Cured, Lunch Meat, Jellied	3	Ounce	85.1	94	0	16	3	1	1
13355	Beef, Cured, Pastrami	3	Ounce	85.1	297	3	15	25	9	12
13357	Beef, Cured, Sausage, Smoked	3	Ounce	85.1	265	2	12	23	10	11
13358	Beef, Cured, Smoked, Chopped Beef	3	Ounce	85.1	105	2	17	4	2	2
13360	Beef, Cured, Thin-sliced Beef	3	Ounce	85.1	151	5	24	3	1	1
13298	Beef, Ground, Extra Lean, Broiled	3	Ounce	85.1	218	0	22	14	5	6
13300	Beef, Ground, Extra Lean, Pan-fried	3	Ounce	85.1	217	0	21	14	5	6
13305	Beef, Ground, Lean, Broiled	3	Ounce	85.1	231	0	21	16	6	7
13307	Beef, Ground, Lean, Pan-fried	3	Ounce	85.1	234	0	21	16	6	7
13312	Beef, Ground, Regular, Broiled	3	Ounce	85.1	246	0	20	18	7	8
13314	Beef, Ground, Regular, Pan-fried	3	Ounce	85.1	260	0	20	19	8	8
13326	Beef, Liver, Ckd, Braised	3	Ounce	85.1	137	3	21	4	2	1

Polyunsaturated Fat (gm)	Fiber (gm)	Cholesterol (mg)	Folate (μg)	Vitamin A (re)	Vitamin B6 (mg)	Vitamin B12 (μg)	Vitamin C (mg)	Vitamin E (mg)	Riboflavin (mg)	Thiamin (mg)	Calcium (mg)	Iron (mg)	Magnesium (mg)	Niacin (mg)	Phosphorus (mg)	Potassium (mg)	Sodium (mg)	Zinc (mg)
0	-	0	11	0	0	0	0	-	0.2	0.3	13	2.5	20	2.9	68	72	379	0.6
-	-	55	-	60	-	-	36	-	0.3	0.1	160	0.8	-	1.1	-	380	590	-
-	-	20	-	500	-	-	5	-	0.3	0.3	200	1.5	-	1.9	240	590	420	-
-	-	15	-	350	-	-	30	-	0.3	0.2	160	0.6	-	1.1	-	900	570	-
0	2	0	2	1	0.1	0	1	-	0	0	5	0.2	3	0.1	16	52	5	0.4
0	2	0	5	2	0.2	0	3	-	0.1	0.1	10	0.4	2	0.5	45	402	3	0.8
0	2	0	4	2	0.1	0	2	-	0	0	5	0.4	22	0.2	16	152	2	0.2
5	-	75	16	104	0.2	0.4	2	-	0.3	0.2	111	1.5	24	1.6	136	244	355	0.7
3	-	0	-	-	-	-	-	-	0.1	0.2	80	1	-	0.8	160	250	80	-
4	-	0	6	89	0.1	0.5	1	-	0.4	0.1	253	0.4	24	0.5	206	328	584	0.8
0	3	0	22	9	0.7	0	10	0.3	0.1	0.1	7	0.4	33	0.6	23	451	1	0.2
1	1	0	5	109	0.1	0	9	-	0	0	24	1.1	22	1.1	25	217	1019	0.2
0	0	9	2	2	0.1	0.4	4	-	0.1	0.1	13	0.3	4	0.5	30	76	307	0.6
1	0	74	14	30	0.1	2	2	-	0.1	0.1	88	1.6	32	1.3	218	388	77	0.7
1	0	88	9	26	0.3	3.8	0	-	0	0.1	16	0.9	43	2.2	216	279	75	0.4
1	-	5	-	60	-	-	2	-	0.2	0.2	48	1	-	1.1	220	630	480	-
0	6	0	30	22	0.2	0	4	-	0.1	0.2	64	0.4	41	0.5	132	376	504	1.8
0	-	29	58	28	0.1	0	2	-	0.1	0.1	60	2.1	33	1.3	108	426	632	1.6
1	9	8	39	19	0.1	0	3	-	0.1	0.1	62	2.2	36	1.2	134	302	553	2.4
0	7	9	46	23	0.1	0	3	-	0	0.1	67	2.2	43	0.6	137	391	524	1.8
1	7	6	61	0	0.1	0	1	-	0.1	0.2	77	2.5	54	0.5	138	453	534	0.9
0	-	0	128	1	0.1	0	0	-	0.1	0.2	23	1.8	60	0.4	120	305	204	1
0	1	0	22	24	0	0	3	-	0	0	18	0.6	9	0.1	13	74	171	0.2
0	2	0	20	37	0	0	9	-	0.1	0	20	0.6	14	0.4	21	115	3	0.1
0	2	0	6	36	0	0	6	-	0	0	30	0.6	14	0.3	16	76	9	0.4
0	-	0	63	0	0.1	0	2	-	0.1	0.1	35	1.6	40	0.6	134	329	444	0.7
0	6	0	61	0	0.1	0	0	-	0	0.1	25	2.2	47	0.3	89	265	405	0.8
0	-	0	14	15	0.1	0	5	-	0	0.1	25	1.8	50	0.7	101	370	26	0.5
0	7	0	82	0	0.1	0	1	-	0.1	0.2	62	2.4	62	0.6	176	377	587	1
0	4	0	72	0	0.1	0	1	-	0.1	0.1	44	1.9	32	0.4	110	361	499	0.8
0	7	0	106	0	0.1	0	8	-	0.1	0.1	58	2.2	49	0.6	106	497	536	1.7
0	1	0	22	7	0	0	3	-	0	0	18	0.6	9	0.1	13	74	171	0.2
0	1	0	20	6	0	0	9	-	0.1	0	20	0.6	14	0.4	21	115	3	0.1
3	-	15	-	20	-	-	4	-	0.2	0.4	48	1.5	-	1.9	180	270	520	-
2	-	10	-	20	-	-	1	-	0.2	0.4	32	2	-	2.9	130	330	450	-
1	-	45	-	80	-	-	6	-	0.3	0.2	80	1	-	1.9	-	470	480	-
-	-	20	-	-	-	-	2	-	-	0	-	0.2	-	0.4	-	100	550	-
0	-	0	8	24	0	0.1	2	-	0.1	0	20	1.1	5	0.3	24	176	240	0
-	-	25	-	350	-	-	6	-	0.2	0.1	120	1.5	-	2.9	-	800	490	-
2	-	30	-	250	-	-	24	-	0.3	0.3	120	1	-	1.9	260	600	450	-
0	0	96	14	0	0.4	3.4	0	-	0.8	0.1	9	4.7	43	7.8	323	508	2445	6.9
-	-	-	-	700	-	-	2	-	0.4	0.3	32	1.5	-	3.8	-	300	1130	-
-	-	-	-	250	-	-	-	-	0.2	0.2	16	1.5	-	2.9	-	-	730	-
1	-	20	-	100	-	-	11	-	0.3	0.2	48	0.9	28	2.5	-	359	920	1.1
2	-	65	-	700	-	-	42	-	0.2	0.2	16	1	-	2.9	190	520	360	-
-	-	45	-	320	-	-	2	-	0.1	0	16	0.9	21	2.3	-	487	1140	2.4
-	-	-	-	40	-	-	1	-	0.3	0.1	48	1.5	-	2.9	-	300	1090	-
1	0	83	5	0	0.2	1.4	14	-	0.1	0	7	1.6	10	2.6	106	123	964	3.9
0	0	29	6	0	0.2	4.4	15	-	0.2	0.1	9	2.9	15	4.1	118	342	1124	3
1	0	79	6	0	0.2	1.5	3	-	0.1	0.1	8	1.6	15	4.3	128	194	1044	3.6
1	0	57	3	0	0.1	1.6	10	-	0.1	0	6	1.5	11	2.7	89	150	962	2.4
0	0	39	7	0	0.3	1.5	18	-	0.1	0.1	7	2.4	18	3.9	154	321	1070	3.3
0	0	35	9	0	0.3	2.2	12	-	0.2	0.1	9	2.3	16	4.5	143	365	1224	3.4
1	0	71	8	0	0.2	1.8	0	-	0.2	0.1	6	2	18	4.2	137	266	60	4.6
1	0	69	8	0	0.2	1.7	0	-	0.2	0.1	6	2	18	4	136	265	60	4.6
1	0	74	8	0	0.2	2	0	-	0.2	0	9	1.8	18	4.4	134	256	65	4.6
1	0	71	8	0	0.2	1.9	0	-	0.2	0	9	1.9	17	4.1	135	254	65	4.4
1	0	77	8	0	0.2	2.5	0	-	0.2	0	9	2.1	17	4.9	145	248	71	4.4
1	0	76	8	0	0.2	2.3	0	-	0.2	0	9	2.1	17	5	145	255	71	4.3
1	0	331	185	9017	0.8	60.4	20	-	3.5	0.2	6	5.8	17	9.1	344	200	60	5.2

Code	Food Name	Amount	Unit	Grams	kCalories	Carbohydrate (gm)	Protein (gm)	Fat (gm)	Saturated Fat (gm)	Monounsaturated Fat (gm)
13327	Beef, Liver, Ckd, Pan-fried	3	Ounce	85.1	185	7	23	7	2	1
7042	Beef, Loaved, Lunch Meat	1	Slice	28.4	87	1	4	7	3	3
13504	Beef, Steaks and Roasts, Ckd, ½ in. Fat	3	Ounce	85.1	297	0	21	23	9	10
13361	Beef, Steaks and Roasts, Ckd, Fat Trimmed	3	Ounce	85.1	232	0	23	15	6	6
13004	Beef, Steaks and Roasts,Ckd., ¼ in. Fat	3	Ounce	85.1	259	0	22	18	7	8
7043	Beef, Thin Sliced	1	Slice	4.2	7	0	1	0	0	0
14006	Beer, Light	12	Fl Oz	354	99	5	1	0	0	0
14003	Beer, Regular	12	Fl Oz	356.4	146	13	1	0	0	0
11081	Beets, Ckd	½	Cup	85	37	8	1	0	0	0
18009	Biscuits, Plain or Buttermilk	1	Each	35	127	17	2	6	1	2
14008	Bloody Mary	1	Fl Oz	29.7	23	1	0	0	0	0
9052	Blueberries, Cnd, Heavy Syrup	½	Cup	128	113	28	1	0	-	-
9050	Blueberries, Fresh	½	Cup	72.5	41	10	0	0	-	-
9055	Blueberries, Frozen, Sweetened	½	Cup	115	93	25	0	0	-	-
9054	Blueberries, Frozen, Unsweetened	½	Cup	77.5	40	9	0	0	-	-
41241	Blueberry Muffin-Healthy Choice	1	Each	70.9	190	39	3	4	-	-
18305	Blueberry Pie	1	Slice	125	290	44	2	13	2	7
15189	Bluefish, Ckd, Dry Heat	3	Ounce	85.1	135	0	22	5	1	2
10126	Bologna	1	Slice	23	57	0	4	5	2	2
7007	Bologna, Beef	1	Slice	28.4	88	0	3	8	3	4
41286	Boneless Beef Ribs w/ Barbecue Sauce-Healthy Choice	1	Each	311.8	330	40	28	6	2	-
14413	Bourbon and Soda	1	Fl Oz	29	26	0	0	0	0	0
12078	Brazilnuts, Dried, Unblanched	½	Cup	70	459	9	10	46	11	16
19167	Bread Pudding	1	Cup	252	423	62	13	15	6	5
18080	Bread Sticks, Plain	1	Stick	10	41	7	1	1	0	0
18083	Bread Stuffing, Plain	1	Cup	232	390	52	9	17	3	7
18020	Bread, Banana	1	Slice	60	203	33	3	7	2	3
18024	Bread, Cornbread	1	Piece	65	173	28	4	5	1	1
18025	Bread, Cracked-wheat	1	Slice	25	65	12	2	1	0	0
18026	Bread, Cracked-wheat, Toasted	1	Slice	23	65	12	2	1	0	0
18344	Bread, Dinner Roll, Egg	1	Each	35	107	18	3	2	1	1
18349	Bread, Dinner Roll, French	1	Each	38	105	19	3	2	0	1
18345	Bread, Dinner Roll, Oat Bran	1	Each	33	78	13	3	2	0	0
18342	Bread, Dinner Roll, Plain	1	Each	35	105	18	3	3	1	1
18346	Bread, Dinner Roll, Rye	1	Each	35	100	19	4	1	0	0
18347	Bread, Dinner Roll, Wheat	1	Each	33	90	15	3	2	1	1
18348	Bread, Dinner Roll, Whole-wheat	1	Each	33	88	17	3	2	0	0
18027	Bread, Egg	1	Slice	40	115	19	4	2	1	1
18028	Bread, Egg, Toasted	1	Slice	37	117	19	4	2	1	1
18029	Bread, French or Vienna	1	Slice	25	69	13	2	1	0	0
18030	Bread, French or Vienna, Toasted	1	Slice	23	69	13	2	1	0	0
18033	Bread, Italian	1	Slice	30	81	15	3	1	0	0
18034	Bread, Italian, Toasted	1	Slice	27	80	15	3	1	0	0
18049	Bread, Lo Cal, Oat Bran	1	Slice	23	46	9	2	1	0	0
18050	Bread, Lo Cal, Oat Bran, Toasted	1	Slice	19	45	9	2	1	0	0
18051	Bread, Lo Cal, Oatmeal	1	Slice	23	48	10	2	1	0	0
18052	Bread, Lo Cal, Oatmeal, Toasted	1	Slice	19	48	10	2	1	0	0
18053	Bread, Lo Cal, Rye	1	Slice	23	47	9	2	1	0	0
18054	Bread, Lo Cal, Rye, Toasted	1	Slice	19	46	9	2	1	0	0
18055	Bread, Lo Cal, Wheat	1	Slice	23	46	10	2	1	0	0
18056	Bread, Lo Cal, Wheat, Toasted	1	Slice	19	45	10	2	1	0	0
18057	Bread, Lo Cal, White	1	Slice	23	48	10	2	1	0	0
18058	Bread, Lo Cal, White, Toasted	1	Slice	19	47	10	2	1	0	0
18035	Bread, Mixed-grain	1	Slice	26	65	12	3	1	0	0
18036	Bread, Mixed-grain, Toasted	1	Slice	24	65	12	3	1	0	0
18037	Bread, Oat Bran	1	Slice	30	71	12	3	1	0	0
18038	Bread, Oat Bran, Toasted	1	Slice	27	70	12	3	1	0	0
18039	Bread, Oatmeal	1	Slice	27	73	13	2	1	0	0
18040	Bread, Oatmeal, Toasted	1	Slice	25	73	13	2	1	0	0
18041	Bread, Pita, White, Enriched	1	Pita	60	165	33	5	1	0	0

Polyunsaturated Fat (gm)	Fiber (gm)	Cholesterol (mg)	Folate (µg)	Vitamin A (re)	Vitamin B6 (mg)	Vitamin B12 (µg)	Vitamin C (mg)	Vitamin E (mg)	Riboflavin (mg)	Thiamin (mg)	Calcium (mg)	Iron (mg)	Magnesium (mg)	Niacin (mg)	Phosphorus (mg)	Potassium (mg)	Sodium (mg)	Zinc (mg)
1	0	410	187	9125	1.2	95.1	20	-	3.5	0.2	9	5.3	20	12.3	392	310	90	4.6
0	0	18	1	0	0.1	1.1	4	-	0.1	0	3	0.7	4	1	34	59	377	0.7
1	0	77	6	0	0.3	2	0	-	0.2	0.1	9	2.2	18	2.9	164	244	50	4.7
1	0	74	6	0	0.3	2.1	0	-	0.2	0.1	8	2.3	20	3.1	179	275	53	5.2
1	0	75	6	0	0.3	2.1	0	-	0.2	0.1	9	2.2	19	3.1	173	266	53	5
0	0	2	0	0	0	0.1	1	-	0	0	0	0.1	1	0.2	7	18	60	0.2
0	0	0	15	0	0.1	0	0	-	0.1	0	18	0.1	18	1.4	42	64	11	0.1
0	1	0	21	0	0.2	0.1	0	-	0.1	0	18	0.1	21	1.6	43	89	18	0.1
0	1	0	68	3	0.1	0	3	-	0	0	14	0.7	20	0.3	32	259	65	0.3
2	-	0	2	0	0	0	0	-	0.1	0.1	17	1.2	6	1.2	151	78	368	0.2
0	-	0	4	10	0	0	4	-	0	0	2	0.1	2	0.1	4	43	67	0
-	2	0	2	8	0	0	1	-	0.1	0	6	0.4	5	0.1	13	51	4	0.1
-	2	0	5	7	0	0	9	-	0	0	4	0.1	4	0.3	7	65	4	0.1
-	2	0	8	5	0.1	0	1	-	0.1	0	7	0.4	2	0.3	8	69	1	0.1
-	2	0	5	6	0	0	2	-	0	0	6	0.1	4	0.4	9	42	1	0.1
2	-	0	-	-	-	-	4	-	0.2	0.2	80	0.8	-	0.8	160	200	110	-
2	-	0	5	43	0	0	3	-	0	0	10	0.4	6	0.4	26	63	406	0.2
1	0	65	2	117	0.4	5.3	0	-	0.1	0.1	8	0.5	36	6.2	247	406	65	0.9
0	0	14	1	0	0.1	0.2	8	-	0	0.1	3	0.2	3	0.9	32	65	272	0.5
0	0	16	1	0	0	0.4	6	-	0	0	3	0.5	3	0.7	25	45	278	0.6
2	-	70	-	60	-	-	5	-	0.3	0.2	48	1	-	2.9	220	670	530	-
0	-	0	0	0	0	0	0	-	0	0	1	0	0	0	1	1	4	0
17	4	0	3	0	0.2	0	0	-	0.1	0.7	123	2.4	158	1.1	420	420	1	3.2
2	-	166	33	164	0.2	-	2	-	0.6	0.2	287	2.8	48	1.6	275	564	582	1.3
0	-	0	3	0	0	0	0	-	0.1	0.1	2	0.4	3	0.5	12	12	66	0.1
5	-	0	39	160	0.1	0	4	-	0.3	0.4	148	3.8	35	3.7	114	304	1070	0.7
2	-	26	7	14	0.1	0.1	1	-	0.1	0.1	11	0.8	8	0.9	34	79	119	0.2
2	-	26	12	35	0.1	0.1	0	-	0.2	0.2	162	1.6	16	1.5	110	96	428	0.4
0	1	0	10	0	0.1	0	0	-	0.1	0.1	11	0.7	13	0.9	38	44	135	0.3
0	-	0	7	0	0.1	0	0	-	0.1	0.1	11	0.7	13	0.8	38	44	135	0.3
0	1	18	19	8	0	0.1	0	-	0.2	0.2	21	1.2	9	1.2	35	37	191	0.3
0	-	0	13	0	0	0	0	-	0.1	0.2	35	1	8	1.7	32	43	231	0.3
1	1	10	0	0	0	0	0	-	0.1	0.1	28	1.4	10	1.6	34	36	136	0.3
0	1	0	11	0	0	0	0	-	0.1	0.2	42	1.1	8	1.4	41	47	182	0.3
0	-	0	8	0	0	0	0	-	0.1	0.1	11	0.9	19	1.4	56	63	312	0.4
0	-	0	5	0	0	0	0	-	0.1	0.1	58	1.2	14	1.3	39	44	112	0.3
1	-	0	10	0	0.1	0	0	-	0.1	0.1	35	0.8	28	1.2	74	90	158	0.7
0	-	20	28	9	0	0	0	-	0.2	0.2	37	1.2	8	1.9	42	46	197	0.3
0	-	21	20	9	0	0	0	-	0.2	0.1	38	1.2	8	1.8	43	47	200	0.3
0	1	0	8	0	0	0	0	-	0.1	0.1	19	0.6	7	1.2	26	28	152	0.2
0	-	0	6	0	0	0	0	-	0.1	0.1	19	0.6	7	1.1	26	28	152	0.2
0	1	0	9	0	0	0	0	-	0.1	0.1	23	0.9	8	1.3	31	33	175	0.3
0	-	0	6	0	0	0	0	-	0.1	0.1	23	0.9	8	1.2	31	33	173	0.3
0	-	0	8	0	0	0	0	-	0	0.1	13	0.7	11	0.9	28	23	81	0.2
0	-	0	5	0	0	0	0	-	0	0.1	13	0.7	10	0.8	27	23	79	0.2
0	-	0	8	0	0	-	0	-	0.1	0.1	26	0.5	7	0.7	27	35	89	0.2
0	-	0	5	0	0	0	0	-	0.1	0.1	26	0.5	6	0.6	27	35	88	0.2
0	-	0	5	0	0	0	0	-	0.1	0.1	17	0.7	4	0.6	19	23	93	0.2
0	-	0	4	0	0	0	0	-	0	0.1	17	0.7	4	0.5	19	22	92	0.2
0	3	0	6	-	0	0	0	-	0.1	0.1	18	0.7	6	0.9	-	29	118	0.2
0	-	0	4	0	0	0	0	-	0.1	0.1	18	0.7	6	0.8	21	28	116	0.2
0	2	0	8	-	0	0.1	0	-	0.1	0.1	22	0.7	6	0.8	31	17	104	0.3
0	-	0	6	0	0	0.1	0	-	0.1	0.1	21	0.7	6	0.7	30	17	102	0.3
0	2	0	12	0	0.1	0	0	-	0.1	0.1	24	0.9	14	1.1	46	53	127	0.3
0	-	0	9	0	0.1	0	0	-	0.1	0.1	24	0.9	14	1	46	53	127	0.3
1	1	0	8	0	0	0	0	-	0.1	0.2	20	0.9	9	1.4	32	34	122	0.3
1	-	0	5	-	0	0	0	-	0.1	0.1	19	0.9	9	1.3	31	33	121	0.3
0	1	0	7	1	0	-	0	-	0.1	0.1	18	0.7	10	0.8	34	38	162	0.3
0	-	0	5	1	0	0	0	-	0.1	0.1	18	0.7	10	0.8	34	39	163	0.3
0	1	0	14	0	0	0	0	-	0.2	0.4	52	1.6	6	2.8	58	72	322	0.5

Code	Food Name	Amount	Unit	Grams	kCalories	Carbohydrate (gm)	Protein (gm)	Fat (gm)	Saturated Fat (gm)	Monounsaturated Fat (gm)
18042	Bread, Pita, Whole-wheat	1	Pita	64	170	35	6	2	0	0
18044	Bread, Pumpernickel	1	Slice	32	80	15	3	1	0	0
18045	Bread, Pumpernickel, Toasted	1	Slice	29	80	15	3	1	0	0
18046	Bread, Pumpkin	1	Slice	60	199	31	2	8	1	2
18047	Bread, Raisin	1	Slice	26	71	14	2	1	0	1
18048	Bread, Raisin, Toasted	1	Slice	24	71	14	2	1	0	1
18059	Bread, Rice Bran	1	Slice	27	66	12	2	1	0	0
18384	Bread, Rice Bran, Toasted	1	Slice	25	66	12	2	1	0	0
18353	Bread, Rolls, Hard (includes Kaiser)	1	Each	57	167	30	6	2	0	1
18060	Bread, Rye	1	Slice	32	83	15	3	1	0	0
18061	Bread, Rye, Toasted	1	Slice	29	82	15	3	1	0	0
18064	Bread, Wheat (includes Wheat Berry)	1	Slice	25	65	12	2	1	0	0
18066	Bread, Wheat Bran	1	Slice	36	89	17	3	1	0	1
18067	Bread, Wheat Bran, Toasted	1	Slice	33	90	17	3	1	0	1
18065	Bread, Wheat, Toasted	1	Slice	23	65	12	2	1	0	0
18069	Bread, White	1	Slice	25	67	12	2	1	0	0
18070	Bread, White, Toasted	1	Slice	23	67	13	2	1	0	0
41348	Breaded Fish-Healthy Choice	1	Stick	9.8	15	2	1	1	-	-
43400	Breast of Chicken w/ Spanish Rice, Top Shelf-Hormel	1	Each	283.5	400	38	27	15	7	4
41252	Breast of Turkey-Healthy Choice	1	Each	297.7	290	39	21	5	2	-
62616	Broccoli and Cheese Baked Potato-Weight Watchers	1	Each	283.5	230	34	12	7	2	-
11091	Broccoli, Ckd	½	Cup	78	22	4	2	0	0	0
11740	Broccoli, Flower Clusters, Fresh	½	Cup	44	12	2	1	0	0	0
11093	Broccoli, Frz, Chopped, Ckd	½	Cup	92	26	5	3	0	0	0
18151	Brownies	1	Each	56	227	36	3	9	2	5
11099	Brussels Sprouts, Ckd	½	Cup	78	30	7	2	0	0	0
62601	Buffalo (Chicken) Wings	4	Each	91	190	2	18	12	3	-
18351	Buns, Hamburger or Hot Dog, Mixed-grain	1	Each	43	113	19	4	3	1	1
18350	Buns, Hamburger or Hot Dog, Plain	1	Each	43	123	22	4	2	1	1
18155	Butter Cookies, Enriched	1	Each	5	23	3	0	1	1	0
4136	Butter, w/ Salt	1	Pat	5	36	0	0	4	3	1
1145	Butter, w/o Salt	1	Pat	5	36	0	0	4	3	1
1002	Butter, Whipped	1	Tbsp.	11	79	0	0	9	6	3
19069	Butterfinger Bar	1	Bar	61	267	41	5	11	5	4
19070	Butterscotch Candy	1	Piece	6	24	6	0	0	0	0
18307	Butterscotch Pudding Pie	1	Slice	127	354	42	6	18	5	8
11110	Cabbage, Ckd	½	Cup	75	17	3	1	0	0	0
11749	Cabbage, Fresh	1	Cup	70	17	4	1	0	0	0
18086	Cake, Angelfood	1	Slice	28.4	73	16	2	0	0	0
18090	Cake, Boston Cream Pie	1	Slice	92	232	39	2	8	2	4
18094	Cake, Carrot, w/ Cream Cheese Frosting	1	Slice	111	484	52	5	29	5	7
18096	Cake, Chocolate w/ Chocolate Frosting	1	Slice	64	235	35	3	10	3	6
18110	Cake, Fruitcake	1	Piece	43	139	26	1	4	0	2
18113	Cake, German Chocolate, w/ Frosting	1	Slice	111	404	55	4	21	5	9
18115	Cake, Gingerbread	1	Slice	67	207	34	3	7	2	4
18119	Cake, Pineapple Upside-down	1	Slice	115	367	58	4	14	3	6
18120	Cake, Pound	1	Slice	28.4	110	14	2	6	3	2
18133	Cake, Sponge	1	Slice	38	110	23	2	1	0	0
18102	Cake, White, w/ Coconut Frosting	1	Slice	112	399	71	5	12	4	4
18139	Cake, White, w/B289o Frosting	1	Slice	74	264	42	4	9	2	4
18140	Cake, Yellow, w/ Chocolate Frosting	1	Slice	64	243	35	2	11	3	6
18141	Cake, Yellow, w/ Vanilla Frosting	1	Slice	64	239	38	2	9	2	4
55177	Canadian Style Bacon, French Bread Pizzas-Stouffer's	1	Each	163	370	40	18	15	-	-
19074	Caramels	1	Piece	8	31	6	0	1	1	0
11655	Carrot Juice, Cnd	¾	Cup	184.5	74	17	2	0	0	0
11960	Carrots, Baby, Fresh	1	Medium	10	4	1	0	0	0	0
11125	Carrots, Ckd	½	Cup	78	35	8	1	0	0	0
11128	Carrots, Cnd, Reg Pk	½	Cup	73	17	4	0	0	0	0
11124	Carrots, Fresh	1	Medium	60	26	6	1	0	0	0
11131	Carrots, Frz, Ckd	½	Cup	73	26	6	1	0	0	0

Polyunsaturated Fat (gm)	Fiber (gm)	Cholesterol (mg)	Folate (μg)	Vitamin A (re)	Vitamin B6 (mg)	Vitamin B12 (μg)	Vitamin C (mg)	Vitamin E (mg)	Riboflavin (mg)	Thiamin (mg)	Calcium (mg)	Iron (mg)	Magnesium (mg)	Niacin (mg)	Phosphorus (mg)	Potassium (mg)	Sodium (mg)	Zinc (mg)
1	5	0	22	0	0.1	0	0	-	0.1	0.2	10	1.8	44	1.8	115	109	340	1
0	2	0	11	0	0	0	0	-	0.1	0.1	22	0.9	17	1	57	67	215	0.5
0	-	0	8	0	0	0	0	-	0.1	0.1	21	0.9	17	0.9	57	66	214	0.5
4	-	26	7	334	0	0	1	-	0.1	0.1	11	1	8	0.8	32	55	188	0.2
0	1	0	9	0	0	0	0	-	0.1	0.1	17	0.8	7	0.9	28	59	101	0.2
0	-	0	6	0	0	0	0	-	0.1	0.1	17	0.8	7	0.8	28	59	102	0.2
0	-	0	8	-	0.1	0	0	-	0.1	0.2	19	1	19	1.8	43	53	119	0.3
0	-	0	6	0	0.1	0	0	-	0.1	0.1	19	1	19	1.7	44	53	120	0.3
1	-	0	9	0	0	0	0	-	0.2	0.3	54	1.9	15	2.4	57	62	310	0.5
0	2	0	16	0	0	0	-	-	0.1	0.1	23	0.9	13	1.2	40	53	211	0.4
0	-	0	11	-	0	0	0	-	0.1	0.1	23	0.9	12	1.1	40	53	210	0.4
0	1	0	10	0	0	0	0	-	0.1	0.1	26	0.8	12	1	38	50	133	0.3
0	3	0	9	0	0.1	0	0	-	0.1	0.1	27	1.1	29	1.6	67	82	175	0.5
0	-	0	7	0	0.1	0	0	-	0.1	0.1	27	1.1	29	1.4	67	82	176	0.5
0	-	0	7	0	0	0	0	-	0.1	0.1	26	0.8	12	0.9	37	50	132	0.3
0	1	0	9	0	0	-	0	-	0.1	0.1	27	0.8	6	1	24	30	135	0.2
0	-	0	6	0	0	0	0	-	0.1	0.1	27	0.8	6	0.9	24	30	136	0.2
0	3	-	-	-	-	-	-	-	0	0	-	0.1	-	0.1	-	20	31	-
3	-	75	-	100	-	-	4	-	0.3	0.1	80	0.4	35	7.6	-	584	810	1.7
-	-	45	-	40	-	-	48	-	0.3	0.5	32	1	-	5.7	270	540	420	-
-	6	10	-	200	-	-	9	-	-	-	300	0.8	-	-	-	830	510	-
0	2	0	39	108	0.1	0	58	-	0.1	0	36	0.7	19	0.4	46	228	20	0.3
0	-	0	31	132	0.1	0	41	-	0.1	0	21	0.4	11	0.3	29	143	12	0.2
0	3	0	52	174	0.1	0	37	-	0.1	0.1	47	0.6	18	0.4	51	166	22	0.3
1	1	10	7	11	0	0.1	0	-	0.1	0.1	16	1.3	17	1	57	83	175	0.4
0	3	0	47	56	0.1	0	48	-	0.1	0.1	28	0.9	16	0.5	44	247	16	0.3
-	-	100	-	60	-	-	1	-	-	-	24	0.4	-	-	-	-	900	-
0	2	0	12	0	0	0	0	-	0.1	0.2	41	1.7	21	1.9	52	65	197	0.5
0	-	0	12	0	0	0	0	-	0.1	0.2	60	1.4	9	1.7	38	61	241	0.3
0	0	4	0	8	0	0	0	-	0	0	1	0.1	1	0.2	5	6	18	0
0	0	11	0	38	0	0	0	0.1	0	0	1	0	0	0	1	1	41	0
0	0	11	0	38	0	0	0	0.1	0	0	1	0	0	0	1	1	1	0
0	0	24	0	83	0	0	0	-	0	0	3	0	0	0	3	3	91	0
2	2	1	19	12	0	0.1	2	-	0	0.1	15	0.6	27	2	58	129	83	0.4
0	0	1	0	2	0	0	0	-	0	0	0	0	0	0	0	0	3	0
4	-	77	14	107	0.1	0.4	1	-	0.3	0.2	128	1.6	22	1.3	135	221	335	0.7
0	2	0	15	10	0.1	0	15	-	0	0	23	0.1	6	0.2	11	73	6	0.1
0	-	0	40	9	0.1	0	36	-	0	0	33	0.4	11	0.2	16	172	13	0.1
0	0	0	1	0	0	-	0	-	0.1	0	40	0.1	3	0.3	66	26	212	0
1	1	34	7	21	0	0.1	0	-	0.2	0.4	21	0.3	6	0.2	45	36	132	0.1
15	-	60	13	426	0.1	0.1	1	-	0.2	0.2	28	1.4	20	1.1	79	124	273	0.5
1	2	29	5	18	-	0.1	0	-	0.1	0.1	28	1.4	22	0.4	78	128	214	0.4
1	2	2	1	8	0	0	0	-	0	0	14	0.9	7	0.3	22	66	116	0.1
5	-	53	4	23	0	0.1	0	-	0.1	0.1	53	1.2	19	1.1	173	151	369	0.5
1	2	23	7	11	0	0	0	-	0.1	0.1	46	2.2	11	1	113	161	307	0.3
4	-	25	8	75	0	0.1	1	-	0.2	0.2	138	1.7	15	1.4	94	129	367	0.4
0	-	63	3	44	0	0.1	0	-	0.1	0	10	0.4	3	0.4	39	34	113	0.1
0	-	39	5	17	0	0.1	0	-	0.1	0.1	27	1	4	0.7	52	38	93	0.2
2	-	1	6	12	0	0.1	0	-	0.2	0.1	101	1.3	13	1.2	78	111	318	0.4
2	-	1	5	12	0	0.1	0	-	0.2	0.1	96	1.1	9	1.1	69	70	242	0.2
1	1	35	5	17	0	0.1	0	-	0.1	0.1	24	1.3	19	0.8	103	114	216	0.4
3	-	36	6	12	0	0.1	0	-	0	0.1	40	0.7	4	0.3	92	34	220	0.2
-	-	-	-	80	-	-	6	-	0.4	0.6	160	1	-	3.8	-	300	1070	-
0	0	1	0	1	0	0	0	-	0	0	11	0	1	0	9	17	20	0
0	1	0	7	4751	0.4	0	16	-	0.1	0.2	44	0.8	26	0.7	77	539	54	0.3
0	-	0	3	20	0	0	1	-	0	0	2	0.1	1	0.1	4	28	4	0
0	3	0	11	1915	0.2	0	2	-	0	0	24	0.5	10	0.4	23	177	51	0.2
0	1	0	7	1005	0.1	0	2	-	0	0	18	0.5	6	0.4	18	131	176	0.2
0	2	0	8	1688	0.1	0	6	-	0	0.1	16	0.3	9	0.6	26	194	21	0.1
0	3	0	8	1292	0.1	0	2	-	0	0	20	0.3	7	0.6	19	115	43	0.2

Code	Food Name	Amount	Unit	Grams	kCalories	Carbohydrate (gm)	Protein (gm)	Fat (gm)	Saturated Fat (gm)	Monounsaturated Fat (gm)
12585	Cashew Dry Roasted	½	Cup	68.5	393	22	10	32	6	19
12586	Cashew Oil Roasted	½	Cup	65	374	19	10	31	6	18
15235	Catfish, Channel, Farmed, Ckd, Dry Heat	3	Ounce	85.1	129	0	16	7	2	4
15233	Catfish, Channel, Wild, Ckd, Dry Heat	3	Ounce	85.1	89	0	16	2	1	1
15011	Catfish, Fried	3	Ounce	85.1	195	7	15	11	3	5
11935	Catsup	1	Tbsp.	15	16	4	0	0	0	0
11949	Catsup, Low Sodium	1	Tbsp.	15	16	4	0	0	0	0
11136	Cauliflower, Ckd, Boiled	½	Cup	62	14	3	1	0	0	0
11135	Cauliflower, Fresh	½	Cup	50	13	3	1	0	0	0
11138	Cauliflower, Frz, Ckd	½	Cup	90	17	3	1	0	0	0
15012	Caviar, Black and Red, Granular	1	Tbsp.	16	40	1	4	3	1	1
11144	Celery, Ckd	½	Cup	75	14	3	1	0	0	0
11143	Celery, Fresh	½	Cup	60	10	2	0	0	0	0
8053	Cereals, 100% Bran	1	Cup	66	178	48	8	3	1	1
8054	Cereals, 100% Natural Cereal, Plain	1	Cup	104	489	65	12	22	15	4
8055	Cereals, 100% Natural Cereal, w/ Apple and Cinn.	1	Cup	104	477	70	11	20	15	2
8056	Cereals, 100% Natural Cereal, w/ Raisins and Dates	1	Cup	110	496	72	11	20	14	4
8028	Cereals, 40% Bran Flakes, Kellogg's	1	Cup	39	127	31	5	1	-	-
8029	Cereals, 40% Bran Flakes, Post	1	Cup	47	152	37	5	1	-	-
8153	Cereals, 40% Bran Flakes, Ralston Purina	1	Cup	49	159	39	6	1	-	-
8001	Cereals, All-bran	1	Cup	85.2	212	63	12	2	-	-
8006	Cereals, Bran Chex	1	Cup	49	156	39	5	1	-	-
8008	Cereals, C.W. Post, Plain	1	Cup	97	432	69	9	15	11	2
8009	Cereals, C.W. Post, w/ Raisins	1	Cup	103	446	74	9	15	11	2
8010	Cereals, Cap'n Crunch	1	Cup	37	156	30	2	3	2	0
8011	Cereals, Cap'n Crunch's Crunchberries	1	Cup	35	146	29	2	3	2	0
8012	Cereals, Cap'n Crunch's Peanut Butter	1	Cup	35	154	26	3	5	2	1
8013	Cereals, Cheerios	1	Cup	22.7	89	16	3	1	0	1
8014	Cereals, Cocoa Krispies	1	Cup	36	139	32	2	1	-	-
8017	Cereals, Cookie-crisp, Choc Chip and Van.	1	Cup	30	120	26	2	1	-	-
8018	Cereals, Corn Bran	1	Cup	36	125	30	2	1	-	-
8019	Cereals, Corn Chex	1	Cup	28.4	111	25	2	0	-	-
8020	Cereals, Corn Flakes, Kellogg's	1	Cup	22.7	88	20	2	0	-	-
8022	Cereals, Corn Flakes, Low Sodium	1	Cup	25	100	22	2	0	-	-
8021	Cereals, Corn Flakes, Ralston Purina	1	Cup	25	98	22	2	0	-	-
8023	Cereals, Cracklin' Bran	1	Cup	60	229	41	6	9	-	-
8168	Cereals, Cream Of Rice, Ckd	1	Cup	244	127	28	2	0	-	-
8171	Cereals, Cream Of Wheat, Instant	1	Cup	241	154	32	4	0	-	-
8170	Cereals, Cream Of Wheat, Quick	1	Cup	239	129	27	4	0	-	-
8169	Cereals, Cream Of Wheat, Regular	1	Cup	251	133	28	4	1	-	-
8024	Cereals, Crisp Rice, Low Sodium	1	Cup	26	105	24	1	0	-	-
8025	Cereals, Crispy Rice	1	Cup	28	111	25	2	0	-	-
8026	Cereals, Crispy Wheats 'n Raisins	1	Cup	43	150	35	3	1	-	-
8027	Cereals, Fortified Oat Flakes	1	Cup	48	177	35	9	1	-	-
8030	Cereals, Fruit Loops	1	Cup	28.4	111	25	2	1	-	-
8035	Cereals, Golden Grahams	1	Cup	39	150	33	2	1	1	0
8036	Cereals, Graham Crackos	1	Cup	30	108	26	2	0	-	-
8037	Cereals, Granola, Homemade	1	Cup	122	594	67	15	33	6	9
8038	Cereals, Grape-nuts	1	Cup	113.6	406	93	13	0	-	-
8039	Cereals, Grape-nuts Flakes	1	Cup	32.5	116	27	3	0	-	-
8040	Cereals, Heartland Natural Cereal, Plain	1	Cup	115	499	79	12	18	-	-
8041	Cereals, Heartland Natural Cereal, w/ Cocnt	1	Cup	105	463	71	11	17	-	-
8042	Cereals, Heartland Natural Cereal, w/ Raisins	1	Cup	110	468	76	11	16	-	-
8043	Cereals, Honey and Nut Corn Flakes	1	Cup	37.9	151	31	2	2	-	-
8045	Cereals, Honey Nut Cheerios	1	Cup	33	125	26	4	1	0	0
8044	Cereals, Honeybran	1	Cup	35	119	29	3	1	-	-
8046	Cereals, Honeycomb	1	Cup	22	86	20	1	0	-	-
8048	Cereals, Kix	1	Cup	18.9	74	16	2	0	0	0
8049	Cereals, Life, Plain and Cinn Products	1	Cup	44	162	32	8	1	-	-
8050	Cereals, Lucky Charms	1	Cup	32	125	26	3	1	0	0

Polyunsaturated Fat (gm)	Fiber (gm)	Cholesterol (mg)	Folate (µg)	Vitamin A (re)	Vitamin B6 (mg)	Vitamin B12 (µg)	Vitamin C (mg)	Vitamin E (mg)	Riboflavin (mg)	Thiamin (mg)	Calcium (mg)	Iron (mg)	Magnesium (mg)	Niacin (mg)	Phosphorus (mg)	Potassium (mg)	Sodium (mg)	Zinc (mg)
5	2	0	47	0	0.2	0	0	-	0.1	0.1	31	4.1	178	1	336	387	438	3.8
5	2	0	44	0	0.2	0	0	-	0.1	0.3	27	2.7	166	1.2	277	345	407	3.1
1	0	54	6	13	0.1	2.4	1	-	0.1	0.4	8	0.7	22	2.1	208	273	68	0.9
1	0	61	9	13	0.1	2.5	1	-	0.1	0.2	9	0.3	24	2	259	356	43	0.5
3	-	69	14	7	0.2	1.6	0	-	0.1	0.1	37	1.2	23	1.9	184	289	238	0.7
0	0	0	2	15	0	0	2	-	0	0	3	0.1	3	0.2	6	72	178	0
0	0	0	2	15	0	0	2	-	0	0	3	0.1	3	0.2	6	72	3	0
0	2	0	27	1	0.1	0	27	-	0	0	10	0.2	6	0.3	20	88	9	0.1
0	1	0	29	1	0.1	0	23	-	0	0	11	0.2	8	0.3	22	152	15	0.1
0	2	0	37	2	0.1	0	28	-	0	0	15	0.4	8	0.3	22	125	16	0.1
1	0	94	8	90	0.1	3.2	0	-	0.1	0	44	1.9	48	0	57	29	240	0.2
0	1	0	17	10	0.1	0	5	-	0	0	32	0.3	9	0.2	19	213	68	0.1
0	1	0	17	8	0.1	0	4	-	0	0	24	0.2	7	0.2	15	172	52	0.1
2	20	0	47	0	2.1	6.3	63	-	1.8	1.6	46	8.1	312	20.9	801	824	457	5.7
2	9	1	31	-	0.2	0.1	0	-	0.6	0.3	181	3.1	125	2.4	383	514	45	2.4
1	7	1	17	-	0.1	0.3	1	-	0.6	0.3	157	2.9	72	1.9	350	514	52	2
2	7	1	45	-	0.2	0.1	0	-	0.6	0.3	160	3.1	124	2.1	348	538	47	2.1
-	5	0	138	516	0.7	2.1	0	-	0.6	0.5	19	24.8	71	6.9	192	248	303	5.1
-	9	0	166	622	0.8	2.5	0	-	0.7	0.6	21	7.5	102	8.3	296	251	431	2.5
-	7	0	173	649	0.9	2.6	26	-	0.7	0.6	23	7.8	118	8.6	273	286	456	2
-	30	0	301	1128	1.5	0	45	-	1.3	1.1	69	13.5	318	15	794	1051	961	11.2
-	8	0	173	11	0.9	2.6	26	-	0.3	0.6	29	7.8	126	8.6	327	394	455	2.1
1	7	0	342	1284	1.7	5.1	0	-	1.5	1.3	47	15.4	67	17.1	224	198	167	1.6
1	14	0	364	1364	1.9	5.5	0	-	1.5	1.3	50	16.4	74	18.1	232	261	161	1.6
1	1	0	238	5	1	2.3	0	-	0.7	0.7	6	9.8	15	8.6	47	48	278	4
0	1	0	128	5	0.9	2.5	0	-	0.7	0.6	11	9	14	8.1	47	49	244	3.6
1	0	0	244	6	1	2.3	0	-	0.7	0.6	7	9.1	19	9	49	57	268	3.8
1	2	0	5	301	0.4	1.2	12	-	0.3	0.3	39	3.6	31	4	107	81	246	0.6
-	0	0	127	477	0.6	0	19	-	0.5	0.5	6	2.3	12	6.3	47	53	275	1.9
-	0	0	3	397	0.5	1.6	16	-	0.4	0.4	6	4.8	8	5.3	24	29	207	0.3
-	7	0	232	8	0.9	1.4	0	-	0.7	0.4	41	12.2	18	10.9	52	70	310	4
-	1	0	100	14	0.5	1.5	15	-	0.1	0.4	3	1.8	4	5	11	23	272	0.1
-	1	0	80	301	0.4	0	12	-	0.3	0.3	1	1.4	3	4	14	21	232	0.1
-	0	0	2	10	0	0	0	-	0	0	11	0.6	3	0.1	12	18	3	0.1
-	0	0	2	10	0	0	0	-	0	0.1	2	0.6	3	1.1	10	22	239	0.1
-	10	0	212	794	1.1	0	32	-	0.9	0.8	40	3.8	116	10.6	241	355	487	3.2
-	-	0	7	0	0.1	0	0	-	0	0	7	0.5	7	1	41	49	422	0.4
-	-	0	10	0	0	0	0	-	0	0.2	60	12.1	14	1.7	43	48	364	0.4
-	-	0	10	0	0	0	0	-	0	0.2	50	10.3	12	1.4	100	45	464	0.3
-	-	0	10	0	0	0	0	-	0	0.3	50	10.3	10	1.5	43	43	336	0.3
-	-	0	3	0	0	0	0	-	0	0	17	0.8	10	0.4	27	20	3	0.4
-	0	0	3	0	0	0.1	1	-	0	0.1	5	0.7	12	2	31	27	206	0.5
-	3	0	15	569	0.8	2.3	0	-	0.6	0.6	71	6.8	34	7.6	117	174	204	0.5
-	1	0	169	636	0.9	2.5	0	-	0.7	0.6	68	13.7	58	8.4	176	343	429	1.5
-	1	0	100	376	0.5	0	15	-	0.4	0.4	3	4.5	7	5	24	26	145	3.7
0	1	0	6	516	0.7	2.1	21	-	0.6	0.5	24	6.2	16	6.9	56	86	385	0.3
-	2	0	106	397	0.5	0	16	-	0.4	0.4	14	1.9	25	5.3	66	108	196	1.6
17	13	0	99	-	0.4	0	1	-	0.3	0.7	76	4.8	142	2.1	494	612	12	4.5
-	11	0	401	1504	2	6	0	-	1.7	1.5	11	4.9	76	20	285	379	790	2.5
-	3	0	115	430	0.6	1.7	0	-	0.5	0.4	13	9.3	36	5.7	97	113	183	0.6
-	7	0	64	-	0.2	0	1	-	0.2	0.4	75	4.3	147	1.6	416	385	293	3
-	7	0	57	-	0.2	0	1	-	0.1	0.3	66	5.4	138	1.8	380	384	213	2.7
-	6	0	44	-	0.2	0	1	-	0.1	0.3	66	4	141	1.5	376	415	226	2.8
-	0	0	134	501	0.7	0	20	-	0.6	0.5	5	2.4	8	6.7	17	48	301	0.1
0	1	0	21	437	0.6	1.7	17	-	0.5	0.4	23	5.2	39	5.8	122	115	299	0.9
-	4	0	23	463	0.6	1.9	19	-	0.5	0.5	16	5.6	46	6.2	132	151	202	0.9
-	1	0	78	291	0.4	1.2	0	-	0.3	0.3	4	2.1	7	3.9	22	70	124	1.2
0	0	0	67	251	0.3	1	10	-	0.3	0.2	24	5.4	8	3.3	26	30	194	0.2
-	3	0	37	-	0.1	0	-	-	1	1	154	11.6	14	11.6	238	197	229	1.5
0	1	0	6	424	0.6	1.7	17	-	0.5	0.4	36	5.1	27	5.6	89	166	227	0.6

Code	Food Name	Amount	Unit	Grams	kCalories	Carbohydrate (gm)	Protein (gm)	Fat (gm)	Saturated Fat (gm)	Monounsaturated Fat (gm)
8178	Cereals, Malt-o-meal, Plain and Choc	1	Cup	240	122	26	4	0	-	-
8179	Cereals, Maypo, Ckd w/ water, w/ Salt	1	Cup	240	170	32	6	2	-	-
8119	Cereals, Maypo, Ckd w/ water, w/o Salt	1	Cup	240	170	32	6	2	-	-
8051	Cereals, Most Brand	1	Cup	52	175	40	7	1	-	-
8052	Cereals, Nature Valley Granola	1	Cup	113	503	75	12	20	13	3
8149	Cereals, Nutri-grain, Barley	1	Cup	41	153	34	4	0	-	-
8150	Cereals, Nutri-grain, Corn	1	Cup	42	160	35	3	1	-	-
8151	Cereals, Nutri-grain, Rye	1	Cup	40	144	34	3	0	-	-
8152	Cereals, Nutri-grain, Wheat	1	Cup	44	158	37	4	0	-	-
8123	Cereals, Oats, Instant, Plain	1	Pkt.	177	104	18	4	2	-	-
8125	Cereals, Oats, Instant, w/ Apples and cinn	1	Pkt.	149	136	26	4	2	-	-
8127	Cereals, Oats, Instant, w/ bran&rsns	1	Pkt.	195	158	30	5	2	-	-
8129	Cereals, Oats, Instant, w/ cinn and spice	1	Pkt.	161	177	35	5	2	-	-
8131	Cereals, Oats, Instant, w/ mapl&brn sug flav	1	Pkt.	155	163	32	5	2	-	-
8133	Cereals, Oats, Instant, w/ raisins and spice	1	Pkt	158	161	32	4	2	-	-
8180	Cereals, Oats, Reg and Quick and Instant	1	Cup	234	145	25	6	2	0	1
8058	Cereals, Product 19	1	Cup	33	126	27	3	0	-	-
8059	Cereals, Quisp	1	Cup	30	124	25	2	2	1	0
8060	Cereals, Raisin Bran, Kellogg's	1	Cup	49.2	154	37	5	1	-	-
8061	Cereals, Raisin Bran, Post	1	Cup	56.8	174	43	5	1	-	-
8062	Cereals, Raisin Bran, Ralston Purina	1	Cup	56	178	46	4	0	-	-
8063	Cereals, Raisins, Rice and Rye	1	Cup	46	155	39	3	0	-	-
8064	Cereals, Rice Chex	1	Cup	25.2	100	23	1	0	-	-
8065	Cereals, Rice Krispies	1	Cup	28.4	112	25	2	0	-	-
8156	Cereals, Rice, Puffed	1	Cup	14	56	13	1	0	-	-
8067	Cereals, Special K	1	Cup	21.3	83	16	4	0	-	-
8068	Cereals, Sugar Corn Pops	1	Cup	28.4	108	26	1	0	-	-
8069	Cereals, Sugar Frosted Flakes	1	Cup	35	133	32	2	0	-	-
8074	Cereals, Tasteeos	1	Cup	24	94	19	3	1	-	-
8075	Cereals, Team	1	Cup	42	164	36	3	1	-	-
8077	Cereals, Total	1	Cup	33	116	26	3	1	0	0
8078	Cereals, Trix	1	Cup	28	108	25	2	0	-	-
8080	Cereals, Wheat 'n Raisin Chex	1	Cup	54	185	43	5	0	-	-
8082	Cereals, Wheat Chex	1	Cup	46	169	38	5	1	-	-
8147	Cereals, Wheat, Shredded, Large Biscuit	1	Biscuit	23.6	83	19	3	0	-	-
8148	Cereals, Wheat, Shredded, Small Biscuit	1	Cup	33.1	119	26	4	1	-	-
8143	Cereals, Wheatena, Ckd w/ water	1	Cup	243	136	29	5	1	-	-
8182	Cereals, Wheatena, Ckd w/ water, w/ Salt	1	Cup	243	136	29	5	1	-	-
8089	Cereals, Wheaties	1	Cup	29	101	23	3	0	0	0
8183	Cereals, Whole Wheat Hot Natural Cereal	1	Cup	242	150	33	5	1	-	-
55832	Cheddar Cheese Sauce-Stouffer's	1	Cup	283.9	731	22	26	60	-	-
55764	Cheddar Cheese Soup-Stouffer's	1	Cup	283.9	441	18	21	31	-	-
55772	Cheddar Cheese, Heat'n Serve Soup -Stouffer's	1	Cup	307.6	488	22	22	36	-	-
55196	Cheese Cannelloni, Lean Cuisine-Stouffer's	1	Each	258.7	270	27	23	8	4	-
55108	Cheese Enchiladas-Stouffer's	1	Each	276.4	490	33	23	29	-	-
41331	Cheese French Bread Pizza-Healthy Choice	1	Each	159.5	290	46	19	4	2	-
41300	Cheese Manicotti-Healthy Choice	1	Each	262.2	220	34	15	3	2	-
55796	Cheese Manicotti-Stouffer's	1	Ounce	28.4	29	3	2	1	-	-
55822	Cheese Ravioli-Stouffer's	1	Ounce	28.4	54	6	3	2	-	-
1150	Cheese Spread, Past. Processed, American	2	Ounce	56.7	165	5	9	12	8	4
55808	Cheese Stuffed Shells-Stouffer's	1	Ounce	28.4	28	3	2	1	-	-
55819	Cheese Tortellini w/ Egg Pasta-Stouffer's	1	Each	145.3	212	22	11	8	-	-
55821	Cheese Tortellini w/ Spinach Pasta-Stouffer's	1	Ounce	28.4	56	6	3	2	-	-
1147	Cheese, American, Pastuerized Processed	2	Ounce	56.7	213	1	13	18	11	5
1004	Cheese, Blue	1½	Ounce	42.5	150	1	9	12	8	3
1005	Cheese, Brick	1½	Ounce	42.5	158	1	10	13	8	4
1006	Cheese, Brie	1½	Ounce	42.5	142	0	9	12	7	3
1008	Cheese, Caraway	1½	Ounce	42.5	160	1	11	12	8	4
1009	Cheese, Cheddar, American Domestic	1½	Ounce	42.5	171	1	11	14	9	4
62577	Cheese, Cheddar, Reduced Fat	1½	Ounce	42.5	120	2	12	8	5	-

Polyunsaturated Fat (gm)	Fiber (gm)	Cholesterol (mg)	Folate (μg)	Vitamin A (re)	Vitamin B6 (mg)	Vitamin B12 (μg)	Vitamin C (mg)	Vitamin E (mg)	Riboflavin (mg)	Thiamin (mg)	Calcium (mg)	Iron (mg)	Magnesium (mg)	Niacin (mg)	Phosphorus (mg)	Potassium (mg)	Sodium (mg)	Zinc (mg)
-	-	0	5	0	0	0	0	-	0.2	0.5	5	9.6	5	5.8	24	31	324	0.2
-	-	0	10	703	1	2.9	29	-	0.7	0.7	125	8.4	50	9.4	247	211	259	1.5
-	6	0	10	703	1	2.9	29	-	0.7	0.7	125	8.4	50	9.4	247	211	10	1.5
-	7	0	734	2754	3.7	11	110	-	3.1	2.8	79	33	103	36.7	361	340	276	2.8
3	6	0	85	-	0.1	0	0	-	0.2	0.4	71	3.8	115	0.8	354	389	233	2.2
-	2	0	145	543	0.7	2.2	22	-	0.6	0.5	11	1.4	32	7.2	126	108	277	5.4
-	3	0	148	556	0.8	2.2	22	-	0.6	0.5	1	0.9	27	7.4	121	98	276	5.5
-	3	0	141	530	0.7	2.1	21	-	0.6	0.5	8	1.1	30	7	104	72	272	5.3
-	3	0	155	583	0.8	2.3	23	-	0.7	0.6	12	1.2	34	7.7	165	120	299	5.8
-	3	0	150	453	0.7	0	0	-	0.3	0.5	163	6.3	42	5.5	133	99	285	0.9
-	-	0	137	435	0.7	0	0	-	0.3	0.5	158	6.1	34	5.1	118	107	222	0.7
-	-	0	156	480	0.8	0	0	-	0.6	0.6	174	7.6	57	8.1	207	236	248	1.3
-	3	0	153	473	0.8	0	0	-	0.3	0.6	172	6.6	52	5.7	145	105	280	1
-	-	0	146	451	0.7	0	0	-	0.3	0.5	161	6.4	42	5.3	143	102	279	0.9
-	2	0	150	441	0.7	0	0	-	0.4	0.5	166	6.6	36	5.5	133	150	226	0.7
1	1	0	9	-	0	0	0	-	0	0.3	19	1.6	56	0.3	178	131	374	1.1
-	1	0	466	1748	2.3	7	70	-	2	1.7	4	21	12	23.3	47	51	378	0.5
0	1	0	8	5	0.9	2.6	0	-	0.8	0.5	9	6.3	12	5.8	25	45	241	0.2
-	5	0	133	500	0.7	2	0	-	0.6	0.5	17	22.3	63	6.7	183	256	273	5
-	8	0	201	752	1	3	0	-	0.9	0.7	27	9	97	10	238	350	370	3
-	8	0	148	556	0.7	2.2	2	-	0.6	0.6	27	27.3	85	7.4	248	287	486	1.7
-	3	0	125	468	0.6	1.9	0	-	0.6	0.5	10	5.6	20	6.3	50	144	350	4.7
-	0	0	89	2	0.5	1.3	13	-	0	0.3	4	1.6	6	4.4	25	29	211	0.3
-	0	0	100	376	0.5	0	15	-	0.4	0.4	4	1.8	10	5	34	30	341	0.5
-	-	0	3	0	0	0	0	-	0.3	0.4	1	4.4	4	4.9	14	16	0	0.1
-	1	0	75	282	0.4	0	11	-	0.3	0.3	6	3.4	12	3.7	41	37	199	2.8
-	0	0	100	376	0.5	0	15	-	0.4	0.4	1	1.8	2	5	28	17	104	1.5
-	1	0	124	463	0.6	0	19	-	0.5	0.5	1	2.2	3	6.2	26	22	284	0
-	3	0	9	318	0.4	1.3	13	-	0.4	0.3	11	3.8	26	4.2	96	71	183	0.7
-	1	0	7	556	0.8	2.2	22	-	0.6	0.5	6	2.6	18	7.4	65	71	260	0.6
0	4	0	466	1748	2.3	7	70	-	2	1.7	282	21	37	23.3	137	123	326	0.8
-	0	0	3	371	0.5	1.5	15	-	0.4	0.4	6	4.5	6	4.9	19	26	179	0.1
-	4	0	143	0	0.7	2.2	2	-	0.6	0.5	24	7.7	53	7.1	163	227	306	1.2
-	4	0	162	0	0.8	2.4	24	-	0.2	0.6	18	7.3	58	8.1	182	173	308	1.2
-	2	0	12	0	0.1	0	0	-	0.1	0.1	10	0.7	40	1.1	86	77	0	0.6
-	3	0	17	0	0.1	0	0	-	0.1	0.1	13	1.4	44	1.7	117	120	3	1.1
-	7	0	17	0	0	0	0	-	0	0	10	1.4	49	1.3	146	187	5	1.7
-	-	0	17	0	0	0	0	-	0	0	10	1.4	49	1.3	146	187	578	1.7
0	3	0	102	384	0.5	1.5	15	-	0.4	0.4	44	4.6	32	5.1	100	108	276	0.6
-	-	0	27	0	0.2	0	0	-	0.1	0.2	17	1.5	53	2.2	167	172	564	1.2
-	-	130	-	-	-	-	0	-	0	0	6329	0.1	-	0	-	341	1392	-
-	-	70	-	-	-	-	0	-	0	0	4967	0	-	0.2	-	511	681	-
-	-	98	-	-	-	-	0	-	0	0	4947	0.1	-	0.2	-	553	770	-
-	-	25	60	-	-	-	21	-	0.3	0.1	240	0.4	-	1.5	-	400	590	-
-	-	-	150	-	-	-	6	-	0.3	0.1	480	0.8	-	1.5	-	400	550	-
1	-	15	-	20	-	-	0	-	0.3	0.5	240	2	-	2.9	240	310	390	-
-	-	30	-	250	-	-	6	-	0.3	0.3	120	1.5	-	1.9	210	590	310	-
-	-	4	-	-	-	-	2	-	0	0	296	0	-	0	-	45	108	-
-	-	14	-	-	-	-	0	-	0	0	336	0	-	0	-	16	52	-
0	0	31	4	107	0.1	0.2	0	-	0.2	0	319	0.2	16	0.1	496	137	921	1.5
-	-	3	-	-	-	-	1	-	0	0	248	0	-	0.1	-	53	59	-
-	-	63	-	-	-	-	0	-	0	0	1524	0.1	-	0.2	-	71	272	-
-	-	19	-	-	-	-	0	-	0	0	456	0	-	0.1	-	26	79	-
1	0	54	4	164	0	0.4	0	-	0.2	0	349	0.2	13	0	252	92	369	1.7
0	0	32	15	97	0.1	0.5	0	-	0.2	0	224	0.1	10	0.4	165	109	593	1.1
0	0	40	9	128	0	0.5	0	-	0.1	0	286	0.2	10	0.1	192	58	238	1.1
0	0	43	28	77	0.1	0.7	0	-	0.2	0	78	0.2	9	0.2	80	65	268	1
0	0	40	8	123	0	0.1	0	-	0.2	0	286	0.3	9	0.1	208	40	293	1.3
0	0	45	8	129	0	0.4	0	-	0.2	0	307	0.3	12	0	218	42	264	1.3
-	0	23	-	90	-	-	-	-	-	-	360	0	-	-	-	35	270	-

Code	Food Name	Amount	Unit	Grams	kCalories	Carbohydrate (gm)	Protein (gm)	Fat (gm)	Saturated Fat (gm)	Monounsaturated Fat (gm)
1011	Cheese, Colby	1½	Ounce	42.5	167	1	10	14	9	4
1012	Cheese, Cottage, Creamed	1½	Ounce	42.5	44	1	5	2	1	1
1013	Cheese, Cottage, Creamed, w/ Fruit	1½	Ounce	42.5	53	6	4	1	1	0
1016	Cheese, Cottage, Lowfat, 1% Fat	1½	Ounce	42.5	31	1	5	0	0	0
1015	Cheese, Cottage, Lowfat, 2% Fat	1½	Ounce	42.5	38	2	6	1	1	0
1014	Cheese, Cottage, Uncreamed, Dry	1½	Ounce	42.5	36	1	7	0	0	0
1017	Cheese, Cream	1½	Ounce	42.5	148	1	3	15	9	4
62554	Cheese, Cream, Fat Free	2	Tbsp.	35	35	2	5	0	0	-
62553	Cheese, Cream, Light	2	Tbsp.	32	70	2	3	5	4	-
1018	Cheese, Edam	1½	Ounce	42.5	152	1	11	12	7	3
62579	Cheese, Fat Free Slices, White	1	Slice	21.3	30	2	5	0	0	-
62578	Cheese, Fat Free Slices, Yellow	1	Slice	21.3	30	2	5	0	0	-
1019	Cheese, Feta	1½	Ounce	42.5	112	2	6	9	6	2
1020	Cheese, Fontina	1½	Ounce	42.5	165	1	11	13	8	4
1156	Cheese, Goat, Hard Type	1½	Ounce	42.5	192	1	13	15	10	3
1157	Cheese, Goat, Semisoft Type	1½	Ounce	42.5	155	1	9	13	9	3
1159	Cheese, Goat, Soft Type	1½	Ounce	42.5	114	0	8	9	6	2
1022	Cheese, Gouda	1½	Ounce	42.5	152	1	11	12	7	3
1023	Cheese, Gruyere	1½	Ounce	42.5	176	0	13	14	8	4
1024	Cheese, Limburger	1½	Ounce	42.5	139	0	9	12	7	4
1025	Cheese, Monterey	1½	Ounce	42.5	159	0	10	13	8	4
62576	Cheese, Monterey, Reduced Fat	1½	Ounce	42.5	120	2	12	8	5	-
1028	Cheese, Mozzarella, Part Skim Milk	1½	Ounce	42.5	108	1	10	7	4	2
1029	Cheese, Mozzarella, Part Skim Milk, Low Moisture	1½	Ounce	42.5	119	1	12	7	5	2
1026	Cheese, Mozzarella, Whole Milk	1½	Ounce	42.5	120	1	8	9	6	3
1027	Cheese, Mozzarella, Whole Milk, Low Moisture	1½	Ounce	42.5	135	1	9	10	7	3
1161	Cheese, Mozzarella, Substitute	1½	Ounce	42.5	105	10	5	5	2	3
1030	Cheese, Muenster	1½	Ounce	42.5	157	0	10	13	8	4
1032	Cheese, Parmesan, Grated	1	Tbsp.	5	23	0	2	2	1	0
62608	Cheese, Parmesan, Grated, Fat Free	1	Tbsp.	5	5	1	1	0	0	0
1033	Cheese, Parmesan, Piece	1½	Ounce	42.5	167	1	15	11	7	3
1146	Cheese, Parmesan, Shredded	1½	Ounce	42.5	176	1	16	12	7	4
1035	Cheese, Provolone	1½	Ounce	42.5	149	1	11	11	7	3
1037	Cheese, Ricotta, Part Skim Milk	1½	Ounce	42.5	59	2	5	3	2	1
1036	Cheese, Ricotta, Whole Milk	1½	Ounce	42.5	74	1	5	6	4	2
1038	Cheese, Romano	1½	Ounce	42.5	164	2	14	11	7	3
1039	Cheese, Roquefort	1½	Ounce	42.5	157	1	9	13	8	4
1040	Cheese, Swiss, Domestic	1½	Ounce	42.5	160	1	12	12	8	3
1044	Cheese, Swiss, Pasteurized Processed	2	Ounce	56.7	189	1	14	14	9	4
18147	Cheesecake, Commercially Prepared	1	Slice	85	273	22	5	19	10	7
18149	Cheesecake, Homemade	1	Slice	85	303	21	6	22	12	7
18148	Cheesecake, No-bake Type	1	Slice	80	219	28	4	10	6	3
18382	Cheesecake, Plain, w/ Cherry Topping	1	Slice	90	258	24	5	17	9	5
9066	Cherries, Sour, Red, Cnd, Heavy Syrup Pack	½	Cup	128	116	30	1	0	0	0
9065	Cherries, Sour, Red, Cnd, Light Syrup Pack	½	Cup	126	95	24	1	0	0	0
9064	Cherries, Sour, Red, Cnd, Water Pack	½	Cup	122	44	11	1	0	0	0
9067	Cherries, Sour, Red, Cnd, X-heavy Syrup Pack	½	Cup	130.5	149	38	1	0	0	0
9063	Cherries, Sour, Red, Fresh	½	Cup	51.5	26	6	1	0	0	0
9074	Cherries, Sweet, Cnd, Heavy Syrup Pack	½	Cup	128.5	107	27	1	0	0	0
9072	Cherries, Sweet, Cnd, Juice Pack	½	Cup	125	67	17	1	0	0	0
9073	Cherries, Sweet, Cnd, Light Syrup Pack	½	Cup	126	84	22	1	0	0	0
9071	Cherries, Sweet, Cnd, Water Pack	½	Cup	124	57	15	1	0	0	0
9075	Cherries, Sweet, Cnd, X-heavy Syrup Pack	½	Cup	130.5	133	34	1	0	0	0
9070	Cherries, Sweet, Fresh	½	Cup	72.5	52	12	1	1	0	0
9076	Cherries, Sweet, Frozen, Sweetened	½	Cup	129.5	115	29	1	0	0	0
18308	Cherry Pie	1	Slice	125	325	50	3	14	3	7
18444	Cherry Pie, Fried	1	Pie	128	404	55	4	21	3	10
19163	Chewing Gum	1	Stick	3	10	3	0	0	-	-
19033	Chex Mix	1	Cup	42.5	181	28	5	7	-	-
55109	Chicken a la King w/ Rice-Stouffer's	1	Each	269.3	270	38	18	5	-	-

Polyunsaturated Fat (gm)	Fiber (gm)	Cholesterol (mg)	Folate (µg)	Vitamin A (re)	Vitamin B6 (mg)	Vitamin B12 (µg)	Vitamin C (mg)	Vitamin E (mg)	Riboflavin (mg)	Thiamin (mg)	Calcium (mg)	Iron (mg)	Magnesium (mg)	Niacin (mg)	Phosphorus (mg)	Potassium (mg)	Sodium (mg)	Zinc (mg)
0	0	40	8	117	0	0.4	0	-	0.2	0	291	0.3	11	0	194	54	257	1.3
0	0	6	5	20	0	0.3	0	-	0.1	0	26	0.1	2	0.1	56	36	172	0.2
0	0	5	4	15	0	0.2	0	-	0.1	0	20	0	2	0	44	28	172	0.1
0	0	2	5	5	0	0.3	0	-	0.1	0	26	0.1	2	0.1	57	36	173	0.2
0	0	4	6	9	0	0.3	0	-	0.1	0	29	0.1	3	0.1	64	41	173	0.2
0	0	3	6	3	0	0.4	0	-	0.1	0	13	0.1	2	0.1	44	14	5	0.2
1	0	47	6	186	0	0.2	0	-	0.1	0	34	0.5	3	0	44	51	126	0.2
-	-	5	-	100	-	-	0	-	-	-	120	0	-	-	-	-	180	-
-	-	15	-	80	-	-	0	-	-	-	48	0	-	-	-	-	150	-
0	0	38	7	108	0	0.7	0	-	0.2	0	311	0.2	13	0	228	80	410	1.6
-	0	0	-	40	-	-	0	-	-	-	120	0	-	-	-	18	310	-
-	0	0	-	40	-	-	0	-	-	-	120	0	-	-	-	18	310	-
0	0	38	14	54	0.2	0.7	0	-	0.4	0.1	209	0.3	8	0.4	143	26	475	1.2
1	0	49	3	123	0	0.7	0	-	0.1	0	234	0.1	6	0.1	147	27	340	1.5
0	-	45	2	663	0	0.1	0	-	0.5	0.1	381	0.8	23	1	310	20	147	0.7
0	0	34	1	702	0	0.1	0	-	0.3	0	127	0.7	12	0.5	159	67	219	0.3
0	0	20	5	578	0.1	0.1	0	-	0.2	0	60	0.8	7	0.2	109	11	156	0.4
0	0	48	9	74	0	0.7	0	-	0.1	0	298	0.1	12	0	232	51	348	1.7
1	0	47	4	128	0	0.7	0	-	0.1	0	430	0.1	15	0	257	34	143	1.7
0	0	38	24	134	0	0.4	0	-	0.2	0	211	0.1	9	0.1	167	54	340	0.9
0	0	38	8	108	0	0.4	0	-	0.2	0	317	0.3	11	0	189	34	228	1.3
-	0	23	-	90	-	-	0	-	-	-	360	0	-	-	-	27	270	-
0	0	25	4	75	0	0.3	0	-	0.1	0	275	0.1	10	0	197	36	198	1.2
0	0	23	4	81	0	0.4	0	-	0.1	0	311	0.1	11	0.1	223	40	224	1.3
0	0	33	3	102	0	0.3	0	-	0.1	0	220	0.1	8	0	158	29	159	0.9
0	0	38	3	117	0	0.3	0	-	0.1	0	244	0.1	9	0	175	32	176	1
1	0	0	5	186	0	0.3	0	-	0.2	0	259	0.2	17	0.1	248	193	291	0.8
0	0	41	5	134	0	0.6	0	-	0.1	0	305	0.2	12	0	199	57	267	1.2
0	0	4	0	9	0	0.1	0	-	0	0	69	0	3	0	40	5	93	0.2
0	0	2	-	0	-	-	0	-	-	-	16	0	-	-	-	10	15	-
0	0	29	3	63	0	0.5	0	-	0.1	0	503	0.3	19	0.1	295	39	681	1.2
0	0	31	3	74	0	0.6	0	-	0.1	0	533	0.4	22	0.1	313	41	721	1.4
0	0	29	4	112	0	0.6	0	-	0.1	0	321	0.2	12	0.1	211	59	372	1.4
0	0	13	6	48	0	0.1	0	-	0.1	0	116	0.2	6	0	78	53	53	0.6
0	0	22	5	57	0	0.1	0	-	0.1	0	88	0.2	5	0	67	44	36	0.5
0	0	44	3	60	0	0.5	0	-	0.2	0	452	0.3	17	0	323	37	510	1.1
1	0	38	21	127	0.1	0.3	0	-	0.2	0	281	0.2	13	0.3	167	39	769	0.9
0	0	39	3	108	0	0.7	0	-	0.2	0	409	0.1	15	0	257	47	111	1.7
0	0	48	3	130	0	0.7	0	-	0.2	0	438	0.3	17	0	432	122	777	2
1	2	47	13	137	0	0.1	1	-	0.2	0	43	0.5	9	0.2	79	77	176	0.4
2	-	103	10	273	0	0.2	0	-	0.2	0	49	1.1	7	0.3	82	87	241	0.5
1	2	34	14	79	0	0.2	0	-	0.2	0.1	138	0.4	15	0.4	187	169	304	0.4
1	-	77	9	217	0	0.2	1	-	0.1	0	39	1.1	6	0.3	64	84	183	0.4
0	1	0	10	91	0.1	0	3	-	0	0	13	1.7	8	0.2	13	119	9	0.1
0	-	0	10	92	0.1	0	3	-	0	0	13	1.7	8	0.2	13	120	9	0.1
0	1	0	10	92	0.1	0	3	-	0.1	0	13	1.7	7	0.2	12	120	9	0.1
0	-	0	10	91	0.1	0	2	-	0	0	13	1.6	7	0.2	12	119	9	0.1
0	1	0	4	66	0	0	5	0.1	0	0	8	0.2	5	0.2	8	89	2	0.1
0	1	0	5	19	0	0	5	-	0.1	0	12	0.4	12	0.5	23	186	4	0.1
0	1	0	5	16	0	0	3	-	0	0	17	0.7	15	0.5	27	164	4	0.1
0	1	0	5	20	0	0	5	-	0.1	0	11	0.5	11	0.5	23	186	4	0.1
0	1	0	5	20	0	0	3	-	0.1	0	14	0.4	11	0.5	19	162	1	0.1
0	-	0	5	20	0	0	5	-	0.1	0	12	0.5	10	0.5	22	185	4	0.1
0	2	0	3	15	0	0	5	-	0	0	11	0.3	8	0.3	14	162	0	0.1
0	1	0	5	25	0	0	1	-	0.1	0	16	0.5	13	0.2	21	258	1	0.1
3	1	0	10	-	0.1	0	1	-	0	0	15	0.6	10	0.3	36	101	308	0.2
7	-	-	4	22	0	0.1	2	-	0.1	0.2	28	1.6	13	1.8	55	83	479	0.3
-	0	0	0	0	0	0	0	-	0	0	0	0	0	0	0	0	0	0
-	-	0	0	6	0.7	5.3	20	-	0.2	0.7	15	10.5	27	7.2	80	114	432	0.9
-	-	-	-	20	-	-	1	-	0.2	0.1	160	0.8	-	2.9	32	260	800	-

Code	Food Name	Amount	Unit	Grams	kCalories	Carbohydrate (gm)	Protein (gm)	Fat (gm)	Saturated Fat (gm)	Monounsaturated Fat (gm)
43397	Chicken a la King, Top Shelf-Hormel	1	Each	283.5	360	49	18	10	4	4
57799	Chicken a la King-Swanson	1	Each	250	319	15	17	20	-	-
55197	Chicken a la Orange, Lean Cuisine-Stouffer's	1	Each	226.8	280	33	27	4	1	-
41301	Chicken a la Orange-Healthy Choice	1	Each	255.1	240	36	20	2	2	-
55792	Chicken and Dumplings-Stouffer's	1	Each	220	303	24	15	16	-	-
57801	Chicken and Dumplings-Swanson	1	Each	200	207	18	10	10	-	-
41253	Chicken and Pasta Divan-Healthy Choice	1	Each	340.2	300	41	25	4	2	-
55794	Chicken and Veg. Oriental-Stouffer's	1	Each	220	186	14	12	9	-	-
55198	Chicken and Veg. w/ Vermicelli, Lean Cuisine-Stouffer's	1	Each	333.1	240	30	18	5	1	-
41302	Chicken and Vegetables-Healthy Choice	1	Each	326	210	31	20	1	-	-
55199	Chicken Cacciatore, Lean Cuisine-Stouffer's	1	Each	308.3	280	31	22	7	2	-
43398	Chicken Cacciatore, Top Shelf-Hormel	1	Each	283.5	210	25	21	3	-	-
55200	Chicken Chow Mein w/ Rice, Lean Cuisine-Stouffer's	1	Each	255.1	240	34	14	5	1	-
55110	Chicken Chow Mein w/ Rice-Stouffer's	1	Each	304.8	250	39	13	5	-	-
41303	Chicken Chow Mein-Healthy Choice	1	Each	241	220	31	18	3	1	-
62611	Chicken Chow Mein-Weight Watchers	1	Each	255.2	200	34	12	2	1	-
55807	Chicken Classica -Stouffer's	1	Ounce	28.4	22	2	2	1	-	-
41336	Chicken Con Queso Burritos (mild)-Healthy Choice	1	Each	148.8	280	40	15	8	2	-
41254	Chicken Dijon-Healthy Choice	1	Each	311.8	250	40	21	3	1	-
55111	Chicken Divan-Stouffer's	1	Each	226.8	220	11	24	10	-	-
62618	Chicken Enchiladas Suiza-Weight Watchers	1	Each	255.2	250	28	15	8	3	-
55201	Chicken Enchiladas, Lean Cuisine-Stouffer's	1	Each	280	290	34	17	9	3	-
41304	Chicken Enchiladas-Healthy Choice	1	Each	269.3	310	44	14	9	3	-
55112	Chicken Enchiladas-Stouffer's	1	Each	283.5	490	31	21	31	-	-
41305	Chicken Fajitas-Healthy Choice	1	Each	198.5	200	25	17	3	1	-
55203	Chicken Fettucini, Lean Cuisine-Stouffer's	1	Each	255.1	280	33	23	6	3	-
41306	Chicken Fettucini-Healthy Choice	1	Each	241	240	29	22	4	2	-
62620	Chicken Fettucini-Weight Watchers	1	Each	233.9	280	25	22	9	3	-
55763	Chicken Gumbo Soup-Stouffer's	1	Cup	283.9	110	9	7	5	-	-
55202	Chicken in BBQ Sauce, Lean Cuisine-Stouffer's	1	Each	248.1	260	32	20	6	1	-
55204	Chicken Italiano, Lean Cuisine-Stouffer's	1	Each	255.1	270	33	22	6	1	-
55789	Chicken Italienne-Stouffer's	1	Ounce	28.4	22	1	2	1	-	-
55755	Chicken Noodle Soup-Stouffer's	1	Cup	283.9	130	10	7	7	-	-
55768	Chicken Noodle, Heat'n Serve Soup-Stouffer's	1	Cup	283.9	320	28	13	17	-	-
55205	Chicken Oriental, Lean Cuisine-Stouffer's	1	Each	255.1	280	31	22	7	2	-
41256	Chicken Oriental-Healthy Choice	1	Each	318.9	200	32	19	1	-	-
41257	Chicken Parmigiana-Healthy Choice	1	Each	326	280	45	22	4	2	-
41271	Chicken Pasta Soup-Healthy Choice	1	Each	212.6	100	13	7	2	-	-
55113	Chicken Pie-Stouffer's	1	Each	283.5	440	32	16	27	-	-
57807	Chicken Pot Pie-Swanson	1	Each	198.5	380	35	11	22	-	-
55790	Chicken Primavera-Stouffer's	1	Ounce	28.4	17	1	2	1	-	-
5280	Chicken Roll, Light Meat	3	Ounce	85.1	135	2	17	6	2	3
5283	Chicken Salad Sandwich Spread	3	Ounce	85.1	170	6	10	11	3	3
5281	Chicken Spread, Cnd	3	Ounce	85.1	163	5	13	10	3	4
41295	Chicken Stir Fry w/ Broccoli-Healthy Choice	1	Each	340.2	280	35	21	6	3	-
55206	Chicken Tenderloins, Lean Cuisine-Stouffer's	1	Each	269.3	240	19	29	5	2	-
55820	Chicken Tortellini w/ Egg Pasta-Stouffer's	1	Ounce	28.4	51	6	3	2	-	-
41248	Chicken w/ Barbeque Sauce-Healthy Choice	1	Each	361.5	410	65	24	6	2	-
41277	Chicken w/ Rice Soup-Healthy Choice	1	Each	212.6	90	14	5	1	-	-
5054	Chicken, Back, Meat Only, Ckd, Fried	3	Ounce	85.1	245	5	26	13	4	5
5055	Chicken, Back, Meat Only, Ckd, Roasted	3	Ounce	85.1	203	0	24	11	3	4
5056	Chicken, Back, Meat Only, Ckd, Stewed	3	Ounce	85.1	178	0	22	10	3	3
5049	Chicken, Back, Meat&skin, Ckd, Fried, Batter	3	Ounce	85.1	282	9	19	19	5	8
5050	Chicken, Back, Meat&skin, Ckd, Fried, Flr	3	Ounce	85.1	282	6	24	18	5	7
5051	Chicken, Back, Meat&skin, Ckd, Roasted	3	Ounce	85.1	255	0	22	18	5	7
5052	Chicken, Back, Meat&skin, Ckd, Stewed	3	Ounce	85.1	219	0	19	15	4	6
5063	Chicken, Breast, Meat Only, Ckd, Fried	3	Ounce	85.1	159	0	28	4	1	1
5064	Chicken, Breast, Meat Only, Ckd, Roasted	3	Ounce	85.1	140	0	26	3	1	1
5065	Chicken, Breast, Meat Only, Ckd, Stewed	3	Ounce	85.1	128	0	25	3	1	1
5058	Chicken, Breast, Meat&skin, Ckd, Fried, Batter	3	Ounce	85.1	221	8	21	11	3	5

Polyunsaturated Fat (gm)	Fiber (gm)	Cholesterol (mg)	Folate (µg)	Vitamin A (re)	Vitamin B6 (mg)	Vitamin B12 (µg)	Vitamin C (mg)	Vitamin E (mg)	Riboflavin (mg)	Thiamin (mg)	Calcium (mg)	Iron (mg)	Magnesium (mg)	Niacin (mg)	Phosphorus (mg)	Potassium (mg)	Sodium (mg)	Zinc (mg)
2	-	37	-	250	-	-	1	-	0.2	0.1	48	0.2	28	8.6	-	476	890	1.2
-	-	-	-	-	-	-	-	-	0.2	0.1	54	0.3	-	3.2	-	-	1159	-
-	-	55	-	80	-	-	12	-	0.2	0.2	32	0.4	-	9.5	-	490	290	-
-	-	45	-	150	-	-	27	-	0.1	0.2	16	0.8	-	5.7	230	430	220	-
-	-	70	-	-	-	-	0	-	0	0	1055	0.2	-	0.4	-	248	660	-
-	-	-	-	75	-	-	-	-	0.1	0	15	0.4	-	1.8	-	-	922	-
1	-	50	-	800	-	-	72	-	0.3	0.4	120	1	-	4.8	270	500	520	-
-	-	31	-	-	-	-	5	-	0	0	372	0.1	-	0.6	-	349	1079	-
1	-	30	-	150	-	-	6	-	0.3	0.3	64	1	-	5.7	-	500	500	-
-	-	35	-	150	-	-	9	-	0.2	0.3	32	1.5	-	3.8	190	390	490	-
1	-	45	-	100	-	-	9	-	0.2	0.2	32	0.8	-	5.7	-	560	570	-
-	-	50	-	100	-	-	2	-	0.3	0.2	80	1	-	6.7	-	-	810	-
1	-	30	-	60	-	-	6	-	0.2	0.2	32	0.6	-	4.8	-	350	530	-
-	-	-	-	80	-	-	12	-	0.2	0	16	0.4	-	1.9	-	340	720	-
1	-	45	-	80	-	-	4	-	0.1	0.2	16	0.8	-	3.8	290	290	440	-
-	3	25	-	300	-	-	36	-	-	-	48	0.4	-	-	-	360	430	-
-	-	5	-	-	-	-	1	-	0	0	112	0	-	0.1	-	50	83	-
3	-	20	-	20	-	-	6	-	0.3	0.5	80	1.5	-	2.9	170	260	500	-
-	-	40	-	100	-	-	9	-	0.1	0.2	16	1	-	9.5	300	350	470	-
-	-	-	-	60	-	-	4	-	0.2	0.5	200	2	-	3.8	32	490	610	-
-	4	25	-	40	-	-	1	-	-	-	360	0.8	-	-	-	470	570	-
2	-	55	-	250	-	-	6	-	0.3	0.2	120	1.5	-	2.9	-	450	500	-
1	-	35	-	80	-	-	21	-	0.2	0.2	80	0.8	-	4.8	160	380	480	-
-	-	-	-	60	-	-	2	-	0.3	0.1	240	0.6	-	2.9	-	420	860	-
1	-	35	-	150	-	-	9	-	0.2	0.2	64	1.5	-	3.8	210	360	310	-
-	-	35	-	-	-	-	-	-	0.4	0.3	120	0.8	-	5.7	-	420	500	-
2	-	45	-	-	-	-	-	-	0.2	0.2	64	1	-	2.9	210	190	370	-
-	2	40	-	40	-	-	0	-	-	-	240	1	-	-	-	730	590	-
-	-	20	-	-	-	-	0	-	0	0	160	0.1	-	0.2	-	180	1422	-
2	-	50	-	250	-	-	18	-	0.2	0.2	48	0.8	-	5.7	-	650	500	-
2	-	40	-	100	-	-	24	-	0.3	0.3	80	0.8	-	5.7	-	600	590	-
-	-	7	-	-	-	-	1	-	0	0	48	0	-	0.1	-	57	128	-
-	-	20	-	-	-	-	0	-	0	0	80	0.1	-	0.2	-	140	1282	-
-	-	60	-	-	-	-	6	-	0	0	240	0.2	-	0.6	-	310	1793	-
2	-	35	-	40	-	-	6	-	0.2	0.2	32	1	-	6.7	-	470	480	-
-	-	35	-	250	-	-	36	-	0.1	0.2	32	0.8	-	7.6	200	400	440	-
-	-	45	-	900	-	-	12	-	0.2	0.2	80	1	-	9.5	260	500	370	-
-	-	15	-	60	-	-	-	-	-	0	-	-	-	0.4	-	70	560	-
-	-	-	-	500	-	-	1	-	0.4	0.3	80	1	-	4.8	-	320	750	-
-	-	-	-	400	-	-	-	-	0.2	0.2	16	1	-	2.9	-	-	760	-
-	-	5	-	-	-	-	1	-	0	0	48	0	-	0.1	-	40	119	-
1	0	43	2	20	0.2	0.1	0	-	0.1	0.1	37	0.8	16	4.5	134	194	497	0.6
5	0	26	4	36	0.1	0.3	1	-	0.1	0	9	0.5	9	1.4	28	156	321	0.9
2	0	44	3	21	0.1	0.1	0	-	0.1	0	106	2	10	2.3	76	90	328	1
-	-	55	-	20	-	-	-	-	0.3	0.2	48	1.5	-	2.9	260	630	500	-
1	-	60	-	200	-	-	5	-	0.3	0.2	120	0.4	-	7.6	-	750	490	-
-	-	20	-	-	-	-	0	-	0	0	72	0	-	0.1	-	31	57	-
2	-	55	-	100	-	-	12	-	0.1	0.1	48	1.5	-	8.6	250	670	550	-
-	-	10	-	80	-	-	6	-	0.1	0	16	0.2	-	1.9	70	140	510	-
3	0	79	8	25	0.3	0.3	0	-	0.2	0.1	22	1.4	21	6.5	150	213	84	2.4
3	0	77	6	24	0.3	0.3	0	-	0.2	0.1	20	1.2	19	6	140	202	82	2.3
2	0	72	6	23	0.2	0.2	0	-	0.1	0	18	1.1	14	3.9	111	134	57	2
4	-	75	8	31	0.2	0.2	0	-	0.2	0.1	22	1.3	16	5	117	153	270	1.7
4	-	76	7	31	0.3	0.2	0	-	0.2	0.1	20	1.4	20	6.2	141	192	77	2.1
4	0	75	5	84	0.2	0.2	0	-	0.2	0.1	18	1.2	17	5.7	131	179	74	1.9
3	0	66	4	75	0.1	0.2	0	-	0.1	0	15	1	14	3.7	102	123	54	1.6
1	0	77	3	6	0.5	0.3	0	-	0.1	0.1	14	1	26	12.6	209	235	67	0.9
1	0	72	3	5	0.5	0.3	0	-	0.1	0.1	13	0.9	25	11.7	194	218	63	0.9
1	0	65	3	5	0.3	0.2	0	-	0.1	0	11	0.7	20	7.2	140	159	54	0.8
3	0	72	5	17	0.4	0.3	0	-	0.1	0.1	17	1.1	20	8.9	157	171	234	0.8

Code	Food Name	Amount	Unit	Grams	kCalories	Carbohydrate (gm)	Protein (gm)	Fat (gm)	Saturated Fat (gm)	Monounsaturated Fat (gm)
5059	Chicken, Breast, Meat&skin, Ckd, Fried, Flr	3	Ounce	85.1	189	1	27	8	2	3
5060	Chicken, Breast, Meat&skin, Ckd, Roasted	3	Ounce	85.1	168	0	25	7	2	3
5061	Chicken, Breast, Meat&skin, Ckd, Stewed	3	Ounce	85.1	156	0	23	6	2	2
5044	Chicken, Dark Meat, Meat Only, Ckd, Fried	3	Ounce	85.1	203	2	25	10	3	4
5045	Chicken, Dark Meat, Meat Only, Ckd, Roasted	3	Ounce	85.1	174	0	23	8	2	3
5046	Chicken, Dark Meat, Meat Only, Ckd, Stewed	3	Ounce	85.1	163	0	22	8	2	3
5035	Chicken, Dark Meat, Meat&skin, Ckd, Fried, Batter	3	Ounce	85.1	253	8	19	16	4	6
5036	Chicken, Dark Meat, Meat&skin, Ckd, Fried, Flr	3	Ounce	85.1	242	3	23	14	4	6
5037	Chicken, Dark Meat, Meat&skin, Ckd, Roasted	3	Ounce	85.1	215	0	22	13	4	5
5038	Chicken, Dark Meat, Meat&skin, Ckd, Stewed	3	Ounce	85.1	198	0	20	12	3	5
5072	Chicken, Drumstick, Meat Only, Ckd, Fried	3	Ounce	85.1	166	0	24	7	2	3
5073	Chicken, Drumstick, Meat Only, Ckd, Roasted	3	Ounce	85.1	146	0	24	5	1	2
5074	Chicken, Drumstick, Meat Only, Ckd, Stewed	3	Ounce	85.1	144	0	23	5	1	2
5067	Chicken, Drumstick, Meat&skin, Ckd, Fried, Batter	3	Ounce	85.1	228	7	19	13	4	5
5068	Chicken, Drumstick, Meat&skin, Ckd, Fried, Flr	3	Ounce	85.1	208	1	23	12	3	5
5069	Chicken, Drumstick, Meat&skin, Ckd, Roasted	3	Ounce	85.1	184	0	23	9	3	4
5070	Chicken, Drumstick, Meat&skin, Ckd, Stewed	3	Ounce	85.1	174	0	22	9	2	3
5021	Chicken, Giblets, Ckd, Fried	3	Ounce	85.1	236	4	28	11	3	4
5022	Chicken, Giblets, Ckd, Simmered	3	Ounce	85.1	134	1	22	4	1	1
5026	Chicken, Heart, Ckd, Simmered	3	Ounce	85.1	157	0	22	7	2	2
5081	Chicken, Leg, Meat Only, Ckd, Fried	3	Ounce	85.1	177	1	24	8	2	3
5082	Chicken, Leg, Meat Only, Ckd, Roasted	3	Ounce	85.1	162	0	23	7	2	3
5083	Chicken, Leg, Meat Only, Ckd, Stewed	3	Ounce	85.1	157	0	22	7	2	2
5076	Chicken, Leg, Meat&skin, Ckd, Fried, Batter	3	Ounce	85.1	232	7	19	14	4	6
5077	Chicken, Leg, Meat&skin, Ckd, Fried, Flour	3	Ounce	85.1	216	2	23	12	3	5
5078	Chicken, Leg, Meat&skin, Ckd, Roasted	3	Ounce	85.1	197	0	22	11	3	4
5079	Chicken, Leg, Meat&skin, Ckd, Stewed	3	Ounce	85.1	187	0	21	11	3	4
5028	Chicken, Liver, Ckd, Simmered	3	Ounce	85.1	134	1	21	5	2	1
5012	Chicken, Meat Only, Ckd, Fried	3	Ounce	85.1	186	1	26	8	2	3
5013	Chicken, Meat Only, Roasted	3	Ounce	85.1	162	0	25	6	2	2
5014	Chicken, Meat Only, Stewed	3	Ounce	85.1	151	0	23	6	2	2
5097	Chicken, Thigh, Meat Only, Ckd, Fried	3	Ounce	85.1	185	1	24	9	2	3
5098	Chicken, Thigh, Meat Only, Ckd, Roasted	3	Ounce	85.1	178	0	22	9	3	4
5099	Chicken, Thigh, Meat Only, Ckd, Stewed	3	Ounce	85.1	166	0	21	8	2	3
5092	Chicken, Thigh, Meat&skin, Ckd, Fried, Batter	3	Ounce	85.1	236	8	18	14	4	6
5093	Chicken, Thigh, Meat&skin, Ckd, Fried, Flr	3	Ounce	85.1	223	3	23	13	3	5
5094	Chicken, Thigh, Meat&skin, Ckd, Roasted	3	Ounce	85.1	210	0	21	13	4	5
5095	Chicken, Thigh, Meat&skin, Ckd, Stewed	3	Ounce	85.1	197	0	20	13	3	5
5106	Chicken, Wing, Meat Only, Ckd, Fried	3	Ounce	85.1	179	0	26	8	2	3
5107	Chicken, Wing, Meat Only, Ckd, Roasted	3	Ounce	85.1	173	0	26	7	2	2
5108	Chicken, Wing, Meat Only, Ckd, Stewed	3	Ounce	85.1	154	0	23	6	2	2
5101	Chicken, Wing, Meat&skin, Ckd, Fried, Batter	3	Ounce	85.1	276	9	17	19	5	8
5102	Chicken, Wing, Meat&skin, Ckd, Fried, Flr	3	Ounce	85.1	273	2	22	19	5	8
5103	Chicken, Wing, Meat&skin, Ckd, Roasted	3	Ounce	85.1	247	0	23	17	5	6
5104	Chicken, Wing, Meat&skin, Ckd, Stewed	3	Ounce	85.1	212	0	19	14	4	6
16058	Chickpeas, Cnd	½	Cup	120	143	27	6	1	0	0
41272	Chili Beef Soup-Healthy Choice	1	Each	212.6	150	22	11	1	-	-
55114	Chili Con Carne w/ Beans-Stouffer's	1	Each	248.1	280	28	20	10	-	-
43411	Chili Mac, Micro Cup-Hormel	1	Each	212.6	192	18	10	9	4	4
43408	Chili no Beans, Micro Cup-Hormel	1	Each	209.1	290	15	18	17	8	8
55767	Chili w/ Beans Soup-Stouffer's	1	Cup	283.9	240	25	14	9	-	-
16059	Chili w/ Beans, Cnd	½	Cup	127.5	143	15	7	7	3	3
43409	Chili w/ Beans, Micro Cup-Hormel	1	Each	209.1	250	23	15	11	4	4
43369	Chili w/ Beans-Hormel	1	Cup	253.2	357	32	18	18	6	7
43368	Chili w/o Beans-Hormel	1	Cup	253.2	429	17	19	32	13	15
18198	Chocolate Chip Cookies, Dietary	1	Each	7	32	5	0	1	1	0
18159	Chocolate Chip Cookies, Higher Fat, Enr	1	Each	10	48	7	1	2	1	1
18158	Chocolate Chip Cookies, Lower Fat	1	Each	10	45	7	1	2	0	1
18160	Chocolate Chip Cookies, Soft-type	1	Each	15	69	9	1	4	1	2
18310	Chocolate Creme Pie	1	Slice	113	344	38	3	22	6	12

Polyunsaturated Fat (gm)	Fiber (gm)	Cholesterol (mg)	Folate (µg)	Vitamin A (re)	Vitamin B6 (mg)	Vitamin B12 (µg)	Vitamin C (mg)	Vitamin E (mg)	Riboflavin (mg)	Thiamin (mg)	Calcium (mg)	Iron (mg)	Magnesium (mg)	Niacin (mg)	Phosphorus (mg)	Potassium (mg)	Sodium (mg)	Zinc (mg)
2	-	76	3	13	0.5	0.3	0	-	0.1	0.1	14	1	26	11.7	198	220	65	0.9
1	0	71	3	23	0.5	0.3	0	-	0.1	0.1	12	0.9	23	10.8	182	208	60	0.9
1	0	64	3	20	0.2	0.2	0	-	0.1	0	11	0.8	19	6.6	133	151	53	0.8
2	0	82	8	20	0.3	0.3	0	-	0.2	0.1	15	1.3	21	6	159	215	82	2.5
2	0	79	7	19	0.3	0.3	0	-	0.2	0.1	13	1.1	20	5.6	152	204	79	2.4
2	0	75	6	18	0.2	0.2	0	-	0.2	0	12	1.2	17	4	122	154	63	2.3
4	-	76	8	26	0.2	0.2	0	-	0.2	0.1	18	1.2	17	4.8	123	157	251	1.8
3	-	78	7	26	0.3	0.3	0	-	0.2	0.1	14	1.3	20	5.8	150	196	76	2.2
3	0	77	6	49	0.3	0.2	0	-	0.2	0.1	13	1.2	19	5.4	143	187	74	2.1
3	0	70	5	46	0.1	0.2	0	-	0.2	0	12	1.1	15	3.8	113	141	60	1.9
2	0	80	8	15	0.3	0.3	0	-	0.2	0.1	10	1.1	20	5.2	158	212	82	2.7
1	0	79	8	15	0.3	0.3	0	-	0.2	0.1	10	1.1	20	5.2	156	209	81	2.7
1	0	75	7	14	0.2	0.2	0	-	0.2	0	9	1.2	18	3.7	128	169	68	2.6
3	-	73	8	22	0.2	0.2	0	-	0.2	0.1	14	1.1	17	4.3	125	158	229	2
3	-	77	7	21	0.3	0.3	0	-	0.2	0.1	10	1.1	20	5.1	150	195	76	2.5
2	0	77	7	26	0.3	0.3	0	-	0.2	0.1	10	1.1	20	5.1	149	195	77	2.4
2	0	71	6	23	0.2	0.2	0	-	0.2	0	9	1.1	17	3.6	120	156	65	2.3
3	0	379	322	3044	0.5	11.3	7	-	1.3	0.1	15	8.8	21	9.3	243	281	96	5.3
1	0	334	320	1896	0.3	8.6	7	-	0.8	0.1	10	5.5	17	3.5	195	134	49	3.9
2	0	206	68	8	0.3	6.2	2	-	0.6	0.1	16	7.7	17	2.4	169	112	41	6.2
2	0	84	8	17	0.3	0.3	0	-	0.2	0.1	11	1.2	21	5.7	164	216	82	2.5
2	0	80	7	16	0.3	0.3	0	-	0.2	0.1	10	1.1	20	5.4	156	206	77	2.4
2	0	76	7	15	0.2	0.2	0	-	0.2	0.1	9	1.2	18	4.1	127	162	66	2.4
3	-	77	8	23	0.2	0.2	0	-	0.2	0.1	15	1.2	17	4.6	129	161	237	1.8
3	-	80	7	24	0.3	0.3	0	-	0.2	0.1	11	1.2	20	5.6	155	198	75	2.3
3	0	78	6	33	0.3	0.3	0	-	0.2	0.1	10	1.1	20	5.3	148	191	74	2.2
2	0	71	5	31	0.2	0.2	0	-	0.2	0	9	1.1	17	3.9	118	150	62	2.1
1	0	537	655	4179	0.5	16.5	13	-	1.5	0.1	12	7.2	18	3.8	265	119	43	3.7
2	0	80	6	15	0.4	0.3	0	-	0.2	0.1	14	1.1	23	8.2	174	219	77	1.9
1	0	76	5	14	0.4	0.3	0	-	0.2	0.1	13	1	21	7.8	166	207	73	1.8
1	0	71	5	13	0.2	0.2	0	-	0.1	0	12	1	18	5.2	128	153	60	1.7
2	0	87	8	18	0.3	0.3	0	-	0.2	0.1	11	1.2	22	6.1	169	220	81	2.4
2	0	81	7	17	0.3	0.3	0	-	0.2	0.1	10	1.1	20	5.5	156	202	75	2.2
2	0	77	6	16	0.2	0.2	0	-	0.2	0.1	9	1.2	18	4.4	127	156	64	2.2
3	-	79	8	25	0.2	0.2	0	-	0.2	0.1	15	1.2	18	4.9	132	163	245	1.7
3	-	82	7	25	0.3	0.3	0	-	0.2	0.1	12	1.3	21	5.9	159	202	75	2.1
3	0	79	6	41	0.3	0.2	0	-	0.2	0.1	10	1.1	19	5.4	148	189	71	2
3	0	71	5	37	0.1	0.2	0	-	0.2	0	9	1.2	16	4.2	118	145	60	1.9
2	0	71	3	15	0.5	0.3	0	-	0.1	0	13	1	18	6.2	139	177	77	1.8
2	0	72	3	15	0.5	0.3	0	-	0.1	0	14	1	18	6.2	141	179	78	1.8
1	0	63	3	14	0.3	0.2	0	-	0.1	0	11	1	15	4.4	114	130	62	1.7
4	-	67	5	29	0.3	0.2	0	-	0.1	0.1	17	1.1	14	4.5	103	117	272	1.2
4	-	69	3	32	0.3	0.2	0	-	0.1	0	13	1.1	16	5.7	128	151	65	1.5
4	0	71	3	40	0.4	0.2	0	-	0.1	0	13	1.1	16	5.7	128	156	70	1.5
3	0	60	3	34	0.2	0.2	0	-	0.1	0	10	1	14	3.9	103	118	57	1.4
1	5	0	80	2	0.6	0	5	-	0	0	38	1.6	35	0.2	108	206	359	1.3
-	-	15	-	20	-	-	6	-	0	0.1	16	0.6	-	0.4	-	290	560	-
-	-	-	-	200	-	-	15	-	0.3	0.2	64	2	-	2.9	-	700	910	-
-	-	22	-	210	-	-	-	-	0.2	0.1	-	1.5	35	2.1	-	443	977	2.1
1	-	60	-	400	-	-	-	-	0.2	0.1	48	1.6	35	2.5	-	507	830	3.9
-	-	30	-	-	-	-	0	-	0	0	721	0.3	-	0.6	-	711	991	-
0	6	22	29	43	0.2	0	2	-	0.1	0.1	60	4.4	57	0.5	196	465	666	2.6
-	-	49	-	190	-	-	-	-	0.2	0.1	48	1.9	46	1.7	-	677	977	2.7
1	-	65	-	250	-	-	-	-	0.2	0.1	57	1.9	58	2	-	913	1226	2.5
1	-	71	-	786	-	-	-	-	0.3	0.1	48	1.7	42	2.9	-	592	1024	3.2
0	-	0	0	0	0	0	0	-	0	0	2	0.2	2	0.2	6	14	1	0
0	0	0	1	0	0	0	0	-	0	0	3	0.3	3	0.3	11	14	32	0.1
0	0	0	1	0	0	0	0	-	0	0	2	0.3	3	0.3	8	12	38	0.1
0	0	0	1	0	0	0	0	-	0	0	2	0.4	5	0.2	8	14	49	0.1
3	2	6	8	-	0	0	0	-	0.1	0	41	1.2	24	0.8	77	144	154	0.3

Code	Food Name	Amount	Unit	Grams	kCalories	Carbohydrate (gm)	Protein (gm)	Fat (gm)	Saturated Fat (gm)	Monounsaturated Fat (gm)
18312	Chocolate Mousse Pie	1	Slice	95	247	28	3	15	8	5
19183	Chocolate Pudding	1	Cup	298.1	396	68	8	12	2	5
18157	Chocolate Wafers	1	Each	6	26	4	0	1	0	0
19119	Chunky Bar	1	Bar	35	173	20	3	10	8	0
43370	Chunky Chili w/ Beans-Hormel	1	Cup	253.2	345	30	18	17	-	-
14187	Clam and Tomato Juice, Cnd	¾	Cup	181.1	83	20	1	0	0	0
15158	Clam, Ckd, Breaded and Fried	3	Ounce	85.1	172	9	12	9	2	4
15159	Clam, Ckd, Moist Heat	3	Ounce	85.1	126	4	22	2	0	0
15160	Clam, Cnd, Drained Solids	3	Ounce	85.1	126	4	22	2	0	0
15162	Clam, Cnd, Solids and Liquids	3	Ounce	85.1	2	0	0	0	0	0
14121	Club Soda	12	Fl Oz	355.2	0	0	0	0	0	0
19219	Coconut Cream Pudding	1	Cup	280	291	50	9	7	5	1
18313	Coconut Creme Pie	1	Slice	64	191	24	1	11	5	4
18316	Coconut Custard Pie	1	Slice	104	270	31	6	14	6	6
15016	Cod, Atlantic, Ckd, Dry Heat	3	Ounce	85.1	89	0	19	1	0	0
15017	Cod, Atlantic, Cnd	3	Ounce	85.1	89	0	19	1	0	0
14209	Coffee, Brewed	6	Fl Oz	177.6	4	1	0	0	0	0
14219	Coffee, Instant, Decaffeinated	6	Fl Oz	179.2	4	1	0	0	0	0
14215	Coffee, Instant, Regular	6	Fl Oz	179.2	4	1	0	0	0	0
18104	Coffeecake	1	Slice	63	263	29	4	15	4	8
18103	Coffeecake, Cheese	1	Slice	76	258	34	5	12	4	6
18106	Coffeecake, Fruit	1	Slice	50	156	26	3	5	1	3
14400	Cola	12	Fl Oz	369.6	152	38	0	0	0	-
62530	Cola, Diet	12	Fl Oz	355.2	0	0	0	0	-	-
11159	Coleslaw	½	Cup	64	44	8	1	2	0	0
11162	Collards, Ckd	½	Cup	64	17	4	1	0	-	-
11161	Collards, Fresh	1	Cup	36	11	3	1	0	-	-
11164	Collards, Frz, Chopped, Ckd	½	Cup	85	31	6	3	0	-	-
19049	Combos Snacks Cheddar Pretzel	1	Ounce	28.4	136	18	3	6	-	-
55799	Confetti Rice-Stouffer's	1	Ounce	28.4	24	5	1	0	-	-
55824	Corn Pudding-Stouffer's	1	Ounce	28.4	38	5	1	2	-	-
55168	Corn Souffle-Stouffer's	1	Each	170.1	240	27	7	11	-	-
20092	Corn, Ckd	½	Cup	70	88	20	2	1	0	0
11901	Corn, Sweet, White, Ckd	½	Cup	82	89	21	3	1	0	0
11905	Corn, Sweet, White, Cnd	½	Cup	82	66	15	2	1	0	0
11906	Corn, Sweet, White, Cnd, Cream Style	½	Cup	128	92	23	2	1	0	0
11900	Corn, Sweet, White, Fresh	½	Cup	77	66	15	2	1	0	0
11168	Corn, Sweet, Yellow, Ckd	½	Cup	82	89	21	3	1	0	0
11172	Corn, Sweet, Yellow, Cnd, Brine Pk	½	Cup	82	66	15	2	1	0	0
11174	Corn, Sweet, Yellow, Cnd, Cream Style	½	Cup	128	92	23	2	1	0	0
11167	Corn, Sweet, Yellow, Fresh	½	Cup	77	66	15	2	1	0	0
43366	Corned Beef Hash-Hormel	1	Cup	253.2	420	18	27	27	9	18
7020	Corned Beef Loaf, Jellied	1	Slice	28.4	43	0	6	2	1	1
19401	Cornnuts, Barbecue-flavor	1	Ounce	28.4	124	20	3	4	1	2
19402	Cornnuts, Nacho-flavor	1	Ounce	28.4	124	20	3	4	1	2
19009	Cornnuts, Plain	1	Ounce	28.4	124	21	2	4	1	2
41278	Country Vegetable Soup-Healthy Choice	1	Each	212.6	120	23	3	1	-	-
15137	Crab, Alaska King, Ckd, Moist Heat	3	Ounce	85.1	82	0	16	1	0	0
15138	Crab, Alaska King, Imitation	3	Ounce	85.1	87	9	10	1	0	0
15140	Crab, Blue, Ckd, Moist Heat	3	Ounce	85.1	87	0	17	2	0	0
15141	Crab, Blue, Cnd	3	Ounce	85.1	84	0	17	1	0	0
15142	Crab, Blue, Crab Cakes	3	Ounce	85.1	132	0	17	6	1	2
15226	Crab, Dungeness, Ckd, Moist Heat	3	Ounce	85.1	94	1	19	1	0	0
15227	Crab, Queen, Ckd, Moist Heat	3	Ounce	85.1	98	0	20	1	0	0
9077	Crabapples, Fresh	½	Cup	55	42	11	0	0	0	0
18214	Crackers, Cheese, Regular	1	Each	1	5	1	0	0	0	0
18215	Crackers, Cheese, w/ Peanut Butter Filling	1	Each	7	34	4	1	2	0	1
18216	Crackers, Crispbread, Rye	1	Each	10	37	8	1	0	0	0
18218	Crackers, Matzo, Egg	1	Each	28.4	111	22	3	1	0	0
18400	Crackers, Matzo, Egg and Onion	1	Each	28.4	111	22	3	1	0	0

Polyunsaturated Fat (gm)	Fiber (gm)	Cholesterol (mg)	Folate (µg)	Vitamin A (re)	Vitamin B6 (mg)	Vitamin B12 (µg)	Vitamin C (mg)	Vitamin E (mg)	Riboflavin (mg)	Thiamin (mg)	Calcium (mg)	Iron (mg)	Magnesium (mg)	Niacin (mg)	Phosphorus (mg)	Potassium (mg)	Sodium (mg)	Zinc (mg)
1	-	21	3	96	0	0.2	0	-	0.1	0	73	1	30	0.6	219	271	437	0.6
4	3	9	9	33	0.1	0	5	-	0.5	0.1	268	1.5	63	1	238	537	385	1.3
0	-	0	1	0	0	0	0	-	0	0	2	0.2	3	0.2	8	13	35	0.1
2	2	4	8	4	0	0.1	0	-	0.1	0	50	0.4	26	0.7	73	187	19	0.6
-	-	60	-	-	-	-	-	-	-	-	-	-	-	-	-	-	929	-
0	-	0	29	40	0.2	55.4	7	-	0.1	0.1	22	1.1	40	0.3	141	163	724	2
2	-	52	15	77	0.1	34.2	9	-	0.2	0.1	54	11.8	12	1.8	160	277	310	1.2
0	0	57	24	145	0.1	84.1	19	-	0.4	0.1	78	23.8	15	2.9	287	534	95	2.3
0	0	57	24	145	0.1	84.1	19	-	0.4	0.1	78	23.8	15	2.9	287	534	95	2.3
0	0	3	2	8	0	4.3	1	-	0	0	11	0.3	9	0.2	97	127	183	0.1
0	0	0	0	0	0	0	0	-	0	0	18	0	4	0	0	7	75	0.4
0	-	20	11	140	0.4	0.7	2	-	0.4	0.1	316	0.6	45	0.3	249	445	456	1
1	-	0	3	13	0	-	0	-	0.1	0	19	0.5	13	0.1	54	42	163	0.4
1	2	36	4	28	0	0.1	0	-	0.2	0.1	84	0.8	19	0.4	127	182	348	0.7
0	0	47	7	12	0.2	0.9	1	-	0.1	0.1	12	0.4	36	2.1	117	208	66	0.5
0	0	47	7	12	0.2	0.9	1	-	0.1	0.1	18	0.4	35	2.1	221	449	185	0.5
0	0	0	0	0	0	0	0	-	0	0	4	0.1	9	0.4	2	96	4	0
0	-	0	0	0	0	0	0	-	0	0	5	0.1	7	0.5	5	63	5	0.1
0	-	0	0	0	0	0	0	-	0	0	5	0.1	7	0.5	5	64	5	0.1
2	2	20	20	18	0	0.1	0	-	0.1	0.1	34	1.2	14	1.1	68	77	221	0.5
1	1	26	44	54	0	0.1	0	-	0.1	0.1	45	0.5	11	0.5	75	220	258	0.4
1	1	11	10	10	0	0	0	-	0.1	0	23	1.2	9	1.3	59	45	193	0.3
-	0	0	0	0	0	0	0	-	0	0	11	0.1	4	0	44	4	15	0
-	0	-	-	-	-	-	-	-	-	-	-	-	-	-	-	-	30	-
1	-	5	17	52	0.1	0	21	-	0	0	29	0.4	6	0.2	20	116	15	0.1
-	1	0	4	175	0	0	8	-	0	0	15	0.1	4	0.2	5	84	10	0.1
-	1	0	4	120	0	0	8	-	0	0	10	0.1	3	0.1	4	61	7	0
-	-	0	65	508	0.1	0	22	-	0.1	0	179	1	26	0.5	23	213	43	0.2
-	-	3	2	2	0	0	0	-	0.2	0	54	0.9	6	0.9	41	37	317	0.2
-	1	-	-	-	-	0	-	-	0	0	24	0	-	0	-	14	136	-
-	-	15	-	-	-	-	1	-	0	0	88	0	-	0.1	-	51	125	-
-	-	-	-	60	-	-	-	-	0.3	0.2	48	0.4	-	1.1	-	200	760	-
0	3	0	4	4	0	0	0	-	0	0	1	0.2	25	0.4	53	22	0	0.4
0	5	0	38	0	0	0	5	-	0.1	0.2	2	0.5	26	1.3	84	204	14	0.4
0	1	0	40	0	0	0	7	-	0.1	0	4	0.7	16	1	53	160	265	0.3
0	2	0	57	0	0.1	0	6	-	0.1	0	4	0.5	22	1.2	65	172	365	0.7
0	2	0	35	0	0	0	5	-	0	0.2	2	0.4	28	1.3	69	208	12	0.3
0	2	0	38	18	0	0	5	-	0.1	0.2	2	0.5	26	1.3	84	204	14	0.4
0	2	0	40	13	0	0	7	-	0.1	0	4	0.7	16	1	53	160	265	0.3
0	2	0	57	13	0.1	0	6	-	0.1	0	4	0.5	22	1.2	65	172	365	0.7
0	2	0	35	22	0	0	5	-	0	0.2	2	0.4	28	1.3	69	208	12	0.3
-	-	80	-	-	-	-	-	-	0.2	-	71	1.8	31	3.4	-	625	991	4
0	0	13	2	0	0	0.4	2	-	0	0	3	0.6	3	0.5	21	29	270	1.2
1	2	0	0	10	0.1	0	0	-	0	0.1	5	0.5	31	0.4	80	81	277	0.5
1	2	1	4	1	0.1	0	4	-	0	0.1	10	0.5	31	0.3	88	88	180	0.5
1	2	0	0	0	0.1	0	0	-	0	0	3	0.5	32	0.5	78	79	156	0.5
-	-	0	-	200	-	-	6	-	0.1	0.1	32	0.4	-	1.5	100	380	540	-
0	0	45	43	8	0.2	9.8	6	-	0	0	50	0.6	54	1.1	238	223	912	6.5
1	0	17	1	17	0	1.4	0	-	0	0	11	0.3	37	0.2	240	77	715	0.3
1	0	85	43	2	0.2	6.2	3	-	0	0.1	88	0.8	28	2.8	175	276	237	3.6
0	0	76	36	2	0.1	0.4	2	-	0.1	0.1	86	0.7	33	1.2	221	318	283	3.4
2	0	128	35	69	0.1	5	2	-	0.1	0.1	89	0.9	28	2.5	181	276	281	3.5
0	0	65	36	26	0.1	8.8	3	-	0.2	0	50	0.4	49	3.1	149	347	321	4.7
0	0	60	36	44	0.1	8.8	6	-	0.2	0.1	28	2.4	54	2.5	109	170	588	3.1
0	-	0	-	2	-	0	4	-	0	0	10	0.2	4	0.1	8	107	1	-
0	0	0	0	0	0	0	0	-	0	0	2	0	0	0	2	1	10	0
0	0	0	2	-	0.1	0	0	-	0	0	6	0.2	4	0.5	23	17	69	0.1
0	2	0	2	0	0	0	0	-	0	0	3	0.2	8	0.1	27	32	26	0.2
0	-	25	8	4	0	0.1	0	-	0.2	0.2	11	0.8	7	1.4	45	43	6	0.2
0	1	15	3	5	0	0.1	0	-	0.1	0.2	10	1.2	9	1.4	25	24	81	0.2

Code	Food Name	Amount	Unit	Grams	kCalories	Carbohydrate (gm)	Protein (gm)	Fat (gm)	Saturated Fat (gm)	Monounsaturated Fat (gm)
18217	Crackers, Matzo, Plain	1	Each	28.4	112	24	3	0	0	0
18219	Crackers, Matzo, Whole-wheat	1	Each	28.4	100	22	4	0	0	0
18220	Crackers, Melba Toast, Plain	1	Each	5	20	4	1	0	0	0
18424	Crackers, Melba Toast, Plain, w/o Salt	1	Each	5	20	4	1	0	0	0
18221	Crackers, Melba Toast, Rye	1	Each	5	19	4	1	0	0	0
18222	Crackers, Melba Toast, Wheat	1	Each	5	19	4	1	0	0	0
18229	Crackers, Ritz	1	Each	3	15	2	0	1	0	0
18427	Crackers, Ritz, Low Sodium	1	Each	3	15	2	0	1	0	0
18225	Crackers, Rye, w/ Cheese Filling	1	Each	7	34	4	1	2	0	1
18226	Crackers, Rye, Wafers, Plain	1	Each	25	84	20	2	0	0	0
18227	Crackers, Rye, Wafers, Seasoned	1	Each	22	84	16	2	2	0	1
18228	Crackers, Saltines	1	Each	3	13	2	0	0	0	0
18425	Crackers, Saltines, Low Salt	1	Each	3	13	2	0	0	0	0
18230	Crackers, Snack-type, w/ Cheese Filling	1	Each	7	33	4	1	1	0	1
18231	Crackers, Snack-type, w/ Peanut Butter Filling	1	Each	7	34	4	1	2	0	1
18428	Crackers, Wheat, Low Salt	1	Each	2	9	1	0	0	0	0
18232	Crackers, Wheat, Regular	1	Each	2	9	1	0	0	0	0
18233	Crackers, Wheat, w/ Cheese Filling	1	Each	7	35	4	1	2	0	1
18234	Crackers, Wheat, w/ Peanut Butter Filling	1	Each	7	35	4	1	2	0	1
18235	Crackers, Whole-wheat	1	Each	4	18	3	0	1	0	0
18429	Crackers, Whole-wheat, Low Salt	1	Each	4	18	3	0	1	0	0
9078	Cranberries, Fresh	½	Cup	47.5	23	6	0	0	-	-
9080	Cranberry Juice Bottled	¾	Cup	189.4	108	27	0	0	-	-
9081	Cranberry Sauce, Cnd, Sweetened	½	Cup	138.5	209	54	0	0	-	-
14238	Cranberry-apple Juice Drink, Bottled	¾	Cup	183.4	123	31	0	0	0	-
14240	Cranberry-apricot Juice Drink, Bottled	¾	Cup	183.4	117	30	0	0	0	-
14241	Cranberry-grape Juice Drink, Bottled	¾	Cup	183.4	103	26	0	0	0	-
9082	Cranberry-orange Relish, Cnd	½	Cup	137.5	245	64	0	0	-	-
15243	Crayfish, Farmed, Ckd, Moist Heat	3	Ounce	85.1	74	0	15	1	0	0
15146	Crayfish, Wild, Ckd, Moist Heat	3	Ounce	85.1	75	0	14	1	0	0
55762	Cream of Broccoli Soup-Stouffer's	1	Cup	283.9	300	16	12	21	-	-
55765	Cream of Potato Soup-Stouffer's	1	Cup	283.9	300	34	11	13	-	-
18238	Cream Puffs, Shell, w/ Custard Filling	1	Each	130	335	30	9	20	5	8
14130	Cream Soda	12	Fl Oz	370.8	189	49	0	0	0	0
1067	Cream Substitute, Nondairy, Liquid	1	Tbsp.	15	20	2	0	1	0	1
1069	Cream Substitute, Nondairy, Powdered	1	Tsp.	2	11	1	0	1	1	0
1049	Cream, Half and Half, Cream and Milk	1	Tbsp.	15	20	1	0	2	1	0
1053	Cream, Heavy Whipping	1	Tbsp.	15	52	0	0	6	3	2
1052	Cream, Light Whipping	1	Tbsp.	15	44	0	0	5	3	1
1050	Cream, Light, Coffee or Table	1	Tbsp.	15	29	1	0	3	2	1
1051	Cream, Medium, 25% Fat	1	Tbsp.	15	37	1	0	4	2	1
1054	Cream, Whipped, Pressurized	1	Tbsp.	3	8	0	0	1	0	0
55788	Creamed Chicken-Stouffer's	1	Ounce	28.4	48	1	3	4	-	-
55777	Creamed Chipped Beef-Stouffer's	1	Ounce	28.4	45	2	2	3	-	-
55169	Creamed Spinach-Stouffer's	1	Each	127.6	190	8	4	16	-	-
55756	Creamy Chicken Soup-Stouffer's	1	Cup	283.9	240	25	17	8	-	-
14034	Creme De Menthe, 72 Proof	1	Fl Oz	33.6	125	14	0	0	0	0
18240	Croissants, Apple	1	Medium	57	145	21	4	5	3	1
18239	Croissants, Butter	1	Medium	57	231	26	5	12	7	3
18241	Croissants, Cheese	1	Medium	57	236	27	5	12	5	4
18242	Croutons, Plain	1	Cup	30	122	22	4	2	0	1
18243	Croutons, Seasoned	1	Cup	40	186	25	4	7	2	4
11205	Cucumber, Fresh	½	Cup	52	7	1	0	0	0	0
14010	Daiquiri	1	Fl Oz	30.2	56	2	0	0	0	0
14009	Daiquiri, Cnd	1	Fl Oz	30.5	38	5	0	0	0	-
18245	Danish Pastry, Cheese	1	Each	71	266	26	6	16	5	8
18244	Danish Pastry, Cinnamon	1	Each	65	262	29	5	15	4	8
18246	Danish Pastry, Fruit,	1	Each	71	263	34	4	13	3	7
18433	Danish Pastry, Lemon	1	Each	71	263	34	4	13	3	7
18247	Danish Pastry, Nut	1	Each	65	280	30	5	16	4	8

Polyunsaturated Fat (gm)	Fiber (gm)	Cholesterol (mg)	Folate (μg)	Vitamin A (re)	Vitamin B6 (mg)	Vitamin B12 (μg)	Vitamin C (mg)	Vitamin E (mg)	Riboflavin (mg)	Thiamin (mg)	Calcium (mg)	Iron (mg)	Magnesium (mg)	Niacin (mg)	Phosphorus (mg)	Potassium (mg)	Sodium (mg)	Zinc (mg)
0	1	0	4	0	0	0	0	-	0.1	0.1	4	0.9	7	1.1	25	32	1	0.2
0	3	0	10	0	0	0	0	-	0.1	0.1	7	1.3	38	1.5	86	90	1	0.7
0	0	0	1	0	0	0	0	-	0	0	5	0.2	3	0.2	10	10	41	0.1
0	-	0	1	0	0	0	0	-	0	0	5	0.2	3	0.2	10	10	1	0.1
0	0	0	1	-	0	0	0	-	0	0	4	0.2	2	0.2	9	10	45	0.1
0	0	0	1	0	0	0	0	-	0	0	2	0.2	3	0.3	8	7	42	0.1
0	0	0	0	0	0	0	0	-	0	0	4	0.1	1	0.1	7	4	25	0
0	0	0	0	0	0	0	0	-	0	0	4	0.1	1	0.1	7	11	11	0
0	-	1	1	0	0	0	0	-	0	0	16	0.2	3	0.2	24	24	73	0
0	-	0	11	1	0.1	0	0	-	0.1	0.1	10	1.5	30	0.4	84	124	199	0.7
0	-	0	11	-	0	0	0	-	0	0.1	10	0.7	23	0.5	68	100	195	0.6
0	0	0	4	0	0	0	0	-	0	0	4	0.2	1	0.2	3	4	39	0
0	-	0	1	0	0	0	0	-	0	0	4	0.2	1	0.2	3	22	19	0
0	-	0	1	0	0	0	0	-	0	0	18	0.2	3	0.3	28	30	98	0
0	-	0	2	0	0	0	0	-	0	0	7	0.2	4	0.4	17	16	66	0.1
0	-	0	0	0	0	0	0	-	0	0	1	0.1	1	0.1	4	4	6	0
0	0	0	0	0	0	0	0	-	0	0	1	0.1	1	0.1	4	4	16	0
0	-	0	1	1	0	0	0	-	0	0	14	0.2	4	0.2	27	21	64	0.1
0	-	0	3	0	0	0	0	-	0	0	12	0.2	3	0.4	24	21	56	0.1
0	0	0	1	0	0	0	0	-	0	0	2	0.1	4	0.2	12	12	26	0.1
0	-	0	1	0	0	0	0	-	0	0	2	0.1	4	0.2	12	12	10	0.1
-	2	0	1	2	0	0	6	-	0	0	3	0.1	2	0	4	34	0	0.1
-	-	0	0	0	0	0	67	-	0	0	6	0.3	4	0.1	4	34	4	0.1
-	1	0	-	3	0	0	3	-	0	0	6	0.3	4	0.1	8	36	40	0.1
-	0	0	0	0	0	0	59	-	0	0	13	0.1	4	0.1	6	50	4	0.1
-	0	0	1	84	0	0	0	-	0	0	17	0.3	6	0.2	9	112	4	0.1
-	0	0	1	0	0.1	0	59	-	0	0	15	0	6	0.2	7	44	6	0.1
-	-	0	-	10	-	0	25	-	0	0	15	0.3	5	0.1	11	52	44	-
0	0	117	9	13	0.1	2.6	0	-	0.1	0	43	0.9	28	1.4	205	202	82	1.3
0	0	113	37	13	0.1	1.8	1	-	0.1	0	51	0.7	28	1.9	230	252	80	1.5
-	-	60	-	-	-	-	0	-	0	0	2484	0	-	0	-	431	791	-
-	-	30	-	-	-	-	0	-	0	0	2083	0.1	-	0.2	-	791	1422	-
5	-	174	20	259	0.1	0.5	0	-	0.4	0.2	86	1.5	16	1.1	142	150	443	0.8
0	0	0	0	0	0	0	0	-	0	0	19	0.2	4	0	0	4	44	0.3
0	0	0	1	0	0	0	0	-	0	0	1	0	0	0	10	29	12	0
0	0	0	0	0	0	0	0	-	0	0	0	0	0	0	8	16	4	0
0	0	6	0	16	0	0	0	-	0	0	16	0	2	0	14	19	6	0.1
0	0	21	1	63	0	0	0	-	0	0	10	0	1	0	9	11	6	0
0	0	17	1	44	0	0	0	-	0	0	10	0	1	0	9	15	5	0
0	0	10	0	27	0	0	0	-	0	0	14	0	1	0	12	18	6	0
0	0	13	0	35	0	0	0	-	0	0	14	0	1	0	11	17	6	0
0	0	2	0	6	0	0	0	-	0	0	3	0	0	0	3	4	4	0
-	-	14	-	-	-	-	0	-	0	0	352	0	-	0.1	-	37	119	-
-	-	13	-	-	-	-	0	-	0	0	184	0	-	0.2	-	57	176	-
-	-	-	-	400	-	-	6	-	0.2	0	80	0.4	-	-	-	400	400	-
-	-	20	-	-	-	-	0	-	0	0	2484	0	-	0.2	-	511	1282	-
0	0	0	0	0	0	0	0	-	0	0	0	0	0	0	0	0	2	0
0	1	29	7	42	0	0.1	0	-	0.1	0.1	17	0.6	7	0.9	33	51	156	0.6
1	2	43	16	78	0	0.2	0	-	0.1	0.2	21	1.2	9	1.2	60	67	424	0.4
2	2	36	19	89	0	0.2	0	-	0.2	0.3	30	1.2	14	1.2	74	75	316	0.5
0	2	0	7	0	0	0	0	-	0.1	0.2	23	1.2	9	1.6	34	37	209	0.3
1	2	1	16	2	0	0	0	-	0.2	0.2	38	1.1	17	1.9	56	72	495	0.4
0	0	0	7	11	0	0	3	-	0	0	7	0.1	6	0.1	10	75	1	0.1
0	0	0	1	0	0	0	0	-	0	0	1	0	1	0	2	6	2	0
-	0	0	0	0	0	0	0	-	0	0	0	0	0	0	1	3	12	0
2	-	32	18	44	0	0.2	0	-	0.2	0.1	25	1.1	11	1.4	77	70	320	0.6
2	1	20	21	7	0	0.1	0	-	0.2	0.2	46	1.3	12	1.9	70	81	241	0.5
2	1	15	11	11	-	0.1	3	-	0.2	0.2	33	1.3	11	1.4	63	59	251	0.4
2	-	-	11	38	-	-	3	-	0.1	0	33	0.5	11	0.5	63	59	251	0.4
4	1	30	18	9	0.1	0.1	1	-	0.2	0.1	61	1.2	21	1.5	72	62	236	0.6

Code	Food Name	Amount	Unit	Grams	kCalories	Carbohydrate (gm)	Protein (gm)	Fat (gm)	Saturated Fat (gm)	Monounsaturated Fat (gm)
18435	Danish Pastry, Raspberry	1	Each	71	263	34	4	13	3	7
9087	Dates, Domestic, Natural and Dry	½	Cup	89	245	65	2	0	-	-
17165	Deer, Ckd, Roasted	3	Ounce	85.1	134	0	26	3	1	1
1073	Dessert Topping, Nondairy	1	Tbsp.	4	13	1	0	1	1	0
43375	Dinty Moore Beef Stew-Hormel	1	Cup	253.2	246	18	12	15	7	6
43376	Dinty Moore Chicken Stew-Hormel	1	Cup	253.2	310	18	13	21	5	7
43377	Dinty Moore Meatball Stew-Hormel	1	Cup	253.2	268	16	12	18	8	8
43378	Dinty Moore Vegetable Stew-Hormel	1	Cup	253.2	173	22	6	7	2	1
19032	Doo Dads Snack Mix, Original Flavor	1	Cup	56.7	259	36	6	10	-	-
18251	Doughnuts, Chocolate, Sugared or Glazed	1	Each	42	175	24	2	8	2	5
18253	Doughnuts, French Crullers, Glazed	1	Each	41	169	24	1	8	2	4
18255	Doughnuts, Glazed	1	Each	60	242	27	4	14	3	8
18248	Doughnuts, Plain	1	Each	47	198	23	2	11	2	5
18249	Doughnuts, Plain, Chocolate-coated or Frosted	1	Each	43	204	21	2	13	4	7
18250	Doughnuts, Plain, Sugared or Glazed	1	Each	45	192	23	2	10	2	5
18254	Doughnuts, w/ Creme Filling	1	Each	85	307	26	5	21	6	11
18256	Doughnuts, w/ Jelly Filling	1	Each	85	289	33	5	16	4	9
18252	Doughnuts, Wheat, Sugared or Glazed	1	Each	45	162	19	3	9	1	4
14153	Dr. Pepper	12	Fl Oz	368.4	151	38	0	0	0	-
5142	Duck, Domesticated, Meat Only, Roasted	3	Ounce	85.1	171	0	20	10	4	3
5140	Duck, Domesticated, Meat&skin, Roasted	3	Ounce	85.1	287	0	16	24	8	11
7021	Dutch Brand Loaf, Lunch Meat	1	Slice	28.4	68	2	4	5	2	2
18257	Eclairs, Custard-filled w/ Chocolate Glaze	1	Each	62	162	15	4	10	3	4
18317	Egg Custard Pie	1	Slice	105	221	22	6	12	3	6
19168	Egg Custards	1	Cup	282	296	30	14	13	7	4
1142	Egg Substitute, Frozen	1	Cup	240	384	8	27	27	5	6
1143	Egg Substitute, Liquid	1	Cup	251	211	2	30	8	2	2
1057	Eggnog	1	Cup	254	342	34	10	19	11	6
11210	Eggplant, Ckd	½	Cup	48	13	3	0	0	0	0
11209	Eggplant, Fresh	½	Cup	41	11	2	0	0	0	0
1128	Eggs, Chicken, Whole, Ckd, Fried	1	Large	46	92	1	6	7	2	3
1129	Eggs, Chicken, Whole, Ckd, Hard-boiled	1	Large	50	78	1	6	5	2	2
1130	Eggs, Chicken, Whole, Ckd, Omelet	1	Large	59	90	1	6	7	2	3
1131	Eggs, Chicken, Whole, Ckd, Poached	1	Large	50	75	1	6	5	2	2
1132	Eggs, Chicken, Whole, Ckd, Scrambled	½	Cup	110	183	2	12	13	4	5
1123	Eggs, Chicken, Whole, Fresh, and Frozen	1	Large	50	75	1	6	5	2	2
41242	English Muffin Sandwich-Healthy Choice	1	Each	120.5	200	30	16	3	1	-
18260	English Muffins, Mixed-grain (includes Granola)	1	Each	66	155	31	6	1	0	1
18261	English Muffins, Mixed-grain, Toasted	1	Each	61	156	31	6	1	0	1
18258	English Muffins, Plain	1	Each	57	134	26	4	1	0	0
18259	English Muffins, Plain, Toasted	1	Each	52	133	26	4	1	0	0
18262	English Muffins, Raisin-cinnamon	1	Each	57	139	28	4	2	0	0
18263	English Muffins, Raisin-cinnamon, Toasted	1	Each	52	137	28	4	2	0	0
18264	English Muffins, Wheat	1	Each	57	127	26	5	1	0	0
18265	English Muffins, Wheat, Toasted	1	Each	52	126	25	5	1	0	0
18266	English Muffins, Whole-wheat	1	Each	66	134	27	6	1	0	0
18267	English Muffins, Whole-wheat, Toasted	1	Each	61	135	27	6	1	0	0
55170	Escalloped Apples-Stouffer's	1	Each	170.1	200	41	0	4	-	-
55117	Escalloped Chicken and Noodles-Stouffer's	1	Each	283.5	420	30	21	24	-	-
62592	Fat Free Cinnamon Graham Snacks-SnackWell	20	Each	13.4	49	12	1	0	0	0
62606	Fat Free Cracked Pepper Crackers-SnackWell	7	Each	15	60	13	2	0	0	0
62589	Fat Free Devils Food Cookie Cakes-SnackWell	1	Each	16	50	13	1	0	0	0
62591	Fat Free Double Fudge Cookie Cakes-SnackWell	1	Each	16	50	12	1	0	0	0
62590	Fat Free Wheat Crackers-SnackWell	5	Each	15	60	12	2	0	0	0
62621	Fettucini Alfredo with Broccoli-Weight Watchers	1	Each	241	220	24	15	6	3	-
55208	Fettucini Alfredo, Lean Cuisine-Stouffer's	1	Each	255.1	280	41	14	7	3	-
55171	Fettucini Alfredo-Stouffer's	1	Each	141.8	245	22	8	14	-	-
55209	Fettucini Primavera, Lean Cuisine-Stouffer's	1	Each	283.5	260	32	14	8	3	-
55831	Fettucini Sauce (Alfredo Style)-Stouffer's	1	Cup	283.9	701	11	14	67	-	-
41288	Fettucini w/ Turkey and Vegetables-Healthy Choice	1	Each	354.4	350	45	29	6	3	-

Polyunsaturated Fat (gm)	Fiber (gm)	Cholesterol (mg)	Folate (μg)	Vitamin A (re)	Vitamin B6 (mg)	Vitamin B12 (μg)	Vitamin C (mg)	Vitamin E (mg)	Riboflavin (mg)	Thiamin (mg)	Calcium (mg)	Iron (mg)	Magnesium (mg)	Niacin (mg)	Phosphorus (mg)	Potassium (mg)	Sodium (mg)	Zinc (mg)
2	-	-	11	43	-	-	3	-	0.1	0	33	0.5	11	0.5	63	59	251	0.4
-	7	0	11	4	0.2	0	0	-	0.1	0.1	28	1	31	2	36	580	3	0.3
1	0	95	-	0	-	-	0	-	0.5	0.2	6	3.8	20	5.7	192	285	46	2.3
0	0	0	0	3	0	0	0	-	0	0	0	0	0	0	0	1	1	0
1	-	33	-	815	-	-	3	-	0.1	0	27	1	23	2.5	-	588	971	2.8
8	-	95	-	476	-	-	2	-	0.3	0.1	38	0.7	25	3.6	-	610	1012	1.3
1	-	33	-	279	-	-	1	-	0.2	0.1	27	1.2	27	3.2	-	586	1094	2.7
2	-	16	-	714	-	-	2	-	0.1	0.1	36	0.7	31	1.7	-	509	949	0.8
-	4	1	23	24	0.1	0	0	-	0.1	0.2	42	1.4	34	3	168	157	721	1.3
1	1	24	7	11	0	0.1	0	-	0	0	89	1	14	0.2	68	50	143	0.2
1	-	5	3	-	0	0	0	-	0.1	0.1	11	0.6	5	0.6	50	32	141	0.1
2	1	4	13	-	0	0.1	0	-	0.1	0.2	26	1.2	13	1.7	56	65	205	0.5
4	1	17	4	8	0	0.1	0	-	0.1	0.1	21	0.9	9	0.9	126	60	257	0.3
2	1	25	7	13	0	0.2	0	-	0	0.1	15	1.1	17	0.6	87	49	184	0.3
1	-	14	5	1	0	0.1	0	-	0.1	0.1	27	0.5	8	0.7	53	46	181	0.2
3	-	20	12	7	0	0.1	0	-	0.1	0.3	21	1.6	17	1.9	65	68	263	0.7
2	-	22	14	7	0	0.1	1	-	0.1	0.3	21	1.5	17	1.8	72	67	249	0.6
3	-	9	7	9	0	0.1	0	-	0.1	0.1	22	0.5	10	0.8	47	67	160	0.3
-	0	0	0	0	0	0	0	-	0	0	11	0.1	0	0	41	4	37	0.1
1	0	76	9	20	0.2	0.3	0	-	0.4	0.2	10	2.3	17	4.3	173	214	55	2.2
3	0	71	5	54	0.2	0.3	0	-	0.2	0.1	9	2.3	14	4.1	133	174	50	1.6
1	0	13	1	0	0.1	0.4	5	-	0.1	0.1	24	0.4	6	0.7	46	107	354	0.5
2	-	79	9	118	0	0.2	0	-	0.2	0.1	39	0.7	9	0.5	66	73	209	0.4
2	1	35	21	53	0.1	0.5	0	-	0.2	0	84	0.6	12	0.3	118	111	252	0.5
1	-	245	28	169	0.1	0.9	1	-	0.6	0.1	316	0.8	39	0.2	319	431	217	1.5
15	0	5	39	324	0.3	0.8	1	-	0.9	0.3	175	4.8	36	0.3	172	512	479	2.4
4	0	3	37	542	0	0.7	0	-	0.8	0.3	133	5.3	22	0.3	304	828	444	3.3
1	0	149	2	203	0.1	1.1	4	-	0.5	0.1	330	0.5	47	0.3	278	420	138	1.2
0	1	0	7	3	0	0	1	-	0	0	3	0.2	6	0.3	11	119	1	0.1
0	1	0	8	3	0	0	1	-	0	0	3	0.1	6	0.2	9	89	1	0.1
1	0	211	17	114	0.1	0.4	0	-	0.2	0	25	0.7	5	0	89	61	162	0.5
1	0	212	22	84	0.1	0.6	0	-	0.3	0	25	0.6	5	0	86	63	62	0.5
1	0	207	17	110	0.1	0.4	0	-	0.2	0	25	0.7	5	0	87	60	159	0.5
1	0	212	18	95	0.1	0.4	0	-	0.2	0	25	0.7	5	0	89	60	140	0.6
2	0	387	33	215	0.1	0.8	0	-	0.5	0.1	78	1.3	13	0	187	152	308	1.1
1	0	213	24	96	0.1	0.5	0	-	0.3	0	25	0.7	5	0	89	61	63	0.6
1	-	20	-	60	-	-	4	-	0.4	0.5	120	2	-	2.9	220	200	510	-
0	-	0	23	1	0.1	0	0	-	0.2	0.3	129	2	29	2.4	98	103	275	0.6
0	-	0	16	1	0.1	0	0	-	0.2	0.2	130	2	29	2.1	99	103	276	0.6
1	-	0	21	0	0	0	0	-	0.2	0.3	99	1.4	12	2.2	76	75	264	0.4
1	-	0	15	0	0	0	0	-	0.1	0.2	98	1.4	11	2	75	74	262	0.4
1	-	0	18	0	0	0	0	-	0.2	0.2	84	1.4	9	2	44	119	255	0.6
1	-	0	13	0	0	0	0	-	0.1	0.2	83	1.4	9	1.8	44	118	253	0.6
0	-	0	22	0	0.1	0	0	-	0.2	0.2	101	1.6	22	1.9	66	106	218	0.6
0	-	0	16	0	0	0	0	-	0.1	0.2	100	1.6	22	1.7	64	105	216	0.6
1	4	0	32	0	0.1	0	0	-	0.1	0.2	175	1.6	47	2.3	186	139	420	1.1
1	-	0	23	0	0.1	0	0	-	0.1	0.2	176	1.6	47	2	187	139	422	1.1
-	-	-	-	-	-	-	30	-	-	0	-	-	-	-	-	90	15	-
-	-	-	20	-	-	-	-	-	0.3	0.2	80	0.8	-	3.8	-	300	840	-
0	0	0	-	0	-	-	0	-	-	-	0	0.3	-	-	-	-	40	-
0	0	0	-	0	-	-	0	-	-	-	24	0.4	-	-	-	-	150	-
0	1	0	-	0	-	-	0	-	-	-	0	0	-	-	-	-	25	-
0	1	0	-	0	-	-	0	-	-	-	0	0.2	-	-	-	-	70	-
0	1	0	-	0	-	-	0	-	-	-	24	0.4	-	-	-	45	170	-
-	6	15	-	60	-	-	1	-	-	-	300	1.5	-	-	-	510	540	-
-	-	15	-	-	-	-	-	-	0.4	0.3	200	0.8	-	1.5	-	270	570	-
-	-	-	-	-	-	-	-	-	0.3	0.2	120	0.4	-	1	-	100	400	-
-	-	45	-	400	-	-	18	-	0.4	0.3	240	0.8	-	1.5	-	400	510	-
-	-	180	-	-	-	-	0	-	0	0	2724	0	-	0	-	341	1813	-
2	-	60	-	150	-	-	-	-	0.5	0.5	120	1.5	-	3.8	310	450	480	-

Code	Food Name	Amount	Unit	Grams	kCalories	Carbohydrate (gm)	Protein (gm)	Fat (gm)	Saturated Fat (gm)	Monounsaturated Fat (gm)
62612	Fiesta Chicken-Weight Watchers	1	Each	241	220	38	12	2	1	-
55773	Fiesta Mexicali Heat'n Serve Soup -Stouffer's	1	Cup	283.9	110	18	3	3	-	-
19098	Fifth Avenue Bar	1	Bar	60	280	41	5	13	-	-
18170	Fig Bars	1	Each	16	56	11	1	1	0	1
55210	Filet of Fish Divan, Lean Cuisine-Stouffer's	1	Each	294.1	210	13	27	5	2	-
55211	Filet of Fish Florentine, Lean Cuisine-Stouffer's	1	Each	272.9	220	13	26	7	3	-
15027	Fish Fillets and Sticks, Fried	3	Ounce	85.1	231	20	13	10	3	4
15029	Flounder, Ckd, Dry Heat	3	Ounce	85.1	100	0	21	1	0	0
55178	French Bread Pizza, Cheese-Stouffer's	1	Each	145.3	350	40	16	14	-	-
41332	French Bread Pizza, Deluxe-Healthy Choice	1	Each	180.7	330	41	23	7	3	-
55181	French Bread Pizza, Deluxe-Stouffer's	1	Each	173.6	420	40	21	19	-	-
55180	French Bread Pizza, Double Cheese-Stouffer's	1	Each	166.6	420	43	22	18	-	-
55182	French Bread Pizza, Hamburger-Stouffer's	1	Each	173.6	410	39	23	18	-	-
55183	French Bread Pizza, Pepperoni-Stouffer's	1	Each	159.5	400	39	19	19	-	-
55185	French Bread Pizza, Sausage-Stouffer's	1	Each	170.1	430	40	20	21	-	-
55187	French Bread Pizza, Vegetable Deluxe-Stouffer's	1	Each	180.7	420	41	18	20	-	-
55761	French Onion Soup-Stouffer's	1	Cup	283.9	100	10	4	4	-	-
18268	French Toast, Frozen, Ready-to-heat	1	Slice	59	126	19	4	4	1	1
18269	French Toast, Made w/ Lowfat (2%) Milk	1	Slice	65	149	16	5	7	2	3
18381	French Toast, Made w/ Whole Milk	1	Slice	65	151	16	5	7	2	3
19226	Frostings, Chocolate, Creamy	1	Ounce	28.4	113	18	0	5	2	3
19713	Frostings, Cream Cheese-flavor	1	Ounce	28.4	117	19	0	5	1	3
19229	Frostings, Sour Cream-flavor	1	Ounce	28.4	117	19	0	5	1	3
19230	Frostings, Vanilla, Creamy	1	Ounce	28.4	119	20	0	5	1	2
41319	Frozen Dessert, Bordeaux Cherry-Healthy Choice	1	Cup	133	240	46	6	4	0	-
41320	Frozen Dessert, Butter Pecan Crunch-Healthy Choice	1	Cup	133	280	52	6	4	-	-
41321	Frozen Dessert, Chocolate Chip-Healthy Choice	1	Cup	133	260	48	6	4	0	-
41322	Frozen Dessert, Coffee Toffee-Healthy Choice	1	Cup	133	260	50	6	4	-	-
41323	Frozen Dessert, Cookies 'n Cream-Healthy Choice	1	Cup	133	260	48	8	4	0	-
41324	Frozen Dessert, Double Fudge Swirl-Healthy Choice	1	Cup	133	260	48	6	4	-	-
41325	Frozen Dessert, Fudge Brownie-Healthy Choice	1	Cup	133	280	54	6	4	0	-
41326	Frozen Dessert, Mint Chocolate Chip-Healthy Choice	1	Cup	133	280	50	6	4	0	-
41327	Frozen Dessert, Neapolitan-Healthy Choice	1	Cup	133	240	44	6	4	0	-
41328	Frozen Dessert, Praline and Caramel-Healthy Choice	1	Cup	133	260	52	6	4	0	-
41329	Frozen Dessert, Rocky Road-Healthy Choice	1	Cup	133	320	64	6	4	0	-
41330	Frozen Dessert, Vanilla-Healthy Choice	1	Cup	133	240	42	8	4	0	-
19263	Fruit and Juice Bars	1	Bar	77	63	16	1	0	-	-
9100	Fruit Hvy Syrup	½	Cup	127.5	93	24	0	0	0	0
9097	Fruit Juice Pack	½	Cup	124	57	15	1	0	0	0
9099	Fruit Lt Syrup	½	Cup	126	72	19	1	0	0	0
18319	Fruit Pie, Fried	1	Pie	128	404	55	4	21	3	10
14267	Fruit Punch Drink, Cnd	¾	Cup	185.8	87	22	0	0	0	0
9105	Fruit Salad, Hvy Syrup	½	Cup	127.5	93	24	0	0	0	0
9103	Fruit Salad, Juice Pack	½	Cup	124.5	62	16	1	0	0	0
9104	Fruit Salad, Lt Syrup	½	Cup	126	73	19	0	0	0	0
9102	Fruit Salad, Water Pack	½	Cup	122.5	37	10	0	0	0	0
9096	Fruit Water Pack	½	Cup	122.5	39	10	1	0	0	0
9188	Fruit, Mixed, Dried	¼	Cup	37.5	91	24	1	0	0	0
9189	Fruit, Mixed, Frzn, Swtnd, Thawd	½	Cup	125	123	30	2	0	0	0
9187	Fruit, Mixed, Hvy Syrup	½	Cup	127.5	92	24	0	0	0	0
19381	Fudge, Brown Sugar w/ Nuts	1	Piece	14	55	11	0	1	0	0
19100	Fudge, Chocolate	1	Piece	17	65	14	0	1	1	0
19101	Fudge, Chocolate w/ Nuts	1	Piece	19	81	14	1	3	1	1
19102	Fudge, Peanut Butter	1	Piece	16	59	13	1	1	0	0
19103	Fudge, Vanilla	1	Piece	16	59	13	0	1	1	0
19104	Fudge, Vanilla w/ Nuts	1	Piece	15	62	11	0	2	1	0
41337	Garden Potato Casserole-Healthy Choice	1	Each	262.2	180	23	12	4	2	-
55774	Garden Tomato Heat'n Serve Soup-Stouffer's	1	Cup	283.9	110	16	4	3	-	-
41273	Garden Vegetable Soup-Healthy Choice	1	Each	212.6	100	18	3	1	-	-
19215	Gelatin Pops	1	Each	44	31	7	1	0	-	-

Polyunsaturated Fat (gm)	Fiber (gm)	Cholesterol (mg)	Folate (µg)	Vitamin A (re)	Vitamin B6 (mg)	Vitamin B12 (µg)	Vitamin C (mg)	Vitamin E (mg)	Riboflavin (mg)	Thiamin (mg)	Calcium (mg)	Iron (mg)	Magnesium (mg)	Niacin (mg)	Phosphorus (mg)	Potassium (mg)	Sodium (mg)	Zinc (mg)
-	5	25	-	450	-	-	42	-	-	-	72	1.5	-	-	-	490	480	-
-	-	10	-	-	-	-	6	-	0	0	2404	1	-	0.2	-	431	711	-
-	-	2	33	5	0.1	0.1	0	-	0.1	0	42	0.6	38	2	90	197	112	0.6
0	1	0	2	1	0	0	0	-	0	0	10	0.5	4	0.3	10	33	56	0.1
1	-	65	-	20	-	-	27	-	0.3	0.2	120	0.4	-	1.9	-	800	490	-
2	-	65	-	500	-	-	1	-	0.3	0.2	120	0.4	-	1.9	-	780	590	-
3	0	95	15	26	0.1	1.5	0	-	0.2	0.1	17	0.6	21	1.8	154	222	495	0.6
0	0	58	8	9	0.2	2.1	0	-	0.1	0.1	15	0.3	49	1.9	246	293	89	0.5
-	-	-	-	60	-	-	4	-	0.3	0.5	200	1.5	-	2.9	-	300	630	-
1	-	35	-	80	-	-	-	-	0.3	0.5	200	2.5	-	3.8	280	350	500	-
-	-	-	-	100	-	-	6	-	0.4	0.5	160	1.5	-	3.8	-	350	950	-
-	-	-	-	40	-	-	6	-	0.5	0.5	360	1.5	-	3.8	-	320	850	-
-	-	-	-	60	-	-	6	-	0.3	0.4	160	1.5	-	3.8	-	340	650	-
-	-	-	-	100	-	-	6	-	0.4	0.5	160	1.5	-	3.8	-	300	880	-
-	-	-	-	80	-	-	6	-	0.4	0.6	160	1.5	-	3.8	-	340	840	-
-	-	-	-	250	-	-	4	-	0.4	0.5	280	1.5	-	3.8	-	230	830	-
-	0	-	-	-	-	-	0	-	0	0	240	0	-	0	-	170	2073	-
1	2	48	14	32	0.3	1	0	-	0.2	0.2	63	1.3	10	1.6	82	79	292	0.5
2	-	75	15	86	0	0.2	0	-	0.2	0.1	65	1.1	11	1.1	76	87	311	0.4
2	-	76	15	81	0	0.2	0	-	0.2	0.1	64	1.1	11	1.1	76	86	311	0.4
1	-	0	0	56	0	0	0	-	0	0	2	0.4	6	0	22	56	52	0.1
1	-	0	0	0	0	0	0	-	0	0	1	0	1	0	1	10	11	0
1	-	0	0	35	0	0	0	-	0	0	1	0	1	0.2	1	55	58	0
1	-	0	0	64	0	0	0	-	0	0	1	0	0	0	11	10	26	0
2	-	10	-	-	-	-	-	-	0.3	0.1	160	-	-	-	200	300	100	-
2	-	10	-	-	-	-	2	-	0.3	0.1	160	-	-	-	160	300	160	-
2	-	10	-	-	-	-	2	-	0.3	0.1	160	0.4	-	-	160	320	140	-
2	-	10	-	-	-	-	2	-	0.3	0.1	160	-	-	-	160	320	160	-
2	-	10	-	-	-	-	-	-	0.3	0.1	240	-	-	-	200	360	160	-
2	-	10	-	-	-	-	-	-	0.3	0.1	160	0.8	-	-	200	420	140	-
2	-	10	-	-	-	-	-	-	0.3	0.1	160	0.4	-	-	160	380	140	-
4	-	10	-	-	-	-	-	-	0.3	0.1	160	0.4	-	-	-	340	160	-
2	-	10	-	-	-	-	-	-	0.3	0.1	160	-	-	-	200	320	120	-
2	-	10	-	-	-	-	-	-	0.3	0.1	160	-	-	-	200	380	140	-
2	-	10	-	-	-	-	-	-	0.5	0.1	240	-	-	-	200	360	120	-
-	-	0	5	2	0	0	7	-	0	0	4	0.1	3	0.1	5	41	3	0
0	1	0	3	26	0.1	0	2	-	0	0	8	0.4	6	0.5	14	112	8	0.1
0	1	0	3	38	0.1	0	3	-	0	0	10	0.3	9	0.5	17	118	5	0.1
0	1	0	3	26	0.1	0	2	-	0	0	8	0.4	6	0.5	14	112	8	0.1
7	3	0	4	4	0	0.1	2	-	0.1	0.2	28	1.6	13	1.8	55	83	479	0.3
0	0	0	2	2	0	0	55	-	0	0	15	0.4	4	0	2	46	41	0.2
0	1	0	3	64	0	0	3	-	0	0	8	0.4	6	0.4	11	102	8	0.1
0	-	0	3	75	0	0	4	-	0	0	14	0.3	10	0.4	17	144	6	0.2
0	-	0	3	54	0	0	3	-	0	0	9	0.4	6	0.5	11	103	8	0.1
0	-	0	3	54	0	0	2	-	0	0	9	0.4	6	0.5	11	96	4	0.1
0	1	0	3	31	0.1	0	3	-	0	0	6	0.3	9	0.4	13	115	5	0.1
0	-	0	1	92	0.1	0	1	-	0.1	0	14	1	15	0.7	29	299	7	0.2
0	2	0	9	40	0	0	94	-	0	0	9	0.3	7	0.5	15	164	4	0.1
0	-	0	4	24	0	0	88	-	0.1	0	1	0.5	6	0.8	13	107	5	0.1
1	-	1	2	2	0	0	0	-	0	0	16	0.3	7	0	12	52	14	0.1
0	0	2	0	8	0	0	0	-	0	0	7	0.1	4	0	10	18	11	0.1
1	0	3	2	9	0	0	0	-	0	0	10	0.1	9	0	18	30	11	0.1
0	-	1	2	2	0	0	0	-	0	0	7	0	4	0.2	10	21	12	0.1
0	0	3	0	8	0	0	0	-	0	0	6	0	1	0	5	8	11	0
1	0	2	2	7	0	0	0	-	0	0	7	0.1	4	0	11	17	9	0.1
-	-	20	-	-	-	-	-	-	-	-	-	-	-	-	-	600	360	-
-	-	10	-	-	-	-	0	-	0	0	240	0.3	-	0.2	-	431	1052	-
-	-	0	-	350	-	-	9	-	0.1	0.1	16	0.4	-	0.8	-	230	560	-
-	0	0	0	0	0	0	0	-	0	0	1	0	0	0	0	1	20	0

Code	Food Name	Amount	Unit	Grams	kCalories	Carbohydrate (gm)	Protein (gm)	Fat (gm)	Saturated Fat (gm)	Monounsaturated Fat (gm)
14011	Gin and Tonic	1	Fl Oz	30	23	2	0	0	0	0
14136	Ginger Ale	12	Fl Oz	366	124	32	0	0	0	-
62532	Ginger Ale, Diet	12	Fl Oz	355.2	0	0	0	0	-	-
18172	Gingersnaps	1	Each	7	29	5	0	1	0	0
43399	Glazed Breast of Chicken, Top Shelf-Hormel	1	Each	283.5	170	19	19	2	1	1
55212	Glazed Chicken w/ Veg. Lean Cuisine-Stouffer's	1	Each	241	250	24	21	7	2	-
41307	Glazed Chicken-Healthy Choice	1	Each	241	220	27	21	3	1	-
55784	Glazed Chicken-Stouffer's	1	Ounce	28.4	26	1	3	1	-	-
19105	Goobers	1	Piece	1	5	0	0	0	0	0
18173	Graham Crackers, Plain or Honey	1	Each	7	30	5	0	1	0	0
19016	Granola Bars, Hard, Almond	1	Each	28.4	140	18	2	7	4	2
19017	Granola Bars, Hard, Chocolate Chip	1	Each	28.4	124	20	2	5	3	1
19019	Granola Bars, Hard, Peanut	1	Each	28.4	136	18	3	6	1	2
19420	Granola Bars, Hard, Peanut Butter	1	Each	28.4	137	18	3	7	1	2
19015	Granola Bars, Hard, Plain	1	Each	28.4	134	18	3	6	1	1
19404	Granola Bars, Soft, Chocolate Chip	1	Each	28.4	119	20	2	5	3	1
19406	Granola Bars, Soft, Nut and Raisin	1	Each	28.4	129	18	2	6	3	1
19021	Granola Bars, Soft, Peanut Butter	1	Each	28.4	121	18	3	4	1	2
19027	Granola Bars, Soft, Peanut Butter and Choc Chip	1	Each	28.4	122	18	3	6	2	2
19020	Granola Bars, Soft, Plain	1	Each	28.4	126	19	2	5	2	1
19022	Granola Bars, Soft, Raisin	1	Each	28.4	127	19	2	5	3	1
14277	Grape Drink, Cnd	¾	Cup	187.6	84	22	0	0	0	0
14282	Grape Juice Drink, Cnd	¾	Cup	187.6	94	24	0	0	0	0
9135	Grape Juice, Cnd or Bottled, Unsweetened	¾	Cup	189.4	116	28	1	0	0	0
14142	Grape Soda	12	Fl Oz	372	160	42	0	0	0	0
9124	Grapefruit Juice, Cnd, Sweetened	¾	Cup	187	86	21	1	0	0	0
9123	Grapefruit Juice, Cnd, Unsweetened	¾	Cup	185.2	70	17	1	0	0	0
9404	Grapefruit Juice, Pink, Fresh	¾	Cup	185.3	72	17	1	0	0	0
9128	Grapefruit Juice, White, Fresh	¾	Cup	185.3	72	17	1	0	0	0
9112	Grapefruit, Fresh, Pink&red	1	Medium	146	44	11	1	0	0	0
9116	Grapefruit, Fresh, White	1	Medium	136	45	11	1	0	0	0
9120	Grapefruit, Sections, Cnd, Juice Pack	½	Cup	124.5	46	11	1	0	0	0
9121	Grapefruit, Sections, Cnd, Light Syrup Pack	½	Cup	127	76	20	1	0	0	0
9119	Grapefruit, Sections, Cnd, Water Pack	½	Cup	122	44	11	1	0	0	0
9131	Grapes, American Type, Fresh	½	Cup	46	29	8	0	0	0	0
6114	Gravy, Au Jus, Cnd	¼	Cup	59.6	10	1	1	0	0	0
6116	Gravy, Beef, Cnd	¼	Cup	58.3	31	3	2	1	1	1
6119	Gravy, Chicken, Cnd	¼	Cup	59.6	47	3	1	3	1	2
6121	Gravy, Mushroom, Cnd	¼	Cup	59.6	30	3	1	2	0	1
6125	Gravy, Turkey, Cnd	¼	Cup	59.6	30	3	2	1	0	1
6527	Gravy, Unspecified Type	¼	Cup	65.4	22	4	1	0	0	0
55172	Green Bean Mushroom Casserole-Stouffer's	1	Each	134.7	160	13	5	10	-	-
55118	Green Pepper Steak w/ Rice-Stouffer's	1	Each	297.7	310	35	20	10	-	-
55780	Green Pepper Steak-Stouffer's	1	Ounce	28.4	28	1	3	1	-	-
62617	Grilled Salisbury Steak-Weight Watchers	1	Each	241	250	24	19	9	3	-
15032	Grouper, Ckd, Dry Heat	3	Ounce	85.1	100	0	21	1	0	0
62534	Guava Juice	¾	Cup	179.9	66	16	-	0	-	-
19106	Gumdrops	1	Each	3.5	14	3	0	0	-	-
15034	Haddock, Ckd, Dry Heat	3	Ounce	85.1	95	0	21	1	0	0
15035	Haddock, Smoked	3	Ounce	85.1	99	0	21	1	0	0
15037	Halibut, Ckd, Dry Heat	3	Ounce	85.1	119	0	23	3	0	1
15196	Halibut, Greenland, Ckd, Dry Heat	3	Ounce	85.1	203	0	16	15	3	9
55159	Ham and Asparagus Bake-Stouffer's	1	Each	269.3	520	32	18	35	-	-
7032	Ham and Cheese Loaf(or Roll), Lunch Meat	1	Slice	28.4	73	0	5	6	2	3
7033	Ham and Cheese Spread, Lunch Meat	1	Tbsp.	15	37	0	2	3	1	1
7031	Ham Salad Spread	1	Tbsp.	15	32	2	1	2	1	1
7029	Ham, Approx 11% Fat, Sliced	1	Slice	28.4	52	1	5	3	1	1
7027	Ham, Chopped, Not Cnd	3	Ounce	85.1	195	0	15	15	5	7
7026	Ham, Chopped, Spiced, Cnd	3	Ounce	85.1	203	0	14	16	5	8
7028	Ham, Extra Lean, Appx 5% Fat	1	Slice	28.4	37	0	5	1	0	1

Polyunsaturated Fat (gm)	Fiber (gm)	Cholesterol (mg)	Folate (µg)	Vitamin A (re)	Vitamin B6 (mg)	Vitamin B12 (µg)	Vitamin C (mg)	Vitamin E (mg)	Riboflavin (mg)	Thiamin (mg)	Calcium (mg)	Iron (mg)	Magnesium (mg)	Niacin (mg)	Phosphorus (mg)	Potassium (mg)	Sodium (mg)	Zinc (mg)
0	-	0	0	0	0	0	0	-	0	0	1	0	0	0	0	2	1	0
-	0	0	0	0	0	0	0	-	0	0	11	0.7	4	0	0	4	26	0.2
-	0	-	-	-	-	-	-	-	-	-	-	-	-	-	-	-	30	-
0	0	0	0	0	0	0	0	-	0	0	5	0.4	3	0.2	6	24	46	0
1	-	35	-	400	-	-	4	-	0.2	0.1	32	0.4	35	7.6	-	804	780	1.1
4	-	50	-	20	-	-	4	-	0.2	0.2	16	0.2	-	7.6	-	580	590	-
1	-	45	-	-	-	-	1	-	0.1	0.2	-	0.6	-	6.7	240	370	510	-
-	-	9	-	-	-	-	0	-	0	0	24	0	-	0.2	-	45	105	-
0	-	0	0	0	0	0	0	-	0	0	1	0	1	0.1	3	5	0	0
0	0	0	1	0	0	0	0	-	0	0	2	0.3	2	0.3	7	9	42	0.1
1	-	0	3	1	0	0	0	-	0	0.1	9	0.7	23	0.2	65	77	73	0.4
0	1	0	4	1	0	0	0	-	0	0.1	22	0.9	20	0.2	58	71	98	0.5
3	-	0	7	1	0	0	0	-	0	0.1	11	0.7	31	0.4	85	86	79	0.6
3	-	0	5	1	0	0	0	-	0	0.1	12	0.7	16	0.6	39	82	80	0.4
3	2	0	7	4	0	0	0	-	0	0.1	17	0.8	27	0.4	79	95	83	0.6
1	1	0	6	1	0	0	0	-	0	0.1	26	0.7	22	0.3	65	96	77	0.4
2	2	0	9	1	0	0.1	0	-	0.1	0.1	24	0.6	26	0.7	68	111	72	0.5
1	1	0	9	1	0	0.1	0	-	0	0.1	26	0.6	24	0.9	71	82	116	0.5
1	1	0	9	1	0	0.1	0	-	0	0	23	0.5	25	0.9	74	107	93	0.5
2	1	0	7	0	0	0.1	0	-	0	0.1	30	0.7	21	0.1	65	92	79	0.4
1	1	0	6	0	0	0.1	0	-	0	0.1	29	0.7	20	0.3	62	103	80	0.4
0	0	0	1	0	0	0	64	-	0	0	6	0.3	4	0	2	9	11	0.2
0	0	0	2	0	0	0	30	-	0	0	6	0.2	8	0.2	8	66	2	0.1
0	0	0	5	2	0.1	0	0	-	0.1	0	17	0.5	19	0.5	21	250	6	0.1
0	0	0	0	0	0	0	0	-	0	0	11	0.3	4	0	0	4	56	0.3
0	0	0	19	0	0	0	50	-	0	0.1	15	0.7	19	0.6	21	303	4	0.1
0	0	0	19	2	0	0	54	0.1	0	0.1	13	0.4	19	0.4	20	283	2	0.2
0	-	0	19	82	0.1	0	70	-	0	0.1	17	0.4	22	0.4	28	300	2	0.1
0	0	0	19	2	0.1	0	70	-	0	0.1	17	0.4	22	0.4	28	300	2	0.1
0	0	0	18	38	0.1	0	56	-	0	0	16	0.2	12	0.3	13	188	0	0.1
0	1	0	14	1	0.1	0	45	-	0	0.1	16	0.1	12	0.4	11	201	0	0.1
0	0	0	11	0	0	0	42	-	0	0	19	0.3	14	0.3	15	210	9	0.1
0	1	0	11	0	0	0	27	-	0	0	18	0.5	13	0.3	13	164	3	0.1
0	0	0	11	0	0	0	27	-	0	0	18	0.5	12	0.3	12	161	2	0.1
0	1	0	2	5	0.1	0	2	-	0	0	6	0.1	2	0.1	5	88	1	0
0	-	0	1	0	0	0.1	1	-	0	0	2	0.4	1	0.5	18	48	30	0.6
0	0	2	1	0	0	0.1	0	-	0	0	3	0.4	1	0.4	17	47	326	0.6
1	0	1	1	66	0	0.1	0	-	0	0	12	0.3	1	0.3	17	65	344	0.5
1	0	0	7	0	0	0	0	-	0	0	4	0.4	1	0.4	9	63	340	0.4
0	0	1	1	0	0	0.1	0	-	0	0	2	0.4	1	0.8	17	65	344	0.5
0	-	0	1	0	0	0	0	-	0	0	9	0.1	3	0.2	12	16	356	0.1
-	-	-	-	40	-	-	2	-	0.2	0.1	64	0.2	-	0.4	-	200	550	-
-	-	-	-	40	-	-	6	-	0.2	0.2	16	1	-	3.8	-	410	700	-
-	-	7	-	-	-	-	4	-	0	0	48	0	-	0.1	-	51	164	-
-	4	30	-	60	-	-	0	-	-	-	120	1.5	-	-	-	450	590	-
0	0	40	9	43	0.3	0.6	0	-	0	0.1	18	1	31	0.3	122	404	45	0.4
-	-	0	-	0	-	-	30	-	-	-	0	0	-	-	-	-	18	-
-	0	0	0	0	0	0	0	-	0	0	0	0	0	0	0	0	2	0
0	0	63	11	16	0.3	1.2	0	-	0	0	36	1.1	43	3.9	205	339	74	0.4
0	0	65	13	19	0.3	1.4	0	-	0	0	42	1.2	46	4.3	213	353	649	0.4
1	0	35	12	46	0.3	1.2	0	-	0.1	0.1	51	0.9	91	6.1	242	490	59	0.5
1	0	50	1	15	0.4	0.8	0	-	0.1	0.1	3	0.7	28	1.6	179	293	88	0.4
-	-	-	-	60	-	-	36	-	0.5	0.5	160	0.8	-	2.9	-	360	1100	-
1	0	16	1	7	0.1	0.2	7	-	0.1	0.2	16	0.3	5	1	72	83	381	0.6
0	0	9	0	14	0	0.1	1	-	0	0	33	0.1	3	0.3	74	24	180	0.3
0	0	6	0	0	0	0.1	1	-	0	0.1	1	0.1	2	0.3	18	22	137	0.2
0	0	16	1	0	0.1	0.2	8	-	0.1	0.2	2	0.3	5	1.5	70	94	373	0.6
2	0	43	1	0	0.3	0.8	17	-	0.2	0.5	6	0.7	14	3.3	132	271	1166	1.6
2	0	42	1	0	0.3	0.6	2	-	0.1	0.5	6	0.8	11	2.7	118	242	1161	1.6
0	0	13	1	0	0.1	0.2	7	-	0.1	0.3	2	0.2	5	1.4	62	99	405	0.5

Code	Food Name	Amount	Unit	Grams	kCalories	Carbohydrate (gm)	Protein (gm)	Fat (gm)	Saturated Fat (gm)	Monounsaturated Fat (gm)
7030	Ham, Minced	3	Ounce	85.1	224	2	14	18	6	8
62626	Hamburger Patty, Meatless	1	Each	90	140	8	18	4	2	-
55809	Heartland Medley-Stouffer's	1	Ounce	28.4	17	2	1	0	-	-
41279	Hearty Beef Soup-Healthy Choice	1	Each	212.6	120	17	9	1	-	-
41280	Hearty Chicken Soup-Healthy Choice	1	Each	212.6	110	17	7	2	-	-
41258	Herb Roasted Chicken-Healthy Choice	1	Each	347.3	300	50	22	5	2	-
15040	Herring, Ckd, Dry Heat	3	Ounce	85.1	173	0	20	10	2	4
15042	Herring, Kippered	3	Ounce	85.1	185	0	21	11	2	4
15197	Herring, Pacific, Ckd, Dry Heat	3	Ounce	85.1	213	0	18	15	4	7
15041	Herring, Pickled	3	Ounce	85.1	223	8	12	15	2	10
41311	Homestyle Turkey w/ Vegetables-Healthy Choice	1	Each	269.3	260	34	26	2	-	-
20030	Hominy, Cnd, White	½	Cup	80	58	11	1	1	0	0
20330	Hominy, Cnd, Yellow	½	Cup	80	58	11	1	1	0	0
19296	Honey	1	Tbsp.	21	64	17	0	0	-	-
7035	Honey Loaf, Lunch Meat	1	Slice	28.4	36	2	4	1	0	1
55214	Honey Mustard Chicken, Lean Cuisine-Stouffer's	1	Each	212.6	230	30	18	4	1	-
41312	Honey Mustard Chicken-Healthy Choice	1	Each	269.3	310	41	26	4	1	-
43371	Hot Chili no Beans-Hormel	1	Each	212.6	360	14	16	27	11	13
43410	Hot Chili w/ Beans, Micro Cup-Hormel	1	Each	209.1	250	24	15	11	4	4
43372	Hot Chili w/ Beans-Hormel	1	Each	212.6	300	27	15	15	5	6
7022	Hot Dog, Beef	1	Each	57	180	1	7	16	7	8
7024	Hot Dog, Chicken	1	Each	45	116	3	6	9	2	4
62605	Hot Dog, Fat Free	1	Each	50	40	2	7	0	0	0
7025	Hot Dog, Turkey	1	Each	45	102	1	6	8	3	3
16137	Hummus, Fresh	½	Cup	123	210	25	6	10	2	4
18270	Hush Puppies	1	Each	22	74	10	2	3	0	1
18271	Ice Cream Cones, Cake or Wafer-type	1	Each	4	17	3	0	0	0	0
18272	Ice Cream Cones, Sugar, Rolled-type	1	Each	10	40	8	1	0	0	0
19270	Ice Cream, Chocolate	½	Cup	66	143	19	3	7	4	2
19090	Ice Cream, French Vanilla, Soft-serve	½	Cup	66.5	143	15	3	9	5	2
19271	Ice Cream, Strawberry	½	Cup	66	127	18	2	6	-	-
19095	Ice Cream, Vanilla	½	Cup	66	133	16	2	7	4	2
19089	Ice Cream, Vanilla, Rich	½	Cup	66.5	160	15	2	11	7	3
19088	Ice Milk, Vanilla	½	Cup	66.5	92	15	3	3	2	1
19096	Ice Milk, Vanilla, Soft Serve	½	Cup	66.5	84	14	3	2	1	1
19283	Ice Pops	1	Bar	52	37	10	0	0	-	-
19717	Ice Pops, w/ Added Ascorbic Acid	1	Bar	52	37	10	0	0	-	-
62547	Iced Tea, Bottled, All Flavors	1	Cup	236.6	118	29	0	0	0	-
62548	Iced Tea, Bottled, All Flavors, Diet	1	Cup	236.6	0	1	0	0	0	-
62622	Italian Cheese Lasagna-Weight Watchers	1	Each	311.9	300	28	29	8	3	-
43395	Italian Lasagna, Top Shelf-Hormel	1	Each	283.5	350	30	23	16	8	5
55798	Italian Style Vegetables-Stouffer's	1	Ounce	28.4	10	2	0	0	-	-
19297	Jams and Preserves	1	Tbsp.	20	48	13	0	0	0	0
19300	Jellies	1	Tbsp.	19	51	13	0	0	-	-
19108	Jellybeans	1	Each	1.1	4	1	0	0	-	-
19109	Kit Kat Wafer Bar	1	Bar	46	235	28	3	13	8	4
9148	Kiwifruit, Fresh	1	Medium	76	46	11	1	0	-	-
19110	Krackel Chocolate Bar	1	Bar	47	236	29	3	13	6	3
17225	Lamb, Ground, Ckd, Broiled	3	Ounce	85.1	241	0	21	17	7	7
17016	Lamb, Leg, Shank, Meat and Fat, Ckd, Rstd	3	Ounce	85.1	191	0	22	11	4	4
17018	Lamb, Leg, Shank, Meat Only, Ckd, Rstd	3	Ounce	85.1	153	0	24	6	2	2
17020	Lamb, Leg, Sirloin, Meat and Fat, Ckd, Rstd	3	Ounce	85.1	248	0	21	18	7	7
17022	Lamb, Leg, Sirloin, Meat Only, Ckd, Rstd	3	Ounce	85.1	174	0	24	8	3	3
17012	Lamb, Leg, Whole, Meat and Fat, Ckd, Rstd	3	Ounce	85.1	219	0	22	14	6	6
17014	Lamb, Leg, Whole, Meat Only, Ckd, Rstd	3	Ounce	85.1	162	0	24	7	2	3
17024	Lamb, Loin, Meat and Fat, Ckd, Broiled	3	Ounce	85.1	269	0	21	20	8	8
17025	Lamb, Loin, Meat and Fat, Ckd, Roasted	3	Ounce	85.1	263	0	19	20	9	8
17027	Lamb, Loin, Meat Only, Ckd, Broiled	3	Ounce	85.1	184	0	26	8	3	4
17028	Lamb, Loin, Meat Only, Ckd, Roasted	3	Ounce	85.1	172	0	23	8	3	3
17002	Lamb, Meat and Fat, Ckd	3	Ounce	85.1	250	0	21	18	8	8

Polyunsaturated Fat (gm)	Fiber (gm)	Cholesterol (mg)	Folate (μg)	Vitamin A (re)	Vitamin B6 (mg)	Vitamin B12 (μg)	Vitamin C (mg)	Vitamin E (mg)	Riboflavin (mg)	Thiamin (mg)	Calcium (mg)	Iron (mg)	Magnesium (mg)	Niacin (mg)	Phosphorus (mg)	Potassium (mg)	Sodium (mg)	Zinc (mg)
2	0	60	1	0	0.2	0.8	26	-	0.2	0.6	9	0.7	14	3.5	134	265	1059	1.6
1	5	0	-	0	-	-	0	-	-	0.3	96	1.5	-	4	-	-	380	7.5
-	-	3	-	-	-	-	1	-	0	0	40	0	-	0.1	-	60	85	-
-	-	20	-	150	-	-	9	-	0.1	0.1	32	0.4	-	1.9	90	280	540	-
-	-	25	-	200	-	-	2	-	0.2	0.1	32	0.4	-	1.9	90	190	520	-
1	-	40	-	250	-	-	24	-	0.1	0.2	32	0.8	-	7.6	280	370	560	-
2	0	65	10	26	0.3	11.2	1	-	0.3	0.1	63	1.2	35	3.5	258	356	98	1.1
2	0	70	12	33	0.4	15.9	1	-	0.3	0.1	71	1.3	39	3.7	276	380	781	1.2
3	0	84	5	30	0.4	8.2	0	-	0.2	0.1	90	1.2	35	2.4	248	461	81	0.6
1	0	11	2	219	0.1	3.6	0	-	0.1	0	65	1	7	2.8	76	59	740	0.5
-	-	30	-	100	-	-	5	-	0.1	0	32	-	-	-	-	100	550	-
0	2	0	1	0	0	0	0	-	0	0	8	0.5	13	0	28	7	168	0.8
0	-	0	1	9	0	0	0	-	0	0	8	0.5	13	0	28	7	168	0.8
-	0	0	0	0	0	0	0	-	0	0	1	0.1	0	0	1	11	1	0
0	0	10	2	0	0.1	0.3	6	-	0.1	0.1	5	0.4	5	0.9	41	97	374	0.7
1	-	40	-	200	-	-	2	-	0.2	0.2	16	0.4	-	3.8	-	340	540	-
-	-	45	-	100	-	-	4	-	0	0.2	16	0.8	-	1.5	-	110	520	-
1	-	60	-	330	-	-	-	-	0.2	0	40	1.4	35	2.5	-	497	860	2.7
-	-	49	-	190	-	-	-	-	0.2	0.1	48	1.9	46	1.7	-	677	977	2.7
1	-	55	-	210	-	-	-	-	0.2	0.1	48	1.8	49	1.7	-	777	1030	2.3
1	0	35	2	0	0.1	0.9	14	-	0.1	0	11	0.8	2	1.4	50	95	585	1.2
2	0	45	2	17	0.1	0.1	0	-	0.1	0	43	0.9	5	1.4	48	38	617	1.4
0	0	15	-	0	-	-	0	-	-	-	0	0.2	-	-	-	-	460	-
2	0	48	4	0	0.1	0.1	0	-	0.1	0	48	0.8	6	1.9	60	81	642	1.4
4	6	0	73	2	0.5	0	10	-	0.1	0.1	61	1.9	36	0.5	138	214	300	1.4
2	1	10	4	9	0	0	0	-	0.1	0.1	61	0.7	5	0.6	42	32	147	0.1
0	0	0	0	0	0	0	0	-	0	0	1	0.1	1	0.2	4	4	6	0
0	0	0	1	0	0	0	0	-	0	0.1	4	0.4	3	0.5	10	15	32	0.1
0	-	22	11	79	0	0.2	0	-	0.1	0	72	0.6	19	0.1	71	164	50	0.4
0	-	61	6	102	0	0.3	1	-	0.1	0	87	0.1	8	0.1	77	118	41	0.3
-	-	19	8	51	0	0.2	5	-	0.2	0	79	0.1	9	0.1	66	124	40	0.2
0	0	29	3	77	0	0.3	0	-	0.2	0	84	0.1	9	0.1	69	131	53	0.5
0	0	41	3	122	0	0.2	0	-	0.1	0	78	0	7	0.1	63	106	37	0.3
0	0	9	4	31	0	0.4	1	-	0.2	0	92	0.1	10	0.1	72	140	57	0.3
0	0	8	4	19	0	0.3	1	-	0.1	0	104	0	9	0.1	80	147	47	0.4
-	0	0	0	0	0	0	0	-	0	0	0	0	1	0	0	2	6	0
-	-	0	0	0	0	0	6	-	0	0	0	0	1	0	0	2	6	0
-	0	0	-	0	-	-	0	-	-	-	0	0	-	-	-	-	10	-
-	0	0	-	0	-	-	0	-	-	-	0	0	-	-	-	-	0	-
-	7	25	-	350	-	-	15	-	-	-	780	1.5	-	-	-	720	560	-
1	-	60	-	100	-	-	2	-	0.5	0.3	240	1.5	49	3.8	-	728	840	3.2
-	-	0	-	-	-	-	2	-	0	0	72	0	-	0	-	62	147	-
0	0	0	7	0	0	0	2	-	0	0	4	0.1	1	0	2	15	8	0
-	0	0	0	0	0	0	0	-	0	0	2	0.1	1	0	1	12	7	0
0	0	0	0	0	0	0	0	-	0	0	0	0	0	0	0	0	0	0
0	0	12	0	14	0	0.3	1	-	0.1	0	83	0.4	20	0.2	80	142	46	0.5
-	3	0	-	14	-	0	74	-	0	0	20	0.3	23	0.4	30	252	4	-
3	-	9	4	6	0	0.3	0	-	0.1	0	84	0.4	26	0.2	104	161	64	0.6
1	0	82	16	0	0.1	2.2	-	0.1	0.2	0.1	19	1.5	20	5.7	171	288	69	4
1	0	77	19	0	0.1	2.3	0	0.1	0.2	0.1	9	1.7	21	5.6	168	277	55	4
0	0	74	20	0	0.1	2.3	0	0.2	0.2	0.1	7	1.8	22	5.4	177	291	56	4.3
1	0	82	14	0	0.1	2.2	0	0.1	0.2	0.1	9	1.7	19	5.6	156	256	58	3.5
1	0	78	18	0	0.1	2.2	0	0.1	0.3	0.1	7	1.9	21	5.3	173	283	60	4.1
1	0	79	17	0	0.1	2.2	0	0.1	0.2	0.1	9	1.7	20	5.6	162	266	56	3.7
0	0	76	20	0	0.1	2.2	0	0.2	0.2	0.1	7	1.8	22	5.4	175	287	58	4.2
1	0	85	15	0	0.1	2.1	0	0.1	0.2	0.1	17	1.5	20	6	167	278	65	3
2	0	81	16	0	0.1	1.9	0	0.1	0.2	0.1	15	1.8	20	6	153	209	54	2.9
1	0	81	20	0	0.1	2.1	0	0.1	0.2	0.1	16	1.7	24	5.8	192	320	71	3.5
1	0	74	21	0	0.1	1.8	0	0.1	0.2	0.1	14	2.1	23	5.8	175	227	56	3.5
1	0	82	15	0	0.1	2.2	0	-	0.2	0.1	14	1.6	20	5.7	160	264	61	3.8

Code	Food Name	Amount	Unit	Grams	kCalories	Carbohydrate (gm)	Protein (gm)	Fat (gm)	Saturated Fat (gm)	Monounsaturated Fat (gm)
17004	Lamb, Meat Only, Ckd	3	Ounce	85.1	175	0	24	8	3	4
17030	Lamb, Rib, Meat and Fat, Ckd, Broiled	3	Ounce	85.1	307	0	19	25	11	10
17031	Lamb, Rib, Meat and Fat, Ckd, Roasted	3	Ounce	85.1	305	0	18	25	11	11
17033	Lamb, Rib, Meat Only, Ckd, Broiled	3	Ounce	85.1	200	0	24	11	4	4
17034	Lamb, Rib, Meat Only, Ckd, Roasted	3	Ounce	85.1	197	0	22	11	4	5
4002	Lard	¼	Cup	51.3	462	0	0	51	20	23
62613	Lasagna Florentine-Weight Watchers	1	Each	283.5	210	37	13	2	1	-
55215	Lasagna w/ Meat Sauce, Lean Cuisine-Stouffer's	1	Each	290.6	280	36	20	6	3	-
41308	Lasagna w/ Meat Sauce-Healthy Choice	1	Each	283.5	260	37	18	5	2	-
62623	Lasagna with Meat Sauce-Weight Watchers	1	Each	290.6	290	34	24	7	3	-
43403	Lasagna, Micro Cup-Hormel	1	Each	212.6	250	25	8	13	6	4
55134	Lasagna-Stouffer's	1	Each	283.5	340	40	18	12	-	-
11247	Leeks, Ckd	½	Cup	52	16	4	0	0	0	0
11246	Leeks, Fresh	½	Cup	52	32	7	1	0	0	0
18320	Lemon Meringue Pie	1	Slice	113	303	53	2	10	2	4
41259	Lemon Pepper Fish-Healthy Choice	1	Each	304.8	300	52	13	5	1	-
18445	Lemon Pie, Fried	1	Pie	128	404	55	4	21	3	10
19380	Lemon Pudding	1	Cup	298.1	373	75	0	9	1	4
14145	Lemon-lime Soda	12	Fl Oz	368.4	147	38	0	0	0	0
62529	Lemon-lime Soda, Diet	12	Fl Oz	355.2	0	0	0	0	-	-
14297	Lemonade Flavor Drink	1	Cup	266	112	29	0	0	0	0
14543	Lemonade, Pink	1	Cup	247.8	99	26	0	0	0	0
14290	Lemonade, Low Calorie	1	Cup	243.7	5	1	0	0	0	-
14293	Lemonade, White	1	Cup	247.8	99	26	0	0	0	0
9150	Lemons, Fresh, w/o Peel	1	Medium	58	17	5	1	0	0	0
41274	Lentil Soup-Healthy Choice	1	Each	212.6	140	23	8	1	-	-
11250	Lettuce, Butterhead, Fresh	1	Cup	56	7	1	1	0	0	0
11252	Lettuce, Iceberg, Fresh	1	Cup	56	7	1	1	0	0	0
11253	Lettuce, Looseleaf, Fresh	1	Cup	56	10	2	1	0	0	0
11251	Lettuce, Romaine, Fresh	1	Cup	56	9	1	1	0	0	0
55216	Linguini w/ Clam Sauce, Lean Cuisine-Stouffer's	1	Each	272.9	280	36	17	8	2	-
14415	Liqueur, Coffee w/ Cream, 34 Proof	1	Fl Oz	31.1	102	6	1	5	3	1
14414	Liqueur, Coffee, 53 Proof	1	Fl Oz	34.8	117	16	0	0	0	0
14534	Liqueur, Coffee, 63 Proof	1	Fl Oz	34.8	107	11	0	0	0	0
14533	Liquor, Distilled, All 100 Proof	1	Fl Oz	27.8	82	0	0	0	0	0
14037	Liquor, Distilled, All 80 Proof	1	Fl Oz	27.8	64	0	0	0	0	0
14550	Liquor, Distilled, All 86 Proof	1	Fl Oz	27.8	70	0	0	0	0	0
14551	Liquor, Distilled, All 90 Proof	1	Fl Oz	27.8	73	0	0	0	0	0
14532	Liquor, Distilled, All 94 Proof	1	Fl Oz	27.8	76	0	0	0	0	0
15148	Lobster, Northern, Ckd, Moist Heat	3	Ounce	85.1	83	1	17	1	0	0
15228	Lobster, Spiny, Ckd, Moist Heat	3	Ounce	85.1	122	3	22	2	0	0
19107	Lollipop	1	Each	6	22	6	0	0	-	-
19140	M&M's Peanut	1	Pkg	49	243	29	5	13	-	-
19141	M&M's Plain	1	Pkg	48	228	33	3	11	-	-
12131	Macadamia Dried	½	Cup	67	470	9	6	49	7	39
12633	Macadamia Oil Roasted	½	Cup	67	481	9	5	51	8	40
55217	Macaroni and Beef in Sauce, Lean Cuisine-Stouffer's	1	Each	283.5	250	35	14	6	1	-
55137	Macaroni and Beef w/ Tomatoes-Stouffer's	1	Each	326	340	38	21	12	-	-
41338	Macaroni and Beef-Healthy Choice	1	Each	241	200	32	12	3	1	-
62533	Macaroni and Cheese	1	Cup	111.9	360	44	1	13	8	-
57808	Macaroni and Cheese Pot Pie-Swanson	1	Each	198.5	200	24	7	8	-	-
55218	Macaroni and Cheese, Lean Cuisine-Stouffer's	1	Each	255.1	290	37	15	9	4	-
43406	Macaroni and Cheese, Micro Cup-Hormel	1	Each	212.6	260	28	12	11	6	3
41339	Macaroni and Cheese-Healthy Choice	1	Each	255.1	280	45	12	6	3	-
55155	Macaroni and Cheese-Stouffer's	1	Each	170.1	250	23	11	13	-	-
62624	Macaroni and Cheese-Weight Watchers	1	Each	255.2	260	43	15	6	2	-
20100	Macaroni, Ckd, Enriched	1	Cup	140	197	40	7	1	0	0
20400	Macaroni, Ckd, Unenriched	1	Cup	140	197	40	7	1	0	0
20106	Macaroni, Vegetable, Ckd, Enriched	1	Cup	134	172	36	6	0	0	0
20108	Macaroni, Whole-wheat, Ckd	1	Cup	140	174	37	7	1	0	0

Polyunsaturated Fat (gm)	Fiber (gm)	Cholesterol (mg)	Folate (µg)	Vitamin A (re)	Vitamin B6 (mg)	Vitamin B12 (µg)	Vitamin C (mg)	Vitamin E (mg)	Riboflavin (mg)	Thiamin (mg)	Calcium (mg)	Iron (mg)	Magnesium (mg)	Niacin (mg)	Phosphorus (mg)	Potassium (mg)	Sodium (mg)	Zinc (mg)
1	0	78	20	0	0.1	2.2	0	0.2	0.2	0.1	13	1.7	22	5.4	179	293	65	4.5
2	0	84	12	0	0.1	2.2	0	0.1	0.2	0.1	16	1.6	20	6	151	230	65	3.4
2	0	82	13	0	0.1	1.9	0	0.1	0.2	0.1	19	1.4	17	5.7	141	230	62	3
1	0	77	18	0	0.1	2.2	0	0.2	0.2	0.1	14	1.9	25	5.6	181	266	72	4.5
1	0	75	19	0	0.1	1.8	0	0.1	0.2	0.1	18	1.5	20	5.2	166	268	69	3.8
6	0	49	0	0	0	0	0	0.6	0	0	0	0	0	0	0	0	0	0.1
-	5	10	-	300	-	-	15	-	-	-	300	1.5	-	-	-	440	420	-
-	-	25	-	100	-	-	6	-	0.3	0.2	120	1	-	2.9	-	700	560	-
1	-	20	-	150	-	-	2	-	0.3	0.3	80	1.5	-	1.9	210	500	420	-
-	7	15	-	250	-	-	12	-	-	-	480	1.5	-	-	-	720	580	-
2	-	23	-	100	-	-	2	-	0.2	0.1	40	0.8	25	1.9	-	331	949	1.1
-	-	-	-	150	-	-	6	-	0.3	0.2	200	1	-	6.7	-	570	840	-
0	-	0	13	3	0.1	0	2	-	0	0	16	0.6	7	0.1	9	45	5	0
0	1	0	33	5	0.1	0	6	-	0	0	31	1.1	15	0.2	18	94	10	0.1
3	1	51	9	59	0	0.2	4	-	0.2	0.1	63	0.7	17	0.7	119	101	165	0.6
2	-	40	-	80	-	-	48	-	0.1	0.2	32	0.6	-	1.1	180	410	370	-
7	-	4	4	0	0.1	0	-	-	0.1	0.2	28	1.6	13	1.8	55	83	479	0.3
3	-	0	0	0	0	0	0	-	0	0	6	0.2	3	0	15	3	417	0.1
0	0	0	0	0	0	0	0	-	0	0	7	0.3	4	0.1	0	4	41	0.2
-	0	-	-	-	-	-	-	-	-	-	-	-	-	-	-	-	30	-
0	-	0	0	0	0	0	34	-	0	0	29	0.1	3	0	3	3	19	0.1
0	-	0	5	0	0	0	10	-	0.1	0	7	0.4	5	0	5	37	7	0.1
-	0	0	0	0	0	0	6	-	0	0	51	0.1	2	0	24	0	7	0.1
0	-	0	5	5	0	0	10	-	0.1	0	7	0.4	5	0	5	37	7	0.1
0	2	0	6	2	0	0	31	-	0	0	15	0.3	5	0.1	9	80	1	0
-	-	0	-	60	-	-	2	-	0	0.1	-	0.6	-	0.4	-	160	480	-
0	1	0	41	54	0	0	4	-	0	0	18	0.2	7	0.2	13	144	3	0.1
0	1	0	31	18	0	0	2	-	0	0	11	0.3	5	0.1	11	88	5	0.1
0	1	0	28	106	0	0	10	-	0	0	38	0.8	6	0.2	14	148	5	0.2
0	1	0	76	146	0	0	13	-	0.1	0.1	20	0.6	3	0.3	25	162	4	0.1
2	-	30	-	-	-	-	-	-	0.2	0.3	32	1.5	-	1.9	-	90	560	
0	0	5	0	13	0	0	0	-	0	0	5	0	1	0	16	10	29	0
0	0	0	0	0	0	0	0	-	0	0	0	0	1	0.1	2	10	3	0
0	-	0	0	0	0	0	0	-	0	0	0	0	1	0.1	2	10	3	0
0	-	0	0	0	0	0	0	-	0	0	0	0	0	0	1	1	0	0
0	0	0	0	0	0	0	0	-	0	0	0	0	0	0	1	1	0	0
0	0	0	0	0	0	0	0	-	0	0	0	0	0	0	1	1	0	0
0	0	0	0	0	0	0	0	-	0	0	0	0	0	0	1	1	0	0
0	-	0	0	0	0	0	0	-	0	0	0	0	0	0	1	1	0	0
0	0	61	9	22	0.1	2.6	0	-	0.1	0	52	0.3	30	0.9	157	299	323	2.5
1	0	77	1	5	0.1	3.4	2	-	0	0	54	1.2	43	4.2	195	177	193	6.2
-	0	0	0	0	0	0	0	-	0	0	0	0	0	0	0	0	2	0
-	2	6	27	4	0.1	0.2	0	-	0.1	0	65	0.7	40	1.6	134	191	46	0.7
-	1	7	4	12	0	0.2	0	-	0.1	0	81	0.7	32	0.3	94	188	49	0.6
1	6	0	11	0	0.1	0	0	-	0.1	0.2	47	1.6	78	1.4	91	247	3	1.1
1	6	0	11	1	0.1	0	0	-	0.1	0.1	30	1.2	78	1.4	134	220	174	0.7
1	-	25	-	100	-	-	4	-	0.2	0.2	48	1.5	-	2.9	-	450	540	-
-	-	-	-	60	-	-	6	-	0.1	0.1	32	0.8	-	1.9	-	300	1440	-
-	-	15	-	200	-	-	15	-	0.3	0.3	32	1	-	0	-	530	420	-
-	16	40	-	100	-	-	0	-	-	-	240	1.5	-	-	-	-	1029	-
-	-	-	-	80	-	-	-	-	0.2	0.1	120	0.6	-	0.8	-	-	740	-
-	-	30	-	-	-	-	-	-	0.4	0.3	200	0.8	-	1.5	-	160	550	-
1	-	45	-	80	-	-	6	-	0.3	0.1	80	0.6	25	1.1	-	209	650	1.1
1	-	20	-	-	-	-	-	-	0.3	0.3	120	1	-	1.1	230	220	520	-
-	-	-	-	20	-	-	-	-	0.3	0.2	160	0.4	-	0.4	-	140	640	-
-	7	20	-	100	-	-	0	-	-	-	300	1	-	-	-	410	550	-
0	2	0	10	0	0	0	0	-	0.1	0.3	10	2	25	2.3	76	43	1	0.7
0	2	0	10	-	0	0	0	-	0	0	10	0.7	25	0.6	76	43	1	0.7
0	6	0	8	7	0	0	0	-	0.1	0.2	15	0.7	25	1.4	67	42	8	0.6
0	6	0	7	0	0.1	0	0	-	0.1	0.2	21	1.5	42	1	125	62	4	1.1

Code	Food Name	Amount	Unit	Grams	kCalories	Carbohydrate (gm)	Protein (gm)	Fat (gm)	Saturated Fat (gm)	Monounsaturated Fat (gm)
41309	Mandarin Chicken-Healthy Choice	1	Each	311.8	260	39	23	2	-	-
62535	Mango Juice	¾	Cup	179.9	66	16	-	0	-	-
9176	Mangos, Fresh	½	Cup	82.5	54	14	0	0	0	0
14012	Manhattan	1	Fl Oz	28.5	64	1	0	0	0	0
4067	Margarine, Hard, Corn&sybn	1	Tsp.	4.7	34	0	0	4	1	2
4071	Margarine, Hard, Corn(hydr)	1	Tsp.	4.7	34	0	0	4	1	2
4128	Margarine, Imitation (appx 40% Fat)	1	Tsp.	4.8	17	0	0	2	0	1
4132	Margarine, Regular, w/ Salt Added	1	Tsp.	4.7	34	0	0	4	1	2
4131	Margarine, Regular, w/o Added Salt	1	Tsp.	4.7	34	0	0	4	1	2
4130	Margarine, Soft, w/ Salt Added	1	Tsp.	4.7	34	0	0	4	1	1
4129	Margarine, Soft, w/o Added Salt	1	Tsp.	4.7	34	0	0	4	1	2
11256	Marinara Sauce	½	Cup	125	85	13	2	4	1	2
55830	Marinara Sauce-Stouffer's	1	Cup	283.9	180	18	3	11	-	-
19303	Marmalade, Orange	1	Tbsp.	20	49	13	0	0	-	-
19116	Marshmallows	1	Cup	46	146	37	1	0	-	-
14014	Martini	1	Fl Oz	28.2	63	0	0	0	0	0
4018	Mayonnaise	1	Tbsp.	14.7	57	4	0	5	1	1
62610	Mayonnaise, Fat Free	1	Tbsp.	15	10	3	0	0	0	-
62609	Mayonnaise, Light	1	Tbsp.	15	25	1	0	2	0	-
55219	Meatloaf w/ Mac. and Cheese, Lean Cuisine-Stouffer's	1	Each	265.8	280	26	26	8	3	-
41260	Meatloaf-Healthy Choice	1	Each	340.2	340	48	17	8	3	-
55779	Meatloaf-Stouffer's	1	Ounce	28.4	57	2	4	3	-	-
9185	Melon Balls, Frozen, Unthawed	½	Cup	86.5	29	7	1	0	-	-
9181	Melons, Cantaloup, Fresh	1	Wedge	80	28	7	1	0	-	-
9183	Melons, Casaba, Fresh	1	Wedge	164	43	10	1	0	-	-
9184	Melons, Honeydew, Fresh	1	Wedge	129	45	12	1	0	-	-
55812	Mexicali Chicken-Stouffer's	1	Ounce	28.4	20	2	1	1	-	-
19120	Milk Chocolate	1	Bar	44	226	26	3	13	8	4
19126	Milk Chocolate Coated Peanuts	1	Ounce	28.4	147	14	4	9	4	4
19127	Milk Chocolate Coated Raisins	1	Ounce	28.4	111	19	1	4	2	1
19132	Milk Chocolate w/ Almonds	1	Bar	41	216	22	4	14	7	6
1110	Milk Shakes, Thick Chocolate	1	Cup	345.4	410	73	11	9	6	3
1111	Milk Shakes, Thick Vanilla	1	Cup	345.4	386	61	13	10	7	3
1075	Milk Substitutes, Fluid w/ hydr Vegetable Oils	1	Cup	244	150	15	4	8	2	5
1076	Milk Substitutes, Fluid, w/ lauric Acid Oil	1	Cup	244	150	15	4	8	7	0
1088	Milk, Buttermilk	1	Cup	245	99	12	8	2	1	1
1104	Milk, Chocolate Drink, Lowfat, 1% Fat	1	Cup	250	158	26	8	2	2	1
1103	Milk, Chocolate Drink, Lowfat, 2% Fat	1	Cup	250	179	26	8	5	3	1
1102	Milk, Chocolate Drink, Whole	1	Cup	250	208	26	8	8	5	2
1105	Milk, Chocolate Homemade Hot Cocoa	1	Cup	250	218	26	9	9	6	3
1095	Milk, Cnd, Condensed, Sweetened	¼	Cup	76.3	245	42	6	7	4	2
1153	Milk, Cnd, Evaporated	¼	Cup	63	85	6	4	5	3	1
1097	Milk, Cnd, Evaporated, Skim	¼	Cup	63.8	50	7	5	0	0	0
1082	Milk, Lowfat, 1% Fat	1	Cup	244	102	12	8	3	2	1
1079	Milk, Lowfat, 2% Fat	1	Cup	244	121	12	8	5	3	1
1099	Milk, Malted, Beverage	1	Cup	265	236	27	10	10	6	3
1101	Milk, Malted, Chocolate Flavor, Beverage	1	Cup	265	228	30	9	9	6	3
1085	Milk, Skim	1	Cup	245	86	12	8	0	0	0
1077	Milk, Whole, 3.3% Fat	1	Cup	244	150	11	8	8	5	2
1078	Milk, Whole, 3.7% Fat	1	Cup	244	157	11	8	9	6	3
19135	Milky Way Bar	1	Bar	60	251	44	3	9	5	3
18322	Mince Meat Pie	1	Slice	165	477	79	4	18	4	8
55770	Minestrone Heat'n Serve Soup-Stouffer's	1	Cup	283.9	130	18	5	4	-	-
41281	Minestrone Soup-Healthy Choice	1	Each	212.6	160	30	6	1	-	-
55760	Minestrone Soup-Stouffer's	1	Cup	283.9	140	20	6	3	-	-
12635	Mixed w/ Peanuts, Dry Roasted	½	Cup	68.5	407	17	12	35	5	22
12637	Mixed w/ Peanuts, Oil Roasted	½	Cup	71	438	15	12	40	6	23
12638	Mixed w/o Peanuts, Oil Roasted	½	Cup	72	443	16	11	40	7	24
18177	Molasses Cookies	1	Each	15	65	11	1	2	0	1
19142	Mounds Candy Bar	1	Bar	20	72	12	1	4	2	1

Polyunsaturated Fat (gm)	Fiber (gm)	Cholesterol (mg)	Folate (µg)	Vitamin A (re)	Vitamin B6 (mg)	Vitamin B12 (µg)	Vitamin C (mg)	Vitamin E (mg)	Riboflavin (mg)	Thiamin (mg)	Calcium (mg)	Iron (mg)	Magnesium (mg)	Niacin (mg)	Phosphorus (mg)	Potassium (mg)	Sodium (mg)	Zinc (mg)
-	-	50	-	250	-	-	9	-	0.2	0.2	16	1	-	4.8	200	400	400	-
-	-	0	-	0	-	-	30	-	-	-	0	0	-	-	-	-	18	-
0	1	0	-	321	0.1	0	23	0.9	0	0	8	0.1	7	0.5	9	129	2	0
0	-	0	0	0	0	0	0	-	0	0	1	0	1	0	2	7	1	0
1	0	0	0	47	0	0	0	0.5	0	0	1	0	0	0	1	2	44	0
1	0	0	0	47	0	0	0	0.5	0	0	1	0	0	0	1	2	44	-
1	0	0	0	48	0	0	0	0.2	0	0	1	0	0	0	1	1	46	0
1	0	0	0	47	0	0	0	0.4	0	0	1	0	0	0	1	2	44	0
1	0	0	0	47	0	0	0	0.4	0	0	1	0	0	0	1	1	0	0
2	0	0	0	47	0	0	0	0.3	0	0	1	0	0	0	1	2	51	0
1	0	0	0	47	0	0	0	0.3	0	0	1	0	0	0	1	2	1	0
1	-	0	17	120	0.3	0	16	-	0.1	0.1	22	1	30	2	44	530	786	0.3
-	-	0	-	-	-	-	66	-	0	0	721	0.2	-	0.4	-	681	1222	-
-	0	0	7	1	0	0	1	-	0	0	8	0	0	0	1	7	11	0
-	0	0	0	0	0	0	0	-	0	0	1	0.1	1	0	4	2	22	0
0	-	0	0	0	0	0	0	-	0	0	1	0	1	0	1	5	1	0
3	0	4	1	12	0	0	0	0.6	0	0	2	0	0	0	4	1	104	0
-	0	0	-	0	-	-	0	-	-	-	0	0	-	-	-	10	105	-
-	-	5	-	0	-	-	0	-	-	-	0	0	-	-	-	5	130	-
1	-	55	-	60	-	-	9	-	0.4	0.2	120	2	-	3.8	-	550	540	-
1	-	40	-	-	-	-	-	-	-	-	-	-	-	-	240	690	560	-
-	-	15	-	-	-	-	0	-	0	0	48	0.1	-	0.1	-	4	193	-
-	1	0	22	153	0.1	0	5	-	0	0.1	9	0.3	12	0.6	10	242	27	0.1
-	1	0	14	258	0.1	0	34	0.1	0	0	9	0.2	9	0.5	14	247	7	0.1
-	1	0	-	5	-	0	26	-	0	0.1	8	0.7	13	0.7	11	344	20	-
-	1	0	-	5	0.1	0	32	-	0	0.1	8	0.1	9	0.8	13	350	13	-
-	-	5	-	-	-	-	4	-	0	0	88	0	-	0.1	-	68	48	-
0	2	10	3	21	0	0.2	0	-	0.1	0	84	0.6	26	0.1	95	169	36	0.6
1	1	3	2	0	0.1	0.1	0	-	0	0	29	0.4	26	1.2	60	112	12	0.5
0	1	1	1	2	0	0.1	0	-	0	0	24	0.5	13	0.1	41	146	10	0.2
1	3	8	5	6	0	0.2	0	-	0.2	0	92	0.7	37	0.3	108	182	30	0.5
0	1	36	17	73	0.1	1.1	0	-	0.8	0.2	456	1.1	55	0.4	435	774	383	1.7
0	0	41	23	97	0.1	1.8	0	-	0.7	0.1	505	0.3	41	0.5	398	631	330	1.3
1	0	0	0	0	0	0	0	-	0.2	0	79	1	16	0	181	279	191	2.9
0	0	0	0	0	0	0	0	-	0.2	0	79	1	16	0	181	279	191	2.9
0	0	9	12	20	0.1	0.5	2	-	0.4	0.1	285	0.1	27	0.1	219	371	257	1
0	0	7	12	147	0.1	0.9	2	-	0.4	0.1	287	0.6	33	0.3	256	425	152	1
0	4	17	12	142	0.1	0.8	2	-	0.4	0.1	284	0.6	33	0.3	254	422	150	1
0	4	30	12	72	0.1	0.8	2	-	0.4	0.1	280	0.6	33	0.3	251	417	149	1
0	4	33	12	85	0.1	0.9	2	-	0.4	0.1	298	0.8	55	0.4	270	480	123	1.2
0	0	26	9	62	0	0.3	2	-	0.3	0.1	216	0.1	20	0.2	193	284	97	0.7
0	0	19	5	34	0	0.1	1	-	0.2	0	164	0.1	15	0.1	127	191	67	0.5
0	0	2	5	75	0	0.2	1	-	0.2	0	185	0.2	17	0.1	124	211	73	0.6
0	0	10	12	144	0.1	0.9	2	-	0.4	0.1	300	0.1	34	0.2	235	381	123	1
0	0	18	12	139	0.1	0.9	2	-	0.4	0.1	297	0.1	33	0.2	232	377	122	1
1	0	37	22	95	0.2	1	3	-	0.6	0.2	355	0.3	53	1.3	302	530	223	1.1
0	0	34	16	80	0.1	0.9	3	-	0.4	0.1	305	0.6	48	0.6	265	498	172	1.1
0	0	4	13	149	0.1	0.9	2	-	0.3	0.1	302	0.1	28	0.2	247	406	126	1
0	0	33	12	76	0.1	0.9	2	-	0.4	0.1	291	0.1	33	0.2	228	370	120	0.9
0	0	35	12	83	0.1	0.9	4	-	0.4	0.1	290	0.1	33	0.2	227	368	119	0.9
0	1	12	5	28	0	0.3	1	-	0.1	0	78	0.5	20	0.2	98	145	144	0.4
5	-	0	8	3	0.1	0	10	-	0.2	0.2	36	2.5	23	2	69	335	419	0.4
-	-	0	-	-	-	-	0	-	0	0	481	0.2	-	0	-	310	1192	-
-	-	0	-	60	-	-	15	-	0.1	0.1	32	0.6	-	1.5	130	440	520	-
-	-	10	-	-	-	-	0	-	0	0	721	0.2	-	0.2	-	371	1282	-
7	6	0	35	1	0.2	0	0	-	0.1	0.1	48	2.5	154	3.2	298	409	458	2.6
9	6	0	59	1	0.2	0	0	-	0.2	0.4	77	2.3	167	3.6	329	413	463	3.6
8	4	0	41	1	0.1	0	0	-	0.3	0.4	76	1.9	181	1.4	323	392	504	3.4
0	-	0	1	0	0	0	0	-	0	0.1	11	1	8	0.5	14	52	69	0.1
0	1	0	1	0	0	0	0	-	0	0	5	0.8	14	0	24	42	25	0.2

Code	Food Name	Amount	Unit	Grams	kCalories	Carbohydrate (gm)	Protein (gm)	Fat (gm)	Saturated Fat (gm)	Monounsaturated Fat (gm)
19143	Mr. Goodbar Chocolate Bar	1	Bar	50	257	26	6	16	9	6
18274	Muffins, Blueberry	1	Large	65	180	31	4	4	1	2
18279	Muffins, Corn	1	Large	65	198	33	4	5	1	2
18283	Muffins, Oat Bran	1	Large	65	176	31	5	5	1	1
18273	Muffins, Plain	1	Large	65	192	27	4	7	1	2
18287	Muffins, Wheat Bran	1	Large	65	184	27	5	8	1	2
15056	Mullet, Striped, Ckd, Dry Heat	3	Ounce	85.1	128	0	21	4	1	1
41313	Mushroom Gravy over Beef Sirloin Tips-Healthy Choice	1	Each	269.3	310	43	22	5	2	-
11261	Mushrooms, Ckd	½	Cup	78	21	4	2	0	0	0
11264	Mushrooms, Cnd, Drained Solids	½	Cup	78	19	4	1	0	0	0
11950	Mushrooms, Enoki, Fresh	1	Medium	3	1	0	0	0	0	0
11260	Mushrooms, Fresh	½	Cup	35	9	2	1	0	0	0
11269	Mushrooms, Shiitake, Ckd	½	Cup	72.5	40	10	1	0	0	0
11268	Mushrooms, Shiitake, Dried	1	Medium	3.6	11	3	0	0	0	0
15165	Mussel, Blue, Ckd, Moist Heat	3	Ounce	85.1	146	6	20	4	1	1
62619	Nacho Grande Chicken Enchiladas-Weight Watchers	1	Each	255.2	290	42	15	8	3	-
41340	Nacho Macaroni and Cheese-Healthy Choice	1	Each	255.1	280	44	13	5	3	-
55754	Navy Bean w/ Ham Soup-Stouffer's	1	Cup	283.9	240	31	11	8	-	-
19145	Nestle Crunch	1	Bar	40	198	26	2	10	6	4
55757	New England Clam Chowder Soup-Stouffer's	1	Cup	283.9	341	21	14	23	-	-
55829	Newburg Sauce Supreme-Stouffer's	1	Cup	283.9	481	20	7	41	-	-
43407	Noodles and Chicken, Micro Cup-Hormel	1	Each	212.6	174	19	7	7	2	3
55804	Noodles Romanoff-Stouffer's	1	Cup	283.9	441	36	17	25	-	-
20113	Noodles, Chinese, Chow Mein	½	Cup	22.5	119	13	2	7	1	2
20310	Noodles, Egg, Ckd, Enriched	½	Cup	80	106	20	4	1	0	0
20510	Noodles, Egg, Ckd, Unenriched	½	Cup	80	106	20	4	1	0	0
20112	Noodles, Egg, Spinach, Ckd, Enriched	½	Cup	80	106	19	4	1	0	0
20115	Noodles, Japanese, Soba, Ckd	½	Cup	57	56	12	3	0	0	0
18200	Oatmeal Cookies, Dietary	1	Each	7	31	5	0	1	1	1
18178	Oatmeal Cookies, Regular	1	Each	18	81	12	1	3	1	2
18179	Oatmeal Cookies, Soft-type	1	Each	15	61	10	1	2	0	1
15058	Ocean Perch, Atlantic, Ckd, Dry Heat	3	Ounce	85.1	103	0	20	2	0	1
4053	Oil, Olive	1	Tbsp.	13.5	119	0	0	14	2	10
4042	Oil, Peanut	1	Tbsp.	13.5	119	0	0	14	2	6
4058	Oil, Sesame	1	Tbsp.	13.6	121	0	0	14	2	5
4044	Oil, Soybean	1	Tbsp.	13.6	121	0	0	14	2	3
4034	Oil, Soybean, (hydr)	1	Tbsp.	13.6	121	0	0	14	2	6
4543	Oil, Soybean, (hydr)&cttnsd	1	Tbsp.	13.6	121	0	0	14	2	4
4518	Oil, Vegetable Corn	1	Tbsp.	13.6	121	0	0	14	2	3
4582	Oil, Vegetable, Canola	1	Tbsp.	13.6	121	0	0	14	1	8
4501	Oil, Vegetable, Cocoa Butter	1	Tbsp.	13.6	121	0	0	14	8	4
4502	Oil, Vegetable, Cottonseed	1	Tbsp.	13.6	121	0	0	14	4	2
4055	Oil, Vegetable, Palm	1	Tbsp.	13.6	121	0	0	14	7	5
4513	Oil, Vegetable, Palm Kernel	1	Tbsp.	13.6	118	0	0	14	11	2
4510	Oil, Vegetable, Safflower, Linoleic	1	Tbsp.	13.6	121	0	0	14	1	2
4511	Oil, Vegetable, Safflower, Oleic	1	Tbsp.	13.6	121	0	0	14	1	10
4584	Oil, Vegetable, Sunflower	1	Tbsp.	13.6	121	0	0	14	1	11
11279	Okra, Ckd	½	Cup	80	26	6	1	0	0	0
11278	Okra, Fresh	½	Cup	50	19	4	1	0	0	0
11281	Okra, Frz, Ckd	½	Cup	92	34	8	2	0	0	0
11280	Okra, Frz, Unprepared	½	Cup	71.3	21	5	1	0	0	0
41282	Old Fashioned Chicken Noodle Soup-Healthy Choice	1	Each	212.6	90	11	5	2	-	-
55806	Old-Fashion Stuff'n-Stouffer's	½	Cup	142	310	31	6	19	-	-
10161	Olive Loaf, Lunch Meat	1	Slice	28.4	67	3	3	5	2	2
7051	Olive Loaf, Pork, Lunch Meat	1	Slice	28.4	67	3	3	5	2	2
9194	Olives, Ripe, Canned (jumbo-super colossal)	1	Jumbo	8.3	7	0	0	1	0	0
9193	Olives, Ripe, Canned (small-extra large)	1	Small	3.2	4	0	0	0	0	0
11283	Onions, Ckd	½	Cup	119.9	53	12	2	0	0	0
11285	Onions, Cnd, Sol&liq	½	Cup	112	21	4	1	0	0	0
11282	Onions, Fresh	½	Cup	79.9	30	7	1	0	0	0

Polyunsaturated Fat (gm)	Fiber (gm)	Cholesterol (mg)	Folate (µg)	Vitamin A (re)	Vitamin B6 (mg)	Vitamin B12 (µg)	Vitamin C (mg)	Vitamin E (mg)	Riboflavin (mg)	Thiamin (mg)	Calcium (mg)	Iron (mg)	Magnesium (mg)	Niacin (mg)	Phosphorus (mg)	Potassium (mg)	Sodium (mg)	Zinc (mg)
1	2	10	36	5	0.1	0.2	0	-	0.1	0	56	0.6	48	2.4	140	225	17	0.9
1	2	20	10	-	0	0.4	1	-	0.1	0.1	37	1	10	0.7	128	80	291	0.3
2	-	33	22	23	0.1	0.1	0	-	0.2	0.2	48	1.8	24	1.3	185	45	339	0.5
3	5	0	12	-	0.1	0	0	-	0.1	0.2	41	2.7	102	0.3	244	330	255	1.2
4	2	25	8	26	0	0.1	0	-	0.2	0.2	130	1.6	11	1.5	99	79	304	0.4
4	-	21	34	163	0.2	0.1	5	-	0.3	0.2	122	2.7	51	2.6	185	207	382	1.8
1	0	54	8	36	0.4	0.2	1	-	0.1	0.1	26	1.2	28	5.4	208	390	60	0.7
-	-	35	-	60	-	-	2	-	0	-	-	0.2	-	0.4	-	80	500	-
0	2	0	14	0	0.1	0	3	-	0.2	0.1	5	1.4	9	3.5	68	278	2	0.7
0	2	0	10	0	0	0	0	-	0	0.1	9	0.6	12	1.2	51	101	332	0.6
0	-	0	1	0	0	0	0	-	0	0	0	0	0	0.1	3	11	0	0
0	0	0	7	0	0	0	1	-	0.2	0	2	0.4	4	1.4	36	130	1	0.3
0	2	0	15	0	0.1	0	0	-	0.1	0	2	0.3	10	1.1	21	85	3	1
0	0	0	6	0	0	0	0	-	0	0	0	0.1	5	0.5	11	55	0	0.3
1	0	48	64	77	0.1	20.4	12	-	0.4	0.3	28	5.7	31	2.6	242	228	314	2.3
-	4	20	-	300	-	-	12	-	-	-	360	0.6	-	-	-	600	560	-
-	-	20	-	0	-	-	0	-	0.5	0.6	160	0.8	-	0	-	420	560	-
-	-	20	-	-	-	-	0	-	0	0	70	3	-	0.2	-	571	1252	-
0	1	8	4	6	0	0.2	0	-	0.1	0	68	0.3	18	0.2	71	138	59	0.4
-	-	40	-	-	-	-	0	-	0	0	2484	0.1	-	0.2	-	571	961	-
-	-	120	-	-	-	-	0	-	0	0	1843	0	-	0	-	371	1052	-
2	-	29	-	270	-	-	8	-	0.1	0.1	32	0.7	21	1.7	-	254	1009	0.8
-	-	40	-	-	-	-	0	-	0	0	1602	0.2	-	0.2	-	260	1993	-
4	1	0	5	2	0	0	0	-	0.1	0.1	5	1.1	12	1.3	36	27	99	0.3
0	-	26	6	5	0	0.1	0	-	0.1	0.1	10	1.3	15	1.2	55	22	132	0.5
0	-	26	6	5	0	0.1	0	-	0	0	10	0.5	15	0.3	55	22	132	0.5
0	2	26	17	11	0.1	0.1	0	-	0.1	0.2	15	0.9	19	1.2	46	30	10	0.5
0	-	0	4	0	0	0	0	-	0	0.1	2	0.3	5	0.3	14	20	34	0.1
0	-	0	1	0	0	0	0	-	0	0	3	0.2	2	0.1	10	12	1	0
0	1	0	1	0	0	0	0	-	0	0	7	0.5	6	0.4	25	26	69	0.1
0	0	1	1	1	0	0	0	-	0	0	14	0.4	5	0.3	31	20	52	0.1
0	0	46	9	12	0.2	1	1	-	0.1	0.1	117	1	33	2.1	236	298	82	0.5
1	0	0	0	0	0	0	0	1.6	0	0	0	0.1	0	0	0	0	0	0
4	0	0	0	0	0	0	0	1.6	0	0	0	0	0	0	0	0	0	0
6	0	0	0	0	0	0	0	0.2	0	0	0	0	0	0	0	0	0	0
8	0	0	0	0	0	0	0	1.5	0	0	0	0	0	0	0	0	0	0
5	0	0	0	0	0	0	0	1.1	0	0	0	0	0	0	0	0	0	0
7	0	0	0	0	0	0	0	1.7	0	0	0	0	0	0	0	0	0	0
8	0	0	0	0	0	0	0	2	0	0	0	0	0	0	0	0	0	0
4	0	-	0	0	0	0	0	-	0	0	0	0	0	0	0	0	0	0
0	0	0	0	0	0	0	0	0.2	0	0	0	0	0	0	0	0	0	0
7	0	0	0	0	0	0	0	4.8	-	0	0	0	0	0	0	0	0	0
1	0	0	0	0	0	0	0	2.6	0	0	0	0	0	0	0	0	0	-
0	0	0	0	0	0	0	0	-	0	0	0	0	0	0	0	0	0	0
10	0	0	0	0	0	0	0	4.7	0	0	0	0	0	0	0	0	0	0
2	0	0	0	0	0	0	0	4.7	0	0	0	0	0	0	0	0	0	0
1	0	-	0	0	0	0	0	-	0	0	0	0	0	0	0	0	0	0
0	2	0	37	46	0.1	0	13	-	0	0.1	50	0.4	46	0.7	45	258	4	0.4
0	1	0	44	33	0.1	0	11	-	0	0.1	41	0.4	29	0.5	32	152	4	0.3
0	3	0	134	47	0	0	11	-	0.1	0.1	88	0.6	47	0.7	42	215	3	0.6
0	2	0	105	33	0	0	9	-	0.1	0.1	58	0.4	31	0.5	30	150	2	0.4
-	-	20	-	80	-	-	12	-	0.1	0	16	0.2	-	1.9	60	130	540	-
-	-	5	-	-	-	-	0	-	0	0	361	0.2	-	0.4	-	100	561	-
1	0	11	1	6	0.1	0.4	2	-	0.1	0.1	31	0.2	5	0.5	36	84	421	0.4
1	0	11	1	0	0.1	0.4	3	-	0.1	0.1	31	0.2	5	0.5	36	84	421	0.4
0	-	0	0	3	0	0	0	-	0	0	8	0.3	0	0	0	1	75	0
0	-	0	0	1	0	0	0	-	0	0	3	0.1	0	0	0	0	28	0
0	2	0	18	0	0.2	0	6	-	0	0.1	26	0.3	13	0.2	42	199	4	0.3
0	1	0	11	0	0.2	0	5	-	0	0	50	0.1	7	0.1	31	124	416	0.3
0	1	0	15	0	0.1	0	5	0.2	0	0	16	0.2	0	0.1	26	125	2	0.2

Code	Food Name	Amount	Unit	Grams	kCalories	Carbohydrate (gm)	Protein (gm)	Fat (gm)	Saturated Fat (gm)	Monounsaturated Fat (gm)
14327	Orange and Apricot Juice Drink, Cnd	¾	Cup	187	95	24	1	0	0	0
14323	Orange Drink, Cnd	¾	Cup	185.8	95	24	0	0	0	0
9206	Orange Juice, Fresh	¾	Cup	186	84	19	1	0	0	0
9215	Orange Juice, From Concentrate	¾	Cup	186.4	84	20	1	0	0	0
62558	Orange Juice, w/ Added Calcium	¾	Cup	186.4	84	20	1	0	0	0
9200	Oranges, Fresh	1	Medium	131	62	15	1	0	0	0
9205	Oranges, Fresh, w/ Peel	1	Medium	159	64	25	2	0	0	0
18199	Oreos, Dietary	1	Each	10	46	7	0	2	1	1
18166	Oreos, Regular	1	Each	10	47	7	0	2	0	1
18168	Oreos, w/ Extra Creme Filling	1	Each	13	65	9	0	3	1	2
55220	Oriental Beef w/ Veg., Lean Cuisine-Stouffer's	1	Each	244.5	290	31	20	9	2	-
41314	Oriental Chicken w/ Spicy Peanut Sauce-Healthy Choice	1	Each	269.3	340	40	33	5	1	-
19031	Oriental Mix, Rice-based	1	Ounce	28.4	155	9	6	12	5	3
55221	Oven Baked Chicken, Lean Cuisine-Stouffer's	1	Each	226.8	200	21	17	5	2	-
15168	Oyster, Eastern, Breaded and Fried	3	Ounce	85.1	168	10	7	11	3	4
15170	Oyster, Eastern, Cnd	3	Ounce	85.1	59	3	6	2	1	0
18288	Pancakes Plain, Frozen	1	4 In.	9	21	4	0	0	0	0
18294	Pancakes, Blueberry	1	4 In.	9.5	21	3	1	1	0	0
18390	Pancakes, Buttermilk	1	4 In.	9.5	22	3	1	1	0	0
18298	Pancakes, Dietary	1	3 In.	22	44	9	1	0	0	0
18293	Pancakes, Plain	1	4 In.	9.5	22	3	1	1	0	0
18300	Pancakes, Whole-wheat	1	4 In.	44	92	13	4	3	1	1
9229	Papaya Nectar, Cnd	¾	Cup	187	107	27	0	0	0	0
9226	Papayas, Fresh	1	Medium	304	119	30	2	0	0	0
11808	Parsnips, Ckd, w/ Salt	½	Cup	78	63	15	1	0	0	0
11299	Parsnips, Ckd, w/o Salt	½	Cup	78	63	15	1	0	0	0
11298	Parsnips, Fresh	½	Cup	66.5	50	12	1	0	0	0
9232	Passion-fruit Juice, Purple, Fresh	¾	Cup	185.2	94	25	1	0	-	-
9233	Passion-fruit Juice, Yellow, Fresh	¾¾	Cup	185.2	111	27	1	0	-	-
55800	Pasta Florentine-Stouffer's	½	Cup	142	190	16	8	11	-	-
41294	Pasta Italiano-Healthy Choice	1	Each	340.2	350	59	16	5	2	-
55810	Pasta Roma-Stouffer's	½	Cup	142	130	16	8	4	-	-
41292	Pasta Shells w/ Tomato Sauce-Healthy Choice	1	Each	340.2	330	53	24	3	2	-
55142	Pasta Shells, Cheese w/ Sauce-Stouffer's	1	Each	262.2	300	28	17	13	-	-
41287	Pasta w/ Cacciatore Chicken-Healthy Choice	1	Each	354.4	310	47	26	3	-	-
41293	Pasta w/ Teriyaki Chicken-Healthy Choice	1	Each	357.9	350	58	24	3	1	-
20321	Pasta, Ckd, Enriched, w/ Added Salt	½	Cup	70	99	20	3	0	0	0
20121	Pasta, Ckd, Enriched, w/o Added Salt	½	Cup	70	99	20	3	0	0	0
20094	Pasta, Fresh-refrigerated, Plain, Ckd	½	Cup	73	96	18	4	1	0	0
20096	Pasta, Fresh-refrigerated, Spinach, Ckd	½	Cup	73	95	18	4	1	0	0
20097	Pasta, Homemade, Made w/ Egg, Ckd	½	Cup	73.6	96	17	4	1	0	0
20098	Pasta, Homemade, Made w/o Egg, Ckd	½	Cup	73.6	91	18	3	1	0	0
20127	Pasta, Spinach, Ckd	½	Cup	70	91	18	3	0	0	0
20125	Pasta, Whole-wheat, Ckd	½	Cup	70	87	19	4	0	0	0
9251	Peach Nectar, Cnd, w/o Added Vit C	¾	Cup	186.4	101	26	1	0	0	0
9241	Peaches, Cnd, Heavy Syrup Pack	½	Cup	128	95	26	1	0	0	0
9238	Peaches, Cnd, Juice Pack	½	Cup	124	55	14	1	0	0	0
9240	Peaches, Cnd, Light Syrup Pack	½	Cup	125.5	68	18	1	0	0	0
9237	Peaches, Cnd, Water Pack	½	Cup	122	29	7	1	0	0	0
9242	Peaches, Cnd, X-heavy Syrup Pack	½	Cup	131	126	34	1	0	0	0
9239	Peaches, Cnd, X-light Syrup	½	Cup	123.5	52	14	0	0	0	0
9244	Peaches, Dehydrated, Sulfured	¼	Cup	29	94	24	1	0	0	0
9246	Peaches, Dried, Sulfured	¼	Cup	40	96	25	1	0	0	0
9236	Peaches, Fresh	1	Medium	87	37	10	1	0	0	0
9250	Peaches, Frozen, Sliced, Sweetened	½	Cup	125	118	30	1	0	0	0
19147	Peanut Bar	1	Bar	40	209	19	6	13	2	7
19148	Peanut Brittle	1	Ounce	28.4	128	20	2	5	1	2
18185	Peanut Butter Cookies, Regular	1	Each	15	72	9	1	4	1	1
18186	Peanut Butter Cookies, Soft-type	1	Each	15	69	9	1	4	1	2
18201	Peanut Butter Sandwich Cookies, Dietary	1	Each	10	54	5	1	3	1	2

Polyunsaturated Fat (gm)	Fiber (gm)	Cholesterol (mg)	Folate (µg)	Vitamin A (re)	Vitamin B6 (mg)	Vitamin B12 (µg)	Vitamin C (mg)	Vitamin E (mg)	Riboflavin (mg)	Thiamin (mg)	Calcium (mg)	Iron (mg)	Magnesium (mg)	Niacin (mg)	Phosphorus (mg)	Potassium (mg)	Sodium (mg)	Zinc (mg)
0	0	0	11	108	0.1	0	37	-	0	0	9	0.2	7	0.4	15	150	4	0.1
0	0	0	4	4	0	0	63	-	0	0	11	0.5	4	0.1	2	33	30	0.2
0	0	0	56	37	0.1	0	93	0.1	0.1	0.2	20	0.4	20	0.7	32	372	2	0.1
0	0	0	82	15	0.1	0	73	-	0	0.1	17	0.2	19	0.4	30	354	2	0.1
0	0	0	82	15	0.1	0	73	-	0	0.1	223731	0.2	19	0.4	30	354	2	0.1
0	3	0	40	28	0.1	0	70	0.3	0.1	0.1	52	0.1	13	0.4	18	237	0	0.1
0	4	0	-	40	0.1	0	113	-	0.1	0.2	111	1.3	22	0.8	35	312	3	-
0	-	0	1	0	0	0	0	-	0	0	6	0.5	7	0.3	18	30	24	0.1
0	0	0	1	0	0	0	0	-	0	0	3	0.4	5	0.2	10	18	60	0.1
0	-	0	1	0	0	0	0	-	0	0	3	0.4	4	0.2	12	16	64	0.1
-	-	40	-	150	-	-	1	-	0.2	0.1	16	1	-	2.9	-	400	590	-
1	-	45	-	-	-	-	2	-	-	-	-	0.2	-	0.4	-	50	470	-
3	4	0	25	1	0.1	0	0	-	0	0.1	22	0.8	40	3	112	147	235	1.3
-	-	35	-	350	-	-	6	-	0.2	0.2	16	0.8	-	7.6	-	550	480	-
3	-	69	12	77	0.1	13.3	3	-	0.2	0.1	53	5.9	49	1.4	135	208	355	74.1
1	0	47	8	77	0.1	16.3	4	-	0.1	0.1	38	5.7	46	1.1	118	195	95	77.4
0	-	1	1	3	0	0	0	-	0	0	6	0.3	1	0.4	33	7	46	0.1
0	-	5	1	5	0	0	0	-	0	0	20	0.2	2	0.1	14	13	39	0.1
0	-	6	1	3	0	0	0	-	0	0	15	0.2	1	0.1	13	14	50	0.1
0	-	0	1	2	0	0	0	-	0	0	13	0.4	6	0.4	75	85	58	0.2
0	-	6	1	5	0	0	0	-	0	0	21	0.2	2	0.1	15	13	42	0.1
1	-	27	9	28	0	0.1	0	-	0.2	0.1	110	1.4	20	1	164	123	252	0.5
0	1	0	4	21	0	0	6	-	0	0	19	0.6	6	0.3	0	58	9	0.3
0	5	0	116	85	0.1	0	188	-	0.1	0.1	73	0.3	30	1	15	781	9	0.2
0	-	0	45	0	0.1	0	10	-	0	0.1	29	0.5	23	0.6	54	286	192	0.2
0	3	0	45	0	0.1	0	10	-	0	0.1	29	0.5	23	0.6	54	286	8	0.2
0	3	0	44	0	0.1	0	11	-	0	0.1	24	0.4	19	0.5	47	249	7	0.4
-	0	0	133	-		0	55	-	0.2	0	7	0.4	31	2.7	24	515	11	-
-	0	0	-	446	-	0	34	-	0.2	0	7	0.7	31	4.1	46	515	11	-
-	-	25	-	-	-	-	0	-	0	0	1723	0.1	-	0.1	-	200	446	-
3	-	30	-	60	-	-	-	-	0.5	0.5	48	2	-	2.9	180	540	530	-
-	-	15	-	-	-	-	3	-	0	0.1	521	0.2	-	0.5	-	300	391	-
-	-	35	-	100	-	-	21	-	0.4	0.5	320	1.5	-	2.9	240	640	470	-
-	-	-	-	150	-	-	9	-	0.3	0.1	280	1	-	1.9	-	480	820	-
1	-	35	-	100	-	-	6	-	0.4	0.5	32	1.5	-	6.7	250	660	430	-
2	-	45	-	100	-	-	6	-	0.3	0.3	48	1.5	-	3.8	200	390	370	-
0	-	0	5	-	0	0	0	-	0.1	0.1	5	1	13	1.2	38	22	70	0.4
0	1	0	5	-	0	0	0	-	0.1	0.1	5	1	13	1.2	38	22	1	0.4
0	-	24	5	4	0	0.1	0	-	0.1	0.2	4	0.8	13	0.7	46	18	4	0.4
0	-	24	13	10	0.1	0.1	0	-	0.1	0.1	13	0.8	18	0.7	42	27	4	0.5
0	-	30	14	13	0	0.1	0	-	0.1	0.1	7	0.9	10	0.9	38	15	61	0.3
0	-	0	13	0	0	0	0	-	0.1	0.1	4	0.8	10	1	29	14	54	0.3
0	-	0	8	11	0.1	0	0	-	0.1	0.1	21	0.7	43	1.1	76	41	10	0.8
0	3	0	4	0	0.1	0	0	-	0	0.1	11	0.7	21	0.5	62	31	2	0.6
0	1	0	3	48	0	0	10	-	0	0	9	0.4	7	0.5	11	75	13	0.1
0	1	0	4	42	0	0	4	-	0	0	4	0.3	6	0.8	14	118	8	0.1
0	1	0	4	47	0	0	4	-	0	0	7	0.3	9	0.7	21	159	5	0.1
0	1	0	4	44	0	0	3	-	0	0	4	0.5	6	0.7	14	122	6	0.1
0	1	0	4	65	0	0	4	-	0	0	2	0.4	6	0.6	12	121	4	0.1
0	-	0	4	17	0	0	2	-	0	0	4	0.4	7	0.7	14	109	10	0.1
0	-	0	4	33	0	0	4	-	0	0	6	0.4	6	1	14	91	6	0.1
0	-	2	41				3	-	0	0	11	1.6	17	1.4	47	392	3	0.2
0	3	0	0	86	0	0	2	-	0.1	0	11	1.6	17	1.8	48	398	3	0.2
0	2	0	3	47	0	0	6	-	0	0	4	0.1	6	0.9	10	171	0	0.1
0	2	0	4	35	0	0	118	-	0	0	4	0.5	6	0.8	14	162	7	0.1
4	1	3	24	20	0	0	0	-	0.1	0	31	0.4	30	3.2	61	163	96	0.5
1	1	4	20	13	0	0	0	-	0	0.1	9	0.4	14	1	31	59	128	0.3
1	-	0	5	1	0	0	0	-	0	0	5	0.4	7	0.6	13	25	62	0.1
1	0	0	1	0	0	0	0	-	0	0	2	0.1	5	0.3	13	16	50	0.1
1	-	0	3	0	0	0	0	-	0	0	5	0.2	5	0.5	19	29	41	0.2

Code	Food Name	Amount	Unit	Grams	kCalories	Carbohydrate (gm)	Protein (gm)	Fat (gm)	Saturated Fat (gm)	Monounsaturated Fat (gm)
18190	Peanut Butter Sandwich Cookies, Regular	1	Each	14	67	9	1	3	1	2
16097	Peanut Butter, Chunk Style, w/ Salt	2	Tbsp.	32.3	190	7	8	16	3	8
16397	Peanut Butter, Chunk Style, w/o Salt	2	Tbsp.	32.3	190	7	8	16	3	8
16098	Peanut Butter, Smooth Style, w/ Salt	2	Tbsp.	32.3	190	7	8	16	3	8
16398	Peanut Butter, Smooth Style, w/o Salt	2	Tbsp.	32.3	190	7	8	16	3	8
12681	Peanut Kernels, Oil Roasted	½	Cup	72	418	14	19	35	5	18
16088	Peanuts, All Types, Ckd, Boiled, w/ Salt	½	Cup	31.5	100	7	4	7	1	3
16090	Peanuts, All Types, Dry-roasted, w/ Salt	½	Cup	73	427	16	17	36	5	18
16390	Peanuts, All Types, Dry-roasted, w/o Salt	½	Cup	73	427	16	17	36	5	18
16087	Peanuts, All Types, Fresh	½	Cup	73	414	12	19	36	5	18
16089	Peanuts, All Types, Oil-roasted, w/ Salt	½	Cup	72	418	14	19	35	5	18
16389	Peanuts, All Types, Oil-roasted, w/o Salt	½	Cup	72	418	14	19	35	5	18
16091	Peanuts, Spanish, Fresh	½	Cup	73	416	12	19	36	6	16
16092	Peanuts, Spanish, Oil-roasted, w/ Salt	½	Cup	73.5	426	13	21	36	6	16
16392	Peanuts, Spanish, Oil-roasted, w/o Salt	½	Cup	73.5	426	13	21	36	6	16
16093	Peanuts, Valencia, Fresh	½	Cup	73	416	15	18	35	5	16
16094	Peanuts, Valencia, Oil-roasted, w/ Salt	½	Cup	72	424	12	19	37	6	17
16394	Peanuts, Valencia, Oil-roasted, w/o Salt	½	Cup	72	424	12	19	37	6	17
16095	Peanuts, Virginia, Fresh	½	Cup	73	411	12	18	36	5	18
16096	Peanuts, Virginia, Oil-roasted, w/ Salt	½	Cup	71.5	413	14	18	35	5	18
16396	Peanuts, Virginia, Oil-roasted, w/o Salt	½	Cup	71.5	413	14	18	35	5	18
9340	Pears, Asian, Fresh	1	Medium	122	51	13	1	0	0	0
9257	Pears, Cnd, Heavy Syrup Pack	½	Cup	127.5	94	24	0	0	0	0
9254	Pears, Cnd, Juice Pack	½	Cup	124	62	16	0	0	0	0
9256	Pears, Cnd, Light Syrup Pack	½	Cup	125.5	72	19	0	0	0	0
9253	Pears, Cnd, Water Pack	½	Cup	122	35	10	0	0	0	0
9258	Pears, Cnd, X-heavy Syrup Pack	½	Cup	130.5	127	33	0	0	0	0
9255	Pears, Cnd, X-light Syrup Pack	½	Cup	123.5	58	15	0	0	0	0
9252	Pears, Fresh	1	Medium	166	98	25	1	1	0	0
11318	Peas and Carrots, Cnd	½	Cup	76	29	6	2	0	0	0
11323	Peas and Carrots, Frz, Ckd	½	Cup	80	38	8	2	0	0	0
11324	Peas and Onions, Cnd	½	Cup	60	31	5	2	0	0	0
11327	Peas and Onions, Frz, Ckd	½	Cup	90	41	8	2	0	0	0
11300	Peas, Edible-podded, Fresh	½	Cup	72.5	30	5	2	0	0	0
11305	Peas, Green, Ckd	½	Cup	80	67	13	4	0	0	0
11308	Peas, Green, Cnd	½	Cup	85	59	11	4	0	0	0
11310	Peas, Green, Cnd, Seasoned	½	Cup	85	43	8	3	0	0	0
11304	Peas, Green, Fresh	½	Cup	72.5	59	10	4	0	0	0
11313	Peas, Green, Frz, Ckd	½	Cup	80	62	11	4	0	0	0
18324	Pecan Pie	1	Slice	113	452	65	5	21	4	12
12142	Pecans, Dried	½	Cup	54	360	10	4	37	3	23
41333	Pepperoni French Bread Pizza-Healthy Choice	1	Each	170.1	310	38	20	7	3	-
62625	Pepperoni Pizza-Weight Watchers	1	Each	157.6	390	46	23	12	4	-
11329	Peppers, Hot Chili, Green, Cnd	1	Each	73	18	4	1	0	0	0
11670	Peppers, Hot Chili, Green, Fresh	1	Each	45	18	4	1	0	0	0
11820	Peppers, Hot Chili, Red, Cnd	1	Each	73	18	4	1	0	0	0
11819	Peppers, Hot Chili, Red, Fresh	1	Each	45	18	4	1	0	0	0
11632	Peppers, Jalapeno, Cnd	¼	Cup	34	8	2	0	0	0	0
11333	Peppers, Sweet, Green, Fresh	1	Medium	74	20	5	1	0	0	0
11821	Peppers, Sweet, Red, Fresh	1	Medium	74	20	5	1	0	0	0
11951	Peppers, Sweet, Yellow, Fresh	1	Medium	74	20	5	1	0	-	-
15061	Perch, Ckd, Dry Heat	3	Ounce	85.1	100	0	21	1	0	0
55827	Pesto Sauce-Stouffer's	¼	Cup	71	193	5	9	15	-	-
10162	Pickle and Pimento Loaf, Lunch Meat	1	Slice	28.4	74	2	3	6	2	3
7058	Pickle and Pimiento Loaf, Pork, Lunch Meat	1	Slice	28.4	74	2	3	6	2	3
11958	Pickle Relish, Hamburger	1	Tbsp.	15	19	5	0	0	0	0
11944	Pickle Relish, Hot Dog	1	Tbsp.	15	14	4	0	0	0	0
11945	Pickle Relish, Sweet	1	Tbsp.	15	19	5	0	0	0	0
11941	Pickle, Cucumber ,Sour	1	Slice	7	1	0	0	0	0	0
11937	Pickle, Cucumber, Dill	1	Slice	6	1	0	0	0	0	0

Polyunsaturated Fat (gm)	Fiber (gm)	Cholesterol (mg)	Folate (µg)	Vitamin A (re)	Vitamin B6 (mg)	Vitamin B12 (µg)	Vitamin C (mg)	Vitamin E (mg)	Riboflavin (mg)	Thiamin (mg)	Calcium (mg)	Iron (mg)	Magnesium (mg)	Niacin (mg)	Phosphorus (mg)	Potassium (mg)	Sodium (mg)	Zinc (mg)
1	-	0	2	0	0	0	0	-	0	0	7	0.4	7	0.5	26	27	52	0.1
5	2	0	30	0	0.1	0	0	-	0	0	13	0.6	51	4.4	102	241	157	0.9
5	2	0	30	0	0.1	0	0	-	0	0	13	0.6	51	4.4	102	241	5	0.9
5	2	0	25	0	0.1	0	0	-	0	0	11	0.5	51	4.2	104	233	154	0.8
5	-	0	25	0	0.1	0	0	-	0	0	11	0.5	51	4.2	104	233	5	0.8
11	6	0	91	0	0.2	0	0	-	0.1	0.2	63	1.3	133	10.3	372	491	312	4.8
2	3	0	23	0	0	0	0	-	0	0.1	17	0.3	32	1.7	62	57	237	0.6
11	6	0	106	0	0.2	0	0	5.7	0.1	0.3	39	1.6	128	9.9	261	480	593	2.4
11	6	0	106	0	0.2	0	0	-	0.1	0.3	39	1.6	128	9.9	261	480	4	2.4
11	6	0	175	0	0.3	0	0	6.1	0.1	0.5	67	3.3	123	8.8	274	515	13	2.4
11	7	0	91	0	0.2	0	0	5	0.1	0.2	63	1.3	133	10.3	372	491	312	4.8
11	7	0	91	0	0.2	0	0	-	0.1	0.2	63	1.3	133	10.3	372	491	4	4.8
13	7	0	175	0	0.3	0	0	-	0.1	0.5	77	2.9	137	11.6	283	543	16	1.5
13	-	0	93	0	0.2	0	0	-	0.1	0.2	74	1.7	123	11	284	570	318	1.5
13	-	0	93	0	0.2	0	0	-	0.1	0.2	74	1.7	123	11	284	570	4	1.5
12	-	0	179	0	0.2	0	0	-	0.2	0.5	45	1.5	134	9.4	245	242	1	2.4
13	-	0	90	0	0.2	0	0	-	0.1	0.1	39	1.2	115	10.3	230	441	556	2.2
13	-	0	90	0	0.2	0	0	-	0.1	0.1	39	1.2	115	10.3	230	441	4	2.2
11	-	0	174	0	0.3	0	0	-	0.1	0.5	65	1.9	125	9	277	504	7	3.2
10	-	0	90	0	0.2	0	0	-	0.1	0.2	61	1.2	134	10.5	362	466	310	4.7
10	-	0	90	0	0.2	0	0	-	0.1	0.2	61	1.2	134	10.5	362	466	4	4.7
0	4	0	10	0	0	0	5	-	0	0	5	0	10	0.3	13	148	0	0
0	3	0	2	0	0	0	1	-	0	0	6	0.3	5	0.3	9	83	6	0.1
0	2	0	1	1	0	0	2	-	0	0	11	0.4	9	0.2	15	119	5	0.1
0	3	0	2	0	0	0	1	-	0	0	6	0.4	5	0.2	9	83	6	0.1
0	2	0	1	0	0	0	1	-	0	0	5	0.3	5	0.1	9	65	2	0.1
0	-	0	2	0	0	0	1	-	0	0	7	0.3	5	0.3	9	84	7	0.1
0	-	0	1	0	0	0	2	-	0	0	9	0.2	6	0.5	9	56	2	0.1
0	4	0	12	3	0	0	7	-	0.1	0	18	0.4	10	0.2	18	208	0	0.2
0	3	0	14	438	0.1	0	5	-	0	0.1	17	0.6	11	0.4	35	76	197	0.4
0	3	0	21	621	0.1	0	6	-	0.1	0.2	18	0.8	13	0.9	39	126	54	0.4
0	-	0	16	10	0.1	0	2	-	0	0.1	10	0.5	10	0.8	31	58	265	0.3
0	3	0	18	32	0.1	0	6	-	0.1	0.1	13	0.8	12	0.9	31	105	33	0.3
0	2	0	30	10	0.1	0	44	-	0.1	0.1	31	1.5	17	0.4	38	145	3	0.2
0	4	0	51	48	0.2	0	11	-	0.1	0.2	22	1.2	31	1.6	94	217	2	1
0	3	0	38	65	0.1	0	8	-	0.1	0.1	17	0.8	14	0.6	57	147	186	0.6
0	-	0	24	37	0.1	0	10	-	0.1	0.1	13	1	13	0.6	46	104	216	0.6
0	4	0	47	46	0.1	0	29	0.1	0.1	0.2	18	1.1	24	1.5	78	177	4	0.9
0	4	0	47	54	0.1	0	8	-	0.1	0.2	19	1.3	23	1.2	72	134	70	0.8
3	4	36	7	53	0	0.1	1	-	0.1	0.1	19	1.2	20	0.3	87	84	479	0.6
9	4	0	21	7	0.1	0	1	-	0.1	0.5	19	1.2	69	0.5	157	212	1	3
1	-	30	-	150	-	-	-	-	0.3	0.5	160	2.5	-	3.8	240	350	470	-
-	4	45	-	80	-	-	5	-	-	-	540	1	-	-	-	320	650	-
0	1	0	7	45	0.1	0	50	-	0	0	5	0.4	10	0.6	12	137	856	0.1
0	1	0	11	35	0.1	0	109	-	0	0	8	0.5	11	0.4	21	153	3	0.1
0	1	0	7	868	0.1	0	50	-	0	0	5	0.4	10	0.6	12	137	856	0.1
0	1	0	11	484	0.1	0	109	-	0	0	8	0.5	11	0.4	21	153	3	0.1
0	-	0	5	58	0.1	0	4	-	0	0	9	1	4	0.2	6	46	497	0.1
0	1	0	16	47	0.2	0	66	0.5	0	0	7	0.3	7	0.4	14	131	1	0.1
0	2	0	16	422	0.2	0	141	0.5	0	0	7	0.3	7	0.4	14	131	1	0.1
-	-	0	19	18	0.1	0	136	-	0	0	8	0.3	9	0.7	18	157	1	0.1
0	0	98	5	9	0.1	1.9	1	-	0.1	0.1	87	1	32	1.6	219	293	67	1.2
-	-	18	-	-	-	-	3	-	0	0	1422	0.1	-	0.1	-	155	341	-
1	0	10	1	2	0.1	0.3	4	-	0.1	0.1	27	0.3	5	0.6	40	96	394	0.4
1	0	10	1	8505	0.1	0.3	4	-	0.1	0.1	27	0.3	5	0.6	40	96	394	0.4
0	0	0	0	4	0	0	0	-	0	0	1	0.2	1	0.1	3	11	164	0
0	-	0	0	3	0	0	0	-	0	0	1	0.2	3	0.1	6	12	164	0
0	0	0	0	2	0	0	0	-	0	0	0	0.1	1	0	2	4	122	0
0	0	0	0	1	0	0	0	-	0	0	0	0	0	0	1	2	85	0
0	0	0	0	2	0	0	0	-	0	0	1	0	1	0	1	7	77	0

Code	Food Name	Amount	Unit	Grams	kCalories	Carbohydrate (gm)	Protein (gm)	Fat (gm)	Saturated Fat (gm)	Monounsaturated Fat (gm)
11947	Pickle, Cucumber, Dill, Low Sodium	1	Slice	6	1	0	0	0	0	0
11946	Pickle, Cucumber, Sour, Low Sodium	1	Slice	7	1	0	0	0	0	0
11940	Pickle, Cucumber, Sweet	1	Slice	6	7	2	0	0	0	0
11948	Pickle, Cucumber, Sweet, Low Sodium	1	Slice	6	7	2	0	0	0	0
7062	Picnic Loaf, Lunch Meat	1	Slice	28.4	66	1	4	5	2	2
15063	Pike, Northern, Ckd, Dry Heat	3	Ounce	85.1	96	0	21	1	0	0
15204	Pike, Walleye, Ckd, Dry Heat	3	Ounce	85.1	101	0	21	1	0	0
14017	Pina Colada	1	Fl Oz	31.4	58	9	0	1	0	0
12147	Pine Nuts	1	Tbsp.	10	52	1	2	5	1	2
14334	Pineapple and Grapefruit Juice Drink, Cnd	¾	Cup	187.6	88	22	0	0	0	0
14341	Pineapple and Orange Juice Drink, Cnd	¾	Cup	187.6	94	22	2	0	0	0
9273	Pineapple Juice, Cnd	¾	Cup	187.6	105	26	1	0	0	0
9270	Pineapple, Cnd, Heavy Syrup Pack	½	Cup	127.5	99	26	0	0	0	0
9268	Pineapple, Cnd, Juice Pack	½	Cup	125	75	20	1	0	0	0
9269	Pineapple, Cnd, Light Syrup Pack	½	Cup	126	66	17	0	0	0	0
9267	Pineapple, Cnd, Water Pack	½	Cup	123	39	10	1	0	0	0
9271	Pineapple, Cnd, X-heavy Syrup Pack	½	Cup	130	108	28	0	0	0	0
9266	Pineapple, Fresh	1	Slice	84	41	10	0	0	0	0
12151	Pistachio Dried	½	Cup	64	369	16	13	31	4	21
12652	Pistachio Dry Roasted	½	Cup	64	388	18	10	34	4	23
9284	Plums, Cnd, Purple, Heavy Syrup Pack	½	Cup	129	115	30	0	0	0	0
9282	Plums, Cnd, Purple, Juice Pack	½	Cup	126	73	19	1	0	0	0
9283	Plums, Cnd, Purple, Light Syrup Pack	½	Cup	126	79	21	0	0	0	0
9281	Plums, Cnd, Purple, Water Pack	½	Cup	124.5	51	14	0	0	0	0
9285	Plums, Cnd, Purple, X-heavy Syrup Pack	½	Cup	130.5	132	34	0	0	0	0
9279	Plums, Fresh	1	Medium	66	36	9	1	0	0	0
15205	Pollock, Atlantic, Ckd, Dry Heat	3	Ounce	85.1	100	0	21	1	0	0
15069	Pompano, Florida, Ckd, Dry Heat	3	Ounce	85.1	179	0	20	10	4	3
19034	Popcorn, Air-popped	1	Cup	8	31	6	1	0	0	0
19806	Popcorn, Air-popped, White Popcorn	1	Cup	8	31	6	1	0	0	0
19036	Popcorn, Cakes	1	Cake	10	38	8	1	0	0	0
19038	Popcorn, Caramel-coated, w/ Peanuts	1	Cup	35.2	141	28	2	3	0	1
19039	Popcorn, Caramel-coated, w/o Peanuts	1	Cup	35.2	152	28	1	5	1	1
19040	Popcorn, Cheese-flavor	1	Cup	11	58	6	1	4	1	1
19035	Popcorn, Oil-popped	1	Cup	11	55	6	1	3	1	1
19807	Popcorn, Oil-popped, White Popcorn	1	Cup	11	55	6	1	3	1	1
62602	Popsicles	1	Each	56	40	11	0	0	0	0
19408	Pork Skins, Barbecue-flavor	1	Ounce	28.4	153	0	16	9	3	4
19041	Pork Skins, Plain	1	Ounce	28.4	155	0	17	9	3	4
10193	Pork, Backribs	3	Ounce	85.1	315	0	21	25	9	11
10127	Pork, Braunschweiger	3	Ounce	85.1	305	3	11	27	9	13
7045	Pork, Cnd, Lunch Meat	1	Slice	21	70	0	3	6	2	3
10220	Pork, Ground, Ckd	3	Ounce	85.1	253	0	22	18	7	8
10154	Pork, Ham and Cheese Loaf or Roll	3	Ounce	85.1	220	1	14	17	6	8
10147	Pork, Ham Patties, Grilled	3	Ounce	85.1	291	1	11	26	9	12
10148	Pork, Ham Salad Spread	3	Ounce	85.1	184	9	7	13	4	6
10143	Pork, Ham, Chopped, Cnd	3	Ounce	85.1	203	0	14	16	5	8
10138	Pork, Ham, Cnd, Extra Lean (appx 4% Fat), Roasted	3	Ounce	85.1	116	0	18	4	1	2
10185	Pork, Ham, Cnd, Extra Lean and Reg, Roasted	3	Ounce	85.1	142	0	18	7	2	3
10184	Pork, Ham, Cnd, Extra Lean and Reg, Unheated	3	Ounce	85.1	122	0	15	6	2	3
10140	Pork, Ham, Cnd, Regular (approx 13% Fat), Roasted	3	Ounce	85.1	192	0	17	13	4	6
10134	Pork, Ham, Extra Lean (5% Fat), Roasted	3	Ounce	85.1	123	1	18	5	2	2
10133	Pork, Ham, Extra Lean (5% Fat), Unheated	3	Ounce	85.1	111	1	16	4	1	2
10183	Pork, Ham, Extra Lean and Reg, Roasted	3	Ounce	85.1	140	0	19	7	2	3
10182	Pork, Ham, Extra Lean and Reg, Unheated	3	Ounce	85.1	138	2	16	7	2	3
10151	Pork, Ham, Meat and Fat, Roasted	3	Ounce	85.1	207	0	18	14	5	7
10153	Pork, Ham, Meat Only, Roasted	3	Ounce	85.1	134	0	21	5	2	2
10136	Pork, Ham, Regular (11% Fat), Roasted	3	Ounce	85.1	151	0	19	8	3	4
10135	Pork, Ham, Regular (11% Fat), Unheated	3	Ounce	85.1	155	3	15	9	3	4
10172	Pork, Smoked Link Sausage, Grilled	3	Ounce	85.1	331	2	19	27	10	12

Polyunsaturated Fat (gm)	Fiber (gm)	Cholesterol (mg)	Folate (µg)	Vitamin A (re)	Vitamin B6 (mg)	Vitamin B12 (µg)	Vitamin C (mg)	Vitamin E (mg)	Riboflavin (mg)	Thiamin (mg)	Calcium (mg)	Iron (mg)	Magnesium (mg)	Niacin (mg)	Phosphorus (mg)	Potassium (mg)	Sodium (mg)	Zinc (mg)
0	-	0	0	2	0	0	0	-	0	0	1	0	1	0	1	7	1	0
0	0	0	-	1	-	0	0	-	0	0	0	0	0	0	1	2	1	0
0	0	0	0	1	0	0	0	-	0	0	0	0	0	0	1	2	56	0
0	0	0	0	1	0	0	0	-	0	0	0	0	0	0	1	2	1	0
1	0	11	1	0	0.1	0.4	5	-	0.1	0.1	13	0.3	4	0.7	35	76	330	0.6
0	0	43	15	20	0.1	2	3	-	0.1	0.1	62	0.6	34	2.4	240	282	42	0.7
0	0	94	14	20	0.1	2	0	-	0.2	0.3	120	1.4	32	2.4	229	424	55	0.7
0	-	0	3	0	0	0	1	-	0	0	3	0.1	3	0	2	22	2	0
2	0	0	6	0	0	0	0	-	0	0.1	3	0.9	23	0.4	51	60	0	0.4
0	0	0	20	8	0.1	0	86	-	0	0.1	13	0.6	11	0.5	11	114	26	0.1
0	0	0	20	99	0.1	0	42	-	0	0.1	9	0.5	11	0.4	8	86	6	0.1
0	0	0	43	0	0.2	0	20	-	0	0.1	32	0.5	24	0.5	15	251	2	0.2
0	1	0	6	1	0.1	0	9	-	0	0.1	18	0.5	20	0.4	9	133	1	0.2
0	1	0	6	5	0.1	0	12	-	0	0.1	17	0.3	17	0.4	7	152	1	0.1
0	1	0	6	1	0.1	0	9	-	0	0.1	18	0.5	20	0.4	9	132	1	0.2
0	1	0	6	2	0.1	0	9	-	0	0.1	18	0.5	22	0.4	5	156	1	0.1
0	-	0	6	1	0.1	0	9	-	0	0.1	18	0.5	20	0.4	9	133	1	0.1
0	1	0	9	2	0.1	0	13	0.1	0	0.1	6	0.3	12	0.4	6	95	1	0.1
5	7	0	37	15	0.2	0	5	-	0.1	0.5	86	4.3	101	0.7	322	700	4	0.9
5	7	0	38	15	0.2	0	5	-	0.2	0.3	45	2	83	0.9	305	621	499	0.9
0	1	0	3	34	0	0	1	-	0	0	12	1.1	6	0.4	17	117	25	0.1
0	1	0	3	127	0	0	4	-	0.1	0	13	0.4	10	0.6	19	194	1	0.1
0	1	0	3	33	0	0	1	-	0	0	11	1.1	6	0.4	16	117	25	0.1
0	1	0	3	113	0	0	3	-	0.1	0	9	0.2	6	0.5	16	157	1	0.1
0	-	0	3	33	0	0	1	-	0	0	12	1.1	7	0.4	16	116	25	0.1
0	1	0	1	21	0.1	0	6	-	0.1	0	3	0.1	5	0.3	7	114	0	0.1
1	0	77	3	10	0.3	3.1	0	-	0.2	0	65	0.5	73	3.4	241	388	94	0.5
1	0	54	15	31	0.2	1	0	-	0.1	0.6	37	0.6	26	3.2	290	541	65	0.6
0	1	0	2	2	0	0	0	-	0	0	1	0.2	10	0.2	24	24	0	0.3
0	-	0	2	0	0	0	0	-	0	0	1	0.2	10	0.2	24	24	0	0.3
0	0	0	2	1	0	0	0	-	0	0	1	0.2	16	0.6	28	33	29	0.4
1	1	0	6	2	0.1	0	0	-	0	0	23	1.4	28	0.7	45	125	104	0.4
2	2	2	1	4	0	0	0	-	0	0	15	0.6	12	0.8	29	38	73	0.2
2	1	1	1	5	0	0.1	0	-	0	0	12	0.2	10	0.2	40	29	98	0.2
1	1	0	2	2	0	0	0	-	0	0	1	0.3	12	0.2	27	25	97	0.3
1	-	0	2	0	0	0	0	-	0	0	1	0.3	12	0.2	27	25	97	0.3
0	0	0	-	0	-	-	1	-	-	-	0	0	-	-	-	-	10	-
1	-	33	9	52	0	0	0	-	0.1	0	12	0.3	0	1	62	51	756	0.2
1	-	27	0	11	0	0.2	0	-	0.1	0	9	0.2	3	0.4	24	36	521	0.2
2	-	100	3	3	0.3	0.5	0	-	0.2	0.4	38	1.2	18	3	166	268	86	2.9
3	0	133	37	3589	0.3	17.1	8	-	1.3	0.2	8	8	9	7.1	143	169	972	2.4
1	0	13	1	0	0	0.2	0	-	0	0.1	1	0.2	2	0.7	17	45	271	0.3
2	0	80	5	2	0.3	0.5	1	-	0.2	0.6	19	1.1	20	3.6	192	308	62	2.7
2	0	48	3	20	0.2	0.7	21	-	0.2	0.5	49	0.8	14	2.9	215	250	1142	1.7
3	0	61	3	0	0.1	0.6	0	-	0.2	0.3	8	1.4	9	2.8	86	208	904	1.6
2	0	31	1	0	0.1	0.6	5	-	0.1	0.4	7	0.5	9	1.8	102	128	776	0.9
2	0	42	1	0	0.3	0.6	2	-	0.1	0.5	6	0.8	11	2.7	118	242	1161	1.6
0	0	26	4	0	0.4	0.6	23	-	0.2	0.9	5	0.8	18	4.2	178	296	965	1.9
1	0	35	4	0	0.3	0.7	19	-	0.2	0.8	6	0.9	17	4.3	188	299	908	2
1	0	32	5	0	0.4	0.7	21	-	0.2	0.7	5	0.8	14	3.9	176	284	1085	1.6
2	0	53	4	0	0.3	0.9	12	-	0.2	0.7	7	1.2	14	4.5	207	304	800	2.1
0	0	45	3	0	0.3	0.6	18	-	0.2	0.6	7	1.3	12	3.4	167	244	1023	2.4
0	0	40	3	0	0.4	0.6	22	-	0.2	0.8	6	0.6	14	4.1	185	298	1215	1.6
1	0	48	3	0	0.3	0.6	19	-	0.2	0.6	7	1.2	16	4.5	211	308	1178	2.2
1	0	45	3	0	0.3	0.7	23	-	0.2	0.8	6	0.8	15	4.3	201	253	1087	1.7
2	0	53	3	0	0.3	0.5	-	-	0.2	0.6	6	0.7	16	3.8	182	243	1010	2
1	0	47	3	0	0.4	0.6	-	-	0.2	0.6	6	0.8	19	4.3	193	269	1129	2.2
1	0	50	3	0	0.3	0.6	19	-	0.3	0.6	7	1.1	19	5.2	239	348	1276	2.1
1	0	48	3	0	0.3	0.7	24	-	0.2	0.7	6	0.8	16	4.5	210	282	1120	1.8
3	0	58	4	0	0.3	1.4	2	-	0.2	0.6	26	1	16	3.9	138	286	1276	2.4

Code	Food Name	Amount	Unit	Grams	kCalories	Carbohydrate (gm)	Protein (gm)	Fat (gm)	Saturated Fat (gm)	Monounsaturated Fat (gm)
10089	Pork, Spareribs, Meat and Fat, Ckd, Braised	3	Ounce	85.1	338	0	25	26	9	11
10221	Pork, Tenderloin, Meat and Fat, Ckd, Broiled	3	Ounce	85.1	171	0	25	7	2	3
10223	Pork, Tenderloin, Meat Only, Ckd, Broiled	3	Ounce	85.1	159	0	26	5	2	2
19042	Potato Chips, Barbecue-flavor	1	Ounce	28.4	139	15	2	9	2	2
19421	Potato Chips, Cheese-flavor	1	Ounce	28.4	141	16	2	8	2	2
19422	Potato Chips, Light	1	Ounce	28.4	134	19	2	6	1	1
19411	Potato Chips, Plain, Salted	1	Ounce	28.4	152	15	2	10	3	3
19811	Potato Chips, Plain, Unsalted	1	Ounce	28.4	152	15	2	10	3	3
19412	Potato Chips, Pringles, Cheese-flavor	1	Ounce	28.4	156	14	2	10	3	2
19045	Potato Chips, Pringles, Light	1	Ounce	28.4	142	18	2	7	1	2
19410	Potato Chips, Pringles, Plain	1	Ounce	28.4	158	14	2	11	3	2
19046	Potato Chips, Pringles, Sour-cream&onion-flavor	1	Ounce	28.4	155	15	2	10	3	2
19043	Potato Chips, Sour-cream-and-onion-flavor	1	Ounce	28.4	151	15	2	10	3	2
11920	Potato Chips, w/o Salt Added	1	Ounce	28.4	148	15	2	10	3	2
11672	Potato Pancakes, Home-prepared	1	Ounce	28.4	77	8	2	4	1	1
11399	Potato Puffs, Frz, Prepared	1	Each	7	16	2	0	1	0	0
11414	Potato Salad	½	Cup	125	179	14	3	10	2	3
19415	Potato Sticks	1	Ounce	28.4	148	15	2	10	3	2
55174	Potatoes Au Gratin-Stouffer's	1	Each	163	170	17	5	9	-	-
11843	Potatoes, Au Gratin, Home-prepared	½	Cup	122.5	162	14	6	9	4	3
11363	Potatoes, Baked w/o Skin	1	Medium	202	188	44	4	0	0	0
11364	Potatoes, Baked, Skin only	1	Each	58	115	27	2	0	0	0
11674	Potatoes, Baked, w/ Skin	1	Medium	202	220	51	5	0	0	0
11365	Potatoes, Boiled, Ckd In Skin w/o Skin	1	Medium	202	176	41	4	0	0	0
11367	Potatoes, Boiled, Ckd w/o Skin	1	Medium	202	174	40	3	0	0	0
11366	Potatoes, Boiled, Skin only	1	Each	34	27	6	1	0	0	0
11376	Potatoes, Cnd, Drained Solids	½	Cup	90	54	12	1	0	0	0
11374	Potatoes, Cnd, Solids and Liquids	½	Cup	150	60	13	2	0	0	0
11370	Potatoes, Hashed Brown	½	Cup	78	119	6	2	11	4	5
11657	Potatoes, Mashed, Home-prepared	½	Cup	105	81	18	2	1	0	0
11930	Potatoes, Mashed, Prepared From Flakes	½	Cup	105	119	16	2	6	2	2
11368	Potatoes, Microwaved w/o Skin	½	Cup	78	78	18	2	0	0	0
11369	Potatoes, Microwaved, Skin only	1	Each	58	77	17	3	0	0	0
11675	Potatoes, Microwaved, w/ Skin	1	Medium	202	212	49	5	0	0	0
11671	Potatoes, O'brien, Home-prepared	½	Cup	97	79	15	2	1	1	0
11844	Potatoes, Scalloped	½	Cup	122.5	105	13	4	5	2	2
19216	Praline	1	Piece	39	177	24	1	9	1	6
19047	Pretzels, Hard, Plain, Salted	1	Ounce	28.4	108	22	3	1	0	0
19814	Pretzels, Hard, Plain, Unsalted	1	Ounce	28.4	108	22	3	1	0	0
19050	Pretzels, Hard, Whole-wheat	1	Ounce	28.4	103	23	3	1	0	0
9294	Prune Juice, Cnd	¾	Cup	191.8	136	33	1	0	0	0
9289	Prunes, Dehydrated	¼	Cup	33	112	29	1	0	0	0
9293	Prunes, Dried, Stewed, w/ Added Sugar	¼	Cup	59.5	74	20	1	0	0	0
9292	Prunes, Dried, Stewed, w/o Added Sugar	¼	Cup	53	57	15	1	0	0	0
9291	Prunes, Dried, Uncooked	¼	Cup	40.3	96	25	1	0	0	0
19072	Pudding Pops, Chocolate	1	Each	47	72	12	2	2	-	-
19073	Pudding Pops, Vanilla	1	Each	47	75	13	2	2	-	-
18326	Pumpkin Pie	1	Slice	109	229	30	4	10	2	5
11423	Pumpkin, Ckd	½	Cup	122.5	24	6	1	0	0	0
11424	Pumpkin, Cnd, w/o Salt	½	Cup	122.5	42	10	1	0	0	0
11429	Radishes, Fresh	½	Cup	58	10	2	0	0	0	0
11431	Radishes, Oriental, Ckd	½	Cup	73.5	12	3	0	0	0	0
11432	Radishes, Oriental, Dried	½	Cup	58	157	37	5	0	0	0
11430	Radishes, Oriental, Fresh	½	Cup	44	8	2	0	0	0	0
11637	Radishes, White Icicle, Fresh	½	Cup	50	7	1	1	0	0	0
18191	Raisin Cookies, Soft-type	1	Each	15	60	10	1	2	1	1
19149	Raisinets	10	Piece	10	41	7	0	2	1	1
9297	Raisins, Golden Seedless	½	Cup	72.5	219	58	2	0	0	0
9299	Raisins, Seeded	½	Cup	72.5	215	57	2	0	0	0
9298	Raisins, Seedless	½	Cup	72.5	218	57	2	0	0	0

Polyunsaturated Fat (gm)	Fiber (gm)	Cholesterol (mg)	Folate (µg)	Vitamin A (re)	Vitamin B6 (mg)	Vitamin B12 (µg)	Vitamin C (mg)	Vitamin E (mg)	Riboflavin (mg)	Thiamin (mg)	Calcium (mg)	Iron (mg)	Magnesium (mg)	Niacin (mg)	Phosphorus (mg)	Potassium (mg)	Sodium (mg)	Zinc (mg)
2	0	103	3	3	0.3	0.9	-	-	0.3	0.3	40	1.6	20	4.7	222	272	79	3.9
1	-	80	5	2	0.4	0.8	1	-	0.3	0.8	4	1.2	30	4.3	247	378	54	2.5
0	-	80	5	2	0.4	0.9	1	-	0.3	0.8	4	1.2	31	4.4	251	384	55	2.5
5	1	0	24	6	0.2	0	10	-	0.1	0.1	14	0.5	21	1.3	53	357	213	0.3
3	-	1	0	2	0.1	0	15	-	0	0	20	0.5	21	1.4	85	433	225	0.3
3	-	0	8	0	0.2	0	7	-	0.1	0.1	6	0.4	25	2	55	494	139	0
3	1	0	13	0	0.2	0	9	-	0.1	0	7	0.5	19	1.1	47	361	168	0.3
3	-	0	13	0	0.2	0	9	-	0.1	0	7	0.5	19	1.1	47	361	2	0.3
5	1	5	0	0	0.1	0	2	-	0	0.1	31	0.5	15	0.7	46	108	214	0.2
4	1	0	7	0	0.2	0	3	-	0	0.1	10	0.4	18	1.2	44	285	121	0.2
6	1	0	2	0	0	0	2	-	0	0.1	7	0.4	16	0.9	45	286	186	0.2
5	-	1	7	28	0.1	0	3	-	0	0.1	18	0.4	16	0.7	48	141	204	0.2
5	1	2	18	6	0.2	0.3	11	-	0.1	0.1	20	0.5	21	1.1	50	377	177	0.3
5	1	0	13	0	0.1	0	12	-	0	0	7	0.3	17	1.2	43	368	2	0.3
2	1	27	7	4	0.1	0.1	6	-	0	0	7	0.4	9	0.6	31	223	144	0.2
0	0	0	1	0	0	0	0	-	0	0	2	0.1	1	0.3	3	27	52	0
5	-	85	8	41	0.2	0	12	-	0.1	0.1	24	0.8	19	1.1	65	317	661	0.4
5	1	0	11	0	0.1	0	13	-	0	0	5	0.6	18	1.4	49	351	71	0.3
-	-	-	-	20	-	-	4	-	0.1	-	48	0.8	-	0.8	-	260	670	-
1	-	18	10	17	0.2	0	12	-	0.1	0.1	146	0.8	24	1.2	138	485	530	0.8
0	3	0	18	0	0.6	0	26	-	0	0.2	10	0.7	51	2.8	101	790	10	0.6
0	2	0	13	0	0.4	0	8	-	0.1	0.1	20	4.1	25	1.8	59	332	12	0.3
0	5	0	22	0	0.7	0	26	-	0.1	0.2	20	2.7	55	3.3	115	844	16	0.6
0	4	0	20	0	0.6	0	26	-	0	0.2	10	0.6	44	2.9	89	766	8	0.6
0	4	0	18	0	0.5	0	15	-	0	0.2	16	0.6	40	2.7	81	663	10	0.5
0	-	0	3	0	0.1	0	2	-	0	0	15	2.1	10	0.4	18	138	5	0.1
0	-	0	6	0	0.2	0	5	-	0	0.1	4	1.1	13	0.8	25	206	234	0.3
0	2	0	7	0	0.2	0	19	-	0	0.1	45	1.5	21	1.3	33	364	451	0.6
1	2	-	6	0	0.2	0	4	-	0	0.1	6	0.6	16	1.6	33	250	19	0.2
0	2	2	9	20	0.2	0	7	-	0	0.1	27	0.3	19	1.2	50	314	318	0.3
2	-	4	8	22	0	0	10	-	0.1	0.1	51	0.2	19	0.7	59	245	349	0.2
0	-	0	10	0	0.2	0	12	-	0	0.1	4	0.3	20	1.3	85	321	5	0.3
0	-	0	10	0	0.3	0	9	-	0	0	27	3.4	21	1.3	48	377	9	0.3
0	-	0	24	0	0.7	0	31	-	0.1	0.2	22	2.5	55	3.5	212	903	16	0.7
0	-	4	8	55	0.2	0	16	-	0.1	0.1	35	0.5	17	1	49	258	210	0.3
1	-	7	11	23	0.2	0	13	-	0.1	0.1	70	0.7	23	1.3	77	463	410	0.5
2	-	0	5	2	0	0	0	-	0	0.1	12	0.5	20	0.1	43	82	24	0.8
0	1	0	24	0	0	0	0	-	0.2	0.1	10	1.2	10	1.5	32	41	486	0.2
0	1	0	24	0	0	0	0	-	0.2	0.1	10	1.2	10	1.5	32	41	82	0.2
0	-	0	15	0	0.1	0	0	-	0.1	0.1	8	0.8	9	1.9	35	122	58	0.2
0	2	0	1	0	0.4	0	8	-	0.1	0	23	2.3	27	1.5	48	529	8	0.4
0	-	0	1	58	0.2	0	0	-	0.1	0	24	1.2	21	1	37	349	2	0.2
0	2	0	0	17	0.1	0	2	-	0.1	0	12	0.6	11	0.4	20	186	1	0.1
0	3	0	0	16	0.1	0	2	-	0.1	0	12	0.6	11	0.4	19	177	1	0.1
0	3	0	1	80	0.1	0	1	-	0.1	0	21	1	18	0.8	32	300	2	0.2
-	0	1	1	16	0	0.3	0	-	0.1	0	66	0.2	10	0.1	53	105	78	0.2
-	0	1	2	24	0	0.2	0	-	0.1	0	61	0	5	0	47	65	50	0.2
2	3	22	16	523	0.1	0.4	2	-	0.2	0.1	65	0.9	16	0.2	77	168	307	0.5
0	-	0	10	132	0.1	0	6	-	0.1	0	18	0.7	11	0.5	37	282	1	0.3
0	3	0	15	2702	0.1	0	5	-	0.1	0	32	1.7	28	0.4	43	252	6	0.2
0	1	0	16	1	0	0	13	-	0	0	12	0.2	5	0.2	10	135	14	0.2
0	1	0	13	0	0	0	11	-	0	0	12	0.1	7	0.1	18	209	10	0.1
0	-	0	171	0	0.4	0	0	-	0.4	0.2	365	3.9	99	2	118	2027	161	1.2
0	1	0	12	0	0	0	10	-	0	0	12	0.2	7	0.1	10	100	9	0.1
0	-	0	7	0	0	0	15	-	0	0	14	0.4	5	0.2	14	140	8	0.1
0	-	0	1	2	0	0	0	-	0	0	7	0.3	3	0.3	12	21	51	0
0	-	0	1	1	0	0	0	-	0	0	11	0.1	5	0	14	51	4	0.1
0	3	0	2	3	0.2	0	2	-	0.1	0	38	1.3	25	0.8	83	541	9	0.2
0	5	0	2	0	0.1	0	4	-	0.1	0.1	20	1.9	22	0.8	54	598	20	0.1
0	3	0	2	1	0.2	0	2	-	0.1	0.1	36	1.5	24	0.6	70	544	9	0.2

Code	Food Name	Amount	Unit	Grams	kCalories	Carbohydrate (gm)	Protein (gm)	Fat (gm)	Saturated Fat (gm)	Monounsaturated Fat (gm)
9304	Raspberries, Cnd, Red, Heavy Syrup Pack	½	Cup	128	116	30	1	0	0	0
9302	Raspberries, Fresh	½	Cup	61.5	30	7	1	0	0	0
9306	Raspberries, Frozen, Red, Sweetened	½	Cup	125	129	33	1	0	0	0
62536	Ravioli, Beef	1	Cup	243.9	230	36	9	5	2	-
62537	Ravioli, Cheese	1	Cup	243.9	220	38	9	3	1	-
62557	Red Beans and Rice	2	Ounce	56.7	189	40	8	1	0	-
62607	Reduced Fat Chocolate Chip Cookies	13	Each	5.8	26	4	0	1	0	0
62595	Reduced Fat Chocolate Sandwich Cookies-SnackWell	2	Each	25	100	-	1	3	1	1
62593	Reduced Fat Classic Golden Crackers-SnackWell	6	Each	14	60	11	1	1	0	0
62594	Reduced Fat Creme Sandwich Cookies-SnackWell	2	Each	26	110	21	1	3	1	1
62597	Reduced Fat French Onion Snack Crackers-SnackWell	32	Each	30	120	23	2	2	0	1
62598	Reduced Fat Oatmeal Raisin Cookies-SnackWell	2	Each	27	110	20	2	3	0	1
62525	Reduced Fat Zesty Cheese Snack Crackers-SnackWell	32	Each	30	120	23	3	2	1	1
19150	Reese's Peanut Butter Cups	1	Each	7	34	3	1	2	2	0
19151	Reese's Pieces Candy	1	Pkg	55	258	34	7	11	-	-
19052	Rice Cakes, Brown Rice, Buckwheat	1	Cake	9	34	7	1	0	0	0
19817	Rice Cakes, Brown Rice, Buckwheat, Unsalted	1	Cake	9	34	7	1	0	0	0
19413	Rice Cakes, Brown Rice, Corn	1	Cake	9	35	7	1	0	0	0
19414	Rice Cakes, Brown Rice, Multigrain	1	Cake	9	35	7	1	0	0	0
19818	Rice Cakes, Brown Rice, Multigrain, Unsalted	1	Cake	9	35	7	1	0	0	0
19051	Rice Cakes, Brown Rice, Plain	1	Cake	9	35	7	1	0	0	0
19816	Rice Cakes, Brown Rice, Plain, Unsalted	1	Cake	9	35	7	1	0	0	0
19416	Rice Cakes, Brown Rice, Rye	1	Cake	9	35	7	1	0	0	0
19193	Rice Pudding	1	Cup	298.1	486	66	6	22	3	10
20037	Rice, Brown, Long-grain, Ckd	½	Cup	97.5	108	22	3	1	0	0
20041	Rice, Brown, Medium-grain, Ckd	½	Cup	97.5	109	23	2	1	0	0
20045	Rice, White, Long-grain, Ckd	½	Cup	79	103	22	2	0	0	0
20049	Rice, White, Long-grain, Instant, Enriched	½	Cup	82.5	81	18	2	0	0	0
20051	Rice, White, Medium-grain, Ckd	½	Cup	93	121	27	2	0	0	0
20053	Rice, White, Short-grain, Ckd	½	Cup	93	121	27	2	0	0	0
20057	Rice, White, w/ Pasta, Ckd	½	Cup	101	123	22	3	3	1	1
55222	Rigatoni Bake, Lean Cuisine-Stouffer's	1	Each	276.4	250	27	18	8	3	-
41341	Rigatoni in Meat Sauce-Healthy Choice	1	Each	269.3	260	34	16	6	2	-
55782	Rigatoni w/ Meat Sauce-Stouffer's	½	Cup	142	145	16	8	6	-	-
62614	Roast Turkey Medallions-Weight Watchers	1	Each	241	190	34	10	2	1	-
41310	Roasted Turkey and Mushrooms in Gravy-Healthy Choice	1	Each	241	200	26	18	3	1	-
15071	Rockfish, Pacific, Ckd, Dry Heat	3	Ounce	85.1	103	0	20	2	0	0
15207	Roe, Ckd, Dry Heat	3	Ounce	85.1	174	2	24	7	2	2
14157	Root Beer	12	Fl Oz	369.6	152	39	0	0	0	0
62531	Root Beer, Diet	12	Fl Oz	355.2	0	0	0	0	-	-
15232	Roughy, Orange, Ckd, Dry Heat	3	Ounce	85.1	76	0	16	1	0	1
62541	Salad Dressing, Blue Cheese	2	Tbsp.	32	90	5	1	7	4	-
62542	Salad Dressing, Blue Cheese, Fat Free	2	Tbsp.	35	50	12	1	0	0	-
4120	Salad Dressing, French	2	Tbsp.	31.3	134	5	0	13	3	3
62545	Salad Dressing, French, Fat Free	2	Tbsp.	35	50	12	0	0	0	-
4020	Salad Dressing, French, Lo Fat	2	Tbsp.	32.5	44	7	0	2	0	0
4114	Salad Dressing, Italian	2	Tbsp.	29.4	137	3	0	14	2	3
62543	Salad Dressing, Italian, Fat Free	2	Tbsp.	31	10	2	0	0	0	-
4021	Salad Dressing, Italian, Lo Cal	2	Tbsp.	30	32	1	0	3	0	1
62539	Salad Dressing, Ranch	2	Tbsp.	29	170	2	0	18	3	-
62540	Salad Dressing, Ranch, Fat Free	2	Tbsp.	35	50	11	0	0	0	-
4015	Salad Dressing, Russian	2	Tbsp.	30.7	151	3	0	16	2	4
4022	Salad Dressing, Russian, Low Cal	2	Tbsp.	32.5	46	9	0	1	0	0
4016	Salad Dressing, Sesame Seed	2	Tbsp.	30.7	136	3	1	14	2	4
4017	Salad Dressing, Thousand Island	2	Tbsp.	31.3	118	5	0	11	2	3
4023	Salad Dressing, Thousand Island, Lo Cal	2	Tbsp.	30.7	49	5	0	3	0	1
62544	Salad Dressing, Thousnad Island, Fat Free	2	Tbsp.	35	45	11	0	0	0	-
4135	Salad Dressing, Vinegar and Oil	2	Tbsp.	31.3	140	1	0	16	3	5
41290	Salisbury Steak w/ Mushroom Gravy-Healthy Choice	1	Each	311.8	280	35	21	6	3	-
43402	Salisbury Steak, Top Shelf-Hormel	1	Each	283.5	320	22	25	15	7	8

Polyunsaturated Fat (gm)	Fiber (gm)	Cholesterol (mg)	Folate (µg)	Vitamin A (re)	Vitamin B6 (mg)	Vitamin B12 (µg)	Vitamin C (mg)	Vitamin E (mg)	Riboflavin (mg)	Thiamin (mg)	Calcium (mg)	Iron (mg)	Magnesium (mg)	Niacin (mg)	Phosphorus (mg)	Potassium (mg)	Sodium (mg)	Zinc (mg)
0	4	0	13	4	0.1	0	11	-	0	0	14	0.5	15	0.6	12	120	4	0.2
0	4	0	16	8	0	0	15	0.2	0.1	0	14	0.4	11	0.6	7	93	0	0.3
0	5	0	32	7	0	0	21	-	0.1	0	19	0.8	16	0.3	21	142	1	0.2
-	4	20	-	150	-	-	2	-	-	-	0	1.5	-	-	-	-	1150	-
-	4	15	-	60	-	-	1	-	-	-	24	1.5	-	-	-	-	1280	-
-	7	0	-	99	-	-	6	-	-	0.2	48	1.5	-	2.8	-	-	786	-
0	0	0	-	0	-	-	0	-	-	-	0	0.1	-	-	-	-	34	-
0	1	0	-	0	-	-	0	-	-	-	0	0.4	-	-	-	-	190	-
0	0	0	-	0	-	-	0	-	-	-	24	0.4	-	-	-	-	140	-
0	1	0	-	0	-	-	0	-	-	-	24	0.2	-	-	-	-	95	-
-	1	23	-	0	-	-	0	-	-	-	48	0.6	-	-	-	-	290	-
1	1	0	-	0	-	-	0	-	-	-	24	0.4	-	-	-	-	135	-
0	1	5	0	0	0	0	0	0	0	0	48	0.6	0	0	0	0	350	0
0	0	1	2	1	0	0	0	-	0	0	5	0.1	6	0.3	17	28	20	0.1
-	2	2	31	2	0.1	0.2	0	-	0.1	0	73	0.8	45	3.1	127	242	83	0.6
0	0	0	2	0	0	0	0	-	0	0	1	0.1	14	0.7	34	27	10	0.2
0	-	0	2	0	0	0	0	-	0	0	1	0.1	14	0.7	34	27	0	0.2
0	0	0	2	0	0	0	0	-	0	0	1	0.1	10	0.6	29	25	26	0.2
0	0	0	2	0	0	0	0	-	0	0	2	0.2	12	0.6	33	26	23	0.2
0	-	0	2	0	0	0	0	-	0	0	2	0.2	12	0.6	33	26	0	0.2
0	0	0	2	0	0	0	0	-	0	0	1	0.1	12	0.7	32	26	29	0.3
0	0	0	2	0	0	0	0	-	0	0	1	0.1	12	0.7	32	26	2	0.3
0	0	0	0	0	0	0	0	-	0	0	2	0.2	13	0.6	34	28	10	0.3
8	-	3	9	104	0.1	0.6	1	-	0.2	0.1	155	0.9	24	0.5	203	179	253	1.5
0	2	0	4	0	0.1	0	0	-	0	0.1	10	0.4	42	1.5	81	42	5	0.6
0	-	0	4	0	0.1	0	0	-	0	0.1	10	0.5	43	1.3	75	77	1	0.6
0	0	0	2	0	0.1	0	0	-	0	0.1	8	0.9	9	1.2	34	28	1	0.4
0	0	0	3	0	0	0	0	-	0	0.1	7	0.5	4	0.7	12	3	2	0.2
0	0	0	2	0	0	0	0	-	0	0.2	3	1.4	12	1.7	34	27	0	0.4
0	-	0	2	0	0.1	0	0	-	0	0.2	1	1.4	7	1.4	31	24	0	0.4
1	4	1	7	0	0.1	0.1	0	-	0.1	0.1	8	0.9	12	1.8	37	42	574	0.3
1	-	25	-	200	-	-	6	-	0.3	0.2	160	1.5	-	3.8	-	620	430	-
-	-	30	-	200	-	-	2	-	0.3	0.3	120	1.5	-	2.9	200	700	540	-
-	-	15	-	-	-	-	24	-	0	0	1042	0.2	-	0.4	-	310	426	-
-	4	20	-	100	-	-	5	-	-	-	24	1	-	-	-	220	530	-
1	-	40	-	200	-	-	-	-	0.1	0.1	16	0.8	-	2.9	150	260	380	-
1	0	37	9	56	0.2	1	0	-	0.1	0	10	0.5	29	3.3	194	442	65	0.5
3	0	407	78	77	0.2	9.8	14	-	0.8	0.2	24	0.7	22	1.9	438	241	100	1.1
0	0	0	0	0	0	0	0	-	0	0	18	0.2	4	0	0	4	48	0.3
-	0	-	-	-	-	-	-	-	-	-	-	-	-	-	-	-	30	-
0	0	22	7	20	0.3	2	0	-	0.2	0.1	32	0.2	32	3.1	218	327	69	0.8
-	0	10	-	0	-	-	0	-	-	-	24	0	-	-	-	-	470	-
-	0	0	-	0	-	-	0	0.4	-	-	0	0	-	-	-	-	340	-
7	0	18	1	6	0	0	0	1.6	0	0	3	0.1	0	0	4	25	428	0
-	0	0	-	100	-	-	0	-	-	-	0	0	-	-	-	-	300	-
1	0	2	0	0	0	0	0	0.3	0	0	4	0.1	0	0	5	26	256	0.1
8	0	0	1	7	0	0	0	1.5	0	0	3	0.1	0	0	1	4	231	0
-	0	0	-	0	-	-	0	-	-	-	0	0	-	-	-	-	290	-
2	0	2	0	0	0	0	0	0.3	0	0	1	0.1	0	0	2	5	236	0
-	0	5	-	0	-	-	0	-	-	-	0	0	-	-	-	-	270	-
-	0	0	-	0	-	-	0	0.6	-	-	0	0	-	-	-	-	310	-
9	0	6	3	63	0	0.1	2	1.8	0	0	6	0.2	0	0.2	11	48	266	0.1
1	0	2	1	5	0	0	2	0.1	0	0	6	0.2	0	0	12	51	282	0
8	-	0	0	63	0	0	0	1.5	0	0	6	0.2	0	0	11	48	307	0
6	1	8	2	30	0	0.1	0	1.3	0	0	3	0.2	1	0	5	35	219	0
2	0	5	2	29	0	0.1	0	0.3	0	0	3	0.2	0	0	5	35	307	0
-	0	0	-	0	-	-	0	-	-	-	0	0	-	-	-	-	300	-
8	0	0	0	0	0	0	0	1.3	0	0	0	0	0	0	0	2	0	0
-	-	55													260	630	500	-
1	-	70	-	0	-	-	4	-	0.3	0	16	1.5	35	4.8	-	801	910	5.7

Code	Food Name	Amount	Unit	Grams	kCalories	Carbohydrate (gm)	Protein (gm)	Fat (gm)	Saturated Fat (gm)	Monounsaturated Fat (gm)
15209	Salmon, Atlantic, Wild, Ckd, Dry Heat	3	Ounce	85.1	155	0	22	7	1	2
15210	Salmon, Chinook, Ckd, Dry Heat	3	Ounce	85.1	196	0	22	11	3	5
15211	Salmon, Chum, Ckd, Dry Heat	3	Ounce	85.1	131	0	22	4	1	2
15239	Salmon, Coho, Farmed, Ckd, Dry Heat	3	Ounce	85.1	151	0	21	7	2	3
15247	Salmon, Coho, Wild, Ckd, Dry Heat	3	Ounce	85.1	118	0	20	4	1	1
15082	Salmon, Coho, Wild, Ckd, Moist Heat	3	Ounce	85.1	156	0	23	6	1	2
15212	Salmon, Pink, Ckd, Dry Heat	3	Ounce	85.1	127	0	22	4	1	1
62546	Salsa	2	Tbsp.	33	20	5	0	0	0	-
41262	Salsa Chicken-Healthy Choice	1	Each	318.9	240	36	20	2	1	-
2047	Salt, Table	1	Tsp.	6	0	0	0	0	0	0
15088	Sardine, Atlantic, Cnd In Oil	3	Ounce	85.1	177	0	21	10	1	3
6313	Sauce, White	½	Cup	131.9	120	11	5	7	3	2
11439	Sauerkraut, Cnd, Sol&liq	½	Cup	118	22	5	1	0	0	0
7003	Sausage, Beerwurst, Pork	1	Slice	23	55	0	3	4	1	2
7006	Sausage, Bockwurst	1	Link	65	200	0	9	18	7	8
7013	Sausage, Bratwurst	1	Link	85	256	2	12	22	8	10
7089	Sausage, Italian, Ckd	1	Link	83	268	1	17	21	8	10
7037	Sausage, Kielbasa, Kolbassy	1	Link	85	264	2	11	23	8	11
7038	Sausage, Knockwurst	1	Link	68	209	1	8	19	7	9
7075	Sausage, Link, Pork and Beef	1	Link	68	228	1	9	21	7	10
16107	Sausage, Meatless	1	Link	25	64	2	5	5	1	1
7057	Sausage, Pepperoni	1	Slice	5.5	27	0	1	2	1	1
7059	Sausage, Polish-style	1	Each	227	740	4	32	65	23	31
7064	Sausage, Pork, Links or Bulk, Ckd	1	Link	13	48	0	3	4	1	2
7072	Sausage, Salami, Beef and Pork, Dry	1	Slice	10	42	0	2	3	1	2
7068	Sausage, Salami, Beef, Ckd	1	Slice	23	60	1	3	5	2	2
7074	Sausage, Smoked Link, Pork	1	Link	68	265	1	15	22	8	10
15173	Scallop, Breaded and Fried	3	Ounce	85.1	183	9	15	9	2	4
15174	Scallop, Imitation	3	Ounce	85.1	84	9	11	0	0	0
43412	Scalloped Potatoes and Ham, Micro Cup-Hormel	1	Each	212.6	260	21	8	16	6	8
55175	Scalloped Potatoes-Stouffer's	1	Each	163	130	16	4	6	-	-
14018	Screwdriver	1	Fl Oz	30.4	25	3	0	0	0	0
15092	Sea Bass, Ckd, Dry Heat	3	Ounce	85.1	105	0	20	2	1	0
12036	Seeds, Sunflower, Dried	½	Cup	72	410	14	16	36	4	7
12537	Seeds, Sunflower, Dry Roasted, w/ Salt added	½	Cup	64	372	15	12	32	3	6
12037	Seeds, Sunflower, Dry Roasted, w/o Salt	½	Cup	64	372	15	12	32	3	6
12538	Seeds, Sunflower, Oil Roasted, w/ Salt added	½	Cup	67.5	415	10	14	39	4	7
12038	Seeds, Sunflower, Oil Roasted, w/o Salt	½	Cup	67.5	415	10	14	39	4	7
12539	Seeds, Sunflower, Toasted, w/ Salt added	½	Cup	67	415	14	12	38	4	7
12039	Seeds, Sunflower, Toasted, w/o Salt	½	Cup	67	415	14	12	38	4	7
19418	Sesame Sticks, Wheat-based, Salted	1	Ounce	28.4	153	13	3	10	2	3
19820	Sesame Sticks, Wheat-based, Unsalted	1	Ounce	28.4	153	13	3	10	2	3
14346	Shake, Chocolate	1	Cup	226.4	288	46	8	8	5	2
14428	Shake, Strawberry	1	Cup	226.4	256	43	8	6	4	-
14347	Shake, Vanilla	1	Cup	226.4	251	41	8	7	4	2
11640	Shallots, Freeze-dried	½	Cup	7.2	25	6	1	0	0	0
11677	Shallots, Fresh	½	Cup	79.9	58	13	2	0	0	0
15096	Shark, Ckd, Batter-dipped and Fried	3	Ounce	85.1	194	5	16	12	3	5
19097	Sherbet, All Flavors	1	Cup	192	265	58	2	4	2	1
18193	Shortbread Cookies, Pecan	1	Each	14	76	8	1	5	1	3
18192	Shortbread Cookies, Plain	1	Each	8	40	5	0	2	0	1
41263	Shrimp Marinara-Healthy Choice	1	Each	297.7	260	51	10	1	-	-
62615	Shrimp Marinara-Weight Watchers	1	Each	255.2	190	35	9	2	1	-
15150	Shrimp, Ckd, Breaded and Fried	3	Ounce	85.1	206	10	18	10	2	3
15151	Shrimp, Ckd, Moist Heat	3	Ounce	85.1	84	0	18	1	0	0
15152	Shrimp, Cnd	3	Ounce	85.1	102	1	20	2	0	0
15149	Shrimp, Fresh	3	Ounce	85.1	90	1	17	1	0	0
15153	Shrimp, Imitation	3	Ounce	85.1	86	8	11	1	0	0
55143	Single Serving Stuffed Pepper-Stouffer's	1	Each	283.5	220	28	10	8	-	-
41264	Sirloin Beef w/ Barbecue Sauce-Healthy Choice	1	Each	311.8	280	44	17	4	2	-

Polyunsaturated Fat (gm)	Fiber (gm)	Cholesterol (mg)	Folate (µg)	Vitamin A (re)	Vitamin B6 (mg)	Vitamin B12 (µg)	Vitamin C (mg)	Vitamin E (mg)	Riboflavin (mg)	Thiamin (mg)	Calcium (mg)	Iron (mg)	Magnesium (mg)	Niacin (mg)	Phosphorus (mg)	Potassium (mg)	Sodium (mg)	Zinc (mg)
3	0	60	25	11	0.8	2.6	0	-	0.4	0.2	13	0.9	31	8.6	218	534	48	0.7
2	0	72	30	127	0.4	2.4	3	-	0.1	0	24	0.8	104	8.5	316	430	51	0.5
1	0	81	4	29	0.4	2.9	0	-	0.2	0.1	12	0.6	24	7.3	309	468	54	0.5
2	0	54	12	50	0.5	2.7	1	-	0.1	0.1	10	0.3	29	6.3	282	391	44	0.4
1	0	47	11	33	0.5	4.3	1	-	0.1	0.1	-	0.5	28	6.8	274	369	49	0.5
2	0	48	8	27	0.5	3.8	1	-	0.1	0.1	39	0.6	30	6.6	253	387	45	0.4
1	0	57	4	35	0.2	2.9	0	-	0.1	0.2	14	0.8	28	7.3	251	352	73	0.6
-	0	0	-	80	-	-	4	-	-	-	0	0	-	-	-	-	240	-
-	-	50	-	200	-	-	66	-	0.2	0.2	64	0.6	-	3.8	200	540	450	-
0	0	0	0	0	0	0	0	-	0	0	3	0	0	0	0	0	2325	0
4	0	121	10	57	0.1	7.6	0	-	0.2	0.1	325	2.5	33	4.5	417	338	430	1.1
1	-	17	8	46	0	0.5	1	-	0.2	0	212	0.1	132	0.3	128	222	398	0.3
0	3	0	28	2	0.2	0	17	-	0	0	35	1.7	15	0.2	24	201	780	0.2
1	0	14	1	0	0.1	0.2	7	-	0	0.1	2	0.3	3	0.7	24	58	285	0.4
2	0	38	4	4	0.1	0.5	0	-	0.1	0.3	10	0.4	12	2.7	95	176	718	1
2	0	51	2	0	0.2	0.8	1	-	0.2	0.4	37	1.1	13	2.7	127	180	473	2
3	0	65	4	0	0.3	1.1	2	-	0.2	0.5	20	1.2	15	3.5	141	252	765	2
3	0	57	4	0	0.2	1.4	18	-	0.2	0.2	37	1.2	14	2.4	126	230	915	1.7
2	0	39	1	0	0.1	0.8	18	-	0.1	0.2	7	0.6	7	1.9	67	135	687	1.1
2	0	48	1	0	0.1	1	13	-	0.1	0.2	7	1	8	2.2	73	129	643	1.4
2	1	0	7	16	0.2	0	0	-	0.1	0.6	16	0.9	9	2.8	56	58	222	0.4
0	0	4	0	0	0	0.1	0	-	0	0	1	0.1	1	0.3	7	19	112	0.1
7	0	159	5	0	0.4	2.2	2	-	0.3	1.1	27	3.3	32	7.8	309	538	1989	4.4
0	0	11	0	0	0	0.2	0	-	0	0.1	4	0.2	2	0.6	24	47	168	0.3
0	0	8	0	0	0.1	0.2	3	-	0	0.1	1	0.2	2	0.5	14	38	186	0.3
0	0	15	0	0	0	0.7	4	-	0	0	2	0.5	3	0.7	26	52	270	0.5
3	0	46	3	0	0.2	1.1	1	-	0.2	0.5	20	0.8	13	3.1	110	228	1020	1.9
2	-	52	15	19	0.1	1.1	2	-	0.1	0	36	0.7	50	1.3	201	283	395	0.9
0	0	19	1	17	0	1.4	0	-	0	0	7	0.3	37	0.3	240	88	676	0.3
2	-	33	-	-	-	-	11	-	0.1	0.1	32	0.4	21	2.1	-	425	768	0.9
-	-	-	-	-	-	-	2	-	0.1	0	80	0.2	-	0.8	-	375	610	-
0	-	0	11	2	0	0	9	-	0	0	2	0	2	0	4	47	0	0
1	0	45	5	54	0.4	0.3	0	-	0.1	0.1	11	0.3	45	1.6	211	279	74	0.4
24	8	0	164	4	0.6	0	1	-	0.2	1.6	84	4.9	255	3.2	508	496	2	3.6
21	4	0	152	0	0.5	0	1	-	0.2	0.1	45	2.4	83	4.5	739	544	499	3.4
21	6	0	152	0	0.5	0	1	-	0.2	0.1	45	2.4	83	4.5	739	544	2	3.4
26	5	0	158	3	0.5	0	1	-	0.2	0.2	38	4.5	86	2.8	769	326	407	3.5
26	5	0	158	3	0.5	0	1	-	0.2	0.2	38	4.5	86	2.8	769	326	2	3.5
25	-	0	159	0	0.5	0	1	-	0.2	0.2	38	4.6	86	2.8	776	329	411	3.6
25	-	0	159	0	0.5	0	1	-	0.2	0.2	38	4.6	86	2.8	776	329	2	3.6
5	1	0	6	3	0	0	0	-	0	0	48	0.2	13	0.4	39	50	422	0.3
5	-	0	6	3	0	0	0	-	0	0	48	0.2	13	0.4	39	50	8	0.3
0	-	29	8	52	0.1	0.8	1	-	0.6	0.1	256	0.7	38	0.4	231	453	220	0.9
-	-	25	7	66	0.1	0.7	2	-	0.4	0.1	256	0.2	29	0.4	226	412	188	0.8
0	-	25	7	72	0.1	0.8	2	-	0.4	0.1	276	0.2	27	0.4	231	394	186	0.8
0	-	0	8	404	0.1	0	3	-	0	0	13	0.4	7	0.1	21	119	4	0.1
0	-	0	27	998	0.3	0	6	-	0	0	30	1	17	0.2	48	267	10	0.3
3	0	50	4	46	0.3	1	0	-	0.1	0.1	43	0.9	37	2.4	165	132	104	0.4
0	-	10	8	27	0.1	0.2	8	-	0.1	0	104	0.3	15	0.2	77	184	88	0.9
1	0	5	1	0	0	0	0	-	0	0	4	0.3	3	0.3	12	10	39	0.1
0	-	2	1	1	0	0	0	-	0	0	3	0.2	1	0.3	9	8	36	0
-	-	60	-	100	-	-	114	-	0.1	0.2	48	1.5	-	1.1	130	390	320	-
-	4	40	-	150	-	-	6	-	-	-	120	1	-	-	-	440	400	-
4	-	151	7	48	0.1	1.6	1	-	0.1	0.1	57	1.1	34	2.6	185	191	293	1.2
0	0	166	3	56	0.1	1.3	2	-	0	0	33	2.6	29	2.2	117	155	191	1.3
1	0	147	2	15	0.1	1	2	-	0	0	50	2.3	35	2.3	198	179	144	1.1
1	0	129	3	46	0.1	1	2	-	0	0	44	2	31	2.2	174	157	126	0.9
1	0	31	1	17	0	1.4	0	-	0	0	16	0.5	37	0.1	240	76	600	0.3
-	-	-	-	20	-	-	6	-	0.2	0.2	32	1	-	2.9	-	400	1010	-
1	-	25	-	-	-	-	-	-	-	-	-	-	-	-	190	630	240	-

Code	Food Name	Amount	Unit	Grams	kCalories	Carbohydrate (gm)	Protein (gm)	Fat (gm)	Saturated Fat (gm)	Monounsaturated Fat (gm)
19370	Skittles Bite Size Candies	1	Pkg	65	255	62	0	2	-	-
41291	Sliced Turkey Breast w/ Gravy and Dressing-Healthy Choice	1	Each	283.5	270	30	27	4	2	-
41296	Sliced Turkey Breast w/ Gravy-Healthy Choice	1	Each	340.2	290	46	19	3	1	-
55225	Sliced Turkey w/ Dressing, Lean Cuisine-Stouffer's	1	Each	223.3	200	23	16	5	1	-
19407	Slim Jims, Smoked	1	Ounce	28.4	156	2	6	14	6	6
15100	Smelt, Rainbow, Ckd, Dry Heat	3	Ounce	85.1	105	0	19	3	0	1
15102	Snapper, Ckd, Dry Heat	3	Ounce	85.1	109	0	22	1	0	0
19155	Snickers Bar	1	Bar	61	278	37	6	14	7	4
62599	Sorbet, All Flavors	½	Cup	90	100	25	0	0	0	-
6474	Soup, Bean w/ Bacon	1	Cup	264.9	106	16	5	2	1	1
6007	Soup, Bean w/ Ham	1	Cup	243	231	27	13	9	3	4
6406	Soup, Bean w/ Hot Dogs	1	Cup	250	187	22	10	7	2	3
6404	Soup, Bean w/ Pork	1	Cup	253	172	23	8	6	2	2
6008	Soup, Beef Broth or Boullion	1	Cup	240	17	0	3	1	0	0
6547	Soup, Beef Mushroom	1	Cup	244	73	6	6	3	1	1
6409	Soup, Beef Noodle	1	Cup	244	83	9	5	3	1	1
6070	Soup, Beef, Chunky	1	Cup	240	170	20	12	5	3	2
6402	Soup, Black Bean	1	Cup	247	116	20	6	2	0	1
6478	Soup, Cauliflower	1	Cup	256.1	69	11	3	2	0	1
6411	Soup, Cheese	1	Cup	247	156	11	5	10	7	3
6480	Soup, Chicken Broth or Bouillon	1	Cup	244	22	1	1	1	0	0
6417	Soup, Chicken Gumbo	1	Cup	244	56	8	3	1	0	1
6549	Soup, Chicken Mushroom	1	Cup	244	132	9	4	9	2	4
6419	Soup, Chicken Noodle	1	Cup	241	75	9	4	2	1	1
6018	Soup, Chicken Noodle, Chunky	1	Cup	240	175	17	13	6	1	3
6485	Soup, Chicken Rice	1	Cup	252.8	61	9	2	1	0	1
6022	Soup, Chicken Rice, Chunky	1	Cup	240	127	13	12	3	1	1
6425	Soup, Chicken Vegetable	1	Cup	241	75	9	4	3	1	1
6024	Soup, Chicken Vegetable, Chunky	1	Cup	240	166	19	12	5	1	2
6412	Soup, Chicken w/ Dumplings	1	Cup	241	96	6	6	6	1	3
6423	Soup, Chicken w/ Rice	1	Cup	241	60	7	4	2	0	1
6015	Soup, Chicken, Chunky	1	Cup	251	178	17	13	7	2	3
6426	Soup, Chili Beef	1	Cup	250	170	21	7	7	3	3
6027	Soup, Clam Chowder, Manhattan Style	1	Cup	240	134	19	7	3	2	1
6230	Soup, Clam Chowder, New England	1	Cup	248	164	17	9	7	3	2
6034	Soup, Crab	1	Cup	244	76	10	5	2	0	1
6201	Soup, Cream Of Asparagus	1	Cup	248	161	16	6	8	3	2
6210	Soup, Cream Of Celery	1	Cup	248	164	15	6	10	4	2
6216	Soup, Cream Of Chicken	1	Cup	248	191	15	7	11	5	4
6243	Soup, Cream Of Mushroom	1	Cup	248	203	15	6	14	5	3
6246	Soup, Cream Of Onion	1	Cup	248	186	18	7	9	4	3
6253	Soup, Cream Of Potato	1	Cup	248	149	17	6	6	4	2
6256	Soup, Cream Of Shrimp	1	Cup	248	164	14	7	9	6	3
6501	Soup, Cream Of Vegetable	1	Cup	260.1	107	12	2	6	1	3
6036	Soup, Gazpacho	1	Cup	244	56	1	9	2	0	1
6037	Soup, Lentil w/ ham	1	Cup	248	139	20	9	3	1	1
6440	Soup, Minestrone	1	Cup	241	82	11	4	3	1	1
6039	Soup, Minestrone, Chunky	1	Cup	240	127	21	5	3	1	1
6493	Soup, Mushroom	1	Cup	253	96	11	2	5	1	2
6445	Soup, Onion	1	Cup	241	58	8	4	2	0	1
6249	Soup, Pea, Green	1	Cup	254	239	32	13	7	4	2
6451	Soup, Pea, Split w/ Ham	1	Cup	253	190	28	10	4	2	2
6050	Soup, Pea, Split w/ Ham, Chunky	1	Cup	240	185	27	11	4	2	2
6359	Soup, Tomato	1	Cup	248	161	22	6	6	3	2
6461	Soup, Tomato Beef w/ noodle	1	Cup	244	139	21	4	4	2	2
6463	Soup, Tomato Rice	1	Cup	247	119	22	2	3	1	1
6499	Soup, Tomato Vegetable	1	Cup	253	56	10	2	1	0	0
6465	Soup, Turkey Noodle	1	Cup	244	68	9	4	2	1	1
6466	Soup, Turkey Vegetable	1	Cup	241	72	9	3	3	1	1
6064	Soup, Turkey, Chunky	1	Cup	236	135	14	10	4	1	2

Polyunsaturated Fat (gm)	Fiber (gm)	Cholesterol (mg)	Folate (µg)	Vitamin A (re)	Vitamin B6 (mg)	Vitamin B12 (µg)	Vitamin C (mg)	Vitamin E (mg)	Riboflavin (mg)	Thiamin (mg)	Calcium (mg)	Iron (mg)	Magnesium (mg)	Niacin (mg)	Phosphorus (mg)	Potassium (mg)	Sodium (mg)	Zinc (mg)
-	0	0	0	0	0	0	0	-	0	0	2	0.1	1	0	2	15	30	0
1	-	50	-	150	-	-	-	-	0.3	0.3	48	1	-	7.6	310	590	530	-
1	-	20	-	150	-	-	27	-	0.1	0.2	16	0.6	-	1.5	-	360	520	-
2	-	25	-	500	-	-	6	-	0.3	0.2	32	0.8	-	4.8	-	400	590	-
1	-	38	0	48	0.1	0.3	2	-	0.1	0	19	1	6	1.3	51	73	420	0.7
1	0	77	4	14	0.1	3.4	0	-	0.1	0	65	1	32	1.5	251	316	65	1.8
1	0	40	5	30	0.4	3	1	-	0	0	34	0.2	31	0.3	171	444	48	0.4
1	2	7	24	19	0.1	0.3	0	-	0.1	0	70	0.5	37	1.8	129	199	163	0.7
-	1	0	-	0	-	-	12	-	-	-	0	0	-	-	-	-	10	-
0	9	3	8	5	0	0	1	-	0.3	0.1	56	1.3	29	0.4	90	326	927	0.7
1	11	22	29	396	0.1	0.1	4	-	0.1	0.1	78	3.2	46	1.7	143	425	972	1.1
2	-	12	30	87	0.1	0.1	1	-	0.1	0.1	87	2.3	47	1	165	477	1092	1.2
2	9	3	32	89	0	0.1	2	-	0	0.1	81	2	46	0.6	132	402	951	1
0	0	0	5	0	0	0.2	0	-	0.1	0	14	0.4	5	1.9	31	130	782	0
0	-	7	10	0	0	0.2	5	-	0.1	0	5	0.9	10	1	34	154	942	1.5
0	1	5	4	63	0	0.2	0	-	0.1	0.1	15	1.1	5	1.1	46	100	952	1.5
0	1	14	13	262	0.1	0.6	7	-	0.2	0.1	31	2.3	5	2.7	120	336	866	2.6
0	4	0	25	49	0.1	0	1	-	0.1	0.1	44	2.1	42	0.5	106	274	1198	1.4
1	-	0	3	0	0	0.2	3	-	0.1	0.1	10	0.5	3	0.5	51	105	843	0.3
0	-	30	5	109	0	0	0	-	0.1	0	141	0.7	5	0.4	136	153	958	0.6
0	0	0	2	12	0	0	0	-	0	0	15	0.1	5	0.2	12	24	1484	0
0	2	5	5	15	0.1	0	5	-	0	0	24	0.9	5	0.7	24	76	954	0.4
2	-	10	0	112	0	0	0	-	0.1	0	29	0.9	10	1.6	27	154	942	1
1	1	7	2	72	0	0.1	0	-	0.1	0.1	17	0.8	5	1.4	36	55	1106	0.4
2	4	19	5	122	0	0.3	0	-	0.2	0.1	24	1.4	10	4.3	72	108	850	1
0	1	3	1	0	0	0.1	0	-	0	0	8	0	0	0.4	10	10	981	0.1
1	1	12	4	586	0	0.3	4	-	0.1	0	34	1.9	10	4.1	72	108	888	1
1	1	10	5	265	0	0.1	1	-	0.1	0	17	0.9	7	1.2	41	154	945	0.4
1	-	17	12	600	0.1	0.2	6	-	0.2	0	26	1.5	10	3.3	106	367	1068	2.2
1	1	34	2	53	0	0.2	0	-	0.1	0	14	0.6	5	1.8	60	116	860	0.4
0	1	7	1	65	0	0.1	0	-	0	0	17	0.7	0	1.1	22	101	815	0.3
1	2	30	5	131	0.1	0.3	1	-	0.2	0.1	25	1.7	8	4.4	113	176	889	1
0	9	12	17	150	0.2	0.3	4	-	0.1	0.1	42	2.1	30	1.1	147	525	1035	1.4
0	3	14	9	329	0.3	7.9	12	-	0.1	0.1	67	2.6	19	1.8	84	384	1001	1.7
1	1	22	10	40	0.1	10.2	3	-	0.2	0.1	186	1.5	22	1	156	300	992	0.8
0	1	10	15	51	0.1	0.2	0	-	0.1	0.2	66	1.2	15	1.3	88	327	1235	1.5
2	1	22	30	84	0.1	0.5	4	-	0.3	0.1	174	0.9	20	0.9	154	360	1042	0.9
3	1	32	8	67	0.1	0.5	1	-	0.2	0.1	186	0.7	22	0.4	151	310	1009	0.2
2	0	27	8	94	0.1	0.5	1	-	0.3	0.1	181	0.7	17	0.9	151	273	1047	0.7
5	0	20	10	37	0.1	0.5	2	-	0.3	0.1	179	0.6	20	0.9	156	270	1076	0.6
2	1	32	12	67	0.1	0.5	2	-	0.3	0.1	179	0.7	22	0.6	154	310	1004	0.6
1	0	22	9	67	0.1	0.5	1	-	0.2	0.1	166	0.5	17	0.6	161	322	1061	0.7
0	0	35	10	55	0.4	1	1	-	0.2	0.1	164	0.6	22	0.5	146	248	1037	0.8
1	1	0	8	3	0	0.1	4	-	0.1	1.2	31	0.5	10	0.5	55	96	1170	0.3
1	4	0	10	20	0.1	0	3	-	0	0	24	1	7	0.9	37	224	1183	0.2
0	-	7	50	35	0.2	0.3	4	-	0.1	0.2	42	2.7	22	1.4	184	357	1319	0.7
1	1	2	16	234	0.1	0	1	-	0	0.1	34	0.9	7	0.9	55	313	911	0.7
0	2	5	31	434	0.2	0	5	-	0.1	0.1	60	1.8	14	1.2	110	612	864	1.4
2	1	0	5	0	0	0.3	1	-	0.1	0.3	66	0.5	5	0.5	76	200	1020	0.1
1	1	0	15	0	0	0	1	-	0	0	27	0.7	2	0.6	12	67	1053	0.6
1	3	18	8	58	0.1	0.4	3	-	0.3	0.2	173	2	56	1.3	239	376	1046	1.8
1	-	8	3	46	0.1	0.3	2	-	0.1	0.1	23	2.3	48	1.5	213	400	1007	1.3
1	4	7	5	487	0.2	0.2	7	-	0.1	0.1	34	2.1	38	2.5	178	305	965	3.1
1	0	17	21	109	0.2	0.4	68	-	0.2	0.1	159	1.8	22	1.5	149	449	932	0.3
1	1	5	7	54	0.1	0.2	0	-	0.1	0.1	17	1.1	7	1.9	56	220	917	0.8
1	1	2	14	77	0.1	0	15	-	0	0.1	22	0.8	5	1.1	35	331	815	0.5
0	1	0	10	20	0.1	0	6	-	0	0.1	8	0.6	20	0.8	30	104	1146	0.2
0	1	5	2	29	0	0.1	0	-	0.1	0.1	12	1	5	1.4	49	76	815	0.6
1	0	2	5	243	0	0.2	0	-	0	0	17	0.8	5	1	41	176	906	0.6
1	-	9	11	715	0.3	2.1	6	-	0.1	0	50	1.9	24	3.6	104	361	923	2.1

Code	Food Name	Amount	Unit	Grams	kCalories	Carbohydrate (gm)	Protein (gm)	Fat (gm)	Saturated Fat (gm)	Monounsaturated Fat (gm)
6500	Soup, Vegetable Beef	1	Cup	253.1	53	8	3	1	1	0
6067	Soup, Vegetable, Chunky	1	Cup	240	122	19	4	4	1	2
6468	Soup, Vegetarian Vegetable	1	Cup	241	72	12	2	2	0	1
1056	Sour Cream	1	Tbsp.	12	26	1	0	3	2	1
62556	Sour Cream, Fat Free	1	Tbsp.	16	13	3	1	0	0	-
1055	Sour Cream, Half and Half, Cultured	1	Tbsp.	15	20	1	0	2	1	1
1074	Sour Cream, Imitation, Nondairy, Cultured	1	Tbsp.	14.4	30	1	0	3	3	0
62555	Sour Cream, Light	1	Tbsp.	16	16	1	1	1	1	-
41265	Southwestern Style Chicken-Healthy Choice	1	Each	354.4	340	51	25	5	2	-
6134	Soy Sauce	1	Tbsp.	18	10	2	1	0	0	0
16109	Soybeans, Boiled	½	Cup	86	149	9	14	8	1	2
16111	Soybeans, Dry Roasted	½	Cup	86	387	28	34	19	3	4
43404	Spaghetti and Meatballs, Micro Cup-Hormel	1	Each	212.6	210	27	10	7	3	3
11455	Spaghetti Sauce	½	Cup	124.5	136	20	2	6	1	3
55226	Spaghetti w/ Meat Sauce, Lean Cuisine-Stouffer's	1	Each	326	290	45	15	6	2	-
43396	Spaghetti w/ Meat Sauce, Top Shelf-Hormel	1	Each	283.5	260	37	14	6	2	2
41342	Spaghetti w/ Meat Sauce-Healthy Choice	1	Each	283.5	280	42	14	6	2	-
55247	Spaghetti w/ Meat Sauce-Stouffer's	1	Each	365	320	38	16	12	-	-
55150	Spaghetti w/ Meatballs, -Stouffer's	1	Each	276.4	290	37	14	9	-	-
19164	Special Dark Sweet Chocolate Bar	1	Bar	79	376	49	4	24	-	-
55176	Spinach Souffle-Stouffer's	1	Each	170.1	220	11	9	15	-	-
11458	Spinach, Ckd	½	Cup	90	21	3	3	0	0	0
11461	Spinach, Cnd, Drained Solids	½	Cup	107	25	4	3	1	0	0
11459	Spinach, Cnd, Reg Pk, Sol&liq	½	Cup	117	22	3	2	0	0	0
11457	Spinach, Fresh	1	Cup	56	12	2	2	0	0	0
11464	Spinach, Frz, Ckd	½	Cup	95	27	5	3	0	0	0
11463	Spinach, Frz, Unprepared	½	Cup	78	19	3	2	0	0	0
41283	Split Pea and Ham Soup-Healthy Choice	1	Each	212.6	170	25	10	3	1	-
55766	Split Pea Soup w/ Ham-Stouffer's	1	Cup	283.9	220	35	15	3	-	-
11642	Squash, Summer, Ckd	½	Cup	90	18	4	1	0	0	0
11641	Squash, Summer, Fresh	½	Cup	65	13	3	1	0	0	0
11644	Squash, Winter, Baked	½	Cup	102.5	40	9	1	1	0	0
11643	Squash, Winter, Fresh	½	Cup	58	21	5	1	0	0	0
11953	Squash, Zucchini, Baby, Fresh	1	Medium	11	2	0	0	0	0	0
15176	Squid, Fried	3	Ounce	85.1	149	7	15	6	2	2
9316	Strawberries, Fresh	½	Cup	74.5	22	5	0	0	0	0
9320	Strawberries, Frozen, Sweetened	½	Cup	127.5	122	33	1	0	0	0
9318	Strawberries, Frozen, Unsweetened	½	Cup	74.5	26	7	0	0	0	0
14351	Strawberry Flavor Beverage	1	Cup	266	234	33	8	8	5	2
18354	Strudel, Apple	1	Each	71	195	29	2	8	2	4
55781	Stuffed Cabbage no Sauce-Stouffer's	1	Ounce	28.4	39	3	2	2	-	-
55228	Stuffed Cabbage w/ Meat, Lean Cuisine-Stouffer's	1	Each	269.3	210	26	13	6	2	-
55778	Stuffed Cabbage-Stouffer's	1	Ounce	28.4	29	3	1	1	-	-
55157	Stuffed Green Peppers-Stouffer's	1	Each	219.7	200	22	9	8	-	-
18203	Sugar Cookies, Dietary	1	Each	7	30	5	1	1	0	1
18204	Sugar Cookies, Regular (includes Vanilla)	1	Each	15	72	10	1	3	1	2
15218	Sunfish, Ckd, Dry Heat	3	Ounce	85.1	97	0	21	1	0	0
55229	Swedish Meatballs w/ Pasta, Lean Cuisine-Stouffer's	1	Each	258.7	290	31	23	8	3	-
55148	Swedish Meatballs w/ Pasta-Stouffer's	1	Each	262.2	420	32	24	21	-	-
41266	Sweet and Sour Chicken-Healthy Choice	1	Each	326	280	52	20	2	-	-
18359	Sweet Rolls w/ Raisins and Nuts	1	Each	57	196	30	4	7	1	3
18355	Sweet Rolls, Cheese	1	Each	66	238	29	5	12	4	6
18356	Sweet Rolls, Cinnamon w/ Raisins	1	Each	60	223	31	4	10	3	5
11508	Sweetpotatoes, Baked In Skin	½	Cup	100	103	24	2	0	0	0
11510	Sweetpotatoes, Boiled, w/o Skin	½	Cup	164	172	40	3	0	0	0
11659	Sweetpotatoes, Candied	½	Cup	113.4	155	32	1	4	2	1
11514	Sweetpotatoes, Mashed	½	Cup	127.5	129	30	3	0	0	0
11647	Sweetpotatoes, Syrup Pack, Drained Solids	½	Cup	98	106	25	1	0	0	0
15111	Swordfish, Ckd, Dry Heat	3	Ounce	85.1	132	0	22	4	1	2
19093	Symphony Milk Chocolate Bar	1	Bar	68	355	39	5	22	-	-

Polyunsaturated Fat (gm)	Fiber (gm)	Cholesterol (mg)	Folate (μg)	Vitamin A (re)	Vitamin B6 (mg)	Vitamin B12 (μg)	Vitamin C (mg)	Vitamin E (mg)	Riboflavin (mg)	Thiamin (mg)	Calcium (mg)	Iron (mg)	Magnesium (mg)	Niacin (mg)	Phosphorus (mg)	Potassium (mg)	Sodium (mg)	Zinc (mg)
0	1	0	8	23	0.1	0.3	1	-	0	0	13	0.9	23	0.5	35	76	1002	0.3
1	1	0	17	588	0.2	0	6	-	0.1	0.1	55	1.6	7	1.2	72	396	1010	3.1
1	0	0	11	301	0.1	0	1	-	0	0.1	22	1.1	7	0.9	34	210	822	0.5
0	0	5	1	23	0	0	0	-	0	0	14	0	1	0	10	17	6	0
-	-	3	-	30	-	-	0	-	-	-	36	0	-	-	-	-	18	-
0	0	6	2	17	0	0	0	-	0	0	16	0	2	0	14	19	6	0.1
0	0	0	0	0	0	0	0	-	0	0	0	0.1	1	0	6	23	15	0.2
-	-	5	-	18	-	-	0	-	-	-	22	0	-	-	-	27	9	-
2	-	60	-	-	-	-	-	-	-	-	-	-	-	-	260	560	550	-
0	0	0	3	0	0	0	0	-	0	0	3	0.4	6	0.6	20	32	1029	0.1
4	5	0	46	1	0.2	0	1	-	0.2	0.1	88	4.4	74	0.3	211	443	1	1
10	7	0	176	2	0.2	0	4	-	0.6	0.4	232	3.4	196	0.9	558	1173	2	4.1
1	-	20	-	140	-	-	4	-	0.3	0.1	32	1.1	25	2.3	-	341	930	1.1
2	4	0	27	153	0.4	0	14	-	0.1	0.1	35	0.8	30	1.9	45	478	618	0.3
2	-	20	-	100	-	-	6	-	0.3	0.3	48	2	-	3.8	-	500	500	-
1	-	20	-	100	-	-	2	-	0.3	0.2	48	1.5	46	3.8	-	879	980	2.4
2	-	20	-	250	-	-	5	-	0.3	0.4	48	2	-	1.9	160	540	480	-
12	-	-	-	150	-	-	6	-	0.2	0.2	80	1.5	-	3.8	-	800	560	-
-	-	-	-	100	-	-	6	-	0.3	0.3	64	1.5	-	3.8	-	550	790	-
-	4	0	3	2	0	0	0	-	0.2	0	15	1.7	91	0.5	126	269	8	1.2
-	-	-	-	200	-	-	6	-	0.3	0.1	120	0.4	-	0.4	-	345	820	-
0	2	0	131	737	0.2	0	9	-	0.2	0.1	122	3.2	78	0.4	50	419	63	0.7
0	-	0	105	939	0.1	0	15	-	0.1	0	136	2.5	81	0.4	47	370	29	0.5
0	3	0	68	752	0.1	0	16	-	0.1	0	97	1.8	66	0.3	37	269	373	0.5
0	2	0	109	376	0.1	0	16	-	0.1	0	55	1.5	44	0.4	27	312	44	0.3
0	3	0	102	739	0.1	0	12	-	0.2	0.1	139	1.4	66	0.4	46	283	82	0.7
0	2	0	93	605	0.1	0	19	-	0.1	0.1	87	1.6	45	0.3	32	252	58	0.3
-	-	10	-	100	-	-	6	-	0.1	0.2	16	0.6	-	1.9	190	450	460	-
-	-	10	-	-	-	-	0	-	0	0	240	0.2	-	0.4	-	571	1192	-
0	1	0	18	26	0.1	0	5	-	0	0	24	0.3	22	0.5	35	173	1	0.4
0	1	0	17	13	0.1	0	10	-	0	0	13	0.3	15	0.4	23	127	1	0.2
0	3	0	29	365	0.1	0	10	-	0	0.1	14	0.3	8	0.7	21	448	1	0.3
0	1	0	13	235	0	0	7	-	0	0.1	18	0.3	12	0.5	19	203	2	0.1
0	-	0	2	5	0	0	4	-	0	0	2	0.1	4	0.1	10	50	0	0.1
2	0	221	5	9	0	1	4	-	0.4	0	33	0.9	32	2.2	213	237	260	1.5
0	2	0	13	2	0	0	42	0.1	0	0	10	0.3	7	0.2	14	124	1	0.1
0	2	0	19	3	0	0	53	-	0.1	0	14	0.8	9	0.5	17	125	4	0.1
0	2	0	13	3	0	0	31	0.2	0	0	12	0.6	8	0.3	10	110	1	0.1
0	-	32	12	74	0.1	0.9	2	-	0.4	0.1	293	0.2	32	0.2	229	370	128	0.9
1	2	20	4	6	0	0.1	1	-	0	0	11	0.3	6	0.2	23	69	191	0.1
-	-	5	-	-	-	-	1	-	0	0	72	0	-	0.1	-	48	150	-
1	-	30	-	80	-	-	6	-	0.2	0.1	64	1.5	-	3.8	-	600	560	-
-	-	4	-	-	-	-	3	-	0	0	48	0	-	0.1	-	51	145	-
-	-	-	-	60	-	-	6	-	0.1	0.1	32	0.8	-	2.9	-	380	650	-
0	-	0	0	0	0	0	0	-	0	0	2	0.3	1	0.2	6	7	0	0
0	-	8	2	4	0	0	0	-	0	0	3	0.3	2	0.4	12	9	54	0.1
0	0	73	14	14	0.1	2	1	-	0.1	0.1	88	1.3	32	1.2	196	382	88	1.7
1	-	55	-	20	-	-	-	-	0.3	0.2	48	1.5	-	3.8	-	450	550	-
-	-	-	-	20	-	-	1	-	0.3	0.2	48	1.5	-	2.9	-	350	740	-
-	-	35	-	250	-	-	30	-	0.2	0.2	32	1	-	8.6	220	480	320	-
3	-	13	18	60	0.1	0.1	0	-	0.2	0.2	36	1.5	16	1.3	63	123	185	0.4
1	-	37	20	41	0	0.1	0	-	0.1	0.1	78	0.5	13	0.5	65	87	236	0.4
1	1	40	14	38	0.1	0.1	1	-	0.2	0.2	43	1	10	1.4	46	67	230	0.4
0	3	0	23	2182	0.2	0	25	-	0.1	0.1	28	0.4	20	0.6	55	348	10	0.3
0	4	0	18	2796	0.4	0	28	-	0.2	0.1	34	0.9	16	1	44	302	21	0.4
0	-	9	13	475	0	0	8	-	0	0	29	1.3	12	0.4	29	214	79	0.2
0	-	0	14	1929	0.3	0	7	-	0.1	0	38	1.7	31	1.2	66	268	96	0.2
0	-	0	8	702	0.1	0	11	-	0	0	17	0.9	12	0.3	25	189	38	0.2
1	0	43	2	35	0.3	1.7	1	-	0.1	0	5	0.9	29	10	287	314	98	1.3
-	-	19	5	9	0	0.3	0	-	0.3	0.1	160	0.7	37	0.2	170	262	58	0.8

Code	Food Name	Amount	Unit	Grams	kCalories	Carbohydrate (gm)	Protein (gm)	Fat (gm)	Saturated Fat (gm)	Monounsaturated Fat (gm)
19348	Syrup, Chocolate, Fudge-type	1	Tbsp.	21	73	12	1	3	1	1
19349	Syrup, Corn, Dark	1	Tbsp.	20	56	15	0	0	-	-
19351	Syrup, Corn, High-fructose	1	Tbsp.	19	53	14	0	0	-	-
19350	Syrup, Corn, Light	1	Tbsp.	20	56	15	0	0	-	-
19352	Syrup, Malt	1	Tbsp.	24	76	17	1	0	-	-
19353	Syrup, Maple	1	Tbsp.	20	52	13	0	0	-	-
19128	Syrup, Pancake, Lo Cal	1	Tbsp.	20	33	9	0	0	-	-
19360	Syrup, Pancake, w/ 2% Maple	1	Tbsp.	20	53	14	0	0	-	-
19113	Syrup, Pancake, w/ Butter	1	Tbsp.	20	59	15	0	0	0	0
18360	Taco Shells, Baked	1	Medium	13	61	8	1	3	0	1
18448	Taco Shells, Baked, w/o Added Salt	1	Medium	13	61	8	1	3	0	1
43438	Taco Shells, Chi-Chi's-Hormel	1	Each	20	99	12	1	5	-	-
19382	Taffy	1	Piece	15	56	14	0	0	0	0
9223	Tangerine Juice, Cnd, Sweetened	¾	Cup	186.4	93	22	1	0	0	0
9221	Tangerine Juice, Fresh	¾	Cup	185.2	80	19	1	0	0	0
9219	Tangerines, Cnd, Juice Pack	½	Cup	124.5	46	12	1	0	0	0
9220	Tangerines, Cnd, Light Syrup Pack	½	Cup	126	77	20	1	0	0	0
9218	Tangerines, Fresh	1	Medium	84	37	9	1	0	0	0
19218	Tapioca Pudding	1	Cup	298.1	355	58	6	11	2	5
19524	Taro Chips	1	Ounce	28.4	141	19	1	7	2	1
14355	Tea, Brewed	8	Fl Oz	236.8	2	1	0	0	0	0
14381	Tea, Herb, Brewed	8	Fl Oz	236.8	2	0	0	0	0	0
14371	Tea, Instant, Sweetened	8	Fl Oz	259	88	22	0	0	0	0
14367	Tea, Instant, Unsweetened	8	Fl Oz	236.8	2	0	0	0	0	0
43401	Tender Beef Roast, Top Shelf-Hormel	1	Each	283.5	240	19	28	6	2	2
14020	Tequila Sunrise	1	Fl Oz	31.2	34	3	0	0	0	0
41267	Teriyaki Chicken-Healthy Choice	1	Each	347.3	290	39	24	4	1	-
6112	Teriyaki Sauce	1	Tbsp.	18	15	3	1	0	0	0
55811	Three Bean Chili-Stouffer's	1	Cup	283.9	210	32	10	5	-	-
19159	Three Musketeers Bar	1	Bar	60	250	46	2	8	4	3
14382	Thrist Quencher Drink, Bottled	12	Fl Oz	361.2	90	23	0	0	0	0
18361	Toaster Pastries, Brown-sugar-cinn.	1	Each	52	214	35	3	7	2	4
18362	Toaster Pastries, Fruit	1	Each	52	204	37	2	5	1	2
19383	Toffee	1	Piece	12	65	8	0	4	2	1
16126	Tofu, Fresh, Firm	1	Ounce	28.4	41	1	4	2	0	1
16127	Tofu, Fresh, Regular	1	Ounce	28.4	22	1	2	1	0	0
16129	Tofu, Fried	1	Ounce	28.4	77	3	5	6	1	1
16429	Tofu, Fried, Prepared w/ Calcium Sulfate	1	Ounce	28.4	77	3	5	6	1	1
16130	Tofu, Okara	1	Ounce	28.4	22	4	1	0	0	0
16132	Tofu, Salted and Fermented (fuyu)	1	Ounce	28.4	33	1	2	2	0	1
14023	Tom Collins	1	Fl Oz	29.6	16	0	0	0	0	0
11954	Tomatillos, Fresh	1	Medium	34	11	2	0	0	-	-
41284	Tomato Garden Soup-Healthy Choice	1	Each	212.6	130	22	4	3	1	-
11540	Tomato Juice, Cnd, w/ Salt	¾	Cup	183	31	8	1	0	0	0
11886	Tomato Juice, Cnd, w/o Salt	¾	Cup	183	31	8	1	0	0	0
11530	Tomatoes, Ckd, Boiled	½	Cup	120	32	7	1	0	0	0
11660	Tomatoes, Ckd, Stewed	½	Cup	50.5	40	7	1	1	0	1
11533	Tomatoes, Cnd, Stewed	½	Cup	127.5	33	8	1	0	0	0
11537	Tomatoes, Cnd, w/ Green Chilies	½	Cup	120.5	18	4	1	0	0	0
11535	Tomatoes, Cnd, Wedges In Tomato Juice	½	Cup	130.5	34	8	1	0	0	0
11531	Tomatoes, Cnd, Whole, Reg Pk	½	Cup	120	24	5	1	0	0	0
11529	Tomatoes, Fresh	1	Medium	123	26	6	1	0	0	0
11527	Tomatoes, Green, Fresh	1	Medium	123	30	6	1	0	0	0
11955	Tomatoes, Sun-dried	¼	Cup	13.5	35	8	2	0	0	0
11956	Tomatoes, Sun-dried, Packed In Oil	¼	Cup	27.5	59	6	1	4	1	2
14155	Tonic Water	12	Fl Oz	366	124	32	0	0	0	0
19364	Toppings, Butterscotch or Caramel	1	Tbsp.	20.5	52	14	0	0	0	0
62550	Toppings, Caramel	1	Tbsp.	16.7	52	13	0	-	-	-
62549	Toppings, Hot Fudge	1	Tbsp.	19	70	11	1	2	1	-
19365	Toppings, Marshmallow Cream	1	Tbsp.	20.5	64	16	0	0	-	-

Polyunsaturated Fat (gm)	Fiber (gm)	Cholesterol (mg)	Folate (µg)	Vitamin A (re)	Vitamin B6 (mg)	Vitamin B12 (µg)	Vitamin C (mg)	Vitamin E (mg)	Riboflavin (mg)	Thiamin (mg)	Calcium (mg)	Iron (mg)	Magnesium (mg)	Niacin (mg)	Phosphorus (mg)	Potassium (mg)	Sodium (mg)	Zinc (mg)
1	0	3	1	5	0	0.1	0	-	0	0	21	0.3	10	0	36	45	27	0.2
-	0	0	0	0	0	0	0	-	0	0	4	0.1	2	0	2	9	31	0
-	0	0	0	0	0	0	0	-	0	0	0	0	0	0	0	0	0	0
-	-	0	0	0	0	0	0	-	0	0	1	0	0	0	0	1	24	0
-	-	0	3	0	0.1	0	0	-	0.1	0	15	0.2	17	1.9	57	77	8	0
-	0	0	0	0	0	0	0	-	0	0	13	0.2	3	0	0	41	2	0.8
-	0	0	0	0	0	0	0	-	0	0	0	0	0	0	9	1	40	0
-	0	0	0	0	0	0	0	-	0	0	1	0	0	0	2	1	12	0
0	-	1	0	3	0	0	0	-	0	0	0	0	0	0	2	1	20	0
1	1	0	1	5	0	0	0	-	0	0	21	0.3	14	0.2	32	23	48	0.2
1	-	0	1	-	-	0	0	-	0	0	21	0.3	14	0.2	32	23	2	0.2
-	-	0	-	-	-	-	-	-	0.1	0.1	-	0.1	-	0.5	-	-	4	-
0	-	1	0	5	0	0	0	-	0	0	0	0	0	0	0	1	13	0
0	0	0	9	78	0.1	0	41	-	0	0.1	34	0.4	15	0.2	26	332	2	0.1
0	0	0	9	78	0.1	0	57	-	0	0.1	33	0.4	15	0.2	26	330	2	0.1
0	1	0	6	106	0.1	0	43	-	0	0.1	14	0.3	14	0.6	12	166	6	0.6
0	1	0	6	106	0.1	0	25	-	0.1	0.1	9	0.5	10	0.6	13	98	8	0.3
0	2	0	17	77	0.1	0	26	-	0	0.1	12	0.1	10	0.1	8	132	1	0.2
4	0	3	12	0	0.3	0.3	2	-	0.3	0.1	250	0.7	24	0.9	236	310	352	0.8
4	2	0	6	0	0.1	0	1	-	0	0	17	0.3	24	0.1	37	214	97	0.1
0	0	0	12	0	0	0	0	-	0	0	0	0	7	0	2	88	7	0
0	0	0	1	0	0	0	0	-	0	0	5	0.2	2	0	0	21	2	0.1
0	-	0	10	0	0	0	0	-	0	0	5	0.1	5	0.1	3	49	8	0.1
0	0	0	1	0	0	0	0	-	0	0	5	0	5	0.1	2	47	7	0.1
1	-	60	-	400	-	-	2	-	0.4	0.8	16	1.5	42	5.7	-	933	880	4.5
0	-	0	3	3	0	0	6	-	0	0	2	0.1	2	0.1	3	32	1	0
2	-	55	-	20	-	-	6	-	0.1	0.1	32	0.8	-	7.6	250	520	560	-
0	0	0	4	0	0	0	0	-	0	0	5	0.3	11	0.2	28	41	690	0
-	-	20	-	-	-	-	6	-	0	0	1202	0.4	-	0.6	-	891	861	-
0	1	7	0	16	0	0.1	0	-	0.1	0	50	0.4	17	0.1	55	80	116	0.3
0	0	0	0	0	0	-	0	-	0	0	0	0.2	4	0	33	40	144	0.1
1	-	0	42	116	0.2	0.1	0	-	0.3	0.2	18	2.1	12	2.4	69	59	220	0.3
2	-	0	42	55	0.2	0	0	-	0.2	0.2	14	1.8	9	2	58	58	218	0.3
0	-	13	0	38	0	0	0	-	0	0	4	0	0	0	4	6	22	0
1	1	0	8	5	0	0	0	-	0	0	58	3	27	0.1	54	67	4	0.4
1	0	0	4	3	0	0	0	-	0	0	30	1.5	29	0.1	27	34	2	0.2
3	1	0	8	0	0	0	0	-	0	0	105	1.4	17	0	81	41	5	0.6
3	-	0	8	0	0	0	0	-	0	0	272	1.4	27	0	81	41	5	0.6
0	-	0	7	0	0	0	0	-	0	0	23	0.4	7	0	17	60	3	0.2
1	-	0	8	5	0	0	0	-	0	0	13	0.6	15	0.1	21	21	814	0.4
0	-	0	0	0	0	0	1	-	0	0	1	0	0	0	0	2	5	0
-	1	0	2	4	0	0	4	-	0	0	2	0.2	7	0.6	13	91	0	0.1
-	-	5	-	100	-	-	6	-	0.1	0.1	32	0.4	-	1.1	70	440	510	-
0	1	0	36	102	0.2	0	33	-	0.1	0.1	16	1.1	20	1.2	35	403	661	0.3
0	1	0	36	102	0.2	0	33	-	0.1	0.1	16	1.1	20	1.2	35	403	18	0.3
0	1	0	16	89	0.1	0	27	-	0.1	0.1	7	0.7	17	0.9	37	335	13	0.1
0	1	0	6	34	0	0	9	-	0	0.1	13	0.5	8	0.6	19	125	230	0.1
0	-	0	7	70	0	0	17	-	0	0.1	42	0.9	15	0.9	26	305	324	0.2
0	-	0	11	47	0.1	0	7	-	0	0	24	0.3	13	0.8	17	129	483	0.2
0	-	0	13	76	0.2	0	19	-	0	0.1	34	0.6	14	0.9	30	328	283	0.2
0	1	0	9	72	0.1	0	18	-	0	0.1	31	0.7	14	0.9	23	265	196	0.2
0	1	0	18	76	0.1	0	23	0.4	0.1	0.1	6	0.6	14	0.8	30	273	11	0.1
0	2	0	11	79	0.1	0	29	-	0	0.1	16	0.6	12	0.6	34	251	16	0.1
0	2	0	9	12	0	0	5	-	0.1	0.1	15	1.2	26	1.2	48	463	283	0.3
1	-	0	6	35	0.1	0	28	-	0.1	0.1	13	0.7	22	1	38	430	73	0.2
0	0	0	0	0	0	0	0	-	0	0	4	0	0	0	0	0	15	0.4
0	-	0	6	0	0	0	0	-	0	0	11	0	1	0	10	17	72	0
-	-	-	-	-	-	-	0	-	0	0	9341	-	-	-	5	6	11	0
-	-	0	0	-	-	-	0	-	-	-	36	0.2	-	-	-	-	35	-
-	-	0	0	0	0	0	0	-	0	0	1	0	0	0	2	1	9	0

Code	Food Name	Amount	Unit	Grams	kCalories	Carbohydrate (gm)	Protein (gm)	Fat (gm)	Saturated Fat (gm)	Monounsaturated Fat (gm)
19367	Toppings, Nuts in Syrup	1	Tbsp.	20.5	84	11	1	5	0	1
19366	Toppings, Pineapple	1	Tbsp.	21.3	54	14	0	0	-	-
19137	Toppings, Strawberry	1	Tbsp.	21.3	54	14	0	0	-	-
62538	Tortellini, Beef	1	Cup	257.9	230	46	5	1	0	-
55160	Tortellini-Cheese in Alfredo Sauce-Stouffer's	1	Each	251.6	580	35	26	37	-	-
55161	Tortellini-Cheese w/ Tomato Sauce-Stouffer's	1	Each	262.2	360	39	18	15	-	-
19057	Tortilla Chips, Nacho-flavor	1	Ounce	28.4	141	18	2	7	1	4
19424	Tortilla Chips, Nacho-flavor, Light	1	Ounce	28.4	126	20	2	4	1	3
19056	Tortilla Chips, Plain	1	Ounce	28.4	142	18	2	7	1	4
19058	Tortilla Chips, Ranch-flavor	1	Ounce	28.4	139	18	2	7	1	4
19063	Tortilla Chips, Taco-flavor	1	Ounce	28.4	136	18	2	7	1	4
18363	Tortillas, Corn	1	Medium	25	56	12	1	1	0	0
18449	Tortillas, Corn, w/o Added Salt	1	Medium	25	56	12	1	1	0	0
18364	Tortillas, Flour	1	Medium	35	114	19	3	2	0	1
18450	Tortillas, Flour, w/o Added Salt	1	Medium	35	114	19	3	2	0	1
19059	Trail Mix, Regular	1	Cup	150	693	67	21	44	8	19
19821	Trail Mix, Regular, Unsalted	1	Cup	150	693	67	21	44	8	19
19062	Trail Mix, Regular, w/ Chocolate Chips	1	Cup	146	707	66	21	47	9	20
19061	Trail Mix, Tropical	1	Cup	140	570	92	9	24	12	3
14269	Tropical Fruit Juice, Blend	¾	Cup	185.2	85	22	0	0	0	0
15219	Trout, Ckd, Dry Heat	3	Ounce	85.1	162	0	23	7	1	4
15241	Trout, Rainbow, Farmed, Ckd, Dry Heat	3	Ounce	85.1	144	0	21	6	2	2
15116	Trout, Rainbow, Wild, Ckd, Dry Heat	3	Ounce	85.1	128	0	19	5	1	1
19138	Truffles	1	Piece	12	59	5	1	4	3	1
55162	Tuna Noodle Casserole-Stouffer's	1	Each	283.5	280	33	17	15	-	-
15128	Tuna Salad	3	Ounce	85.1	159	8	14	8	1	2
15183	Tuna, Light Meat, Cnd In Oil	3	Ounce	85.1	168	0	25	7	1	3
15184	Tuna, Light Meat, Cnd In Water	3	Ounce	85.1	111	0	25	0	0	0
15121	Tuna, Light, Cnd In Water	3	Ounce	85.1	99	0	22	1	0	0
15220	Tuna, Skipjack, Ckd, Dry Heat	3	Ounce	85.1	112	0	24	1	0	0
15185	Tuna, White Meat, Cnd In Oil	3	Ounce	85.1	158	0	23	7	1	2
15186	Tuna, White Meat, Cnd In Water	3	Ounce	85.1	116	0	23	2	1	1
15221	Tuna, Yellowfin, Ckd, Dry Heat	3	Ounce	85.1	118	0	25	1	0	0
55814	Turkey and Gravy-Stouffer's	1	Each	255	78	2	12	2	-	-
5297	Turkey Bologna	1	Slice	21	42	0	3	3	1	1
7079	Turkey Breast Meat	1	Slice	21	23	0	5	0	0	0
55232	Turkey Dijon, Lean Cuisine-Stouffer's	1	Each	269.3	210	20	20	6	2	-
55791	Turkey Dijonnaise-Stouffer's	1	Each	260	113	7	8	5	-	-
5287	Turkey Lunch Meat	1	Slice	28.4	36	0	5	1	0	0
5289	Turkey Pastrami	1	Slice	28.4	40	0	5	2	1	1
5292	Turkey Patties, Breaded, Battered, Fried	3	Ounce	85.1	241	13	12	15	4	6
55163	Turkey Pie-Stouffer's	1	Each	283.5	410	33	16	24	-	-
57809	Turkey Pot Pie-Swanson	1	Each	198	191	18	6	11	-	-
5296	Turkey Roast, Roasted	3	Ounce	85.1	132	3	18	5	2	1
5291	Turkey Roll, Light and Dark Meat	3	Ounce	85.1	127	2	15	6	2	2
5290	Turkey Roll, Light Meat	3	Ounce	85.1	125	0	16	6	2	2
5299	Turkey Salami	1	Slice	28.4	56	0	5	4	1	1
41243	Turkey Sausage Omelet on English Muffin-Healthy Choice	1	Each	134.7	210	30	16	4	2	-
5300	Turkey Sticks, Breaded, Battered, Fried	3	Ounce	85.1	237	14	12	14	4	6
41268	Turkey Tetrazzini-Healthy Choice	1	Each	357.9	340	49	23	6	3	-
55164	Turkey Tetrazzini-Stouffer's	1	Each	283.5	400	26	22	23	-	-
5294	Turkey Thigh, Prebasted, Meat&skin, Ckd, Roasted	3	Ounce	85.1	134	0	16	7	2	2
41275	Turkey Vegetable Soup-Healthy Choice	1	Each	212.6	110	17	4	3	1	-
5190	Turkey, Back, Meat&skin, Ckd, Roasted	3	Ounce	85.1	207	0	23	12	4	4
5192	Turkey, Breast, Meat&skin, Ckd, Roasted	3	Ounce	85.1	161	0	24	6	2	2
5164	Turkey, Ckd, Roasted, Meat&skin&giblets&neck	3	Ounce	85.1	174	0	24	8	2	3
5188	Turkey, Dark Meat, Ckd, Roasted	3	Ounce	85.1	159	0	24	6	2	1
5184	Turkey, Dark Meat, Meat&skin, Ckd, Roasted	3	Ounce	85.1	188	0	23	10	3	3
5172	Turkey, Giblets, Ckd, Simmered, Some Giblet Fat	3	Ounce	85.1	142	2	23	4	1	1
5306	Turkey, Ground, Ckd	3	Ounce	85.1	200	0	23	11	3	4

Polyunsaturated Fat (gm)	Fiber (gm)	Cholesterol (mg)	Folate (µg)	Vitamin A (re)	Vitamin B6 (mg)	Vitamin B12 (µg)	Vitamin C (mg)	Vitamin E (mg)	Riboflavin (mg)	Thiamin (mg)	Calcium (mg)	Iron (mg)	Magnesium (mg)	Niacin (mg)	Phosphorus (mg)	Potassium (mg)	Sodium (mg)	Zinc (mg)
3	0	0	4	1	0	0	0	-	0	0	8	0.2	13	0.1	23	43	9	0.2
-	0	0	1	0	0	0	12	-	0	0	5	0.1	0	0	2	67	13	0.1
-	0	0	0	0	0	0	5	-	0	0	5	0.2	1	0.1	3	16	4	0.1
-	9	15	-	150	-	-	4	-	-	-	96	1.5	-	-	-	-	770	-
-	-	-	-	40	-	-	4	-	0.5	0.3	320	0.8	-	1.9	-	270	830	-
-	-	-	-	150	-	-	6	-	0.3	0.2	240	1	-	1.9	-	420	720	-
1	2	1	4	12	0.1	0	1	-	0.1	0	42	0.4	23	0.4	69	61	201	0.3
1	-	1	7	12	0.1	0	0	-	0.1	0.1	45	0.5	27	0.1	90	77	284	-
1	2	0	3	6	0.1	0	0	-	0.1	0	44	0.4	25	0.4	58	56	150	0.4
1	-	0	5	8	0.1	0	0	-	0.1	0	40	0.4	25	0.4	68	69	174	0.4
1	-	1	6	26	0.1	0	0	-	0.1	0.1	44	0.6	25	0.6	68	62	223	0.4
0	1	0	4	6	0.1	0	0	-	0	0	44	0.4	16	0.4	79	39	40	0.2
0	-	0	4	-	0.1	0	0	-	0	0	44	0.4	16	0.4	79	39	3	0.2
1	1	0	4	0	0	0	0	-	0.1	0.2	44	1.2	9	1.3	43	46	167	0.2
1	-	0	4	0	0	0	0	-	0.1	0.2	14	1.2	9	1.3	43	46	167	0.2
14	-	0	107	3	0.4	0	2	-	0.3	0.7	117	4.6	237	7.1	518	1028	344	4.8
14	-	0	107	3	0.4	0	2	-	0.3	0.7	117	4.6	237	7.1	518	1028	15	4.8
16	6	95	7		0.4	0	2	-	0.3	0.6	159	4.9	235	6.4	565	946	177	4.6
7	-	0	59	7	0.5	0	11	-	0.2	0.6	80	3.7	134	2.1	260	993	14	1.6
0	-	0	2	2	0	0	81	-	0	0	7	0.2	4	0	2	24	7	0.1
2	0	63	13	16	0.2	6.4	0	-	0.4	0.4	47	1.6	24	4.9	267	394	57	0.7
2	0	58	20	73	0.3	4.2	3	-	0.1	0.2	-	0.3	27	7.5	226	375	36	0.4
2	0	59	16	13	0.3	5.4	2	-	0.1	0.1	-	0.3	26	4.9	229	381	48	0.4
0	-	6	0	17	0	0	0	-	0	0	19	0.1	6	0	21	37	9	0.1
-	-	-	-	20	-	-		-	0.3	0.2	120	0.6	-	3.8	-	380	1090	-
4	0	11	6	23	0.1	1	2	-	0.1	0	14	0.9	16	5.7	151	151	342	0.5
2	0	15	5	20	0.1	1.9	0	-	0.1	0	11	1.2	26	10.5	265	176	43	0.8
0	0	15	4	20	0.3	1.9	0	-	0.1	0	10	2.7	25	10.5	158	267	43	0.4
0	0	26	3	14	0.3	2.5	0	-	0.1	0	9	1.3	23	11.3	139	202	207	0.7
0	0	51	9	15	0.8	1.9	1	-	0.1	0	31	1.4	37	16	242	444	40	0.9
3	0	26	4	20	0.4	1.9	0	-	0.1	0	3	0.6	29	9.9	227	283	43	0.4
1	0	36	3	20	0.4	1.9	0	-	0	0	3	0.5	29	4.9	227	241	43	0.4
0	0	49	2	17	0.9	0.5	1	-	0	0.4	18	0.8	54	10.2	208	484	40	0.6
-	-	23	-	-	-	-	0	-	0	0	85	0	-	0.9	-	406	296	-
1	0	21	1	0	0	0.1	0	-	0	0	18	0.3	3	0.7	28	42	184	0.4
0	0	9	1	0	0.1	0.4	0	-	0	0	1	0.1	4	1.7	48	58	301	0.2
-	-	45	-	400	-	-	2	-	0.3	0.2	120	0.4	-	4.8	-	640	590	-
-	-	28	-	-	-	-	1	-	0	0	480	0.1	-	0.3	-	176	356	-
0	0	16	2	0	0.1	0.1	0	-	0.1	0	3	0.8	5	1	54	92	282	0.8
0	0	15	1	0	0.1	0.1	0	-	0.1	0	3	0.5	4	1	57	74	296	0.6
4	0	53	7	9	0.2	0.2	0	-	0.2	0.1	12	1.9	13	2	230	234	680	1.2
-	-	-	-	250	-	-	-	-	0.4	0.3	80	1	-	3.8	-	290	750	-
-	-	-	-	176	-	-	-	-	0.1	0.1	8	0.5	-	1.4	-	-	363	-
1	0	45	4	0	0.2	1.3	-	-	0.1	0	4	1.4	19	5.3	208	253	578	2.2
2	0	47	4	0	0.2	0.2	0	-	0.2	0.1	27	1.1	15	4.1	143	230	498	1.7
1	0	37	3	0	0.3	0.2	0	-	0.2	0.1	34	1.1	14	6	156	213	416	1.3
1	0	23	1	0	0.1	0.1	0	-	0	0	6	0.5	4	1	30	69	285	0.5
1	-	20	-	60	-	-	-	-	0.5	0.4	160	2	-	2.9	250	590	470	-
4	-	54	8	10	0.2	0.2	0	-	0.2	0.1	12	1.9	13	1.8	199	221	713	1.2
2	-	40	-	-	-	-	72	-	0.3	0.2	80	1	-	3.8	250	510	490	-
-	-	-	-	20	-	-	-	-	0.4	0.2	80	0.8	-	2.9	-	300	960	-
2	0	53	5	0	0.2	0.2	0	-	0.2	0.1	7	1.3	14	2	145	205	372	3.5
1	-	15	-	150	-	-	5	-	0	0	16	0.2	-	0.4	-	140	540	-
3	0	77	7	0	0.3	0.3	0	-	0.2	0	28	1.9	19	2.9	161	221	62	3.3
2	0	63	5	0	0.4	0.3	0	-	0.1	0	18	1.2	23	5.4	179	245	54	1.7
2	0	81	17	58	0.3	1.1	0	-	0.2	0	22	1.7	20	4.2	170	231	57	2.7
2	0	72	8	0	0.3	0.3	0	-	0.2	0	27	2	20	3.1	174	247	67	3.8
3	0	76	8	0	0.3	0.3	0	-	0.2	0	28	1.9	20	3	167	233	65	3.5
1	0	356	293	1527	0.3	20.4	1	-	0.8	0	11	5.7	14	3.8	174	170	50	3.1
3	0	87	6	0	0.3	0.3	0	-	0.1	0	21	1.6	20	4.1	167	230	91	2.4

Code	Food Name	Amount	Unit	Grams	kCalories	Carbohydrate (gm)	Protein (gm)	Fat (gm)	Saturated Fat (gm)	Monounsaturated Fat (gm)
5194	Turkey, Leg, Meat&skin, Ckd, Roasted	3	Ounce	85.1	177	0	24	8	3	2
5186	Turkey, Light Meat, Ckd, Roasted	3	Ounce	85.1	134	0	25	3	1	0
5182	Turkey, Light Meat, Meat&skin, Ckd, Roasted	3	Ounce	85.1	168	0	24	7	2	2
5168	Turkey, Meat Only, Ckd, Roasted	3	Ounce	85.1	145	0	25	4	1	1
5166	Turkey, Meat&skin, Ckd, Roasted	3	Ounce	85.1	177	0	24	8	2	3
5288	Turkey, Thin Sliced	3	Ounce	85.1	94	0	19	1	0	0
5196	Turkey, Wing, Meat&skin, Ckd, Roasted	3	Ounce	85.1	195	0	23	11	3	4
11565	Turnips, Ckd	½	Cup	78	14	4	1	0	0	0
11564	Turnips, Fresh	½	Cup	65	18	4	1	0	0	0
19160	Twix	1	Each	57	272	37	3	13	-	-
19112	Twizzlers Strawberry Candy	1	Pkg	71	263	66	2	1	0	0
18328	Vanilla Cream Pie	1	Slice	126	350	41	6	18	5	8
19201	Vanilla Pudding	1	Cup	298.1	388	65	7	11	2	5
18210	Vanilla Sandwich Cookies w/ Creme Filling	1	Each	10	48	7	0	2	0	1
18213	Vanilla Wafers, Higher Fat	1	Each	6	28	4	0	1	0	1
18212	Vanilla Wafers, Lower Fat	1	Each	4	18	3	0	1	0	0
17089	Veal, Meat and Fat, Ckd	3	Ounce	85.1	196	0	26	10	4	4
17091	Veal, Meat Only, Ckd	3	Ounce	85.1	167	0	27	6	2	2
41285	Vegetable Beef Soup-Healthy Choice	1	Each	212.6	130	21	8	1	-	-
55759	Vegetable Beef w/ Barley Soup-Stouffer's	1	Cup	283.9	190	15	4	13	-	-
55797	Vegetable Chow Mein-Stouffer's	1	Ounce	28.4	14	2	0	1	-	-
11578	Vegetable Juice Cnd	¾	Cup	181.5	34	8	1	0	0	0
55166	Vegetable Lasagna-Stouffer's	1	Each	274	400	33	23	20	-	-
41343	Vegetable Pasta Italiano-Healthy Choice	1	Each	283.5	220	46	7	1	-	-
11581	Vegetables, Mixed, Cnd	½	Cup	81.5	38	8	2	0	0	0
11584	Vegetables, Mixed, Frz	½	Cup	91	54	12	3	0	0	0
55758	Vegetarian Vegetable Soup-Stouffer's	1	Cup	283.9	120	20	6	2	-	-
55828	Veloute Sauce Supreme-Stouffer's	1	Cup	307.6	564	21	9	50	-	-
62629	Vitamin Supplement, Centrum	1	Each	1	-	-	-	-	-	-
62628	Vitamin Supplement, One-A-Day	1	Each	1	-	-	-	-	-	-
62630	Vitamin Supplement, StressTab	1	Each	1	-	-	-	-	-	-
18392	Waffles, Buttermilk	1	Each	75	217	25	6	10	2	3
18367	Waffles, Plain	1	Each	75	218	25	6	11	2	3
18403	Waffles, Plain, Frozen, Toasted	1	Each	33	87	13	2	3	0	1
12154	Walnuts, Black, Dried	½	Cup	62.5	379	8	15	35	2	8
12155	Walnuts, English or Persian, Dried	½	Cup	60	385	11	9	37	3	9
55167	Welsh Rarebit-Stouffer's	1	Each	141.8	270	9	13	20	-	-
41244	Western Style Omelet on English Muffin-Healthy Choice	1	Each	134.7	200	29	16	3	2	-
55826	Whipped Sweet Potatoes-Stouffer's	½	Cup	142	205	30	2	9	-	-
14032	Whiskey Sour	1	Fl Oz	29.9	41	2	0	0	0	0
15223	Whitefish, Ckd, Dry Heat	3	Ounce	85.1	146	0	21	6	1	2
15131	Whitefish, Smoked	3	Ounce	85.1	92	0	20	1	0	0
20089	Wild Rice, Ckd	½	Cup	82	83	17	3	0	0	0
14536	Wine, Dessert, Dry	3	Fl Oz	90	113	4	0	0	0	0
14057	Wine, Dessert, Sweet	3	Fl Oz	90	138	11	0	0	0	0
14084	Wine, Table, All	3	Fl Oz	88.5	62	1	0	0	0	0
14096	Wine, Table, Red	3	Fl Oz	88.5	64	2	0	0	0	0
14104	Wine, Table, Rose	3	Fl Oz	88.5	63	1	0	0	0	0
14106	Wine, Table, White	3	Fl Oz	88.5	60	1	0	0	0	0
11602	Yam, Baked	½	Cup	68	79	19	1	0	0	0
41269	Yankee Pot Roast-Healthy Choice	1	Each	311.8	260	36	19	4	2	-
15225	Yellowtail, Ckd, Dry Heat	3	Ounce	85.1	159	0	25	6	-	-
15135	Yellowtail, Fresh	3	Ounce	85.1	124	0	20	4	1	2
62552	Yogurt, Frozen, Fat Free	½	Cup	67	100	22	4	0	0	-
62604	Yogurt, Fruit, Fat Free	1	Cup	248	233	48	10	0	0	0
62627	Yogurt, Fruit, Fat Free, Light	1	Cup	248	110	19	10	0	0	0
1121	Yogurt, Fruit, Lowfat, 10 Gm Protein Per 8 Oz	1	Cup	227	231	43	10	2	2	1
1122	Yogurt, Fruit, Lowfat, 11 Gm Protein Per 8 Oz	1	Cup	227	239	42	11	3	2	1
1120	Yogurt, Fruit, Lowfat, 9 Gm Protein Per 8 Oz	1	Cup	227	225	42	9	3	2	1
62603	Yogurt, Plain, Fat Free	1	Cup	248	120	17	13	0	0	0

Polyunsaturated Fat (gm)	Fiber (gm)	Cholesterol (mg)	Folate (µg)	Vitamin A (re)	Vitamin B6 (mg)	Vitamin B12 (µg)	Vitamin C (mg)	Vitamin E (mg)	Riboflavin (mg)	Thiamin (mg)	Calcium (mg)	Iron (mg)	Magnesium (mg)	Niacin (mg)	Phosphorus (mg)	Potassium (mg)	Sodium (mg)	Zinc (mg)
2	0	72	8	0	0.3	0.3	0	-	0.2	0.1	27	2	20	3	169	238	65	3.6
1	0	59	5	0	0.5	0.3	0	-	0.1	0.1	16	1.1	24	5.8	186	259	54	1.7
2	0	65	5	0	0.4	0.3	0	-	0.1	0	18	1.2	22	5.3	177	242	54	1.7
1	0	65	6	0	0.4	0.3	0	-	0.2	0.1	21	1.5	22	4.6	181	253	60	2.6
2	0	70	6	0	0.3	0.3	0	-	0.2	0	22	1.5	21	4.3	173	238	58	2.5
0	0	35	3	0	0.3	1.7	0	-	0.1	0	6	0.3	17	7.1	195	236	1217	1
3	0	69	5	0	0.4	0.3	0	-	0.1	0	20	1.2	21	4.9	168	226	52	1.8
0	2	0	7	0	0.1	0	9	-	0	0	17	0.2	6	0.2	15	105	39	0.2
0	1	0	9	0	0.1	0	14	-	0	0	20	0.2	7	0.3	18	124	44	0.2
-	1	5	4	18	0	0.2	0	-	0.1	0	67	0.4	17	0.2	76	117	115	0.4
-	-	0	0	0	0	0	0	-	0	0	25	0.4	4	0.1	220	45	197	0.1
4	-	78	14	107	0.1	0.4	1	-	0.3	0.2	113	1.3	16	1.2	131	159	328	0.7
4	0	21	0	18	0	0.3	0	-	0.4	0.1	262	0.4	24	0.8	203	337	402	0.7
0	0	0	0	0	-	0	0	-	0	0	3	0.2	1	0.3	8	9	35	0
0	-	0	0	0	0	0	0	-	0	0	2	0.1	1	0.2	4	6	18	0
0	-	2	0	1	0	0	0	-	0	0	2	0.1	1	0.1	4	4	12	0
1	0	97	13	0	0.3	1.3	0	0.3	0.3	0.1	19	1	22	6.8	203	276	74	4
1	0	100	14	0	0.3	1.4	0	0.4	0.3	0.1	20	1	24	7.2	213	287	76	4.3
-	-	15	-	150	-	-	15	-	0.1	0.1	32	0.4	-	1.9	120	360	530	-
-	-	10	-	-	-	-	0	-	0	0	240	0.1	-	0.2	-	341	1252	-
-	-	0	-	-	-	-	1	-	0	0	24	0	-	0	-	26	156	-
0	1	0	38	212	0.3	0	50	-	0.1	0.1	20	0.8	20	1.3	31	350	662	0.4
-	-	-	-	250	-	-	-	-	0.4	0.1	160	0.6	-	0.8	-	350	760	-
-	-	0	-	250	-	-	0	-	0.3	0.5	32	2.5	-	1.5	-	380	330	-
0	-	0	19	949	0.1	0	4	-	0	0	22	0.9	13	0.5	34	237	121	0.3
0	5	0	17	389	0.1	0	3	-	0.1	0.1	23	0.7	20	0.8	46	154	32	0.4
-	-	0	-	-	-	-	0	-	0	0	401	0.1	-	0.2	-	401	911	-
-	-	98	-	-	-	-	0	-	0	0	2257	0	-	0	-	369	1410	-
-	-	-	400	1000	2	6	60	10	1.7	1.5	162	18	100	20	109	40	-	15
-	-	-	400	1000	2	6	60	10	1.7	1.5	-	-	-	20	-	-	-	-
-	-	-	400	-	5	12	500	10	-	10		18	-	100	-	-		
5	-	50	11	26	0	0.2	0	-	0.3	0.2	137	1.6	14	1.5	124	128	451	0.6
5	-	52	11	49	0	0.2	0	-	0.3	0.2	191	1.7	14	1.6	143	119	383	0.5
1	-	8	12	120	0.3	0.8	0	-	0.2	0.1	77	1.5	7	1.5	139	42	260	0.2
23	3	0	41	19	0.3	0	2	-	0.1	0.1	36	1.9	126	0.4	290	328	1	2.1
23	3	0	40	7	0.3	0	2	-	0.1	0.2	56	1.5	101	0.6	190	301	6	1.6
-	-	-	-	40	-	-	-	-	0.3	0	280	0.2	-	-	-	140	460	-
-	-	15	-	100	-	-	4	-	0.5	0.5	160	2	-	1.9	240	220	480	-
-	-	30	-	-	-	-	0	-	0	0	240	0.1	-	0.1	-	200	556	-
0	-	2	0	0	0	0	4	-	0	0.1	2	0	1	0	2	16	3	0
2	0	65	14	33	0.3	0.8	0	-	0.1	0	28	0.4	36	3.3	294	345	55	1.1
0	0	28	6	48	0.3	2.8	0	-	0.1	0	15	0.4	20	2	112	360	867	0.4
0	1	0	21	0	0.1	0	0	-	0.1	0	2	0.5	26	1.1	67	83	2	1.1
0	0	0	0	0	0	0	0	-	0	0	7	0.2	8	0.2	8	83	8	0.1
0	0	0	0	0	0	0	0	-	0	0	7	0.2	8	0.2	8	83	8	0.1
0	0	0	1	0	0	0	0	-	0	0	7	0.4	9	0.1	12	79	7	0.1
0	-	0	2	0	0	0	0	-	0	0	7	0.4	12	0.1	12	99	4	0.1
0	-	0	1	0	0	0	0	-	0	0	7	0.3	9	0.1	13	88	4	0.1
0	-	0	0	0	0	0	0	-	0	0	8	0.3	9	0.1	12	71	4	0.1
0	3	0	11	0	0.2	0	8	-	0	0.1	10	0.4	12	0.4	33	456	5	0.1
-	-	55	-	100	-	-	9	-	0.2	0.2	32	1	-	1.5	150	350	400	-
-	0	60	3	26	0.2	1.1	2	-	0	0.1	25	0.5	32	7.4	171	458	43	0.6
1	0	47	3	25	0.1	1.1	2	-	0	0.1	20	0.4	26	5.8	134	357	33	0.4
-	-	0	-	20	-	-	0	-	-	-	96	0	-	-	-	-	70	-
0	0	7	-	0	-	-	0	-	-	-	438	0	-	-	-	423	153	-
0	0	5	-	0	-	-	15	-	-	-	420	0.2	-	-	-	510	160	-
0	0	10	21	25	0.1	1.1	1	-	0.4	0.1	345	0.2	33	0.2	271	442	133	1.7
0	0	12	24	34	0.1	1.2	2	-	0.4	0.1	383	0.2	37	0.2	301	491	147	1.9
0	0	10	19	27	0.1	1	1	-	0.4	0.1	314	0.1	30	0.2	247	402	121	1.5
0	0	5	-	0	-	-	4	-	0.2	-	480	0	-	-	-	600	170	-

Code	Food Name	Amount	Unit	Grams	kCalories	Carbohydrate (gm)	Protein (gm)	Fat (gm)	Saturated Fat (gm)	Monounsaturated Fat (gm)
1117	Yogurt, Plain, Lowfat, 12 Gm Protein Per 8 Oz	1	Cup	227	144	16	12	4	2	1
1118	Yogurt, Plain, Skim Milk, 13 Gm Protein Per 8 Oz	1	Cup	227	127	17	13	0	0	0
1116	Yogurt, Plain, Whole Milk, 8 Gm Protein Per 8 Oz	1	Cup	227	139	11	8	7	5	2
19393	Yogurt, Soft-serve, Chocolate	1	Cup	144.1	231	36	6	9	5	3
19293	Yogurt, Soft-serve, Vanilla	1	Cup	144.1	229	35	6	8	5	2
1119	Yogurt, Vanilla, Lowfat, 11 Gm Protein Per 8 Oz	1	Cup	227	194	31	11	3	2	1
19091	York Peppermint Pattie	1	Sm Patty	11	38	9	0	1	-	-
55233	Zucchini Lasagna, Lean Cuisine-Stouffer's	1	Each	311.8	260	34	17	6	2	-
41344	Zucchini Lasagna-Healthy Choice	1	Each	326	250	41	14	3	2	-

Restaurants, Including Fast Food (Quick Service)

Code	Food Name	Amount	Unit	Grams	kCalories	Carbohydrate (gm)	Protein (gm)	Fat (gm)	Saturated Fat (gm)	Monounsaturated Fat (gm)
32391	Arby's-Beef'N Cheddar Sandwich	1	Each	194	443	30	35	20	10	4
32433	Arby's-Boston Clam Chowder	1	Each	226.8	207	18	10	11	4	5
32400	Arby's-Chicken Breast Fillet Sandwich	1	Each	204	547	53	26	28	6	11
32434	Arby's-Cream of Broccoli Soup	1	Each	226.8	180	19	9	8	5	2
32413	Arby's-Curly Fries	1	Each	99.2	337	43	4	18	7	8
32405	Arby's-Fish Fillet Sandwich	1	Each	221	526	50	23	27	7	9
32411	Arby's-French Fries	1	Each	70.9	246	30	2	13	3	6
32406	Arby's-Ham'N Cheese Sandwich	1	Each	170.1	411	38	24	19	7	8
32390	Arby's-Regular Roast Beef	1	Each	155.9	388	38	25	16	4	8
32393	Arby's-Super Roast Beef	1	Each	241	516	51	26	23	9	8
32410	Arby's-Turkey Sub	1	Each	277	599	54	33	28	6	7
32438	Arby's-Wisconsin Cheese Soup	1	Each	226.8	287	19	9	19	8	8
34858	Burger King-Bacon Double Cheeseburger	1	Each	202	613	29	34	40	17	15
34856	Burger King-Cheeseburger	1	Each	134.7	360	35	18	16	-	-
34857	Burger King-Double Cheeseburger	1	Each	191.4	537	32	33	30	14	12
34855	Burger King-Hamburger	1	Each	122.9	310	35	16	12	-	-
34843	Burger King-Salad w/ 1000 Island	1	Each	176	145	9	2	12	-	-
34842	Burger King-Salad w/ Bleu Cheese	1	Each	176	184	7	3	16	-	-
34844	Burger King-Salad w/ French	1	Each	176	152	13	2	11	-	-
34845	Burger King-Salad w/ Golden Italian	1	Each	176	162	7	2	14	-	-
34841	Burger King-Salad w/ House Dressing	1	Each	176	159	8	3	13	-	-
34846	Burger King-Salad w/ Reduced-Calorie Italian	1	Each	176	42	7	2	1	-	-
34859	Burger King-Whopper	1	Each	283.5	684	54	28	39	18	15
37167	Dunkin' Donuts-Almond Croissant	1	Each	105	420	38	8	27	-	-
37160	Dunkin' Donuts-Apple 'n Spice Muffin	1	Each	100	300	52	6	8	-	-
37146	Dunkin' Donuts-Apple Filled w/ Cinnamon Sugar	1	Each	79	250	33	5	11	-	-
37159	Dunkin' Donuts-Banana Nut Muffin	1	Each	103	310	49	7	10	-	-
37147	Dunkin' Donuts-Bavarian Fillled /w Chocolate	1	Each	79	240	32	5	11	-	-
37149	Dunkin' Donuts-Blueberry Filled	1	Each	67	210	29	4	8	-	-
37156	Dunkin' Donuts-Blueberry Muffin	1	Each	101	280	46	6	8	-	-
37157	Dunkin' Donuts-Bran Muffin w/ Raisins	1	Each	104	310	51	6	9	-	-
37151	Dunkin' Donuts-Cake Ring, Plain	1	Each	62	270	25	4	17	-	-
37163	Dunkin' Donuts-Chocolate Chunk Cookie	1	Each	43	200	25	3	10	-	-
37164	Dunkin' Donuts-Chocolate Chunk Cookie w/ Nuts	1	Each	43	210	23	3	11	-	-
37168	Dunkin' Donuts-Chocolate Crossant	1	Each	94	440	38	7	29	-	-
37145	Dunkin' Donuts-Chocolate Frosted Yeast Ring	1	Each	55	200	25	4	10	-	-
37158	Dunkin' Donuts-Corn Muffin	1	Each	96	340	51	7	12	-	-
37161	Dunkin' Donuts-Cranberry Nut Muffin	1	Each	98	290	44	6	9	-	-
37166	Dunkin' Donuts-Croissant, Plain	1	Each	72	310	27	7	19	-	-
37153	Dunkin' Donuts-Glazed Buttermilk Ring	1	Each	74	290	37	4	14	-	-

Polyunsaturated Fat (gm)	Fiber (gm)	Cholesterol (mg)	Folate (μg)	Vitamin A (re)	Vitamin B6 (mg)	Vitamin B12 (μg)	Vitamin C (mg)	Vitamin E (mg)	Riboflavin (mg)	Thiamin (mg)	Calcium (mg)	Iron (mg)	Magnesium (mg)	Niacin (mg)	Phosphorus (mg)	Potassium (mg)	Sodium (mg)	Zinc (mg)
0	0	14	25	36	0.1	1.3	2	-	0.5	0.1	415	0.2	40	0.3	326	531	159	2
0	0	4	28	5	0.1	1.4	2	-	0.5	0.1	452	0.2	43	0.3	355	579	174	2.2
0	0	29	17	68	0.1	0.8	1	-	0.3	0.1	274	0.1	26	0.2	215	351	105	1.3
0	-	7	16	62	0.1	0.4	0	-	0.3	0.1	212	1.8	39	0.4	200	376	141	0.7
0	0	3	9	82	0.1	0.4	1	-	0.3	0.1	206	0.4	20	0.4	186	304	125	0.6
0	0	11	24	30	0.1	1.2	2	-	0.5	0.1	389	0.2	37	0.2	306	498	149	1.9
-	-	0	0	0	0	0	0	-	0	0	2	0.2	7	0.1	10	13	4	0.1
-	-	20	-	150	-	-	6	-	0.3	0.2	200	0.8	-	1.9	-	650	520	-
-	-	15	-	350	-	-	6	-	0.3	0.4	200	1.5	-	1.9	250	830	400	-

Polyunsaturated Fat (gm)	Fiber (gm)	Cholesterol (mg)	Folate (μg)	Vitamin A (re)	Vitamin B6 (mg)	Vitamin B12 (μg)	Vitamin C (mg)	Vitamin E (mg)	Riboflavin (mg)	Thiamin (mg)	Calcium (mg)	Iron (mg)	Magnesium (mg)	Niacin (mg)	Phosphorus (mg)	Potassium (mg)	Sodium (mg)	Zinc (mg)
4	1	85	45	64	0.4	2.3	1	0.4	0.5	0.4	202	5.6	44	6.5	442	380	1801	6
2	1	28	9	100	0.1	9.4	4	0.1	0.2	0.1	170	1.4	20	0.9	143	319	1157	0.7
11	2	101	35	17	0.7	0.4	0	2.9	0.4	0.5	123	3.9	51	16.4	322	366	1130	1.9
1	2	3	46	50	0.2	0.6	9	1.4	0.4	0.1	237	0.8	55	0.8	193	455	1113	0.7
2	-	0	-	-	-	-	-	-	0.1	0.1	16	0.8	-	1.9	-	724	167	-
11	-	44	-	-	-	-	1	-	0.3	0.3	72	2.1	-	5.3	-	450	872	-
5	-	0	-	-	-	-	4	-	-	0.1	-	0.6	-	1.9	-	240	114	-
2	1	68	83	112	0.2	0.6	3	1.3	0.6	0.4	151	3.8	19	3.1	177	338	899	1.6
2	1	58	45	71	0.3	1.4	2	0.2	0.3	0.4	61	4.7	35	6.6	268	354	888	3.8
6	2	41	42	0	0.5	4.4	0	0.4	0.6	0.6	118	6.6	60	9.7	414	518	822	11
8	-	82	-	-	-	-	-	-	0.4	0.5	94	3.2	-	9.4	-	-	1432	-
3	2	31	7	90	0.1	0	2	0.4	0.2	0	252	1.3	7	0.7	241	441	1129	1.1
6	1	115	32	74	0.4	3.4	8	1.6	0.4	0.3	162	4.1	39	8.4	386	480	833	6.6
-	-	-	-	-	-	-	-	-	-	-	-	-	-	-	-	-	705	-
2	2	111	34	111	0.3	2	7	2	0.3	0.2	210	3.3	34	5.5	339	383	947	4.5
-	-	-	-	-	-	-	-	-	-	-	-	-	-	-	-	-	560	-
-	-	17	-	-	-	-	26	-	0	0	336	0.1	98	0.2	528	405	251	0.1
-	-	22	-	-	-	-	25	-	0	0	528	0.1	102	0.2	664	382	333	0.1
-	-	0	-	-	-	-	26	-	0	0	320	0.1	98	0.2	480	410	330	0.1
-	-	0	-	-	-	-	25	-	0	0	320	0.1	98	0.2	480	389	292	0.1
-	-	11	-	-	-	-	25	-	0	0	352	0.1	95	0.2	592	402	293	0.1
-	-	0	-	-	-	-	25	-	0	0	320	0.1	105	0.2	472	390	430	0.1
2	3	113	34	209	0.3	3.1	14	4.2	0	0	113	6.5	54	5.6	339	565	1075	5.8
-	3	0	-	-	-	-	-	-	-	-	-	-	-	-	-	-	280	-
-	2	25	-	-	-	-	-	-	-	-	-	-	-	-	-	-	360	-
-	1	0	-	-	-	-	-	-	-	-	-	-	-	-	-	-	280	-
-	3	30	-	-	-	-	-	-	-	-	-	-	-	-	-	-	410	-
-	2	0	-	-	-	-	-	-	-	-	-	-	-	-	-	-	260	-
-	2	0	-	-	-	-	-	-	-	-	-	-	-	-	-	-	240	-
-	2	30	-	-	-	-	-	-	-	-	-	-	-	-	-	-	340	-
-	4	15	-	-	-	-	-	-	-	-	-	-	-	-	-	-	560	-
-	1	0	-	-	-	-	-	-	-	-	-	-	-	-	-	-	330	-
-	1	30	-	-	-	-	-	-	-	-	-	-	-	-	-	-	110	-
-	2	30	-	-	-	-	-	-	-	-	-	-	-	-	-	-	100	-
-	3	0	-	-	-	-	-	-	-	-	-	-	-	-	-	-	220	-
-	1	0	-	-	-	-	-	-	-	-	-	-	-	-	-	-	190	-
-	1	40	-	-	-	-	-	-	-	-	-	-	-	-	-	-	560	-
-	2	25	-	-	-	-	-	-	-	-	-	-	-	-	-	-	360	-
-	2	0	-	-	-	-	-	-	-	-	-	-	-	-	-	-	240	-
-	1	10	-	-	-	-	-	-	-	-	-	-	-	-	-	-	370	-

Code	Food Name	Amount	Unit	Grams	kCalories	Carbohydrate (gm)	Protein (gm)	Fat (gm)	Saturated Fat (gm)	Monounsaturated Fat (gm)
37152	Dunkin' Donuts-Glazed Chocolate Rings	1	Each	71	324	34	4	21	-	-
37144	Dunkin' Donuts-Glazed Coffee Roll	1	Each	81	280	37	5	12	-	-
37155	Dunkin' Donuts-Glazed French Cruller	1	Each	38	140	16	2	8	-	-
37143	Dunkin' Donuts-Glazed Yeast Ring	1	Each	55	200	26	4	9	-	-
37150	Dunkin' Donuts-Jelly Filled	1	Each	67	220	31	4	9	-	-
37148	Dunkin' Donuts-Lemon Filled	1	Each	79	260	33	4	12	-	-
37162	Dunkin' Donuts-Oat Bran Muffin	1	Each	100	330	50	7	11	-	-
37165	Dunkin' Donuts-Oatmeal Pecan Raisin Cookie	1	Each	46	200	28	3	9	-	-
21002	Fast Food-Biscuit w/ Egg	1	Each	136	316	24	11	20	6	8
21003	Fast Food-Biscuit w/ Egg and Bacon	1	Each	150	458	29	17	31	10	13
21004	Fast Food-Biscuit w/ Egg and Ham	1	Each	192	442	30	20	27	8	11
21005	Fast Food-Biscuit w/ Egg and Sausage	1	Each	180	581	41	19	39	15	16
21007	Fast Food-Biscuit w/ Egg, Cheese, and Bacon	1	Each	144	477	33	16	31	11	14
21008	Fast Food-Biscuit w/ Ham	1	Each	113	386	44	13	18	11	5
21009	Fast Food-Biscuit w/ Sausage	1	Each	124	485	40	12	32	14	13
21010	Fast Food-Biscuit w/ Steak	1	Each	141	455	44	13	26	7	11
21001	Fast Food-Biscuit, Plain	1	Each	74	276	34	4	13	9	3
21027	Fast Food-Brownie	1	Each	60	243	39	3	10	3	4
21060	Fast Food-Burrito w/ Beans	1	Each	108.5	224	36	7	7	3	2
21061	Fast Food-Burrito w/ Beans and Cheese	1	Each	93	189	27	8	6	3	1
21062	Fast Food-Burrito w/ Beans and Chili Peppers	1	Each	102	206	29	8	7	4	3
21063	Fast Food-Burrito w/ Beans and Meat	1	Each	115.5	254	33	11	9	4	4
21064	Fast Food-Burrito w/ Beans, Cheese, and Beef	1	Each	101.5	165	20	7	7	4	2
21065	Fast Food-Burrito w/ Beans, Cheese, and Chili Peppers	1	Each	167	329	42	17	11	6	4
21066	Fast Food-Burrito w/ Beef	1	Each	110	262	29	13	10	5	4
21067	Fast Food-Burrito w/ Beef and Chili Peppers	1	Each	100.5	213	25	11	8	4	3
21068	Fast Food-Burrito w/ Beef, Cheese, and Chili Peppers	1	Each	152	316	32	20	12	5	5
21069	Fast Food-Burrito w/ Fruit (Apple or Cherry)	1	Each	74	231	35	3	10	5	3
21100	Fast Food-Cheeseburger, Large, Double Patty	1	Each	258	704	40	38	44	18	17
21098	Fast Food-Cheeseburger, Large, Single Patty	1	Each	219	563	38	28	33	15	13
21097	Fast Food-Cheeseburger, Large, Single Patty w/ Bcn&cond	1	Each	195	608	37	32	37	16	14
21096	Fast Food-Cheeseburger, Large, Single Patty, Plain	1	Each	185	609	47	30	33	15	13
21095	Fast Food-Cheeseburger, Regular, Double Patty	1	Each	228	650	53	30	35	13	13
21091	Fast Food-Cheeseburger, Regular, Single Patty	1	Each	154	359	28	18	20	9	7
21089	Fast Food-Cheeseburger, Regular, Single Patty, Plain	1	Each	102	319	32	15	15	6	6
21101	Fast Food-Cheeseburger, Triple Patty, Plain	1	Each	304	796	27	56	51	22	22
21103	Fast Food-Chicken Fillet Sandwich w/ Cheese	1	Each	228	632	42	29	39	12	14
21102	Fast Food-Chicken Fillet Sandwich, Plain	1	Each	182	515	39	24	29	9	10
21037	Fast Food-Chicken Nuggets, Plain	1	Each	17	48	3	3	3	1	1
21038	Fast Food-Chicken Nuggets, w/ Barb. Sauce	1	Each	17	43	3	2	2	1	1
21039	Fast Food-Chicken Nuggets, w/ Honey	1	Each	17	49	4	2	3	1	1
21040	Fast Food-Chicken Nuggets, w/ Must. Sauce	1	Each	17	42	3	2	2	1	1
21041	Fast Food-Chicken Nuggets, w/ Sweet and Sour	1	Each	17	45	4	2	2	1	1
21042	Fast Food-Chili Con Carne	1	Cup	253	256	22	25	8	3	3
21070	Fast Food-Chimichanga, w/ Beef	1	Each	174	425	43	20	20	9	8
21071	Fast Food-Chimichanga, w/ Beef and Cheese	1	Each	183	443	39	20	23	11	9
21030	Fast Food-Chocolate Chip Cookies	1	Box	55	233	36	3	12	5	5
21043	Fast Food-Clams, Breaded and Fried	3	Ounce	85.1	333	29	9	20	5	8
21128	Fast Food-Corn On The Cob w/ Butter	1	Each	146	155	32	4	3	2	1
21045	Fast Food-Crab, Soft-shell, Fried	1	Each	125	334	31	11	18	4	8
21011	Fast Food-Croissant w/ Egg and Cheese	1	Each	127	368	24	13	25	14	8
21012	Fast Food-Croissant w/ Egg, Cheese, and Bacon	1	Each	129	413	24	16	28	15	9
21013	Fast Food-Croissant w/ Egg, Cheese, and Ham	1	Each	152	474	24	19	34	17	11
21014	Fast Food-Croissant w/ Egg, Cheese, and Sausage	1	Each	160	523	25	20	38	18	14
21015	Fast Food-Danish Pastry, Cheese	1	Each	91	353	29	6	25	5	16
21016	Fast Food-Danish Pastry, Cinnamon	1	Each	88	349	47	5	17	3	11
21017	Fast Food-Danish Pastry, Fruit	1	Each	94	335	45	5	16	3	10
21104	Fast Food-Egg and Cheese Sandwich	1	Each	146	340	26	16	19	7	8
21018	Fast Food-Egg, Scrambled	2	Eggs	94	199	2	13	15	6	6
21074	Fast Food-Enchilada w/ Cheese	1	Each	163	319	29	10	19	11	6

Polyunsaturated Fat (gm)	Fiber (gm)	Cholesterol (mg)	Folate (μg)	Vitamin A (re)	Vitamin B6 (mg)	Vitamin B12 (μg)	Vitamin C (mg)	Vitamin E (mg)	Riboflavin (mg)	Thiamin (mg)	Calcium (mg)	Iron (mg)	Magnesium (mg)	Niacin (mg)	Phosphorus (mg)	Potassium (mg)	Sodium (mg)	Zinc (mg)
-	2	0	-	-	-	-	-	-	-	-	-	-	-	-	-	-	383	-
-	2	0	-	-	-	-	-	-	-	-	-	-	-	-	-	-	310	-
-	0	30	-	-	-	-	-	-	-	-	-	-	-	-	-	-	130	-
-	1	0	-	-	-	-	-	-	-	-	-	-	-	-	-	-	230	-
-	1	0	-	-	-	-	-	-	-	-	-	-	-	-	-	-	230	-
-	1	0	-	-	-	-	-	-	-	-	-	-	-	-	-	-	280	-
-	3	0	-	-	-	-	-	-	-	-	-	-	-	-	-	-	450	-
-	1	25	-	-	-	-	-	-	-	-	-	-	-	-	-	-	100	-
4	-	233	30	178	0.1	0.7	0	-	0.3	0.3	154	3.1	20	0.7	185	160	654	1.1
6	-	353	30	53	0.1	1	3	-	0.2	0.1	189	3.7	24	2.4	239	251	999	1.6
5	-	300	33	240	0.3	1.2	0	-	0.6	0.7	221	4.6	31	2	317	319	1382	2.2
4	-	302	40	164	0.2	1.4	0	-	0.5	0.5	155	4	25	3.6	490	320	1141	2.2
3	-	261	37	166	0.1	1.1	2	-	0.4	0.3	164	2.5	20	2.3	459	230	1260	1.5
1	-	25	8	34	0.1	0	0	-	0.3	0.5	160	2.7	23	3.5	554	197	1433	1.6
3	1	35	9	14	0.1	0.5	0	-	0.3	0.4	128	2.6	20	3.3	446	198	1071	1.6
6	-	25	11	16	0.2	0.9	0	-	0.4	0.4	116	4.3	27	4.2	204	234	795	2.7
1	-	5	6	24	0	0.1	0	-	0.2	0.3	90	1.6	9	1.6	260	87	584	0.3
3	-	10	4	2	0	0.2	3	-	0.1	0.1	25	1.3	16	0.6	88	83	153	0.6
1	-	2	59	16	0.2	0.5	1	-	0.3	0.3	56	2.3	43	2	49	327	493	0.8
1	-	14	41	119	0.1	0.4	1	-	0.4	0.1	107	1.1	40	1.8	90	248	583	0.8
0	-	16	59	10	0.1	0.6	1	-	0.4	0.2	50	2.3	36	2.2	57	290	522	1.7
1	-	24	37	32	0.2	0.9	1	-	0.4	0.4	53	2.4	42	2.7	70	328	668	1.9
1	-	62	30	75	0.1	0.5	3	-	0.4	0.2	65	1.9	25	1.9	70	205	495	1.2
1	-	78	72	190	0.2	1	3	-	0.6	0.3	144	3.8	48	3.8	142	402	1024	3
0	-	32	20	14	0.2	1	1	-	0.5	0.1	42	3	41	3.2	87	370	746	2.4
0	-	27	18	23	0.2	0.6	1	-	0.4	0.2	43	2.2	30	2.5	70	249	558	2.2
1	-	85	29	56	0.2	1	2	-	0.6	0.3	111	3.9	35	4.2	158	333	1046	4
1	-	4	1	37	0.1	0.5	1	-	0.2	0.2	16	1.1	7	1.9	15	104	212	0.4
5	-	142	49	54	0.4	3.4	1	-	0.5	0.4	240	5.9	52	7.2	395	596	1148	6.7
2	-	88	28	129	0.3	2.6	8	1.2	0.5	0.4	206	4.7	44	7.4	311	445	1108	4.6
3	-	111	33	80	0.3	2.3	2	-	0.4	0.3	162	4.7	45	6.6	400	332	1043	6.8
2	-	96	39	148	0.3	2.5	0	-	0.6	0.5	91	5.5	39	11.2	422	644	1589	5.6
6	-	93	34	84	0.3	2.1	3	2	0.4	0.6	169	4.7	36	8.3	349	390	921	4.1
1	-	52	22	71	0.2	1.2	2	-	0.2	0.3	182	2.6	26	6.4	216	229	976	2.6
2	-	50	27	37	0.1	1	0	-	0.4	0.4	141	2.4	21	3.7	196	164	500	2.4
3	-	161	52	85	0.6	5.9	3	-	0.6	0.6	283	8.3	61	11.5	541	821	1213	10.9
10	-	78	46	128	0.4	0.5	3	-	0.5	0.4	258	3.6	43	9.1	406	333	1238	2.9
8	-	60	29	31	0.2	0.4	9	-	0.2	0.3	60	4.7	35	6.8	233	353	957	1.9
0	0	10	2	5	0.1	0.1	0	-	0	0	3	0.2	3	1.1	34	42	90	0.2
0	-	8	4	6	0	0	0	-	0	0	3	0.2	3	0.9	28	42	108	0.1
0	-	9	2	4	0	0	0	-	0	0	3	0.2	3	1	30	38	79	0.2
0	-	8	2	4	0	0	0	-	0	0	3	0.2	3	0.9	29	37	103	0.1
0	-	8	2	10	0	0	0	-	0	0	3	0.2	3	0.9	28	36	89	0.1
1	-	134	30	167	0.3	1.1	2	-	1.1	0.1	68	5.2	46	2.5	197	691	1007	3.6
1	-	9	31	16	0.3	1.5	5	-	0.6	0.5	63	4.5	63	5.8	124	586	910	5
1	-	51	33	126	0.2	1.3	3	-	0.9	0.4	238	3.8	60	4.7	187	203	957	3.4
1	-	12	16	15	0	0.1	1	0.4	0.2	0.1	20	1.5	17	1.4	52	82	188	0.3
5	-	65	7	27	0	0.8	0	-	0.2	0.2	15	2.3	23	2.1	176	196	617	1.2
1	-	6	44	96	0.3	0	7	-	0.1	0.2	4	0.9	41	2.2	108	359	29	0.9
5	-	45	20	4	0.2	4.5	1	-	0.1	0.1	55	1.8	25	1.8	131	163	1118	1.1
1	-	216	37	255	0.1	0.8	0	-	0.4	0.2	244	2.2	22	1.5	348	174	551	1.8
2	-	215	35	120	0.1	0.9	2	-	0.3	0.3	151	2.2	23	2.2	276	201	889	1.9
2	-	213	36	117	0.2	1	11	-	0.3	0.5	144	2.1	26	3.2	336	272	1081	2.2
3	-	216	38	109	0.1	0.9	0	-	0.3	1	144	3	24	4	290	283	1115	2.1
2	-	20	15	43	0.1	0.2	3	-	0.2	0.3	70	1.8	15	2.5	80	116	319	0.6
2	-	27	14	5	0.1	0.2	3	-	0.2	0.3	37	1.8	14	2.2	74	96	326	0.5
2	-	19	15	24	0.1	0.2	2	-	0.2	0.3	22	1.4	14	1.8	69	110	333	0.5
3	-	291	37	181	0.1	1.1	1	-	0.6	0.3	225	3	22	2.1	302	188	804	1.6
2	0	400	53	252	0.2	0.9	3	0.9	0.5	0.1	54	2.4	13	0.2	227	138	211	1.6
1	-	44	34	186	0.4	0.7	1	-	0.4	0.1	324	1.3	51	1.9	134	240	784	2.5

Code	Food Name	Amount	Unit	Grams	kCalories	Carbohydrate (gm)	Protein (gm)	Fat (gm)	Saturated Fat (gm)	Monounsaturated Fat (gm)
21075	Fast Food-Enchilada w/ Cheese and Beef	1	Each	192	323	30	12	18	9	6
21076	Fast Food-Enchirito w/ Cheese, Beef, and Beans	1	Each	193	344	34	18	16	8	7
21019	Fast Food-Eng. Muffin w/ Butter	1	Each	63	189	30	5	6	2	2
21020	Fast Food-Eng. Muffin w/ Cheese and Sausage	1	Each	115	393	29	15	24	10	10
21021	Fast Food-Eng. Muffin w/ Egg, Cheese, and Can. Bacon	1	Each	146	383	31	20	20	9	7
21022	Fast Food-Eng. Muffin w/ Egg, Cheese, and Sausage	1	Each	165	487	31	22	31	12	13
21047	Fast Food-Fish Fillet, Battered and Fried	1	Each	91	211	15	13	11	3	2
21105	Fast Food-Fish Sandwich w/ Tartar Sauce	1	Each	158	431	41	17	23	5	8
21106	Fast Food-Fish Sandwich w/ Tartar Sauce and Cheese	1	Each	183	523	48	21	29	8	9
21023	Fast Food-French Toast w/ Butter	1	Slice	67.5	178	18	5	9	-	-
21031	Fast Food-Fried Pie, Fruit (Apple, Cherry, or Lemon)	1	Each	85	266	33	2	14	7	6
21077	Fast Food-Frijoles w/ Cheese	3	Ounce	85.1	115	15	6	4	2	1
21116	Fast Food-Ham and Cheese Sandwich	1	Each	146	352	33	21	15	6	7
21117	Fast Food-Ham, Egg, and Cheese Sandwich	1	Each	143	347	31	19	16	7	6
21114	Fast Food-Hamburger, Double Patty w/ Cond and Veg	1	Each	226	540	40	34	27	11	10
21111	Fast Food-Hamburger, Double Patty w/ Condiments	1	Each	215	576	39	32	32	12	14
21110	Fast Food-Hamburger, Double Patty, Plain	1	Each	176	544	43	30	28	10	12
21113	Fast Food-Hamburger, Large, Single Patty w/ Cond&veg	1	Each	218	512	40	26	27	10	11
21112	Fast Food-Hamburger, Large, Single Patty, Plain	1	Each	137	426	32	23	23	8	10
21108	Fast Food-Hamburger, Single Patty w/ Condiments	1	Each	107	275	33	14	10	4	4
21107	Fast Food-Hamburger, Single Patty, Plain	1	Each	90	275	31	12	12	4	5
21115	Fast Food-Hamburger, Triple Patty w/ Condiments	1	Each	259	692	29	50	41	16	18
21119	Fast Food-Hot Dog w/ Chili	1	Each	114	296	31	14	13	5	7
21120	Fast Food-Hot Dog w/ Corn Flour Coating (corndog)	1	Each	175	460	56	17	19	5	9
21118	Fast Food-Hot Dog, Plain	1	Each	98	242	18	10	15	5	7
21028	Fast Food-Ice Milk, Vanilla, Soft-serve w/ Cone	1	Each	103	164	24	4	6	4	2
21078	Fast Food-Nachos w/ Cheese	3	Ounce	85.1	260	27	7	14	6	6
21079	Fast Food-Nachos w/ Cheese and Jalapeno Peppers	3	Ounce	85.1	253	25	7	14	6	6
21080	Fast Food-Nachos w/ Cheese, Beans, Ground Beef	3	Ounce	85.1	190	19	7	10	4	4
21081	Fast Food-Nachos w/ Cinnamon and Sugar	3	Ounce	85.1	462	49	6	28	14	9
21130	Fast Food-Onion Rings, Breaded and Fried	1	Each	10	33	4	0	2	1	1
21048	Fast Food-Oysters, Battered or Breaded, and Fried	3	Ounce	85.1	225	24	8	11	3	4
21025	Fast Food-Pancakes w/ Butter and Syrup	1	Each	74	166	29	3	4	2	2
21049	Fast Food-Pizza w/ Cheese	1	Slice	63	140	21	8	3	2	1
21050	Fast Food-Pizza w/ Cheese, Sausage, and Vegetables	1	Slice	79	184	21	13	5	2	3
21051	Fast Food-Pizza w/ Pepperoni	1	Slice	71	181	20	10	7	2	3
21131	Fast Food-Potato, Baked w/ Cheese Sauce	1	Each	296	474	47	15	29	11	11
21132	Fast Food-Potato, Baked w/ Cheese Sauce and Bacon	1	Each	299	451	44	18	26	10	10
21133	Fast Food-Potato, Baked w/ Cheese Sauce and Broccoli	1	Each	339	403	47	14	21	9	8
21134	Fast Food-Potato, Baked w/ Cheese Sauce and Chili	1	Each	395	482	56	23	22	13	7
21135	Fast Food-Potato, Baked w/ Sour Cream and Chives	1	Each	302	393	50	7	22	10	8
21136	Fast Food-Potato, French Fried In Beef Tallow	1	Large	115	359	44	5	19	9	8
21137	Fast Food-Potato, French Fried In Beef Tallow and Veg Oil	1	Large	115	358	44	5	19	8	8
21138	Fast Food-Potato, French Fried In Vegetable Oil	1	Large	115	355	44	5	19	6	9
21139	Fast Food-Potato, Mashed	0.5	Cup	120	100	19	3	1	1	0
21026	Fast Food-Potatoes, Hashed Brown	0.5	Cup	72	151	16	2	9	4	4
21122	Fast Food-Roast Beef Sandwich w/ Cheese	1	Each	176	473	45	32	18	9	4
21121	Fast Food-Roast Beef Sandwich, Plain	1	Each	139	346	33	22	14	4	7
21052	Fast Food-Salad, w/o Dressing	0.5	Cup	69.3	11	2	1	0	0	0
21053	Fast Food-Salad, w/o Dressing, w/ Cheese and Egg	0.5	Cup	72.3	34	2	3	2	1	1
21054	Fast Food-Salad, w/o Dressing, w/ Chicken	0.5	Cup	72.7	35	1	6	1	0	0
21055	Fast Food-Salad, w/o Dressing, w/ Pasta and Seafood	0.5	Cup	139	126	11	5	7	1	2
21056	Fast Food-Salad, w/o Dressing, w/ Shrimp	0.5	Cup	78.7	35	2	5	1	0	0
21058	Fast Food-Scallops, Breaded and Fried	1	Each	24	64	6	3	3	1	2
21059	Fast Food-Shrimp, Breaded and Fried	1	Ounce	28.4	79	7	3	4	1	3
21123	Fast Food-Steak Sandwich	1	Each	140	315	36	21	10	3	4
21124	Fast Food-Submarine Sandwich w/ Coldcuts	1	Each	228	456	51	22	19	7	8
21125	Fast Food-Submarine Sandwich w/ Roast Beef	1	Each	216	410	44	29	13	7	2
21126	Fast Food-Submarine Sandwich w/ Tuna Salad	1	Each	256	584	55	30	28	5	13
21032	Fast Food-Sundae, Caramel	1	Each	155	304	49	7	9	5	3

Polyunsaturated Fat (gm)	Fiber (gm)	Cholesterol (mg)	Folate (μg)	Vitamin A (re)	Vitamin B6 (mg)	Vitamin B12 (μg)	Vitamin C (mg)	Vitamin E (mg)	Riboflavin (mg)	Thiamin (mg)	Calcium (mg)	Iron (mg)	Magnesium (mg)	Niacin (mg)	Phosphorus (mg)	Potassium (mg)	Sodium (mg)	Zinc (mg)
1	-	40	192	142	0.3	1	1	-	0.4	0.1	228	3.1	83	2.5	167	574	1319	2.7
0	-	50	253	133	0.2	1.6	5	-	0.7	0.2	218	2.4	71	3	224	560	1251	2.8
1	-	13	17	33	0	0	1	0.1	0.3	0.3	103	1.6	13	2.6	85	69	386	0.4
3	-	59	18	86	0.1	0.7	1	-	0.3	0.7	168	2.3	24	4.1	186	215	1036	1.7
2	-	234	44	158	0.2	0.8	1	0.6	0.5	0.5	207	3.3	34	3.9	320	213	784	1.8
3	-	274	54	172	0.2	1.4	1	-	0.5	0.8	196	3.5	30	4.5	287	294	1135	2.4
6	-	31	51	11	0.1	1	0	-	0.1	0.1	16	1.9	22	1.9	156	291	484	0.4
8	-	55	44	30	0.1	1.1	3	0.9	0.2	0.3	84	2.6	33	3.4	212	340	615	1
9	-	68	31	97	0.1	1.1	3	1.8	0.4	0.5	185	3.5	37	4.2	311	353	939	1.2
-	-	58	15	73	0	0.2	0	-	0.2	0.3	36	0.9	8	2	73	88	257	0.3
1	-	13	4	33	0	0.1	1	0.4	0.1	0.1	13	0.9	8	1	37	51	325	0.2
0	-	19	57	36	0.1	0.3	1	-	0.2	0.1	96	1.1	43	0.8	89	308	449	0.9
1	-	58	72	76	0.2	0.5	3	0.3	0.5	0.3	130	3.2	16	2.7	152	291	771	1.4
2	-	246	43	149	0.2	1.2	3	-	0.6	0.4	212	3.1	26	4.2	346	210	1005	2
3	-	122	27	11	0.5	4.1	1	-	0.4	0.4	102	5.9	50	7.6	314	570	791	5.7
3	-	103	45	4	0.4	3.3	1	-	0.4	0.3	92	5.5	45	6.7	284	527	742	5.8
2	-	99	37	0	0.3	2.9	0	1.3	0.4	0.3	86	4.6	37	8.3	234	363	554	5.7
2	-	87	37	33	0.3	2.4	3	-	0.4	0.4	96	4.9	44	7.3	233	480	824	4.9
2	-	71	32	0	0.2	2.1	0	-	0.3	0.3	74	3.6	27	6.2	175	267	474	4.1
2	-	43	17	13	0.1	0.8	3	0.4	0.3	0.3	51	2.5	22	4.7	110	215	564	2.1
1	-	35	25	0	0.1	0.9	0	0.5	0.3	0.3	63	2.4	19	3.7	103	145	387	2
3	-	142	31	16	0.6	4.9	1	-	0.5	0.3	65	8.3	54	11	394	785	712	10.7
1	-	51	50	6	0	0.3	3	-	0.4	0.2	19	3.3	10	3.7	192	166	480	0.8
3	-	79	60	37	0.1	0.4	0	-	0.7	0.3	102	6.2	18	4.2	166	263	973	1.3
2	-	44	29	0	0	0.5	0	-	0.3	0.2	24	2.3	13	3.6	97	143	670	2
0	-	28	5	52	0.1	0.2	1	0.4	0.3	0.1	153	0.2	15	0.3	139	169	92	0.6
2	-	14	8	69	0.2	0.6	1	-	0.3	0.1	205	1	42	1.2	208	129	614	1.3
2	-	35	8	196	0.2	0.4	0	-	0.2	0.1	259	1	45	1.2	164	122	724	1.2
2	-	7	13	156	0.1	0.3	2	-	0.2	0.1	128	0.9	32	1.1	129	151	600	1.2
3	-	31	6	9	0.1	1.3	6	-	0.3	0.1	66	2.3	15	3.1	26	61	343	0.5
0	-	2	1	0	0	0	0	0	0	0	9	0.1	2	0.1	10	16	52	0
3	-	66	8	66	0	0.6	3	-	0.2	0.2	17	2.7	14	2.7	120	111	414	9.6
1	-	19	11	22	0	0.1	1	0.4	0.2	0.1	41	0.8	16	1.1	152	80	352	0.3
0	-	9	59	74	0	0.3	1	-	0.2	0.2	117	0.6	16	2.5	113	110	336	0.8
1	-	21	27	101	0.1	0.4	2	-	0.2	0.2	101	1.5	18	2	131	179	382	1.1
1	-	14	53	55	0.1	0.2	2	-	0.2	0.1	65	0.9	9	3	75	153	267	0.5
6	-	18	27	228	0.7	0.2	26	-	0.2	0.2	311	3	65	3.3	320	1166	382	1.9
5	-	30	30	173	0.7	0.3	29	-	0.2	0.3	308	3.1	69	4	347	1178	972	2.2
4	-	20	61	278	0.8	0.3	48	-	0.3	0.3	336	3.3	78	3.6	346	1441	485	2
1	-	32	51	174	0.9	0.2	32	-	0.4	0.3	411	6.1	111	4.2	498	1572	699	3.8
3	-	24	33	278	0.8	0.2	34	-	0.2	0.3	106	3.1	69	3.7	184	1383	181	0.9
1	-	21	38	3	0.3	0.1	6	-	0	0.2	18	1.6	38	2.6	153	819	187	0.6
2	-	16	38	3	0.3	0.1	6	-	0	0.2	18	1.6	38	2.6	153	819	187	0.6
3	-	0	38	3	0.3	0.1	6	-	0	0.2	18	1.6	38	2.6	153	819	187	0.6
0	-	2	10	12	0.3	0.1	0	-	0.1	0.1	25	0.6	22	1.4	66	353	272	0.4
0	-	9	8	3	0.2	0	5	0.1	0	0.1	7	0.5	16	1.1	69	267	290	0.2
4	-	77	40	46	0.3	2.1	0	-	0.5	0.4	183	5.1	40	5.9	401	345	1633	5.4
2	-	51	40	21	0.3	1.2	2	-	0.3	0.4	54	4.2	31	5.9	239	316	792	3.4
0	-	0	26	79	0.1	0	16	-	0	0	9	0.4	8	0.4	27	119	18	0.1
0	-	33	28	38	0	0.1	3	-	0.1	0	33	0.2	8	0.3	44	124	40	0.3
0	-	24	23	32	0.1	0.1	6	-	0	0	12	0.4	11	2	57	149	70	0.3
3	-	17	33	213	0.1	0.6	13	-	0.1	0.1	24	1.1	17	1.2	68	200	524	0.6
0	-	60	29	26	0	1.3	3	-	0.1	0	20	0.3	13	0.4	53	135	163	0.4
0	-	18	7	7	0	0.1	0	-	0.1	0	3	0.3	5	0	49	49	153	0.2
0	-	35	8	6	0	0	0	-	0.2	0	14	0.5	7	0	60	32	250	0.2
2	-	50	62	31	0.3	1.1	4	-	0.3	0.3	63	3.5	34	5	204	360	547	3.1
2	-	36	55	80	0.1	1.1	12	-	0.8	1	189	2.5	68	5.5	287	394	1651	2.6
3	-	73	45	50	0.3	1.8	6	-	0.4	0.4	41	2.8	67	6	192	330	845	4.4
7	-	49	56	41	0.2	1.6	4	-	0.3	0.5	74	2.6	79	11.3	220	335	1293	1.9
1	0	25	12	68	0	0.6	3	0.9	0.3	0.1	189	0.2	22	0.9	217	318	195	0.8

Code	Food Name	Amount	Unit	Grams	kCalories	Carbohydrate (gm)	Protein (gm)	Fat (gm)	Saturated Fat (gm)	Monounsaturated Fat (gm)
21033	Fast Food-Sundae, Hot Fudge	1	Each	158	284	48	6	9	5	2
21034	Fast Food-Sundae, Strawberry	1	Each	153	268	45	6	8	4	3
21082	Fast Food-Taco	1	Large	263	568	41	32	32	17	10
21083	Fast Food-Taco Salad	0.5	Cup	66	93	8	4	5	2	2
21084	Fast Food-Taco Salad w/ Chili Con Carne	0.5	Cup	87	97	9	6	4	2	2
21088	Fast Food-Tostada w/ Guacamole	1	Ounce	28.4	39	3	1	3	1	1
21085	Fast Food-Tostada, w/ Beans and Cheese	1	Each	144	223	27	10	10	5	3
21086	Fast Food-Tostada, w/ Beans, Beef, and Cheese	1	Each	225	333	30	16	17	11	4
21087	Fast Food-Tostada, w/ Beef and Cheese	1	Each	163	315	23	19	16	10	3
40349	Hardee's-Big Cheese	1	Each	141.8	4950	280	300	300	-	-
40350	Hardee's-Big Deluxe	1	Each	248.1	6751	460	310	410	-	-
40356	Hardee's-Big Fish Sandwich	1	Each	191.4	514	49	20	26	-	-
40353	Hardee's-Big Roast Beef	1	Each	163	365	39	22	13	6	6
40351	Hardee's-Big Twin	1	Each	141.8	369	28	19	20	9	7
40358	Hardee's-Biscuit	1	Each	78	275	35	5	13	-	-
40348	Hardee's-Cheeseburger	1	Each	100.6	335	29	17	17	-	-
40357	Hardee's-Chicken Fillet	1	Each	191.4	510	42	27	26	-	-
40347	Hardee's-Hamburger	1	Each	100.1	305	29	17	13	-	-
40354	Hardee's-Hot Dog	1	Each	50	346	26	11	22	-	-
40355	Hardee's-Hot Ham & Cheese	1	Each	141.8	376	37	23	15	-	-
40352	Hardee's-Roast Beef Sandwich	1	Each	141.8	323	39	19	11	5	5
44118	Jack In The Box-Bacon Cheeseburger	1	Each	242	705	41	35	45	15	16
44101	Jack In The Box-Breakfast Jack	1	Each	126	313	29	19	14	5	5
44141	Jack In The Box-Cheesecake	1	Each	99	309	29	8	18	9	7
44115	Jack In The Box-Jumbo Jack	1	Each	222	497	41	25	26	10	11
44116	Jack In The Box-Jumbo Jack w/ Cheese	1	Each	242	559	40	28	31	13	11
44136	Jack In The Box-Regular French Fries	1	Each	109	351	45	4	17	4	7
44135	Jack In The Box-Small French Fries	1	Each	68	219	28	3	11	3	7
47265	K.F.C.-Colonel's Chicken Sandwich	1	Each	166	482	39	21	27	6	4
47261	K.F.C.-French Fries	1	Each	77	244	31	3	12	3	7
47260	K.F.C.-Mashed Potatoes and Gravy	1	Each	98	71	12	2	2	1	0
47239	K.F.C.-Original Recipe Center Breast	1	Each	103	261	9	25	15	4	4
47240	K.F.C.-Original Recipe Drumstick	1	Each	57	169	5	12	12	2	3
47241	K.F.C.-Original Recipe Thigh	1	Each	95	324	11	16	24	6	6
47237	K.F.C.-Original Recipe Wing	1	Each	53	172	5	12	11	3	6
48215	McDonald's-Apple Danish	1	Each	115	390	51	6	17	4	11
48204	McDonald's-Bacon, Egg and Cheese Biscuit	1	Each	153	432	32	18	26	8	16
48174	McDonald's-Big Mac	1	Each	215	560	43	25	32	10	20
48205	McDonald's-Biscuit w/ Spread	1	Each	75	260	32	5	13	3	9
48170	McDonald's-Cheeseburger	1	Each	116	310	30	15	13	5	8
48187	McDonald's-Chef Salad	1	Each	265	215	7	20	12	6	6
48181	McDonald's-Chicken McNuggets	1	Each	18.5	45	3	3	3	1	2
48226	McDonald's-Chocolate Lowfat Milk Shake	1	Each	294.1	321	66	11	2	1	1
48189	McDonald's-Chunky Chicken Salad	1	Each	255	143	5	23	3	1	2
48217	McDonald's-Cinnamon Raisin Danish	1	Each	110	440	58	6	21	5	13
48198	McDonald's-Egg McMuffin	1	Each	135	284	27	18	11	4	6
48201	McDonald's-English Muffin w/ Spread	1	Each	58	170	26	5	4	2	2
48175	McDonald's-Filet O' Fish	1	Each	141	437	38	14	26	5	10
48188	McDonald's-Garden Salad	1	Each	189	50	6	4	2	1	1
48169	McDonald's-Hamburger	1	Each	102	255	30	12	9	3	5
48209	McDonald's-Hash Brown Potatoes	1	Each	53	130	15	1	7	1	4
48210	McDonald's-Hotcakes w/ Margarine and Syrup	1	Each	174	440	74	8	12	2	5
48216	McDonald's-Iced Cheese Danish	1	Each	110	390	42	7	21	6	13
48180	McDonald's-Large French Fries	1	Each	122	400	46	6	22	5	15
48176	McDonald's-McChicken	1	Each	187	415	39	19	20	4	9
48223	McDonald's-McDonaldland Cookies	1	Each	56.7	290	47	4	9	1	7
48172	McDonald's-McLean Deluxe	1	Each	206	320	35	22	10	4	5
48179	McDonald's-Medium French Fries	1	Each	97	320	36	4	17	4	12
48171	McDonald's-Quarter Pounder	1	Each	166	410	34	23	20	8	11
48218	McDonald's-Raspberry Danish	1	Each	117	410	62	6	16	3	11

Polyunsaturated Fat (gm)	Fiber (gm)	Cholesterol (mg)	Folate (µg)	Vitamin A (re)	Vitamin B6 (mg)	Vitamin B12 (µg)	Vitamin C (mg)	Vitamin E (mg)	Riboflavin (mg)	Thiamin (mg)	Calcium (mg)	Iron (mg)	Magnesium (mg)	Niacin (mg)	Phosphorus (mg)	Potassium (mg)	Sodium (mg)	Zinc (mg)
1	0	21	9	57	0.1	0.6	2	0.7	0.3	0.1	207	0.6	33	1.1	228	395	182	0.9
1	0	21	18	58	0.1	0.6	2	0.8	0.3	0.1	161	0.3	24	0.9	155	271	92	0.7
1	-	87	37	226	0.4	1.6	3	-	0.7	0.2	339	3.7	108	4.9	313	729	1233	6
1	-	15	13	26	0.1	0.2	1	-	0.1	0	64	0.8	17	0.8	48	139	254	0.9
1	-	2	21	71	0.2	0.2	1	-	0.2	0.1	82	0.9	17	0.8	51	130	295	1.1
0	-	4	12	24	0	0.1	0	-	0.1	0	46	0.2	8	0.2	25	71	87	0.4
1	-	30	75	85	0.2	0.7	1	-	0.3	0.1	210	1.9	59	1.3	117	403	543	1.9
1	-	74	97	173	0.2	1.1	4	-	0.5	0.1	189	2.5	68	2.9	173	491	871	3.2
1	-	41	15	96	0.2	1.2	3	-	0.6	0.1	217	2.9	64	3.1	179	572	897	3.7
-	-	-	-	-	-	-	-	-	-	-	-	-	-	-	-	-	12510	-
-	-	-	-	-	-	-	-	-	-	-	-	-	-	-	-	-	10632	-
-	-	-	-	-	-	-	-	-	-	-	-	-	-	-	-	-	314	-
2	1	55	29	0	0.3	3	0	0.2	0.4	0.4	80	4.5	40	6.6	280	389	1071	7.4
4	1	45	28	14	0.2	1.9	2	0.7	0.3	0.2	66	3.3	29	5.5	161	229	475	3.8
-	-	-	-	-	-	-	-	-	-	-	-	-	-	-	-	-	650	-
-	-	-	-	-	-	-	2	-	0.3	0.5	-	-	-	5.5	-	-	789	-
-	-	-	-	-	-	-	-	-	-	-	-	-	-	-	-	-	360	-
-	-	-	-	-	-	-	2	-	0.6	0.6	-	-	-	6.4	-	-	682	-
-	-	-	-	-	-	-	-	-	-	-	-	-	-	-	-	-	744	-
-	-	-	-	-	-	-	-	-	-	-	-	-	-	-	-	-	1067	-
2	1	44	25	0	0.3	2.6	0	0.2	0.4	0.3	70	3.9	35	5.7	244	323	908	6.5
9	-	113	-	70	-	-	8	-	0.5	0.2	200	2.8	-	8.4	-	-	1240	-
3	-	190	-	138	0.1	1.1	3	-	0.5	0.4	184	2.6	25	5.3	323	198	1080	1.9
2	-	63	-	-	-	-	-	-	0.2	0	88	0.3	-	1.9	-	-	208	-
2	-	72	-	67	0.3	2.4	4	-	0.3	0.4	121	4.1	40	10.5	236	444	1023	3.8
2	-	98	-	196	0.3	2.7	4	-	0.3	0.5	243	4.1	44	10.1	366	444	1482	4.3
-	-	0	-	-	-	-	26	-	0	0.2	-	0.7	-	3.6	-	-	194	-
-	-	0	-	-	-	-	16	-	-	0.1	-	0.4	-	2.3	-	-	121	-
9	1	47	29	14	0.6	0.3	0	2.3	0.3	0.4	100	3.1	41	10.6	261	297	1060	1.5
1	-	2	-	-	-	-	16	-	0.1	0.2	-	0.3	-	1.9	-	-	139	-
0	-	-	-	-	-	-	-	-	0	-	16	0.2	-	1.1	-	-	339	-
2	0	87	4	15	0.6	0.4	0	0.5	0.1	0.1	16	1.2	31	14	238	265	603	1.1
2	-	59	5	14	0.2	0.2	0	0.4	0.1	0	7	0.7	13	3.4	99	130	268	1.7
3	0	103	8	28	0.3	0.3	0	0.5	0.2	0.1	13	1.4	23	6.5	176	224	549	2.4
2	-	59	-	-	-	-	-	-	0.1	0	24	0.3	-	2.9	-	-	383	-
2	2	25	3	35	0	0	15	3.8	0.2	0.3	14	1.4	8	2.2	31	69	370	0.2
2	1	248	18	157	0.2	0.6	0	1.5	0.3	0.4	181	2.6	30	2.5	442	232	1206	1.7
2	-	103	21	106	0.3	1.8	2	-	0.4	0.5	256	4	38	6.8	314	237	950	4.7
1	1	1	6	0	0	0.1	0	1.8	0.1	0.2	75	1.3	14	1.5	168	100	730	0.7
1	-	50	18	118	0.1	0.9	2	0.5	0.2	0.3	199	2.3	21	3.9	177	223	750	2.1
1	-	120	-	385	-	-	13	-	0.3	0.3	240	1.4	-	3.4	-	-	459	-
0	-	9	-	-	-	-	-	-	0	0	-	0.1	-	1.3	-	-	97	-
0	-	10	-	92	-	-	0	-	0.5	0.1	333	0.8	-	0.4	-	-	241	-
1	1	80	28	373	0.6	0.6	20	11	0.2	0.2	35	1	38	8.7	262	445	235	3
2	-	34	-	33	-	-	4	-	0.3	0.3	32	1	-	2.9	-	-	430	-
1	1	221	43	147	0.2	0.8	1	1.8	0.3	0.5	250	2.7	32	3.6	312	208	724	1.8
1	2	9	51	37	0.1	-	0	0.1	0.1	0.3	151	1.6	12	2.5	60	74	285	0.4
11	1	50	20	44	0.1	0.8	-	-	0.1	0.3	164	1.8	27	2.7	227	149	1023	0.9
0	-	65	-	900	-	-	21	-	0.1	0.1	32	0.8	-	0.4	-	-	70	-
1	-	37	-	40	-	-	2	-	0.2	0.3	80	1.5	-	3.8	-	-	490	-
2	-	0	-	-	-	-	1	-	-	0.1	-	-	-	0.8	-	-	330	-
5	-	8	-	40	-	-	-	-	0.3	0.3	80	1	-	2.9	-	-	685	-
2	-	47	-	40	-	-	-	-	0.3	0.3	32	0.8	-	1.9	-	-	420	-
2	-	0	-	-	-	-	15	-	-	0.2	-	0.6	-	2.9	-	-	20	-
7	-	50	-	20	-	-	2	-	0.2	0.9	120	1.5	-	8.6	-	-	830	-
1	-	0	-	-	-	-	-	-	0.2	0.2	-	1	-	1.9	-	-	300	-
1	-	60	-	100	-	-	6	-	0.3	0.4	120	2	-	6.7	-	-	670	-
2	-	0	-	-	-	-	12	-	-	0.2	-	0.4	-	2.9	-	-	150	-
1	-	85	-	40	-	-	4	-	0.3	0.4	120	2	-	6.7	-	-	645	-
2	-	26	-	-	-	-	4	-	0.2	0.3	-	0.8	-	1.9	-	-	310	-

Code	Food Name	Amount	Unit	Grams	kCalories	Carbohydrate (gm)	Protein (gm)	Fat (gm)	Saturated Fat (gm)	Monounsaturated Fat (gm)
48207	McDonald's-Sausage Biscuit	1	Each	118	420	32	12	28	8	17
48203	McDonald's-Sausage Biscuit w/ Egg	1	Each	175	505	33	19	33	10	20
48199	McDonald's-Sausage McMuffin	1	Each	135	345	27	15	20	7	11
48200	McDonald's-Sausage McMuffin w/ Egg	1	Each	159	430	27	21	25	8	14
48208	McDonald's-Scrambled Eggs	1	Each	100	140	1	12	10	3	5
48190	McDonald's-Side Salad	1	Each	106	30	4	2	1	0	1
48178	McDonald's-Small French Fries	1	Each	68	220	26	3	12	3	8
48227	McDonald's-Strawberry Lowfat Milk Shake	1	Each	294.1	320	67	11	1	1	1
48225	McDonald's-Vanilla Lowfat Milk Shake	1	Each	294.1	290	60	11	1	1	1
52366	Pizza Hut-Cheese Pizza, Hand Tossed	1	Slice	70	259	28	17	10	7	3
52359	Pizza Hut-Cheese Pizza, Pan	1	Slice	70	246	29	15	9	5	5
53322	Pizza Hut-Cheese Pizza, Thin'n Crispy	1	Slice	70	199	19	14	9	5	3
52363	Pizza Hut-Peperoni Pizza, Thin'n Crispy	1	Slice	70	207	18	13	10	5	5
52370	Pizza Hut-Pepperoni Personal Pan Pizza	1	Each	250	675	76	37	29	13	17
52367	Pizza Hut-Pepperoni Pizza, Hand Tossed	1	Slice	70	250	25	14	12	6	5
52360	Pizza Hut-Pepperoni Pizza, Pan	1	Slice	70	270	31	15	11	5	7
52365	Pizza Hut-Super Sprm Pizza, Thin'n Crispy	1	Slice	70	232	22	15	11	5	5
52362	Pizza Hut-Super Supreme Pizza, Pan	1	Slice	70	282	27	17	13	6	7
52369	Pizza Hut-Super Supreme, Hand Tossed	1	Slice	70	278	27	17	13	7	6
52371	Pizza Hut-Supreme Personal Pan Pizza	1	Each	250	647	76	33	28	11	17
52368	Pizza Hut-Supreme Pizza, Hand Tossed	1	Slice	70	270	25	16	13	6	7
52361	Pizza Hut-Supreme Pizza, Pan	1	Slice	70	295	27	16	15	7	8
52364	Pizza Hut-Supreme Pizza, Thin'n Crispy	1	Slice	70	230	21	14	11	6	6
54494	Red Lobster-Atlantic Ocean Perch, Lunch	1	Each	141.8	130	1	24	4	1	-
54506	Red Lobster-Calamari, Brded and Fried, Lunch	1	Each	141.8	360	30	13	21	6	-
54486	Red Lobster-Catfish, Lunch Portion	1	Each	141.8	170	0	20	10	3	-
54514	Red Lobster-Chicken Breast, Skinless, Lunch	1	Each	113.4	140	0	26	3	1	-
54487	Red Lobster-Cod, Atlantic, Lunch Portion	1	Each	141.8	100	0	23	1	0	-
54510	Red Lobster-Deep Sea Scallops, Lnch Portion	1	Each	141.8	130	2	26	2	0	-
54488	Red Lobster-Flounder, Lunch Portion	1	Each	141.8	100	1	21	1	0	-
54489	Red Lobster-Grouper, Lunch Portion	1	Each	141.8	110	0	26	1	0	-
54490	Red Lobster-Haddock, Lunch Portion	1	Each	141.8	110	2	24	1	0	-
54491	Red Lobster-Halibut, Lunch Portion	1	Each	141.8	110	1	25	1	0	-
54513	Red Lobster-Hamburger, Lunch Portion	1	Each	151.2	410	0	37	28	11	-
54504	Red Lobster-King Crab Legs, Lunch Portion	1	Each	453.6	170	6	32	2	1	-
54507	Red Lobster-Langostino, Lunch Portion	1	Each	141.8	120	2	26	1	0	-
54500	Red Lobster-Lemon Sole, Lunch Portion	1	Each	141.8	120	1	27	1	0	-
54524	Red Lobster-Live Maine Lobster	1	Each	510.3	240	5	36	8	2	-
54492	Red Lobster-Mackerel, Lunch Portion	1	Each	141.8	190	1	20	12	4	-
54493	Red Lobster-Monkfish, Lunch Portion	1	Each	141.8	110	0	24	1	0	-
54498	Red Lobster-Norwegian Salmon, Lunch	1	Each	141.8	230	3	27	12	3	-
54495	Red Lobster-Pollock, Lunch Portion	1	Each	141.8	120	1	28	1	0	-
54502	Red Lobster-Rainbow Trout, Lunch Portion	1	Each	141.8	170	0	23	9	3	-
54496	Red Lobster-Red Rockfish, Lunch Portion	1	Each	141.8	90	0	21	1	0	-
54497	Red Lobster-Red Snapper, Lunch Portion	1	Each	141.8	110	0	25	1	0	-
54509	Red Lobster-Rock Lobster, Lunch Portion	1	Each	368.5	230	2	49	3	1	-
54511	Red Lobster-Shrimp, Lunch Portion	1	Each	198.5	120	0	25	2	1	-
54505	Red Lobster-Snow Crab Legs, Lunch Portion	1	Each	453.6	150	1	33	2	1	-
54499	Red Lobster-Sockeye Salmon, Lunch Portion	1	Each	141.8	160	3	28	4	1	-
54512	Red Lobster-Strip Steak, Lunch Portion	1	Each	255.1	560	0	47	40	17	-
54501	Red Lobster-Swordfish, Lunch Portion	1	Each	141.8	100	0	17	4	1	-
54503	Red Lobster-Yellow Fin Tuna, Lunch Portion	1	Each	141.8	180	6	32	2	1	-
62527	Subway-BMT, on Honey Wheat Bread	1	12 In.	220	1011	88	45	57	20	25
62559	Subway-BMT, on Italian Roll	1	12 In.	213	982	83	44	55	20	24
62560	Subway-Club Sandwich, on Honey Wheat Roll	1	12 In.	220	722	89	47	23	7	9
62561	Subway-Club Sandwich, on Italian Roll	1	12 In.	213	693	83	46	22	7	8
62562	Subway-Cold Cut Combo, on Italian Roll	1	12 In.	184	853	83	46	40	12	15
62563	Subway-Cold Cut Combo, on Wheat Roll	1	12 In.	184	853	88	48	41	12	15
62564	Subway-Ham and Cheese, on Italian Roll	1	12 In.	184	643	81	38	18	7	8
62526	Subway-Ham and Cheese, on Wheat	1	12 In.	194	673	86	39	22	7	8

Polyunsaturated Fat (gm)	Fiber (gm)	Cholesterol (mg)	Folate (µg)	Vitamin A (re)	Vitamin B6 (mg)	Vitamin B12 (µg)	Vitamin C (mg)	Vitamin E (mg)	Riboflavin (mg)	Thiamin (mg)	Calcium (mg)	Iron (mg)	Magnesium (mg)	Niacin (mg)	Phosphorus (mg)	Potassium (mg)	Sodium (mg)	Zinc (mg)
3	-	44	-	-	-	-	-	-	0.2	0.5	64	1	-	3.8	-	-	1040	-
3	-	260	-	60	-	-	-	-	0.3	0.5	80	2	-	3.8	-	-	1210	-
2	-	57	-	40	-	-	-	-	0.3	0.5	160	1.5	-	4.8	-	-	770	-
3	-	270	-	100	-	-	-	-	0.4	0.5	200	2	-	4.8	-	-	920	-
2	-	425	-	100	-	-	-	-	0.3	0.1	48	1	-	-	-	-	290	-
0	-	33	-	800	-	-	12	-	0.1	0.1	16	0.4	-	-	-	-	35	-
1	-	0	-	-	-	-	9	-	-	0.2	-	0.2	-	1.9	-	-	110	-
0	-	10	-	60	-	-	-	-	0.5	0.1	280	-	-	0.4	-	-	170	-
0	-	10	-	60	-	-	-	-	0.5	0.1	280	-	-	-	-	-	170	-
-	-	28	-	50	-	0.3	5	-	0.2	0.2	300	1.5	32	2.6	220	198	638	2.3
-	-	17	-	45	-	0.3	4	-	0.3	0.3	252	1.5	26	2.5	188	160	470	2
-	-	17	-	35	-	0.3	2	-	0.2	0.2	264	0.9	21	2.3	188	131	434	1.8
-	-	23	-	35	-	0.3	3	-	0.2	0.2	180	0.9	19	2.5	148	144	493	1.7
-	-	53	-	120	-	0.4	10	-	0.7	0.6	584	3.2	53	7.8	360	408	1335	3.8
-	-	25	-	50	-	0.3	4	-	0.3	0.3	176	1.4	26	2.7	156	208	634	1.9
-	-	21	-	50	-	0.3	4	-	0.2	0.3	208	1.8	25	2.6	176	203	564	2.1
-	-	28	-	50	-	0.4	4	-	0.2	0.3	184	1.4	26	2.6	168	232	668	2.3
-	-	28	-	60	-	0.4	5	-	0.3	0.4	216	1.9	32	3	188	266	724	2.7
-	-	27	-	55	-	0.4	6	-	0.3	0.4	176	1.9	33	3.5	168	258	824	2.4
-	-	49	-	120	-	0.5	11	-	0.7	0.6	416	3.7	53	7.6	320	487	1313	3.8
-	-	28	-	55	-	0.4	6	-	0.3	0.3	192	2.3	35	3.4	184	289	735	2.9
-	-	24	-	60	-	0.4	5	-	0.4	0.4	200	1.4	33	2.9	184	290	832	2.8
-	-	21	-	50	-	0.3	5	-	0.2	0.3	172	1.7	30	2.6	160	272	664	2.3
1	-	75	-	-	-	0.3	-	-	0.1	0.1	-	-	21	1.5	160	-	190	0.3
2	-	140	-	-	-	2	-	-	0.1	0.2	-	0.6	21	1.5	360	-	1150	0.9
2	-	85	-	-	-	0	-	-	0.1	0.3	-	-	21	1.9	160	-	50	0.3
1	-	70	-	-	-	0.1	-	-	0.1	0.1	-	0.4	21	11.4	160	-	60	0.9
1	-	70	-	-	-	0.6	-	-	0.1	0	-	-	28	0.8	200	-	200	0.3
2	-	50	-	-	-	0.4	-	-	0.1	-	-	-	53	1.9	240	-	260	1.5
1	-	70	-	-	-	0.3	-	-	-	0	16	-	21	1.5	48	-	95	0.3
1	-	65	-	-	-	0.1	-	-	0	0.1	32	-	28	1.5	200	-	70	0.3
1	-	85	-	-	-	0.2	-	-	0.1	0	-	-	21	2.9	160	-	180	0.3
1	-	60	-	-	-	0.3	-	-	-	0.2	-	-	28	2.9	240	-	105	-
1	-	130	-	-	-	1.2	-	-	0.3	0.1	-	1.5	28	7.6	200	-	115	7.5
2	-	100	-	-	-	1.6	-	-	0.2	0.1	48	-	70	1.9	320	-	900	6
1	-	210	-	-	-	2	-	-	-	0.1	16	0.8	35	1.1	160	-	410	1.5
0	-	65	-	-	-	0.4	-	-	0.1	0.1	-	-	21	0.4	64	-	90	0.3
4	-	310	-	-	-	2	-	-	0.2	0.2	320	0.8	53	2.9	320	-	550	6.8
5	-	100	-	-	-	0.8	-	-	0.4	0.2	16	0.8	21	5.7	200	-	250	1.2
1	-	80	-	40	-	0.2	-	-	0.1	0.1	-	1	14	0.8	64	-	95	0.3
5	-	80	-	-	-	0.2	-	-	0.1	0.2	16	-	35	6.7	240	-	60	0.3
1	-	90	-	-	-	1	-	-	0.2	0.1	-	-	28	0.4	160	-	90	0.3
4	-	90	-	-	-	1	-	-	0.2	0.1	80	-	21	2.9	200	-	90	0.9
1	-	85	-	-	-	0.6	-	-	0.1	0.1	-	-	21	0.8	120	-	95	0.3
1	-	70	-	-	-	0.3	-	-	0	0.1	-	-	21	4.8	120	-	140	0.3
1	-	200	-	-	-	0.5	-	-	0.1	-	48	-	88	3.8	400	-	1090	6
1	-	230	-	-	-	0.5	-	-	0	-	32	-	35	1.9	120	-	110	1.5
2	-	130	-	-	-	1.6	-	-	0.1	0	80	0.2	70	1.9	200	-	1630	6
2	-	50	-	-	-	2	-	-	0.1	0.4	-	-	35	7.6	280	-	60	0.3
2	-	150	-	-	-	1.2	-	-	0.3	0.2	-	2	35	7.6	280	-	115	9
1	-	100	-	20	-	0.3	-	-	0.1	0.1	-	-	28	3.8	80	-	140	0.6
2	-	70	-	-	-	1.6	-	-	0	0.1	-	0.6	35	13.3	240	-	70	0.3
7	6	133	-	-	-	-	-	-	-	-	-	-	-	-	-	1002	3199	-
7	5	133	63	67	0.5	2.3	5	5.1	0.3	0.3	64000	4.3	66	5.1	308	917	3139	6.1
4	6	84	43	83	0.5	0.4	15	4.2	0.4	0.5	96000	3.2	40	9.3	247	1055	2777	1.4
4	5	84	47	74	0.6	1	20	1.3	0.3	0.5	58000	3.1	66	12.5	384	971	2717	2.5
10	5	166	39	87	0.2	1.2	17	0.9	0.3	0.4	227000	2.9	28	3.8	315	876	2218	2.7
10	6	166	41	90	0.2	1.3	18	0.9	0.4	0.4	235000	3	29	3.9	327	1010	2278	2.8
4	5	73	45	174	0.3	0.8	17	3.8	0.4	0.5	304000	2.2	50	3.6	527	834	1710	2.8
4	6	73	-	-	-	-	-	-	-	-	-	-	-	-	-	918	2508	-

Code	Food Name	Amount	Unit	Grams	kCalories	Carbohydrate (gm)	Protein (gm)	Fat (gm)	Saturated Fat (gm)	Monounsaturated Fat (gm)
62565	Subway-Meat Ball Sandwich, on Italian Roll	1	12 In.	215	918	96	42	44	17	17
62566	Subway-Meat Ball Sandwich, on Wheat Roll	1	12 In.	224	947	101	44	45	17	18
62567	Subway-Roast Beef, on Italian Roll	1	12 In.	184	689	84	42	23	8	9
62568	Subway-Roast Beef, on Wheat Roll	1	12 In.	189	717	89	41	24	8	9
62569	Subway-Seafood, on Italian Roll	1	12 In.	210	986	94	29	57	11	15
62570	Subway-Seafood, on Wheat Roll	1	12 In.	219	1015	100	31	58	11	16
62571	Subway-Spicy Italian, on Italian Roll	1	12 In.	213	1043	83	42	63	23	28
62572	Subway-Steak and Cheese, on Italian Roll	1	12 In.	213	765	83	43	32	12	12
62573	Subway-Turkey Breast, on Wheat Roll	1	12 In.	192	674	88	42	20	6	7
58318	Taco Bell-Bean Burrito	1	Each	206	387	63	15	14	4	-
58319	Taco Bell-Beef Burrito	1	Each	206	431	48	25	21	8	-
58321	Taco Bell-Burrito Supreme	1	Each	198	440	55	20	22	8	-
62585	Taco Bell-Light 7-Layer Burrito	1	Each	276	440	67	19	9	-	-
62583	Taco Bell-Light Bean Burrito	1	Each	198	330	55	14	6	-	-
62586	Taco Bell-Light Burrito Supreme	1	Each	248	350	50	20	8	-	-
62584	Taco Bell-Light Chicken Burrito	1	Each	170	290	45	12	6	-	-
62587	Taco Bell-Light Chicken Burrito Supreme	1	Each	248	410	62	18	10	-	-
62582	Taco Bell-Light Chicken Soft Taco	1	Each	120	180	26	9	5	-	-
62575	Taco Bell-Light Soft Taco	1	Each	99	180	19	13	5	4	-
62581	Taco Bell-Light Soft Taco Supreme	1	Each	128	200	23	14	5	-	-
62574	Taco Bell-Light Taco	1	Each	78	140	11	11	5	4	-
62588	Taco Bell-Light Taco Salad	1	Each	464	330	35	30	9	-	-
62580	Taco Bell-Light Taco Supreme	1	Each	106	160	23	14	5	-	-
58328	Taco Bell-Mexican Pizza	1	Each	223	575	40	21	37	11	-
58325	Taco Bell-Nachos	1	Each	106	346	37	7	18	6	-
58323	Taco Bell-Nachos Bell Grande	1	Each	287	649	61	22	35	12	-
58329	Taco Bell-Pintos 'N Cheese	1	Each	128	190	19	9	9	4	-
58337	Taco Bell-Salsa	1	Each	10	18	4	1	0	0	-
58314	Taco Bell-Soft Taco	1	Each	92	225	18	12	12	5	-
58313	Taco Bell-Taco	1	Each	78	183	11	10	11	5	-
58332	Taco Bell-Taco Salad	1	Each	575	905	55	34	61	19	-
58333	Taco Bell-Taco Salad w/o Shell	1	Each	520	484	22	28	31	14	-
58316	Taco Bell-Tostada	1	Each	156	243	27	9	11	4	-
61273	Wendy's-Big Classic	1	Each	251	480	44	27	23	7	8
62322	Wendy's-Bkd Potato w/ Bacon and Cheese	1	Each	380	510	75	17	17	4	3
61287	Wendy's-Bkd Potato w/ Broccoli and Cheese	1	Each	411	450	77	9	14	2	3
62524	Wendy's-Bkd Potato w/ Cheese	1	Each	383	550	74	14	24	8	6
61281	Wendy's-Chicken Club Sandwich	1	Each	220	520	44	30	25	6	7
61292	Wendy's-Chili, Large	1	Each	340	290	31	28	9	4	2
61291	Wendy's-Chili, Small	1	Each	227	190	21	19	6	2	1
61285	Wendy's-French Fries, Biggie	1	Each	170	450	62	6	22	5	15
61284	Wendy's-French Fries, Medium	1	Each	136	360	50	5	17	4	12
61283	Wendy's-French Fries, Small	1	Each	91	240	33	3	12	2	8
61302	Wendy's-Frosty Dairy Dessert, Large	1	Each	402.2	570	95	15	17	9	4
61301	Wendy's-Frosty Dairy Dessert, Medium	1	Each	321.8	460	76	12	13	7	3
61300	Wendy's-Frosty Dairy Dessert, Small	1	Each	241.3	340	57	9	10	5	3
61271	Wendy's-Plain Single	1	Each	133	350	31	25	15	6	7
61272	Wendy's-Single w/ everything	1	Each	219	440	36	26	23	7	7
62477	White Castle-Cheeseburger Sandwich	1	Each	64.8	200	16	8	11	-	-
62481	White Castle-Chicken Sandwich	1	Each	63.8	186	20	8	7	-	-
62478	White Castle-Fish Sandwich, w/o Tartar	1	Each	59.3	155	21	6	5	-	-
62483	White Castle-French Fries	1	Each	96.9	301	38	2	15	-	-
62476	White Castle-Hamburger Sandwich	1	Each	58.5	161	15	6	8	-	-
62485	White Castle-Onion Chips	1	Each	92.1	329	39	4	17	-	-
62484	White Castle-Onion Rings	1	Each	60.2	245	27	3	13	-	-
62479	White Castle-Sausage and Egg Sandwich	1	Each	96.3	322	16	13	22	-	-
62480	White Castle-Sausage Sandwich	1	Each	48.7	196	13	7	12	-	-

Polyunsaturated Fat (gm)	Fiber (gm)	Cholesterol (mg)	Folate (μg)	Vitamin A (re)	Vitamin B6 (mg)	Vitamin B12 (μg)	Vitamin C (mg)	Vitamin E (mg)	Riboflavin (mg)	Thiamin (mg)	Calcium (mg)	Iron (mg)	Magnesium (mg)	Niacin (mg)	Phosphorus (mg)	Potassium (mg)	Sodium (mg)	Zinc (mg)
4	3	88	35	72	0.4	3.2	19	1	0.4	0.3	78000	5	47	9.4	263	1210	2022	6.2
4	-	88	-	-	-	-	-	-	-	-	-	-	-	-	-	1498	2082	-
4	5	83	54	58	0.4	2	5	4.4	0.3	0.2	55000	3.7	57	4.4	266	910	2288	5.3
4	6	75	56	59	0.4	2.1	5	4.5	0.3	0.2	56000	3.8	59	4.5	273	994	2348	5.4
28	-	56	91	107	0.3	6.5	5	2.5	0.4	0.5	230000	4.4	32	7	336	641	2027	5.3
28	3	56	-	-	-	-	-	-	-	-	-	-	-	-	-	557	1967	-
7	5	137	-	-	-	-	-	-	-	-	-	-	-	-	-	880	2282	-
4	6	82	36	119	0.4	2.5	6	0.8	0.5	0.3	231000	4.2	43	5.1	456	909	1556	6.8
7	7	67	-	-	-	-	-	-	-	-	-	-	-	-	-	605	2520	-
2	3	9	-	-	-	-	53	-	2	0.4	190	4	-	2.8	-	495	1148	-
2	2	57	-	-	-	-	2	-	0.3	0.4	150	3	-	3.2	-	380	1311	-
2	3	33	-	-	-	-	26	-	2.1	0.4	190	4	-	3.6	-	501	1181	-
-	-	5	-	350	-	-	5	-	-	-	300	2.5	-	-	-	-	1130	-
-	-	5	-	300	-	-	2	-	-	-	120	2	-	-	-	-	1340	-
-	-	25	-	600	-	-	9	-	-	-	96	1.5	-	-	-	-	1160	-
-	-	30	-	200	-	-	4	-	-	-	72	1.5	-	-	-	-	900	-
-	-	65	-	250	-	-	5	-	-	-	72	1.5	-	-	-	-	1190	-
-	-	30	-	150	-	-	5	-	-	-	48	0.8	-	-	-	-	570	-
1	2	25	-	40	-	-	0	-	0.2	0.4	48	0.6	-	2.8	-	196	554	-
-	-	25	-	100	-	-	2	-	-	-	48	0.6	-	-	-	-	610	-
1	1	20	-	40	-	-	0	-	0.1	0.1	0	0	-	1.2	-	159	276	-
-	-	50	-	1200	-	-	27	-	-	-	120	1.5	-	-	-	-	1610	-
-	-	20	-	100	-	-	2	-	-	-	0	0	-	-	-	-	340	-
10	3	52	-	-	-	-	31	-	0.3	0.3	257	4	-	3	-	408	1031	-
2	1	9	-	-	-	-	2	-	0.2	-	191	1	-	0.6	-	159	399	-
3	4	36	-	-	-	-	58	-	0.3	0.1	297	3	-	2.2	-	674	997	-
1	2	16	-	-	-	-	52	-	0.2	0.1	156	1	-	0.4	-	384	642	-
0	0	0	-	-	-	-	-	-	0.1	-	36	1	-	-	-	376	376	-
1	2	32	-	-	-	-	1	-	0.2	0.4	116	2	-	2.8	-	196	554	-
1	1	32	-	-	-	-	1	-	0.1	0.1	84	1	-	1.2	-	159	276	-
12	4	80	-	-	-	-	75	-	0.6	0.5	320	6	-	4.8	-	673	910	-
2	3	80	-	-	-	-	74	-	0.4	0.2	290	4	-	3.2	-	612	680	-
1	2	16	-	-	-	-	45	-	0.2	0.1	180	2	-	0.6	-	401	596	-
7	-	75	-	60	-	-	12	-	0.3	0.5	120	3.5	-	6.7	-	500	850	-
8	-	15	-	100	-	-	36	-	0.2	0.5	80	2.5	-	6.7	-	1370	1170	-
7	-	0	-	200	-	-	60	-	0.1	0.3	80	2.5	-	4.8	-	1310	450	-
7	-	30	-	150	-	-	36	-	0.2	0.3	240	2	-	3.8	-	1210	640	-
9	-	75	-	20	-	-	9	-	0.4	0.6	80	8	-	15.2	-	470	980	-
1	-	60	-	150	-	-	12	-	0.2	0.2	80	4.5	-	2.9	-	660	1000	-
1	-	40	-	100	-	-	6	-	0.1	0.1	64	3	-	1.9	-	440	670	-
1	-	0	-	-	-	-	12	-	0.1	0.3	16	0.8	-	3.8	-	950	280	-
1	-	0	-	-	-	-	9	-	0	0.2	16	0.6	-	2.9	-	760	220	-
1	-	0	-	-	-	-	6	-	0	0.2	-	0.4	-	1.9	-	510	150	-
1	-	70	-	100	-	-	-	-	1.4	0.2	400	1	-	0.8	-	1040	330	-
1	-	55	-	100	-	-	-	-	1	0.2	320	0.8	-	0.8	-	830	260	-
-	-	40	-	80	-	-	-	-	0.8	0.1	240	0.6	-	0.4	-	630	200	-
2	-	70	-	-	-	-	-	-	0.2	0.4	80	3	-	5.7	-	280	510	-
7	-	75	-	60	-	-	9	-	0.2	0.4	80	3	-	6.7	-	430	850	-
-	3	-	-	-	-	-	-	-	-	-	-	-	-	-	-	-	361	-
-	2	-	-	-	-	-	-	-	-	-	-	-	-	-	-	-	497	-
-	1	-	-	-	-	-	-	-	-	-	-	-	-	-	-	-	201	-
-	5	-	-	-	-	-	-	-	-	-	-	-	-	-	-	-	193	-
-	2	-	-	-	-	-	-	-	-	-	-	-	-	-	-	-	266	-
-	4	-	-	-	-	-	-	-	-	-	-	-	-	-	-	-	823	-
-	3	-	-	-	-	-	-	-	-	-	-	-	-	-	-	-	566	-
-	3	-	-	-	-	-	-	-	-	-	-	-	-	-	-	-	698	-
-	2	-	-	-	-	-	-	-	-	-	-	-	-	-	-	-	488	-

EXCHANGE LISTS

Groups/Lists	Carbohydrate (grams)	Protein (grams)	Fat (grams)	kCalories
CARBOHYDRATE GROUP				
Starch	15	3	1 or less	80
Fruit	15	—	—	60
Milk				
Skim	12	8	0–3	90
Low-fat	12	8	5	120
Whole	12	8	8	150
Other carbohydrates	15	varies	varies	varies
Vegetables	5	2	—	25
MEAT AND MEAT SUBSTITUTE GROUP				
Very lean	—	7	0–1	35
Lean	—	7	3	55
Medium-fat	—	7	5	75
High-fat	—	7	8	100
FAT GROUP	—	—	5	45

From American Diabetes Association, American Dietetic Association: *Exchange lists for meal planning*, rev, Chicago, 1995, ADA/ADA.

common measurements

3 tsp = 1 Tbsp	4 oz = ½ cup
4 Tbsp = ¼ cup	8 oz = 1 cup
5⅓ Tbsp = ⅓ cup	1 cup = ½ pint

Starch

One starch exchange equals 15 g carbohydrate, 3 g protein, 0-1 g fat, and 80 kcalories.

Bread

Bagel	½ (1 oz)
Bread, reduced-calorie	2 slices (1½ oz)
Bread, white, whole-wheat, pumpernickel, rye	1 slice (1 oz)
Bread sticks, crisp, 4 in long × ½ in	2 (⅔ oz)
English muffin	½
Hot dog or hamburger bun	½ (1 oz)
Pita, 6 in across	½
Roll, plain, small	1 (1 oz)
Raisin bread, unfrosted	1 slice (1 oz)
Tortilla, corn, 6 in across	1
Tortilla, flour, 7 to 8 in across	1
Waffle, 4½ in square, reduced-fat	1

Cereals and grains

Bran cereals	½ cup
Bulgur	½ cup
Cereals	½ cup
Cereals, unsweetened, ready-to-eat	¾ cup
Cornmeal (dry)	3 Tbsp

Couscous	⅓ cup
Flour (dry)	3 Tbsp
Granola, low-fat	¼ cup
Grape-Nuts	¼ cup
Grits	½ cup
Kasha	½ cup
Millet	¼ cup
Muesli	¼ cup
Oats	½ cup
Pasta	½ cup
Puffed cereal	1½ cups
Rice milk	½ cup
Rice, white or brown	⅓ cup
Shredded wheat	½ cup
Sugar-frosted cereal	½ cup
Wheat germ	3 Tbsp

Starchy vegetables

Baked beans	⅓ cup
Corn	½ cup
Corn on cob, medium	1 (5 oz)
Mixed vegetables with corn, peas, or pasta	1 cup
Peas, green	½ cup
Plantain	½ cup
Potato, baked or boiled	1 small (3 oz)
Potato, mashed	½ cup
Squash, winter (acorn, butternut)	1 cup
Yam, sweet potato, plain	½ cup

Crackers and snacks

Animal crackers	8
Graham crackers, 2½ in square	3
Matzoh	¾ oz
Melba toast	4 slices
Oyster crackers	24
Popcorn (popped, no fat added or low-fat microwave)	3 cups
Pretzels	¾ oz
Rice cakes, 4 in across	2
Saltine-type crackers	6
Snack chips, fat-free (tortilla, potato)	15-20 (¾ oz)
Whole-wheat crackers, no fat added	2-5 (¾ oz)

Dried beans, peas, and lentils

Count as 1 starch exchange, plus 1 very lean meat exchange.

Beans and peas (garbanzo, pinto, kidney, white, split, black-eyed)	½ cup
Lima beans	⅔ cup
Lentils	½ cup
Miso 🖋	3 Tbsp

Starchy foods prepared with fat

Count as 1 starch exchange, plus 1 fat exchange.

Biscuit, 2½ in across	1
Chow mein noodles	½ cup
Corn bread, 2 in-cube	1 (2 oz)

🖋 = 400 mg or more of sodium per serving.

Crackers, round butter type	6
Croutons	1 cup
French-fried potatoes	16-25 (3 oz)
Granola	¼ cup
Muffin, small	1 (1½ oz)
Pancake, 4 in across	2
Popcorn, microwave	3 cups
Sandwich crackers, cheese or peanut butter filling	3
Stuffing, bread (prepared)	⅓ cup
Taco shell, 6 in across	2
Waffle, 4½ in square	1
Whole-wheat crackers, fat added	4-6 (1 oz)

Food (Starch Group)	Uncooked	Cooked
Oatmeal	3 Tbsp	½ cup
Cream of Wheat	2 Tbsp	½ cup
Grits	3 Tbsp	½ cup
Rice	2 Tbsp	⅓ cup
Spaghetti	¼ cup	½ cup
Noodles	⅓ cup	½ cup
Macaroni	¼ cup	½ cup
Dried beans	¼ cup	½ cup
Dried peas	¼ cup	½ cup
Lentils	3 Tbsp	½ cup

Fruits

One fruit exchange equals 15 g carbohydrate and 60 kcalories. The weight includes skin, core, seeds, and rind.

Fruit

Apple, unpeeled, small	1 (4 oz)
Applesauce, unsweetened	½ cup
Apples, dried	4 rings
Apricots, fresh	4 whole (5½ oz)
Apricots, dried	8 halves
Apricots, canned	½ cup
Banana, small	1 (4 oz)
Blackberries	¾ cup
Blueberries	¾ cup
Cantaloupe, small	⅓ melon (11 oz) or 1 cup cubes
Cherries, sweet, fresh	12 (3 oz)
Cherries, sweet, canned	½ cup
Dates	3
Figs, fresh	1½ large or 2 medium (3½ oz)
Figs, dried	1½
Fruit cocktail	½ cup
Grapefruit, large	½ (11 oz)
Grapefruit sections, canned	¾ cup
Grapes, small	17 (3 oz)
Honeydew melon	1 slice (10 oz) or 1 cup cubes
Kiwi	1 (3½ oz)
Mandarin oranges, canned	¾ cup
Mango, small	½ fruit (5½ oz) or ½ cup
Nectarine, small	1 (5 oz)
Orange, small	1 (6½ oz)
Papaya	½ fruit (8oz) or 1 cup cubes

Peach, medium, fresh	1 (6 oz)
Peaches, canned	½ cup
Pear, large, fresh	½ (4 oz)
Pears, canned	½ cup
Pineapple, fresh	¾ cup
Pineapple, canned	½ cup
Plums, small	2 (5 oz)
Plums, canned	½ cup
Prunes, dried	3
Raisins	2 Tbsp
Raspberries	1 cup
Strawberries	1¼ cup whole berries
Tangerines, small	2 (8 oz)
Watermelon	1 slice (13½ oz) or 1¼ cup cubes

Fruit juice

Apple juice/cider	½ cup
Cranberry juice cocktail	⅓ cup
Cranberry juice cocktail, reduced-calorie	1 cup
Fruit juice blends, 100% juice	⅓ cup
Grape juice	⅓ cup
Grapefruit juice	½ cup
Orange juice	½ cup
Pineapple juice	½ cup
Prune juice	⅓ cup

Milk

One milk exchange equals 12 g carbohydrate and 8 g protein.

	Carbohydrate (grams)	Protein (grams)	Fat (grams)	Calories
Skim/very low-fat	12	8	0-3	90
Low-fat	12	8	5	120
Whole	12	8	8	150

Skim and very low-fat milk

0–3 g fat per serving

Skim milk	1 cup
½% milk	1 cup
1% milk	1 cup
Nonfat or low-fat buttermilk	1 cup
Evaporated skim milk	½ cup
Nonfat dry milk	⅓ cup dry
Plain nonfat yogurt	¾ cup
Nonfat or low-fat fruit-flavored yogurt sweetened with aspartame or with a nonnutritive sweetener	1 cup

Low fat

5 g fat per serving

2% milk	1 cup
Plain low-fat yogurt	¾ cup
Sweet acidophilus milk	1 cup

Whole milk

8 g fat per serving

Whole milk	1 cup
Evaporated whole milk	½ cup
Goat's milk	1 cup
Kefir	1 cup

Other Carbohydrates

Substitutes for a starch, fruit, or milk exchange. One exchange equals 15 g carbohydrate, or 1 starch, or 1 fruit, or 1 milk.

Food	Serving Size	Exchanges Per Serving
Angel food cake, unfrosted	¹⁄₁₂th cake	2 carbohydrates
Brownie, small, unfrosted	2 in square	1 carbohydrate, 1 fat
Cake, unfrosted	2 in square	1 carbohydrate, 1 fat
Cake, frosted	2 in square	2 carbohydrates, 1 fat
Cookie, fat-free	2 small	1 carbohydrate
Cookie or sandwich cookie with creme filling	2 small	1 carbohydrate, 1 fat
Cupcake, frosted	1 small	2 carbohydrates, 1 fat
Cranberry sauce, jellied	¼ cup	2 carbohydrates
Doughnut, plain cake	1 medium (1½ oz)	1½ carbohydrates, 2 fats
Doughnut, glazed	3¾ in across (2 oz)	2 carbohydrates, 2 fats
Fruit juice bars, frozen, 100% juice	1 bar (3 oz)	1 carbohydrate
Fruit snacks, chewy (pureed fruit concentrate	1 roll (¾ oz)	1 carbohydrate
Fruit spreads, 100% fruit	1 Tbsp	1 carbohydrate
Gelatin, regular	½ cup	1 carbohydrate
Gingersnaps	3	1 carbohydrate
Granola bar	1 bar	1 carbohydrate, 1 fat
Granola bar, fat-free	1 bar	2 carbohydrates
Hummus	⅓ cup	1 carbohydrate, 1 fat
Ice cream	½ cup	1 carbohydrate, 2 fats
Ice cream, light	½ cup	1 carbohydrate, 1 fat
Ice cream, fat-free, no sugar added	½ cup	1 carbohydrate
Jam or jelly, regular	1 Tbsp	1 carbohydrate
Milk, chocolate, whole	1 cup	2 carbohydrates, 1 fat
Pie, fruit, 2 crusts	⅙ pie	3 carbohydrates, 2 fats
Pie, pumpkin or custard	⅛ pie	1 carbohydrate, 2 fats
Potato chips	12-18 (1 oz)	1 carbohydrate, 2 fats
Pudding, regular (made with low-fat milk)	½ cup	2 carbohydrates
Pudding, sugar-free (made with low-fat milk)	½ cup	1 carbohydrate
Salad dressing, fat-free 🖊	¼ cup	1 carbohydrate
Sherbet, sorbet	½ cup	2 carbohydrates
Spaghetti or pasta sauce, canned 🖊	½ cup	1 carbohydrate, 1 fat
Sweet roll or Danish	1 (2½ oz)	2½ carbohydrates, 2 fats
Syrup, light	2 Tbsp	1 carbohydrate
Syrup, regular	1 Tbsp	1 carbohydrate
Syrup, regular	¼ cup	4 carbohydrates
Tortilla chips	6-12 (1oz)	1 carbohydrate, 2 fats
Yogurt, frozen, low-fat, fat-free	⅓ cup	1 carbohydrate, 0-1 fat
Yogurt, frozen, fat-free, no sugar added	½ cup	1 carbohydrate
Yogurt, low-fat with fruit	1 cup	3 carbohydrates, 0-1 fat
Vanilla wafers	5	1 carbohydrate, 1 fat

Vegetables

One vegetable exchange equals 5 g carbohydrate, 2 g protein, 0 g fat, and 25 kcalories.

Artichoke
Artichoke hearts
Asparagus
Beans (green, wax, Italian)
Bean sprouts
Beets
Broccoli
Brussels sprouts
Cabbage
Carrots
Cauliflower
Celery
Cucumber
Eggplant
Green onions or scallions
Greens (collard, kale, mustard, turnip)
Kohlrabi
Leeks
Mixed vegetables (without corn, peas, or pasta

Mushrooms
Okra
Onions
Pea pods
Peppers (all varieties)
Radishes
Salad greens (endive, escarole, lettuce, romaine, spinach)
Sauerkraut ✒
Spinach
Summer squash
Tomato
Tomatoes, canned
Tomato sauce ✒
Tomato/vegetable juice ✒
Turnips
Water chestnuts
Watercress
Zucchini

Meat and Meat Substitutes

	Carbohydrate (grams)	Protein (grams)	Fat (grams)	Calories
Very lean	0	7	0-1	35
Lean	0	7	3	55
Medium-fat	0	7	5	75
High-fat	0	7	8	100

Very lean meat and meat substitutes list

One exchange equals 0 g carbohydrate, 7 g protein, 0-1 g fat, and 35 kcalories.

Poultry: Chicken or turkey (white meat, no skin),
Cornish hen (no skin)   1 oz

Fish: Fresh or frozen cod, flounder, haddock,
halibut, trout, tuna, fresh or canned in water   1 oz

Shellfish: Clams, crab, lobster, scallops, shrimp,
imitation shellfish   1 oz

Game: Duck or pheasant (no skin), venison,
buffalo, ostrich   1 oz

Cheese with 1 g or less fat per ounce:
Nonfat or low-fat cottage cheese   ¼ cup
Fat-free cheese   1 oz

Other: Processed sandwich meats with 1 g or less
fat per ounce, such as deli thin, shaved meats,
chipped beef ✒ , turkey ham   1 oz
Egg whites   2
Egg substitutes, plain   ¼ cup
Hot dogs with 1 g or less fat per ounce ✒   1 oz
Kidney (high in cholesterol)   1 oz
Sausage with 1 g or less fat per ounce   1 oz
Count as one very lean meat and one starch exchange.
Dried beans, peas, lentils (cooked)   ½ cup

Lean meat and meat substitutes list

One exchange equals 0 g carbohydrate, 7 g protein, 3 g fat, and 55 kcalories.

Beef: USDA Select or Choice grades of lean beef trimmed of fat, such as round, sirloin, and flank steak; tenderloin; roast (rib, chuck, rump); steak (T-bone, porterhouse, cubed), ground round	1 oz
Pork: Lean pork, such as fresh ham; canned, cured, or boiled ham; Canadian bacon ✎ ; tenderloin, center loin chop	1 oz
Lamb: Roast, chop, leg	1 oz
Veal: Lean chop, roast	1 oz
Poultry: Chicken, turkey (dark meat, no skin), chicken white meat (with skin), domestic duck or goose (well-drained of fat, no skin)	1 oz
Fish:	
Herring (uncreamed or smoked)	1 oz
Oysters	6 medium
Salmon (fresh or canned), catfish	1 oz
Sardines (canned)	2 medium
Tuna (canned in oil, drained)	1 oz
Game: Goose (no skin), rabbit	1 oz
Cheese:	
4.5%-fat cottage cheese	¼ cup
Grated Parmesan	2 Tbsp
Cheeses with 3 g or less fat per ounce	1 oz
Other:	
Hot dogs with 3 g or less fat per ounce ✎	1½ oz
Processed sandwich meat with 3 g or less fat per ounce, such as turkey pastrami or kielbasa	1 oz
Liver, heart (high in cholesterol)	1 oz

Medium-fat meat and meat substitutes list

One exchange equals 0 g carbohydrate, 7 g protein, 5 g fat, and 75 kcalories.

Beef: Most beef products fall into this category (ground beef, meatloaf, corned beef, short ribs, prime grades of meat trimmed of fat, such as prime rib)	1 oz
Pork: Top loin, Boston butt, cutlet	1 oz
Lamb: Rib roast, ground	1 oz
Veal: Cutlet (ground or cubed, unbreaded)	1 oz
Poultry: Chicken dark meat (with skin), ground turkey or ground chicken, fried chicken (with skin)	1 oz
Fish: Any fried fish product	1 oz
Cheese: With 5 g or less fat per ounce	
Feta	1 oz
Mozzarella	1 oz
Ricotta	¼ cup (2 oz)
Other:	
Egg (high in cholesterol, limit to 3 per week)	1
Sausage with 5 g or less fat per ounce	1 oz
Soy milk	1 cup
Tempeh	¼ cup
Tofu	4 oz or ½ cup

High-fat meat and meat substitutes list

One exchange equals 0 g carbohydrate, 7 g protein, 8 g fat, and 100 kcalories.

Pork: Spareribs, ground pork, pork sausage	1 oz
Cheese: All regular cheeses, such as American 🖋 , cheddar, Monterey Jack, Swiss	1 oz
Other: Processed sandwich meats with 8 g or less fat per ounce, such as bologna, pimento loaf, salami	1 oz
Sausage, such as bratwurst, Italian, knockwurst, Polish, smoked	1 oz
Hot dog (turkey or chicken) 🖋	1 (10/lb)
Bacon	3 slices (20 slices/lb)

Count as one high-fat meat plus one fat exchange.

Hot dog (beef, pork, or combination) 🖋	1 (10/lb)
Peanut butter (contains unsaturated fat)	2 Tbsp

Fats

Monounsaturated fats list

One fat exchange equals 5 g fat and 45 kcalories.

Avocado, medium	⅛ (1 oz)
Oil (canola, olive, peanut)	1 tsp
Olives: ripe (black)	8 large
green, stuffed 🖋	10 large
Nuts	
almonds, cashews	6 nuts
mixed (50% peanuts)	6 nuts
peanuts	10 nuts
pecans	4 halves
Peanut butter, smooth or crunchy	2 tsp
Sesame seeds	1 Tbsp
Tahini paste	2 tsp

Polyunsaturated fats list

One fat exchange equals 5 g fat and 45 kcalories.

Margarine: stick, tub, or squeeze	1 tsp
lower-fat (30% to 50% vegetable oil)	1 Tbsp
Mayonnaise: regular	1 tsp
reduced-fat	1 Tbsp
Nuts, walnuts, English	4 halves
Oil (corn, safflower, soybean)	1 tsp
Salad dressing: regular 🖋	1 Tbsp
reduced-fat	2 Tbsp
Miracle Whip Salad Dressing: regular	2 tsp
reduced-fat	1 Tbsp
Seeds: pumpkin, sunflower	1 Tbsp

Saturated fats list

One fat exchange equals 5 g of fat and 45 kcalories.

Bacon, cooked	1 slice (20 slices/lb)
Bacon, grease	1 tsp
Butter: stick	1 tsp
whipped	2 tsp
reduced-fat	1 Tbsp
Chitterlings, boiled	2 Tbsp (½ oz)

Coconut, sweetened, shredded	2 Tbsp
Cream, half and half	2 Tbsp
Cream cheese: regular	1 Tbsp (1/2 oz)
reduced-fat	2 Tbsp (1 oz)
Fatback or salt pork, see below*	
Shortening or lard	1 tsp
Sour cream: regular	2 Tbsp
reduced-fat	3 Tbsp

Free Foods

>20 kcalories or >5 g carbohydrates per serving

Fat-free or reduced-fat foods

Limit to 3 servings/day	
Cream cheese, fat-free	1 Tbsp
Creamers, nondairy, liquid	1 Tbsp
Creamers, nondairy, powdered	2 tsp
Mayonnaise, fat-free	1 Tbsp
Mayonnaise, reduced-fat	1 tsp
Margarine, fat-free	4 Tbsp
Margarine, reduced-fat	1 tsp
Miracle Whip, nonfat	1 Tbsp
Miracle Whip, reduced-fat	1 tsp
Nonstick cooking spray	
Salad dressing, fat-free	1 Tbsp
Salad dressing, fat-free, Italian	2 Tbsp
Salsa	¼ cup
Sour cream, fat-free, reduced-fat	1 Tbsp
Whipped topping, regular or light	2 Tbsp

Sugar-free or low-sugar foods

Candy, hard, sugar-free	1 candy
Gelatin dessert, sugar-free	
Gelatin, unflavored	
Gum, sugar-free	
Jam or jelly, low-sugar or light	2 tsp
Sugar substitutes†	
Syrup, sugar-free	2 Tbsp

Drinks

Bouillon, broth, consommé 📝	
Bouillon or broth, low-sodium	
Carbonated or mineral water	
Cocoa powder, unsweetened	1 Tbsp
Coffee	

---

*Use a piece 1 inch × 1 inch × ¼ inch if you plan to eat the fatback cooked with vegetables. Use a piece 2 inches × 1 inch × ½ inch when eating only the vegetables with the fatback removed.

†Sugar substitutes, alternatives, or replacements that are approved by the Food and Drug Administration (FDA) are safe to use. Common brand names include: Equal (aspartame), Sprinkle Sweet (saccharin), Sweet One (acesulfame K), Sweet-10 (saccharin), Sugar Twin (saccharin), Sweet 'n Low (saccharin).

Club soda
Diet soft drinks, sugar-free
Drink mixes, sugar-free
Tea
Tonic water, sugar-free

Condiments

Catsup	1 Tbsp
Horseradish	
Lemon juice	
Lime juice	
Mustard	
Pickles, dill ✐	1½ large
Soy sauce, regular or light ✐	
Taco sauce	1 Tbsp
Vinegar	

Seasonings

Be careful with seasonings that contain sodium or are salts, such as garlic or celery salt, and lemon pepper.

Flavoring extracts
Garlic
Herbs, fresh or dried
Pimento
Spices
Tabasco or hot pepper sauce
Wine, used in cooking
Worcestershire sauce

Combination Foods

Food	Serving Size	Exchanges Per Serving
Entrees		
Tuna noodle casserole, lasagna, spaghetti with meatballs, chili with beans, macaroni and cheese ✐	1 cup (8 oz)	2 carbohydrates, 2 medium-fat meats
Chow mein (without noodles or rice)	2 cups (16 oz)	1 carbohydrate, 2 lean meats
Pizza, cheese, thin crust ✐	¼ of 10 in (5 oz)	2 carbohydrates, 2 medium-fat meats, 1 fat
Pizza, meat topping, thin crust ✐	¼ of 10 in (5 oz)	2 carbohydrates, 2 medium-fat meats, 2 fats
Pot pie ✐	1 (7oz)	2 carbohydrates, 1 medium-fat meat, 4 fats
Frozen entrees		
Salisbury steak with gravy, mashed potato ✐	1 (11 oz)	2 carbohydrates, 3 medium-fat meats, 3-4 fats
Turkey with gravy, mashed potato, dressing ✐	1 (11 oz)	2 carbohydrates, 2 medium-fat meats, 2 fats
Entree with less than 300 calories ✐	1 (8 oz)	2 carbohydrates, 3 lean meats
Soups		
Bean ✐	1 cup	1 carbohydrate, 1 very lean meat
Cream (made with water) ✐	1 cup (8 oz)	1 carbohydrate, 1 fat
Split pea (made with water) ✐	½ cup (4 oz)	1 carbohydrate
Tomato (made with water) ✐	1 cup (8 oz)	1 carbohydrate
Vegetable beef, chicken noodle, or other broth type ✐	1 cup (8 oz)	1 carbohydrate

Fast Foods

Food	Serving Size	Exchanges Per Serving
Burritos with beef	2	4 carbohydrates, 2 medium-fat meats, 2 fats
Chicken nuggets	6	1 carbohydrate, 2 medium-fat meats, 1 fat
Chicken breast and wing, breaded and fried	1 each	1 carbohydrate, 4 medium-fat meats, 2 fats
Fish sandwich/tartar sauce	1	3 carbohydrates, 1 medium-fat meat, 3 fats
French fries, thin	20-25	2 carbohydrates, 2 fats
Hamburger, regular	1	2 carbohydrates, 2 medium-fat meats
Hamburger, large	1	2 carbohydrates, 3 medium-fat meats, 1 fat
Hot dog with bun	1	1 carbohydrate, 1 high-fat meat, 1 fat
Individual pan pizza	1	5 carbohydrates, 3 medium-fat meats, 3 fats
Soft-serve cone	1 medium	2 carbohydrates, 1 fat
Submarine sandwich	1 sub (6 in.)	3 carbohydrates, 1 vegetable, 2 medium-fat meats, 1 fat
Taco, hard shell	1 (6 oz)	2 carbohydrates, 2 medium-fat meats, 2 fats
Taco, soft shell	1 (3 oz)	1 carbohydrate, 1 medium-fat meat, 1 fat

Meal Plan

Meal Plan for: _____   Date: _____

Dietitian: _____   Phone: _____

Carbohydrate
Protein
Fat
Calories

Grams   Percent
_____   _____
_____   _____
_____   _____

Time	Number of Exchanges/Choices	Menu Ideas	Menu Ideas
	Carbohydrate group _____ Starch _____ Fruit _____ Milk _____ Vegetables _____ Meat group _____ Fat group _____		
	_____ _____		
	Carbohydrate group _____ Starch _____ Fruit _____ Milk _____ ✓ Vegetables _____ Meat group _____ Fat group _____		
	_____ _____		
	Carbohydrate group _____ Starch _____ Fruit _____ Milk _____ ✓ Vegetables _____ Meat group _____ Fat group _____		
	_____ _____		

PLANNING INDIVIDUALIZED DIETS USING EXCHANGE LISTS

Step 1: Conduct Nutrition History

A 24-hour or 3-day recall (see Chapter 14) can be used to determine usual food intake. Categorize intake into exchanges (or servings) from each list at each meal and snack. Translate into kcalories and grams of carbohydrate, protein, and fat from exchanges. Round off kcalorie level to the nearest 50 or 100 kcalories. Calculations of food intake are not precise enough to allow more accuracy, and patients may consume an extra 50 to 60 kcalories/day from free foods (see Exchange Lists). When in doubt, round up instead of down. Determine percentages of carbohydrates, protein, and fat in current intake.

To determine total kcalories, add up the number of exchanges actually consumed from each Exchange Group. Multiply the number of exchanges by the number of kcalories in each Exchange Group.

Number of exchanges from starch list	= ____	×	80 kcal	= ____
Number of exchanges from fruit list	= ____	×	60 kcal	= ____
Number of exchanges from milk list	= ____	×	80 kcal (skim)	= ____
	= ____	×	120 kcal (low-fat)	= ____
	= ____	×	150 kcal (whole)	= ____
Number of exchanges from vegetable list	= ____	×	25 kcal	= ____
Number of exchanges from meat groups	= ____	×	35 kcal (very lean)	= ____
	= ____	×	55 kcal (lean)	= ____
	= ____	×	75 kcal (medium fat)	= ____
	= ____	×	100 kcal (high-fat)	= ____
Number of exchanges from fat list	= ____	×	45 kcal	= ____
			Total kcal	____

Using the total number of each Exchange Group, calculate the grams of carbohydrate (CHO), protein (PRO) and fat (FAT).

	Number of Exchanges CHO	Number of Exchanges PRO	Number of Exchanges FAT
Bread list	____ × 15g = ____g	____ × 2g = ____g	____ × 0-3g = ____g
Fruit list	____ × 15g = ____g	____ × 0g = ____g	____ × 0g = ____g
Milk list			
Skim	____ × 12g = ____g	____ × 8g = ____g	____ × 0g = ____g
Low fat	____ × 12g = ____g	____ × 8g = ____g	____ × 5g = ____g
Whole	____ × 12g = ____g	____ × 8g = ____g	____ × 8g = ____g
Vegetable list	____ × 5g = ____g	____ × 2g = ____g	____ × 0g = ____g
Meat list			
Very lean	____ × 0g = ____g	____ × 7g = ____g	____ × 0-1g = ____g
Lean	____ × 0g = ____g	____ × 7g = ____g	____ × 3g = ____g
Medium-fat	____ × 0g = ____g	____ × 7g = ____g	____ × 5g = ____g
High-fat	____ × 0g = ____g	____ × 7g = ____g	____ × 8g = ____g
Fat group	____ × 0g = ____g	____ × 0g = ____g	____ × 5g = ____g
	Total ____	Total ____	Total ____

Take total kcalories from above and determine the percentage of the diet that is carbohydrate, protein, and fat:

A.   Multiply total grams CHO × 4 kcal = ____kcal
   Multiply total grams PRO × 4 kcal = ____kcal
   Multiply total grams FAT × 9 kcal = ____kcal
   Total   ____kcal

B. Divide each nutrient's total kcalories by the total kcalories for the day, and multiply by 100 to get the percentage of kcalories.

Kcal from CHO × 100 = % kcal from CHO   ___ × 100 = ___
Total kcal

Kcal from PRO × 100 = % kcal from PRO   ___ × 100 = ___
Total kcal

Kcal from FAT × 100 = % kcal from FAT   ___ × 100 = ___
Total kcal

Step 2: Calculate Daily Kilocalorie Requirements

Kcalorie needs are based on age, weight, and activity level. Use the Harris-Benedict equation to calculate energy needs. Round figure to nearest 100 kcalories. Subtract kcalories if weight loss is desired. Reducing kcaloric intake by 500 kcal/day will theoretically produce a 1 lb weight loss per week. Never reduce kcaloric level to below that required for basal energy needs.

Example: CG is a 62-year-old female with NIDDM. She is 5′5″ tall (medium frame), and weighs 140 lb. CG walks 10-12 miles per week at the mall.

$$655.1 + [9.6 \times \text{wt (kg)}] + [1.8 \times \text{ht (cm)}] - [4.7 \times \text{age (yrs)}]$$
$$655.1 + [9.6 \times 63.6 \text{ kg}] + [1.8 \times 165.1 \text{ cm}] - [4.7 \times 62]$$
$$655.1 + 610.6 + 297.2 - 291.4 = 1271.5 \text{ kcalories}$$
$$1271.5 \text{ kcalories} \times 1.3 \text{ (activity factor)} = 1652.95 \text{ kcalories}$$
Round off to 1700 kcalories

If weight loss is desired, subtract 500 kcalories: 1700 − 500 = 1200 kcalories, which is below her basal energy needs of 1271.5 kcalories. Adjust to 1300 kcalories if weight loss is determined to be a treatment goal.

Step 3: Determine Distribution of Carbohydrate, Protein, and Fat Kcalories

This should be based on the patient's usual intake, blood glucose levels, blood lipid levels, and treatment goals.

Example: CG's 24-hr recall indicates an intake of approximately 1500 kcalories distributed into 17% protein, 30% fat, and 53% carbohydrate. Her pertinent lab values: glycosylated hemoglobin is 6%, cholesterol 210 mg/dl, LDL-cholesterol 179 mg/dl, HDL-cholesterol 55 mg/dl. Although her lipid levels are at the high end of normal or just slightly above normal, her exercise and eating habits appear to be sufficient to control her blood glucose levels. In this case, you would distribute her kcalories in the same pattern as found in her diet recall:

Carbohydrate: 1500 kcalories × .53 = 795 kcal ÷ 4 kcal/gm = 199 gm
Protein: 1500 kcal × .17 = 255 kcal ÷ 4 kcal/gm = 64 gm
Fat: 1500 kcal × .30 = 450 kcal ÷ 9 kcal/gm = 50 gm

Step 4: Determine Servings From Each Exchange List

These calculations are based on the amount of carbohydrate, protein, and fat in each exchange list and the patient's preferences for foods within each list or group. The type of milk the patient uses should be calculated into the meal plan. Skim milk and low-fat milks are recommended, but whole milk can be used if the patient will not drink the others. Although lean meats should be encouraged, when calculating fat grams per meat serving, use the fat value that best represents actual intake. People do not need to add or subtract fat exchanges when using different meat categories.

Example: CG's usual eating pattern indicates she uses the following amounts from the milk, vegetable, and fruit exchange groups:

	Servings	Carbohydrates (gm)	Protein (gm)	Fat (gm)	Kcal
Milk, skim	1	12	8	1	90
Vegetables	4	20	8	0	100
Fruits	4	60	0	0	240
Carbohydrate Subtotal		92	16	1	430

The starch exchange list is the only group remaining that provides carbohydrates. To determine the number of servings to be used from this group, subtract the total grams of carbohydrate (92 gm) from the milk, vegetable, and fruit lists from the total grams of carbohydrate (199 gm) in the meal plan. This amount is divided by 15 gm carbohydrate/serving in the starch list.

	Servings	Carbohydrates (gm)	Protein (gm)	Fat (gm)	Kcal
Carbohydrate Subtotal		92	24	1	460
Starches	7	105	21	7	560
Protein Subtotal		197	45	8	1020

The meat exchange list is the only group remaining that provides protein. To determine the number of servings to be used from this group, subtract the total grams of protein (48 gm) from the milk, vegetable, and starch lists from the total grams of protein (56 gm) in the meal plan. This amount is divided by 7 gm protein/serving in the meat list.

	Servings	Carbohydrates (gm)	Protein (gm)	Fat (gm)	Kcal
Protein Subtotal		197	45	8	1020
Meat/lean	4	0	28	12	220
Fat Subtotal		197	73	20	1240

The fat exchange list is the only group remaining that provides fat. To determine the number of servings to be used from this group, subtract the total grams of fat (20 gm) from the milk, starch, and meat lists from the total grams of fat (50 gm) in the meal plan. This amount is divided by 5 gm fat/serving in the fat list.

	Servings	Carbohydrates (gm)	Protein (gm)	Fat (gm)	Kcal
Fat Subtotal		197	73	20	1240
Fats	6	0	0	30	270
TOTAL		197	73	50	1510

Note: When calculating the number of servings from each exchange list, round to the nearest whole number. It is usually impractical to calculate and plan half servings from the lists.

The daily distribution of servings from the exchange lists is as follows. These servings can now be divided into the appropriate number of meals and snacks per day.

Exchange List Group	Servings	Carbohydrates (gm)	Protein (gm)	Fat (gm)	Kcalories
Carbohydrates	12				
Starches	7	105	21	7	560
Fruit	4	60	0	0	240
Milk (skim)	1	0	0	30	270
Vegetables	4	20	8	1	90
Meats/lean	4	0	28	12	220
Fats	6	0	0	30	270

Modified from American Dietetic Association: *Exchange lists for meal planning*, Alexandria Va, 1995, American Diabetes Association; American Dietetic Association, *Handbook of clinical dietetics*, ed 2, New Haven, 1992, Yale University Press; Davis JR, Sherer K: *Applied nutrition and diet therapy for nurses*, ed 2, Philadelphia, 1994, Saunders; American Dietetic Association: Nutrition recommendations and principles for people with diabetes mellitus, *J Am Diet Assoc* 94:504-506, 1994; and Tinker LF, Heins JM, Holler HJ: Commentary and translation: 1994 nutrition recommendations for diabetes, *J AM Diet Assoc* 94:507-511, 1994.

NUTRITION AND HEALTH ORGANIZATIONS: SOURCES OF NUTRITION INFORMATION

Journals of Professional Organizations

This list only includes nutrition journals. A number of nursing and medical journals also feature nutrition-related articles and studies. The asterisked (*) journals are most recommended based on the applicability of their subject content to the nursing setting and/or ease of availability in most libraries.

American Journal of Clinical Nutrition
*American Journal of Public Health**
Annual Review of Nutrition
British Journal of Nutrition
*FDA Consumer**
Human Nutrition: Allied Nutrition
Human Nutrition: Clinical Nutrition
Journal of the American College of Nutrition
*Journal of the American Dietetic Association**

*Journal of the Canadian Dietetic Association**
Journal of Food Service
Journal of Food Technology
Journal of Nutrition
*Journal of Nutrition Education**
Journal of Nutrition for the Elderly
Journal of Nutrition Reviews
*Journal of Nutrition Today**

Newsletters

Contemporary Nutrition
General Mills, Inc.
Production Manager
P.O. Box 1112, Department 65
Minneapolis, MN 55440
(inexpensive)

CNI Nutrition Week
Community Nutrition Institute
2001 South St. N.W.
Washington, DC 20009

Dairy Council Digest
National Dairy Council
6300 River Rd.
Rosemont, IL 60018
(inexpensive)

Dietetic Currents
Ross Laboratories
Director of Professional Services
625 Cleveland Ave.
Columbus, OH 43216
(free)

Environmental Nutrition
52 Riverside Dr.
New York, NY 10024

Food and Nutrition News
National Livestock and Meat Board
444 Michigan Ave.
Chicago, IL 60610
(free)

Harvard Medical School Health Letter
Department of Continuing Education
25 Shattuck St.
Boston, MA 02115

Healthline
830 Menlo Ave. #100
Menlo Park, CA 94025

National Council Against Health Fraud Newsletter (NCAHF)
P.O. Box 1276
Loma Linda, CA 92354

Nutrition Forum
George Stickley Co.
210 Washington Square
Philadelphia, PA 19106

Nutrition & the M.D.
P.O. Box 2160
Van Nuys, CA 91404

Nutrition Research Newsletter
P.O. Box 700
Pallisades, NY 10964

*Tufts University Diet & Nutrition
Letter*
P.O. Box 10948
Des Moines, IA 50940

Professional Association Organizations

American Academy of Pediatrics
P.O. Box 1034
Evanston, IL 60204

American Cancer Society
777 Third Ave.
New York, NY 10017

American Dental Association
211 E. Chicago Ave.
Chicago, IL 60611

American Diabetes Association
2 Park Ave.
New York, NY 10016

American Dietetic Association
216 W. Jackson Blvd.
Suite 800
Chicago, IL 60606

American Geriatrics Society
770 Lexington Ave.
Suite 400
New York, NY 10021

American Heart Association
7320 Greenville Ave.
Dallas, TX 75231

American Home Economics Association
2010 Massachusetts Ave. N.W.
Washington, DC 20036

American Institute of Nutrition
9650 Rockville Pike
Bethesda, MD 20014

American Medical Association
Nutrition Information Section
535 N. Dearborn St.
Chicago, IL 60610

American Public Health Association
1015 Fifteenth St. N.W.
Washington, DC 20005

American Society for Clinical
Nutrition
9650 Rockville Pike
Bethesda, MD 20014

The Canadian Diabetes Association
123 Edward St.
Suite 601
Toronto, Ontario M5G 1E2 Canada

The Canadian Dietetic Association
480 University Ave.
Suite 601
Toronto, Ontario M5G 1V2 Canada

The Canadian Society for Nutritional
Sciences
Department of Foods and Nutrition
University of Manitoba
Winnipeg, Manitoba, R3T 2N2 Canada

Food and Nutrition Board
National Research Council
National Academy of Sciences
2101 Constitution Ave. N.W.
Washington, DC 20418

Institute of Food Technologies
211 N. LaSalle St.
Chicago, IL 60601

National Council on the Aging
1828 L St. N.W.
Washington, DC 20036

National Institute of Nutrition
1335 Carling Ave.
Suite 210
Ottawa, Ontario K1Z 0L2 Canada

Nutrition Foundation, Inc.
1126 Sixteenth St. N.W.
Suite 111
Washington, DC 20036

Nutrition Today Society
428 E. Preston St.
Baltimore, MD 21202

Society for Nutrition Education
2001 Killebrew Dr. #340
Minneapolis, MN 55425-1882

Professional or Lay Advocacy Organizations

Bread for the World
802 Rhode Island Ave. N.E.
Washington, DC 20018

Center for Science in the Public Interest
  (CSPI)
1755 S. Street N.W.
Washington, DC 20009

California Council Against Health
  Fraud, Inc.
P.O. Box 1276
Loma Linda, CA 92354

Children's Foundation
1420 New York Ave. N.W.
Suite 800
Washington, DC 20005

Food Research and Action Center
  (FRAC)
1875 Connecticut Ave. N.W. #540
Washington, DC 20009

Institute for Food and Development
  Policy
1885 Mission St.
San Francisco, CA 94103

La Leche League International, Inc.
9616 Minneapolis Ave.
Franklin Park, IL 60131

March of Dimes Birth Defects Foundation
  (National Headquarters)
1275 Mamaroneck Ave.
White Plains, NY 10605

Overeaters Anonymous (OA)
2190 190th St.
Torrance, CA 90504

Oxfam America
115 Broadway
Boston, MA 02116

Local Resources

Cooperative extension agents in county extension offices
Dietitians (contact the state or local Dietetics Association)
Nutrition faculty affiliated with department of food and nutrition, home economics, and dietetics
Registered dieticians (RDs) in city, county, or state agencies

Government Agencies

United States
The Consumer Information Center
Department 609K
Pueblo, CO 81009

Department of Agriculture (USDA)
Extension Services
3 South Building
Room 6007
Washington, DC 20250

Food and Drug Administration (FDA)
5600 Fishers Lane
Rockville, MD 20852

Food and Nutrition Information and
  Education Resources Center
National Library of Congress
Beltsville, MD 20705

Human Nutrition Research Division
Agricultural Research Center
Beltsville, MD 20705

Office of Cancer Communications
National Cancer Institute
Building 31
Room 10A18
90 Rockville Pike
Bethesda, MD 20205

National Agricultural Library
10301 Baltimore Blvd.
Room 304
Beltsville, MD 20705

National Center for Health Statistics
3700 East-West
Hyattsville, MD 20782

US Government Printing Office
The Superintendent of Documents
Washington, DC 20402

Canada

Department of Community Health
1075 Ste-Foy Rd.
Seventh Floor
Quebec, Quebec G1S 2M1

Home Economics Directorate
880 Portage Ave.
Second Floor
Winnipeg, Manitoba R3G 0P1

Nutrition Programs
446 Jeanne Mance Building
Tunney's Pasture
Ottawa, Ontario K1A 1B4

Nutrition Services
P.O. Box 488
Halifax, Nova Scotia B3J 3R8

Nutrition Services
P.O. Box 6000
Fredericton, New Brunswick
 E3B 5H1

Public Health Resource Service
15 Overlea Blvd.
Fifth Floor
Toronto, Ontario M4H 1A9

United Nations

Food and Agriculture Organization
 (FAO)
North American Regional Office
1325 C St. S.W.
Washington, DC 20025
  or
Via della Terma di Caracella
0100 Rome, Italy

World Health Organization (WHO)
1211 Geneva 27
Switzerland

Trade Organizations and Companies

American Egg Board
1460 Renaissance St.
Park Ridge, IL 60068

American Institute of Baking
P.O. Box 1148
Manhattan, KS 66502

American Meat Institute
P.O. Box 3556
Washington, D.C. 20007

Best Foods
Consumer Service Department
Division of CPC International
International Plaza
Englewood Cliffs, NJ 07632

Borden Farm Products
Bordon Co.
Consumer Affairs
180 E. Broad St.
Columbus, OH 43215

Campbell Soup Co.
Food Service Products Division
375 Memorial Ave.
Camden, NJ 08101

Del Monte Teaching Aids
P.O. Box 9075
Clinton, IA 52736

Fleischman's Margarines
Standard Brands, Inc.
625 Madison Ave.
New York, NY 10022

General Foods Consumer Center
250 North St.
White Plains, NY 10625

General Mills
P.O. Box 113
Minneapolis, MN 55440

Gerber Products Co.
445 State St.
Fremont, MI 49412

H.J. Heinz
Consumer Relations
P.O. Box 57
Pittsburgh, PA 15230

Hunt-Wesson Foods
Education Services
1654 W. Valencia Dr.
Fullerton, CA 92634

Kellogg Co.
Department of Home Economics
  Services
Battle Creek, MI 49016

Mead Johnson Nutritionals
2404 Pennsylvania Ave.
Evansville, IN 47721

National Dairy Council
6300 N. River Rd.
Rosemont, IL 60018-4233

Oscar Mayer Co.
Consumer Service
P.O. Box 1409
Madison, WI 53701

Pillsbury Co.
1177 Pillsbury Building
608 Second Ave. S.
Minneapolis, MN 55402

The Potato Board
1385 S. Colorado Blvd.
Suite 512
Denver, CO 80222

Rice Council
P.O. Box 22802
Houston, TX 77027

Ross Laboratories
Director of Professional Services
625 Cleveland Ave.
Columbus, OH 43216

Sunkist Growers Consumer Service
Division BB, P.O. Box 7888
Valley Annex
Van Nuys, CA 91409

Vitamin Nutrition Information Service
  (VNIS)
Hoffmann-LaRoche
340 Kingsland Ave.
Nutley, NJ 07110

United Fresh Fruit and Vegetables
  Association
727 N. Washington St.
Alexandria, VA 22314

LIFETIME MANAGEMENT OF BODY FAT LEVELS: RESOURCES

Organizations

Association for the Health Enrichment of Large People: A clinical organization for professionals who work with large people. Contact Joe McVoy, PhD, P.O. Drawer C, Radford, VA 24143; 1-800-368-3468, Ext. 501.

Council on Size & Weight Discrimination: An organization dedicated to influencing public policy and opinion in order to end oppression related to body weight, size, or shape. Contact the Council at P.O. Box 238, Columbia, MD 21045.

National Association for the Advancement of Fat Acceptance: An organization that provides information, support, and leadership in advocacy regarding the needs and rights of fat persons. Contact NAAFA, P.O. Box 188620, Sacramento, CA 95818; 916-443-0303.

Society for Nutrition Education: A professional association of nutrition educators and other health professionals with involvement in nutrition education. Within this organization the Division of Nutrition and Weight Realities addresses size acceptance and nondiet approaches. Contact SNE, 2001 Killebrew Drive, Suite 340, Minneapolis, MN 55425-1882; 612-854-0035.

In addition to these organizations there is an ever-increasing number of more geographically localized groups. In most cases you can learn of these through one of the organizations above.

Magazines

BBW, a fashion magazine for large women that promotes self acceptance and expanded definitions of beauty. *BBW Magazine,* P.O. Box 16958, North Hollywood, CA 91615.

Radiance, a magazine devoted to the positive health and well-being of women of all sizes of large. *Radiance,* P.O. Box 30246, Oakland, CA 94604.

Self-help Books

There have been numerous helpful books published in the last few years; these listed are only a representative sampling. Check the health and psychology sections of your favorite bookstores (but beware of the many traditional diet books there).

Fanning P: *Lifetime weight control,* Oakland, Calif, 1990, New Harbinger.

Foreyt JP, Goodrick GK: *Living without dieting,* Houston, 1992, Harrison Publishing.

Hall L: *Full lives: Women who have freed themselves from food & weight obsession,* Carlsbad, Calif, 1993, Gürze Books.

Hirschmann JR, Munter CH: *Overcoming overeating,* Reading, Mass, 1988, Addison-Wesley Publishing.

Omichinski L: *You count, calories don't,* Winnipeg, Manitoba, 1993, Tamos Books.

Roth G: *Why weight? A guide to ending compulsive eating,* New York, 1989, Penguin Books.

Materials for Professionals

Ciliska D: *Beyond dieting: Psychoeducational interventions for chronically obese women,* New York, 1990, Brunner/Mazel.

Healthy Weight Journal (formerly *Obesity & Health*). A bimonthly review journal. Healthy Living Institute, Route 2, Box 905, Hettinger, ND 58639; 701-567-2845.

EATING DISORDERS

Organizations (for professionals and the public)

AABA-American Anorexia/Bulimia Association, 293 Central Park West, New York, NY 10024; (212) 501-8351.

ANAD-National Association of Anorexia Nervosa and Associated Disorders, P.O. Box 7, Highland Park, IL 60035; (847) 831-3438.

Anorexia Nervosa and Related Eating Disorders, Inc, P.O. Box 5102, Eugene, OR 97405; (503)-344-1144.

Professional Organization (membership for health professionals only)

Academy for Eating Disorders, Business Office—c/o Division of Adolescent Medicine, Montefiore Medical Center, 111 East 210th St, Bronx, NY 10467; (718)-920-6782.

LACTOSE CONTENT OF FOODS

L actose contents are approximate, depending on portion size and product preparation. Foods not listed do not usually contain lactose. Most individuals can experiment with different lactose-containing foods to determine their level of tolerance. Although dairy products all contain lactose, the lactose in some products is reduced by processing.

Low-Lactose Foods

Lactose-reduced milk
  (nonfat, skim, low-fat, whole)
Sherbert
Processed foods containing dry
  milk solids or whey
Aged cheese (cheddar, Swiss)
Processed cheese (depending on
  milk solids added)
Butter/margarine

Commercial bread or cake products
  (bread, muffins, pancakes,
  waffles, biscuits)
Ready-to-eat cereals containing
  milk/lactose
Yogurt (may be tolerated)
Drug preparations (tablets) may
  contain lactose as filler
  (usually tolerated)

High-Lactose Foods

Milk (nonfat, skim, low-fat, whole)
  powdered milk
  evaporated milk
  half and half
  cream
  buttermilk
Cream cheese
Sour cream
Milk-related products
  ice cream (regular and low-fat),
   ice milk, frozen yogurt
  pudding, custard
  cheese cake, cream pies

creamy sauces (white sauce,
  Alfredo sauce, vegetables
  au gratin)
salad dressings with milk
cream or milk soups
cottage cheese (nonfat, low-fat,
  regular)
ricotta cheese
yogurt
cold cuts and wieners/frankfurters
  (some may contain varying amounts
  of lactose)

From Nelson JK et al: *Mayo Clinic diet manual,* ed 7, St. Louis, 1994, Mosby; and Dietary Department, University of Iowa Hospital and Clinics, Iowa City: *Recent advances in therapeutic diets,* ed 4, Ames, Iowa, 1989, Iowa State University Press.

Appendix E

VALUES FOR COMMON LABORATORY TESTS

Assessment of Iron Status

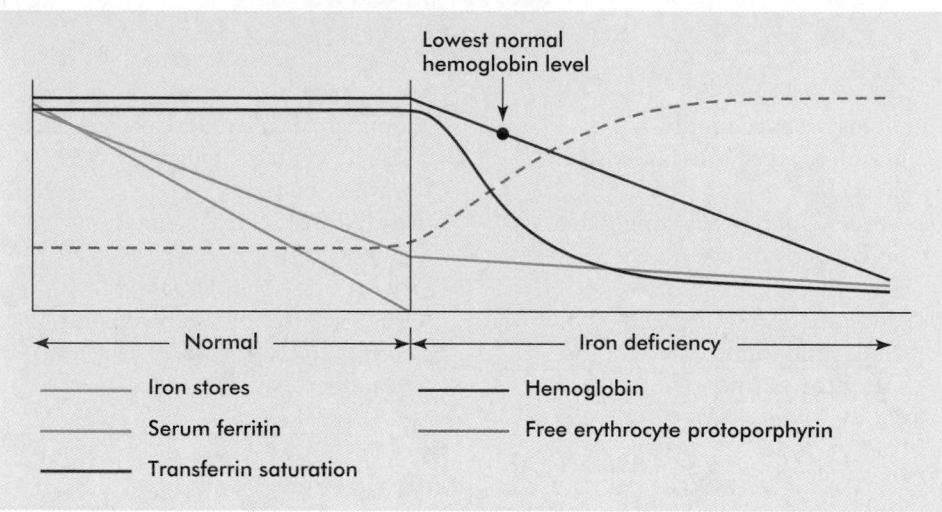

Fig. E-1 Relationship between various indicators of iron status and the body's level of iron stores.

Table E-1 Criteria for Assessment of Iron Status With Levels Indicative of Deficiency					
Age (Years)	Hemoglobin (g/dl)	Serum Ferritin (pg/ml)	Transferrin Saturation (%)	Erythrocyte Protoporphyrin (µg/dl Red Blood Cells)	Mean Corpuscular Volume (cu µ)
1–2	<9	<10	<10	>100	<73
3–4	<10	<10	<14	>100	<75
5–10	<10	<10	<15	>100	<76
11–14	<12 (male)	<10	<16	>100	<78
	<10 (female)	<10	<10	>100	<78
15–74	<12 (male)	<12	<16	>100	<80
	<10 (female)	<12	<12	>100	<80

Table E-2   Changes in Measures of Iron Status Indicative of Developing Iron Deficiency

Measures of Iron Status	Normal	Iron Depletion	Iron-Deficient Erythropoiesis	Iron-Deficient Anemia
Iron stores (bone marrow, liver, spleen)	Adequate	Very low	0	0
Erythron iron (iron in red blood cells)	Normal	Normal	Slightly reduced	Less than half of normal
TIBC (µg/dl)	330	360	390	410
Iron absorption	Normal	Increased	Increased	Increased
Plasma iron (µg/dl)	115-50	115	60	40
Transferrin saturation (%)	35	35	16	16
Red blood cell protoporphyrin (µg/dl in red blood cell)	30	30	100	100
Erythrocytes	Normal	Normal	Normal	Microcytic hypochromic
Hemoglobin (g/dl)	12	12	12	<12

TIBC, Total iron binding capacity.

VITALITY—A FRESH APPROACH

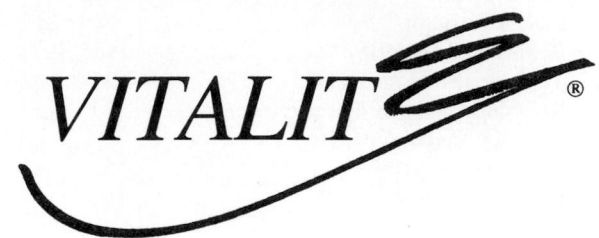

Vitality. It's an approach to life that promotes the idea of personal choice—of taking charge of how you eat, how you can stay active daily and how you can feel good about yourself. Most of all, *Vitality* is about enjoying life.

Vitality is a new concept that has evolved from consensus-building initiated in 1986 by Health and Welfare Canada, to promote healthy body weights. This work pointed out that a broad range of body weights and sizes can be "healthy." It depends on the individual. What was needed was a broader view of well-being and healthy living. Hence, *Vitality* was born—a fresh approach to living that corresponds with enjoying eating well, being active, and feeling good about yourself.

Eating well means choosing from a wide variety of foods that you enjoy. This includes emphasizing breads, other grain products, vegetables, and fruit. It also includes lower-fat dairy products, leaner meats, and foods prepared with little or no fat. If you eat a treat, balance it by staying active and eating a wide variety of foods for the rest of the day. Health and Welfare Canada's new *Guidelines for Healthy Eating* can help you make enjoyable choices.

Enjoying being active, "your way, every day," is the key to "active living." This concept, developed under the leadership of Fitness and Amateur Sport, means finding ways to enjoy being active every day, at home, at work or within your community. It may be walking to the store, taking the kids to the park, mowing the lawn, or going dancing with someone special. The only thing better than personal activity is sharing it with family and friends you care about.

Feeling good about yourself starts with accepting who you are and how you look. Healthy, good-looking bodies come in a broad range of sizes. Being proud of how your body looks and moves and believing in your own self-worth are more important than societal pressures to be perfect. *Vitality* suggests taking charge of your life and enjoying time with family and friends.

One of the key partners in promoting *Vitality* is ParticipACTION. Its *Vitality* commercials, public service announcements, and articles appear on television, and in magazines and newspapers. Health and Welfare Canada and Fitness and Amateur Sport are developing programs to help Canadians make *Vitality* part of their daily lives. They also are inviting professionals, educators, and other social influencers to encourage an environment that can make *Vitality* happen. For further information, please call (613) 941-2648.

Summary Examples of Recommended Nutrient Intake Based on Age and Body Weight Expressed as Daily Rates

Age	Gender	Weight (kg)	Protein (g)	Vit. A (RE)*	Vit. D (µg)	Vit. E (mg)	Vit. C (mg)	Folate (µg)	Vit. B_{12} (µg)	Calcium (mg)	Phosphorus (mg)	Magnesium (mg)	Iron (mg)	Iodine (µg)	Zinc (mg)
Months															
0–4	Both	6.0	12†	400	10	3	20	25	0.3	250‡	150	20	0.3§	30	2
5–12	Both	9.0	12	400	10	3	20	40	0.4	400	200	32	7	40	3
Years															
1	Both	11	13	400	10	3	20	40	0.5	500	300	40	6	55	4
2–3	Both	14	16	400	5	4	20	50	0.6	550	350	50	6	65	4
4–6	Both	18	19	500	5	5	25	70	0.8	600	400	65	8	85	5
7–9	M	25	26	700	2.5	7	25	90	1.0	700	500	100	8	110	7
7–9	F	25	26	700	2.5	6	25	90	1.0	700	500	100	8	95	7
10–12	M	34	34	800	2.5	8	25	120	1.0	900	700	130	8	125	9
10–12	F	36	36	800	2.5	7	25	130	1.0	1100	800	135	8	110	9
13–15	M	50	49	900	2.5	9	30	175	1.0	1100	900	185	10	160	12
13–15	F	48	46	800	2.5	7	30	170	1.0	1000	850	180	13	160	9
16–18	M	62	58	1000	2.5	10	40‖	220	1.0	900	1000	230	10	160	12
16–18	F	53	47	800	2.5	7	30‖	190	1.0	700	850	200	12	160	9
19–24	M	71	61	1000	2.5	10	40‖	220	1.0	800	1000	240	9	160	12
19–24	F	58	50	800	2.5	7	30‖	180	1.0	700	850	200	13	160	9
25–49	M	74	64	1000	2.5	9	40‖	230	1.0	800	1000	250	9	160	12
25–49	F	59	51	800	2.5	6	30‖	185	1.0	700	850	200	13	160	9
50–74	M	73	63	1000	5	7	40‖	230	1.0	800	1000	250	9	160	12
50–74	F	63	54	800	5	6	30‖	195	1.0	800	850	210	8	160	9
75+	M	69	59	1000	5	6	40‖	215	1.0	800	1000	230	9	160	12
75+	F	64	55	800	5	5	30‖	200	1.0	800	850	210	8	160	9
Pregnancy (additional)															
1st Trimester			5	0	2.5	2	0	200	1.2	500	200	15	0	25	6
2nd Trimester			20	0	2.5	2	10	200	1.2	500	200	45	5	25	6
3rd Trimester			24	0	2.5	2	10	200	1.2	500	200	45	10	25	6
Lactation (additional)			20	400	2.5	3	25	100	0.2	500	200	65	0	50	6

From Scientific Review Committee: *Nutrition recommendations*, Ottawa, Canada, 1990, Health and Welfare.

*Retinol equivalents.

†Protein is assumed to be from breast milk and must be adjusted for infant formula.

‡Infant formula with high phosphorus should contain 375 mg calcium.

§Breast milk is assumed to be the source of the mineral.

‖Smokers should increase vitamin C by 50%.

KCALORIE-RESTRICTED DIETARY PATTERNS

The most successful and safest approach to permanent weight loss is to adopt and maintain healthy lifestyle behaviors. Achieving weight loss through these means, as described in Chapter 10, may be a long-term process and for some individuals, regardless of dietary and lifestyle changes, original weight levels may be retained.

Certain medical conditions that are often improved by weight loss may be so detrimental to health that the physical and psychological risks of kcalorie-restricted diets are outweighed by the benefits of faster weight loss. Below are brief reviews of the primary formats of these diets and a guide for comparison of weight-loss programs.

Moderate Restriction of Kcalories

Kcalorie restriction should be at least 500 kcal less than the individual's daily requirement for energy; the amount of daily kcaloric intake should not be lower than about 1200 kcal. Adults, depending on their gender, height, and weight, may lose weight at intakes between 1200 kcal to 1500 kcal. Intake below this level cannot provide sufficient amounts of nutrients unless supplements are prescribed. The diet should still follow general dietary guidelines and provide about 55% kcal from carbohydrates, about 12% to 15% kcal from protein and 20% to 30% kcal from fat.

The Exchange List for Meal Planning is often used to implement kcalorie-restricted diets. By prescribing the number of each exchange allowed, the individual can then design a dietary pattern based on personal taste preference and scheduling. The following exchanges equal about 1200 kcal: 2 carbohydrates as milk, 3 vegetable, 4 fruit, 5 carbohydrate (either as starch, milk, fruit or vegetables), 5 lean meat, and 3 fat.

Formula Diets

Developed by pharmaceutical and food manufacturers, these solutions are available in a variety of forms. Designed to replace meals, they may provide a daily total of about 900 kcal and often contain or may be supplemented by vitamins and minerals. Although helpful for quick weight loss, the loss is rarely maintained, as boredom with the solution and the lack of learning new eating approaches soon leads to the weight being regained.

Very Low Calorie Diets (VLCD)

These diets are intended for use by morbidly obese individuals whose medical condition depends on weight loss for improvement. Containing only 200 kcal to 800 kcal, a VLCD causes rapid weight loss but increases the risk of electrolyte imbalances, gout, gallstones, and other related symptoms. Individuals must be

From American Dietetic Association: Position of the American Dietetic Association: Very-low-calorie weight-loss diets, *J Am Diet Assoc* 90:722, 1990.

under the complete and regular supervision of a physician. ADA has developed medical nutrition intervention procedures for use of VLCD. Maintenance of the weight loss is very difficult and depends on nutritional counseling, exercise, and lifestyle changes.

COMPARISON OF WEIGHT-LOSS* PROGRAMS

Do-It-Yourself Programs

Overeaters Anonymous (OA)

Approach/method. Nonprofit international organization that provides volunteer support groups worldwide patterned after the 12-step Alcoholics Anonymous program. Addresses physical, emotional, and spiritual recovery aspects of compulsive overeating. Members encouraged to seek professional help for individualized diet/nutrition plan and for any emotional or physical problems.

Clients. Individuals who define themselves as compulsive eaters.

Staff. Nonprofessional volunteer group members who meet specific criteria lead meetings, sit on the board, and conduct activities.

Expected weight-loss/length of program. Makes no claims for weight loss. Unlimited length.

Cost. Self-supporting with member contributions and sales of publications (includes workbooks, tapes, newsletters, and sponsor outreach programs. Its international monthly journal, *Lifeline,* costs $12.99/year.

Healthy lifestyle components. Recommends emotional, spiritual, and physical recovery changes. Makes no exercise or food recommendations.

Comments. Inexpensive. Provides group support. No need to follow a specific diet plan to participate. Minimal organization at the group level, so groups vary in approach. No health-care providers on staff.

Availability. 10,500 groups in 47 countries. Headquarters: Rio Rancho, NM; (505) 891-2664.

TOPS (Take Off Pounds Sensibly)

Approach/method. Nonprofit support organization of 310,000 members who meet weekly in groups. Does not prescribe or endorse particular eating or exercise regimen. Mandatory weigh-in at weekly meetings. Provides peer support. Uses award programs for healthy lifestyle changes; special recognition given to best weight losers. Members who maintain their goal weight loss for 3 months become members of KOPS (Keep Off Pounds Sensibly).

Clients. Members must submit weight goals and diets obtained from a health professional in writing.

Staff. Each group elects a volunteer (non-health professional) to direct and organize activities for one year. Health professionals, including RDs and psychologists, may be invited to speak at weekly meetings. Organization consults with a medical advisor.

Expected weight loss/length of program. No claims made for weight loss. Unlimited length.

Cost. First visit free. $16 annual fee ($20 in Canada) for the first 2 years; $14 annually thereafter ($18 in Canada). Includes 40-page quarterly magazine from company headquarters. Weekly meetings cost 50 cents to $1.

Thomas P, ed: *Weighing the Options: Criteria for evaluating weight-management programs,* Washington, DC, 1995, National Academy Press.

Healthy lifestyle components. No official lifestyle or exercise recommendations, but endorses slow, permanent lifestyle changes. Members encouraged to consult health-care provider for an exercise regimen to meet their needs.

Comments. Inexpensive form of continuing group support. Used as adjunct to professional care. Nonprofit and noncommercial, so no purchases required. Encourages long-term participation. Lacks professional guidance at chapter level since meetings run by volunteers. Groups vary widely in approach.

Availability. 11,700 chapters in 20 countries, mostly US and Canada. Headquarters: Milwaukee, WI; (800) 932-8677.

Nonclinical Programs

Diet Center

Approach/method. Focuses on achieving healthy body composition through diet and personalized exercise recommendations under the name *Exclusively You Weight Management Program.* Diet based on regular supermarket food; Diet Center prepackaged cuisine is optional. Body-fat analysis via electrical impedance taken at start of program and every 4 to 6 weeks thereafter. Clients encouraged to visit center daily for weigh-in. Calorie levels individualized to meet client needs and goals. Minimum level: 1200 kcal/day. Four phases: 2-day conditioning phase prepares dieter for reducing. Reducing phase used until goal achieved. Stabilization, the third phase, has clients adjusting calories and physical activity to maintain weight. Maintenance, the fourth phase, lasts for 1 year. One-to-one counseling. Some group meetings available.

Clients. Not allowed to join: pregnant, lactating, anorectic, bulimic, and underweight individuals, and those under 18 years of age. Require physician's written approval: those with more than 50 pounds to lose, kidney or heart disease, diabetes, cancer, or emphysema.

Staff. Clients consult with nonprofessional counselors who typically are program graduates trained by Diet Center. Two staff RDs and scientific advisors made up of a variety of health professionals design program at corporate level.

Expected weight loss/length of program. Not more than 1.5 to 2 lb weekly. Length will vary with individualized client goals, but 1-year maintenance program strongly encouraged.

Cost. Varies. Ranges from about $35 to $50/week. The 1-year maintenance is a one-time flat fee ranging from $50 to $200. Some centers charge additional one-time fee for all body composition analyses and adjustments in diet and exercise goals.

Healthy lifestyle components. *Exclusively Me* behavior management, as an ongoing part of the program, includes an activity book, audio tapes, and counseling. Used in conjunction with regular one-to-one sessions; counselor helps clients design personal solutions to weight-control problems.

Comments. Emphasizes body composition, not pounds, as a measure of health. Does not require the purchase of Diet Center food for preparation. Professional guidance lacking at the client level. Little group support available. Vitamin supplement required.

Availability. 700 centers in US, Canada, Bermuda, Guam, and South America. Headquarters: Pittsburgh, PA; (800) 333-2581.

Jenny Craig

Approach/method. *Personal Weight Management* menu plans based on Jenny Craig's cuisine with additional store-bought foods. Diet ranges from 1000 to 2600 kcal, depending on client needs. Mandatory weekly one-to-one counseling; group workshops. After clients lose half their goal, they begin planning their own meals using their own foods.

Clients. Not allowed to join: individuals who are underweight, pregnant, or those below age 13; those with celiac disease, diabetes (who inject more than twice daily or who are under 18 years of age), or allergies to ubiquitous ingredients in company's food products. Require physician's written permission: individuals with 18 additional conditions. Regardless of condition, clients encouraged to communicate with personal physician throughout program.

Staff. Program developed by corporate RDs and psychologists. Company consults with advisory board of MDs, RDs, and PhDs on program design. Consultants trained by Jenny Craig to implement program and offer support and motivational strategies. Corporate dietitians available for client questions or concerns at no extra charge.

Expected weight loss/length of program. Clients encouraged to set reasonable weight goals based on personal history and healthy weight standards. Program designed to produce weight loss of 1 to 2 lb/week. A separate, 12-month maintenance program is also offered.

Cost. To join: $99 to $299, depending on option. Prices vary per inclusion of home audio- and videocassettes. Most expensive price includes *Lifestyle Maintenance* program. Jenny Craig cuisine costs average $70 weekly.

Healthy lifestyle components. Clients use program guides to learn cognitive behavioral techniques for relapse prevention and problem management for lifestyle changes. Based on individual priorities, clients address major factors involved with weight management (for example, exercise, which is addressed through a physical activity module and a walking program). Individual consultations; group workshops provide motivation and peer exchange. The *Lifestyle Maintenance* program addresses issues such as body image and maintaining motivation to exercise.

Comments. Little food preparation. Vegetarian and kosher meal plans available; also plans for diabetic, hypoglycemic, and breastfeeding clients. Recipes provided. Must rely on Jenny Craig cuisine for participation. Lack of professional guidance at client level.

Availability. 800 centers in five countries; 650 centers in US Headquarters: Del Mar, Calif; (800) 94-JENNY.

Nutri/System

Approach/method. Menu plans based on Nutri/System's prepared meals with additional grocery foods. Clients receive individual calorie levels ranging from 1000 to 2200 kcal/day. Multivitamin-mineral supplement available for clients. Personal counseling and group sessions available.

Clients. Not allowed to join: individuals who are pregnant, under 14 years of age, underweight, or anorectic. Require physician's written permission: lactating women and those with a variety of conditions including diabetes (if require insulin shots), heart disease (that limits normal activity), and kidney disease.

Staff. Staff dietitians, health educators, and PhDs develop program at corporate level. Scientific Advisory Board consisting of MDs and PhDs employed for program design. Counselors with education and experience in psychology, nutrition, counseling, and health-related fields provide weekly guidance to clients. Certified Personal Trainers administer the Personal Trainer Program developed in conjunction with Johnson & Johnson Advanced Behavioral Technologies, Inc. RDs available through a toll-free number to address client questions.

Expected weight loss/length of program. Averages 1.5 to 2 lb/week. Clients select weight goal based on a recommended weight range using standard tables. Program length varies with weight-loss goals.

Cost. Varies. Clients can lose all desired weight for $99. Unlimited service program costs $249. Food costs average $49/week. Vitamin-mineral supplements, at-home cholesterol test, motivational audiotapes, and exercise audio/videocassettes available at additional cost.

Healthy lifestyle components. Wellness and Personal Trainer services developed in conjunction with Johnson & Johnson Health Management have been added to the program.

Comments. Few decisions about what to eat; relatively rigid diet with company foods. Portion-controlled Nutri/System foods allow dieters to focus more on making lifestyle changes than on the reducing diet. Program provides both Wellness and Personal Trainer services. Little contact with health professionals.

Availability. 650 centers in US and Canada. Headquarters: Horsham, PA; (215) 442-5411.

Weight Watchers

Approach/method. Emphasis on portion control and healthy lifestyle habits. Dieters choose from regular supermarket food, *Weight Watchers Personal Cuisine* (available in select markets to members only), or both. Reducing phase: Women average 1250 kcal daily; men 1600 daily. Levels for weight maintenance determined individually. Weekly group meetings with mandatory weigh-in. Must need to lose at least 5 lb to join.

Clients. Not allowed to join: those not weighing at least 5 pounds above the lowest end of their healthy weight range and those with a medically diagnosed eating disorder. Require physician's written approval: pregnant and lactating women and children under 10 years of age.

Staff. Group leaders are non-health professional graduates of program (Lifetime Members) trained by Weight Watchers. Program developed by corporate RDs. Company consults with medical advisor and advisory board consisting of MDs and PhDs on program design. Health professionals at corporate level, including RDs, direct program.

Expected weight loss/length of program. Up to 2 lb weekly. Unlimited length. Special 2-week *Superstart* program offers more rapid initial weight loss. Maintenance plan is 6 weeks.

Cost. $17-$20 to join; $10-$13 weekly. Fee entitles member to unlimited meetings for that week. Monthly meetings are free for Lifetime Members who have completed maintenance plan and maintain their weight goal within 2 lb. *Personal Cuisine* prices vary, averaging about $70 weekly.

Healthy lifestyle components. Emphasizes making positive lifestyle changes, including regular exercise. Encourages daily minimum physical activity level.

Comments. Flexible program offering group support and well-balanced diet. Vegetarian plan available, plus healthy eating plans for pregnant and breastfeeding women. Encourages long-term participation for members to attain their weight-loss goals. Lacks professional guidance at client level. No personalized counseling except in select markets.

Availability. 29,000 weekly meetings in 24 countries. Headquarters: Jericho, NY; (516) 939-0400.

Clinical Programs

Health Management Resources (HMR)

Approach/method. Medically supervised very-low-calorie diet (VLCD) of fortified, high-protein liquid meal replacements (520 to 800 kcal daily) or a low-calorie option consisting of liquid supplements and prepackaged HMR entrees (800 to 1300 kcal daily). Dieters receive HMR Risk Factor Profile that measures and displays an individual's medical and lifestyle health risks. Mandatory weekly 90-minute group meetings. Maintenance meetings are 1 hour per week. One-to-one counseling. Need to have BMI >30 for VLCD.

Clients. Contraindications: pregnancy, lactation, and acute substance abuse. Require physician's written approval: some with acute psychiatric disorders, recent heart disease, cancer, renal or liver disease, insulin-dependent diabetes mellitus, and those who test positive for acquired immunodeficiency syndrome (AIDS).

Staff. Program developed by MDs, RDs, RNs, and psychologists. Each location has at least one MD and health educator on staff. Participants assigned "personal coaches" (RDs, exercise physiologists, health educators) who help dieters learn and practice weight-management skills. Dieters on VLCD see MD or RN weekly.

Expected weight loss/length of program. Averages 2 to 5 lb weekly. Reducing phase varies according to weight-loss needs, but averages 12 weeks; refeeding phase (after liquids only) lasts about 6 weeks. Maintenance program recommended for up to 18 months.

Cost. Varies depending on diet chosen and medical conditions. Ranges from $80 to $130/week including medical visits. Cost may be covered by insurance. Maintenance is $60-$90/month.

Healthy lifestyle components. Recommends every client burn a minimum of 2000 kcal in physical activity weekly. Advocates consuming a diet with no more than 30 percent of calories from fat and at least 35 servings of fruits and vegetables per week. Emphasizes lifestyle issues in weekly classes and in personal coaching.

Comments. Emphasizes exercise as a means for weight loss and control. Few decisions about what to eat. Supervised by a health professional. Requires a strong commitment to physical activity. Side effects of VLCD may include intolerance to cold, constipation, dizziness, dry skin, and headaches. All options include liquid supplement; diet is very high in protein, even at higher calorie levels.

Availability. 180 hospitals and medical settings nationwide. Headquarters: Boston, MA; (617) 357-9876.

Medifast

Approach/method. Medifast is a physician-supervised very-low-calorie diet program of fortified meal replacements containing 450 to 500 kcal/day. *Lifestyles— The Medifast Program of Patient Support* prepares patients to maintain their goal weight after completing the VLCD. Medifast also provides a low-calorie diet of approximately 860 kcal/day for those not indicated for the VLCD.

Clients. Contraindications: those who are not at least 30 percent above ideal body weight, those who have not reached sexual and physical maturation, pregnant and lactating women, those with a history of cerebrovascular accident, and those with conditions such as anorexia nervosa, bulimia, recent myocardial infarction, unstable angina, insulin-dependent diabetes, thrombophlebitis, active cancer, and uncompensated renal or hepatic disease.

Staff. Program supervised by a physician. At the corporate level, a medical advisory board of MDs, PhDs, and RDs is consulted on program development.

Expected weight loss/length of program. Physician and patient arrive at an individualized goal weight. Metropolitan Life Insurance Company tables, Dietary Guidelines for Americans, and BMI charts used as guides. Weight loss varies with individual; average weight loss is 3 to 5 lb/week. Weight Reduction Phase lasts 16 weeks, and Realimentation Phase lasts 4 to 6 weeks. Maintenance strongly encouraged for up to 1 year.

Cost. Cost for office visits, laboratory tests, and Medifast products vary by individual physician. The program ranges from $65 to $85/week. Costs may be covered by insurance.

Healthy lifestyle components. The Medifast program includes a comprehensive education program called *LifeStyles* that includes behavior modification, recommended physical activity, and nutrition education. Instruction booklets and patient guides provided, including quarterly newsletter to patients.

Comments. Close contact with one or more health professionals. Low calorie level promotes quick weight loss. Extensive product line. Company products and regular foods incorporated when VLCD not recommended. Must rely on company products during reducing phase. Maintenance program assists with transition to regular foods.

Availability. 15,000 physicians nationwide, primarily in office-based settings, and in six foreign countries. Headquarters: Jason Pharmaceuticals, Inc., Owings Mills, Md; (410) 581-8042.

New Direction

Approach/method. The New Direction System includes a medically supervised VLCD program of fortified meal replacements with 600 to 840 kcal/day. The OUTLook and ShapeWise programs are moderate-calorie programs of 1000 to 1500 kcal/day and include the use of regular food and fortified bars and beverages.

Clients. Contraindications to VLCD: women with less than 40 pounds to lose and men with less than 50 pounds to lose (except in special cases), those less than 18 years of age, pregnant and lactating women, and those with conditions such as insulin-dependent (type 1) diabetes, metastatic cancer, recent myocardial infarction, liver disease requiring protein restriction, and renal insufficiency.

Staff. Weekly sessions in the New Direction and OUTLook programs are led by health professionals with degrees in dietetics, exercise physiology, behavioral counseling, or related fields. One-on-one counseling in each discipline is part of the program. Each program has a medical director.

Expected weight loss/length of program. In the New Direction program, average weight losses of 3 lb/week after the first few weeks are common. In the OUTLook and ShapeWise programs, losses greater than 2 lb/week are grounds for concern (after the first 2 weeks). The Reducing Phase averages 12 to 16 weeks, the Adapting Phase (with transition to regular food) lasts 5 weeks, and the Sustaining Phase is a minimum of 6 months (12 months preferred). Ongoing care is encouraged.

Cost. Varies with the program chosen, amount of weight to lose, and medical conditions. An approximate range is $40/week in the OUTLook and ShapeWise programs; $110 to $120/week in the Reducing Phase of the VLCD and $0 to $20/week in the later phases. Costs may be covered by insurance.

Healthy lifestyle components. Weekly classes have a strong behavioral component with an emphasis on problem-solving and lifestyle skills development in nutrition and exercise.

Comments. Individualized care and close contact with health professionals. Must rely on company products during the Reducing Phase of VLCD program. Transition from VLCD to regular food requires supervision. Low calorie level promotes quick weight loss, most beneficial for people with certain health problems. Clients make few decisions about what to eat while on the VCLD. OUTLook and ShapeWise programs include regular food.

Availability. Headquarters: Ross Products Division, Abbott Laboratories, Columbus, Ohio; (614) 624-7573.

Optifast

Approach/method. Medically supervised program of fortified liquid meal replacements and/or fortified food bars, eventually including more regular foods. Dieters assigned an 800-, 950-, or 1200-kcal plan. Weekly sessions on how to change eating behavior and one-to-one counseling.

Clients. Not allowed to join: individuals less than 30 percent or less than 50 pounds over desirable weight (corresponding to a BMI of approximately 30 to 32) and those less than 18 years of age. Contraindications for the low-calorie protocol include pregnant and lactating women and individuals with recent acute myocardial infarction or unstable angina, insulin-dependent (type I) diabetes mellitus, and advanced liver or kidney disease.

Staff. Dieters seen regularly by MDs, RNs, RDs, and psychologists at most locations; exercise physiologist used on consulting basis. Group meeting leaders are psychologists or dietitians. Meetings often include RDs. Clients assigned case manager who coordinates care.

Expected weight loss/length of program. Program limits weight loss to 2% of body weight weekly. *Active Weight Loss Plan* lasts for about 13 weeks. Transition phase lasts for about 6 weeks. Maintenance, which begins at 20th week, is encouraged. No time limit on maintenance.

Cost. Varies with type of diet and length of program. Costs range from $1500 to $3000, depending on health status and the amount of weight to lose. Price may include maintenance at some centers. Insurance may cover a portion of cost.

Healthy lifestyle components. Emphasis on behavior modification and diet planning for "real food" in group and counseling sessions. Exercise physiologist available to help design personal exercise plan.

Comments. Close contact with health professionals. Controlled calorie level promotes quick weight loss, most beneficial for people with certain health problems. Clients make few decisions about what to eat. Must rely on Optifast products during reducing phase.

Availability. Numerous hospitals and clinics in US and foreign countries. Headquarters: Sandoz Nutrition, Minneapolis, MN (800) 662-2540.

Physicians in a multidisciplinary program

Approach/method. Multidisciplinary programs may provide a program similar to HMR, New Direction, or Optifast. They may also provide food-based weight-loss programs or modifications of the two approaches. The multidisciplinary aspect implies the coordination of services, availability of individual and/or group counseling, and comprehensive medical supervision.

Staff. Typically physicians, dietitians, behavior therapists, exercise physiologists, psychologists, and counselors working individually and in group settings. Service providers should be licensed and regulated and should have their activities scrutinized by peers.

Expected weight loss/length of program. Variable and adapted to the needs of patient. There should be a maintenance program with continuing patient access to services for sustaining care and reinforcement. Patient use of medications and consequences of surgery will be monitored.

Cost. Varies with approach used and duration. Some programs will use a standard professional fee-for-service schedule of charges; others will use a single charge for a comprehensive set of services for a specified period of time. Potential for reimbursement from health-insurance plans. A packaged set of services may be substantially less expensive than the individual services in a fee-for-service arrangement.

Health lifestyle components. Varies. All recognized factors in weight management will be considered.

Comments. Similar to, but more extensive services than physicians working alone. Professional staff coordinates all aspects of care and long-term management of obesity. Diverse staff is able to adapt care to the needs of patients, including the management of associated medical problems. These are often university-based programs, which have structured peer-review mechanisms and may conduct research. Costs for professional services tend to be high.

Availability. Very limited.

Others

Registered dietitians (RDs)

Approach/method. Highly personalized approach to weight loss and maintenance.

Clients. Those acceptable and not acceptable will vary with the RD.

Staff. RDs have, at a minimum, baccalaureate degrees in nutrition or closely related field and have completed approved or accredited clinical training. Often have advanced degrees. RDs must pass a registration examination given by the Commission on Dietetic Registration of the American Dietetic Association and participate in continuing education.

Expected weight loss/length of program. Varies according to weight goal. Clients rarely encouraged to lose more than 2 lb weekly.

Cost. Varies across the country, but can range from $35 to $150 per hour. Fees for weight-control groups may be substantially less than for individual counseling.

Healthy lifestyle components. Exercise encouraged as part of safe, sensible weight-control program. RDs help clients identify barriers to weight loss and maintenance, and provide education about healthy lifestyles.

Comments. Highly adaptable. Personalized approach to clients' health concerns. Trained health professionals who can address medical history and account for it in diet therapy, if necessary. Appropriate for any age group. Can be expensive.

Availability. Located in every state in private practice, outpatient hospital clinics, health maintenance organizations (HMOs), and in practice with MDs. For a free referral to a local RD, call (800) 366-1655.

Physicians practicing alone

Approach/method. Individualized approach to weight loss and maintenance. Patients able to coordinate the management of their weight with concurrent management of associated medical problems. Services can be adapted to specific needs. Options include medications and surgery to treat obesity.

Staff. Individual physicians possibly working with associates (for example, nurses and physicians' assistants). Provision of services by licensed professional health-care providers.

Expected weight loss/length of program. Varies with patient. Program may be of indefinite length and should be coordinated with care of related or unrelated medical issues.

Cost. Varies. Fees will be comparable to those charged for comparable medical services. Cost may be reduced by reimbursement from health-insurance companies and avoidance of duplication of services in referrals for medical care by nonprofessional programs.

Healthy lifestyle components. Varies with the physician and weight-loss approach. Should include exercise and nutrition counseling.

Comments. Professional care. Coordination with other medical problems. Appropriate for patients with complex or serious associated medical problems. Long-term attention in the context of other medical care can be provided. The potential for using medications and/or surgery expands the opportunities for patients at varying stages of their disease. Individual physicians have the ability to vary the patient's care and intensity of the effort depending on the patient's life circumstances. Physicians often inadequately trained in nutrition and in low-calorie physiology. Cost for services can be high.

Availability. Generally available, but many physicians are reluctant to treat obesity because of their lack of interest or training, recognition that support services that they cannot provide are needed, and concern for the limited usefulness of their intervention.

INFANT AND CHILD GROWTH CHARTS

Girls: birth to 36 months physical growth NCHS percentiles*

Name_____ Record #_____

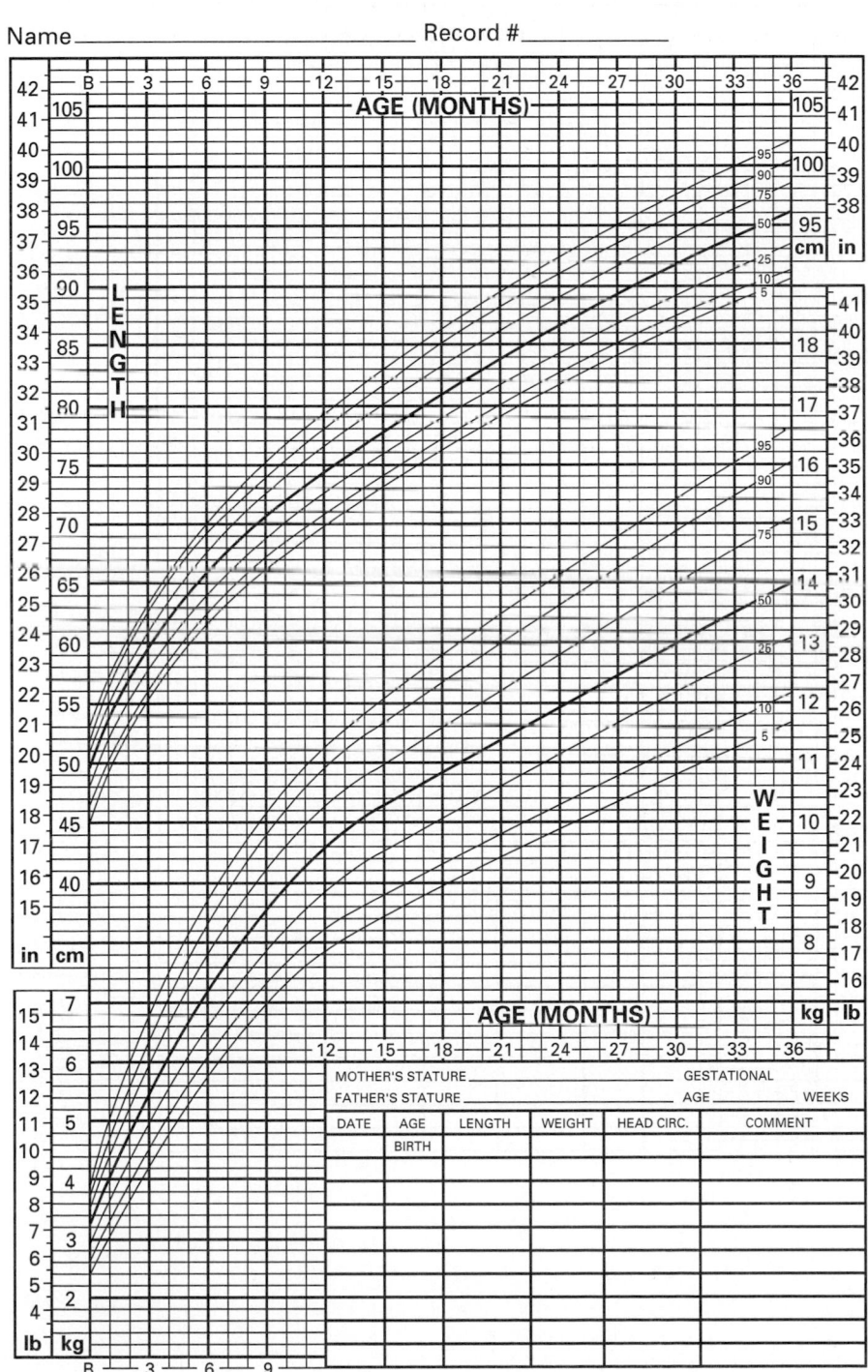

MOTHER'S STATURE_____ GESTATIONAL

FATHER'S STATURE_____ AGE_____ WEEKS

DATE	AGE	LENGTH	WEIGHT	HEAD CIRC.	COMMENT
	BIRTH				

* Adapted from: Hamill PVV, Drizd TA, Johnson CL, Reed RB, Roche AF, Moore WM: Physical growth: National Center for Health Statistics percentiles. AM J CLIN NUTR 32:607-629, 1979. Data from the Fels Research Institute, Wright State University School of Medicine, Yellow Springs, Ohio.
©1982 ROSS LABORATORIES

Boys: birth to 36 months physical growth NCHS percentiles*

Name_____ Record #_____

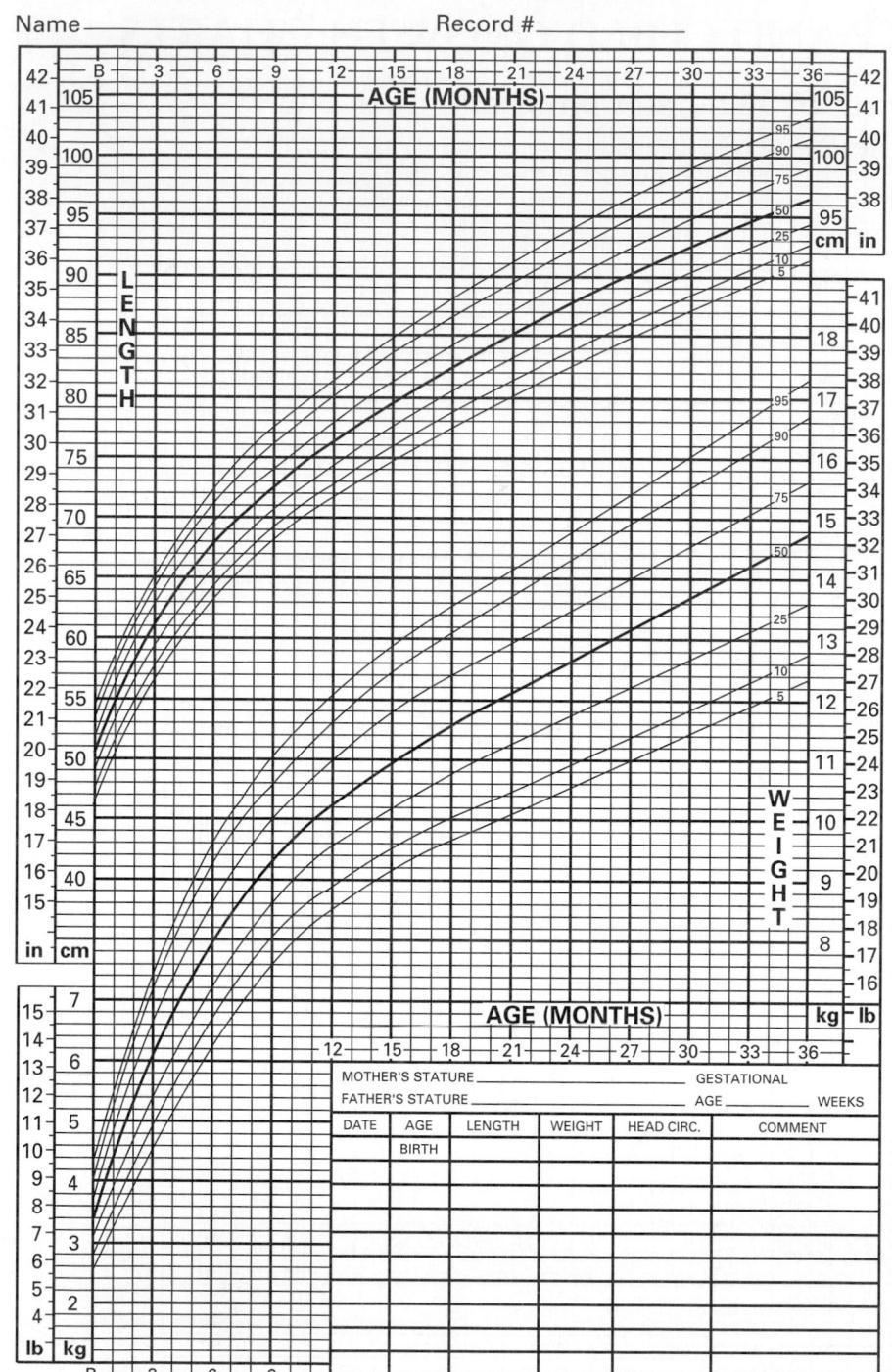

DATE	AGE	LENGTH	WEIGHT	HEAD CIRC.	COMMENT
	BIRTH				

MOTHER'S STATURE_____ GESTATIONAL
FATHER'S STATURE_____ AGE_____ WEEKS

* Adapted from: Hamill PVV, Drizd TA, Johnson CL, Reed RB, Roche AF, Moore WM: Physical growth: National Center for Health Statistics percentiles. AM J CLIN NUTR 32:607-629, 1979. Data from the Fels Research Institute, Wright State University School of Medicine, Yellow Springs, Ohio.
©1982 ROSS LABORATORIES

Girls: birth to 36 months physical growth NCHS percentiles*

Name _____   Record # _____

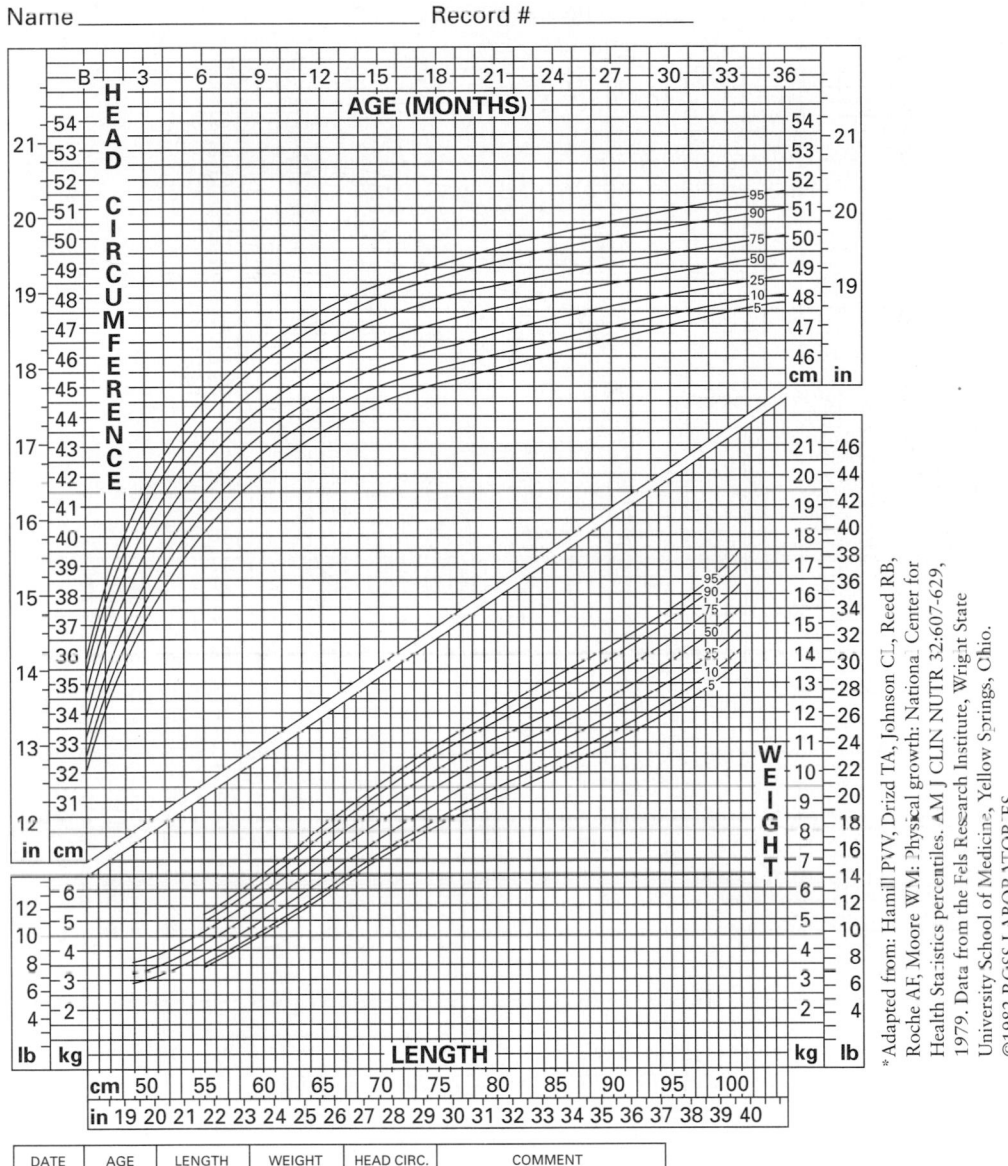

* Adapted from: Hamill PVV, Drizd TA, Johnson CL, Reed RB, Roche AF, Moore WM: Physical growth: National Center for Health Statistics percentiles. AM J CLIN NUTR 32:607-629, 1979. Data from the Fels Research Institute, Wright State University School of Medicine, Yellow Springs, Ohio.
©1982 ROSS LABORATORES

DATE	AGE	LENGTH	WEIGHT	HEAD CIRC.	COMMENT

Boys: birth to 36 months physical growth NCHS percentiles*

Name _____ Record # _____

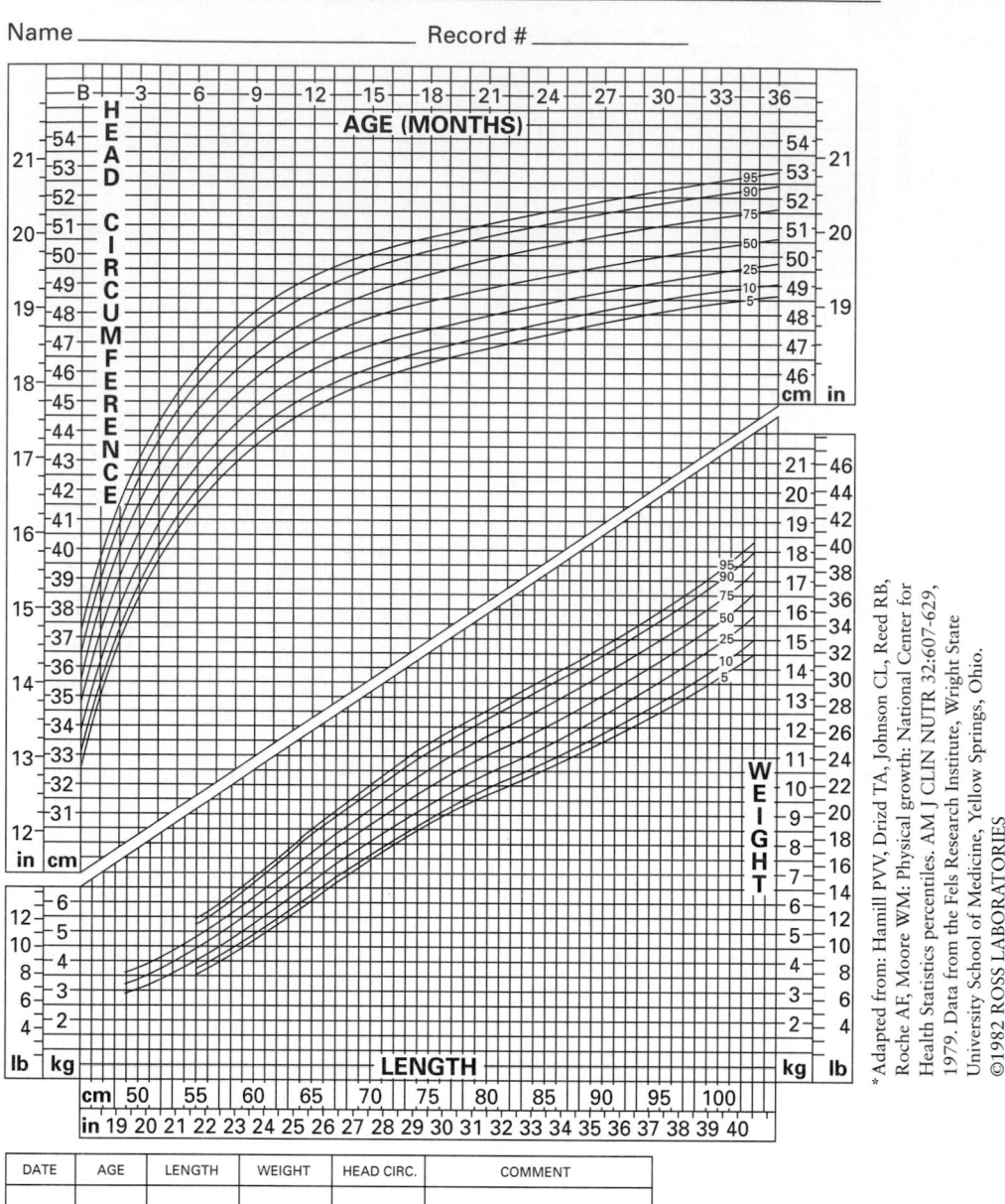

* Adapted from: Hamill PVV, Drizd TA, Johnson CL, Reed RB, Roche AF, Moore WM: Physical growth: National Center for Health Statistics percentiles. AM J CLIN NUTR 32:607-629, 1979. Data from the Fels Research Institute, Wright State University School of Medicine, Yellow Springs, Ohio.
©1982 ROSS LABORATORIES

DATE	AGE	LENGTH	WEIGHT	HEAD CIRC.	COMMENT

Boys: prepubescent physical growth NCHS percentiles*

Name _____   Record # _____

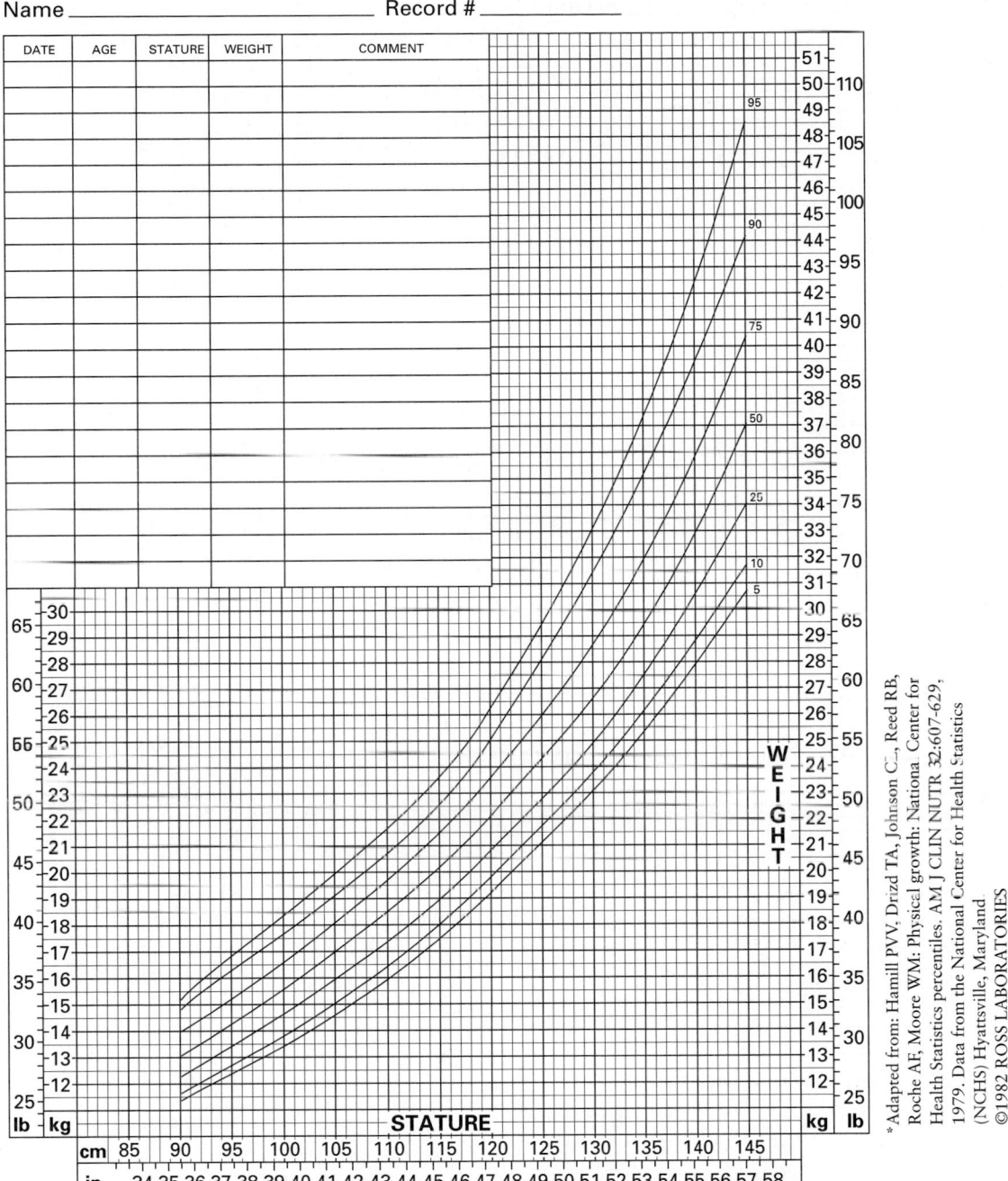

Girls: prepubescent physical growth NCHS percentiles*

Name _____   Record # _____

DATE	AGE	STATURE	WEIGHT	COMMENT

STATURE

cm 85 90 95 100 105 110 115 120 125 130 135 140 145

in 34 35 36 37 38 39 40 41 42 43 44 45 46 47 48 49 50 51 52 53 54 55 56 57 58

WEIGHT

*Adapted from: Hamill PVV, Drizd TA, Johnson CL, Reed RB, Roche AF, Moore WM: Physical growth: National Center for Health Statistics percentiles. AM J CLIN NUTR 32:607-629, 1979. Data from the National Center for Health Statistics (NCHS) Hyattsville, Maryland.
©1982 ROSS LABORATORIES

Girls: 2 to 18 years physical growth NCHS percentiles*

Name_____ Record #_____

| MOTHER'S STATURE_____ | FATHER'S STATURE_____ |
DATE	AGE	STATURE	WEIGHT	COMMENT

AGE (YEARS)

STATURE

WEIGHT

AGE (YEARS)

* Adapted from: Hamill PVV, Drizd TA, Johnson CL, Reed RB, Roche AF, Moore WM: Physical growth: National Center for Health Statistics percentiles. AM J CLIN NUTR 32:607-629, 1979. Data from the National Center for Health Statistics (NCHS) Hyattsville, Maryland.
©1982 ROSS LABORATORIES

Boys: 2 to 18 years physical growth NCHS percentiles*

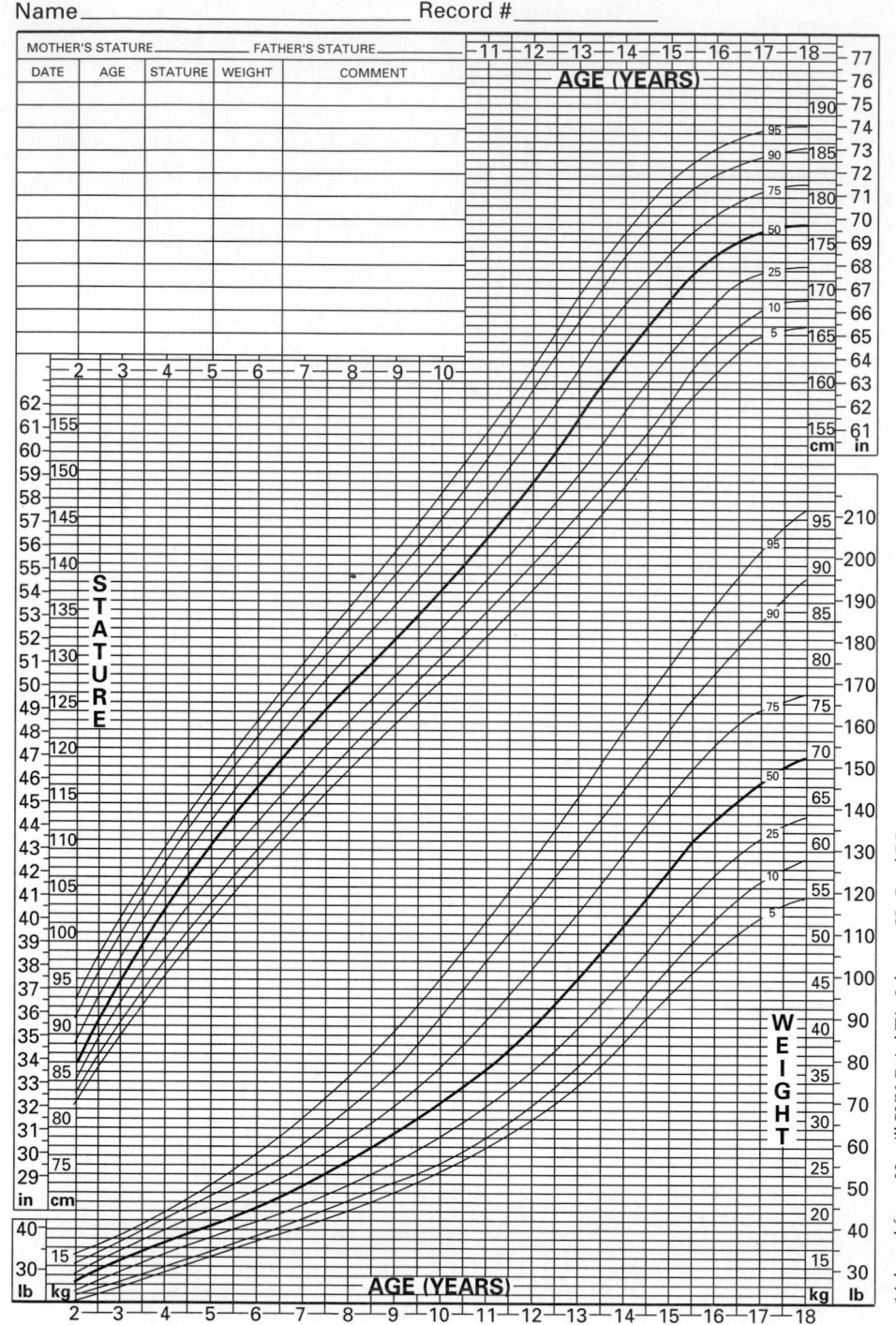

SAMPLE 24-HOUR RECALL FORM

Name _____

Date _____/_____/_____

Day of week (circle):   Sun   Mon   Tue   Wed   Thu   Fri   Sat

Time or meal	Food or beverage	Type or preparation	Amount

Was this intake unusual?   Yes_____   No_____

If so, how? _____

_____

Do you take any vitamin or mineral supplements?   Yes_____   No_____

If yes, describe:

Name or type	Dose (if known)	How often
_____	_____	_____
_____	_____	_____
_____	_____	_____

From American Dietetic Association: *Handbook of clinical dietetics,* ed 2, New Haven, 1992, Yale University Press.

NATIONAL RENAL DIET

Milk choices　　　　　per day

Average per choice: 4 grams protein, 120 kcalories, 80 mg sodium, 100 mg phosphorus

Milk (nonfat, low-fat whole)	½ cup
Lo Pro	1 cup
Buttermilk, cultured	½ cup
Chocolate milk	½ cup
Light cream or half and half	½ cup
Ice milk or ice cream	½ cup
Yogurt, plain or fruit-flavored	½ cup
Evaporated milk	¼ cup
Sweetened condensed milk	¼ cup
Cream cheese	3 Tbsp
Sour cream	4 Tbsp
Sherbet	1 cup

Nondairy milk substitutes　　per day

Average per choice: 0.5 gram protein, 140 kcalories, 40 mg sodium, 30 mg phosphorus

Dessert, nondairy frozen	½ cup
Dessert topping, nondairy frozen	½ cup
Liquid nondairy creamer, polyunsatured	½ cup

From American Dietetic Association: *A healthy food guide: Kidney disease,* 1993, American Dietetic Association.

Meat choices

per day

Average per choice: 7 grams protein, 65 kcalories, 25 mg sodium, 65 mg phosphorus

Prepared without added salt

Beef	1 oz
Round, sirloin, flank, cubed, T-bone, and porterhouse steak; tenderloin, rib, chuck, and rump roast; ground beef or ground chuck	
Pork	1 oz
Fresh ham, tenderloin, chops, loin roast, cutlets	
Lamb	1 oz
Chops, leg, roasts	
Veal	1 oz
Chops, roasts, cutlets	
Poultry	1 oz
Chicken, turkey, Cornish hen, domestic duck and goose	
Fish	
Fresh and frozen fish	1 oz
Lobster, scallops, shrimp, clams	1 oz
Crab, oysters	1½ oz
Canned tuna, canned salmon (canned without salt)	1 oz
Sardines (canned without salt) ✦	1 oz
Wild game	1 oz
Venison, rabbit, squirrel, pheasant, duck, goose	
Egg	
Whole	1 large
Egg white or yolk	2 large
Low-cholesterol egg product	¼ cup
Chitterlings	2 oz
Organ meats ✦	1 oz

Prepared with added salt

Beef	1 oz
Deli-style roast beef ✎	
Pork	1 oz
Boiled or deli-style ham ✎	
Poultry	1 oz
Deli-style chicken or turkey ✎	
Fish	
Canned tuna, canned salmon ✎	1 oz
Sardines ✎ ✦	1 oz
Cheese	
Cottage ✎	¼ cup

✎ High sodium—each serving counts as 1 Starch choice and 1 Salt choice.

✦ High phosphorus.

The following are high in sodium, phosphorus, and/or saturated fat. They should be used in your diet only as advised by your dietitian.

- Bacon
- Black beans, black-eyed peas, great northern beans, lentils, lima beans, navy beans, pinto beans, red kidney beans, soybeans, split peas, turtle beans
- Frankfurters, bratwurst, Polish sausage
- Luncheon meats, including bologna, braunschweiger, liverwurst, picnic loaf, summer sausage, salami
- Nuts and nut butters
- All cheeses except cottage cheese

Starch choices   per day

Average per choice: 2 grams protein, 90 kcalories, 80 mg sodium, 35 mg phosphorus

Breads and rolls

Bread (French, Italian, raisin, light rye, sourdough, white)	1 slice (1 oz)
Bagel	½ small
Bun, hamburger or hot dog type	½
Danish pastry or sweet roll, no nuts	½ small
Dinner roll or hard roll	1 small
Doughnut	1 small
English muffin	½
Muffin, no nuts, bran, or whole-wheat	1 small (1 oz)
Pancake 🖉 ✦	1 small (1 oz)
Pita or "pocket" bread	½ 6-in diameter
Tortilla, corn	2 6-in diameter
Tortilla, flour	1 6-in diameter
Waffle 🖉 ✦	1 small (1 oz)

Cereals and grains
Prepared without added salt

Cereals, ready-to-eat, most brands 🖉	¾ cup
Puffed rice	2 cups
Puffed wheat	1 cup
Cereals, cooked	
Cream of Rice or Wheat, Farina, Malt-O-Meal	½ cup
Oat bran or oatmeal, Ralston	⅓ cup
Cornmeal, cooked	¾ cup
Grits, cooked	½ cup

🖉   High sodium—each serving counts as 1 Starch choice and 1 Salt choice.

✦   High phosphorus.

Flour, all-purpose	2½ Tbsp
Pasta (noodles, macaroni, spaghetti), cooked	½ cup
Pasta made with egg (egg noodles), cooked	⅓ cup
Rice, white or brown, cooked	½ cup

Starchy vegetables
Prepared or canned without added salt

Corn	⅓ cup or ½ ear
Green peas	¼ cup
Potatoes, boiled or mashed	½ cup
Potatoes, baked, white, or sweet	1 small (3 oz)
Potatoes, French fried	½ cup or 10 small
Potatoes, hashed brown	½ cup
Squash, butternut, mashed	½ cup
Squash, winter, baked (all other varieties), cubed	1 cup

Crackers and snacks

Crackers: saltines, round butter	4 crackers
Graham crackers	3 squares
Melba toast	3 oblong
RyKrisp ✎	3 crackers
Popcorn, plain	1½ cup popped
Potato chips	1 oz, 14 chips
Tortilla chips	¾ oz, 9 chips
Pretzels, sticks or rings ✎	¾ oz, 10 sticks
Pretzels, sticks or rings, unsalted	¾ oz, 10 sticks

Desserts

Cake, angel food	1⁄20 cake or 1 oz
Cake	2 × 2-in square or 1½ oz
Sandwich cookie ✎ ✦	4 cookies
Shortbread cookie	4 cookies
Sugar cookie	4 cookies
Sugar wafer	4 cookies
Vanilla wafer	10 cookies
Fruit pie	⅛ pie
Sweetened gelatin	½ cup

The following foods are high in poor-quality protein and/or phosphorus. They should be used only when advised by your dietitian.

- Bran cereal or muffins, Grape-Nuts cereal, granola cereal or bars
- Boxed, frozen, or canned meals, entrees, or side dishes
- Black beans, black-eyed peas, great northern beans, lentils, lima beans, navy beans, pinto beans, red kidney beans, soybeans, split peas, turtle beans
- Pumpernickel, dark rye, whole-wheat, or oatmeal bread
- Whole-wheat cereals
- Whole-wheat crackers

Vegetable choices

See Starch Choices for other vegetables. Average per choice: 1 gram protein, 25 kcalories, 15 mg sodium, 20 mg phosphorus

Prepared or canned without added salt unless otherwise indicated

1-cup serving

Alfalfa sprouts	Escarole
Cabbage	Lettuce, all varieties
Celery	Pepper, green, sweet
Cucumber (or ½ whole)	Radishes, sliced (or 15 small)
Eggplant	Turnips
Endive	Watercress

½-cup serving

Artichoke	Onions
Bamboo shoots	Parsnips ✦
Bean sprouts	Pumpkin
Beans, green or wax	Rutabagas ✦
Beets	Sauerkraut ✎ ✎ ✎
Carrots (or 1 small)	Squash, summer
Cauliflower	Tomato (or 1 medium)
Chard	Tomato juice, unsalted
Chinese cabbage	Tomato juice, canned with salt ✎ ✎
Collards	Tomato puree
Kale	Turnip greens
Kohlrabi	Vegetable juice cocktail, unsalted
Mushrooms, fresh raw (or 4 medium)	Vegetable juice cocktail, canned with salt ✎ ✎

✎   High sodium—each serving counts as 1 Vegetable choice and 1 Salt choice.

✎ ✎   High sodium—each serving counts as 1 Vegetable choice and 2 Salt choices.

✎ ✎ ✎   High sodium—each serving counts as 1 Vegetable choice and 3 Salt choices.

✦   High phosphorus.

¼-cup serving

Asparagus (or 2 spears)	Mushrooms, fresh cooked
Avocado (¼ whole)	Mustard greens
Beet greens	Okra
Broccoli	Snow peas
Brussels sprouts	Spinach
Chili pepper	Tomato sauce

Prepared or canned with salt

Vegetables canned with salt (use serving size listed above) 🖊

Fruit choices

Average per choice: 0.5 gram protein, 70 kcalories, 15 mg phosphorus

1-cup serving

Apple (1 medium)	Papaya nectar
Apple juice	Peach nectar
Applesauce	Pear nectar
Cranberries	Pear, canned or fresh (1 medium)
Cranberry juice cocktail	Tangerine (1 medium)

½-cup serving

Apricot nectar	Lemon (½ medium)
Banana (½ small)	Lemon juice
Blueberries	Mango (½ medium)
Figs, canned	Nectarine (½ medium)
Fruit cocktail	Orange (½ medium)
Grapes (15 small)	Peach, canned or fresh (½ medium)
Grape juice	Pineapple
Grapefruit (½ medium)	Plums, canned or fresh (1 medium)
Grapefruit juice	Rhubarb
Gooseberries	Strawberries
Kiwifruit (½ medium)	Watermelon

¼-cup serving

Apricots (2 halves)	Honeydew melon (⅛ small)
Apricots, dried (2)	Orange juice
Blackberries	Papaya (¼ medium)
Cantaloupe (⅛ small)	Prune juice
Cherries	Prunes, cooked (5)
Dates (2 Tbsp)	Raisins (2 Tbsp)
Figs, dried (1 whole)	Raspberries

Fat choices

Average per choice: trace protein, 45 kcalories, 55 mg sodium, 5 mg phosphorus

Unsaturated Fats

Margarine	1 tsp
Reduced-calorie margarine	1 Tbsp
Mayonnaise	1 tsp
Low-calorie mayonnaise	1 Tbsp
Oil (safflower, sunflower, corn, soybean, olive, peanut, canola)	1 tsp
Salad dressing (mayonnaise-type)	2 tsp
Salad dressing (oil-type)	1 Tbsp
Low-calorie salad dressing (mayonnaise-type)	2 Tbsp
Low-calorie salad dressing (oil-type) ✎	2 Tbsp
Tartar sauce	1½ tsp

Saturated Fats

Butter	1 tsp
Coconut	2 Tbsp
Powdered coffee whitener	1 Tbsp
Solid shortening	1 tsp

✎ High sodium—each serving counts as 1 Fat choice and 1 Salt choice.

High-calorie choices

Average per choice: trace protein, 100 kcalories, 15 mg sodium, 5 mg phosphorus

Beverages

Carbonated beverages (fruit flavors, root beer; colas or pepper-type) ✔	1 cup
Kool-Aid	1 cup
Limeade	1 cup
Lemonade	1 cup
Cranberry juice cocktail	1 cup
Tang	1 cup
Fruit-flavored drink	1 cup
Wine*	½ cup

Frozen desserts

Fruit ice	½ cup
Popsicle (3 oz)	1 bar
Juice bar (3 oz)	1 bar
Sorbet	½ cup

Candy and sweets

Butter mints	14
Candy corn	20 or 1 oz
Chewy fruit snacks	1 pouch
Cranberry sauce or relish	¼ cup
Fruit chews	4
Fruit Roll Ups	2
Gumdrops	15 small
Honey	2 Tbsp
Hard candy	4 pieces
Jam or jelly	2 Tbsp
Jelly beans	10
LifeSavers or cough drops	12
Marmalade	2 Tbsp
Marshmallows	5 large
Sugar, brown or white	2 Tbsp
Sugar, powdered	3 Tbsp
Syrup	2 Tbsp

✔   High phosphorus.
*   Check with your physician before using alcohol.

Special Low-Protein Products

Ask your dietitian for information on how to obtain these products.

Low-protein gelled dessert	½ cup
Low-protein bread	1 slice
Low-protein cookies	2
Low-protein pasta	½ cup
Low-protein rusk	2 slices

The following foods are high in poor-quality protein and/or phosphorus. They should be used only when advised by your dietitian.

- Beer*
- Chocolate
- Nuts and nut butters

Salt choices

Average per choice: 25 mg sodium

Salt	⅛ tsp
Seasoned salts (onion, garlic, etc)	⅛ tsp
Accent	¼ tsp
Barbecue sauce	2 Tbsp
Bouillon	⅓ cup
Catsup	1½ Tbsp
Chili sauce	1½ Tbsp
Dill pickle	⅙ large or ½ oz
Mustard	4 tsp
Olives, green	2 medium or ⅓ oz
Olives, black	3 large or 1 oz
Soy sauce	¾ tsp
Light soy sauce	1 tsp
Steak sauce	2½ tsp
Sweet pickle relish	2½ Tbsp
Taco sauce	2 Tbsp
Tamari sauce	¾ tsp
Teriyaki sauce	1¼ tsp
Worcestershire sauce	1 Tbsp

---

*   Check with your physician before using alcohol.

A Healthy Food Guide: Kidney Disease

Name: _____

Date: _____

Your dietitian is: _____

Telephone number: _____

_____ grams protein

_____ Calories

_____ milligrams phosphorus

_____ milligrams sodium

Your Daily Meal Plan

Breakfast

		Sample Menu
Milk	_____ choices	_____
Nondairy Milk Substitute	_____ choices	_____
Meat	_____ choices	_____
Starch	_____ choices	_____
Fruit	_____ choices	_____
Fat	_____ choices	_____
High-Calorie	_____ choices	_____
Salt	_____ choices	_____

Snack

		Sample Menu
	_____ choices	_____
	_____ choices	_____

Lunch

		Sample Menu
Milk	_____ choices	_____
Nondairy Milk Substitute	_____ choices	_____
Meat	_____ choices	_____
Starch	_____ choices	_____
Vegetable	_____ choices	_____
Fruit	_____ choices	_____
Fat	_____ choices	_____
High-Calorie	_____ choices	_____
Salt	_____ choices	_____

Snack

		Sample Menu
	_____ choices	_____
	_____ choices	_____

Dinner

		Sample Menu
Milk	_____ choices	_____
Nondairy Milk Substitute	_____ choice	_____
Meat	_____ choices	_____
Starch	_____ choices	_____
Vegetable	_____ choices	_____
Fruit	_____ choices	_____
Fat	_____ choices	_____
High-Calorie	_____ choices	_____
Salt	_____ choices	_____

Snack

		Sample Menu
	_____ choices	_____
	_____ choices	_____

Appendix K

Foods High in Purines

HIGH: CONTENT 150–825 mg/100g

Fish/seafood
- Anchovies
- Herring
- Mackeral
- Sardines
- Scallops

Meats
- Brains
- Gravies
- Kidney
- Liver
- Meat extracts
- Sweetbreads
- Wild game
- Goose

MODERATE: CONTENT 50–150 mg/100g

Vegetables
- Asparagus
- Cauliflower
- Green peas
- Mushrooms
- Spinach

Grains and legumes
- Legumes (split peas, beans, lentils)
- Oatmeal
- Wheat bran and germ
- Whole grain breads and cereals

Fish/Seafood
- Crabs
- Eel
- Fish (all kinds)
- Lobsters
- Oysters

Meats and related products
- Beef
- Lamb
- Pork
- Veal

Poultry
- Chicken
- Duck
- Turkey

LOW: CONTENT 0–50 mg/100g

Beverages
- Carbonated beverages
- Coffee
- Tea

Grains
- Breads and cereals (refined white flour)

Food High in Purines, cont'd.

Dairy
   Cheese
   Milk (all fat levels)

Miscellaneous
   Eggs
   Fats
   Fish roe
   Fruits and their juices
   Gelatin
   Nuts
   Sugars (all types) and foods containing sweets
   Vegetables (unless noted in A or B)

Foods High in Oxalate (>10 mg/serving)

VEGETABLES

Beans, wax, green, dried; beets; cassava; celery; chives; collards; cucumbers; dandelion greens; okra; parsley; green peppers; sweet potatoes; rutabagas; spinach; summer squash; Swiss chard

FRUITS AND JUICES

Blackberries; blueberries; red currants; raspberries, black/red; grapes, purple/Concord; strawberries; gooseberries; citrus peel (lemon, lime, orange); fruit cocktail; rhubarb; tangerines; plums

STARCHES/BREADS

Amaranth, breads and pasta; fruit cake; grits; soybean crackers; wheat germ; bran

MEAT AND PROTEIN SOURCES

Tofu, baked beans (tomato sauce)

FATS

Peanuts, almonds, pecans, cashews, walnuts, nut butters, sesame seeds, tahini

BEVERAGES

Beer, Ovaltine, tea, chocolate milk, cocoa, coffee (instant), colas

OTHERS

Chocolate, cocoa powder, vegetable soup, tomato soup

From Nelson JK et al: *Mayo Clinic diet manual,* ed 7, St. Louis, 1994, Mosby; and Dietary Department, University of Iowa Hospital and Clinics, Iowa City: *Recent advances in therapeutic diets,* ed 4, Ames, Iowa, 1989, Iowa State University Press.

CULTURAL DIETARY PATTERNS

Only foods that are specifically associated with these cultural groups are noted. Individuals may also consume typical American foods as well; assumptions of dietary patterns cannot be made, but knowledge of these unique foods provides a common understanding of the range of possible food choices.

Native American

Each tribe may have specific foods; listed here are commonly consumed foods.

1. Bread, cereal, rice, and pasta group:

Blue corn flour (ground dried blue corn kernels) used to make cornbread, mush dumplings; fruit dumplings (walakshi); fry bread (biscuit dough deep fried); ground sweet acorn; tortillas; wheat or rye used to make cornmeal and flours.

2. Vegetable group:

Cabbage, carrots, cassava, dandelion greens, eggplant, milkweed, onions, pumpkin, squash (all varieties), sweet and white potatoes, turnips, wild tullies (a tuber), yellow corn.

3. Fruit group:

Dried wild cherries and grapes; wild banana, berries, and yucca.

4. Milk, yogurt, and cheese group:

None.

5. Meat, poultry, fish, dry beans, eggs, and nuts group:

Duck, eggs, fish eggs (roe), geese, groundhog, kidney beans, lentils, peanuts, pinenuts, pinto beans, all nuts, venison, wild rabbit.

6. Fats, oils, and sweets:

None.

African-American

1. Bread, cereal, rice, and pasta group:

Biscuits, cornbread as spoon bread, cornpone or hush puppies, grits.

2. Vegetable group:

Leafy greens including dandelion greens, kale, mustard greens, collard greens, turnips.

3. Fruit group:

None.

4. Milk, yogurt, and cheese group:

Buttermilk.

5. Meat, poultry, fish, dry beans, eggs, and nuts group:

Pork and pork products, scrapple (cornmeal and pork), chitterlings (pork intestines), bacon, pig's feet, pig ears, souse, pork neck bones, fried meats and poultry, organ meats (kidney, liver, tongue, tripe), venison, rabbit, catfish, buffalo fish, mackerel, legumes (black-eyed peas, kidney, navy, chickpeas).

6. Fats, oils, and sweets:

Lard.

Japanese

1. Bread, cereal, rice, and pasta group:

Rice and rice products, rice flour (mochiko), noodles (comen/soba), seaweed around rice with or without fish (sushi).

2. Vegetable group:

Bamboo shoots (takenoko), burdock (gobo), cabbage (nappa), dried mushrooms (shiitake), eggplant, horseradish (wasabi), Japanese parsley (seri), lotus root (renkon), mustard greens, pickled cabbage (kimchee), pickled vegetables, seaweed (laver, nori, wakame, kombu), vegetable soup (mizutaki), white radish (daikon).

3. Fruit group:

Pear-like apple (nasi), persimimmons.

4. Milk, yogurt, and cheese group:

None.

5. Meat, poultry, fish, dry beans, eggs, and nuts group:

Fish and shellfish including dried fish with bones, raw fish (sashimi), and fish cake (kamaboko); soybeans as soybean curd (tofu), fermented soy bean paste (miso), and sprouts; red beans (azuki).

6. Fats, oils, and sweets:

Soy and rice oil.

Chinese

1. Bread, cereal, rice, and pasta group:

Rice and related products (flour, cakes, and noodles); noodles made from barley, corn and millet; wheat and related products (breads, noodles, spaghetti, stuffed noodles [won ton] and filled buns [bow]).

2. Vegetable group:

Bamboo shoots; cabbage (napa); Chinese celery; Chinese parsley (coriander); Chinese turnips (lo bok); dried day lillies; dry fungus (Black Juda's ear); leafy green vegetables including kale, Chinese cress, Chinese mustard greens (gai choy), Chinese chard (bok choy), amaranth greens (yin choy), wolfberry leaves (gou gay), and Chinese broccoli (gai lan); lotus tubers; okra; snow peas; stir-fried vegetables (chow yuk); taro roots, white radish (daikon).

3. Fruit group:

Kumquat.

4. Milk, yogurt, and cheese group:

None.

5. Meat, poultry, fish, dry beans, eggs, and nuts group:

Fish and seafood (all kinds, dried and fresh), hen, legumes, nuts, organ meats, pigeon eggs, pork and pork products, soybean curd (tofu), steamed stuffed dumplings (dim sum).

6. Fats, oils, and sweets:

Peanut, soy, sesame and rice oil; lard.

Filipino

1. Bread, cereal, rice, and pasta group:

Noodles, rice, rice flour (mochiko), stuffed noodles (won ton), white bread (pan de sal).

2. Vegetable group:

Bamboo shoots, dark green leafy vegetables (malunggay and salvyot), eggplant, sweet potatoes (camotes), okra, palm, peppers, turnips, root crop (gabi).

3. Fruit group:

Avocado, bitter melon (ampalaya), guavas, jackfruit, limes, mangoes, papaya, pod fruit (tamarind), pomelos, tangelo (naranghita).

4. Milk, yogurt, and cheese group:

Custards.

5. Meat, poultry, fish, dry beans, eggs, and nuts group:

Fish in all forms; dried fish (dilis); egg roll (lumpia); fish sauce (alamang and bagoong); legumes such as mung beans, bean sprouts, chickpeas, organ meats (liver, heart, intestines); pork with chicken in soy sauce (adobo); pork sausage; soybean curd (tofu).

6. Fats, oils, and sweets:

None.

Southeastern Asians: (Laos, Cambodia, Thailand, Viet Nam, the Hmong and the Mien)

1. Bread, cereal, rice, and pasta group:

Rice (long and short grain) and related products such as noodles; Hmong cornbread or cake.

2. Vegetable group:

Bamboo shoots, broccoli, Chinese parsley (coriander), mustard greens, pickled vegetables, water chestnuts, Thai chili peppers.

3. Fruit group:

Apple pear (Asian pear), bitter melon, coconut cream and milk, guava, jack fruit, mango.

4. Milk, yogurt, and cheese group:

Sweetened condensed milk.

5. Meat, poultry, fish, dry beans, eggs, and nuts group:

Beef; chicken; deer; eggs; fish and shellfish (all kinds freshwater and saltwater);

legumes including black-eyed peas, peanuts, kidney beans, and soybeans; organ meats (liver, stomach); pork; rabbit; soybean curd (tofu).

6. Fats, oils, and sweets:

Lard, peanut oil.

Mexican

1. Bread, cereal, rice, and pasta group:

Corn and related products; taco shells (fried corn tortillas); tortillas (corn and flour); white bread.

2. Vegetable group:

Cactus (nopoles), chili peppers, salsa, tomatoes, yambean root (jicama), yucca root (cassava or manioc).

3. Fruit group:

Avocado; guacamole (mashed avocado, onion, cilantro [coriander], and chilis); papaya.

4. Milk, yogurt, and cheese group:

Cheese, flan, sour cream.

5. Meat, poultry, fish, dry beans, eggs, and nuts group:

Black or pinto beans (reijoles); refried beans (frijoles refritos); flour tortilla stuffed with beef, chicken, eggs, or beans (burrito); corn tortilla stuffed with chicken, cheese, or beef topped with chili sauce (enchilada); Mexican sausage (chorizo).

6. Fats, oils, and sweets:

Bacon fat, lard (manteca), salt pork.

Puerto Rican and Cuban

1. Bread, cereal, rice, and pasta group:

Rice; starchy green bananas, usually fried (plantain).

2. Vegetable group:

Beets; eggplant; tubers (yucca); white yams (boniato).

3. Fruit group:

Coconuts, guava, mango, oranges (sweet and sour), prune and mango paste.

4. Milk, yogurt, and cheese group:

Flan, hard cheese (queso de mano).

5. Meat, poultry, fish, dry beans, eggs, and nuts group:

Chicken, fish (all kinds and preparations including smoked, salted, canned and fresh), legumes (all kinds especially black beans), pork (fried), sausage (chorizo).

6. Fats, oils, and sweets:

Olive and peanut oil, lard.

JEWISH

The foods below reflect both religious and cultural customs of Jewish people. Adherence to religious dietary patterns by followers of the different forms of Judaism (Orthodox, Conservative, Reform, and Reconstructionist) vary. Generally, Orthodox Jews and many Conservative Jews follow kosher dietary rules both at home and when out. Others may only observe when in their own homes. These rules of "keeping kosher" are reviewed in the next section on religious dietary patterns.

1. Bread, cereal, rice, and pasta group:

Bagel, buckwheat groats (kasha), dumplings made with matzoh meal (matzoh balls or knaidelach), egg bread (challah), noodle or potato pudding (kugel), a crepe filled with farmer cheese and/or fruit (blintz), unleavened bread or large cracker made with wheat flour and water (matzoh).

2. Vegetable group:

Potato pancakes (latkes); a vegetable stew made with sweet potatoes, carrots, prunes and sometimes brisket (tzimmes); beet soup (borscht).

3. Fruit group:

None.

4. Milk, yogurt, and cheese group:

None.

5. Meat, poultry, fish, dry beans, eggs, and nuts group:

A mixture of fish formed into balls and poached (gefilte fish); smoked salmon (lox).

6. Fats, oils, and sweets:

Chicken fat.

RELIGIOUS DIETARY PATTERNS

Beliefs of several major religions include practices that affect or prescribe specific dietary patterns or prohibit consumption of certain types of foods. Individuals practicing these religions may or may not adhere to all of the prescribed customs. Following is a brief review of some of these practices.

Moslem

Pork and pork-related products are not eaten. Meats that are consumed must be slaughtered by prescribed rituals; these procedures are similar to the Judaic kosher slaughtering of animals, so Moslems may eat kosher meats. Coffee, tea, and alcohol are not consumed. During the month of Ramadan, Muslims fast during the day from dawn to sunset.

Christianity

Some sects may not eat meat on holy days; others prohibit alcohol consumption.

Hinduism

Animal foods of beef, pork, lamb, and poultry are not eaten. Followers are lacto-vegetarians or vegans.

Judaism

Food consumption is guided by religious doctrines; no pork or pork-related products nor seafood or fish without scales and fins are eaten. Dairy foods are not consumed with meat or animal-related foods (excludes fish). If meat or dairy is eaten, six hours must pass for the other to be acceptable for consumption. Animals are slaughtered according to a ritual in which blood is drained and the carcass is salted and rinsed; meat prepared in this manner is "kosher." The preparation of all processed foods eaten must also adhere to these guidelines. Since meat and dairy must not mix, two sets of dishes and utensils are used at home and in kosher restaurants. Foods that are neither meat nor dairy are called parve and are often so labeled by food manufacturers. Additional customs affect food consumption on Saturday, the Sabbath, during which no cooking occurs. Special foods are associated with each religious holiday. Fasting (no water or food) for 24 hours occurs during Yom Kippur (Day of Atonement). During Passover, an 8-day holiday, no leavened bread is consumed, only matzoh (made from flour and water) and products made from matzoh flour; other symbolic food restrictions are also observed.

Seventh Day Adventist

General restrictions of pork and pork-related products, shellfish, alcohol, coffee, and tea are followed. Some followers are ovo-lacto-vegetarians, whereas others are vegans.

Chapter 5

1. Before accepting the patient's conclusion that she has lowered her fat intake, the following should be asked: Is the skin from chicken removed before cooking or eating? How is the chicken cooked? Is it breaded or fried in oil or cooked with butter? How is the chicken served? With potentially high-fat sauces? What other low-fat foods do you regularly eat? What kind of milk and dairy products do you use? Can you describe the difference between visible and invisible dietary fats?

2. A friend may always feel he is starving between meals because his fat intake may be too low. A low fat intake causes the stomach to empty quickly. Fat provides satiety and helps prevent hunger between meals because fat slows down the digestion process.

3. Reducing cholesterol intake will not control clogged arteries; the man's statement is incorrect. Clogged arteries are affected by blood cholesterol levels. These levels are most affected by dietary saturated fat. Although dietary cholesterol affects blood levels, saturated fats have a greater effect and should be reduced to possibly keep his problem under control. Dietary restrictions alone may not be sufficient, since dietary sources account for about 25% of the cholesterol in the body; the rest is produced by the liver. His primary health care provider should be consulted.

4. If a child consumes well below the recommended daily amount of fat, the extreme effect could be failure to thrive and impaired brain development. A less extreme effect could be insufficient availability of vitamins A, D, E, and K as well as essential fatty acids; fats provide these nutrients and may transport them in the body.

5. Just drinking skim milk instead of whole milk is not adequate fat control for a teenager. Although the number of fat calories appropriate for her age is higher than an adult's (because of a higher activity and growth), other foods also add significant amounts of fats. Foods to limit or to choose lower-fat versions of are ice cream (if eaten regularly) and other related dairy foods (hard cheeses and cream cheese), hamburgers, hot dogs, luncheon meats, French fries, and other fried foods.

6. It is not possible to eat fats that contain only high-density lipoproteins. High-density lipoproteins are only within the body as part of blood cholesterol along with low-density lipoproteins. High-density lipoproteins are not part of any known dietary fat found in foods.

7. Reducing sugar and carbohydrates is not the most efficient way to reduce kcalories because they contain 4 kcal/gm whereas fat provides 9 kcal/gm; by weight, fat contains more kcalories. Restricting fat intake is a more effective strategy to reduce kcaloric intake.

8. Other assessments to determine appropriate fat intake are to evaluate his blood cholesterol levels (HDL/LDL) and to conduct a 24-hour food intake recall of her husband's dietary intake that could be analyzed with a computer dietary analysis program.

Chapter 11

1. The amount of weight gained during pregnancy often reflects the amount of nutrients consumed. Inadequate nutrient intake can lead to poor weight gain that may result in growth retardation while the fetus is still in the womb. When born, babies who are small for gestational age are more at risk for medical complications that may necessitate prolonged hospitalization. Discussing average weight gain recommendations can assure her that gaining weight during pregnancy is normal and healthy for both her and her baby.

   Rather than trying to "catch up" by gaining weight quickly, she should increase her intake by 300 kcal a day in the form of snacks such as an afternoon sandwich or fruit and cheese with a glass of skim milk.

2. The teenage mother can be referred to the federal government's program, the USDA's Special Supplemental Food Program for Women, Infants, and Children (WIC), which will provide her and her baby with food vouchers and additional nutrition education and counseling services. Local departments of health can provide information on the WIC programs in the area. Since she was comfortable enough to reveal her concerns, follow-up contact is appropriate to be sure she is able to get to the clinic regularly and follows the recommended procedures.

   To ensure that her food money is spent wisely, the concept of nutrient density can be discussed, as well as the idea of planning meals to include the different food groups of the Food Guide Pyramid. The nutrient value of low-cost foods can also be explained in relation to nutrient density. It may be less expensive to buy foods in larger quantities and divide into serving sizes, assuming storage facilities are available. Buying foods in less prepared forms may also be more economical. For example, precooked rice in plastic serving-sized bags is much more expensive than buying a larger bag of uncooked rice. Once she is enrolled in the WIC program, she will receive additional nutrition education about low-cost foods and nutrition.

3. Fortunately, for most women, problems with morning sickness, nausea, and vomiting begin to subside by the beginning of the second trimester. These symptoms are probably caused by hormonal factors as the body adjusts to the pregnancy; it does not reflect a pregnancy-related illness. If the woman begins to lose weight, becomes severely dehydrated, or if she cannot retain foods or fluids for 6 hours or longer, the primary health care provider should be contacted.

    Foods and food patterns that might help reduce symptoms include eating small, frequent meals; consuming liquids between rather than with meals; and avoiding fried and greasy foods. If she is working, she can keep some snacks available such as dried fruit, crackers, and juice.

4. During the first several weeks of life, newborns should be offered the breast at least 10 to 12 times per 24 hours. The fussy newborn is most likely ready to feed, and the mother should be awakened.

5. Criteria to determine if a child is ready for solids include the ability of the baby to sit with some support; move the jaw, lips, and tongue independently; be able to roll the tongue to the back of the mouth to facilitate a food bolus entering the esophagus; and show interest in what the rest of the family is eating.

    The mother will know the amount of food to feed based on the satiety cues of the baby. When full, the baby may turn her head to the side, refuse to open her mouth, or grimace when the spoon comes close to her mouth. The baby should not be forced to eat. If the baby is tired or not interested in eating, the feeding session should end and foods can be offered later.

Chapter 13

1. The VLCD wasn't providing enough protein or energy to maintain her immune function. Healing will be slower because the stress of the injuries from the accident occurred while she was in a debilitated state.

2. M.G. developed pneunomia because of a lack of protein and energy, which depletes visceral protein stores, for example, lung cells. This can lead to deterioration of lung function as well as depression of the immune system.

3. The stresses M.G. was experiencing include infection (pneumonia), trauma (multiple fractures, possible surgery) and poor nutritional status.

4. The pneumonia possibly could have been prevented if an in-depth nutritional assessment had been performed. The information obtained would have alerted the health care team to the following: before admission, her diet did not supply sufficient energy or protein; M.G. needed nutritional support; and her immune system functioning may have been compromised.

Chapter 14

1. Assessment of R.G.'s weight status:
   R.G. has lost 25 lbs during the past year:

   $$\% \text{ wt change from usual wt} = \frac{(\text{usual wt} - \text{actual wt})}{\text{usual wt}} \times 100$$

   $$-13\% \text{ change from usual wt} = \frac{(180 - 155)}{180} \times 100$$

   or R.G. is 87% of his usual weight (a 13% weight loss); a possible cause for alarm.

2. Serum albumin and TIBC are indicators of visceral protein status.

   serum albumin = 2.5 mg/dl (normal = 3.5–5.5 mg/dl)—low
   TIBC = 250 µg/dl (normal = 270–400 µg/dl)—low

   Low values are associated with low dietary protein intake, low energy intake, and stress of surgery. This indicates compromised protein status. Dietary intake before admission was low.

3. Serum creatinine and MAMC are indicators of somatic protein status.

   serum creatinine 0.5 mg/dl (normal = 0.6–1.6 mg/dl)—low

   Arm muscle circumference and triceps skinfold are decreased, therefore resulting in decreased midarm muscle circumference. (Although exact values are not given, this value, taken into consideration with the other indices, can indicate decrease somatic protein stores.)

   Low values are associated with muscle wasting caused by energy deficiency. Energy intake before admission was low.

4.   TLC 1350 cells/mm^3 (normal = > 1500 cells/mm^3)—low

   Low values are associated with protein-energy malnutrition; indicates compromised immune function. Protein and energy intakes before admission were low.

5. Patient has history of inadequate energy and protein intake. These indices also demonstrate somatic and visceral protein depletion. His nutritional status is compromised, which will have a negative impact on his ability to heal properly (increased morbidity and possibly mortality) after surgery.

Chapter 15

These questions are actual court cases. They are presented in this Clinical Application to stimulate students to think about their own beliefs and feelings regarding these matters and to stimulate classroom discussion. Technically, there are no *right* or *wrong* answers. The *answers* given are the court's decisions in these matters and do not reflect the opinion of the authors or the reference listed below.

1. In the case *Plaza Health and Rehabilitation Center v. New York* (1984), the court refused to order tube feedings for this man who wished to starve himself to death. The decision was based on the patient's (presumed) short life expectancy, his immediate family's choice, his physician's recommendation against forced feeding, and a state statute giving competent patients the right to refuse medically necessary treatment.
2. In *Hier v Massachusetts* (1984), the appellate court authorized surgery for the placement of a feeding tube despite the patient's former desires (from a time in her life when she was considered competent) of being allowed to die rather than being kept alive in an incompetent state.
3. In *Corbett v D'Allessandro* (1986), the court allowed the tube to be removed, as a constitutionally protected right.

Chapter 16

1. Common nutrition problems found in patients who have gastrectomies are dumping syndrome, malabsorption, steatorrhea, hypoglycemia, anemia, B_{12} deficiency, folate deficiency, and weight loss.
2. T.E. experienced megaloblastic anemia (folate and B_{12} deficiencies), weight loss, and iron deficiency anemia.
3. Factors accounting for iron deficiency anemia after gastrectomy are blood loss from surgery, poor iron absorption (rapid transit time through duodenum where approximately 50% of iron absorption takes place), lack of HCl to convert iron to more absorbable form, inadequate food intake, and malabsorption. Iron supplements are used to treat this anemia.
4. Compared with normal values, T.E.'s laboratory values are low for hemoglobin, hematocrit, and serum albumin. These values indicate an inadequate intake of protein and foods high in iron content.
5. T.E. is receiving monthly injections of vitamin B_{12} to prevent a vitamin B_{12} deficiency. The main cause of vitamin B_{12} deficiency is pernicious anemia caused by lack of intrinsic factor (produced by specialized cells in the stomach), which leads to B_{12} malabsorption despite adequate dietary intake. Because of the gastrectomy, she cannot produce the intrinsic factor required. Since there is no source of intrinsic factor, she should not be advised to eat more foods high in B_{12}. The vitamin will never be absorbed from food properly, and must be given parenterally.
6. The food groups and/or nutrients lacking in her diet are dairy products (vitamins A and D, calcium, riboflavin, phosphorus), fruits (vitamin C), cereals/grains (complex carbohydrates, fiber), and vegetables, particularly leafy green vegetables (beta carotene, vitamin A).
7. Suggestions to T.E. are to consume fluids separately from meals to slow down transit time, decrease intake of simple carbohydrates and moderately increase complex carbohydrates, increase iron-rich protein sources, and moderately increase fat. Small, frequent meals and lying down after meals are additional beneficial strategies.
8. T.E. should continue to consume six small meals and snacks because larger meals aggravate dumping syndrome, diarrhea, and other symptoms.

Chapter 17

1. Two shots of 80-proof tequila provide 36 grams of alcohol and 252 kcalories.

2 shots = 3 oz or 90 ml
80-proof rum × 0.5 % alcohol = 40 grams of alcohol
90 ml × 40 grams/100 ml = 36 grams alcohol
36 grams alcohol × 7 kcal/gram = 252 kcalories*

2. The best way to obtain information from an individual about his/her alcohol consumption is to ask open-ended questions and phrase them several different ways to double check the accuracy of information. Additionally, double-checking with friends or family members also helps.

3. 176 grams of alcohol are consumed. 1232 kcal are provided by the alcohol.

7.5 oz vodka × 30 ml/oz × 40 g/100ml = 90 g alcohol
72 oz beer × 30 ml/oz × 4 g/100ml = 86 g alcohol
90 g + 86 g = 176 g alcohol × 7 kcal/g = 1232 kcal from alcohol

38.5 percent of the kcalories are provided by alcohol.

1232 kcal from alcohol/3200 kcal total × 100 = 38.5%

Chapter 18

1. D.E.'s blood glucose level could become so high without producing ketones because patients with NIDDM still produce enough insulin to prevent massive fatty acid release, but not enough to stimulate entry of glucose into the cells. The stress of the urinary tract infection probably precipitated the HHNK.

2. If the HHNK is not treated, dehydration secondary to osmotic diuresis can occur, progressing to coma and possibly death.

3. D.E.'s blood glucose and lipid goals are to achieve near normal blood glucose levels (80 to 120 mg/dl before meals and 100 to 140 mg/dl at bedtime) and lipid levels (TC ≤ 200 mg/dl, TG < 200 mg/dl).

4. Lasix and hydrochlorothiazide are antihypertensives that are potassium-depleting diuretics; both may cause anorexia.

To prevent drug-nutrient interactions that may occur, propranolol hydrochloride (Inderal), a beta blocker antihypertensive, should be taken with food to enhance bioavailability, and alcohol should be avoided. It may also mask symptoms of and prolong hypoglycemia in diabetes mellitus. Diabinese (chlorpropamide), a sulfonylurea and oral hypoglycemic, requires elimination of alcohol consumption and may cause an Antabuse-like reaction and anorexia.

5. Frequency of blood sugar monitoring depends on the type of diabetes and therapy. NIDDM: With meal plan/exercise, test once or twice per week; with an oral hypoglycemic agent, test at least once per day, at different times each day (for example, Monday—breakfast, Tuesday—lunch, Wednesday—breakfast and dinner, Thursday—bedtime, Friday—lunch, Saturday—dinner, Sunday—bedtime); if control is good, test one or two times per week; if insulin is used, test at least two times per day, at different times each day.

6. Short-term complications may include: hypoglycemia, ketoacidosis, or hyperosmolar hyperglycemic nonketotic coma.

Long-term complications may include: coronary artery disease, peripheral vascular disease, cerebrovascular accident, nephropathy, retinopathy, peripheral neuropathy (decreased sensation in extremities), and autonomic neuropathy (gastropaesis, neurogenic bladder, impotence, impaired pain sensation).

---

*Any beverages used as mixers should be included in the estimated kcalorie intake.

Chapter 19

1. A myocardial infarction (heart attack) occurs when occlusion of a coronary artery results in necrosis (tissue death) of the cardiac muscle.
2. Risk factors for cardiovascular disease include: tobacco use, physical inactivity, male gender, aging, family history, diabetes mellitus, hypertension, obesity, and hypercholesterolemia.
3. I.C.'s risk factors are: male gender, physical inactivity, hypertension, hypercholesterolemia (TC and LDL-cholesterol), and hypertriglyceridemia (elevated triglycerides).
4. Specific guidelines of the NCEP's Step 1 are: ≤ 30% of total kcal from fat (8% to 10% saturated fats, ≤ 10% polyunsaturated fats, ≤ 10% monounsaturated fats); ≥ 55% of total kcal from carbohydrates; approximately 15% total kcal from protein; < 300 mg cholesterol per day, and achieve and maintain desirable weight.
5. Characteristics of I.C.'s intake that contradict the NCEP Step 1 are: high intake of fats (cheeses, ice cream, potato chips, peanuts, probably the crackers, whole milk, butter), high intake of saturated fats (cheeses, ice cream, potato chips, probably the crackers [likely to contain saturated fats], whole milk, butter), and high dietary cholesterol intake depending on consumption pattern (cheeses, ice cream, whole milk, butter). Typically, a high-fat diet will be high in total kcalories.
6. Alternative snack foods are: fruits, vegetables, pretzels, soda or saltine crackers, air-popped popcorn, low-fat yogurt, low-fat cheeses, ice milk, fat-free ice cream or sorbet, and skim or low-fat milk.

Chapter 20

1. The purpose of hemodialysis is to remove excess fluid and waste products from blood that are normally removed by the kidneys.
2. Metabolic waste products are removed during dialysis by the shunting of blood from the body through a machine for diffusion and ultrafiltration and then returning it to the patient's circulation.
3. Two explanations for the decrease of K.D.'s serum albumin levels are that some protein is lost during dialysis, and poor appetite may decrease the intake of high-protein foods.
4. Renal patients develop anemia because they experience decreased production of the hormone erythropoietin, a hormone that stimulates red blood cell production.
5. Water-soluble vitamin supplements are usually prescribed to replace nutrients lost during dialysis and because of poor intake of foods containing these vitamins.
6. Peritoneal dialysis removes excess fluid and waste products from the blood by using the peritoneum as the dialysis membrane. Dialysate is instilled and removed through a catheter surgically placed into the peritoneal cavity.
7. Possible dietary changes caused by peritoneal dialysis (PD) are: lower energy intake because of absorption of kcalories from the dialysate, higher protein intake caused by greater protein losses during PD, and more liberal potassium and sodium restrictions.

Chapter 21

1. Possible causes of her decreased appetite are the cancer and/or the treatment. M.N. may be experiencing some depression over her diagnosis, which can also affect her appetite.
2. Side effects from her chemotherapy may include: anorexia, nausea, vomiting, stomatitis, diarrhea, and decreased nutrient absorption.
3. Her nutritional status may be affected by her inability to consume adequate energy nutrients. Secondly, she may not be able to absorb the nutrients she does consume. Unfortunately, as her nutritional status declines, her ability to tolerate treatment also declines.

GLOSSARY

A

absorption the process by which substances pass through the intestinal mucosa into the blood or lymph

acesulfame K a nonnutritive sweetener

acetyl coenzyme A important intermediate byproduct in metabolism formed from the breakdown of glucose, fatty acids, and certain amino acids

acute respiratory failure a sudden absence of respirations, with confusion or unresponsiveness caused by obstructed air flow or failure of the pulmonary gas exchange mechanism

adaptive thermogenesis energy (or heat released) used by the body to adjust to changing physical and biological environments

adenosine triphosphate (ATP) an energy-rich compound used for all energy-requiring processes in the body

adipocytes cells specialized for storage of fat

adipose tissue a stored form of fat (mainly triglycerides) in the body

adrenocorticotropic hormone (ACTH) an adrenal cortex hormone that stimulates secretion of more hormones

aerobic glycolysis the conversion of glucose to ATP for energy when oxygen is available

aerobic pathway a form of energy production that depends on oxygen

aerophagia the swallowing of air, usually the result of eating with the mouth open, followed by belching, gastric distress, and/or flatulence

alcoholic cirrhosis a liver disease associated with chronic alcohol abuse, accounts for 50% of all cases of cirrhosis; also called Laennec's cirrhosis

aldosterone a hormone secreted by the adrenal gland in response to sodium levels in kidneys; causes kidneys to balance fluid levels as needed

allowance the amount of a nutrient needed to be consumed to maintain good health

alternative sweeteners nonnutritive sweeteners (or artificial sweeteners) synthetically produced to be sweet-tasting, but which provide no nutrients and few, if any, kcalories; include aspartame, saccharin, and acesulfame K

amenorrhea the lack of menstruation

amino acid an organic compound containing carbon, hydrogen, oxygen, and nitrogen

amino acid pool the assortment of amino acids available to cells

aminopeptidase an intestinal peptidase that releases free amino acids from the amino end of short chain peptides

amylophagia pica of corn and laundry starch

anabolism synthesis

anaerobic glycolysis the conversion of glucose to lactic acid to provide energy in the absence of oxygen

anaerobic pathway a form of energy production that does not require oxygen

anencephaly a congenital defect in which the brain does not develop; death occurs shortly after birth

angina pectoris chest pain that often radiates down the left arm and is frequently accompanied by a feeling of suffocation and impending death

anorexia nervosa a mental disorder characterized by self-imposed starvation; may include binge eating episodes associated with bulimic behaviors

anthropometric measurements measurement of the human body as to height, weight, and size of component parts

antidiuretic hormone (ADH) a hormone secreted by the pituitary gland in response to low fluid levels; causes kidneys to decrease excretion of water; also called vasopressin

antineoplastic therapy a substance, procedure, or measure that prevents the proliferation of malignant cells; usually chemotherapy, radiation therapy, surgery, biologic response modifiers, or bone marrow transplantation

antioxidant a compound that guards other compounds from damaging oxidation

anuria <250 ml urine excretion/24 hr

appetite the desire for food

ariboflavinosis riboflavin deficiency

arteriosclerosis a group of diseases characterized by thickening, loss of elasticity, and calcification of arterial walls, resulting in decreased blood supply

ascites an abnormal intraperitoneal accumulation of fluid containing large amounts of protein and electrolytes usually resulting in abdominal swelling, hemodilution, edema, or a decreased urinary output

aspartame a nonnutritive sweetener formed by bonding the amino acids of phenylalanine and aspartic acid

aspiration usually refers to the inhalation of foreign material into the lungs

ataxia muscle weakness and loss of coordination

atherosclerosis the development of lesions (also called fatty streaks) in the intima of arteries; during aging, the lesions develop into fibrous plaques that project into the vessel lumen and begin to disturb blood flow

athetoid purposeless weaving motions of the body or extremities

atonic lacking normal muscle tone

azotemia the retention of excessive amounts of nitrogenous compounds in the blood caused by the kidney's failure to remove urea from the blood; characterized by uremia

B

barium enema a rectal infusion of a radiopaque contrast medium to diagnose obstruction, tumors, or other abnormalities (for example, ulcerative colitis)

basal metabolism the amount of energy required to maintain life-sustaining activities for a specific period of time

beikost supplemental or weaning foods

benign neoplasm a tumor of limited growth, defined shape; does not spread to surrounding tissue or other body organs

beriberi a severe chronic deficiency of thiamin characterized by muscle weakness and pain, anorexia, mental disorientation, and tachycardia

Beta cells insulin-producing cells situated in the islets of Langerhans of the pancreas

bezoars physical obstacles created by tangles of fibrous material in the gastrointestinal tract that may cause dangerous gastrointestinal obstructions

bile a substance that emulsifies fats to aid the digestion of lipids; produced by the liver and stored in the gallbladder

biliary atresia a congenital condition in which the major bile duct is blocked, limiting the availability of bile for fat digestion

biliary cirrhosis a liver disease associated with obstruction of biliary drainage or biliary disorders; accounts for 15% of all cases of cirrhosis

binders substances occurring in plant foods that combine with minerals to form undigestible compounds that cannot be absorbed.

binge eating disorder (BED) a mental disorder characterized by frequent binge eating behaviors, not accompanied by purging or compensatory behaviors; commonly referred to as compulsive overeating

bingeing feeling out of control when eating, resulting in the consumption of excessive amounts of food

bioavailability the level of absorption of a consumed nutrient

bioelectric impedance analysis (BIA) a method using a very mild electric charge to estimate lean body mass in order to determine body fat composition

biological value a method to determine the quality of food protein by measuring the amount of nitrogen kept in the body after digestion and absorption

body image the perceptions we have of the physical appearance or attractiveness of our bodies

bolus a masticated lump or ball of food ready to be swallowed

branched-chain amino acids (BCAA) leucine, isoleucine, and valine

bulimia nervosa a mental disorder characterized as the binge and purge syndrome; includes experiencing repetitive food binges accompanied by purging or compensatory behaviors

C

cachexia general ill health and malnutrition, marked by weakness and emaciation

calcitonin a hormone that reacts in response to high blood levels of calcium; released by the Special C cells of the thyroid gland

calcitriol active vitamin D hormone that raises blood calcium levels

calcium rigor a condition of hardness or stiffness of muscles when blood calcium levels get too high

calcium tetany a condition of spasms and nerve excitability when blood calcium levels get too low

cancer uncontrolled growth of cells that tend to invade surrounding tissue and metastasize to distant body sites

cancer cachexia a syndrome caused by a malignant tumor characterized by anorexia, alterations in taste sensation, weight loss, anemia, weakness, and emaciation that results in decline of physical and mental functions; reversed only by control of the disease

carbohydrates organic compounds composed of carbon, hydrogen, and oxygen

carboxypeptidase a pancreatic protease that hydrolyzes polypeptides into amino acids

carcinogenesis the process of cancer production

cardiac decompensation impaired cardiac output for which the reasons not entirely understood

cardiovascular endurance the ability of the body to take in, deliver, and obtain oxygen for physical work

catabolism breakdown

cheilosis inflammation of the mucous membrane of the mouth and lips (angular stomatitis) caused by deficiencies of riboflavin and other B vitamins

chemical digestion the chemical altering effects of digestive secretions, gastric juices, and enzymes on food substance composition

cholecystectomy the surgical removal of the gallbladder, performed to treat cholelithiasis and cholecystitis

cholecystitis an acute inflammation of the gallbladder associated with pain, tenderness, and fever

cholecystokinin-pancreozymin (CCK) a hormone that initiates pancreatic exocrine secretions, acts against gastrin, and activates the gallbladder to release bile; secreted by the small intestine

choledocholithiasis gallstones in the common bile duct

cholelithiasis the presence of stones in the gallbladder

chronic dieting syndrome a lifestyle inhibited or controlled by a constant concern about food intake, body shape and/or weight that affects an individual's physical and mental health status

chronic hunger a continual experience of undernutrition

chronic obstructive pulmonary disease (COPD) a progressive and irreversible condition identified by obstruction of air flow; chronic bronchitis, asthma, and emphysema (also called chronic obstructive lung disease)

chronic ulcerative colitis an inflammatory process confined to the mucosa of any or all of the large intestine

chylomicrons the first lipoproteins formed after absorption of lipids from food

chyme a semiliquid mixture of food mass

chymotrypsin a pancreatic protease that hydrolyzes peptides into dipeptides

cis-fatty acids *cis* indicates the configuration of the double bond in a natural oil

coenzyme a substance that activates an enzyme

colic a sharp visceral pain

colonoscopic examination the examination of the mucosal lining of the colon using a colonoscope (an elongated endoscope)

colostomy the surgical creation of an artificial anus on the abdominal wall by incising the colon and bringing it out to the surface; may be single-barreled (one opening) or double-barreled (distal and proximal loops open onto the abdomen

colostrum the fluid secreted from the breast during late pregnancy and first few days postpartum; contains immunologically active substances (maternal antibodies) and essential nutrients

complete proteins proteins containing all nine essential amino acids

complex carbohydrates polysaccharides of starch and fiber

component pureeing each food item is pureed separately (food thickeners may be added to help maintain consistency) then presented in a manner that resembles the original product (for example, a pork chop can be pureed, then molded into a pork-chop shape and served)

comprehensive nutritional assessment a procedure conducted by dietetic professionals to determine appropriate medical nutrition therapy based on identified needs of the patient

computed tomography (CT) an imaging technique that can be used to determine body fat composition

congestive heart failure circulatory congestion resulting in the heart's inability to maintain adequate blood supply to meet oxygen demands

constipation slow movement of feces through the large intestine; straining to pass hard, dry stools

cor pulmonale an abnormal cardiac condition characterized by hypertrophy of the right ventricle as a result of hypertension of the pulmonary circulation

Crohn's disease an inflammatory disorder that involves all layers of the intestinal wall and may involve small or large intestine or both; associated with stricture formation, fistulous tracts, and abscesses

cystic fibrosis (CF) a genetic disorder most common among Caucasian populations in which excessive mucus is produced, primarily affecting respiratory airways; also limits fat-absorption in the digestion system

D

Daily Values a system for food labeling composed of two sets of reference values: Reference Daily Intakes and Daily Reference Values

Daily Reference Values a set of daily nutrient and food constituent values for which there are no RDAs; includes fat, fiber, cholesterol, and sodium

deamination a process through which an amino acid group breaks off from an amino acid molecule, resulting in molecules of ammonia and keto acid

Delaney Clause the 1958 Food Additives Amendment to the Federal Food Drug and Cosmetic Act of 1938 that bans any intentional food additive found to induce cancer in man or animal

denatured a change in the shape of protein structures caused by heat, light, acids, or alcohol

densitometry underwater weighing

diabetes mellitus a disorder of carbohydrate metabolism characterized by hyperglycemia and caused by insulin that is either defective or deficient

diagnostic related groups (DRGs) classifications used to determine Medicare payments for inpatient care, based on primary and secondary diagnosis, primary and secondary procedures, age, and length of hospitalization

dialysate dialysis solution

dialysis a procedure that involves diffusion of particles from an area of high to lower concentration, osmosis of fluid across the membrane from an area of lesser to greater concentration of particles, and the ultrafiltration or movement of fluid across the membrane as a result of an artificially created pressure differential

diarrhea the frequent passing of loose, watery bowel movements

diet manual the reference book (usually in a three-ring binder) that describes the rationale and indications for using a specific diet, lists allowed, and restricted foods and sample menus

dietary fiber polysaccharides in plant foods that cannot be digested by humans

dietary standards a guide to adequate nutrient intake levels against which to compare the nutrient values of foods consumed

digestion the process through which foods are broken down into smaller and smaller units to prepare nutrients for absorption

digestive system a series of organs that function to prepare ingested nutrients for digestion and absorption

dipeptidase an intestinal peptidase that completes the hydrolysis of proteins to amino acids

disaccharide a sugar formed by two single carbohydrate units bound together; sucrose, maltose, and galactose are disaccharides

disease prevention the recognition of a danger to health that could be reduced or alleviated through specific actions or through changes in lifestyle behaviors

diverticulosis the presence of diverticula

diverticulitis inflammation of one or more diverticula

diverticulum pouchlike herniations protruding from the muscular layer of the colon

dry beriberi thiamin deficiency affecting the nervous system producing paralysis and extreme muscle wasting

dry body weight an estimate of actual weight without the weight of ascites fluid

dumping syndrome when contents from the stomach empty too rapidly into the duodenum, causing symptoms of profuse sweating, nausea, dizziness, and weakness

durable power of attorney gives an appointed attorney or patient surrogate the authorization to make certain decisions for an individual under specific circumstances, some include health care decisions; assists in situations where the patient has become incompetent; some states may allow the attorney or surrogate to consent or refuse life-sustaining care

dysphagia the inability to swallow normally or freely or to transfer liquid or solid foods from the oral cavity to the stomach; may be caused by an underlying central neurologic or isolated mechanical dysfunction

E

eating disorders a group of behaviors fueled by unresolved emotional conflicts symptomized by altered food consumption

edema an excess accumulation of fluid in interstitial spaces caused by seepage from the circulatory system

elemental formula a dietary solution that provides ready-to-absorb basic nutrients, requiring minimal digestion

edentulous toothless

eicosapentaenoic acid (EPA) the main omega-3 fatty acid in fish

emetic a substance that causes vomiting

emulsifier a substance that works by being soluble in water and fat at the same time

endogenous originating from within the body or produced internally

endometrium the mucous membrane of the uterus

enrichment returning to their original levels nutrients that were lost because of processing

enteritis infection of the small intestine caused by a virus, bacteria, or protozoa

enterokinase an intestinal hormone that activates trypsinogen into trypsin

enuresis incontinence of urine, especially at bedtime

epinephrine an adrenal gland hormone that enhances the fast conversion of liver glycogen to glucose

ergogenic aids drugs and dietary regimens believed by some, but not proven, to increase strength, power, and endurance

esophageal varices large and swollen veins at the lower end of the esophagus that are especially vulnerable to ulceration and hemorrhage, usually the result of portal hypertension

esophagitis inflammation of the lower esophagus

essential amino acids amino acids that cannot be manufactured by the human body

essential fat certain components of body fat that are essential for life

essential fatty acids polyunsaturated fatty acids that cannot be made in the body and must be consumed in the diet

essential hypertension elevated blood pressure for which the cause is unknown; also called primary hypertension

essential nutrients nutrients that cannot be made by the human body and must be provided by foods

exogenous originating outside the body or produced from external sources

extracellular fluid all fluids outside cells including interstitial fluid, plasma, and watery components of body organs and substances

F

fasting blood glucose level of glucose circulating in blood serum after an 8-hour fast; also called fasting blood sugar (FBS)

fatty infiltration an accumulation of fat (triglycerides) in the liver

feeding relationship the interactions or patterns of behaviors surrounding food preparation and consumption within a family

fetal alcohol syndrome (FAS) a disorder caused by alcohol consumption during pregnancy that may produce a range of specific anatomical and central nervous systems defects; fetal alcohol effects (FAE)

flatus intestinal gas

flexibility the ability to move muscles to their full extent without injury

fluid volume deficit the state in which a person experiences vascular, cellular, or intracellular dehydration

fluid volume excess the state in which a person experiences increased fluid retention and edema

fluorosis a condition of mottling or brown spotting of the tooth enamel caused by excessive intake of fluoride

food choice the specific foods that are convenient to choose when we are actually ready to eat

food cholesterol dietary cholesterol; consumed from food sources

food fat dietary triglycerides; consumed from food sources

food liking the foods that we really like to eat

food preferences the foods we choose to eat when all foods are available at the same time and in the same quantity

fractionation the administration of radiation in smaller doses over time rather than in a single large dose; minimizes tissue damage

G

galactosemia an autosomal recessive disorder that results in an inability to metabolize galactose and lactose milk products

gastrin a hormone that increases the release of gastric juices; secreted by stomach mucosa

gastroesophageal reflux the return of gastric contents into the esophagus that results in a severe burning sensation under the sternum

gastrointestinal (GI) tract the main organs of the digestive system that forms a tube that runs from the mouth to the anus

gastroparesis paralysis of the stomach caused by vagal autonomic neuropathy; causes delayed gastric emptying

geophagia pica of clay and dirt

gerontology the study of aging

gestational diabetes mellitus (GDM) a form of diabetes occurring during pregnancy, most commonly after the 20th week of gestation

glomerulonephritis the name of a group of diseases that damage the renal glomeruli; when the glomerulus is injured, protein and RBCs enter the renal tubule and are excreted in urine; can be acute or chronic

glossitis inflammation of the tongue

glucagon a pancreatic hormone that releases glycogen from the liver

gluconeogenesis the process producing glucose from fat and protein

glucocorticoid an adrenal cortex hormone that affects food metabolism

glycogen a carbohydrate energy stored as a polysaccharide in the liver and in muscles

glycogenesis the process of converting glucose to glycogen

glycogenolysis the process converting glycogen back to glucose

glycolysis the conversion of glucose to carbon compounds

glycosylated hemoglobin ($HgbA_{1c}$) a substance (glycohemoglobin) formed when hemoglobin combines with some of the glucose in the blood stream

goiter the enlargement of the thyroid gland because of iodine deficiency

growth hormone a pituitary hormone that inhibits insulin

H

hard water water that contains high amounts of minerals such as calcium and magnesium

health the merging and balance of five physical and psychological dimensions of health; includes the physical, mental, emotional, social, and spiritual dimensions

health promotion strategies to increase the level of health of individuals, families, and/or communities

heartburn a burning sensation felt in the esophagus caused by stomach reflux

heme iron the dietary iron found in animal foods of meat, fish, and poultry

hemochromatosis a genetic disorder causing excessive dietary iron absorption

hemodialysis a procedure to remove impurities or wastes from the blood in treating renal insufficiency by shunting the blood from the body through a machine for diffusion and ultrafiltration and then returning it to the patient's circulation

hemodilution the dilution of the blood

hemoglobin the oxygen transporting protein in red blood cells

hemosiderosis a condition in which too much iron is stored in the body

heparinized the use of an antithrombin factor to prevent intravascular clotting

hepatic coma a neuropsychiatric symptom of extensive liver damage caused by chronic or acute liver disease

hepatic encephalopathy a type of brain damage caused by liver disease and consequent ammonia intoxication

hepatic steatosis an accumulation of fat (triglycerides) in the liver cells

hepatotoxic potentially destructive to liver cells

hiatal hernia herniation of a portion of the stomach into the chest through the esophageal hiatus of the diaphragm

high-density lipoproteins (HDL) lipoproteins made of large proportions of proteins that carry fats and cholesterol from body cells to the liver

high quality protein a food containing the best balance and assortment of essential and nonessential amino acids for protein synthesis

homeostasis a state of physiological equilibrium produced by a balance of functions and of chemical composition within an organism

hormones substances that act as messengers between organs to cause the release of needed secretions

hunger a physiological need for food

hydrogenation breaking a double bond on a fatty acid carbon chain and saturating it with hydrogen

hydroxyapatite a natural mineral structure of bones and teeth

hyperbilirubinemia a neonatal condition of excessively high levels of bilirubin (red bile pigment) leading to jaundice in which bile is deposited in tissues throughout the body

hypercalcemia high blood levels of calcium

hypercalciuria high levels of calcium excreted in urine

hypercaloric more than one kcalorie per ml

hyperemesis gravidarum severe and unrelenting vomiting in the second trimester of pregnancy or that severely interferes with the mother's life; a serious condition usually requiring intravenous replacement of nutrients and fluids

hyperglycemia elevated blood glucose levels (>120 mg/dl)

hyperlipidemia elevated serum lipid levels

hyperlipidemic excess lipids in the blood

hypermetabolism an increase in BMR above expected levels based on age, sex, and body size

hyperosmolar abnormally increased osmolarity

hyperplasia an increase in the number of cells occurring during the growth spurts accompanying normal development

hypertension an average systolic blood pressure ≥140 mmHg and/or a diastolic pressure ≥90 mmHg (or both)

hypertonic having greater concentration of solute than another solution

hypertrophy an increase in the size of cells

hypoalbuminemia decreased serum albumin

hypoglycemia blood glucose levels that are below normal values

hyponatremia abnormally low concentrations of sodium in circulating blood

hypophosphatemia abnormally low phosphate levels in circulating blood

hyporeflexia a neurologic condition characterized by weakened reflex reactions

hypoxia a lack of oxygen to the cells

I

idiopathic steatorrhea fat malabsorption as a result of unknown causes

ileostomy the removal of the entire colon and rectum; surgical formation of an opening of the ileum onto the surface of the abdomen through which fecal matter is emptied

incidental additives substances that inadvertently contaminate processed foods.

incomplete proteins proteins lacking one or more of the essential amino acids

insensible perspiration water lost invisibly through evaporation from the lungs and skin

ischemia decreased blood supply to a body organ or part

insoluble dietary fibers dietary fibers that do not dissolve in fluids

insulin a hormone produced by the pancreas that regulates blood glucose levels

insulin-dependent diabetes mellitus (IDDM) a form of diabetes mellitus in which the pancreas produces no insulin at all

intentional food additives substances purposely added to food products during manufacturing

intrinsic factor a substance produced by stomach mucosa that is required for vitamin B_{12} absorption

intracellular fluid the fluid within the cells composed of water plus concentrations of potassium and phosphates

interstitial fluid the fluid between the cells containing concentrations of sodium and chloride

irradiation a procedure by which food is exposed to radiation, destroying microorganisms, insect growth, and parasites that could spoil food or cause illness

isotonic having the same concentration of solute as another solution, hence exerting the same amount of osmotic pressure as that solution

J

jaundice the yellow discoloration of the skin, mucous membranes, and sclerae of the eyes caused by greater than normal amounts of bilirubin in the blood

K

keratomalacia a condition caused by vitamin A deficiency in which the cornea becomes dry and thickens from the formation of hard protein tissue

ketone bodies breakdown products of fatty acid catabolism

ketosis a condition in which the absence of plasma glucose results in partial oxidation of fatty acids

kwashiorkor malnutrition caused by a lack of protein while consuming adequate energy

L

lactation the production of breast milk

lactovegetarian dietary pattern a food plan consisting of only plant foods and dairy products

lactose intolerance the inability to digest lactose because of a deficiency of the digestive enzyme lactase

lifestyle a pattern of behaviors

limiting amino acid the essential amino acid or amino acids that incomplete proteins lack

linoleic acid an essential polyunsaturated fatty acid with the first double bond located at the sixth carbon atom from the omega end

linolenic acid an essential polyunsaturated fatty acid with the first double bond located at the third carbon atom from the omega end

lipogenesis anabolism (synthesis) of lipids; triglycerides, phospholipids, cholesterol, and prostaglandin synthesis

locus of control the perception of one's ability to control life events and experiences

low birth weight weighing less than 5.5 lbs (2500 g) at birth

low-density lipoproteins (LDL) lipoproteins made of large proportions of cholesterol that carry fats and cholesterol to body cells

lupus erythematosus a chronic inflammatory disease affecting many systems of the body and whose cause is unknown; pathophysiology includes severe vasculitis, renal involvement, and lesions of the skin and nervous system

M

macrophages cells that are able to surround, engulf, and digest microorganisms and cellular debris; scavenger cells

macrosomia larger body size

macrovascular large blood vessels of the body

major minerals essential nutrient minerals required daily in amounts of 100 mg or higher

malignant neoplasm a tumor that grows in an uncontrolled manner, invading surrounding tissue; metastasizes and may cause death if untreated

malnutrition an imbalanced nutrient and energy intake

management the use of available resources to achieve a predetermined goal

marasmus malnutrition caused by a lack of energy (kcalorie) intake

MCT medium chain triglycerides; distinguished from other triglycerides by having 8 to 10 carbon atoms; are easily digested

MCT fat (oil) specialized modular formulas made of medium chain triglycerides that do not require pancreatic lipase or bile for digestion and absorption; they are absorbed directly into the portal vein (like amino acids and monosaccharides) rather than the lymphatic system like other lipids

mechanical digestion the crushing and twisting effects of teeth and peristalsis that divides foods into smaller pieces

medical nutritional therapy the use of specific nutrition services to treat an illness, injury, or condition

megacolon massive, abnormal dilation of the colon that may be congenital, toxic, or acquired in nature

metabolism a set of processes through which absorbed nutrients are used by the body for energy and to form and maintain body structures and functions

methylxanthines caffeine, theobromine, and theophylline; found in beverages such as coffee, tea, cocoa, and cola drinks; have pharmacologic properties that stimulate the central nervous system

micelles tiny emulsion droplets of fatty acids, monoglycerides, cholesterol, and fat-soluble vitamins mixed with bile salts

microvascular small blood vessels of the body

microvilli hairlike projections on the villi

monocytes white blood cells (large leukocytes)

monosaccharides a sugar composed of a single carbohydrate unit; glucose, fructose, and galactose are monosaccharides

monounsaturated fatty acid a fatty acid containing a carbon chain with one double bond

mucosa the inside gastrointestinal muscle tissue layer composed of mucous membrane

mucositis inflammation of mucous membranes

mutation a spontaneous or induced change in genetic material; changes function of the gene

multifactorial phenotype a characteristic that is the product of numerous genetic and environmental factors

muscularis a thick layer of muscle tissue surrounding the submucosa

muscular strength and endurance the ability of the muscles to perform hard work and/or prolonged work

myocardial infarction an occlusion of a coronary artery, caused by atherosclerosis or an embolus resulting from a necrotic area in the myocardial vasculature; also called heart attack

myoglobin oxygen-transporting protein in muscle

N

necrosis localized tissue death that occurs in response to disease or injury

neoplasm any abnormal growth of new tissue; a tumor, benign or malignant

nephrosclerosis necrosis of the renal arterioles, associated with hypertension

neutropenia abnormally low levels of circulating white blood cells (neutrophils) that remove bacteria

night blindness the inability of the eyes to readjust vision from bright to dim light because of vitamin A deficiency

nitrogen-balance studies measurement of the amount of N entering the body compared to the amount excreted

nocturia urination, especially excessive urination at night

nonessential amino acids (NEAAs) amino acids manufactured by the human body

nonheme iron dietary iron found in plant foods

non–insulin-dependent diabetes mellitus (NIDDM) a form of diabetes mellitus in which the pancreas produces some insulin that is defective and unable to serve the complete needs of the body

nutrients chemicals in foods that are required by the body for energy, growth, maintenance and/or repair

nutrition the study of essential nutrients and the processes by which nutrients are used by the body

nutrition support team a multidisciplinary group of health care professionals who aid in the provision of nutritional support; usually composed of a physician director, dietitian, nurse, and pharmacist

nutritional risk the potential to become malnourished because of factors that are primary (inadequate intake of nutrients) or secondary (caused by iatrogenic or disease affects)

nutritional support although commonly used in reference to enteral and parenteral nutrition delivery systems, it can refer to any nutrition intervention used to minimize patient morbidity, mortality, and complications

nutritionist a professional who has completed academic degrees of BS, MS, EdD or PhD in foods and nutrition

O

oliguria <400 ml urine excretion/24 hr

orthostatic hypotension a sudden drop in blood pressure when changing from a lying to a sitting or a sitting to a standing position; also referred to as postural hypotension

osmolality concentration of electrically charged particles per kilogram of solution

osmotic diarrhea diarrhea associated water retention in the large intestine resulting from an accumulation of nonabsorbable water-soluble solutes

osteodystrophy defective bone development associated with disturbances in calcium and phosphorus metabolism and renal insufficiency

osteomalacia an adult disorder caused by vitamin D or calcium deficiency characterized by soft, demineralized bones

osteoporosis a multifactorial disorder in which bone density is reduced and remaining bone is brittle, breaking easily

overnutrition consumption of too many nutrients and too much energy compared to RDA levels

ovo-lacto-vegetarian dietary pattern a food plan consisting of only plant foods plus dairy products and eggs

oxygen debt the amount of oxygen required to clear lactic acid buildup from the body

oxytocin a hormone that initiates uterine contractions of labor and has a role in the ejection of milk in lactation

P

pagophagia pica of excessive ice consumption

pancreatitis inflammation of the pancreas, may be acute or chronic

paralytic ileus a decrease in or absence of intestinal peristalsis

parathormone a hormone that raises blood calcium levels; secreted by the parathyroid gland in response to low blood calcium levels

parenteral nutrition administration of nutrients by a route other than the gastrointestinal tract, usually intravenously

parturition childbirth

pellagra the niacin deficiency disorder characterized by diarrhea, dermatitis, and dementia

pepsin the gastric protease

pepsinogen the inactive form of pepsin

percutaneous endoscopic placement placement of a feeding tube into the stomach via the esophagus and then drawn through the abdominal skin using a stab incision

peristalsis the rhythmic contractions of muscles causing wave-like motions that move food down the gastrointestinal tract

peritoneal dialysis a dialysis procedure performed to correct an imbalance of fluid or electrolytes in the blood or other wastes by using the peritoneum as the diffusible membrane

pernicious anemia inadequate red blood cell formation caused by a lack of intrinsic factor in the stomach with which to absorb vitamin B_{12}

phenylketonuria (PKU) a genetic protein disorder in which the body cannot break down excess phenylalanine

phospholipids lipid compounds that form part of cell walls and act as a fat emulsifier

physical activity any body movement produced by skeletal muscles that results in energy expenditure

physical fitness the limits on the actions that the body is capable of making

phytochemicals nonnutritive substances in plant-based foods that appear to have disease-fighting properties

pica a condition characterized by a hunger and appetite for nonfood substances

plaque deposits of fatty substances, including cholesterol, that attach to arterial walls

pneumothorax air introduced into the thorax

polydipsia excessive thirst

polymeric formula provides intact nutrients (for example, whole proteins and long-chain triglycerides) that require a normally functioning gastrointestinal tract

polyphagia excessive hunger and eating

polysaccharide a carbohydrate consisting of many units of monosaccharides joined together; starch and fiber are food sources and glycogen is a storage form in the liver and muscles

polyunsaturated fatty acid (PUFA) a fatty acid containing one or more double bonds on the carbon chain

polyuria excessive urination

portal hypertension increased blood pressure in the portal circulation caused by compression or occlusion in the portal or hepatic vascular system

postnecrotic cirrhosis a liver disease associated with history of viral hepatitis, improperly treated hepatitis, or hepatic damage from toxic chemicals; accounts for about 20% of all cases of cirrhosis

postprandial occurring after a meal

precursor a substance that the human body can convert to a nutrient

pregnancy-induced hypertension (PIH) a sudden rise in arterial blood pressure accompanied by rapid weight gain and marked edema during pregnancy; formerly known as toxemia of pregnancy

primary hypertension elevated blood pressure for which the cause is unknown; also called essential hypertension

primary prevention activities to avert the initial development of a disease or poor health

prolactin a hormone responsible for milk synthesis

proteases protein enzymes

protein an organic compound formed from chains of amino acids

protein efficiency ratio (PER) a method to determine the quality of food protein by comparing weight gain to protein intake

protein energy malnutrition (PEM) malnutrition caused by the lack of protein, energy, or both

proteinuria >3 gram to 3.5 gram protein lost in the urine per day

R

reactant a substance that enters into and is altered during a chemical reaction

recombinant EPO recombinant human erythropoietin; a drug used to treat anemia by replacing erythropoietin for patients with CRF who do not produce this hormone in adequate amounts

Recommended Dietary Allowances (RDAs) average daily intake levels of essential nutrients that meet the nutritional needs of almost all healthy individuals

refeeding syndrome the physiological and metabolic complications associated with reintroducing nutrition (refeeding) to a person with PEM too rapidly; these complications can include malabsorption, cardiac insufficiency, congestive heart failure, respiratory distress, convulsions, coma, and perhaps death

Reference Daily Intakes a set of daily nutrient values for protein, vitamins, and minerals based on allowances of the 1968 RDAs

refined grains grains that contain only some of the edible kernel

regional enteritis Crohn's disease

registered dietitian (RD) a professional trained in foods and the management of diets (dietetics) credentialed by the Commission on Dietetic Registration of the American Dietetic Association; credentialing is based on completion of a BS degree from an approved program, clinical and administrative training, and passing a registration examination

renal transplantation the transfer of a kidney from one person to another

requirement the amount of a nutrient that must be consumed to prevent deficiency symptoms

respiratory distress syndrome a respiratory disordered identified by insufficient respiration and abnormally low levels of circulating oxygen in the blood

respiratory quotient (RQ) ratio of CO_2 exhaled to O_2 inhaled; depending on the net metabolic needs of the body, the ratio ranges from 0.7 to 1.0, and averages around 0.8; carbohydrate metabolism produces an RQ = 1; protein metabolism RQ = 0.8; and fat metabolism RQ = 0.7

resting energy expenditure (REE) the energy expended in a normal life situation while at rest, and energy used following meals and exercise

retrovirus an RNA virus that becomes integrated into the DNA of a host cell during replication; HIV is a retrovirus

rickets a childhood disorder caused by vitamin D or calcium deficiency leading to insufficient mineralization of bone and tooth matrix

S

saccharin a nonnutritive sweetener

saliva the secretions of the salivary glands of the mouth

satiety feeling full and satisfied after eating

saturated fatty acid a fatty acid with carbon chains completely saturated or filled with hydrogen

scurvy extreme vitamin C deficiency disorder characterized by inflammation of connective tissues, gingivitis, muscle degeneration, bruising, and hemorrhaging as the vascular system weakens

secondary hypertension elevated blood pressure for which the cause can be identified

secondary prevention early detection to stop or reduce the effects of a disease or illness

secretin a hormone secreted by the small intestine that causes the pancreas to release bicarbonate to the small intestine

segmentation the forward and backward muscular action that assists in controlling food mass movement through the gastrointestinal tract

senescence older adulthood

septicemia systemic infection in the circulating bloodstream

serosa the outermost layer of the gastrointestinal wall made of serous membrane

set point a natural level (of some characteristic) that the body regulates or defends

sickle cell disease a genetic disorder in which red blood cells are curved or "sickled"

simple carbohydrates monosaccharides and disaccharides

small for gestational age (SGA) having a lower birthweight than expected for the length of gestation

soft water water that has been filtered to replace some of the minerals with sodium

solute a substance dissolved in another substance

solvent the liquid in which another substance (the solute) is dissolved to form a solution

soluble dietary fibers dietary fibers that dissolve in fluids

somatic protein skeletal muscle protein

somatic protein stores proteins in skeletal muscle

somatostatin a hormone produced by the pancreas and hypothalamus that inhibits insulin and glucagon

spina bifida a congenital defect of the spinal column causing the spinal cord to be unprotected, resulting in a range of disabilities including paralysis and incontinence

stomatitis inflammation of mucous membranes of the mouth

steroid hormones an adrenal gland hormone that functions against insulin, promoting glucose formation from protein

sterols fat-like class of lipids that serve vital functions in the body

storage fat layers and cushions of fat providing stored energy and protection from extremes of environmental temperatures and of internal organs against physical trauma

submucosa a layer of connective muscle tissue under the mucosa

sugar alcohols nutritive sweeteners related to carbohydrates but which provide 4 kcalories per gram; includes sorbitol, mannitol, and xylitol

T

T cells a small circulating lymphocyte produced in the bone marrow that mediates cellular immune responses

TCA cycle cellular reactions that liberate energy from fragments of carbohydrates, fats, and protein; also known as the tricaboxylic acid cycle or Krebs cycle

tachycardia rapid beating of the heart

teratogen an agent that is capable of producing a malformation or a defect in the unborn fetus

tertiary prevention occurs after a disorder develops to minimize further complications or to assist in the restoration of health

thermic effect of food (TEF) or diet-induced thermogenesis an increase of cellular activity when food is eaten

thrombosis thrombus (blood clot) development within a blood vessel of the body

thrombus blood clot

thyrotoxicosis iodine-induced goiter

thyroxine a thyroid hormone that affects blood glucose levels by increasing glucose absorption and releasing epinephrine

trace minerals essential nutrient minerals required daily in amounts less than or equal to 20 mg

trans-fatty acids fatty acids with unusual double-bond structures caused by hydrogenated unsaturated oils

triglycerides the largest class of lipids found in food and body fat; composed of three fatty acids and one glycerol molecule

trypsin the primary pancreatic protease

trypsinogen the inactive form of trypsin

U

undernutrition the underconsumption of energy or nutrients based on RDA values

unrefined grains grains prepared for consumption containing all edible portions of kernels

urea the product of ammonia conversion produced during deamination

uremia excessive amounts of urea and other nitrogenous waste products in the blood

uremic toxicity a buildup of toxic waste products (urea and other nitrogenous waste products) in the blood; symptoms include anorexia, nausea, metallic taste in the mouth, irritability, confusion, lethargy, restlessness, and pruritus (itching)

V

video fluoroscopy a radiological technique used to visually examine a part of the body or the function of an organ; the technique offers immediate serial images

vegan dietary pattern a food plan consisting of only plant foods

very low calorie diets (VLCD) usually defined as diets containing 800 kcalories a day or less

very low-density lipoproteins (VLDL) lipoproteins made of the largest proportions of cholesterol that carry fats and cholesterol to body cells

villi finger-like projections on the walls of the small intestine

visceral fat fat that is within the abdominal cavity

visceral protein protein other than muscle tissue, (for example, internal organs and blood)

visceral protein stores circulating serum proteins and proteins found in organs, including the liver, kidneys, pancreas, and heart

vitamin an essential organic molecule needed in very small amounts for cellular metabolism

vomiting reverse peristalsis

W

wellness a lifestyle that enhances our level of health

Wernicke-Korsakoff syndrome a cerebral form of beriberi affecting the central nervous system

wet beriberi thiamin deficiency with edema affecting cardiac function by weakening of heart muscle and vascular system

whole grain products food items made using unrefined grains

Wilson's disease a rare, inherited disorder of copper metabolism in which copper accumulates slowly in the liver and is then released and taken up in other parts of the body; as copper accumulates in RBCs, hemolysis, and then hemolytic anemia occurs

X

xerophthalmia a condition caused by vitamin A deficiency with symptoms ranging from night blindness to keratomalacia; may result in complete blindness

CREDITS

Chapter 1 Opener, PhotoDisk; Figs. 1–2, 1–3, 1–4, 1–6, unn. fig. 1–2, Joanne Scott/Tracy McCalla; Figs. 1–1, 1–5, Rolin Graphics; unn. figs. 1–1, 1–3, Barbara Bourne.

Chapter 2 Opener, FPG International/Rob Gage.

Chapter 3 Opener, The Stock Market/Jose L. Pelaez; Fig. 3–1, Lisa Shoemaker. In Thibodeau GA, Patton KT: *Anatomy & physiology,* ed 2, 1993, Mosby; Fig. 3–2, Christy Krames. In Thibodeau GA, Patton KT: *Anatomy & physiology,* ed 2, 1993, St. Louis, Mosby; Fig. 3–3A, Marsha J. Dohrmann, and Figs. 3–3B and C, Kathy Mitchell Grey. In Thibodeau GA, Patton KT: *Anatomy & physiology,* ed 2, 1993, St. Louis, Mosby; Figs. 3–4, 3–5, Pagecrafters; Fig. 3–6, Rolin Graphics.

Chapter 4 Opener, PhotoDisk; Fig. 4–3, Joanne Scott/Tracy McCalla; Fig. 4–2, 4–6, Pagecrafters; Fig. 4–5, William C. Ober and Claire Garrison.

Chapter 5 Opener, PhotoDisk; Fig. 5–1, McLaren DS: *Color atlas and text of diet-related disorders,* London, 1992, Wolfe Medical Publishing; Fig. 5–6, Rolin Graphics. Redrawn from The China-Cornell-Oxford project on nutrition, health, and environment at Cornell University (brochure), p. 5, Cornell University, Division of Nutritional Sciences, N204 MVR Hall, Ithaca, NY 14853-4401; Fig. 5–7, William C. Ober and Claire Garrison; unn. fig. 5–1, National Cancer Institute, Bethesda, Md.

Chapter 6 Opener, PhotoDisk; Figs. 6–3, 6–4, Joanne Scott/Tracy McCalla; Fig. 6–5, Rolin Graphics; Fig 6–7, courtesy Professor R. Hendricksen. In McLaren DS: *Color atlas and text of diet-related disorders,* London, 1992, Wolfe Medical Publishing.

Chapter 7 Opener, PhotoDisk; unn. fig. 7–5, Joanne Scott/Tracy McCalla; Fig. 7–1, courtesy Professor Dame S. Sherlock and JA Summerfield. In McLaren DS: *Color atlas and text of diet-related disorders,* London, 1992, Wolfe Medical Publishing; Figs. 7–2, 7–4, McLaren DS: *Color atlas and text of diet-related disorders,* London, 1992, Wolfe Medical Publishing; Fig. 7–3, The Upjohn Company; unn. figs. 7–1, 7–2, 7–3, 7–4, PhotoDisc.

Chapter 8 Opener, PhotoDisk; Fig. 8–2, Joanne Scott/Tracy McCalla; unn. fig. 8–1, LV Bergman & Associates Inc., Cold Spring, NY; unn. fig. 8–2, Shipley M: *A color atlas of rheumatology,* ed 3, London, 1993, Mosby-Year Book-Europe.

Chapter 9 Opener, Science Source/Photo Researchers/J. Wachter; Fig. 9–3, Pagecrafters; Fig. 9–4, Rolin Graphics; unn. fig. 9–1, Barbara Bourne; unn. fig. 9–2, The Stock Market/Lew Long.

Chapter 10 Opener, The Stock Market/Ariel Skelley; Fig. 10–1, Stunkard AJ, Sorenson T, Schulsinger F: Use of the Danish Adoption Register for the study of obesity and thinness. In *The genetics of neurological and psychiatric disorders,* New York 1983, Raven Press; Fig. 10–2, Pagecrafters; Figs. 10–3, 10–7, 10–8, Rolin Graphics; Fig. 10–5, McLaren DS: *Color atlas and text of diet-related disorders,* London, 1992, Wolfe Medical Publishing; Fig. 10–6A, Ed Reschke. In Thibodeau GA, Patton KT: *Anatomy & physiology,* ed 2, St. Louis, 1993, Mosby; Fig. 10-6B, Thibodeau GA, Patton KT: *Anatomy & physiology,* ed 2, St. Louis, 1993, Mosby.

Chapter 11 Opener, Science Source/Photo Researchers/O. Burriel; Fig. 11–1, courtesy Dr. Ann P. Streissguth. In Williams SR, Worthington-Roberts B: *Nutrition throughout the life cycle,* ed 2, St. Louis, 1992, Mosby; Fig. 11–2, Rolin Graphics; unn. fig. 11–1, La Leche League; unn. fig. 11–2, courtesy of Gerber Products Co.

Chapter 12 Opener, PhotoDisk; Fig. 12–1, Cindy Bambini; unn. fig. 12–1, David Oppenheimer Group; unn. fig. 12–2, Washington Apple Commission; unn. fig. 12–3, PhotoDisc; unn. fig. 12–4, Super Stock.

Chapter 13 Opener, PhotoDisk, Figs. 13–1, 13–2, Weinsier RL, Morgan SL: *Fundamentals of clinical nutrition,* St. Louis, 1993, Mosby; unn. fig. 13–1, Wong D: *Whaley & Wong's nursing care of infants and children,* ed 5, St. Louis, 1995, Mosby.

Chapter 14 Opener, Image Bank/Jay Brousseau; Fig. 14–1, Rolin Graphics; Figs. 14–2, 14–3, Lee R, Neimann D: *Nutritional assessment,* ed 2, St. Louis, 1996, Mosby; Fig. 14–4, Adapted from Brunnstrom S: *Clinical kinesiology,* 1962, FA Davis.

Chapter 15 Opener, Photo Researchers/Simon Fraser-Princess Mary Hospital, Newcastle; Figs. 15–2, 15–4, Rolin Graphics; Fig. 15–3, Nelson JK, Weckwerth JA: Home enteral nutrition. In Skipper A, ed: *Dietitian's handbook of enteral and parenteral nutrition,* Rockville, Md, 1989, Aspen; Figs. 15–5, 15–6, Weinsier RL, Morgan SL: *Fundamentals of clinical nutrition,* St. Louis, 1993, Mosby; unn fig. 15–1, courtesy of Bryan Foods.

Chapter 16 Opener, Photo Researchers/Will & Deni McIntyre; Fig. 16–1, Seeley RR, Stephens TD, Tate PT: *Anatomy & physiology,* ed 3, St. Louis, 1995, Mosby; Figs. 16–2, 16–3, 16–4, Rolin Grahics; Fig. 16–5, Mahan LK, Arlin M: *Krause's food, nutrition and diet therapy,* ed 8, Philadelphia, 1992, Saunders; Fig. 16–6, Rolin Graphics. Adapted from Guyton AC: *Textbook of medical physiology,* ed 8, Philadelphia, 1991, Saunders; unn. figs., Table 16–1, Barbara Cousins. In Gottfried SS: *Human biology,* St. Louis, 1994, Mosby.

Chapter 17 Opener, The Stock Market/Jeff Zaruba; Fig. 17–1, Rolin Graphics. Adapted from Davis J, Sherer K: *Applied nutrition and diet therapy for nurses,* ed 2, Philadelphia, 1994, Saunders; Fig. 17–3, Rolin Graphics; Fig. 17–4, SIU Biomedical Communications/Science Source/Photo Researchers, Inc.

Chapter 18 Opener, Science Source/Photo Researchers/St Bartholomew's Hospital; Fig. 18–1, adapted from *Maximizing the role of nutrition in diabetes management.* A clinical education program of American Diabetes Association in cooperation with Diabetes Care and Education, a practice group of the American Dietetic Association, Alexandria, Va, 1994, American Diabetes Association; unn. figs. 18–1, 18–2, Wong D: *Whaley & Wong's nursing care of infants and children,* ed 5, St. Louis, 1995, Mosby.

Chapter 19 Opener, The Stock Market/Jon Feingersh; Fig. 19–1, Harry Ransom Humanities Research Center. In Gottfried SS: *Human biology,* St. Louis, 1994, Mosby; Fig. 19–2, courtesy of Oldways Preservation & Exchange Trust.

Chapter 20 Opener, PhotoDisk; Fig. 20–1, Rolin Graphics; Fig. 20–2A, Joan M. Beck/Donna Odle, and 20–2B, Barbara Stackhouse. In Thibodeau GA, Patton KT: *Anatomy & physiology,* ed 2, St. Louis, 1993, Mosby.

Chapter 21 Opener, Science Source/Photo Researchers/G. Tompkinson; Fig. 21–1, Rolin Graphics; Fig. 21–2, Weinsier RL, Morgan SL: *Fundamentals of clinical nutrition,* St. Louis, 1993, Mosby; unn. fig. 21–1, Florida Citrus Commission.

INDEX

NOTE: Page numbers in italics indicate illustrations: *t* indicates tables.

Goals
  behavioral changes and, 262–263
  establishing, body composition and, 262–263
  of nutrition therapy, for diabetes mellitus, 463–464, 465t
Goiters, 202, *202*
Government programs, for health promotion, during
      adulthood, 320–323
Graft *versus* host disease (GVHD), bone marrow
      transplantation and, 526
Grains
  consumption trends of, 36
  unrefined *vs.* refined, *91,* 91–92
    health debates over, *92*
Growth and maintenance, protein for, 130
Growth hormones, 96
Growth patterns, of childhood, 303
GVHD, bone marrow transplantation and, 526

H

H. pylori, 418
Haloperidol, 440t
Halothane, related anesthetics and, 440t
Handling procedures, for food safety, 48
Hard water, 180
HDLs, 114
  coronary artery disease and, 483
Health
  defined, 5–6
  dimensions of, 11
  emotional, 6
    hypoglycemia and, 7
    nutrition and, 7
    obesity and, *247*
  intellectual, 6
    nutrition and, 7
  physical, 6
    body fat levels and, *245,* 245–247
    nutrition and, 6
  social, 6
    nutrition and, 7
    obesity and, 247
  spiritual, 6
    nutrition and, 7
Health assessments, of patients, nursing roles and,
      358–359
Health benefits, of exercise, 223–225
Health care
  alternative
    for AIDS, *532*
    for HIV, *532*
  in home, nursing roles in, *522*
Health care facilities, food service systems in, 374–375
  nurses and, 375
Health claims
  Food and Drug Administration approved, 40, 42
  food labeling and, 40, 42, 498
Health debates
  on alcohol, *440*
  on amino acid supplements, *134*
  on exercise, *223*
  on foods as pharmaceuticals, *522–523*

Health debates—cont'd
  on garlic
    blood cholesterol and, *490*
    hypertension and, *490*
  on genetically modified foods, *43*
  on refined *vs.* unrefined grains, *92*
  on use of laxatives, *72*
Health fraud
  AIDS and, *532*
  HIV and, *532*
Health histories, of patients, nursing roles and,
      358–359
Health promotion
  during adolescence, 312–313
    community support for, 313
  during adulthood, 319–323
    community support for, 320–323
    Healthy People 2000 objectives for, *320, 321, 322*
  during childhood, 309–311
  college campuses and, 9
  community support for, 7, 9
  food preferences and, 28
  Healthy People 2000, 7, 8t
  for life span, 275–298, 303–335
  nutrition in, 7, 8t, 9
  during pregnancy, 275–286
Health risks
  of bodybuilding, *227*
  of dieting, *247*
Healthy People 2000
  adult health promotion, *320, 321, 322*
  goals for breastfeeding, 286
  low fat foods and, 110, 117
  nutrition objectives of, 7, 8t
  purpose of, 9
Healthy snacks, 309t
Heart attacks, 495
Heart disease; *see also* Cardiovascular diseases
  congestive heart failure, 495–497
  dietary fibers and, 89
  omega-3 fatty acids and, 107
  predisposition for, 121
  saturated fats and, 121
Heart healthy changes, dietary, 496
Heartburn, 416
  causes of, *417*
  minimizing, 416
  during pregnancy, 286
  prevention of, 68–69
  treatment of, 68–69
    medications for, 417t
Height
  measurements of, *364*
    for nutritional assessments, *364,* 364–365
  in Median Heights and Weights and Recommended Energy
      Intake, 18
  recumbent bed, 365
    measurements of, *365*
Helicobacter pylori, 418
Heme iron, 198
Hemochromatosis, 200, 439

Swallowing problems—cont'd
  Mendelson maneuver for, 414
  supraglottic swallow for, 414
  warning signs for, 411
  weight loss and, nursing roles in treating, *432–433*
Sweeteners, 82–84; *see also* Sugars
  alternative, 80*t*, 82
    benefit/risk analysis of, 84
    Delaney Clause and, 84
  consumption trends of, 36
Synthetic fats, 116–117
  Olestra, 117

T

T cells, 527
Table sugars, 79, 80, 80*t*
Tables, recumbent length, 364–365, *365*
Tachycardia, beriberi and, 154
Target heart rates, for exercise, 225*t*
Taste
  age-related changes in, 60
  drugs altering, 354*t*
Taste acuity, patients with altered, suggestions for, *512*
TC, in risk assessments, for coronary artery disease, 482–483
TCA cycle, in metabolism, 119
α-TE, 171
Teaching tools
  for assisting patients, with menu selections, 374
  for behavioral changes, 263
  for breakfast foods, 305
  for breastfeeding, 293
  for calcium intake, 191
  for calculating, recommended protein intake, 134
  for calculating fat intake, 109
  for carbohydrate requirements, 230
  for coping, with fluid restrictions, 443
  for dietary fiber intake, 90
  for dimensions of health, 11
  for eating well
    with colostomies, 427
    with ileostomies, 427
  for evaluating food labels, 41
  for exercise, 227
  for food choices, 266
  for heart healthy dietary changes, 496
  for lactose intolerance, 96
  for managing dumping syndrome, 421
  for maximizing food intake
    in COPD, 534
    in HIV/AIDS, 531
  for minimizing, gastroesophageal reflux, 416
  for overcoming, drug side effects, 355
  for portion sizes, of protein, 138
  for recognizing, foods high in sodium, 495
  for reducing
    dietary fat intake, 113
    potassium in foods, 507
  for sick day guidelines, for diabetes mellitus, 473
  for tube feedings
    for children, 399
    for infants, 399

Teaching tools—cont'd
  for vegetable victories, 164
Teenagers; *see* Adolescence and adolescents
Teeth, in digestion, 60
Temperature regulators, body fat as, 105
Teratogens, during pregnancy, 281
Tertiary prevention, of diseases, 10
Thermogenesis
  adaptive, energy expenditure and, 220, 222
  diet-induced, energy expenditure and, 220
Thiamin, 15, 152, 153–155, 165*t*
  deficiency, 154–155
    vision loss and, *155*
  function of, 153
  Recommended Dietary Allowances for, 153
  sources of, 154
  toxicity of, 155
Thrombosis, 481
Thrombus, 481
Thyrotoxicosis, 202
Thyroxine, 96
Tin, 205
Tobacco, during pregnancy, 282
Toddlers
  food asphyxiation and, 323
  meals and, 305–306
  nutrition requirements of, 306–307
  self-feeding and, 306, *306*
Tongue, in digestion, 60
Tooth decay, baby bottle, 294–295
Total blood cholesterol (TC), in risk assessments, for coronary artery disease, 482–483
Total lymphocyte count (TLC), for immune function assessments, 370
Total nutrient admixtures (TNAs), in parenteral nutrition solutions, 403, *403*
Total parenteral nutrition (TPN), 400, *401*
Toxemia, during pregnancy, 283–284
  risk factors for, 283*t*
Toxic megacolon, 430
Toxicity
  of biotin, 161
  of calcium, 191
  of chloride, 197
  of chromium, 204
  of copper, 204
  of fluoride, 203
  of folate, 160
  of iodine, 202
  of iron, 200
  of magnesium, 192
  of niacin, 158
  of pantothenic acid, 162
  of phosphorus, 192
  of riboflavin, 156
  of selenium, 204
  of sodium, 195
  of sulfur, 193
  of thiamin, 155
  of vitamin A, 168–169
  of vitamin B_6, 158

Median Heights and Weights and Recommended Energy Intake, 10th Edition RDA

Category	Age (years) or Condition	Weight (kg)	Weight (lb)	Height (cm)	Height (in)	REE[a] (kcal/day)	Multiples of REE	Average Energy Allowance (kcal) Per kg	Average Energy Allowance (kcal) Per day[b]
Infants	0.0-0.5	6	13	60	24	320		108	650
	0.5-1.0	9	20	71	28	500		98	850
Children	1-3	13	29	90	56	740		102	1300
	4-6	20	44	112	44	950		90	1800
	7-10	28	62	132	52	1130		70	2000
Males	11-14	45	99	157	62	1440	1.70	55	2500
	15-18	66	145	176	69	1760	1.67	45	3000
	19-24	72	160	177	70	1780	1.67	40	2900
	25-50	79	174	176	70	1800	1.60	37	2900
	51+	77	170	173	68	1530	1.50	30	2300
Females	11-14	46	101	157	62	1310	1.67	47	2200
	15-18	55	120	163	64	1370	1.60	40	2200
	19-24	58	128	164	65	1350	1.60	38	2200
	25-50	63	138	163	64	1380	1.55	36	2200
	51+	65	143	160	63	1280	1.50	30	1900
Pregnant	1st Trimester								+0
	2nd Trimester								+300
	3rd Trimester								+300
Lactating	1st 6 months								+500
	2nd 6 months								+500

[a]Resting energy expenditure (REE); calculation based on FAO equations, then rounded. This is the same as RMR.
[b]Figure is rounded.

Metropolitan Life Insurance Company Height-Weight Data, Revised 1983

Height-Weight Tables for Adults (1983)

Height Ft	Height In	Women Frame* Small	Women Frame* Medium	Women Frame* Large	Height Ft	Height In	Men Frame* Small	Men Frame* Medium	Men Frame* Large
4	10	102-111	109-121	118-131	5	2	128-134	131-141	138-150
4	11	103-113	111-123	120-134	5	3	130-136	133-143	140-153
5	0	104-115	113-126	122-137	5	4	132-138	135-145	142-156
5	1	106-118	115-129	125-140	5	5	134-140	137-148	144-160
5	2	108-121	118-132	128-143	5	6	136-142	139-151	146-164
5	3	111-124	121-135	131-147	5	7	138-145	142-154	149-168
5	4	114-127	124-138	134-151	5	8	140-148	145-157	152-172
5	5	117-130	127-141	137-155	5	9	142-151	148-160	155-176
5	6	120-133	130-144	140-159	5	10	144-154	151-163	158-180
5	7	113-136	133-147	143-163	5	11	146-157	154-166	161-184
5	8	126-139	136-150	146-167	6	0	149-160	157-170	164-188
5	9	129-142	139-153	149-170	6	1	152-164	160-174	168-192
5	10	132-145	142-156	152-173	6	2	155-168	164-178	172-197
5	11	135-148	156-159	155-176	6	3	158-172	167-182	176-202
6	0	138-151	148-162	158-179	6	4	162-176	171-187	181-207

Based on a weight-height mortality study conducted by the Society of Actuaries and the Association of Life Insurance Medical Directors of America, Metropolitan Life Insurance Company, revised 1983.
*Weights at ages 25 to 59 based on lowest mortality. Height includes 1-in heel. Weight for women includes 3 lb for indoor clothing. Weight for men includes 5 lb for indoor clothing.